I0888775

Multifunctional Nanocarriers for Contemporary Healthcare Applications

Md. Abul Barkat
K.R. Mangalam University, India

Harshita A.B.
K.R. Mangalam University, India

Sarwar Beg
Jubilant Generics, India

Farhan J. Ahmad
Jamia Hamdard, India

A volume in the Advances in Medical Technologies and Clinical Practice (AMTCP) Book Series

IGI Global
DISSEMINATOR OF KNOWLEDGE

Published in the United States of America by
IGI Global
Medical Information Science Reference (an imprint of IGI Global)
701 E. Chocolate Avenue
Hershey PA, USA 17033
Tel: 717-533-8845
Fax: 717-533-8661
E-mail: cust@igi-global.com
Web site: http://www.igi-global.com

Copyright © 2018 by IGI Global. All rights reserved. No part of this publication may be reproduced, stored or distributed in any form or by any means, electronic or mechanical, including photocopying, without written permission from the publisher. Product or company names used in this set are for identification purposes only. Inclusion of the names of the products or companies does not indicate a claim of ownership by IGI Global of the trademark or registered trademark.

Library of Congress Cataloging-in-Publication Data

Names: Barkat, Md. Abul, 1987- editor. | Harshita A. B., 1991- editor. | Beg, Sarwar, 1987- editor. | Ahmad, Farhan J., editor.
Title: Multifunctional nanocarriers for contemporary healthcare applications / Md. Abul Barkat, Harshita A.B., Sarwar Beg, and Farhan J. Ahmad, editors.
Description: Hershey, PA : Medical Information Science Reference, [2018] | Includes bibliographical references.
Identifiers: LCCN 2017032790| ISBN 9781522547815 (hardcover) | ISBN 9781522547822 (ebook)
Subjects: | MESH: Nanoparticles | Drug Carriers | Nanocomposites | Drug Delivery Systems | Technology, Pharmaceutical
Classification: LCC RS199.5 | NLM QV 785 | DDC 615/.6--dc23 LC record available at https://lccn.loc.gov/2017032790

This book is published in the IGI Global book series Advances in Medical Technologies and Clinical Practice (AMTCP) (ISSN: 2327-9354; eISSN: 2327-9370)

British Cataloguing in Publication Data
A Cataloguing in Publication record for this book is available from the British Library.

All work contributed to this book is new, previously-unpublished material. The views expressed in this book are those of the authors, but not necessarily of the publisher.

For electronic access to this publication, please contact: eresources@igi-global.com.

Advances in Medical Technologies and Clinical Practice (AMTCP) Book Series

Srikanta Patnaik
SOA University, India
Priti Das
S.C.B. Medical College, India

ISSN:2327-9354
EISSN:2327-9370

Mission

Medical technological innovation continues to provide avenues of research for faster and safer diagnosis and treatments for patients. Practitioners must stay up to date with these latest advancements to provide the best care for nursing and clinical practices.

The **Advances in Medical Technologies and Clinical Practice (AMTCP) Book Series** brings together the most recent research on the latest technology used in areas of nursing informatics, clinical technology, biomedicine, diagnostic technologies, and more. Researchers, students, and practitioners in this field will benefit from this fundamental coverage on the use of technology in clinical practices.

Coverage

- Clinical High-Performance Computing
- Clinical Studies
- Clinical Data Mining
- Patient-Centered Care
- E-Health
- Nutrition
- Neural Engineering
- Telemedicine
- Biometrics
- Clinical Nutrition

IGI Global is currently accepting manuscripts for publication within this series. To submit a proposal for a volume in this series, please contact our Acquisition Editors at Acquisitions@igi-global.com or visit: http://www.igi-global.com/publish/.

The Advances in Medical Technologies and Clinical Practice (AMTCP) Book Series (ISSN 2327-9354) is published by IGI Global, 701 E. Chocolate Avenue, Hershey, PA 17033-1240, USA, www.igi-global.com. This series is composed of titles available for purchase individually; each title is edited to be contextually exclusive from any other title within the series. For pricing and ordering information please visit http://www.igi-global.com/book-series/advances-medical-technologies-clinical-practice/73682. Postmaster: Send all address changes to above address. Copyright © 2018 IGI Global. All rights, including translation in other languages reserved by the publisher. No part of this series may be reproduced or used in any form or by any means – graphics, electronic, or mechanical, including photocopying, recording, taping, or information and retrieval systems – without written permission from the publisher, except for non commercial, educational use, including classroom teaching purposes. The views expressed in this series are those of the authors, but not necessarily of IGI Global.

Titles in this Series

For a list of additional titles in this series, please visit: www.igi-global.com/book-series

Biomedical Signal and Image Processing in Patient Care
Maheshkumar H. Kolekar (Indian Institute of Technology Patna, India) and Vinod Kumar (Indian Institute of Technology Roorkee, India)
Medical Information Science Reference • copyright 2018 • 312pp • H/C (ISBN: 9781522528296) • US $265.00 (our price)

Next-Generation Mobile and Pervasive Healthcare Solutions
Jose Machado (University of Minho, Portugal) António Abelha (University of Minho, Portugal) Manuel Filipe Santos (University of Minho, Portugal) and Filipe Portela (University of Minho, Portugal)
Medical Information Science Reference • copyright 2018 • 286pp • H/C (ISBN: 9781522528517) • US $245.00 (our price)

Innovative Research in Thermal Imaging for Biology and Medicine
Ricardo Vardasca (University of Porto, Portugal) and Joaquim Gabriel Mendes (University of Porto, Portugal)
Medical Information Science Reference • copyright 2017 • 340pp • H/C (ISBN: 9781522520726) • US $210.00 (our price)

Internet of Things and Advanced Application in Healthcare
Catarina I. Reis (Polytechnic Institute of Leiria, Portugal) and Marisa da Silva Maximiano (Polytechnic Institute of Leiria, Portugal)
Medical Information Science Reference • copyright 2017 • 349pp • H/C (ISBN: 9781522518204) • US $210.00 (our price)

Integrating Biologically-Inspired Nanotechnology into Medical Practice
B.K. Nayak (K.M. Centre for Post Graduate Studies, India) Anima Nanda (Sathyabama University, India) and M. Amin Bhat (Sathyabama University, India)
Medical Information Science Reference • copyright 2017 • 394pp • H/C (ISBN: 9781522506102) • US $190.00 (our price)

Recent Advances in Drug Delivery Technology
Raj K. Keservani (Rajiv Gandhi Proudyogiki Vishwavidyalaya, India) Anil K. Sharma (Delhi Institute of Pharmaceutical Sciences and Research, India) and Rajesh Kumar Kesharwani (National Institute of Technology, Warangal, India)
Medical Information Science Reference • copyright 2017 • 510pp • H/C (ISBN: 9781522507543) • US $215.00 (our price)

701 East Chocolate Avenue, Hershey, PA 17033, USA
Tel: 717-533-8845 x100 • Fax: 717-533-8661
E-Mail: cust@igi-global.com • www.igi-global.com

Table of Contents

Detailed Table of Contents

decades. This profound success of lipid nanocarriers as therapeutic delivery systems is a result of their unique properties, that is, biocompatibility and biodegradability, possible delivery by multiple routes of administration, ease of formulation and scale up, amicable dosage form development, enhanced stability, bioavailability, and possible drug targeting. The chapter aims to give a detailed overview of various types of lipid nanocarriers along with methods of fabrication and characterization. The chapter also describes multiple applications of lipid nanocarriers in advanced therapeutics and elaborates on the current market opportunities and future prospects.

Recent trends in drug delivery indicate a growing trend to utilize nanotechnology to target diseased tissues with minimal adverse effects. However, in such cases, the biggest challenge encountered by the formulator is the intracellular delivery of the actives. Nevertheless, pharmaceutical nanocarriers have proven to possess distinct advantages for intracellular delivery of therapeutics over conventional approaches. They are versatile in terms of engineering and provide attractive options to deliver encapsulated or conjugated cargoes to cellular targets. In this chapter, the authors discuss important aspects of lipid-based nanocarriers for intracellular drug targeting. The chapter provides insight of different pathways to internalize lipid nanocarriers and the physicochemical factors affecting the intracellular fate of nanocarriers. Further, the chapter provides details of different types of lipid-based nanocarriers that have been explored for intracellular delivery in infectious diseases as well as cancer.

Nanotechnology is that sphere of technology that involves the participation of biology, chemistry, physics, and engineering sciences. Nanoscale science defines the chemistry and physics of structures lying in the range of 1-100 nm. Among the nanosystems researched, magnetic nanosystems are highlighted due their unique ability, which enables their targeting to specific locations on application of an external magnetic field. The exhibited property of these magnetic nanosystems being super-paramagnetism, there is no retention of magnetic property on removal of the magnetic field, thus enabling a reversion of the targeting process. For effective utilization of these nanosystems, they should be reduced to nanosizes, layered with biocompatible entities, stabilized, and functionalized. In the chapter, synthesis and functionalization and stabilization are elucidated. The biomedical applications such as targeted delivery, MRI, magnetic hyperthermia, tissue engineering, gene delivery, magnetic immunotherapy, magnetic detoxification, and nanomagnetic actuation are discussed.

Integration of nanotechnology and biomedicine has offered great opportunities for the development of nanoscaled therapeutic platforms. Amongst various nanocarriers, mesoporous silica nanoparticles (MSNs) is one of the most developed and promising inorganic materials-based drug delivery system for clinical translations due to their simple composition and nanoporous structure. MSNs possess unique structural features, for example, well-defined morphology, large surface areas, uniform size, controllable structure, flexible pore volume, tunable pore sizes, extraordinarily high loading efficiency, and excellent biocompatibility. Progress in structure control and functionalization may endow MSNs with functionalities that enable medical applications of these integrated nanoparticles such as molecularly targeted drug delivery, multicomponent synergistic therapy, in vivo imaging and therapeutic capability, on-demand/stimuli-responsive drug release, etc. In this chapter, the authors overview MSNs' characteristics and the scientific efforts developed till date involving drug delivery and biomedical applications.

Microsponges, a patented technology for chronotherapeutic topical drug delivery, has evolved for oral, pulmonary, and parenteral drug delivery. Various advances have been made with this carrier particle resulting in the development of novel carrier particles, namely nanosponges, nanoferrosponges, and porous microbeads. This chapter deals with the application for topical delivery of pharmaceuticals and for cosmetic purpose; potential of the delivery system for oral drug delivery, pulmonary, and parenteral purpose; and also provides an insight on the recent advances made in this field and future prospect. While many commercial products are available for topical purpose, the use of the technology for sustained/controlled/targeted delivery of pharmaceuticals/biopharmaceuticals via alternative routes is still in infancy. Extensive research inputs are required to resolve preclinical and clinical intricacies before the technology can be put into use for alternative administrative routes and for tissue engineering.

Multicomponent systems provide the option of combining drugs at the supramolecular level. Among these, co-crystals have gained a widespread interest in pharmaceutical industry as US Food and Drug Administration (FDA) recently introduced new regulatory guidelines regarding this solid form that is anticipated to expand patent portfolios. Apart from co-crystals, other multi-component adducts such as co-amorphous system and eutectics are also a topic of interest for pharmaceutical researchers as they provide therapeutic advantages along with improved the aqueous solubility, dissolution, and bioavailability of poorly soluble drugs. This chapter provides a brief overview of multicomponent solid forms, their preparation methodologies, characterization, evaluation, biopharmaceutical aspects, scale up issues, and regulatory perspectives related to these solid forms. In addition, a section on future perspectives that sheds light on new therapeutic hybrids deploying drug-drug and drug-neutraceuticals combinations with improved pharmaceutical and biopharmaceutical attributes is also included.

The drug delivery to the cancer sites, with maintained effective drug concentration for longer duration, using low dose of drug, with minimum side effects is the prime concern of formulation scientist today. In the recent times, the nanocarrier systems are not only being utilized for achieving targeted, sustained and controlled release of drug to the disease site, but also are used in imaging of diseases. An attempt has been made through this chapter to give a brief outline about the cancer and elaborate details on the various multifunctional nanocarriers researched till date for effective delivery of drugs in cancer treatment. Further, functionalization and surface modification of nanocarrier with various ligands like folate, transferrin, TPGS (d-α- Tocopheryl Polyethylene Glycol 1000 Succinate), trastuzumab and hyaluronic acid etc., that have specific receptor in the proximity of disease site have been explained along with pros and cons of such carrier systems.

The rationale for administering a drug is usually related to the increase of the drug bioavailability with the aim to achieve a therapeutic effect at a predetermined time. A drug delivery system consists of a formulation or even a device that introduces a drug into the organism being capable of assuring the efficacy and safety by controlling the rate, time, and place of release. With the field of multifunctional nanocomposites, crucial factors such as the improvement on the medicine's efficacy, reduced economic implications, extended life of product patent, better safety and efficacy profile, and increased compliance are the aim. Nowadays, nanocomposites and nanostructured materials are important for several biotherapeutic applications, including their use in drug delivery, in orthopaedics, and in dentistry.

Gene therapy is the emerging trend in biomedical science for treatment of life-threatening diseases. This involves delivery of a therapeutic gene to the nucleus of an affected cell by a suitable vector. Gene delivery using non-viral vectors such as cationic polymer and lipid is gaining attention due to their favourable properties, including lack of immunogenicity, low toxicity, and potential for tissue specificity when compared with viral vectors. A variety of non-viral vectors have been proposed, most of which facilitate gene delivery by electrostatic interactions, encapsulation, and in some cases, condensing nucleic acids into nano-sized particles which can then be taken up by cells. Successful gene delivery within a cell is the nanocarrier's ability to protect its contents from degradation in the extracellular environment. A well-designed nanocarrier will promote cellular uptake and intracellular release of the nucleic acid. This chapter highlights different polymers, lipids, and their nanocarriers employed for gene delivery along with clinical trials.

Nanocarriers with various compositions and biological properties are frequently used systems for in-vitro/in-vivo vaccination and gene transfer. In recent years, developments in nanotechnology have focused on the design and synthesis of nanocarriers that have new properties and can be modified for gene and vaccine delivery. In the favorable results obtained from in-vivo studies performed, they increase interest in these developments and pave the way for their therapeutic use. Nanocarriers have become increasingly important because they can stabilize vaccine antigens and serve as adjuvants, with the advantage of easily transporting genetic material to the target site. In nanocarriers, the molecules involved are adsorbed to the surface or encapsulated in particulates. At the same time, surface modification of nanoparticles allows these systems to carry cargo molecules easily to target site. Among the most studied nanocarriers, lipidic and polymeric systems dendrimers, inorganic nanoparticles, cyclodextrins, cell penetration peptides, and ISCOMs are attracting attention.

Nanocomposites are a class of materials in which one or more phases with nanoscale dimensions are embedded in a metal, ceramic, or polymer matrix. The properties of nanocomposites depend on matrix, loading, degree of dispersion, size, shape, and orientation of the nanoscale phase and interaction between the matrix and the nanoscale phase. Nanocomposites are generally prepared using direct melt intercalation. The formation of nanocomposite is ascertained by XRD pattern, FTIR spectra, electron microscopy, and thermal analysis like DSC and TGA. Nanocomposites have properties of nanoparticles, multifunctional capabilities, chemical functionalization, huge interphase zone. Novel nanomaterials offer a new chemotherapeutic route for cancer treatment by combining cell imaging and hyperthermia in a synergistic way. In spite of toxicity and safety concerns, multifunctional nanocomposite still interest the researchers because of emergence of versatile properties, better understanding of disease biomarkers, and quest for ways to improve biocompatibility.

Nanomaterials have revolutionized the drug delivery and therapeutic industry due to their unique physical characteristics, which render them extremely manipulative at nano-scale. One such category of nanomaterials is mesoporous silica nanoparticles. Due to their small size and rigid honeycomb-like structure, they are highly conducive for packaging of drugs, dyes, antibodies, etc. In addition, they show excellent biocompatibility. These new generation nanomaterials can be further functionalized by incorporating surface modifications, thus increasing their acceptability as carriers for drugs and molecules. In this chapter, a brief and comprehensive review covering various aspects of the recent advancements in synthesis of mesoporous nanomaterials and post-synthesis strategies for functionalization has been presented. Further, it also sheds light on how efficiently these smart nano-carriers are involved in transport and site-specific delivery of highly toxic drugs, like chemotherapeutic agents for cancer treatment, and their biocompatibility evaluation from a biosafety point of view.

Nanotechnology has drawn the attention of many researchers for the delivery of therapeutics used in various medical applications. Liposomes and polymeric nanoparticles represent promising nanocarriers that efficiently encapsulate drugs, which prevents their degradation along with the control and sustained drug release. Despite the many advantages of these formulations, some of the drawbacks associated with them limit their application to a certain extent. Therefore, there is need for a novel nanocarrier that possesses all of their individual advantages and excludes their drawbacks. Currently, researchers are focused on developing a novel platform that is a hybrid of a polymeric and liposomal-based carrier that combines the peculiarity of both and excludes their shortcomings. Lipid hybrid polymer nanoparticles (LPNs) contain the hydrophobic biodegradable polymeric core surrounded by a lipid layer for intensification of biocompatibility. This chapter includes an introduction of LPNs along with their advantages, composition, and method of preparation.

Foreword

It gives me immense pleasure to scribble this foreword for the book titled *Multifunctional Nanocarriers for Contemporary Healthcare Applications*. At the onset, I compliment and congratulate the editors and authors of the book for their voluminous compilations on the aforementioned title. I personally and professionally know the Editors of the book, where in my close association with them, I have found them highly motivated, enthusiastic and dynamic for undertaking key initiatives towards innovation and excellence in this particular area of research interest.

I have gone through the book chapters submitted by a gamut of authors from various premier universities of India and overseas are the well-known experts working in the domain of nanomedicines for drug delivery and biomedical applications. The chapters have been very aptly selected, thus well justifying the theme of the book. Highly illustrative descriptions of contents on various key disciplines of nanomedicines including fabrication, characterization and multifaceted applications of polymeric, lipidic, lipid-polymer hybrids and metallic nanoparticulate systems for diverse therapeutic drug applications along with updated bibliography of references are the unique selling features of the book.

Based on my professional experience in the domain of pharmaceutical sciences, I can greatly vouch the humble endeavors and appreciate the untiring efforts of the editors of the book in bringing a meaningful textual repertoire for the benefit of scientific community for the purpose.

At the outset, I wish the editors for all the very best of their efforts for successful completion of the book and anticipate their activeness in bringing more such assignments in the near future.

Ahmed Kamal
Jamia Hamdard, India

Preface

In the contemporary era, the approach of disease treatment employing the available health care tools has been highly thwarted. With the involvement of complex etiology and progression of disease, the reliance on available drugs as well as dosage forms is considered to be quite less effective. The key challenges encounter during dosage form designing include issues of poor biopharmaceutical characteristics like inept solubility, permeability, lack of targeting ability, off-target side effects, etc. In this regard, the modern healthcare system demands the availability of smart drug delivery systems for catering the healthcare needs. Despite tremendous efforts for developing new drug candidates, the approach of designing newer drug delivery systems is considered to be the best and effective alternative for augmenting the therapeutic performance. In the last few decades, use of nanotechnology-based systems have gained immense promise due to their miniscule size, high aspect ratio, ability of carrying multiple therapeutic agents, excellent opportunities for surface modification, functionalization and tunability with ligands, protein/peptides and antibodies, not only for improvement of therapeutic performance of the drugs for disease treatment, but also for ultimately improving the quality of life. Instances of such nanotherapeutic systems include lipidic and polymeric nanoparticles, nanomaterials, nanocomposites, and many more.

Notwithstanding the benefits of nanosystems, extensive research efforts have been poured on exploring the possibility of active targeting to specific sites of body using surface-engineering techniques. The present book endeavors to cater the current demands on providing knowledge and know-how to the pharmaceutical and biomedical scientists to keep them abreast with versatile applications of nanocarriers as the next generation jargons for providing customized therapeutic solutions. Moreover, the book will provide an updated account on recent advancements and progress in the field of nanostructured systems with special emphasis on the application of such systems in diverse healthcare application in drug delivery and biomedical field for tissue engineering, imaging, biosensing and multi-therapeutic application. A brief account on various chapters submitted for the book pertaining to the application of nanocarriers for multifunctional drug delivery applications has been enumerated below.

Chapter 1, "Advanced Nanotherapeutic Systems for Drug Delivery and Imaging in Cancer," provides overview knowledge on recent progress in nanotechnology application, where nanocarriers have paved the way for development of new tools for cancer treatment. As conventional drug delivery approaches suffer from multiple biopharmaceutical challenges, thus usage of nanotechnology tools have greatly addressed such limitations and provides immense scope for early diagnosis, tumor targeted delivery via passive or active targeting mechanisms, personalized drug delivery, etc. This chapter summarizes various merits of nanotechnology with emphasis on different types of nanocarriers that are presently being used for drug delivery and imaging.

Chapter 2 deals with the topic "Application Potential of Polymeric Nanoconstructs for Colon-Specific Drug Delivery." In brief, the chapter describes innumerous applications of colon-specific drug delivery for the treatment of a wide array of diseases like irritable bowel syndrome (IBS), inflammatory bowel diseases (Ulcerative colitis and Crohn's disease), colorectal cancer, diverticulitis, etc. Drug delivery to colon possesses myriad anatomical and pathophysiological barriers and challenges with respect to the delivery of drugs to a particular site of it. With the advent of biodegradable polymeric nanoconstructs or similar systems, multiple therapeutic advantages could be achieved with minimal systemic adverse effects. Such nanosystems can be administered through oral route and precisely deliver the drug molecules to the target location of colon. Overall, the present chapter summarizes colon specific drug delivery application of polymeric nanoconstructs for the purpose.

Chapter 3, "Fabrication and Morphological Characterization of Barium Titanate-Based Polymeric Nanocomposite Thin Films," describes a critical review on the development of composite films of Barium Titanate (BaTiO3) and Poly (methyl methacrylate). Detailed characterization including flow of experimental work and microscopic imaging studies were performed for exploring the biomedical applications of such therapeutic nanostructures for the purpose.

Chapter 4, "Innovative Strategies for Lipid-Based Drug Delivery," endeavors to provide a succinct overview on current progress in lipid-based formulations and their utility in delivery of poorly water soluble drugs. The lipidic formulations also provide opportunities to tackle the poor bioavailability problems. The chapter has particularly stressed upon different lipidic formulations and their manufacturing techniques, mechanistic responsible for drug absorption along with advantages and limitations in commercial scale-up feasibility point-of-view. Moreover, the chapter has also gathered information as a guide for selection of excipients for developing the lipidic formulations.

Chapter 5, "Lipid Nanocarriers for Advanced Therapeutic Applications," highlights current progress in the development and evaluation of lipid nanocarriers as the mainstream nanotechnology-based tools for healthcare applications. Moreover, the chapter emphasizes profound success of lipidic nanocarriers as therapeutic delivery systems for their ultimate biocompatibility and biodegradability characteristics, route of administration, scalability, and suitability for possible drug targeting along with current market opportunities and future prospects.

Chapter 6, "Lipid Nanocarriers for Intracellular Delivery," provides information on specialized application of lipidic nanoformulations for drug targeting to intracellular systems for therapeutic applications. They are versatile in terms of their tunability and surface engineering ability to provide attractive options for delivery of cargos to cellular targets. The chapter has also covered underlying basic with respect to the plausible cellular pathways for internalization of lipid nanocarriers along with physicochemical and pharmaceutical factors affecting the intracellular targeting of nanocarriers.

Chapter 7 summarizes the topic "Magnetic Nano-Systems in Drug Delivery and Biomedical Applications." Since magnetic nanosystems are well known due to their unique physiochemical and material characteristics, which enables them for targeting to deliver the loaded cargos to specific location of the body with the application of an external magnetic field. The super-paramagnetism behavior also helps them to provide zero retention ability, where after removal of magnetic field they exhibit a reversion of targeting process. Moreover, the said chapter particularly emphasizes on the synthesis, functionalization and stabilization of magnetic nanomaterials for biomedical applications in targeted delivery, magnetic resonance imaging, magnetic hyperthermia, tissue engineering, gene delivery, magnetic immunotherapy, magnetic detoxification and nanomagnetic actuation.

Chapter 8, "Mesoporous Silica Nanoparticles: A Multifunctional Nanocarrier for Therapeutic Applications," provides an insight on integration of nanotechnology and biomedicine for the development of nanoscale platforms for exploring therapeutic opportunities. Amongst various nanocarriers, mesoporous silica nanoparticles (MSNs) are the most developed and promising inorganic materials extensively investigated in clinical research due to their nanoporous structure. Progress in structure control and functionalization have now endowed MSNs for medical applications for targeted drug delivery at molecular level, multicomponent synergistic therapy, on-demand/stimuli-responsive drug release ability, *in vivo* imaging, etc. The chapter compiled on the aforesaid topic has holistically covered functional use of MSNs in drug delivery and biomedical applications.

Chapter 9 emphasizes on "Micro- and Nanosponges-Based Carriers in Advanced Drug Delivery Applications," where detailed insight on application of these functional supramolecular materials have been discussed for oral, pulmonary, topical and parenteral drug delivery applications. Various advances have been made on carrier particles resulting in the development of novel materials *viz.* nanosponges, nanoferrosponges, and porous microbeads. The chapter has also provided information on applications beyond pharmaceuticals drug delivery, i.e., in cosmetic technology along with recent advances in preclinical and clinical studies, and future prospect for the purpose.

Chapter 10, "Multicomponent Solid Forms: A New Boost to Pharmaceuticals," provides newer therapeutic avenues for delivery of drugs at supramolecular level to augment their potential. Among these, co-crystals have gained a wide spread interest in pharmaceutical industry as US Food and Drug Administration (FDA) recently introduced new regulatory guidelines regarding this solid form which is anticipated to expand patent portfolios. Apart from cocrystals, other multicomponent adducts such as co-amorphous system and eutectic mixtures have also been discussed as a topic of interest in the present chapter for improving aqueous solubility, dissolution behavior and bioavailability of poorly soluble drugs. In addition, a section on future perspectives which shed light on new therapeutic hybrids deploying drug–drug combinations and drug–neutraceuticals combinations with improved pharmaceutical and biopharmaceutical attributes have also been described here.

Chapter 11 is on the topic "Multifunctional Nanocarrier Systems for Effective Delivery of Drugs in Cancer Treatment." The drug delivery to the cancer sites, with maintained effective drug concentration for longer duration, using low dose of drug, with minimum side effects is the prime concern of formulation scientist today. In the recent times, the nanocarrier systems are not only being utilized for achieving targeted, sustained and controlled release of drug to the disease site, but also are used in imaging of diseases. An attempt has been made through this chapter to give a brief outline about the cancer and elaborate details on the various multifunctional nanocarriers researched till date for effective delivery of drugs in cancer treatment. Further, functionalization and surface modification of nanocarrier with various ligands like folate, transferrin, TPGS (d-α-Tocopheryl Polyethylene Glycol 1000 Succinate), trastuzumab and hyaluronic acid etc., that have specific receptor in the proximity of disease site have been explained. This also includes the multifunctional nanocarrier systems of lipid, polymeric, nanotubes etc. and along with pros and cons of such carrier systems.

Chapter 12, "Multifunctional Nanocomposites for Biotherapeutic Applications," summarizes an overview account on newer therapeutic avenues for disease treatment using nanomedicines. The rationale for administering a drug is usually related to the increase of the drug bioavailability with the aim to achieve a therapeutic effect, at a pre-determined time. With the presence of multifunctional nanocomposites in place, several crucial factors like improvement on the medicine's efficacy, reduced economic implications, extended life of product patent, better safety and efficacy profile and increased compliance have been effectively monitored.

Chapter 13, "Nanocarriers as Non-Viral Vectors in Gene Delivery Application," provides information on emerging biomedical application of gene therapy for treatment of life-threatening diseases. This involves delivery of a therapeutic gene to the nucleus of an affected cell by a suitable vector. Gene delivery using non-viral vectors such as cationic polymer and lipid is gaining attention due to their favorable properties, including lack of immunogenicity, low toxicity, and potential for tissue specificity when compared with viral vectors. A variety of non-viral vectors have been proposed, most of which facilitate gene delivery by electrostatic interactions, encapsulation, and in some cases, condensing nucleic acids into nanosized particles which can be taken up by cells. A well-designed nanocarrier system promote cellular uptake and intracellular release of the nucleic acid. This chapter highlights different polymers, lipids and their nanocarriers employed for gene delivery application along with information on clinical trials.

Chapter 14, "Nanocarriers for Vaccine and Gene Delivery Application," provides information on composition and biological properties of nanocarriers for vaccination and gene delivery application. In recent years, developments in nanotechnology have focused on the design and synthesis of nanocarriers that have new properties and can be modified for gene and vaccine delivery. Nanocarriers have become increasingly important because they can stabilize vaccine antigens and serve as adjuvants, with the advantage of easily transporting genetic material to the target site. The chapter in general covers the application of nanocarriers like lipidic and polymeric systems, dendrimers, inorganic nanoparticles and nanocyclodextrins for vaccine and gene delivery applications.

Chapter 15, "Nanocomposites in Drug Delivery and Imaging Applications," discusses the fundamental characteristic properties of nanomaterials (like matrix structure, size, shape, and orientation, degree of dispersion, drug loading ability, etc. Nanocomposites are generally prepared using direct melt intercalation. The formation of nanocomposite is ascertained by XRD pattern, FTIR spectra, electron microscopy and thermal analysis like DSC and TGA. Nanocomposites have properties of nanoparticles, multifunctional capabilities, chemical functionalization and huge interphase zone. Novel nanomaterials offer a new chemotherapeutic route for cancer treatment by combining cell imaging and hyperthermia in a synergistic way. In spite of toxicity and safety concerns, multifunctional nanocomposite still charm the researchers because of emergence of versatile properties, better understanding of disease biomarkers and quest for ways to improve biocompatibility.

Chapter 16, "Smart Mesoporous Nanomaterials With Improved Therapeutic Applications," discusses on nanomaterials which have greatly revolutionized therapeutic drug delivery due to their unique physical characteristics that render them extremely manipulative at nanoscale level. One such category of nanomaterials is mesoporous silica nanoparticles. Due to their small size and rigid honeycomb like structure, they are highly conducive for packaging of drugs, dyes, antibodies, etc. These new generation nanomaterials can be further functionalized by incorporating surface modifications, thus increasing their acceptability as carriers for drugs and biomolecules. In this chapter, a brief and comprehensive review covering various aspects of the recent advancements in synthesis of mesoporous nanomaterials and post synthesis strategies for functionalization has been presented. Further, the chapter also throws light on how efficiently these smart nanocarriers are involved in transport and site-specific delivery of highly toxic chemotherapeutic agents for treatment of cancer, and their biocompatibility evaluation from safety point of view.

Chapter 17, "Emergence of Polymer-Lipid Hybrid Systems in Healthcare Scenario," provides insight on nanotechnology tools for variegated medicinal applications. Liposomes and polymeric nanoparticles are the promising nanocarriers of all the time which are highly efficient to encapsulate drugs by preventing their degradation along with control and sustained drug release characteristics. Despite many advantages of these nanoformulations, the presence of some of the drawbacks have limited their application to certain extent. Researchers, therefore, are focusing on development of novel nanohybrid structures with combined characteristics of polymeric and liposomal carriers. In this context, lipid hybrid polymer nanoparticles (LPNs) contain hydrophobic biodegradable polymeric core surrounded by a lipid layer for intensification of biocompatibility and biopharmaceutical attributes of the drugs. The book chapter compiled on the aforementioned topic particularly provides discussion on fundamentals of LPNs along with their advantages, composition and method of preparation for diverse therapeutic applications.

Acknowledgment

In the continued pursuit of earnest research endeavors of the Editors for compilation of the book titled *Multifunctional Nanocarriers for Contemporary Healthcare Applications*. At the very onset, the Editors are highly thankful to the authors for their sincere efforts in compiling the book chapters and greatly acknowledge the contributions for the present book. This book, in this regard, will certainly act as a repertoire of knowledge for disseminating the concept of nanotechnology applications in drug delivery, biomedicine and healthcare benefits.

Chapter 1
Advanced Nanotherapeutic Systems for Drug Delivery and Imaging in Cancer

Sanjeeb Sahoo
Institute of Life Sciences, India

Deepika Singh
Institute of Life Sciences, India

Priya Singh
Institute of Life Sciences, India

Aliva Prity Minz
Institute of Life Sciences, India

ABSTRACT

Recent progress in nanotechnology has paved the way for development of new tools for cancer imaging and treatment. Failure of early diagnosis is one of the major hurdles in cancer treatment. In addition, conventional treatment approaches suffer from problems of non-specific bio distribution of chemotherapeutic agent, low aqueous solubility, poor bioavailability, narrow therapeutic window, and rapid clearance. Nanotechnology addresses many of the aforementioned limitations and provides scope for early diagnosis, tumor-targeted delivery via passive or active targeting mechanisms, personalized treatment utilizing nanotheranostics, controlled drug release, and co-delivery of multiple therapeutic agents. This chapter summarizes various merits of nanotechnology with emphasis on different types of nanocarriers that are presently being used for drug delivery and imaging. As per these studies, the fruition of nanotechnology may make the disease curable by early diagnosis and specific drug delivery.

DOI: 10.4018/978-1-5225-4781-5.ch001

Copyright © 2018, IGI Global. Copying or distributing in print or electronic forms without written permission of IGI Global is prohibited.

INTRODUCTION

Cancer is one of the most dreaded diseases characterized by abnormal growth of cell with metastatic potential. As per World Health Organization (WHO) report around 7.8 million people die of this malignant disease every year, making it the second leading cause of death globally. There are around hundred different types of cancers of which, breast, colorectal, cervix, lung and stomach cancer are the most common among women, while lung, colorectal, prostate, stomach and liver cancer are the most common types in men. For over half a century cancer has been in forefront of biomedical research entailing great progress in fundamental cancer biology, however, little has been translated into clinics. This discrepancy is invariably due to cancer heterogeneity.

There are several challenges in cancer treatment, one of them being diagnosis. Despite technical advances in diagnostic radiology, early detection of neoplastic lesions remains an elusive task. In majority of the cases, tumor is detected only after it has metastasized, leaving grim chances of treatment and subsequent survival. Data from Cancer Research UK, suggests that early diagnosis results in three times higher cancer survival rate. Thus, strategies to improve diagnosis can have discernible impact on cancer morbidity and mortality.

Following diagnosis, the next gigantic challenge for cancer therapy is identification of ideal regime for elimination of cancerous cells. Oncologists have primarily depended on three treatment options viz. surgical excision, irradiation and chemotherapy. While surgery and irradiation are predominantly used for local and non-metastatic cancer, chemotherapy is the major therapeutic approach for both localized and metastatic cancer (Chidambaram, Manavalan, & Kathiresan, 2011). Chemotherapy is administration of single or multiple cytotoxic drugs to inhibit growth and division of malignant cells. Different types of chemotherapeutic agents being used are alkylating agents, neoplastic antibiotics (doxorubicin, daunorubicin, etc.), plant alkaloids (vincristine, vinblastine, paclitaxel, etc.), antimetabolites, and other miscellaneous antitumor agents. The principle idea behind using these cytotoxic agents is that they have most deleterious effect on rapidly proliferating cells. However, apart from cancer cells there are other rapidly dividing cells in the body like hair follicles, bone marrow and intestinal epithelial cells. So, these agents also have severe side effects on these tissues. This nonspecific bio distribution of existing therapeutic agents is major concern in cancer treatment. Besides, low solubility, poor bioavailability, inconsistent stability, inability to penetrate tumor cells, narrow therapeutic window, development of multi drug resistance and rapid clearance by reticuloendothelial cells are other bottlenecks in conventional chemotherapy (D. Singh, Minz, & Sahoo, 2017; Steichen, Caldorera-Moore, & Peppas, 2013) .Thus, there is an extensive need for development of new strategies which can overcome above mentioned limitations and specifically target cancer cells, thereby reducing toxicity to normal tissues.

Nanotechnology: A One Step Solution

Nanotechnology fabricated with established cancer research is being harnessed to address and rectify many of the aforementioned cross-cutting problems. It offers unique approaches in diagnostics, therapeutics and prognostics (Figure 1). In diagnostics, it finds its application in imaging which is pivotal to clinical cancer care. All the available imaging modalities require contrast agents to discern malignancies based on their molecular expression profiles. Non-targeted exogenous contrast agents routinely used in clinics are either non-specific to cancer tissue or are relatively insensitive to diagnose cancer in the early stage. Nanocarriers are being greatly explored for the development of targeted exogenous agents with the

Figure 1. Diagram illustrates the potential application of nanoparticles in various aspects of drug delivery and imaging

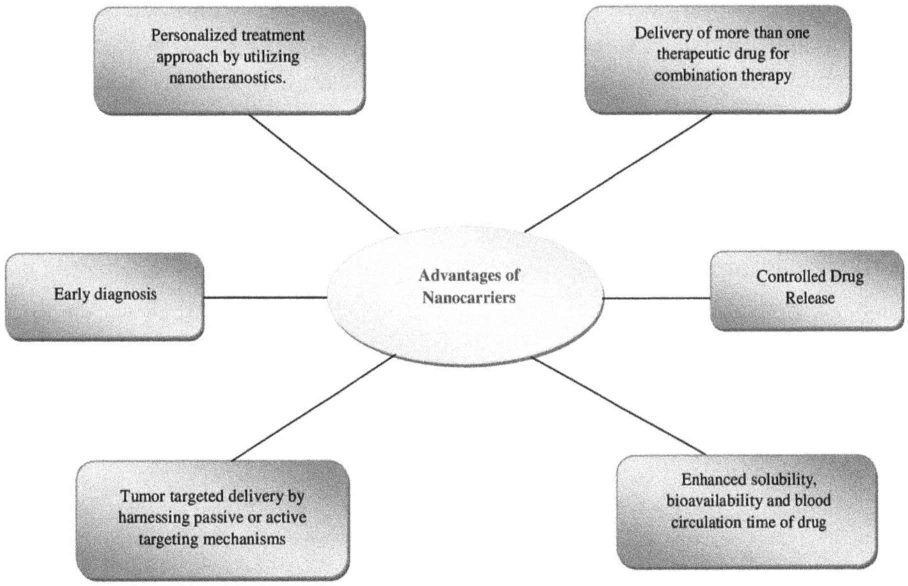

objective of identifying early stage tumors, detecting molecular expressions and microenvironment of neoplasms (Frangioni, 2008). Magnetic nanoparticles like iron oxide nanoparticles are efficient contrast agents for magnetic resonance imaging (MRI) owing to their high sensitivity, high tissue resolution, longer blood retention time, ability for functionalizing tumor targeting agents on surface, biodegradability and biocompatibility (Peng, X. H., Qian, X., Mao, H., Wang, A. Y., Chen, Z. G., Nie, S., 2008). One such example is resovist, an organ specific superparamagnetic iron oxide-carboxydextran coated nanoparticle which has been approved in European market for detection and characterization of early stage small focal liver lesions. Cross-linked iron-oxide nanoparticle conjugated with annexin-V has been tested for MRI detection of camptothecin -induced Jurkat T-cell *in vitro*. The specificity and sensitivity of these nanoparticles show potential for future clinical applications (Ferrari, 2005).

Nanotechnology has paved its way into therapeutics as drug delivery systems showing immense potential in developing formulations with targeting selectivity and ability to overcome biological barriers (Sahoo & Labhasetwar, 2003). Liposomes, micelles, carbon nanotubes, dendrimers, polymeric and magnetic nanoparticles are the different types of nanocarriers being used as nanomedicines (Parhi, Mohanty, & Sahoo, 2012). These nanocarriers are excellent delivering entities because they offer benefits of co-delivery of multiple anti-cancer agents, protect the drug from degradation, enhance aqueous solubility, reduce renal clearance, increase blood circulation time and deploy controlled drug release (Misra, Acharya, & Sahoo, 2010; Weissleder, Kelly, Sun, Shtatland, & Josephson, 2005). Moreover, nanotechnology offers unique platform for designing tumor targeted delivery vehicles by utilizing either passive or active targeting mechanisms (Parveen & Sahoo, 2008). In passive targeting, the Enhanced Permeability and Retention (EPR) effect in cancer tissues is exploited to preferentially accumulate nanoscale particles in tumor interstitium (Iyer, Khaled, Fang, & Maeda, 2006). In contrast to normal vessels, tumor vasculature is abnormal in organization and structure and is heterogeneous. Tumor cells have rapid growth rate and to support this, they are equipped with vascular permeability and angiogenesis mediators that bestow these vessels with hyperpermeability and leakiness. Furthermore, tumor has poor lymphatic drainage due to lack of functional lymphatic vessels which leads to longer retention (Figure 2). These architectural defects lead to the EPR effect which is used as gold standard in targeting nanoparticles to tumor (Jain & Stylianopoulos, 2010). However, this strategy leads to localization of nanoparticles in tumor microenvironment, but it does not promote their uptake into cancer cells. Thus, active targeting mechanisms are being investigated. For this, surface functionalization of nanoparticles is done by attaching different ligands that are specific to receptors or surface markers, over expressed on cancer cells, thereby promoting their internalization by receptor-mediated endocytosis (Mohanty, Das, & Sahoo, 2012). Various targeting ligands like albumin, biotin, transferrin, folate, antibodies, peptides

Figure 2. Diagram showing enhanced permeability and retention effect for passive targeting of nanomedicines. Near the tumor the vasculature is leaky drainage is poor. Hence, nanoparticles get easily accumulated in tumor and gain access to the tumor cell.

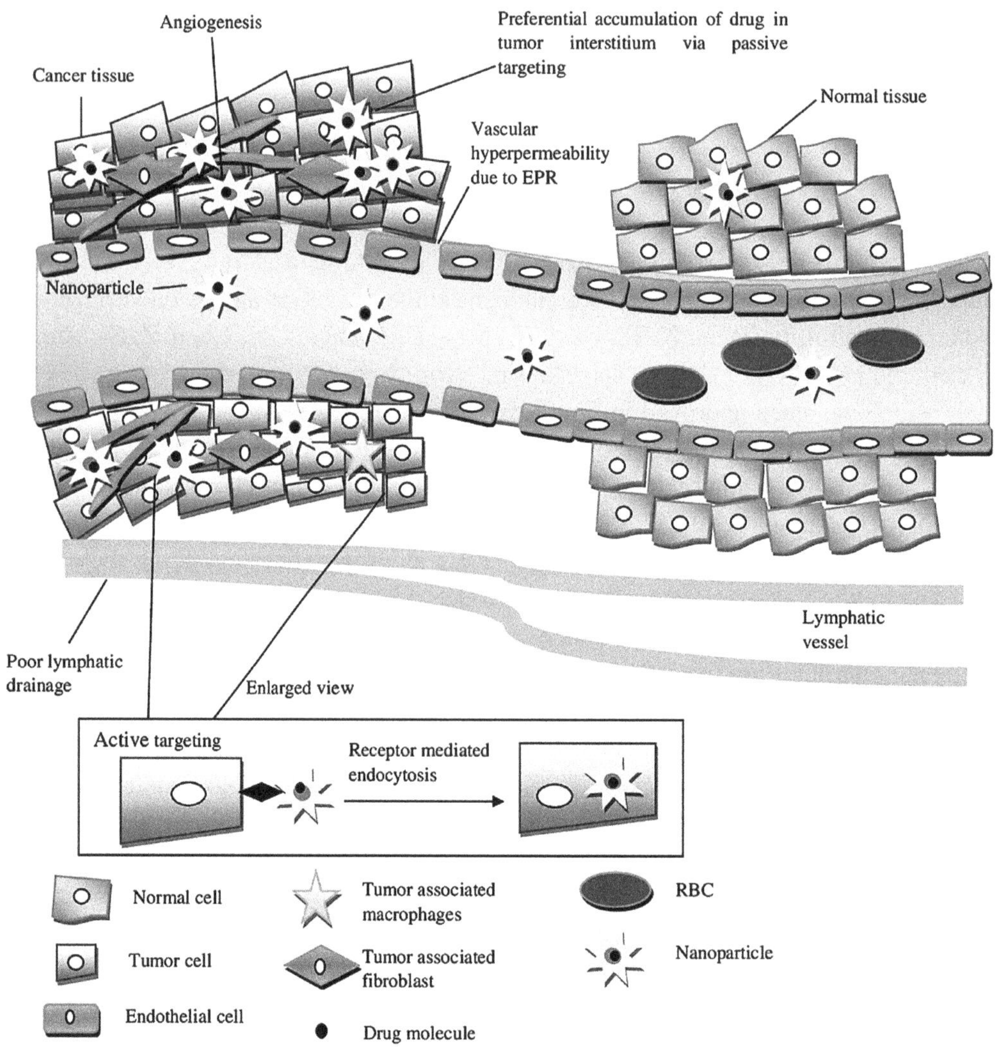

and aptamers are being extensively used for the same. Active targeting improves therapeutic efficacy of cytotoxic drugs and reduces occurrence of drug resistance (Perez-Herrero & Fernandez-Medarde, 2015).

Besides this, nanotechnology also finds its application in the new arena of personalized cancer management as nanotheranostics. It is the amalgamation of therapeutic and diagnostic function in nanoscale formulations. This technology has distinctive applications ranging from patient stratification to patient subpopulation screening, early detection, disease staging, monitoring therapy response and detecting adverse effects at early stage. This is essential to grapple with tumor heterogeneity, which requires individualized approach. Every tumor is different, even the ones with same origin, thus we have to leave the one-for-all approach and adopt technologies that help to cater the hope for tailoring therapy for personalized management of cancer. Nanotheranostics is an emerging field that has the potential to transfigure clinical oncology (Chen Hongmin, 2017; T. H. Kim, Lee, & Chen, 2013; A. Singh & Sahoo, 2014). This review focusses on various types of nanodelivery systems available, or being researched for therapy and imaging in cancer.

Different nanocarriers presently being used for drug delivery are either polymeric or inorganic nanoparticles (Figure 3). Recently, viral proteins are the new addition as delivery vehicles.

Figure 3. Different types of nanoparticles which can be loaded with chemotherapeutic and imaging agent simultaneously. These nanoparticles can be further conjugated with targeting moiety to achieve targeting.

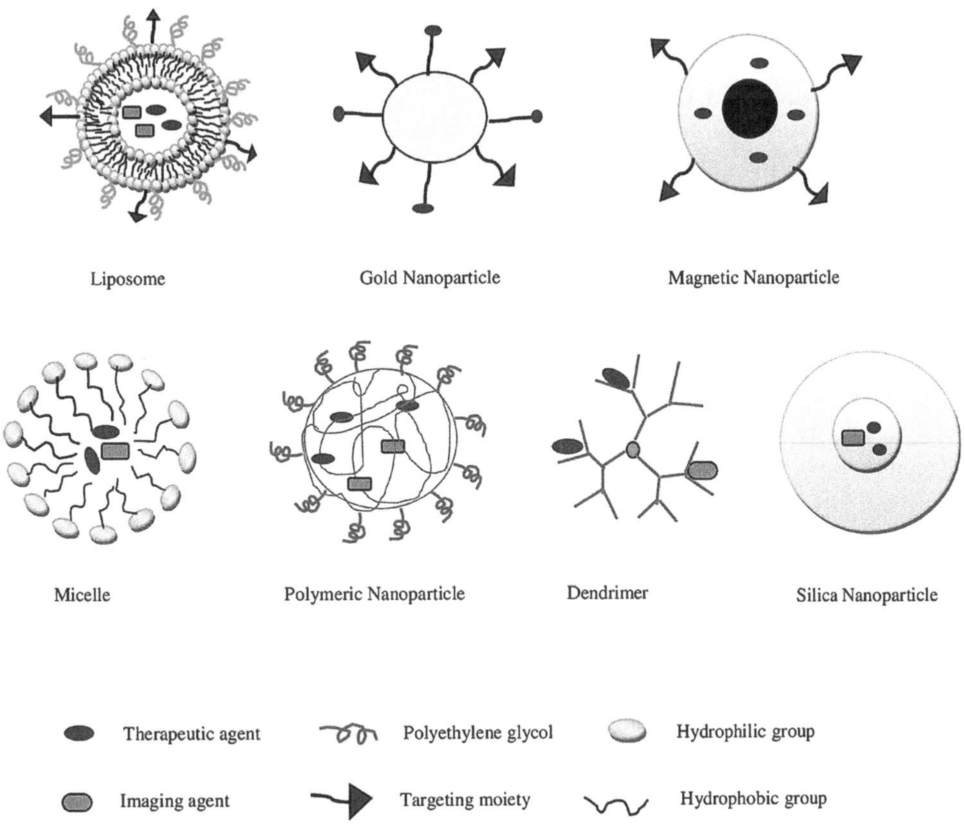

POLYMER BASED NANOPARTICLES

Liposomes

Liposomes are self-assembled, sphere shaped vesicles that can be of a single or bilayer membrane with size ranging from 0.25µm to 2.5µm. Liposomes gained much attention as a delivery vehicle as they can mimic the cell structure, are highly biocompatible and can entrap both hydrophobic and lipophilic compounds simultaneously (Riehemann, K., Schneider, S. W., Luger, T. A., Godin, B., Ferrari, M., & Fuchs, H., 2009). The circulating half-life and drug encapsulation efficiency of liposomes varies with change in its size, surface charge and method of preparation.

Recently Wu *et al.* formulated liposomes with light triggered contrast agents (IR820, iohexol and Gd- chelates) which showed enhanced Computed Tomography (CT), Magnetic Resonance Imaging (MRI) and Fluorescence Imaging (FI) multimodal imaging. *In vitro* studies demonstrated complete inhibition of C6 tumor growth with this formulation as IR820 has high photothermal conversion efficiency. Hence, the formulated theranostic liposome is a potential candidate for NIR-activated imaging and photothermal therapy (Wu, B., Wan, B., Lu, S. T., Deng, K., Li, X. Q., Wu, B. L., 2017).Similar work by Grange et al. (2010) showed that incorporation of gadolinium into doxorubicin loaded liposomes conjugated with Neural Cell Adhesion Molecule (NCAM)-peptide for site specific targeting enhances *in vitro* drug internalization. Gd-labelled liposomes allowed the MRI visualization of drug delivery in the tumor region along with enhanced apoptosis (Grange, C., Geninatti-Crich, S., Esposito, G., Alberti, D., Tei, L., Bussolati, B., 2010).

Solid Lipid Nanoparticles (SLNs)

SLNs are lipid emulsions of submicron- size in which the liquid lipid (oil) is replaced by a solid lipid (Cavalli Roberta, 1993). They show low systemic toxicity, high stability and biocompatibility, low cost of production, ease of preparation and high hydrophobic drug entrapment efficiency. Due to these advantages, pharmaceutical researchers have shown much interest in the area of SLNs based drug delivery from the last decade (Han, Zhang, Chen, Sun, & Kong, 2014). Kuang et al. (2017) formulated SLNs conjugated with an arginyl-glycyl-aspartic acid (RGD) based targeting moiety for example c(RGDyK) for site specific targeting and loaded it with IR-780 for imaging. Results indicated that their formulated nanotheranostic not only improved targeted delivery of IR-780 for imaging but also eradicated tumors by photothermal therapy after application of laser irradiation (Kuang, Y., Zhang, K., Cao, Y., Chen, X., Wang, K., Liu, M., 2017). Recently, it has been found that SLNscan also be exploited for oral delivery of theranostics. In this regard, SLNs were encapsulated with iron oxide nanoparticles and coated with heparin. These theranostic tools showed higher cellular internalisation *in vitro* indicating that it can be a promising tool for oral delivery of theranostic into the lymphatic circulation (Truzzi, E., Bongio, C., Sacchetti, F., Maretti, E., Montanari, M., Iannuccelli, V., 2017). It has also been reported that N-carboxymethyl chitosan (NCC) coated SLNs loaded with curcumin can inhibit burst release of the drug in acidic environment of stomach when given orally to experimental animals. Moreover, SLNs demonstrated enhanced intestinal delivery, increased cellular and lymphatic uptake and can enhance oral bioavailability with high antitumor efficacy (Baek & Cho, 2017).

Polymeric Nanoparticles

Polymeric nanoparticles are solid colloidal particles made of polymers. Drug delivery system using biodegradable polymeric nanoparticle promises a controlled drug release property, biocompatibility with cells, maintains its integrity in blood, non thrombogenic, and is applicable to carry molecules like peptides, nucleic acid, proteins and drug (des Rieux, Fievez, Garinot, Schneider, & Preat, 2006; Gref, R., Minamitake, Y., Peracchia, M. T., Trubetskoy, V., Torchilin, V., & Langer, R., 1994). The drugs can be entrapped, encapsulated or attached to the carrier matrix of polymeric nanoparticles depending upon the methods of preparation used (Rawat, Singh, Saraf, & Saraf, 2006).For example, BIND-014 which is a prostate-specific membrane antigen (PSMA) targeted polymeric nanoparticle loaded with docetaxel has reached phase II clinical trial as it showed unique pharmacokinetic profile with manageable toxicity (Von Hoff, D. D., Mita, M. M., Ramanathan, R. K., Weiss, G. J., Mita, A. C., LoRusso, P. M., 2016).

Recently it has been found that curcumin loaded polymeric nanoparticle, surface decorated with quantum dots as imaging agent displayed significantly improved cellular effect of curcumin via inhibition of JAK/STAT pathway in primary effusion lymphoma. Moreover, it was reported that the localization of nanoparticles and the released drug could be visualised *in vitro*. Hence, this bifunctional nanoparticle could be a promising theranostic in near future (Belletti, D., Riva, G., Luppi, M., Tosi, G., Forni, F., Vandelli, M. A., 2017). In another study, Dumoga et al. (2017) designed polymeric nanoparticles by encapsulating methotrexate and further conjugating with folic acid for specific targeting of cervical carcinoma. These nanoparticles were radiolabelled with ^{99m}Tc to perform Gamma-Single Photon Emission Computed Tomography (SPECT) imaging in animal models. Anti-proliferative effect of these theranostic nanoparticles were established and could be a potential theranostic tool for cervical carcinoma (Dumoga, S., Rai, Y., Bhatt, A. N., Tiwari, A. K., Singh, S., Mishra, A. K., 2017). A similar study carried out by Liu *et al.* showed formulation of Fe_3O_4@mSiO_2@lipid-PEG-methotrexatenanoparticle (FMLM) encapsulated with doxorubicin as a chemotherapeutic, where the Fe_3O_4 core was used for magnet-stimulate-response drug release, MRI and early-phase magnet targeting ability. Further, zinc phthalocyanine was loaded on FMLM for simultaneous near-infrared fluorescence imaging and photodyanamic therapy. This nanotheranostic exhibited increased cellular uptake, enhanced anticancer activity and tumor accumulation in animal model (Liu, G., Ma, J., Li, Y., Li, Q., Tan, C., Song, H., 2017).It has also been shown recently that oral delivery of chitosan coated poly (lactide-co-glycolide) (PLGA) nanoparticles co-delivering polyphenolic bio-enhancers with oleanolic acid can have enhanced anticancerous effect while preserving the female fertility in a metastatic breast cancer rat models (Sharma, M., Sharma, S., Sharma, V., Sharma, K., Yadav, S. K., Dwivedi, P., 2017).

Polymeric Micelles

Polymeric micelles are self-assembled colloidal nanostructure formed by amphiphilic block copolymers. They have both inherent and easy modifiable properties which makes them favourable for drug delivery (Croy & Kwon, 2006). Polymeric micelles have proven to be a potential platform for delivery of drug, gene and imaging agent. Further, it can also be designed to respond to external stimuli like temperature, pH etc. and undergo change in their structure and morphology.

Recently, He et al. (2017) reported the use of IR-780 loaded polymeric micelles (IPM) for photothermal therapy against metastatic breast cancer. Both *in vitro* and *in vivo* studies demonstrated that IPM exhibited higher heat generating capability under laser irradiation, inhibited primary growth of tumor and reduced lymphatic metastasis, proving themselves to be an encouraging theranostic platform (He, B., Hu, H. Y., Tan, T., Wang, H., Sun, K. X., Li, Y. P., 2017). Similarly, Lin et al. (2017) developed pH-responsive theranostic unimolecular micelles where they encapsulated doxorubicin as anti-cancer therapeutic in gold nanoparticles for Computed Tomography (CT). Both *in vitro* and *in vivo* studies revealed enhanced anticancer efficacy and superior imaging properties of nanocomposite for theranostic applications (Lin, W., Yao, N., Qian, L., Zhang, X., Chen, Q., Wang, J., 2017). In another study by Hao *et al.* polymeric micelles was loaded with anticancer drug doxorubicin and conjugated with aggregation-induced emission (AIE) molecule for cellular imaging and Forster Resonance Energy Transfer (FRET) effect for monitoring drug delivery. These polymeric micelles exhibited promising novel nanoplatform for tracing of drug delivery, high quality intracellular imaging and chemotherapy (Hao, N., Sun, C., Wu, Z., Xu, L., Gao, W., Cao, J., 2017).

The fact that polymeric micelles are very well suited for exploiting EPR effect was utilised by Kenmotsu et al.(2010) They formulated polymeric micelles by incorporating 7-ehtyl-10-hydroxycamptothecin (SN-38) which was named NK012. Animal studies revealed that combination therapy of NK012 with bevacizumab shows enhanced pharmacokinetics and greater antitumor efficacy against lung cancer in a xenograft model (Kenmotsu, H., Yasunaga, M., Goto, K., Nagano, T., Kuroda, J., Koga., 2010). Present records suggest that NK012 has reached phase II clinical trial for colorectal cancer, lung cancer and breast cancer (Matsumura, 2011). Another polymeric micelles NC-6004 which is loaded with cisplatin showed delayed and sustained release of the drug with low toxicity as compared to native drug in phase I clinical trial (Cabral & Kataoka, 2014). Presently, different formulations of NC-6004 are in clinical trials. The efficacy of NC-6004 is further increased by combination of gemcitabine which is also in phase III clinical trial.

Hydrogels

Hydrogels are three-dimensional structure of water-swollen polymeric materials and are capable of holding large amount of water within their structure. They are the first biomaterials that are formulated for use in human body (J. Kopecek, Yang, J, 2007). Block and graft copolymers self-assemble into hydrogels at physiological conditions in aqueous environment provide immense opportunities for development of hydrogels as sensitive delivery system(J. Kopecek, 2007).

Recently Cho et al. (2017) developed an injectable and photo responsive composite hydrogel loaded with anti-cancer drug doxorubicin, imaging contrast agent indocyanine green, bio-derived collagen and multifaceted anionic polypeptide, poly (γ-glutamic acid) (γ-PGA). Further, $MnFe_2O_4$ magnetic nanoparticles were incorporated into this hydrogel. It is shown by animal experiments that by NIR light irradiation, release kinetics of doxorubicin and magnetic relaxation of magnetic nanoparticles could be modulated for theranostic purpose (Cho, S. H., Kim, A., Shin, W., Heo, M. B., Noh, H. J., Hong, K. S., 2017). In another study, hydrogels were used for photothermal therapy (PTT) of glioblastomas. RADA16-I, which is a synthetic amphiphilic peptide that can self-assemble into a hydrogel, was conjugated to melittin and loaded with indocyanine green for imaging. Upon treatment in an animal model it shrunk the tumor size and reduced tumor recurrence rate, providing safe and efficient tumor treatment (Jin, H., Zhao, G., Hu, J., Ren, Q., Yang, K., Wan, C., 2017).

Dendrimers

Dendrimers are nano sized, extensively branched 3Dimentional polymeric macromolecules with radial symmetry and monodispersity which can provide large surface functionality and versatility. Dendrimers have attracted researchers' due to their broad applications in chemical reactions, mainly host-guest chemistry. They can be ideal theranostic vehicles mainly due to their poly valency which provides versatile functionalisation and can be advantageous for multiple biological interactions (Abbasi, E., Aval, S. F., Akbarzadeh, A., Milani, M., Nasrabadi, H. T., Joo, S. W., 2014; Nanjwade Basavaraj K., 2009).Wang et al. (2016) developed polyamidoamine (PAMAM) dendrimer functionalised with PEG and conjugated with nonographene oxide (NGO-PEG-dendrimer) for delivery of anti-miR-21 (microRNA) to non-small-cell lung cancer. NGO-PEG-dendrimerled to inhibition of cell migration and invasion along with enhanced bioluminescence signal within the tumor area. This nanotheranostic platform allows image-guided monitoring of nucleotide delivery highlighting the RNA based cancer treatments (Wang, Y., Strohm, E. M., Sun, Y., Wang, Z., Zheng, Y., Wang, Z., 2016). Similarly, Gu et al (2017) designed PAMAM dendrimers functionalised with graphene oxide for co-delivery of doxorubicin and MMP-9 shRNA plasmid for breast cancer treatment (Gu, Y., Guo, Y., Wang, C., Xu, J., Wu, J., Kirk, T. B., 2017).Another study showed formulation of generation five PEG conjugated PAMAM dendrimers radiolabelled with ^{131}I. Further, the targeting moietychlorotoxin and 3-(4'-hydroxyphenyl) propionic acid-OSu (HPAO) was attached to form human glioma targeted nanotheranostic.Results from animal studies indicates that these dendrimers have capability to be used for targeted SPECT imaging and radiation therapy against gliomas (Zhao, L., Zhu, J., Cheng, Y., Xiong, Z., Tang, Y., Guo, L., 2015). As not much clinical success is obtained with dendrimers due to various limitations, Li et al. (2016) have tried to overcome these limitations by formulating supramolecular dendritic system loaded with doxorubicin that mimics virus capsid. This nanomedicine improved the drug location to tumor site, capsid-like structure of nanoparticles improved drug penetration and showed site specific delivery in tumor bearing mouse models (Li, Y., Lai, Y., Xu, X., Zhang, X., Wu, Y., Hu, C., 2016).

Natural Polymeric Nanocarriers

Protein-based nanoparticles are found to be very interesting among the other colloidal drug carrier systems currently available. These nanoparticles show greater stability upon storage and *in vitro* drug delivery. They are also non-toxic, non-antigenic and could be easily scaled up at the time of manufacturing (Elzoghby, Samy, & Elgindy, 2012). Albumin is biodegradable, non-immunogenic, easily purified and hydrophilic which allows easy drug delivery, thus proving itself to be ideal as a drug delivery vehicle (Rahimnejad M, 2006). Studies carried out by Khandelia et al. (2015) showed that albumin nanoparticle embedded with gold nanoclusters and loaded with doxorubicin can be used for single-photon and two-photon imaging and drug delivery to cancer cells. This nanomedicine is not only capable of bio-imaging but also induce apoptotic cell death which states that it is a potential theranostic (Khandelia, Bhandari, Pan, Ghosh, & Chattopadhyay, 2015).

Chitosan is a deacetylated form of chitin, a polysaccharide present abundantly in crustacean shells. Chitosan being hydrophilic and positively charged polymer can interact with negatively charged cell membrane and hence can be used as a promising material for drug delivery and imaging (Patel JK, 2009). Recently, in a study Lee et al. (2017) have formulated chitosan oligosaccharide conjugated with indomethacin and further loaded it with doxorubicin. This nanomedicine so formed is reported to have enhanced anticancer activity, longer blood circulation and tumor targeting ability in animal models. Hence, it can be a promising candidate for drug delivery and real-time imaging (Lee, J. Y., Termsarasab, U., Lee, M. Y., Kim, D. H., Lee, S. Y., Kim, J. S., 2017).

INORGANIC NANOPARTICLES

Iron Oxide Nanoparticles

Iron oxide nanoparticles have received remarkable attention in various aspects owing to their unique physiochemical properties at nanoscale. Superparamagnetic property of these nanoparticles makes them preferred choice for MRI. Among the various types of iron oxide nanoparticles,Fe_3O_4 is very popular due to its biocompatibility (Lodhia, Mandarano, Ferris, Eu, & Cowell, 2010; Nedyalkova, M., Donkova, B., Romanova, J., Tzvetkov, G., Madurga, S., & Simeonov, V., 2017).Large surface area and small size with quantum confinement and novel optical and magnetic properties of iron oxide nanoparticles could be explored for its vast biomedical applications(Erb RM, 2009).

Ultra small sized Fe_3O_4 nanoparticles showed brilliant T_1 or T_1+T_2 contrast abilities and have gained attention as MRI contrast agents (Saraswathy, A., Nazeer, S. S., Nimi, N., Arumugam, S., Shenoy, S. J., & Jayasree, R. S., 2014).In the current study, Cha et al. (2017) modified Fe_3O_4 nanoparticles with star polymers containing β-cyclodextrin (β-CD) core and poly(2-(dimethylamino) ethyl methacrylate) (PDMAEMA) arms. Star polymers were associated with reduced glutathione as a model drug. This nano-formulation is found to serve as a better T_1 MRI contrast agent and could also be a versatile theranostic (Cha, R., Li, J., Liu, Y., Zhang, Y., Xie, Q., & Zhang, M., 2017). Similarly, Fu et al.(2017) developed a NIR controlled hybrid nanoplatform (carbon nanotubes [CNTs]-iron oxide nanoparticle) with MRI and magnetic targeting properties. Doxorubicin and distearoyl-*sn*-glycero-3-phosphoethanolamine-PEG were conjugated to the hybrid nanoparticles surface and this nanoparticle-drug complex was encapsulated in 1-myristyl alcohol (DOX-NPs).Both *in vitro* and *in vivo* studies of DOX-NPs showed excellent MRI ability, magnetic targeting capability, biocompatibility and enhanced antitumor therapeutic efficacy combining hyperthermia and chemotherapy(Fu, Wang, Zhou, & Zhang, 2017). In another study, it is reported that intra peritoneal (i.p.) delivery of magnetic iron oxide nanoparticles targeted to urokinase plasminogen activator receptor (uPAR) leads to higher intratumoral accumulation of nanoparticles in pancreatic cancer mouse model as depicted by non-invasive optical and MRI. These nanoparticles when loaded with cisplatin or doxorubicin significantly reduced tumor growth and proliferating tumor cells and vessels without systemic toxicity. Also strong optical signals within tumors suggested the compatibility of image-guided surgery for removing of drug resistant tumors (Gao, N., Bozeman, E. N., Qian, W., Wang, L., Chen, H., Lipowska., 2017).

Recently, Tian et al.(2017) showed that animal experiments depicts paclitaxel loaded iron oxide magnetic nanoparticles modified with methoxy polyethylene glycol (PEG)-lysine-oleic acid (PTX-MNPs-PLO) had improved pharmacokinetic and enhanced anti-cancerous activity as compared to native paclitaxel. Further, this nanomedicine holds great promise for targeted drug delivery, magnetic accumulation and thermal therapy (Tian, J., Yan, C., Liu, K., Tao, J., Guo, Z., Liu, J., 2017). As per the recent reports, ferumoxytol which is an iron oxide nanoparticle delivering iron to anaemic patients, has now reached early phase I clinical trials for use as an MRI agent for head and neck cancer. Hence, iron oxide nanoparticles can prove to be a novel nanoplatform for theranostic purpose.

Carbon Nanotubes

Carbon nanotubes (CNTs) are cylindrical structure made up of layers of graphene with either opened or closed ends. Single graphene layer is denoted as single-wall carbon nanotubes (SWCNT) while multiple graphene layers denote multiwall carbon nanotubes (MWCNT) (Sumio, 1991). CNTs are compatible with biomolecules like DNA and proteins, in addition they enable fluorescent and photoacoustic imaging along with NIR mediated localised heating (De Volder, Tawfick, Baughman, & Hart, 2013; Kam, O'Connell, Wisdom, & Dai, 2005).In a recent study, Liang et al.(2016) prepared SWCNT conjugated to Cy5.5 to target breast tumor by PTT. *In vitro* studies using this nanoformulation depicted shrunken tumor after irradiation with NIR laser. Hence this data supports the fact that photothermal-responsive SWCNT-Cy5.5 can be a promising theranostic agent for PTT (Liang, X., Shang, W., Chi, C., Zeng, C., Wang, K., Fang, C., 2016). Another study by Zhao et al. (2016) shows that SWCNT when coated with polydopamine and further modified by PEG offers enhanced T1 and T2 contrast MRI. Further, these nanoparticles when labelled with radionuclide ^{131}I enabled nuclear imaging and radioisotope cancer therapy. SWNT@PDA-^{131}I-PEG showed efficient tumor accumulation as depicted by MRI and gamma imaging.Synergistic antitumor therapeutic effect was obtained by combination of NIR triggered PTT with ^{131}I based radiotherapy in animal experiments (Zhao, H., Chao, Y., Liu, J., Huang, J., Pan, J., Guo, W., 2016) thereby, presenting themselves to be a promising theranostic agents.

Silica/Hybrid Nanoparticles

Silica nanoparticles (SNPs) are widely studied and applied for drug delivery and biosensing due to their high rigidity, thermal stability and the property of physical and chemical resistance. To enhance the benefits of SNPs, they are modified on their surface with organic material such as polymers, which are also known as polymer-grafted SNPs (Wu L, 2016). The hybrid nanomaterial so formed combines rigidity and stability of SNPs along with flexibility, processability, and functionality of organic polymers which opens wide application routes of SNPs (Zou, Wu, & Shen, 2008).

In a study, Zeiderman et al.(2016) formulated acidic pH targeted nanomedicine for Multispectral Optoacoustic Tomography (MSOT). They designed gold nanorods, coated with mesoporous silica and capped with chitosan which was further loaded with gemcitabine. This formulation was found suitable for simultaneous tumor imaging and drug delivery (Zeiderman, M. R., Morgan, D. E., Christein, J. D., Grizzle, W. E., McMasters, K. M., & McNally, L. R., 2016). A similar work was carried out by Zao et al. (2017) who showed that their formulated redox and enzyme responsive doxorubicin loaded nanomedicine (HMSN-SS-CD_{PEI}@HA) with hollow mesoporous SNPs capped with carbon dots improved tracking function and conjugation with hyaluronic acid improved their targeted delivery. This nanomedicine can be a promising platform for real-time imaging and targeted drug delivery (Zhao, H., Chao, Y., Liu, J., Huang, J., Pan, J., Guo, W., 2017). Recently Kang et al.(2017) showed that carbon dot created mesoporous hollow organosilica nanoparticles loaded with doxorubicin can be an efficient theranostic for drug delivery and *in vitro* imaging. This nanomedicine exhibits high optical stability of the optical signals (Kang, M. S., Singh, R. K., Kim, T. H., Kim, J. H., Patel, K. D., & Kim, H. W., 2017).

Recently, Sun et al. (2017) formulated core-shell hierarchical mesoporous silica/ organosilica nanoparticles wherein large molecules like siRNA and small molecules like doxorubicin could be encapsulated and released independently. Firstly, large siRNA released from the nanosystem and downregulated the release of P-gp in cell membrane which reverses the Multi Drug Resistance (MDR) effect of cancer cells, followed by release of doxorubicin for cytotoxicity to cancer cells. Both *in vitro* and *in vivo* studies demonstrated the synergistic inhibition of MDR and tumor growth (Sun, L., Wang, D., Chen, Y., Wang, L., Huang, P., Li, Y., 2017). In another study, it has been found that silica containing redox nanoparticles with reactive oxygen species scavenging capacity, loaded with BNS-22 (anticancer compound) was formulated for oral dose against colitis-associated colon cancer. This nanomedicine showed enhanced stability in acidic conditions, improved bioavailability of drug, inhibited tumor progression and reduced toxicity of drug in animal studies (Vong, Kimura, & Nagasaki, 2017)

Gold Nanoparticles

Gold nanoparticles (AuNPs) can be readily synthesised, easily surface modified and exhibits unique optical properties. Based on these advantages, AuNPs are widely used as a carrier for delivery of intracellular therapeutics and molecular nanoprobes for imaging (Jeong, Jung, Hong, & Lee, 2014). Wang et al. (2016) formulated optically triggered multifunctional AuNPs for photoacoustic/fluorescent imaging and chemotherapy. For this, AuNPs were stabilized by PLGA and loaded with paclitaxel. When this nanomedicine was taken up by cancer cells and excited by laser pulses, vaporisation of the nanoparticles takes place reducing the cell viability. Hence, these particles show great potential for photoacoustic imaging and drug delivery in cancer therapy (Wang, Y., Strohm, E. M., Sun, Y., Wang, Z., Zheng, Y., Wang, Z., 2016). Similarly, Manivasagan et al. (2016) synthesised multifunctional doxorubicin encapsulated AuNPs and capped with fucoidan which also acts as a reducing agent. The DOX-Fu AuNPs so formed showed apoptosis in a concentration dependent manner. Therefore, this nanomedicine is capable of efficient drug delivery and photoacoustic imaging (Manivasagan, P., Bharathiraja, S., Bui, N. Q., Jang, B., Oh, Y. O., Lim, I. G., 2016). Researchers have also synthesised highly fluorescent anticancerous gold quantum clusters. These quantum clusters are prepared by etching AuNPs by ethylenediamine and surface stabilized by transferrin. This nanomedicine showed bright photoluminescence indicating high cellular uptake and cytotoxicity within 24 hrs of incubation (J. H. Kim, Eguchi, & Ishikawa, 2017).

Quantum Dots

Quantum dots (QDs) are semiconductor nanocrystals varying from 2-10 nm capable of exhibiting size-dependent optical properties, absorbance and photoluminescence (Xu, G., Zeng, S., Zhang, B., Swihart, M. T., Yong, K. T., & Prasad, P. N., 2016). They are powerful fluorescent probes designed especially for quantitative imaging and detection. QDs are excellent material for studying therapeutic functionalities, imaging and targeting both *in vitro* and *in vivo* (Qi & Gao, 2008). Nigam et al. (2014) formulated human serum albumin nanoparticles labelled with green fluorescent graphene quantum dots and functionalized with hyaluronic acid. This nanoparticle was loaded with gemcitabine. In *in vitro* the nanomedicine so formed enhanced the bioavailability and sustained drug release profile for pancreatic cancer therapy (Nigam P, 2014). Recently, Aizik et al. (2017) developed a nanosystem where QDs are present inside the liposomes and could be engulfed by the phagocytic cells of the innate immune system and carried to the site of inflammation. Treatment with these nanoparticles through intra venous (i.v.) administration showed high accumulation and retention along with enhanced optical properties, proving themselves to be promising strategy for *in vitro* imaging (Aizik, G., Waiskopf, N., Agbaria, M., Levi-Kalisman, Y., Banin, U., & Golomb, G., 2017). In another study by Wu et al.(2017) it was shown that fluorescent indium phosphide QDs modified with vascular endothelial growth factor receptor 2 (VEGFR2) antibody achieved targeted drug delivery. Further miR-92a inhibitor was attached to the nanoformulation which enhanced the expression of tumor suppressor p63. This functionalized nanomedicine induced apoptosis by active targeting and also allowed infrared imaging in animal models. Hence, this nanomedicine can be a potent chemotherapy strategy against cancer in future (Wu, Y. Z., Sun, J., Zhang, Y., Pu, M., Zhang, G., He, N., 2017).

Viral Nanocarriers

Study of virus-derived materials and its impact in the medical sector is an emerging field of interest and many novel viruses from bacteria, plants and mammals are in the process of development. Viral nanoparticles are discrete and monodisperse with precise shape and size (Steinmetz, 2013). Polyomaviruses (PVLP) are efficient delivery vehicles for cargoes like nucleic acid, therapeutics and imaging probes. By surface engineering of PVLP capsid, its targeted delivery to cancer cells over expressing transferring receptors can be achieved. This artificially modified structure of surface protein of PVLP shows higher cellular uptake and selective targeting to cancer cells(Zackova Suchanova, Neburkova, Spanielova, Forstova, & Cigler, 2017). Recently, Li et al.(2017) have explored the potential of plant viral nanoparticles for chemotherapeutic delivery. They used potato virus X for delivery of doxorubicin to ovarian, breast and cervical cancer cells and breast cancer xenografts, which resulted in improved tumor homing and tumor penetration with reduced tumor growth (Le, Lee, Shukla, Commandeur, & Steinmetz, 2017).

In another study, Marino et al. (2017) showed that oncolytic viruses could be genetically modified for therapeutic gene expression and augmenting their anti-cancerous activity. They modified the genome of an oncolytic adenovirus, enadenotucirev by cloning of synthesised transgene cassettes. This modified virus which encodes transgene protein was successfully expressed in tumor both *in vitro* and *in vivo*. Full length anti-VEGF antibodies could be encoded by inserting multiple gene into the genome of the virus, which finally leads to synthesis and secretion of full length functional antibodies. Animal experiments also showed that these viral nanomedicines are capable of disseminating into orthotopic tumor when delivered intravenously (Marino, N., Illingworth, S., Kodialbail, P., Patel, A., Calderon, H., Lear, R., 2017).

CONCLUSION

In this chapter, we have discussed the major challenges associated with cancer treatments, the primary being early diagnosis. Studies have found that early diagnosis of cancer makes it more curable and easy to treat. Secondly, delivery of therapeutic to the actual site of tumor by preventing systemic toxicity is again very challenging. In order to overcome these issues, researchers have diverted their attention to nanoformulations which holds immense opportunities for early detection of tumor and targeted delivery of therapeutics to the tumor site. Nanoparticles can be simultaneously loaded with imaging agent for monitoring drug accumulation in tumor tissues and chemotherapeutic drugs for site specific delivery. A variety of nanotheranostic platforms have been exploited for this purpose. The specificity of these nanotheranostics could be further enhanced by conjugation of targeting moiety for cancer cell specific targeting. Further, the use of various different nanoformulations as theranostics have been discussed. Although studies have reported the vast potential of nanotheranostics, yet much effort is required to bring these nanomedicines out from laboratories to bed side. The unique features of nanoparticles have been exploited for many biomedical applications. However, understanding their toxicity cellular internalization mechanism, environmental fate and impact on long term human health remains as an urgent issue which needs to be addressed by the scientific community. Literature shows success of nanotheranostics in animal studies but most of them fails when translating to clinics. Overall, theranostic approach by nanomedicine with specific targeted delivery to cancer cells is a big hope to contribute towards cancer therapy.

REFERENCES

Abbasi, E., Aval, S. F., Akbarzadeh, A., Milani, M., Nasrabadi, H. T., Joo, S. W., ... Pashaei-Asl, R. (2014). Dendrimers: Synthesis, applications, and properties. *Nanoscale Research Letters*, *9*(1), 247. doi:10.1186/1556-276X-9-247 PMID:24994950

Aizik, G., Waiskopf, N., Agbaria, M., Levi-Kalisman, Y., Banin, U., & Golomb, G. (2017). Delivery of Liposomal Quantum Dots via Monocytes for Imaging of Inflamed Tissue. *ACS Nano*, *11*(3), 3038–3051. doi:10.1021/acsnano.7b00016 PMID:28196324

Baek, J. S., & Cho, C. W. (2017). Surface modification of solid lipid nanoparticles for oral delivery of curcumin: Improvement of bioavailability through enhanced cellular uptake, and lymphatic uptake. *European Journal of Pharmaceutics and Biopharmaceutics*, *117*, 132–140. doi:10.1016/j.ejpb.2017.04.013 PMID:28412471

Belletti, D., Riva, G., Luppi, M., Tosi, G., Forni, F., Vandelli, M. A., ... Pederzoli, F. (2017). Anticancer drug-loaded quantum dots engineered polymeric nanoparticles: Diagnosis/therapy combined approach. *European Journal of Pharmaceutical Sciences*, *107*, 230–239. doi:10.1016/j.ejps.2017.07.020 PMID:28728978

Cabral, H., & Kataoka, K. (2014). Progress of drug-loaded polymeric micelles into clinical studies. *Journal of Controlled Release*, *190*, 465–476. doi:10.1016/j.jconrel.2014.06.042 PMID:24993430

Cavalli Roberta, C. (1993). Solid lipospheres of doxorubicin and idarubicin. *International Journal of Pharmaceutics*, *89*(1), R9–R12. doi:10.1016/0378-5173(93)90313-5

Cha, R., Li, J., Liu, Y., Zhang, Y., Xie, Q., & Zhang, M. (2017). Fe3O4 nanoparticles modified by CD-containing star polymer for MRI and drug delivery. *Colloids and Surfaces. B, Biointerfaces*, *158*, 213–221. doi:10.1016/j.colsurfb.2017.06.049 PMID:28697436

Chen, Guizhi, Jin, & Xiaoyuan. (2017). Rethinking cancer nanotheranostics. *Nature Reviews Materials, 2.*

Chidambaram, M., Manavalan, R., & Kathiresan, K. (2011). Nanotherapeutics to overcome conventional cancer chemotherapy limitations. *Journal of Pharmacy & Pharmaceutical Sciences*, *14*(1), 67–77. doi:10.18433/J30C7D PMID:21501554

Cho, S. H., Kim, A., Shin, W., Heo, M. B., Noh, H. J., Hong, K. S., ... Lim, Y. T. (2017). Photothermal-modulated drug delivery and magnetic relaxation based on collagen/poly(gamma-glutamic acid) hydrogel. *International Journal of Nanomedicine*, *12*, 2607–2620. doi:10.2147/IJN.S133078 PMID:28408827

Croy, S. R., & Kwon, G. S. (2006). Polymeric micelles for drug delivery. *Current Pharmaceutical Design*, *12*(36), 4669–4684. doi:10.2174/138161206779026245 PMID:17168771

De Volder, M. F., Tawfick, S. H., Baughman, R. H., & Hart, A. J. (2013). Carbon nanotubes: Present and future commercial applications. *Science*, *339*(6119), 535–539. doi:10.1126cience.1222453 PMID:23372006

des Rieux, A., Fievez, V., Garinot, M., Schneider, Y. J., & Preat, V. (2006). Nanoparticles as potential oral delivery systems of proteins and vaccines: A mechanistic approach. *Journal of Controlled Release*, *116*(1), 1–27. doi:10.1016/j.jconrel.2006.08.013 PMID:17050027

Dumoga, S., Rai, Y., Bhatt, A. N., Tiwari, A. K., Singh, S., Mishra, A. K., & Kakkar, D. (2017). Block Copolymer Based Nanoparticles for Theranostic Intervention of Cervical Cancer: Synthesis, Pharmacokinetics, and in Vitro/in Vivo Evaluation in HeLa Xenograft Models. *ACS Applied Materials & Interfaces*, *9*(27), 22195–22211. doi:10.1021/acsami.7b04982 PMID:28608677

Elzoghby, A. O., Samy, W. M., & Elgindy, N. A. (2012). Albumin-based nanoparticles as potential controlled release drug delivery systems. *Journal of Controlled Release*, *157*(2), 168–182. doi:10.1016/j.jconrel.2011.07.031 PMID:21839127

Erb, R. M. Y. B. (2009). Magnetic Manipulation of Colloidal Particles. Nanoscale Magnetic Materials and Applications, 19, 563-590.

Ferrari, M. (2005). Cancer nanotechnology: Opportunities and challenges. *Nature Reviews. Cancer*, *5*(3), 161–171. doi:10.1038/nrc1566 PMID:15738981

Frangioni, J. V. (2008). New technologies for human cancer imaging. *Journal of Clinical Oncology*, *26*(24), 4012–4021. doi:10.1200/JCO.2007.14.3065 PMID:18711192

Fu, X., Wang, X., Zhou, S., & Zhang, Y. (2017). IONP-doped nanoparticles for highly effective NIR-controlled drug release and combination tumor therapy. *International Journal of Nanomedicine*, *12*, 3751–3766. doi:10.2147/IJN.S113963 PMID:28553112

Gao, N., Bozeman, E. N., Qian, W., Wang, L., Chen, H., Lipowska, M., ... Yang, L. (2017). Tumor Penetrating Theranostic Nanoparticles for Enhancement of Targeted and Image-guided Drug Delivery into Peritoneal Tumors following Intraperitoneal Delivery. *Theranostics*, *7*(6), 1689–1704. doi:10.7150/thno.18125 PMID:28529645

Grange, C., Geninatti-Crich, S., Esposito, G., Alberti, D., Tei, L., Bussolati, B., ... Camussi, G. (2010). Combined delivery and magnetic resonance imaging of neural cell adhesion molecule-targeted doxorubicin-containing liposomes in experimentally induced Kaposi's sarcoma. *Cancer Research*, *70*(6), 2180–2190. doi:10.1158/0008-5472.CAN-09-2821 PMID:20215497

Gref, R., Minamitake, Y., Peracchia, M. T., Trubetskoy, V., Torchilin, V., & Langer, R. (1994). Biodegradable long-circulating polymeric nanospheres. *Science*, *263*(5153), 1600–1603. doi:10.1126cience.8128245 PMID:8128245

Gu, Y., Guo, Y., Wang, C., Xu, J., Wu, J., Kirk, T. B., ... Xue, W. (2017). A polyamidoamne dendrimer functionalized graphene oxide for DOX and MMP-9 shRNA plasmid co-delivery. *Materials Science and Engineering C*, *70*(Pt 1), 572–585. doi:10.1016/j.msec.2016.09.035 PMID:27770930

Han, Y., Zhang, P., Chen, Y., Sun, J., & Kong, F. (2014). Co-delivery of plasmid DNA and doxorubicin by solid lipid nanoparticles for lung cancer therapy. *International Journal of Molecular Medicine*, *34*(1), 191–196. doi:10.3892/ijmm.2014.1770 PMID:24804644

Hao, N., Sun, C., Wu, Z., Xu, L., Gao, W., Cao, J., ... He, B. (2017). Fabrication of Polymeric Micelles with Aggregation-Induced Emission and Forster Resonance Energy Transfer for Anticancer Drug Delivery. *Bioconjugate Chemistry*, *28*(7), 1944–1954. doi:10.1021/acs.bioconjchem.7b00274 PMID:28570043

He, B., Hu, H. Y., Tan, T., Wang, H., Sun, K. X., Li, Y. P. (2017). IR-780-loaded polymeric micelles enhance the efficacy of photothermal therapy in treating breast cancer lymphatic metastasis in mice. *Acta Pharmacol Sin*.

Iyer, A. K., Khaled, G., Fang, J., & Maeda, H. (2006). Exploiting the enhanced permeability and retention effect for tumor targeting. *Drug Discovery Today*, *11*(17-18), 812–818. doi:10.1016/j.drudis.2006.07.005 PMID:16935749

Jain, R. K., & Stylianopoulos, T. (2010). Delivering nanomedicine to solid tumors. *Nature Reviews. Clinical Oncology*, *7*(11), 653–664. doi:10.1038/nrclinonc.2010.139 PMID:20838415

Jeong, E. H., Jung, G., Hong, C. A., & Lee, H. (2014). Gold nanoparticle (AuNP)-based drug delivery and molecular imaging for biomedical applications. *Archives of Pharmacal Research*, *37*(1), 53–59. doi:10.100712272-013-0273-5 PMID:24214174

Jin, H., Zhao, G., Hu, J., Ren, Q., Yang, K., Wan, C., ... Zou, Z. (2017). Melittin-Containing Hybrid Peptide Hydrogels for Enhanced Photothermal Therapy of Glioblastoma. *ACS Applied Materials & Interfaces*, *9*(31), 25755–25766. doi:10.1021/acsami.7b06431 PMID:28714303

Kam, N. W., O'Connell, M., Wisdom, J. A., & Dai, H. (2005). Carbon nanotubes as multifunctional biological transporters and near-infrared agents for selective cancer cell destruction. *Proceedings of the National Academy of Sciences of the United States of America*, *102*(33), 11600–11605. doi:10.1073/pnas.0502680102 PMID:16087878

Kang, M. S., Singh, R. K., Kim, T. H., Kim, J. H., Patel, K. D., & Kim, H. W. (2017). Optical imaging and anticancer chemotherapy through carbon dot created hollow mesoporous silica nanoparticles. *Acta Biomaterialia*, *55*, 466–480. doi:10.1016/j.actbio.2017.03.054 PMID:28373086

Kenmotsu, H., Yasunaga, M., Goto, K., Nagano, T., Kuroda, J., Koga, Y., ... Matsumura, Y. (2010). The antitumor activity of NK012, an SN-38-incorporating micelle, in combination with bevacizumab against lung cancer xenografts. *Cancer*, *116*(19), 4597–4604. doi:10.1002/cncr.25233 PMID:20572031

Khandelia, R., Bhandari, S., Pan, U. N., Ghosh, S. S., & Chattopadhyay, A. (2015). Gold Nanocluster Embedded Albumin Nanoparticles for Two-Photon Imaging of Cancer Cells Accompanying Drug Delivery. *Small*, *11*(33), 4075–4081. doi:10.1002mll.201500216 PMID:25939342

Kim, J. H., Eguchi, H., & Ishikawa, Y. (2017). Anticancer luminescent gold quantum clusters for in situ cancer-selective marking-imaging-targeting. *Nanoscale*, *9*(26), 9071–9082. doi:10.1039/C7NR02229H PMID:28639680

Kim, T. H., Lee, S., & Chen, X. (2013). Nanotheranostics for personalized medicine. *Expert Review of Molecular Diagnostics*, *13*(3), 257–269. doi:10.1586/erm.13.15 PMID:23570404

Kopecek, J. (2007). Hydrogel biomaterials: A smart future? *Biomaterials*, *28*(34), 5185–5192. doi:10.1016/j.biomaterials.2007.07.044 PMID:17697712

Kopecek, J., & Yang, J. (2007). Hydrogels as smart biomaterials. *Polymer International*, *56*(9), 1078–1098. doi:10.1002/pi.2253

Kuang, Y., Zhang, K., Cao, Y., Chen, X., Wang, K., Liu, M., & Pei, R. (2017). Hydrophobic IR-780 Dye Encapsulated in cRGD-Conjugated Solid Lipid Nanoparticles for NIR Imaging-Guided Photothermal Therapy. *ACS Applied Materials & Interfaces*, *9*(14), 12217–12226. doi:10.1021/acsami.6b16705 PMID:28306236

Le, D. H., Lee, K. L., Shukla, S., Commandeur, U., & Steinmetz, N. F. (2017). Potato virus X, a filamentous plant viral nanoparticle for doxorubicin delivery in cancer therapy. *Nanoscale*, *9*(6), 2348–2357. doi:10.1039/C6NR09099K PMID:28144662

Lee, J. Y., Termsarasab, U., Lee, M. Y., Kim, D. H., Lee, S. Y., Kim, J. S., ... Kim, D.-D. (2017). Chemosensitizing indomethacin-conjugated chitosan oligosaccharide nanoparticles for tumor-targeted drug delivery. *Acta Biomaterialia*, *57*, 262–273. doi:10.1016/j.actbio.2017.05.012 PMID:28483700

Li, Y., Lai, Y., Xu, X., Zhang, X., Wu, Y., & Hu, C. (2016). Capsid-like supramolecular dendritic systems as pH-responsive nanocarriers for drug penetration and site-specific delivery. *Nanomedicine (London)*, *12*(2), 355–364. doi:10.1016/j.nano.2015.09.015 PMID:26711961

Liang, X., Shang, W., Chi, C., Zeng, C., Wang, K., Fang, C., ... Tian, J. (2016). Dye-conjugated single-walled carbon nanotubes induce photothermal therapy under the guidance of near-infrared imaging. *Cancer Letters*, *383*(2), 243–249. doi:10.1016/j.canlet.2016.09.006 PMID:27693557

Lin, W., Yao, N., Qian, L., Zhang, X., Chen, Q., Wang, J., & Zhang, L. (2017). pH-responsive unimolecular micelle-gold nanoparticles-drug nanohybrid system for cancer theranostics. *Acta Biomaterialia*, *58*, 455–465. doi:10.1016/j.actbio.2017.06.003 PMID:28583900

Liu, G., Ma, J., Li, Y., Li, Q., Tan, C., Song, H., ... Zhu, X. (2017). Core-interlayer-shell Fe3O4@mSiO2@lipid-PEG-methotrexate nanoparticle for multimodal imaging and multistage targeted chemo-photodynamic therapy. *International Journal of Pharmaceutics*, *521*(1-2), 19–32. doi:10.1016/j.ijpharm.2017.01.068 PMID:28163230

Lodhia, J., Mandarano, G., Ferris, N., Eu, P., & Cowell, S. (2010). Development and use of iron oxide nanoparticles (Part 1): Synthesis of iron oxide nanoparticles for MRI. *Biomed Imaging Interv J*, *6*(2), e12. doi:10.2349/biij.6.2.e12 PMID:21611034

Manivasagan, P., Bharathiraja, S., Bui, N. Q., Jang, B., Oh, Y. O., Lim, I. G., & Oh, J. (2016). Doxorubicin-loaded fucoidan capped gold nanoparticles for drug delivery and photoacoustic imaging. *International Journal of Biological Macromolecules*, *91*, 578–588. doi:10.1016/j.ijbiomac.2016.06.007 PMID:27267570

Marino, N., Illingworth, S., Kodialbail, P., Patel, A., Calderon, H., Lear, R., ... Brown, A. C. N. (2017). Development of a versatile oncolytic virus platform for local intra-tumoural expression of therapeutic transgenes. *PLoS One*, *12*(5), e0177810. doi:10.1371/journal.pone.0177810 PMID:28542292

Matsumura, Y. (2011). Preclinical and clinical studies of NK012, an SN-38-incorporating polymeric micelles, which is designed based on EPR effect. *Advanced Drug Delivery Reviews*, *63*(3), 184–192. doi:10.1016/j.addr.2010.05.008 PMID:20561951

Misra, R., Acharya, S., & Sahoo, S. K. (2010). Cancer nanotechnology: Application of nanotechnology in cancer therapy. *Drug Discovery Today*, *15*(19-20), 842–850. doi:10.1016/j.drudis.2010.08.006 PMID:20727417

Mohanty, C., Das, M., & Sahoo, S. K. (2012). Emerging role of nanocarriers to increase the solubility and bioavailability of curcumin. *Expert Opinion on Drug Delivery*, *9*(11), 1347–1364. doi:10.1517/17425247.2012.724676 PMID:22971222

Nanjwade Basavaraj, K. (2009). Dendrimers: Emerging polymers for drug-delivery systems. *European Journal of Pharmaceutical Sciences*, *38*(3), 185–196. doi:10.1016/j.ejps.2009.07.008 PMID:19646528

Nedyalkova, M., Donkova, B., Romanova, J., Tzvetkov, G., Madurga, S., & Simeonov, V. (2017). Iron oxide nanoparticles - In vivo/in vitro biomedical applications and in silico studies. *Advances in Colloid and Interface Science*, *249*, 192–212. doi:10.1016/j.cis.2017.05.003 PMID:28499604

Nigam, P. W. S., Louis, M., Wangnoo, S., Chavanb, P., & Sarkar, D. (2014). Graphene quantum dots conjugated albumin nanoparticles for targeted drug delivery and imaging of pancreatic cancer. *Journal of Materials Chemistry. B, Materials for Biology and Medicine*, *2*(21), 3190–3195. doi:10.1039/C4TB00015C

Parhi, P., Mohanty, C., & Sahoo, S. K. (2012). Nanotechnology-based combinational drug delivery: An emerging approach for cancer therapy. *Drug Discovery Today*, *17*(17-18), 1044–1052. doi:10.1016/j.drudis.2012.05.010 PMID:22652342

Parveen, S., & Sahoo, S. K. (2008). Polymeric nanoparticles for cancer therapy. *Journal of Drug Targeting*, *16*(2), 108–123. doi:10.1080/10611860701794353 PMID:18274932

Patel, J. N. (2009). Chitosan based Nanoparticles inDrug Delivery. *International Journal of Pharmaceutical Sciences and Nanotechnology, 2*(2).

Peng, X. H., Qian, X., Mao, H., Wang, A. Y., Chen, Z. G., & Nie, S. (2008). Targeted magnetic iron oxide nanoparticles for tumor imaging and therapy. *International Journal of Nanomedicine*, *3*(3), 311–321. PMID:18990940

Perez-Herrero, E., & Fernandez-Medarde, A. (2015). Advanced targeted therapies in cancer: Drug nanocarriers, the future of chemotherapy. *European Journal of Pharmaceutics and Biopharmaceutics*, *93*, 52–79. doi:10.1016/j.ejpb.2015.03.018 PMID:25813885

Qi, L., & Gao, X. (2008). Emerging application of quantum dots for drug delivery and therapy. *Expert Opinion on Drug Delivery*, *5*(3), 263–267. doi:10.1517/17425247.5.3.263 PMID:18318649

Rahimnejad,, M., & Najafpour. (2006). Production of biological nanoparticles from bovine serum albumin for drug delivery. *African Journal of Biotechnology*, *5*(20), 1918–1923.

Rawat, M., Singh, D., Saraf, S., & Saraf, S. (2006). Nanocarriers: Promising vehicle for bioactive drugs. *Biological & Pharmaceutical Bulletin*, *29*(9), 1790–1798. doi:10.1248/bpb.29.1790 PMID:16946487

Riehemann, K., Schneider, S. W., Luger, T. A., Godin, B., Ferrari, M., & Fuchs, H. (2009). Nanomedicine--challenge and perspectives. *Angewandte Chemie International Edition in English*, *48*(5), 872–897. doi:10.1002/anie.200802585 PMID:19142939

Sahoo, S. K., & Labhasetwar, V. (2003). Nanotech approaches to drug delivery and imaging. *Drug Discovery Today*, *8*(24), 1112–1120. doi:10.1016/S1359-6446(03)02903-9 PMID:14678737

Saraswathy, A., Nazeer, S. S., Nimi, N., Arumugam, S., Shenoy, S. J., & Jayasree, R. S. (2014). Synthesis and characterization of dextran stabilized superparamagnetic iron oxide nanoparticles for in vivo MR imaging of liver fibrosis. *Carbohydrate Polymers*, *101*, 760–768. doi:10.1016/j.carbpol.2013.10.015 PMID:24299836

Sharma, M., Sharma, S., Sharma, V., Sharma, K., Yadav, S. K., Dwivedi, P., ... Rawat, A. K. S. (2017). Oleanolic-bioenhancer coloaded chitosan modified nanocarriers attenuate breast cancer cells by multimode mechanism and preserve female fertility. *International Journal of Biological Macromolecules*, *104*, 1345–1358. doi:10.1016/j.ijbiomac.2017.06.005 PMID:28591594

Singh, A., & Sahoo, S. K. (2014). Magnetic nanoparticles: A novel platform for cancer theranostics. *Drug Discovery Today*, *19*(4), 474–481. doi:10.1016/j.drudis.2013.10.005 PMID:24140592

Singh, D., Minz, A. P., & Sahoo, S. K. (2017). Nanomedicine-mediated drug targeting of cancer stem cells. *Drug Discovery Today*, *22*(6), 952–959. doi:10.1016/j.drudis.2017.04.005 PMID:28435061

Steichen, S. D., Caldorera-Moore, M., & Peppas, N. A. (2013). A review of current nanoparticle and targeting moieties for the delivery of cancer therapeutics. *European Journal of Pharmaceutical Sciences*, *48*(3), 416–427. doi:10.1016/j.ejps.2012.12.006 PMID:23262059

Steinmetz, N. F. (2013). Viral nanoparticles in drug delivery and imaging. *Molecular Pharmaceutics*, *10*(1), 1–2. doi:10.1021/mp300658j PMID:23294244

Sumio, I. (1991). Helical microtubules of graphitic carbon. *Nature*, 354.

Sun, L., Wang, D., Chen, Y., Wang, L., Huang, P., Li, Y., ... Shi, J. (2017). Core-shell hierarchical mesostructured silica nanoparticles for gene/chemo-synergetic stepwise therapy of multidrug-resistant cancer. *Biomaterials*, *133*, 219–228. doi:10.1016/j.biomaterials.2017.04.028 PMID:28441616

Tian, J., Yan, C., Liu, K., Tao, J., Guo, Z., Liu, J., ... Gu, N. (2017). Paclitaxel-Loaded Magnetic Nanoparticles: Synthesis, Characterization, and Application in Targeting. *Journal of Pharmaceutical Sciences*, *106*(8), 2115–2122. doi:10.1016/j.xphs.2017.04.023 PMID:28456728

Truzzi, E., Bongio, C., Sacchetti, F., Maretti, E., Montanari, M., Iannuccelli, V., ... Leo, E. (2017). Self-Assembled Lipid Nanoparticles for Oral Delivery of Heparin-Coated Iron Oxide Nanoparticles for Theranostic Purposes. *Molecules (Basel, Switzerland)*, *22*(6), 963. doi:10.3390/molecules22060963 PMID:28598368

Von Hoff, D. D., Mita, M. M., Ramanathan, R. K., Weiss, G. J., Mita, A. C., LoRusso, P. M., ... Sachdev, J. C. (2016). Phase I Study of PSMA-Targeted Docetaxel-Containing Nanoparticle BIND-014 in Patients with Advanced Solid Tumors. *Clinical Cancer Research*, *22*(13), 3157–3163. doi:10.1158/1078-0432.CCR-15-2548 PMID:26847057

Vong, L. B., Kimura, S., & Nagasaki, Y. (2017). Newly Designed Silica-Containing Redox Nanoparticles for Oral Delivery of Novel TOP2 Catalytic Inhibitor for Treating Colon Cancer. *Adv Healthc Mater*.

Wang, F., Zhang, B., Zhou, L., Shi, Y., Li, Z., Xia, Y., & Tian, J. (2016). Imaging Dendrimer-Grafted Graphene Oxide Mediated Anti-miR-21 Delivery With an Activatable Luciferase Reporter. *ACS Applied Materials & Interfaces*, *8*(14), 9014–9021. doi:10.1021/acsami.6b02662 PMID:27010367

Wang, Y., Strohm, E. M., Sun, Y., Wang, Z., Zheng, Y., Wang, Z., & Kolios, M. C. (2016). Biodegradable polymeric nanoparticles containing gold nanoparticles and Paclitaxel for cancer imaging and drug delivery using photoacoustic methods. *Biomedical Optics Express*, *7*(10), 4125–4138. doi:10.1364/BOE.7.004125 PMID:27867720

Weissleder, R., Kelly, K., Sun, E. Y., Shtatland, T., & Josephson, L. (2005). Cell-specific targeting of nanoparticles by multivalent attachment of small molecules. *Nature Biotechnology*, *23*(11), 1418–1423. doi:10.1038/nbt1159 PMID:16244656

Wu, B., Wan, B., Lu, S. T., Deng, K., Li, X. Q., Wu, B. L., ... Xu, H.-B. (2017). Near-infrared light-triggered theranostics for tumor-specific enhanced multimodal imaging and photothermal therapy. *International Journal of Nanomedicine*, *12*, 4467–4478. doi:10.2147/IJN.S137835 PMID:28670120

Wu, L. G. U., & Boker, A. (2016). Synthesis of Hybrid Silica Nanoparticles Densely Grafted with Thermo and pH Dual-Responsive Brushes via Surface-Initiated ATRP. *Macromolecules*, *49*(24), 9586–9596. doi:10.1021/acs.macromol.6b01792

Wu, Y. Z., Sun, J., Zhang, Y., Pu, M., Zhang, G., He, N., & Zeng, X. (2017). Effective Integration of Targeted Tumor Imaging and Therapy Using Functionalized InP QDs with VEGFR2 Monoclonal Antibody and miR-92a Inhibitor. *ACS Applied Materials & Interfaces*, *9*(15), 13068–13078. doi:10.1021/acsami.7b02641 PMID:28358188

Xu, G., Zeng, S., Zhang, B., Swihart, M. T., Yong, K. T., & Prasad, P. N. (2016). New Generation Cadmium-Free Quantum Dots for Biophotonics and Nanomedicine. *Chemical Reviews*, *116*(19), 12234–12327. doi:10.1021/acs.chemrev.6b00290 PMID:27657177

Zackova Suchanova, J., Neburkova, J., Spanielova, H., Forstova, J., & Cigler, P. (2017). Retargeting Polyomavirus-Like Particles to Cancer Cells by Chemical Modification of Capsid Surface. *Bioconjugate Chemistry*, *28*(2), 307–313. doi:10.1021/acs.bioconjchem.6b00622 PMID:28035816

Zeiderman, M. R., Morgan, D. E., Christein, J. D., Grizzle, W. E., McMasters, K. M., & McNally, L. R. (2016). Acidic pH-targeted chitosan capped mesoporous silica coated gold nanorods facilitate detection of pancreatic tumors via multispectral optoacoustic tomography. *ACS Biomater Sci Eng*, *2*(7), 1108–1120. doi:10.1021/acsbiomaterials.6b00111 PMID:28626793

Zhao, H., Chao, Y., Liu, J., Huang, J., Pan, J., Guo, W., ... Liu, Z. (2016). Polydopamine Coated Single-Walled Carbon Nanotubes as a Versatile Platform with Radionuclide Labeling for Multimodal Tumor Imaging and Therapy. *Theranostics*, *6*(11), 1833–1843. doi:10.7150/thno.16047 PMID:27570554

Zhao, L., Zhu, J., Cheng, Y., Xiong, Z., Tang, Y., Guo, L., ... Zhao, J. (2015). Chlorotoxin-Conjugated Multifunctional Dendrimers Labeled with Radionuclide 131I for Single Photon Emission Computed Tomography Imaging and Radiotherapy of Gliomas. *ACS Applied Materials & Interfaces*, *7*(35), 19798–19808. doi:10.1021/acsami.5b05836 PMID:26291070

Zhao, Q., Wang, S., Yang, Y., Li, X., Di, D., Zhang, C., ... Wang, S. (2017). Hyaluronic acid and carbon dots-gated hollow mesoporous silica for redox and enzyme-triggered targeted drug delivery and bioimaging. *Materials Science and Engineering C*, *78*, 475–484. doi:10.1016/j.msec.2017.04.059 PMID:28576012

Zou, H., Wu, S., & Shen, J. (2008). Polymer/silica nanocomposites: Preparation, characterization, properties, and applications. *Chemical Reviews*, *108*(9), 3893–3957. doi:10.1021/cr068035q PMID:18720998

Chapter 2
Application Potential of Polymeric Nanoconstructs for Colon-Specific Drug Delivery

Sanjay Kumar Jain
Dr. Harisingh Gour University, India

Amit Verma
Dr. Harisingh Gour University, India

Ankita Tiwari
Dr. Harisingh Gour University, India

Shivani Saraf
Dr. Harisingh Gour University, India

Ankit Jain
GLA University, India

Pritish Kumar Panda
Dr. Harisingh Gour University, India

Gaytri Gour
Dr. Harisingh Gour University, India

ABSTRACT

Numerous applications of colon-specific drug delivery have been found in a wide array of diseases like irritable bowel syndrome (IBS), inflammatory bowel diseases (ulcerative colitis and Crohn's disease), colorectal cancer, and diverticulitis. Drug delivery to the colon has different anatomic and patho-physiological barriers. In recent advancements, these barriers were overcome by using biodegradable polymeric nanoconstructs, which are exhibiting minimal systemic adverse effects. Various polymeric nanoconstructs (PNCs) such as nanoparticles, micelles, and dendrimers have been exploited for effective targeting to pathological sites of colon. PNCs on oral administration not only protect the bioactive from physicochemical degradation but also prevent premature leakage in the upper parts of gastrointestinal tract. The chapter summarizes various PNCs-based approaches for colon-specific drug delivery.

DOI: 10.4018/978-1-5225-4781-5.ch002

Copyright © 2018, IGI Global. Copying or distributing in print or electronic forms without written permission of IGI Global is prohibited.

INTRODUCTION

Drug delivery to colon is a challenging task as drug has to traverse all the ways from buccal cavity to large intestine on oral administration or it has to be administered via rectal route which is not convenient to the patient. Hence, various strategies have been adopted for the specific drug delivery to colon on oral administration to achieve effective drug concentration in the colon and to get better therapeutic effect. Colon specific drug delivery is desired for the treatment of various local colon associated diseases like ulcerative colitis, Crohn's disease, amoebiasis, colon cancer, diverticulitis, diverticulosis and irritable bowel syndrome (Jain & Jain, 2015; Vyas & Khar, 2002). A variety of drugs like proteins, peptides, and vaccines etc. has been exploited for specific delivery to the colon. Proteins and peptides are preferably delivered other than oral route due to the less chances of enzymatic activity, low proteolytic activity and longer residence time (Chourasia & Jain, 2003; Hardy, Wilson, & Wood, 1985; Mackay & Tomlinson, 1993). There are various factors like formulation factors, retention time, and spreading capacity etc. which influence the concentration of drug reaching to the colon.. For the development of efficient colon targeted drug delivery systems, a meticulous understanding of the anatomy and physiology of colon is necessitated.

ANATOMY AND PHYSIOLOGY OF THE COLON

Parts of the Colon

The large intestine is approximately 1.5 m and divided into various segments such as caecum, ascending colon, hepatic flexure, transverse colon, splenic flexure, appendix, descending colon, sigmoid colon, rectum and anus. The caecum has out-pouching in the interior; extends beyond ileocaecal junction and is in continuation with the ascending colon superiorly. There is a narrow diverticulum called vermiform appendix at the angle between the caecum and terminal part of ileum. The colon is covered by a pink lining known as mucosa. The ascending colon transcends upwards from the caecum and it bends to the left at the hepatic flexure to form transverse colon. Hepatic flexure is located inferior to the lobe of the liver (Mitchell, Vogl, & Adam, 2009). Splenic flexure is located just inferior to the spleen, higher and more posterior than the right colic flexure and is connected to the diaphragm by phrenicocolic ligament (Mitchell, R. D., Vogl, A. W., & Adam, W. M., 2009). The descending colon transcends down from the left side of the abdominal cavity then folds towards the midline. Sigmoid colon is a S-shaped curve situated in the pelvic region near the left iliac crest which continues downwards to form the rectum.

Layers of the Colon

The colon comprises of four distinct layers of tissues namely: (1) Serosa; (2) Muscularis externa; (3) Sub mucosa and; (4) Mucosa. Serosa is the exterior coat which consists of areolar tissue covered by simple squamous epithelium known as mesothelium. It is made up of loose connective tissue, white adipose tissue, blood vessels, lymphatic vessels and nerves (Waugh & Grant, 2010). Muscularis externa is further subdivided into two layers of smooth muscles. These layers carry out the functions of segmentation and propulsion. Inner layer is made up of the circular muscles which provide the segmentation via wall contractions and consequently leading to the formation of haustra. The outer layer of longitudinal muscles is involved in the peristaltic movement which pushes forward the contents of the intestine. The muscularis externa which is the outer longitudinal layer shows three equally placed bands known as taenia coli. Taenia converges at the base of the appendix proximally and spread out on the sigmoid colon distally to be in continuation with the longitudinal muscle coat of the rectum (Pawar, V. K., Meher, J. G., Singh, Y., Chaurasia, M., Surendar Reddy, B., & Chourasia, M. K P., 2014). The submucosa consists of moderately dense irregular connective tissue, blood vessels, lymphatic vessels, nerve network and ganglion neurons (Meissner's plexus), and white adipose tissue (Waugh & Grant, 2010). The inner mucosa layer is further divided into three more layers known as muscularis mucosa, lamina propria and epithelium. Muscularis mucosa is comparatively thin inner circular and outer longitudinal layer of smooth muscle.

pH

The GI pH influences the release and absorption rate of drugs administered by oral route. Various pH sensitive drugs are subject to degradation by the acidic pH of the stomach. In order to prevent this degradation, coating is done with enteric coating polymers. In small intestine, the pH is slightly rised from 4.5 in the proximal part of duodenum to 7.5 in the ileum. A substantial fall in the pH takes place from the ileum to the colon. The pH falls to 6.4 ± 0.6 in the right colon. The pH in the mid colon is 6.6 ± 0.8 and in the left colon is 7.0 ± 0.7 (Watson, Meldrum, Riddle, Brown, & Sladen, 1972). Inter and intra individual variability in pH is also observed in the GIT. It is also affected by disease, for example during acute stage of inflammatory bowel disease the colonic pH has been noticed to be considerably lower than that in normal condition. In ulcerative colitis, pH of the proximal colon ranges from 2.3-4.7 (Tiwari, Jain, Verma, & Jain, 2017).

Transit Time

After oral administration, drug first reaches the stomach, small intestine and finally colon. To reach the colon safely, the drug delivery systems need to bypass the barriers present in the stomach and small intestine. The mean transit time of the dosage form is nearly 3-4 hrs to reach the ileocecal junction. In comparison to the other region of GIT, movement of material through the colon is quite slow. Total time taken for the transit is found to be highly variable and affected by numerous factors like diet especially dietary fiber content, mobility, stress, disease conditions and few drugs (Coupe, Davis, & Wilding, 1991). The transit time of a capsule through colon is about 20-35 hrs.

Luminal Contents

Due to the high-water absorption capacity of the colon, the colonic contents are substantially viscous and inefficient mixing occurs, thus availability of majority of the drugs to the absorptive membrane is quite low. Table 1 summarizes drugs used for colon targeting (Head & Jurenka, 2003; Jain, Gupta, & Jain, 2007; Modest, D., Kasper, S., Stintzing, S., Prasnikar, N., Müller, L., Caca, K., . . . Trarbach, T., 2016; Stollman & Raskin, 2004).

Table 1. Drugs used for colon targeting

Disease	Symptoms	Drugs Employed
Inflammatory Bowel Disease (Crohn's disease	Abdominal pain, loss in appetite, abscesses, fistulas, stenosis, blood in stool, ulcers and weight loss	Hydrocortisone, Budenoside, Prednisolone, Sulfasalazine
Ulcerative Colitis	Inflammation in the rectum, rectal bleeding, rectal pain	Mesalamine, Balsalazide, Sulfasalazine, and mercaptopurine
Irritable Bowel Syndrome	Abdominal pain or cramping, a bloated feeling, flatulence, diarrhea or constipation people with IBS may also experience alternating bouts of constipation & diarrhea, mucus in stool	Dicyclomine, Hyoscine, Propantheline, Cimetropium, Alosetron, Tegaserod
Colorectal Cancer	Worsening constipation, bowel changes, rectal bleeding or blood in stool, persistent abdominal pain, weight loss, blood in the stool, decreased stool thickness, loss of appetite.	5 - Flourouracil, Leucovorin, and Cetuximab, Irinotecan, Oxaliplatin, Capecitabine
Diverticulitis	It is a condition brought on by infection or rupture of diverticula, which are bulges forming in the lower part of the large intestine or colon.	Sulfamethoxazole and trimethoprim, Metronidazole
Antibiotic Associated Colitis	Overgrowth of *Clostridium difficileandits* subsequent Toxin production	Clindamycin, broad spectrum penicillins (e.g., ampicillin, amoxicillin) and cephalosporins
Diverticulosis	Refers to small out-pouchings (multiple diverticula) from the colonic lumen due to mucosal herniation through the colonic wall at sites of vascular perforation. Abnormal colonic motility and inadequate intake of dietary fiber have been implicated in its pathogenesis.	Metronidazole, Sulfamethoxazole and trimethoprim, Ciprofloxacin, Amoxicillin Clavulanate
Hirschsprung's Disease	Severe form of constipation in which bowel movement occurs only once or twice a week	Metronidazole, Vancomycin, Loperamide, Botulinum toxin

Polymers Employed for Colon Specific Delivery

Polymers are macromolecules consisting of repeating units called monomers or co-monomers with various functional groups. Various polymers can be chosen as efficient drug carriers which are capable of solving the problem of local colon specific drug delivery. The drug/polymer ratio plays an important role in polymeric carrier system. The particle size and entrapment efficiency of polymeric carriers are enhanced by enhancing the drug/polymer ratio, while drug release was increased by decreasing the drug/polymer ratio (Jain, Jain, Ganesh, Barve, & Beg, 2010). Polymers commonly employed in the colon specific targeting belong to the polysaccharides and polyesters family. Moreover, acrylic acid based and other allied polymers are also used which provide important properties to the polymeric vehicles. A brief outline of major polymers used for the colon targeted drug delivery, their monomeric units, type of linkages, sources, advantages and need of modifications associated with them are discussed in the tables below (Dar, Ali, Khan, & Khan, 2017). Polymers are of various types i.e. natural, synthetic, mixed type, biodegradable, non-biodegradable, hydrophilic and/or hydrophobic in nature. Table 2 indicates the basic differences among three types of polymer i.e. natural, synthetic and mixed type of polymer (Averous & Pollet, 2012; Kaur & Kaur, 2014). Table 3 summarizes polymers employed for colon drug delivery system.

Carbohydrate polymers like starch, pectin, guar gum, chitosan (chitin derivatives), gellan gum, and dextran etc. show great importance as they are easily available, very low cost, and flexible for modifications to develop colon targeted drug delivery systems. Thus, by crosslinking of the polymer, the drug

Table 2. Differentiating natural, synthetic, and mixed type of polymer

Natural Polymers	Synthetic Polymers	Mixed Polymers
Natural polymers are most abundant but are difficult to reproduce and purify.	Synthetic polymers are produced on a large scale and have extensive properties and uses.	It is the combination of both natural and synthetic polymers.
May be bio-degradable or non- biodegradable.	It may also degradable or non-biodegradable.	May be degradable or non-biodegradable.
High biocompatibility and less immunogenicity.	High immunogenicity and hence prevent long term use.	The composites of natural polymers with synthetic polymers give added advantages as carriers for drug delivery by complimenting the properties of each other.
Examples: Collagen, starch, chitosan, alginate, gelatine, karkaya gum, psyllium, starch, husk, pectin, casein, cellulose and cellulose derivatives etc.	Examples: Polyvinyl pyrrolidone(PVP), polyethylene glycol acrylate (PGA) etc.	Examples: Collagen with biodegradable polyethylene glycol 6000 and polyvinyl pyrrolidone were developed for the controlled released of the drug etc.

Table 3. Polymers employed for colon drug delivery system

For Improving Physical Characteristics	For Controlled Drug Delivery	For Miscellaneous Uses
Poly (Methyl Methacrylate): Physical Strength.	Poly (Acrylic Acid)	Poly Anhydride
Poly (Vinyl Alcohol): Hydrophilicity and Strength.	Polyacrylamide	Polylactide (PLA)
Poly (Urethanes): Elasticity.	Poly (Ethylene-Co-Vinyl Acetate)	Polyorthoesters
Poly (Ethylene): Toughness and Lack of Swelling.	Poly (Methyl Methacrylate)	Poly (Lactide-Co-Glycolides) (PLGA)
Poly (Siloxanes) or Silicones: Insulating Ability.	Poly (Vinyl Alcohol)	Polyglycolides (PGA)
Poly (Vinyl Pyrrolidone): Suspension Capabilities.	Poly (N-Vinyl Pyrrolidone)	
	Poly (2-Hydroxy Ethyl Methacrylate)	
	Poly (Methacrylic Glycol)	
	Poly (Ethylene Glycol)	

release can be enhanced in a desired manner. Carbohydrate polymers are highly chosen as they are stable in gastric media of the upper GIT. Besides other strongest reason of the unique quality of the natural polymer is that the colonic mucosa contains anaerobic bacteria and degrade the substrates with enzymes released by these bacteria. But the single use of natural polymer or saccharide polymer never permitted the desired effect of release of targeted drug delivery to colon. The pH conditions and the colonic transit time depend upon the individual and various disease states. In this situations drug release violates. Hence combinations of natural polymers are used or modified the polymers chemically by cross linking and sort out the problems (Shukla & Tiwari, 2012). Tables 4 and 5 indicate the sources from which the polymers were collected, structural linkages among the monomer units, drug delivery systems, specify the modifications with different polymers, and their uses and the need of modifications with advantages.

Nanoconstructs Exploited for Colon Specific Delivery

Polymeric nanoconstructs intended for targeted drug release into the lower GI tract is beneficial for the localized treatment of several colonic diseases and conditions, mainly inflammatory bowel diseases

Table 4. Natural polymers for colon specific drug targeting

Natural Polymers	Obtained From Various Sources	Structural Linkages	Reference
Agar	Red algae (Rhodophycea) Obtained from Gelidium and Dracilaria.	(1/3)-β-D-galactopyranose-(1/4)-3,6-anhydro-α-L-galactopyranose.	Mano et al., (2007)
Alginic Acid	Brown algae (Phaeophyceae, mainly Laminaria); Microbial (bacteria *Pseudomonas mendocina, Azotobactervinelandii)*	β-(1/4)-linked D-mannuronic acid and α-(1/4)-linked L-guluronic acid.	Mano et al., (2007)
Arabinogalactan	Plant sources: (extracted from the heartwood of the *Larix occidentalis*).	β-(1/3)-linked D-galactose linkages	Mano et al., (2007)
Chitin	Animal sources: Exoskeleton of crustaceans, arthropods, various insects and fungal cell walls	β-(1/4)-linked N-acetyl-d-glucosamine linkages	Mano et al., (2007)
Dextran	Microbial sources: Bacterium (*Leuconostoc mesenteroides*).	α-(1/6)-linked d-glucose residues with some degree of branching via -β(1/3) linkages	(Naessens, Cerdobbel, Soetaert, & Vandamme, 2005)
Guar Gum	Plant sources: Seeds of *Cyamopsis tetragonolobus.*	(1→4)-β-D- mannopyranosyl units with α-D-galactopyranosyl units attached by (1→6) linkages.	(Prabaharan, 2011)
Gellan Gum	Microbial sources: From bacterium (*Sphingomonas elodea*)	(1/4)-L-rhamnose-α-(1/3)-D-glucose-β-(1/4)-D-glucuronic acid-β-(1/4)-D-glucose linkages	(Ogaji, Nep, & Audu-Peter, 2012)
Hyaluronic Acid	Animal sources: Umbilical tissues, vitreous humour of eye, synovial fluids etc. From bacterium (*Bacillus subtilis*)	D-glucuronic acid and N-acetyl-D-glucosamine (GlcNAc) linked by β-(1/3) bond linkages.	(Kogan, Soltes, Stern, & Gemeiner, 2007)
Inulin	Plant sources: Wide ranges of plants like diascorea plant etc.	Fructan type oligosaccharides (2→1) linked-D- fructosyl backbone linkages.	Apolinario et al., (2014)
Moringa Gum	Plant sources: Stem of the plant *Moringa oleifera* Lam. (family Moringaceae)	D-galactose residues having the presence of linkage of (1→6)-β, (1→3)-β and (1→5)-α-type linkages.	(R. Singh, 2016)
Pectin	Dried peel of citrus fruits and/or pulp of apple	(1→4) linked α D galacturonic acid linkages	Itoh et al., (2007)
Pullulan	Microbial source: From fungus (*Aureobasidium pullulans*).	α-(1/4)-linked) joined by α-(1/6) linkages.	(Oguzhan & Yangilar, 2013)
Starch	Plant sources: Corn plants, rice, potato, wheat, tapioca etc.	α-(1/4)-linked glucose linkages	(Jayakody & Hoover, 2008)

(IBDs; UC, Crohn's disease), irritable bowel syndrome and colon cancer (Gupta, Kshirsagar, Bhalekar, & Saldanha, 2013). The application of targeted drug delivery systems may offer important improvement in current cancer therapy by limiting toxic side effects, increasing circulation half-lives and allowing higher specificity in the delivery of the drug to the targeted site (Koning, Kamps, & Scherphof, 2002). Some nanoconstructs used for colon targeting are listed in the Table 6.

Liposomes

Liposomes are biocompatible bilayer phospholipid vesicles introduced in 1965 as a new drug delivery system (Jain & Jain, 2016a). Hydrophilic drugs are incorporated into core and hydrophobic drugs are

Table 5. Modified polymers for colon specific drug targeting

Polymers	Desired Modifications in Polymers	Drug Delivery Systems	Need of Modifications With Advantages	References
Arabinogalactan	Combination with folic acid	Bio-macromolecular nano-vehicle (BMNV)	Folic acid and the anticancer drug methotrexate (MTX) were combined with arabinogalactan (AG), having unusual water solubility property, a targeted BMNV is formed, which can differentially deliver a cytotoxic cargo into folate receptor-overexpressing cells and help in targeting of colon cancer.	Pinhassi et al., (2010)
Cellulose	Cellulose cross-linked with polyurethanes (PUs) based on poly ε-caprolactone with lactic acid/ glycolic acid/ dimethylol-propionic acid.	Matrix system of drug delivery.	It was done for enhancing the drug release modifying properties and also used as chain extenders purposes. It also represents the highest release rate at pH 7.4, which helps in colon specific drug targeting.	(Solanki & Thakore, 2015)
(A) Chitosan	Complex formation with folate.	Microcapsule	The chitosan–folate microcapsules represented a promising system to selectively target hydrophobic drugs, such as camptothecin and target the cancer cells overexpressing the folic acid receptor. It also significantly reduces the proliferation of HeLa tumor cells, while they have a negligible effect on fibroblasts.	Galbiati et al., (2011)
(B) Chitosan	Bio-reducible chitosan with hyaluronic acid. Hyaluronic acid (HA) is a negatively charged glycosaminoglycan composed of N-acetyl-D-glucosamine and glucuronic acid. It shows high-affinity binding to CD44, an adhesion/homing molecule involved in cancer cell invasion and metastasis.	Nanoparticles	The prepared nanoparticles (NPs) can release drugs in response to changes in the external pH temperature, ultrasound, and magnetic field to reduce multiple-drug resistance and enhance therapeutic efficiencies.	(Lin, Lu, Wang, Sung, & Mi, 2016)
(C) Chitosan	Chitosan (CHI) alone or different ratios of chitosan and Kollicoat Smart seal 30 D (KCSS) were applied to form film-coated tablets.	Film-coated tablet system.	It is intended for enhancing the properties like swelling, drug dissolution, stability and sharp increase of drug release in the colon. In order to clarify whether the colon release is mainly enzyme-driven or pressure controlled the coated tablets were both tested in the colon micro flora test (CMT).	(Drechsler, Garbacz, Thomann, & Schubert, 2014)
(D) Chitosan	Hydroxyethylacryl chitosan (HC) and sodium alginate (SA), the hydrogels were cross-linked by dipping method using different ionic cross linkers (e.g., Ca^{2+}, Zn^{2+} and Cu^{2+}).	Hydrogel system	The result indicated that the mixed polymer system could delay the degradation time of the hydrogels. Calcium crosslinking system showed higher stability than that of zinc or copper crosslinking system. This formulation also represents the linearity of drug release profile and its potential in the application of colon specific oral drug delivery system.	(Treenate & Monvisade, 2017)

continued on following page

Table 5. Continued

Polymers	Desired Modifications in Polymers	Drug Delivery Systems	Need of Modifications With Advantages	References
(E) Chitosan	Chitosan (CH)/ carboxymethyl cellulose (CMC) polyelectrolyte complexes were prepared by spray-drying process.	Microparticles system	These microparticles were prepared in terms of yield, encapsulation efficiency, drug loading, morphology and mucoadhesion properties. Microparticles water-uptake and drug release as well as its protection against gastric pepsin degradation were also investigated.	Cerchiara et al., (2016)
(F) Chitosan	Surface Molecularly Imprinted Chitosan grafted poly (methyl methacrylate) were prepared by free radical polymerization reaction.	Matrix system, microsphere drug delivery system.	It was intended to develop for pH-dependent and time delayed studies. The release system showed that the drugs did not release in simulated gastric fluid having pH = 1 and the drug release was small in the simulated small intestinal fluid (pH = 6.8), and drug abrupt release will be produced in the simulated colon fluid (pH = 7.4), indicating excellent colon-specific drug targeting.	(Zheng, Lian, Yang, & Wang, 2016)
Cyclodextrin	B-Cyclodextrin & azobenzene grafted poly (glycidyl methacrylate).	Polymersomes or polymeric vesicles.	The polymeric vesicles are formed for enhancing the stability under the treatment of ultraviolet radiation, competitive binding or acidic conditions and heating process, on account of the multivalent inter Polymer interaction and drug polymer complexion for excellent biocompatibility having their great potentials in colon-specific macromolecular drug delivery systems.	Gu et al., (2015)
(A) Dextran	Enteric coated (Eudragit S-100) coated microspheres (Eudragit L-100) cross linked with epichlorohydrin using emulsification method.	.	This system was employed for the treatment of colon cancer as it was investigated that designed enteric coated dextran microspheres of 5-FU protected drug release in an acidic pH while a controlled release of the drug from the microspheres was observed, once the coating layer of enteric polymer dissolved at a higher pH (pH 6.8 and 7.4). The results exhibit that the drug concentration was found higher in the colon, with low systemic exposure of the drug.	(Rai, Yadav, Jain, & Agrawal, 2015)
(B) Dextran	Methacrylated and Succinic acid derivative	Hydrogel system.	It is intended for representing the potential mucoadhesive behavior of the hydrogel promoted drug release in the site of action for a prolonged time in colon specific drug targeting approach.	(Casadei, Pitarresi, Calabrese, Paolicelli, & Giammona, 2008)
Guar-Gum	Guar gum was reacted with glutaraldehyde under acidic conditions to obtain different products.	Microparticles.	The modification was done for increasing crosslinking densities to prevent premature drug release.	(Seeli & Prabaharan, 2016)

continued on following page

Table 5. Continued

Polymers	Desired Modifications in Polymers	Drug Delivery Systems	Need of Modifications With Advantages	References
Hydroxypropyl Methyl Cellulose (HPMC)	Hydroxypropyl methyl cellulose (HPMC) has been modified by grafting synthetic polyacrylamide chains [g-HPMC (M)] in presence of microwave irradiation which has used as carrier for controlled release of 5-amino salicylic acid (5-ASA).	Matrix system of drug delivery	It is used as a carrier for controlled release of 5-amino salicylic acid (5-ASA).	(Das & Pal, 2015)
Hydrophilic Polyethylene Glycol (PEG)	Water soluble gold nanoparticles stabilized by a mixed monolayer of a hydrophobic zinc phthalocyanine photosensitizer (C11Pc) and hydrophilic polyethylene glycol (PEG) has been prepared.	Nanoparticles	The water soluble gold nanoparticles stabilized by mixing the hydrophilic PEG and hydrophobic c11pc polymer for desired colon specific targeting.	Girgis et al., (2013)
Katira Gum	Poly acrylamide-grafted Katira gum was synthesized by grafting acrylamide onto katira gum in presence of varying concentration of ceric ammonium nitrate (CAN) as initiator.	Matrix tablet system of drug delivery.	This polymer modification was intended to provide high swelling index and treated as a potential formulation in delivering the drug to the colon and the more susceptible for enzymatic degradation.	(Bharaniraja, Jayaram Kumar, Prasad, & Sen, 2011)
Polymethacrylic Acid (PMAA)	Konjac gluco-mannan (KGM) and poly methacrylic acid) (PMAA) were prepared by immersion of a solution of methacrylic acid (MAA)monomer with cross-linker N,N-methylene bis acrylamide (MBAAm) and initiating into a pre-fabricated dried KGM gel.	Novel pH sensitive interpenetrating polymer networks (IPN) hydrogels	The swelling behaviour of IPN hydrogels were studied for their sensitive response to environment pH value. It was possible to modulate the degree of swelling of the IPN gels by changing the KGM/PMAA ratio and the cross-linking density of the PMAA component.	Q. Xu et al., (2013)
Psyllium	Psyllium and polyacrylic acid (PAA) based polymeric networks by radiation-induced cross-linked co-polymerization.	Hydrogel based drug delivery system.	The hydrogels were developed from the modification of psyllium with acrylic acid through radiation method are pH responsive and have shown good degree of swelling in the pH 7.4 buffer and have potential to deliver the drug in the colon with controlled and sustained form.	(B. Singh, Chauhan, & Kumar, 2008)
Starch	Novel starch based nano scale enteric coatings from soybean meal.	Nano particle drug delivery.	It is employed for potential coating materials for colonic nutrient and drug deliveries as for encapsulating colon-targeted bioactive drugs.	Sivapragasam et al., (2014)

incorporated into lipophilic bilayer. Scientists have developed many liposomes like pegylated liposomes (avoid RES uptake), ligand targeted liposomes, stimuli sensitive liposomes for treatment of various disease such as fungal disorder, ulcerative colitis, IBDs as well as targeting different diseases like cancer. Liposomes equipped with selective targeting molecules on the surface of liposomes such as ligand or antibody can improve the colon targeting performance of liposomes. Most cancer cells show some anomalous features compared with the normal host cells which could be utilized for the selective targeting of anticancer drugs with the help of ligand(s). These ligands bind specifically to the tumor-associated or specific proteins expressed on the cancer cell surface (Allen & Cullis, 2013; Jain, A., Gulbake, A., Jain, A., Shilpi, S., Hurkat, P., & Jain, S. K.., 2013). Nanoliposomes are used for the delivery of topotecan (TPT) and vincristine (VCR) combination that act synergistically against cancer. VCR and TPT combination was entrapped into the nanoliposomes (LipoViTo) using the ammonium sulphate gradient method.

Table 6. Examples of nanoconstructs exploited for colon targeting

System	Structure	Characteristics	Examples of Compounds	References
Dendrimers	Radially emerging Hyper-branched synthetic polymer with regular pattern and repeated units	• Biodistribution and pharmacokinetics properties can be tuned • High structural and chemical homogeneity • Ease of functionalization, • high ligand density • Controlled degradation • Multi-functionality	PAMAM-MTX, PAMAM-platinate, Lauryl-modified G3 PAMAM dendrimer conjugated with paclitaxel, MUC1 and AS1411 aptamers functionalized dendrimers (Epirubicin).	(Kukowska-Latallo, J. F., Candido, K. A., Cao, Z., Nigavekar, S. S., Majoros, I. J., Thomas, T. P., . . . Baker, J. R., Jr., 2005; Malik, N., Evagorou, E. G., & Duncan, R., 1999; Taghdisi, S. M., Danesh, N. M., Ramezani, M., Lavaee, P., Jalalian, S. H., Robati, R. Y., & Abnous, K., 2016; Teow, H. M., Zhou, Z., Najlah, M., Yusof, S. R., Abbott, N. J., & D'Emanuele, A., 2013)
Liposomes	Self-assembling closed phospholipid bilayer structure	• Amphiphilic, biocompatible and nontoxic • Ease to modify according to disease • Targeting potential	Pegylated liposomal DOX (Doxil), Non-pegylated liposomal, DOX (Myocet), Liposomal daunorubicin (DaunoXome), Nanoliposomes (LipoViTo), Anti-RON antibody-directed doxorubicin (Dox) immunoliposomes (IL), TfR targeted immunoliposomes.	(Guin, S., Ma, Q., Padhye, S., Zhou, Y. Q., Yao, H. P., & Wang, M. H., 2011; Jain & Jain, 2016b; Markman, 2006; Rivera, 2003; Rosenthal, E., Poizot-Martin, I., Saint-Marc, T., Spano, J. P., Cacoub, P., & Group, D. N. X. S., 2002; Saraf, Jain, Hurkat, & Jain, 2016)
Polymeric Micelles	Amphiphilic block copolymers assemble and form a micelle with a hydrophobic core and hydrophilic shell	• Suitable carrier for water-insoluble drug • Biocompatible, self-assembling, biodegradable • Ease of functional modification • Targeting potential	Self-assembled polymeric micelles from PEG-b-poly (amino acid) copolymer. Polymer star-PCL-azo-mPEG (sPCEG-azo), α-tocopheryl succinate (α-TOS)-doxorubicin.	(Cabral & Kataoka 2014; Ma, Z. G., Ma, R., Xiao, X. L., Zhang, Y. H., Zhang, X. Z., Hu, N., . . . Sun, Z. J., 2016; Lee, K.-Y., Chiang, Y.-T., Hsu, N.-Y., Yang, C.-Y., Lo, C.-L., & Ku, C.-A., 2015)
Polymeric Nanoparticles (Polymer-Drug Conjugates)	Drug are conjugated to the side chain of a linear polymer with a linker (cleavable bond)	• Water soluble, nontoxic biodegradable • Surface modification (pegylation) • Selective accumulation and retention in tumor tissue (EPR effect) • Specific targeting of cancer cells while sparing normal cells—receptor-mediated targeting with a ligand	Eudragit S100 coated Citrus Pectin Nanoparticles of 5-Fluorouracil (5-FU). Doxorubicin- Mesoporous silica nanoparticles. B-lactoglobulin–pectin nanoparticles of platinum complex (bipyridine ethyl di-thiocarbamate Pt (II) nitrate).	(Izadi, Divsalar, Saboury, & Sawyer, 2016; Subudhi, M., Jain, A., Jain, A., Hurkat, P., Shilpi, S., Gulbake, A., & Jain, S., 2015; Zhang, M., Xu, C., Wen, L., Han, M. K., Xiao, B., Zhou, J., . . . Merlin, D., 2016)

LipoViTo maintained a fixed drug ratio *in vivo* by controlling drug release and was better than the free drugs and liposomal formulation with a single drug in the human cell lines Daoy (medulloblastoma) and SW480 (colon cancer) tumor models in mice (Saraf, S., Jain, A., Hurkat, P., & Jain, S. K., 2016). Guin et al. (2010) formulated the anti-RON antibody-directed doxorubicin (Dox) immunoliposomes (IL) for colon cancer. RON is a potential targeting molecule for delivering anticancer drug to colon cancer which is expressed by hypoxic colon cancer cells. Drug resistance in various anticancer drugs involves the hypoxic region of cancer. Hypoxic tumor cells are highly malignant and increase resistance to apoptosis, increase the matrix invasiveness and angiogenesis. RON and hypoxia inducible factors (HIF-1) expression were observed in hypoxic colon HCT116 and SW620 cells. RON is a suitable moiety for delivery of chemo-drugs to hypoxic cancer cells for enhanced drug cytotoxicity. Such targeted approach is also able to partially overcome the resistance of tumor cells acquired under acute hypoxic conditions (Guin, Yao, & Wang, 2010). Kamps et al. (2000) prepared Pegylated immunoliposomes prepared by random coupling of a tumor cell-specific antibody, CC52, via a thio-ether bond. *In vivo* studied were performed on rat liver CC52 metastasis model. CC52 Immunoliposomes show higher uptake in hepatic cells and lower uptake in splenic cells as compare to simple liposomes (Kamps, J. A., Koning, G. A., Velinova, M. J., Morselt, H. W., Wilkens, M., Gorter, A., . . . Scherphof, G. L., 2000). Local delivery to bowel tissue through oral administration is a challenging but a desirable goal to treat diseases like inflammatory bowel disease (IBD). Colon specific drug delivery system should be capable of protecting the drug en route colon (Kumari, Jain, Hurkat, Verma, & Jain, 2016). Liposomes have shown potential to specific accumulation at inflammation site thus reduce toxicity; hence it can be used for effective treatment of IBD (Jain & Jain, 2015).

Gupta et al., (2013) prepared liposomes and encapsulated into enteric coated capsules. Particle size and entrapment efficiency of liposomes were between 200 and 300 nm and 40 and 60%, respectively. *In vivo* and *ex vivo* study indicates higher accumulation of liposomes in colonic region as compared to pure drug. Enteric coated capsules delivered the drug after 5 h lag time. Higher accumulation of liposomal drug and selectively release in inflammatory area by enteric coated capsules provide better alternative for the treatment of colonic disease (Guin, S., Yao, H. P., & Wang, M. H., 2013).

Dendrimers

Dendrimers are the most promising drug delivery system due to some unique features such as well-defined structure, biocompatible and multivalency. Structurally dendrimers are hyper-branched macromolecule and have potential application in drug delivery system. They enhance solubility and loading capacity of drugs and show controlled bio-distribution. Now-a-days, dendrimers are investigated for their applications in delivery of chemotherapeutic agents in leukemia, lymphoma and different types of solid tumor. Alibolandi et al. (2017) investigated camptothecin-loaded pegylated PAMAM dendrimers for site-specific targeting against colorectal cancer cells using AS1411 nucleolin aptamers as a targeting ligand (Figure 1). Nucleolin is a nucleus membrane protein receptor that is over-expressed on plasma membrane of various cancer cells comprising colorectal cancer, breast cancer, non-small cell lung cancer, and pancreatic carcinoma (Alibolandi, M., Taghdisi, S. M., Ramezani, P., Hosseini Shamili, F., Farzad, S. A., Abnous, K., & Ramezani, M., 2017; Taghdisi, S. M., Danesh, N. M., Ramezani, M., Lavaee, P., Jalalian, S. H., Robati, R. Y., & Abnous, K., 2016). Aptamers are single-strand RNA or DNA which can bind to various molecular targets with high affinity and specificity. The *in vitro* release profile shows the sustain release of drug for 4 days and *in vitro* cytotoxicity study exhibits higher antiproliferation activity, towards nucleolin-positive HT29 and C26 colorectal cancer cells than nucleolin-negative CHO cell line. MUC1 and AS1411 aptamers functionalized dendrimers were increase the therapeutic efficacy of Epirubicin. AS1411 aptamers selectively bind to nucleus membrane protein receptor nucleolin whereas MUC1 selectively bind to abnormally glycosylated mucin-1 (a trans membrane glycoprotein) both are overexpressed on various cancer cells (Alibolandi, M., Taghdisi, S. M., Ramezani, P., Hosseini Shamili, F., Farzad, S. A., Abnous, K., & Ramezani, M., 2017). Xu et al. (2015) have developed target specific coumarin-containing telodendrimers for delivery of 7-ethyl-10-hydroxy camptothecin (SN-38), a prominent and efficacious chemotherapeutic agent, for the treatment of colon cancers. The *in vitro*

Figure 1. Schematic representation of (I) synthesis of pegylated PAMAM dendrimer (PEG-PAMAM); (II) camptothecin (CPT) loading in the cavities of PEG-PAMAM; (III) conjugation of thiolated AS1411 aptamers to the maleimide groups of MAL-PEG-PAMAM-CPT and preparation of Apt-PEG-PAMAM-CPT

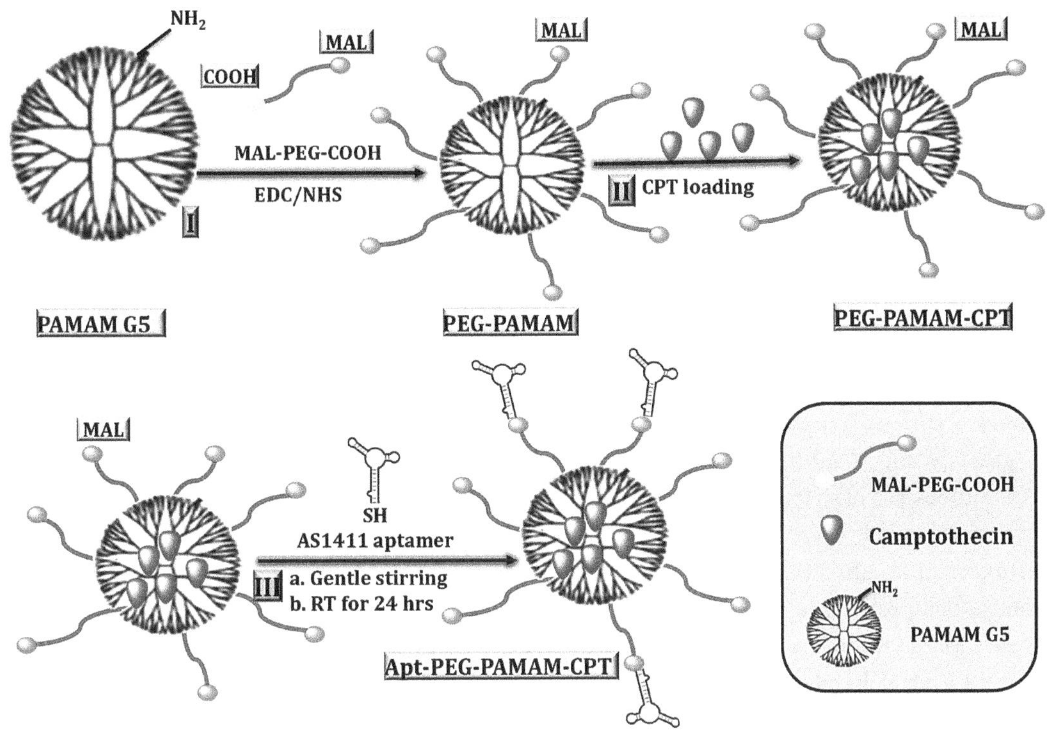

cytotoxicity experiments show the similar cytotoxic activity against colon cancer cells as the free drug and were 500-fold more potent than irinotecan (a prodrug of SN-38) (Xu, G., Shi, C., Guo, D., Wang, L., Ling, Y., Han, X., & Luo, J., 2015). Lauryl-modified G3 PAMAM dendrimer conjugated with paclitaxel were synthesized and cytotoxicity of dendrimer carriers was investigated using Caco-2 cells. A glutaric anhydride linker was selected to attach to paclitaxel via an ester bond and then conjugated with PAMAM dendrimer via an amide bond. Cytotoxicity studies showed that the conjugation of lauryl chains and paclitaxel on G3 dendrimer significantly ($p < 0.05$) increased the cytotoxicity against Caco-2 cell (Teow, H. M., Zhou, Z., Najlah, M., Yusof, S. R., Abbott, N. J., & D'Emanuele, A., 2013).

Ulcerative colitis (UC) is a severe inflammatory disease in colon. G5-NH-acetamide (Ac)-TOS system for the treatment of UC was prepared by conjugating alpha-tocopheryl succinate (α-TOS) to generation 5 (G5) poly (amidoamine) (PAMAM) dendrimer. *In vivo* evaluation was performed in dextran sulfate sodium induced UC mouse model, The G5-NH-Ac-TOS exhibits greater inhibitive effects on UC than free α-TOS due to inhibition of expression of nuclear translocation of NF-κB, phosphorylation of Akt, and reduction of reactive oxygen species production in the macrophages (Wang, Y., Shen, W., Shi, X., Fu, F., Fan, Y., Shen, W., . . . Qi, R., 2017). 5-aminosalicylic acid was bound to PAMAM dendrimers using p-aminobenzoic acid (PABA) and p-aminohippuric acid (PAH) as a spacer contains the azo-bond. The dendrimer conjugates were incubated in homogenate of the stomach or phosphate buffer, pH 1.2 and 6.8 and homogenate of the small intestine. It was observed that dendrimer conjugates which were incubated with homogenate of the stomach or phosphate buffer, pH 1.2 and 6.8showed no drug detection, while dendrimer conjugates incubated with homogenate of the small intestine for 12 h shown small amount of 5- aminosalicylic acid. Thus PAMAM dendrimers may be a promising carrier for colon targeting (Wiwattanapatapee, Lomlim, & Saramunee, 2003).

Carbon Nanotubes (CNTs)

Carbon nanotubes (CNTs) show some unique features such as quasi-one-dimensional nanostructure which have been widely investigated as an excellent candidate for drug delivery carrier. It has good thermal and chemical stability, ultra-high cargo loading capacity, and structure flexibility. In recent years, CNTs widely investigated for their application in fields of biology, drug delivery, sensing and detection, and imaging. CNTs can penetrate cell membrane and deliver drug molecules into cytoplasm efficiently also reduce the side toxic effect (Zhang, X., Hui, Z., Wan, D., Huang, H., Huang, J., Yuan, H., & Yu, J., 2010; Zhou, Peng, Liao, Li, & Li, 2014). Multi-walled carbon nanotubes decrease the expression and transport activity of ABC transporter such as ABCB1/Pgp and ABCC4/ MRP4 in human colon adenocarcinoma Caco-2 cells due to decrease Myc (Proto-oncogene c) that regulates the expression of ABC gene (Wang, Z., Xu, Y., Meng, X., Watari, F., Liu, H., & Chen, X., 2015). Irinotecan loaded carbon nanotubes (CNTs)-based colon-specific microspheres were synthesized and cytotoxicity study was performed on HT-29 cells. Folate–chitosan conjugate and irinotecan attached to CNTs via non-covalent interaction, after that microencapsulated into Eudragit S-100. Eudragit coated microspheres show control drug release at pH 7.4 while no drug release was found at pH below 7. Irinotecan loaded CNTs were more cytotoxic as compare to drug free FA-CS decorated CNTs (Figure 2) (Zhou, M., Peng, Z., Liao, S., Li, P., & Li, S., 2014).

Nanoparticles

Nanoparticles can be defined as the small object that behaves like a whole unit with respect to its transport, comes in the range of 1 to 100nm (Soppimath, Aminabhavi, Kulkarni, & Rudzinski, 2001). In current scenario nanoparticle-based oral formulations protect drugs from the harsh gastrointestinal environment, and selectively raise drug concentration inside diseased colon cells, therefore elevating therapeutic efficacy while reducing systemic toxicity (Lu, L., Chen, G., Qiu, Y., Li, M., Liu, D., Hu, D., . . . Xiao, Z., 2016). As nanoparticles bind to specific receptors, they are generally enveloped by endosomes via receptor-mediated endocytosis, thus bypassing the recognition of P-glycoprotein, which is responsible for drug resistance mechanisms (Cho, Wang, Nie, Chen, & Shin, 2008). For targeting the tumor cell, ligand conjugated nanoparticles (such as antibodies, peptides, aptamers and other small molecules) were used which enhance *in vivo* specificity and cell recognition. The incorporation of these ligands is usually achieved by chemical modification during nanoparticle synthesis (Cisterna, B. A., Kamaly, N., Choi, W. I., Tavakkoli, A., Farokhzad, O. C., & Vilos, C., 2016). Nanoparticles can be used as a targeting therapy for colon cancer, inflammatory bowel disease like ulcerative colitis and Crohn's disease. Hyaluronidase-responsive nanoparticle specifically prepared for colon cancer cells. In this study, mesoporous silica nanoparticles (MSN) were fabricated for targeted drug delivery system that is responsive to hyaluronidase (HAase). Desthiobiotin engraftment onto the surface of MSN generated a streptavidin complex, which was functionalized with biotin-modified hyaluronic acid (HA) to enable controlled drug release at cancer cells expressing HAase. *In vitro* study revealed that the release of doxorubicin hydrochloride (Dox) was enhanced considerably in the presence of biotin or HAase and

Figure 2. (a) Encapsulation of multi walled carbon nanotubes (MWCNTs) with folate- chitosan (FA-CS) conjugate and irinotecan, (b) Microencapsulation of carbon nano tubes based drug carrier with eudragit S-100 and its probable mechanism of drug release from the eudragit microencapsulated nanotubes microcores

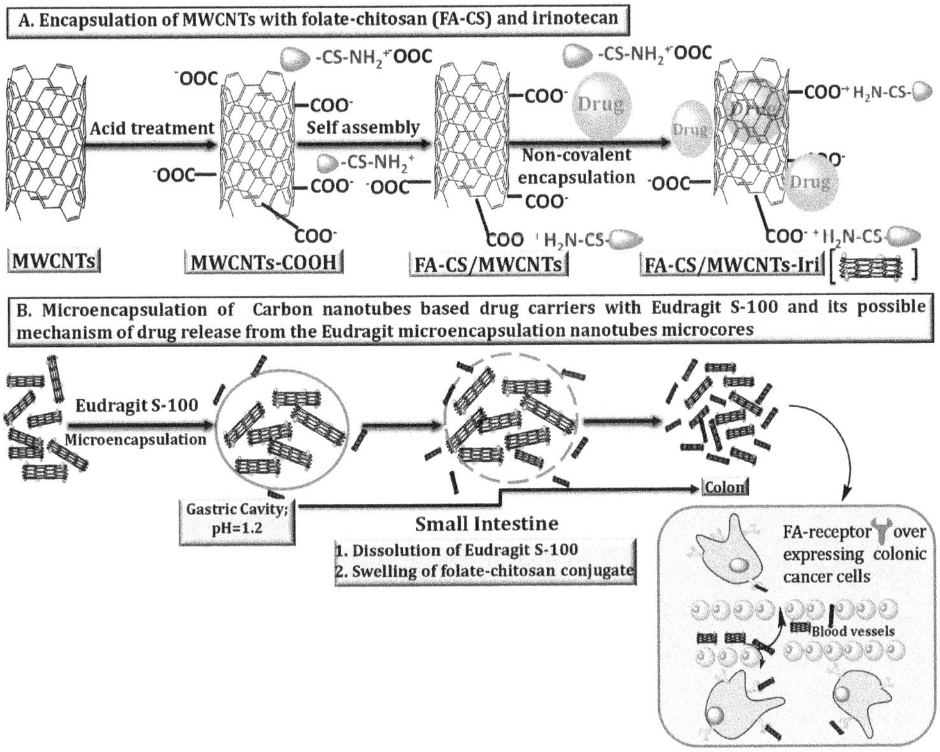

uptake by cancer cells was mediated efficiently by CD44 receptor–mediated endocytosis (Figure 3). This study concluded that apoptosis of cancer cells by MSN-HA/Dox Nanoparticles was more efficient than free doxorubicin and inhibited tumor growth with minimal systemic toxicity *in vivo* (Zhang, M., Xu, C., Wen, L., Han, M. K., Xiao, B., Zhou, J., . . . Merlin, D., 2016).

Propyl amine-functionalized silica (MSN-NH2) was first reformed with desthiobiotin to obtain MSN-desthiobiotin, then by employing biotin (or desthiobiotin)–SA interaction, SA and biotinylated HA were self-assembled on the external surface of MSN to yield MSN-HA then therapeutic drug, doxorubicin, was able to load to obtain MSN-HA/Dox., in figure 3 B is showing that CD44 receptor–mediated endocytosis and triggering of drug release in tumor cells. MSN-HA/Dox were taken up by cancer cell via receptor-mediated endocytosis (HA–CD44 interaction), then loaded doxorubicin was released from the pore of MSN by t triggering of HAase and intracellular biotin. In another application, mesoporous Silica nanoparticles (MSN) based on enzyme responsive materials were developed for colon specific drug delivery. In this study 5-flurouracil (5FU) was incorporated as a model drug with Guar gum, a natural carbohydrate polymer as a capping layer. Non-covalent interaction through guar gum capping shows identical nanoparticles. The release of 5FU from guar gum capped MSN (GG-MSN) was specifically triggered via enzymatic biodegradation of guar gum by colonic enzymes in the simulated colonic microenvironment (Kumar, B., Kulanthaivel, S., Mondal, A., Mishra, S., Banerjee, B., Bhaumik, A.,

Figure 3. MSN-HA nanoparticles mediated delivery of the, doxorubicin (Dox), to tumor cells. (A) Drug loading steps to yield MSN-HA/Dox delivery system. (B) Diagram demonstrating the CD44 receptor–mediated endocytosis and triggering of drug release in tumor cells.

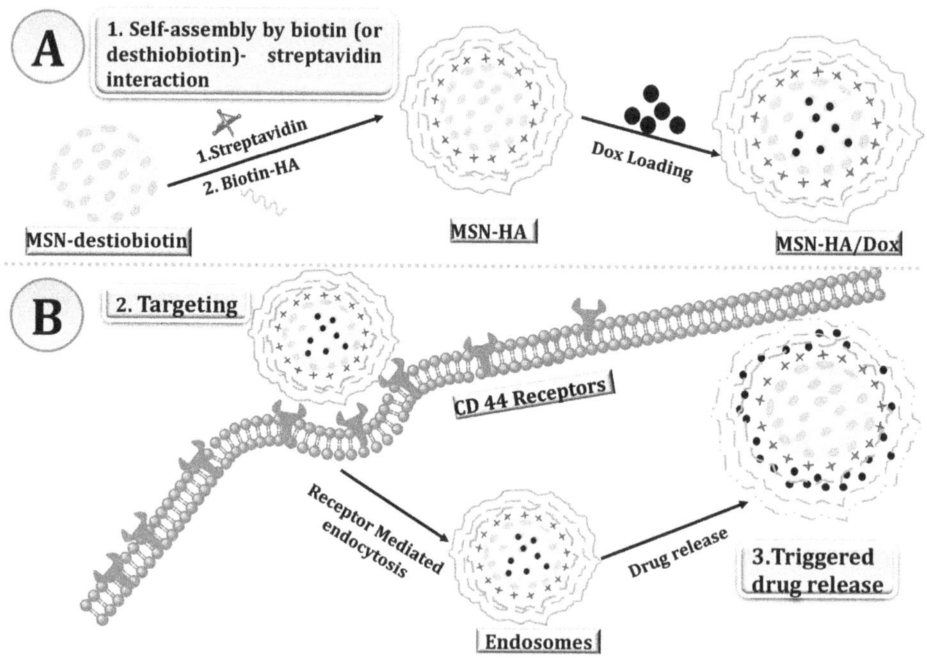

. . . Giri, S. , 2017). Izadi et al. (2016) developed β-lacto globulin–pectin nanoparticle that hold great potential as an effective drug delivery system. Various physicochemical properties of β-lacto globulin (whey protein of cow's milk) such as its stability at low pH, its resistance to gastric protease, and its ability to bind hydrophobic ligands, provide it potential for transporting drugs specifically for colon cancer. β- lactoglobulin–pectin nanoparticles was prepared to transfer a newly synthesized, anticancer platinum complex (bipyridine ethyl dithiocarbamate Pt(II) nitrate), to the colon. The drug release profile in simulated gastrointestinal conditions demonstrated that β-lacto globulin with a secondary coating is stable in acidic conditions but is able to release its cargo at pH 7. Hence, these nanoparticles have potential to serve as novel and effective vehicles for oral drug delivery (Izadi, Z., Divsalar, A., Saboury, A. A., & Sawyer, L., 2016). Eudragit S100 coated Citrus Pectin Nanoparticles (E-CPNs) containing 5-Fluorouracil (5-FU) were prepared for the colon targeting. Citrus pectin also acts as a ligand for galectin-3 receptors that are over expressed on colorectal cancer cells. *In vitro* drug release studies revealed selective drug release more than 70% in 24 h in the colonic region in the case of E-CPNs. *In vitro* cytoxicity assay (Sulphorhodamine B assay) was performed against HT-29 cancer cells and exhibited 1.5 fold greater cytotoxicity potential of nanoparticles compared to 5-FU solution. Therefore, a multifaceted strategy is introduced here in terms of receptor mediated uptake and pH-dependent release using E-CPNs for effective chemotherapy of colorectal cancer with uncompromised safety and efficacy (Subudhi, M., Jain, A., Jain, A., Hurkat, P., Shilpi, S., Gulbake, A., & Jain, S., 2015). More efficient treatment could be achieved by preparing copper oxide nanoparticles (CuO NPs) from the leaves of *O. cochinchinense (Ormocarpum cochinchinense)* whichwas screened for anticancer activity on human colon cancer cell lines (HCT-116) by MTT (3-(4,5-dimethyl-2-tiazolyl)-2,5-diphenyl-2-tetrazolium bromide) assay. The synthesized CuO NPs showed high anticancer cytotoxicity on human colon cancer cell lines (HCT-116) with IC50 value of 40 μg/ml (Gnanavel, Palanichamy, & Roopan, 2017). Solid lipid nanoparticle (SLNs) containing 5-flurouracil (5-FU) were prepared by double emulsion-solvent evaporation technique (w/o/w) using triglyceride esters, Dynasan™ 114 or Dynasan™ 118 along with soya lecithin as the lipid parts for local treatment of colon cancer. Incomplete biphasic prolonged release profile of the drug was observed in phosphate buffer pH 6.8 as well as simulated colonic medium containing rat caecal contents (Yassin, A. E., Alsarra, I. A., Alanazi, F. K., Al-Mohizea, A. M., Al-Robayan, A. A., & Al-Obeed, O. A., 2010). Further study was done for the treatment of inflammatory bowel disease by targeted drug delivery system through biodegradable nanoparticles. In this study male wistar rats was used to induce an experimental colitis with trinitro- benzene sulfonic. Rolipram (anti- inflammatory) was combined within poly (lactic-co-glycolic acid) nanoparticles. Myeloperoxidase activity was determined to assess the inflammation, while an adverse effect index reflected the remaining neurotropic effect of rolipram resulting from its systemic absorption. Myeloperoxidase activity decreased considerably after the oral administration of rolipram nanoparticles or solution (Lamprecht, A., Ubrich, N., Yamamoto, H., Schafer, U., Takeuchi, H., Maincent, P., . . . Lehr, C. M. , 2001).

Micelles

Block copolymer micelles are usually made by the self-assembly of either amphiphilic or oppositely charged copolymers in aqueous medium. Corona and core of the micelles is formed by the hydrophilic and hydrophobic blocks, respectively. The presence of a non-ionic water-soluble shell as well as the range (10–100 nm) of polymeric micelles are expected to restrict their uptake by the mononuclear phagocyte system and permit for passive targeting of cancerous or inflamed tissues through the greater permeation and retention effect. Research in the field has been increasingly intensive on achieving greater stability of the micellar assembly, prolonged circulation times and controlled release of the drug for ideal targeting. Block copolymers developed with various applications, including amphiphilic micelles for passive targeting of chemotherapeutic agents and environment-sensitive micelles for the oral delivery of poorly bioavailable compounds for the treatment of various diseased conditions such as colon cancer, ulcerative colitis or Crohn's disease (Gaucher, G., Dufresne, M. H., Sant, V. P., Kang, N., Maysinger, D., & Leroux, J. C., 2005). For targeting therapy, ligands are an imperative part of targeted drug delivery systems. A 12-residue peptide (TK) specifically binds with integrin α6β1 overexpressed on colonic cancer cells. Due to its high binding affinity with integrin α6β1, it increases not only Caco-2 cells uptake but also increases penetration of the tumor spheroids. A novel PEG-PLA micelles loading DOX or coumarin-6 (TK-MS/DOX or TK-MS/C6) was prepared with the conjugation of PEG-PLA and TK. TK-MS/DOX exhibited significantly stronger cytotoxicity for Caco-2 as compared to MS/DOX. Therefore, TK peptide appears to be fit as a targeting ligand with potential applications in colonic targeted therapy (Ren, Y., Mu, Y., Song, Y., Xie, J., Yu, H., Gao, S., . . . Lu, W., 2016). Di-block copolymer micellar system of α-tocopheryl succinate (α-TOS) containing doxorubicin (Dox), was prepared with the conjugation of α-TOS molecules and mPEG-b-PHEMA hydrophilic di-block copolymer by ester bonds for HCT116 colon cancer therapy. The release pattern of drug from this system was dependent on acidic surroundings such as endosomes or secondary lysosomes. *In vitro* study revealed that Dox-loaded polymeric micelles enhanced the cytotoxicity of Dox and α-TOS to cancer cells. Dox-loaded polymeric micelles also showed an exceptional tumor inhibiting effect *in vivo*. The α-TOS containing polymeric micelle system can be used as a drug carrier for colon cancer (Lee, K.-Y., Chiang, Y.-T., Hsu, N.-Y., Yang, C.-Y., Lo, C.-L., &

Ku, C.-A., 2015). Photo thermal therapy by EGFR-targeted micelles containing near-infrared dye is good for treatment in colorectal cancer. The aim of this research was to explore the effectiveness of epidermal growth factor receptor (EGFR) targeted micelles loaded with IR-780 (Cetuximab/IR-780/micelles) for producing colon targeting, multimodal images, and photo thermal therapy (PTT). Biodistribution and antitumor effects of Cetuximab/IR-780/micelles was observed in HCT-116 (high expression of EGFR) and SW-620 (low expression of EGFR) cell lines. HCT-116 tumors in tumor-bearing mice exhibited significantly higher accumulations of Cetuximab/IR-780/^{111}In-micelles than SW-620 tumors in Micro-SPECT/CT imaging. Dual-radioisotope Nano-SPECT/CT imaging of Cetuximab/^{131}I-IR-780/^{111}In-micelles demonstrated simultaneous high accumulation of both IR-780 and micelles in HCT-116 tumors, but not in SW-620 tumors. Regarding antitumor effects, following the Cetuximab/IR-780/micelles with PPT on day 6, all HCT-116 tumor-bearing mice were cured. In contrast, SW-620 tumors relapsed at 13 days after treatment. Hence the results showed that Cetuximab/IR-780/micelles could improve the antitumor effects by PTT in EGFR overexpressed colorectal cancers (Shih, Y. H., Luo, T. Y., Chiang, P. F., Yao, C. J., Lin, W. J., Peng, C. L., & Shieh, M. J., 2017) (depicted in Figure 4). Thermo-responsive polymer micelles were prepared by conjugation of thermo-responsive di-block copolymers with the covalently bound cancerostatic drug pirarubicin (PIR) as a reversible micelles forming drug delivery system.The di- block copolymer carriers were composed of hydrophilic poly (N-(2- hydroxypropyl) methacrylamide) based block containing a small amount (~ 5 mol. %) of comonomer units with reactive hydrazide groups and a thermo-responsive poly (2-(2- methoxyethoxy) ethyl methacrylate) block. Drug was attached to the hydrophilic block of the copolymer through the pH-sensitive hydrazone bond designed to be stable in the blood stream at pH 7.4 but to be degraded in the intratumoral/intracellular environment at pH 5 - 6. The temperature induced conformational change of the thermo-responsive block (coil-globule transition) followed by self-assembly of the copolymer into a micellar structure. The process was controlled by the thermo-responsive block length and PIR content. The human colon adenocarcinoma (DLD-1) cell lines (*in vitro* study) was used to evaluate the cytotoxicity and intracellular transport of the conjugates as well as the release of PIR from the conjugates inside the cells, followed by its accumulation in the cell nuclei. It was demonstrated that the studied conjugates have a great potential to become efficacious *in vivo*(Laga, R., Janoušková, O., Ulbrich, K., Pola, R., Blažková, J., Filippov, S. K., . . . Pechar, M., 2015). Colon-targeted drug delivery and circumventing drug resistance are extremely important for colon cancer chemotherapy. Dimethyl fumarate (DMF), for the treatment of multiple sclerosis, shows anti-tumor activity on colon cancer cells. Based on the pharmacological properties of DMF and azo-bond in olsalazine chemical structure, azo polymeric micelles was delivered for colon-targeted dimethyl fumarate delivery by synthesized the star-shape amphiphilic polymer with azo bond and fabricated the DMF-loaded azo polymeric micelles. The four arm polymer star-PCL-azo-mPEG (sPCEG-azo) (constituted by star shape PCL (polycaprolactone) and mPEG (methoxypolyethylene glycols)-olsalazine) showed self-assembly ability. *In vitro* drug release study reveals that the cumulative release of DMF from the DMF-loaded sPCEG-azo polymeric micelles in rat gastric fluid was compared with rat colonic fluids; the cumulative release of DMF reached 60% in the initial 2 h and 100% within 10 h in rat colonic fluids, indicating that the DMF-loaded sPCEG-azo polymeric micelles had excellent colon-targeted property. In conclusion, the DMF-loaded sPCEG-azo polymeric micelles show colon-targeted DMF release and anti-tumor activity, providing a novel approach potential for colon cancer therapy (Ma, Z. G., Ma, R., Xiao, X. L., Zhang, Y. H., Zhang, X. Z., Hu, N., . . . Sun, Z. J., 2016). Chronic inflammation on the digestive system causes the inflammatory bowel disease either ulcerative colitis (affected only colonic mucosa) or chron's disease (affected entire digestive tract) can be treated by budesonide (BUD),a glucocorticoid (Gionchetti,

P., Rizzello, F., Annese, V., Armuzzi, A., Biancone, L., Castiglione, F., . . . Daperno, M., 2017). A new pharmaceutical formulation for the treatment of ulcerative colitis was developed by BUD-HP-β-CD inclusion complex incorporating PL 407 and PL407-PL403. Phase solubility study (1:1 stoichiometry, Kc = 8662.8 M−1) confirmed complexation between BUD and HP-β-CD. BUD solubility was improved with the association of HP-β-CD and PL 407 or PL407-PL403 (Santos Akkari, A. C., Ramos Campos, E. V., Keppler, A. F., Fraceto, L. F., de Paula, E., Tofoli, G. R., & de Araujo, D. R., 2016).

Advancements

The formulation of colon specific drug delivery systems has been a matter of keen interest among various scientists in the past few years. Colon targeted drug delivery systems provide remarkable therapeutic advantages to the patients like safety, efficacy, and patient compliance. Few recent researches in the polymer based drug delivery systems for colon targeting in the last two years have been elucidated below. Ribeiro et al. (2014) developed 5-ASA encapsulated pectin-coated chitosan–LDH bio-nanocomposite beads for targeted delivery to colon. The formulated pectin coated composite beads were found to be stable to water swelling and depicted a controlled release in *in vitro* experiments, due to their pH resistant nature (Ribeiro, L. N., Alcântara, A. C., Darder, M., Aranda, P., Araújo-Moreira, F. M., & Ruiz-Hitzky,

Figure 4. Cetuximab conjugated, 131I-IR-780-loaded and 111In-labeled fabricated micelles (Cetuximab/131I-IR-780/111In-micelles)

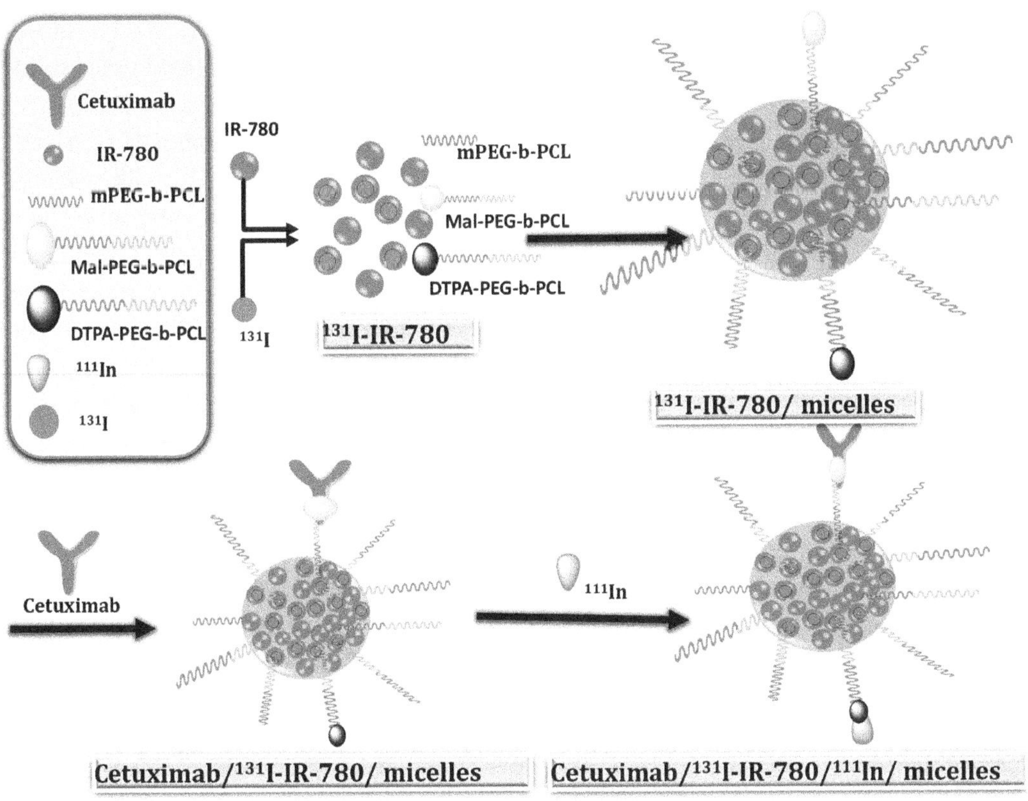

E., 2014). Xie *et al.* performed a modification of doxorubicin (DOX)-loaded mesoporous silica (MSNs) nanoparticles with the help of aptamer (Ap) against the epithelial cell adhesion molecule (EpCAM). The study depicted an increase in the binding capacity of Ap-MSN-DOX with EpCAM overexpressing SW620 colon cancer cells due to EpCAM conjugation although the same was not observed in the case of EpCAM-negative Ramos cells. This led to raised cellular uptake and enhanced cytotoxicity of the DOX in SW620 cells in comparison to non-Ap-modified nanoparticles (MSNDOX). Thus, it was demonstrated that Ap-MSN-DOX possessed the potential for the targeting the EpCAM positive colon cancer cells with reduced side effects and enhanced efficacy (Xie, X., Li, F., Zhang, H., Lu, Y., Lian, S., Lin, H., . . . Jia, L., 2016). Liang et al. (2016) developed gemcitabine (GEM)-conjugated methoxy poly (ethylene glycol)-poly (lactic acid) (GEM-PL) biodegradable polymeric drug carriers which demonstrated a controlled release of drug. The developed GEM-PL efficiently killed the HT29 cancers cells in a typical time dependent manner. GEM-PL formulation showed a remarkable greater apoptosis of tumor cells (~25%). mPEG-PLA conjugated GEM showed an enhanced blood circulation potential as observed in animal model when compared to free GEM. GEM-PL depicted a significant tumor regression in HT-29 containing tumor model. The formulated mPEG-PLA/GEM conjugates demonstrated that polymer-based drug targeting and could be of clinical significance in the treating colon cancers (Liang, T.-J., Zhou, Z.-M., Cao, Y.-Q., Ma, M.-Z., Wang, X.-J., & Jing, K., 2016). 5-ASA loaded silicon dioxide nanoparticles (5-ASA-SiO_2 NPs) were prepared by Tang *et al.* for the targeted treatment of ulcerative colitis. Cytotoxicity of 5-ASA-SiO_2 NPs was determined *in vitro*. The therapeutic efficacy of 5-ASA-SiO_2 NPs was evaluated on the basis of their disease activity index (DAI), colon histopathology and tumor necrosis factor-α (TNF-α) and interleukin-6 (IL-6) levels. Colonic mucosal IL-6 and TNF-α mRNA expression in the groups given a high dose and 5-ASA-SiO_2 NP groups was substantially lower as compared to that in the normal dosage group ($P<0.05$) (Tang, H., Xiang, D., Wang, F., Mao, J., Tan, X., & Wang, Y., 2017). Nguyen et al. formulated an oral system by loading prednisolone in 3-aminopropyl-functionalized mesoporous silica nanoparticles (MCM-NH2) and coated them with pH responsive succinylated ε-polylysine (SPL) for targeted release in colon (Nguyen, C. T., Webb, R. I., Lambert, L. K., Strounina, E., Lee, E. C., Parat, M.-O., . . . Ross, B. P., 2017). Tian et al.(2017) developed a novel pH-triggered oral drug delivery system by cresting mesoporous silica SBA-15 with a pH-sensitive polymer poly (acrylic acid) (PAA). The mesoporous SBA-15 (PAA/SBA-15) capped with PAA demonstrated quite high drug loading capacity (785.7 mg/g), remarkable pH-sensitivity and biocompatibility. In the acidic pH, the drug doxorubicin (DOX) was encapsulated in the pore channels since the collapsed PAA capped the pores .Whereas, in the basic environment of the colon (pH = 7.6), it showed a fast release due to the removal of capping. Besides, the water solubility of DOX in colonic environment was increased after DOX being loaded into PAA/SBA-15. This pH-triggered system for oral drug delivery exhibited quite promising applications in the treatment of colon diseases like colon cancer (Tian, B., Liu, S., Wu, S., Lu, W., Wang, D., Jin, L., . . . Quan, Z., 2017). Hammadi et al. (2017) described the targeting potential of folic acid and pegylated poly(D,L-lactide-co-glycolide) nanoparticles (FOL-PEG-PLGA NPs) for delivering 5-FU to colon and breast cancers. They were discovered to be haemo-compatible, and showed very negligible cytotoxicity in normal (CCD-18 and MCF-10A) and tumour (HT-29 and MCF-7) human cell lines. The cytotoxic studies when conducted *in vitro* in folate-overexpressed HT-29 colon cancer cells and MCF-7 breast cancer cells exhibited that the half maximal inhibitory concentration (IC50) of 5-FU-loaded FOL-PEG-PLGA NPs was about 4-times less than that of the 5-FU-loaded PLGA NPs ($p < 0.05$) (El-Hammadi, Delgado, Melguizo, Prados, & Arias, 2017). Alibolandi et al. (2017) synthesized PAMAM dendrimers loaded with camptothecin and their functionalization was done with the help of AS1411 anti-nucleolin aptamers for specifically targeting those colorectal cancer cells which overexpress the neucleolin receptors. A sustained release of the drug was observed when *in vitro* studies were carried out. Cytotoxicity studies depicted a higher antiproliferative activity of pegylated dendrimers loaded with camptothecin against HT29 and C26 colon cells as compared to nucleolin-negative CHO cells. Conjugation of AS1411 aptamer to the camptothecin loaded-pegylated dendrimer surface provides site-specific delivery of camptothecin, inhibiting C26 tumor growth *in vivo* and significantly decreases systemic toxicity. The outcomes suggested that pegylated PAMAM dendrimers loaded with camptothecin could serve to be a potential delivery system for the treatment of colorectal cancer(Alibolandi, M., Taghdisi, S. M., Ramezani, P., Hosseini Shamili, F., Farzad, S. A., Abnous, K., & Ramezani, M., 2017). Shen et al.(2017) synthesized polylactidestereo complex micelle (cRGD-SCM) decorated with c(RGDfC) for treating the $\alpha v\beta 3$ integrin-positive C26 colon cancer. cRGD-SCM/DOX depicted a sustained release pattern showed prolonged circulation time, increased tumor inhibition, and reduced side effects in comparison to free DOX and non-targeting SCM/DOX *in vivo*. The results obtained clearly indicated that potential of RGD-decorated micelles in the targeted delivery to colon (Shen, K., Li, D., Guan, J., Ding, J., Wang, Z., Gu, J., . . . Chen, X., 2017).

Future Perspectives

The implementation of various approaches for effective colon targeting demands meticulous transformation from laboratory scale outcomes to the industrial level scale up. There are number of issues to be resolved such as stability of the polymeric vehicle, safety aspects, cost-effectiveness, specificity towards inflamed sites, formulation aspects, and drug protection leading to a failure in the accessibility of these products to the market. Taking all these concerns into consideration, safe and effective polymeric nanocarriers systems may be formulated for the targeted delivery to the colon. The application of polymers in colon targeted drug delivery depicts its potential use in the treatment of various colonic diseases. Recent progressions in polymer science have led to an enhancement in the polymer based carrier systems but, further research is necessitated for safer and effective targeting to the colon.

REFERENCES

Alibolandi, M., Taghdisi, S. M., Ramezani, P., Hosseini Shamili, F., Farzad, S. A., Abnous, K., & Ramezani, M. (2017). Smart AS1411-aptamer conjugated pegylated PAMAM dendrimer for the superior delivery of camptothecin to colon adenocarcinoma in vitro and in vivo. *International Journal of Pharmaceutics*, *519*(1-2), 352–364. doi:10.1016/j.ijpharm.2017.01.044 PMID:28126548

Allen, T. M., & Cullis, P. R. (2013). Liposomal drug delivery systems: From concept to clinical applications. *Advanced Drug Delivery Reviews*, *65*(1), 36–48. doi:10.1016/j.addr.2012.09.037 PMID:23036225

Apolinario, A. C., de Lima Damasceno, B. P., de Macedo Beltrao, N. E., Pessoa, A., Converti, A., & da Silva, J. A. (2014). Inulin-type fructans: A review on different aspects of biochemical and pharmaceutical technology. *Carbohydrate Polymers*, *101*, 368–378. doi:10.1016/j.carbpol.2013.09.081 PMID:24299785

Averous, L., & Pollet, E. (2012). Biodegradable polymers. In *Environmental silicate nano-biocomposites* (pp. 13–39). Springer. doi:10.1007/978-1-4471-4108-2_2

Bharaniraja, B., Jayaram Kumar, K., Prasad, C., & Sen, A. (2011). Modified katira gum for colon targeted drug delivery. *Journal of Applied Polymer Science*, *119*(5), 2644–2651. doi:10.1002/app.32829

Casadei, M. A., Pitarresi, G., Calabrese, R., Paolicelli, P., & Giammona, G. (2008). Biodegradable and pH-sensitive hydrogels for potential colon-specific drug delivery: Characterization and in vitro release studies. *Biomacromolecules*, *9*(1), 43–49. doi:10.1021/bm700716c PMID:18052027

Cerchiara, T., Abruzzo, A., Parolin, C., Vitali, B., Bigucci, F., Gallucci, M. C., ... Luppi, B. (2016). Microparticles based on chitosan/carboxymethylcellulose polyelectrolyte complexes for colon delivery of vancomycin. *Carbohydrate Polymers*, *143*, 124–130. doi:10.1016/j.carbpol.2016.02.020 PMID:27083351

Cho, K., Wang, X., Nie, S., Chen, Z. G., & Shin, D. M. (2008). Therapeutic nanoparticles for drug delivery in cancer. *Clinical Cancer Research*, *14*(5), 1310–1316. doi:10.1158/1078-0432.CCR-07-1441 PMID:18316549

Chourasia, M. K., & Jain, S. K. (2003). Pharmaceutical approaches to colon targeted drug delivery systems. *Journal of Pharmacy & Pharmaceutical Sciences*, *6*(1), 33–66. PMID:12753729

Cisterna, B. A., Kamaly, N., Choi, W. I., Tavakkoli, A., Farokhzad, O. C., & Vilos, C. (2016). Targeted nanoparticles for colorectal cancer. *Nanomedicine (London)*, *11*(18), 2443–2456. doi:10.2217/nnm-2016-0194 PMID:27529192

Coupe, A. J., Davis, S. S., & Wilding, I. R. (1991). Variation in gastrointestinal transit of pharmaceutical dosage forms in healthy subjects. *Pharmaceutical Research*, *8*(3), 360–364. doi:10.1023/A:1015849700421 PMID:2052525

Dar, M. J., Ali, H., Khan, A., & Khan, G. M. (2017). Polymer-based drug delivery: The quest for local targeting of inflamed intestinal mucosa. *Journal of Drug Targeting*, *25*(7), 582–596. doi:10.1080/1061186X.2017.1298601 PMID:28277824

Das, R., & Pal, S. (2015). Modified hydroxypropyl methyl cellulose: Efficient matrix for controlled release of 5-amino salicylic acid. *International Journal of Biological Macromolecules*, *77*, 207–213. doi:10.1016/j.ijbiomac.2015.03.015 PMID:25796452

Drechsler, M., Garbacz, G., Thomann, R., & Schubert, R. (2014). Development and evaluation of chitosan and chitosan/Kollicoat® Smartseal 30 D film-coated tablets for colon targeting. *European Journal of Pharmaceutics and Biopharmaceutics*, *88*(3), 807–815. doi:10.1016/j.ejpb.2014.09.006 PMID:25301294

El-Hammadi, M. M., Delgado, A. V., Melguizo, C., Prados, J. C., & Arias, J. L. (2017). Folic acid-decorated and PEGylated PLGA nanoparticles for improving the antitumour activity of 5-fluorouracil. *International Journal of Pharmaceutics*, *516*(1-2), 61–70. doi:10.1016/j.ijpharm.2016.11.012 PMID:27825867

Galbiati, A., Tabolacci, C., Morozzo Della Rocca, B., Mattioli, P., Beninati, S., Paradossi, G., & Desideri, A. (2011). Targeting tumor cells through chitosan-folate modified microcapsules loaded with camptothecin. *Bioconjugate Chemistry*, *22*(6), 1066–1072. doi:10.1021/bc100546s PMID:21545180

Gaucher, G., Dufresne, M. H., Sant, V. P., Kang, N., Maysinger, D., & Leroux, J. C. (2005). Block copolymer micelles: Preparation, characterization and application in drug delivery. *Journal of Controlled Release*, *109*(1-3), 169–188. doi:10.1016/j.jconrel.2005.09.034 PMID:16289422

Gionchetti, P., Rizzello, F., Annese, V., Armuzzi, A., Biancone, L., Castiglione, F., ... Daperno, M. (2017). Use of corticosteroids and immunosuppressive drugs in inflammatory bowel disease: Clinical practice guidelines of the Italian Group for the Study of Inflammatory Bowel Disease. *Digestive and Liver Disease*, *49*(6), 604–617. doi:10.1016/j.dld.2017.01.161 PMID:28254463

Girgis, M. D., Federman, N., Rochefort, M. M., McCabe, K. E., Wu, A. M., Nagy, J. O., ... Tomlinson, J. S. (2013). An engineered anti-CA19-9 cys-diabody for positron emission tomography imaging of pancreatic cancer and targeting of polymerized liposomal nanoparticles. *The Journal of Surgical Research*, *185*(1), 45–55. doi:10.1016/j.jss.2013.05.095 PMID:23827791

Gnanavel, V., Palanichamy, V., & Roopan, S. M. (2017). Biosynthesis and characterization of copper oxide nanoparticles and its anticancer activity on human colon cancer cell lines (HCT-116). *Journal of Photochemistry and Photobiology. B, Biology*, *171*, 133–138. doi:10.1016/j.jphotobiol.2017.05.001 PMID:28501691

Gu, W. X., Li, Q. L., Lu, H., Fang, L., Chen, Q., Yang, Y. W., & Gao, H. (2015). Construction of stable polymeric vesicles based on azobenzene and beta-cyclodextrin grafted poly(glycerol methacrylate)s for potential applications in colon-specific drug delivery. *Chemical Communications (Cambridge)*, *51*(22), 4715–4718. doi:10.1039/C5CC00628G PMID:25692460

Guin, S., Ma, Q., Padhye, S., Zhou, Y. Q., Yao, H. P., & Wang, M. H. (2011). Targeting acute hypoxic cancer cells by doxorubicin-immunoliposomes directed by monoclonal antibodies specific to RON receptor tyrosine kinase. *Cancer Chemotherapy and Pharmacology*, *67*(5), 1073–1083. doi:10.100700280-010-1408-8 PMID:20658288

Guin, S., Yao, H. P., & Wang, M. H. (2010). RON receptor tyrosine kinase as a target for delivery of chemodrugs by antibody directed pathway for cancer cell cytotoxicity. *Molecular Pharmaceutics*, *7*(2), 386–397. doi:10.1021/mp900168v PMID:20039696

Gupta, A. S., Kshirsagar, S. J., Bhalekar, M. R., & Saldanha, T. (2013). Design and development of liposomes for colon targeted drug delivery. *Journal of Drug Targeting*, *21*(2), 146–160. doi:10.3109/1061186X.2012.734311 PMID:23373543

Hardy, J. G., Wilson, C. G., & Wood, E. (1985). Drug delivery to the proximal colon. *The Journal of Pharmacy and Pharmacology*, *37*(12), 874–877. doi:10.1111/j.2042-7158.1985.tb04992.x PMID:2868094

Head, K. A., & Jurenka, J. S. (2003). Inflammatory bowel disease Part 1: Ulcerative colitis--pathophysiology and conventional and alternative treatment options. *Alternative Medicine Review*, *8*(3), 247–283. PMID:12946238

Itoh, K., Hirayama, T., Takahashi, A., Kubo, W., Miyazaki, S., Dairaku, M., ... Attwood, D. (2007). In situ gelling pectin formulations for oral drug delivery at high gastric pH. *International Journal of Pharmaceutics*, *335*(1), 90–96. doi:10.1016/j.ijpharm.2006.10.042 PMID:17141988

Izadi, Z., Divsalar, A., Saboury, A. A., & Sawyer, L. (2016). beta-lactoglobulin-pectin Nanoparticle-based Oral Drug Delivery System for Potential Treatment of Colon Cancer. *Chemical Biology & Drug Design*, *88*(2), 209–216. doi:10.1111/cbdd.12748 PMID:26896377

Jain, A., Gulbake, A., Jain, A., Shilpi, S., Hurkat, P., & Jain, S. K. (2013). Dual drug delivery using "smart" liposomes for triggered release of anticancer agents. *Journal of Nanoparticle Research, 15*(7), 1–12. doi:10.100711051-013-1772-5

Jain, A., Gupta, Y., & Jain, S. K. (2007). Perspectives of biodegradable natural polysaccharides for site-specific drug delivery to the colon. *Journal of Pharmacy & Pharmaceutical Sciences, 10*(1), 86–128. PMID:17498397

Jain, A., & Jain, S. K. (2015). Colon Targeted Liposomal Systems (CTLS): Theranostic Potential. *Current Molecular Medicine, 15*(7), 621–633. doi:10.2174/1566524015666150831131320 PMID:26321756

Jain, A., & Jain, S. K. (2016a). Liposomes in Cancer Therapy. In *Nanocarrier Systems for Drug Delivery* (pp. 1–42). Nova Science Publishers. Retrieved from https://www.novapublishers.com/catalog/product_info.php?products_id=59761&osCsid=e7d37031 8f328e75748328a1e44e48aa

Jain, A., & Jain, S. K. (2016b). Multipronged, strategic delivery of paclitaxel-topotecan using engineered liposomes to ovarian cancer. *Drug Development and Industrial Pharmacy, 42*(1), 136–149. doi:10.3109/03639045.2015.1036066 PMID:26006330

Jain, A., Jain, S. K., Ganesh, N., Barve, J., & Beg, A. M. (2010). Design and development of ligand-appended polysaccharidic nanoparticles for the delivery of oxaliplatin in colorectal cancer. *Nanomedicine (London), 6*(1), 179–190. doi:10.1016/j.nano.2009.03.002 PMID:19447205

Jayakody, L., & Hoover, R. (2008). Effect of annealing on the molecular structure and physicochemical properties of starches from different botanical origins–A review. *Carbohydrate Polymers, 74*(3), 691–703. doi:10.1016/j.carbpol.2008.04.032

Kamps, J. A., Koning, G. A., Velinova, M. J., Morselt, H. W., Wilkens, M., Gorter, A., ... Scherphof, G. L. (2000). Uptake of long-circulating immunoliposomes, directed against colon adenocarcinoma cells, by liver metastases of colon cancer. *Journal of Drug Targeting, 8*(4), 235–245. doi:10.3109/10611860008997902 PMID:11144234

Kaur, R., & Kaur, S. (2014). Role of polymers in drug delivery. *Journal of Drug Delivery and Therapeutics, 4*(3), 32–36.

Kogan, G., Soltes, L., Stern, R., & Gemeiner, P. (2007). Hyaluronic acid: A natural biopolymer with a broad range of biomedical and industrial applications. *Biotechnology Letters, 29*(1), 17–25. doi:10.100710529-006-9219-z PMID:17091377

Koning, G. A., Kamps, J. A., & Scherphof, G. L. (2002). Efficient intracellular delivery of 5-fluorodeoxyuridine into colon cancer cells by targeted immunoliposomes. *Cancer Detection and Prevention, 26*(4), 299–307. doi:10.1016/S0361-090X(02)00087-9 PMID:12430634

Kukowska-Latallo, J. F., Candido, K. A., Cao, Z., Nigavekar, S. S., Majoros, I. J., Thomas, T. P., ... Baker, J. R. Jr. (2005). Nanoparticle targeting of anticancer drug improves therapeutic response in animal model of human epithelial cancer. *Cancer Research, 65*(12), 5317–5324. doi:10.1158/0008-5472.CAN-04-3921 PMID:15958579

Kumar, B., Kulanthaivel, S., Mondal, A., Mishra, S., Banerjee, B., Bhaumik, A., ... Giri, S. (2017). Mesoporous silica nanoparticle based enzyme responsive system for colon specific drug delivery through guar gum capping. *Colloids and Surfaces. B, Biointerfaces*, *150*, 352–361. doi:10.1016/j.colsurfb.2016.10.049 PMID:27847225

Kumari, A., Jain, A., Hurkat, P., Verma, A., & Jain, S. K. (2016). Microsponges: A Pioneering Tool for Biomedical Applications. *Critical Reviews in Therapeutic Drug Carrier Systems*, *33*(1), 77–105. doi:10.1615/CritRevTherDrugCarrierSyst.v33.i1.40 PMID:27279339

Laga, R., Janoušková, O., Ulbrich, K., Pola, R., Blažková, J., Filippov, S. K., ... Pechar, M. (2015). Thermoresponsive Polymer Micelles as Potential Nanosized Cancerostatics. *Biomacromolecules*, *16*(8), 2493–2505. doi:10.1021/acs.biomac.5b00764 PMID:26153904

Lamprecht, A., Ubrich, N., Yamamoto, H., Schafer, U., Takeuchi, H., Maincent, P., ... Lehr, C. M. (2001). Biodegradable nanoparticles for targeted drug delivery in treatment of inflammatory bowel disease. *The Journal of Pharmacology and Experimental Therapeutics*, *299*(2), 775–781. PMID:11602694

Lee, K.-Y., Chiang, Y.-T., Hsu, N.-Y., Yang, C.-Y., Lo, C.-L., & Ku, C.-A. (2015). Vitamin E containing polymer micelles for reducing normal cell cytotoxicity and enhancing chemotherapy efficacy. *Acta Biomaterialia*, *24*, 286–296. doi:10.1016/j.actbio.2015.06.014 PMID:26087112

Liang, T.-J., Zhou, Z.-M., Cao, Y.-Q., Ma, M.-Z., Wang, X.-J., & Jing, K. (2016). Gemcitabine-based polymer-drug conjugate for enhanced anticancer effect in colon cancer. *International Journal of Pharmaceutics*, *513*(1), 564–571. doi:10.1016/j.ijpharm.2016.09.018 PMID:27613255

Lin, C.-W., Lu, K.-Y., Wang, S.-Y., Sung, H.-W., & Mi, F.-L. (2016). CD44-specific nanoparticles for redox-triggered reactive oxygen species production and doxorubicin release. *Acta Biomaterialia*, *35*, 280–292. doi:10.1016/j.actbio.2016.02.005 PMID:26853764

Lu, L., Chen, G., Qiu, Y., Li, M., Liu, D., Hu, D., ... Xiao, Z. (2016). Nanoparticle-based oral delivery systems for colon targeting: Principles and design strategies. *Science Bulletin*, *61*(9), 670–681. doi:10.100711434-016-1056-4

Ma, Z. G., Ma, R., Xiao, X. L., Zhang, Y. H., Zhang, X. Z., Hu, N., ... Sun, Z. J. (2016). Azo polymeric micelles designed for colon-targeted dimethyl fumarate delivery for colon cancer therapy. *Acta Biomaterialia*, *44*, 323–331. doi:10.1016/j.actbio.2016.08.021 PMID:27544813

Mackay, M., & Tomlinson, E. (1993). Colonic delivery of therapeutic peptides and proteins. *Drugs and the Pharmaceutical Sciences*, *60*, 159–176.

Malik, N., Evagorou, E. G., & Duncan, R. (1999). Dendrimer-platinate: A novel approach to cancer chemotherapy. *Anti-Cancer Drugs*, *10*(8), 767–776. doi:10.1097/00001813-199909000-00010 PMID:10573209

Mano, J., Silva, G., Azevedo, H. S., Malafaya, P., Sousa, R., Silva, S., ... Marques, A. (2007). Natural origin biodegradable systems in tissue engineering and regenerative medicine: Present status and some moving trends. *Journal of the Royal Society, Interface*, *4*(17), 999–1030. doi:10.1098/rsif.2007.0220 PMID:17412675

Markman, M. (2006). Pegylated liposomal doxorubicin in the treatment of cancers of the breast and ovary. *Expert Opinion on Pharmacotherapy, 7*(11), 1469–1474. doi:10.1517/14656566.7.11.1469 PMID:16859430

Mitchell, R. D., Vogl, A. W., & Adam, W. M. (2009). *Gray's Anatomy for Students E-Book*. Academic Press.

Modest, D., Kasper, S., Stintzing, S., Prasnikar, N., Müller, L., Caca, K., . . . Trarbach, T. (2016). Randomized phase II study of maintenance treatment with 5-FU/FA plus panitumumab vs 5-FU/FA alone after induction (mFOLFOX6 plus panitumumab) in patients with RAS WT metastatic colorectal cancer. *Annals of Oncology, 27*(suppl 6), 605TiP.

Naessens, M., Cerdobbel, A., Soetaert, W., & Vandamme, E. J. (2005). Leuconostoc dextransucrase and dextran: Production, properties and applications. *Journal of Chemical Technology and Biotechnology (Oxford, Oxfordshire), 80*(8), 845–860. doi:10.1002/jctb.1322

Nguyen, C. T., Webb, R. I., Lambert, L. K., Strounina, E., Lee, E. C., Parat, M.-O., ... Ross, B. P. (2017). Bifunctional Succinylated ε-Polylysine-Coated Mesoporous Silica Nanoparticles for pH-Responsive and Intracellular Drug Delivery Targeting the Colon. *ACS Applied Materials & Interfaces, 9*(11), 9470–9483. doi:10.1021/acsami.7b00411 PMID:28252278

Ogaji, I. J., Nep, E. I., & Audu-Peter, J. D. (2012). *Advances in natural polymers as pharmaceutical excipients*. Academic Press.

Oguzhan, P., & Yangilar, F. (2013). Pullulan: Production and usage in food industry. *African Journal of Food Science and Technology, 4*(3), 57–63.

Pawar, V. K., Meher, J. G., Singh, Y., Chaurasia, M., Surendar Reddy, B., & Chourasia, M. K. (2014). Targeting of gastrointestinal tract for amended delivery of protein/peptide therapeutics: Strategies and industrial perspectives. *Journal of Controlled Release, 196*, 168–183. doi:10.1016/j.jconrel.2014.09.031 PMID:25305562

Pinhassi, R. I., Assaraf, Y. G., Farber, S., Stark, M., Ickowicz, D., Drori, S., ... Livney, Y. D. (2010). Arabinogalactan-folic acid-drug conjugate for targeted delivery and target-activated release of anticancer drugs to folate receptor-overexpressing cells. *Biomacromolecules, 11*(1), 294–303. doi:10.1021/bm900853z PMID:20014825

Prabaharan, M. (2011). Prospective of guar gum and its derivatives as controlled drug delivery systems. *International Journal of Biological Macromolecules, 49*(2), 117–124. doi:10.1016/j.ijbiomac.2011.04.022 PMID:21596058

Rai, G., Yadav, A. K., Jain, N. K., & Agrawal, G. P. (2015). Enteric-coated epichlorohydrin crosslinked dextran microspheres for site-specific delivery to colon. *Drug Development and Industrial Pharmacy, 41*(12), 2018–2028. doi:10.3109/03639045.2015.1044901 PMID:26006331

Ren, Y., Mu, Y., Song, Y., Xie, J., Yu, H., Gao, S., ... Lu, W. (2016). A new peptide ligand for colon cancer targeted delivery of micelles. *Drug Delivery, 23*(5), 1763–1772. doi:10.3109/10717544.2015.1077293 PMID:26289214

Ribeiro, L. N., Alcântara, A. C., Darder, M., Aranda, P., Araújo-Moreira, F. M., & Ruiz-Hitzky, E. (2014). Pectin-coated chitosan–LDH bionanocomposite beads as potential systems for colon-targeted drug delivery. *International Journal of Pharmaceutics*, *463*(1), 1–9. doi:10.1016/j.ijpharm.2013.12.035 PMID:24374607

Rivera, E. (2003). Current status of liposomal anthracycline therapy in metastatic breast cancer. *Clinical Breast Cancer*, *4*(Suppl 2), S76–S83. doi:10.3816/CBC.2003.s.019 PMID:14667278

Rosenthal, E., Poizot-Martin, I., Saint-Marc, T., Spano, J. P., Cacoub, P., & Group, D. N. X. S. (2002). Phase IV study of liposomal daunorubicin (DaunoXome) in AIDS-related Kaposi sarcoma. *American Journal of Clinical Oncology*, *25*(1), 57–59. doi:10.1097/00000421-200202000-00012 PMID:11823698

Santos Akkari, A. C., Ramos Campos, E. V., Keppler, A. F., Fraceto, L. F., de Paula, E., Tofoli, G. R., & de Araujo, D. R. (2016). Budesonide-hydroxypropyl-beta-cyclodextrin inclusion complex in binary poloxamer 407/403 system for ulcerative colitis treatment: A physico-chemical study from micelles to hydrogels. *Colloids and Surfaces. B, Biointerfaces*, *138*, 138–147. doi:10.1016/j.colsurfb.2015.11.048 PMID:26674842

Saraf, S., Jain, A., Hurkat, P., & Jain, S. K. (2016). Topotecan Liposomes: A Visit from a Molecular to a Therapeutic Platform. *Critical Reviews in Therapeutic Drug Carrier Systems*, *33*(5), 401–432. doi:10.1615/CritRevTherDrugCarrierSyst.2016015926 PMID:27910741

Seeli, D. S., & Prabaharan, M. (2016). Guar gum succinate as a carrier for colon-specific drug delivery. *International Journal of Biological Macromolecules*, *84*, 10–15. doi:10.1016/j.ijbiomac.2015.12.002 PMID:26675135

Shen, K., Li, D., Guan, J., Ding, J., Wang, Z., Gu, J., ... Chen, X. (2017). Targeted sustained delivery of antineoplastic agent with multicomponent polylactide stereocomplex micelle. *Nanomedicine (London)*, *13*(3), 1279–1288. doi:10.1016/j.nano.2016.12.022 PMID:28064009

Shih, Y. H., Luo, T. Y., Chiang, P. F., Yao, C. J., Lin, W. J., Peng, C. L., & Shieh, M. J. (2017). EGFR-targeted micelles containing near-infrared dye for enhanced photothermal therapy in colorectal cancer. *Journal of Controlled Release*, *258*, 196–207. doi:10.1016/j.jconrel.2017.04.031 PMID:28445743

Shukla, R. K., & Tiwari, A. (2012). Carbohydrate polymers: Applications and recent advances in delivering drugs to the colon. *Carbohydrate Polymers*, *88*(2), 399–416. doi:10.1016/j.carbpol.2011.12.021

Singh, B., Chauhan, N., & Kumar, S. (2008). Radiation crosslinked psyllium and polyacrylic acid based hydrogels for use in colon specific drug delivery. *Carbohydrate Polymers*, *73*(3), 446–455. doi:10.1016/j.carbpol.2007.12.009

Singh, R. (2016). Confirmation of gum polysaccharide structure from Moringa oleifera Lam. plant by periodate oxidation studies. *IJCS*, *4*(2), 40–41.

Sivapragasam, N., Thavarajah, P., Ohm, J. B., Ohm, J. B., Margaret, K., & Thavarajah, D. (2014). Novel starch based nano scale enteric coatings from soybean meal for colon-specific delivery. *Carbohydrate Polymers*, *111*, 273–279. doi:10.1016/j.carbpol.2014.04.091 PMID:25037352

Solanki, A., & Thakore, S. (2015). Cellulose crosslinked pH-responsive polyurethanes for drug delivery: A-hydroxy acids as drug release modifiers. *International Journal of Biological Macromolecules*, *80*, 683–691. doi:10.1016/j.ijbiomac.2015.07.003 PMID:26188306

Soppimath, K. S., Aminabhavi, T. M., Kulkarni, A. R., & Rudzinski, W. E. (2001). Biodegradable polymeric nanoparticles as drug delivery devices. *Journal of Controlled Release*, *70*(1), 1–20. doi:10.1016/S0168-3659(00)00339-4 PMID:11166403

Stollman, N., & Raskin, J. B. (2004). Diverticular disease of the colon. *Lancet*, *363*(9409), 631–639. doi:10.1016/S0140-6736(04)15597-9 PMID:14987890

Subudhi, M., Jain, A., Jain, A., Hurkat, P., Shilpi, S., Gulbake, A., & Jain, S. (2015). Eudragit S100 Coated Citrus Pectin Nanoparticles for Colon Targeting of 5-Fluorouracil. *Materials (Basel)*, *8*(3), 832–849. doi:10.3390/ma8030832 PMID:28787974

Taghdisi, S. M., Danesh, N. M., Ramezani, M., Lavaee, P., Jalalian, S. H., Robati, R. Y., & Abnous, K. (2016). Double targeting and aptamer-assisted controlled release delivery of epirubicin to cancer cells by aptamers-based dendrimer in vitro and in vivo. *European Journal of Pharmaceutics and Biopharmaceutics*, *102*, 152–158. doi:10.1016/j.ejpb.2016.03.013 PMID:26987703

Tang, H., Xiang, D., Wang, F., Mao, J., Tan, X., & Wang, Y. (2017). 5-ASA-loaded SiO2 nanoparticles-a novel drug delivery system targeting therapy on ulcerative colitis in mice. *Molecular Medicine Reports*, *15*(3), 1117–1122. doi:10.3892/mmr.2017.6153 PMID:28138699

Teow, H. M., Zhou, Z., Najlah, M., Yusof, S. R., Abbott, N. J., & D'Emanuele, A. (2013). Delivery of paclitaxel across cellular barriers using a dendrimer-based nanocarrier. *International Journal of Pharmaceutics*, *441*(1), 701–711. doi:10.1016/j.ijpharm.2012.10.024 PMID:23089576

Tian, B., Liu, S., Wu, S., Lu, W., Wang, D., Jin, L., ... Quan, Z. (2017). pH-responsive poly (acrylic acid)-gated mesoporous silica and its application in oral colon targeted drug delivery for doxorubicin. *Colloids and Surfaces. B, Biointerfaces*, *154*, 287–296. doi:10.1016/j.colsurfb.2017.03.024 PMID:28351801

Tiwari, A., Jain, A., Verma, A., & Jain, S. K. (2017). Exploitable Signaling Pathways for the treatment of Inflammatory Bowel Disease. *Current Signal Transduction Therapy*, 12.

Treenate, P., & Monvisade, P. (2017). In vitro drug release profiles of pH-sensitive hydroxyethylacryl chitosan/sodium alginate hydrogels using paracetamol as a soluble model drug. *International Journal of Biological Macromolecules*, *99*, 71–78. doi:10.1016/j.ijbiomac.2017.02.061 PMID:28219689

Vyas, S. P., & Khar, R. K. (2002). Controlled drug delivery concepts and advances. *Vallabh prakashan*, *1*, 411-447.

Wang, Y., Shen, W., Shi, X., Fu, F., Fan, Y., Shen, W., ... Qi, R. (2017). Alpha-Tocopheryl Succinate-Conjugated G5 PAMAM Dendrimer Enables Effective Inhibition of Ulcerative Colitis. *Advanced Healthcare Materials*, *6*(14), 1700276. doi:10.1002/adhm.201700276 PMID:28474434

Wang, Z., Xu, Y., Meng, X., Watari, F., Liu, H., & Chen, X. (2015). Suppression of c-Myc is involved in multi-walled carbon nanotubes' down-regulation of ATP-binding cassette transporters in human colon adenocarcinoma cells. *Toxicology and Applied Pharmacology*, *282*(1), 42–51. doi:10.1016/j.taap.2014.11.002 PMID:25461681

Watson, B., Meldrum, S., Riddle, H., Brown, R., & Sladen, G. (1972). pH profile of gut as measured by radiotelemetry capsule. *British Medical Journal*, *2*(5805), 104–106. doi:10.1136/bmj.2.5805.104 PMID:5018285

Waugh, A., & Grant, A. (2010). *Ross & Wilson anatomy and physiology in health and illness*. Elsevier Health Sciences.

Wiwattanapatapee, R., Lomlim, L., & Saramunee, K. (2003). Dendrimers conjugates for colonic delivery of 5-aminosalicylic acid. *Journal of Controlled Release*, *88*(1), 1–9. doi:10.1016/S0168-3659(02)00461-3 PMID:12586498

Xie, X., Li, F., Zhang, H., Lu, Y., Lian, S., Lin, H., ... Jia, L. (2016). EpCAM aptamer-functionalized mesoporous silica nanoparticles for efficient colon cancer cell-targeted drug delivery. *European Journal of Pharmaceutical Sciences*, *83*, 28–35. doi:10.1016/j.ejps.2015.12.014 PMID:26690044

Xu, G., Shi, C., Guo, D., Wang, L., Ling, Y., Han, X., & Luo, J. (2015). Functional-segregated coumarin-containing telodendrimer nanocarriers for efficient delivery of SN-38 for colon cancer treatment. *Acta Biomaterialia*, *21*, 85–98. doi:10.1016/j.actbio.2015.04.021 PMID:25910639

Xu, Q., Huang, W., Jiang, L., Lei, Z., Li, X., & Deng, H. (2013). KGM and PMAA based pH-sensitive interpenetrating polymer network hydrogel for controlled drug release. *Carbohydrate Polymers*, *97*(2), 565–570. doi:10.1016/j.carbpol.2013.05.007 PMID:23911486

Yassin, A. E., Alsarra, I. A., Alanazi, F. K., Al-Mohizea, A. M., Al-Robayan, A. A., & Al-Obeed, O. A. (2010). New targeted-colon delivery system: In vitro and in vivo evaluation using X-ray imaging. *Journal of Drug Targeting*, *18*(1), 59–66. doi:10.3109/10611860903165022 PMID:19653868

Zhang, M., Xu, C., Wen, L., Han, M. K., Xiao, B., Zhou, J., ... Merlin, D. (2016). A Hyaluronidase-Responsive Nanoparticle-Based Drug Delivery System for Targeting Colon Cancer Cells. *Cancer Research*, *76*(24), 7208–7218. doi:10.1158/0008-5472.CAN-16-1681 PMID:27742685

Zhang, X., Hui, Z., Wan, D., Huang, H., Huang, J., Yuan, H., & Yu, J. (2010). Alginate microsphere filled with carbon nanotube as drug carrier. *International Journal of Biological Macromolecules*, *47*(3), 389–395. doi:10.1016/j.ijbiomac.2010.06.003 PMID:20600269

Zheng, X. F., Lian, Q., Yang, H., & Wang, X. (2016). Surface Molecularly Imprinted Polymer of Chitosan Grafted Poly(methyl methacrylate) for 5-Fluorouracil and Controlled Release. *Scientific Reports*, *6*(1), 21409. doi:10.1038rep21409 PMID:26892676

Zhou, M., Peng, Z., Liao, S., Li, P., & Li, S. (2014). Design of microencapsulated carbon nanotube-based microspheres and its application in colon targeted drug delivery. *Drug Delivery*, *21*(2), 101–109. doi:10.3109/10717544.2013.834413 PMID:24044613

Chapter 3
Fabrication and Morphological Characterization of Barium Titanate-Based Polymeric Nanocomposite Thin Films

Sudhanshu Singh
Amity University, India

Umesh Kumar Dwivedi
Amity University, India

ABSTRACT

In this critical review chapter, the authors explain the development of composite films of Barium Titanate (BaTiO3) and Poly (methyl methacrylate) prepared by solution casting technique. Different weight percentage composition of BaTiO3 has been selected to find out the best optimization condition for further investigation and correlate the results. The structural properties have been carried out at room temperature using XRD. Efforts have been made to correlate the results with investigated XRD results of pure BaTiO3 and its composites as observed by other workers at room temperature. The flow of experimental work and microscopic images are explained.

INTRODUCTION

The main focus of this chapter is to familiarize the nanostructures materials [BaTiO3 (Barium Titanate) + PMMA (Poly Methacrylate) + TiO2 (Titanium Oxide)] for energy storage (embedded capacitor and super capacitor) in our case. We also show how the hierarchical strategy has been adopted by scientist in the area of energy storage device and structural applications. The structural properties have been carried out at room temperature using XRD (X-ray powder diffraction). The average crystallite size of the BaTiO3 (Barium Titanate) particles in the composite films has been found to be lies in between ~ 20 - 30nm. It has been found that the peak intensities increases with increasing the wt. % of BaTiO3 in the composite films. The XRD (X-ray powder diffraction) analysis revealed that the addition of TiO_2

DOI: 10.4018/978-1-5225-4781-5.ch003

Copyright © 2018, IGI Global. Copying or distributing in print or electronic forms without written permission of IGI Global is prohibited.

has played a crucial role to enhance the crystalline nature of the composite films at room temperature. Normally the value of percentage of Barium titanate varies from zero to fifty (0 to 50), which means by keeping the weight percentage of Titanium oxide and poly methacrylate as constant, also the ambient condition throughout the experiment also fixed.

During last one decade, the advance research work has been carried out on pure $BaTiO_3$ (Barium titanate). Various elements from alkaline earth metal group (such as Ba and Sr etc) and different metal oxides [such as TiO_2 (Titanium Dioxide or Titania), $BaTiO_3$ (Barium Titanate), ZnO (Zinc Oxide), SnO (Tin (II) oxide / Stannous Oxide) and PZT (Lead zirconate titanate) etc] have been selected by researchers and numerous group. They have been used in various dielectric, ferroelectric, switching, pyroelectric, optoelectric and piezoelectric applications (Schmidt, H., 2000; May, Gary S., 2007; Lim, J. B., 2008; Morse, Daniel E., 2011; Bruley, John, 2013; Chocat, Noemie, Multimaterial, 2012; Collins, David E., 1999). These metals and elements have well known properties of electrical, structural, thermal, dielectric, electronic, ferroelectric, and morphological (Bhalla, Amar S., 1989; Bhattacharya, Swapan, 2007; Chinchamalatpure, Vijay Ramkrishna, 2010; Zhang, Tianshui, 2014; Cross, L. Eric, 1989). Still there are some problems in addition to these materials lie difficulties to find out the electrical, thermal and physical stability. One of the main problems is its fragile nature.

POLYMERS

Background of Polymers

We intend to choose polymers (such as P V D F - Poly Vinylidene Di Fluoride) [Bobic, J. D., 2008; Abothu, Isaac Robin, 2007; Kumar, Neeaj, 2010; Wang, Hong, 2015; Rajanna, K., 2013; E, Longo, 2013). Therefore the addition of polymer in such materials are use to make in thin film formation. $BaTiO_3$ was discovered during World War II in 1941 and 1944 in the United States, Russia, and Japan. They are very well suited for low power electronic devices (Bertacco, R., 2014). Also, the nano composite film of $BaTiO_3$ found various applications in device fabrication such as super capacitor, Frequency Electro Mechanical System (FEMS), Micro Electro Mechanical System (MEMS), Nano Electro Mechanical System(NEMS), FEMS, Actuators, Embedded capacitors etc (Zhang, Tianshui, 2014; Zhang, Jialiang, 2015; Cross, L. Eric, 1989). In our knowledge and the literature review as carried out be me, is very few work on $BaTiO_3$ and PVDF had been carried out by previous researcher. Now our deep intension is to develop the thin composite films of $BaTiO_3$ and PVDF at room temperature. Structural, Thermal, Electrical, Optoelectronic, Electronic and morphological properties and studies are being started. The flow of advanced and novel work can be shown by the below flow:

APPLICATIONS

Memory development Thin Films → Smart material and Nanocomposite structure → Supercapaciotor → Embedded capacitors → FinFET → MEMS → NEMS → FEMS → Sensor.

Types of Polymers

There are two types of polymers, have found their applications in this work. When alkaline earth metal and metal oxide formed the compound structure in the presence of any polymer, they are called as composite films. In general, the range of such films remains in few nanometre domains. By combining the properties of metals, metal oxides and polymers, scientist found numerous applications of such nano structured composite films. Chemical-routed nanocomposite thin films refer to the methodology of applying chemical reaction methods in nature for design the better composite. Some popular methods are physical, chemical, sol-gel methods (Schmidt, H., 2000; Morse, Daniel E., 2011; Kotov, Nicholas A., 2008).

The versatile and important feature of modern methods comes from the capability of emulating the best feature in nature, specifically chemical vapour deposition and chemical solution deposition evolved from natural selection over several years via two important characteristics, which are selection of the stable compound in materials science domain, and adaptation to the environment (Bhalla, Amar S., 1989; Kotov, Nicholas A., 2008; Rajanna, K., 2013; Collins, David E., 1999).

The main objective of the present investigation is to provide a frame work for selecting and synthesizing the optimize thin layers related to various applications in device fabrication such as Smart materials.

Nature- inspired composite films (such as green nanocomposite film) are more suitable in field of the memory storage, micro electro mechanical system (MEMS), nano electro mechanical system (NEMS), FinFET, CCD (charge coupled devices), Acoustic Amplifier, Spintronics, MOSFET, Medical Imaging, and frequency electro mechanical system (FEMS) at various frequency (Murty, B. S., 2012; Bertacco, R., 2014; E, Longo, 2013).

DESCRIPTION OF THE METAL OXIDES

Barium Titante

Barium titanate ($BaTiO_3$) has superb attraction for research in the domain of electro-ceramics and microelectronics because of its good characteristics. High dielectric constant and low loss characteristics of barium titanate make it as an excellent choice for diverse set of examples, such that in capacitors, multilayer capacitors and energy storage devices. Properly doped barium titanate has found wide application in semiconductors, positive temperature coefficient resistors, ultrasonic transducers, piezoelectric devices. Due to this $BaTiO_3$ become one of the most important ferroelectric ceramics. [Bobic, J. D., 2008; Chinchamalatpure & Vijay Ramkrishna, 2010; Zhang, Tianshui, 2014). The nano powder form is shown in Figure 1.

Salient Features of Barium Titanate

So the basic knowledge of chemical synthesis protocol of $BaTiO_3$ and chemical/physical composition with polymers helps for development of composite films. As the size of these thin layers various within nano domain, so it is well suited to be renamed as nano composite thin films. Depending upon the variation in types of compounds and polymers, applications are changed accordingly. TEM results of Cubic $BaTiO_3$ are shown in Figure 2.

Figure 1. Nano $BaTiO_3$ powder

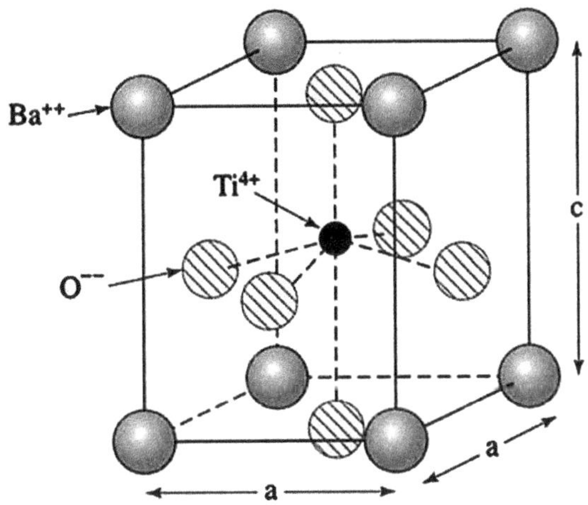

Table 1. Key properties of $BaTiO_3$

Property	Value
Density (g.cm $^{-3}$)	6.02
Melting Point (° C)	1650
Young's Modulus (G Pa)	67
Hardness (Mohs)	5

Figure 2. TEM of $BaTiO_3$

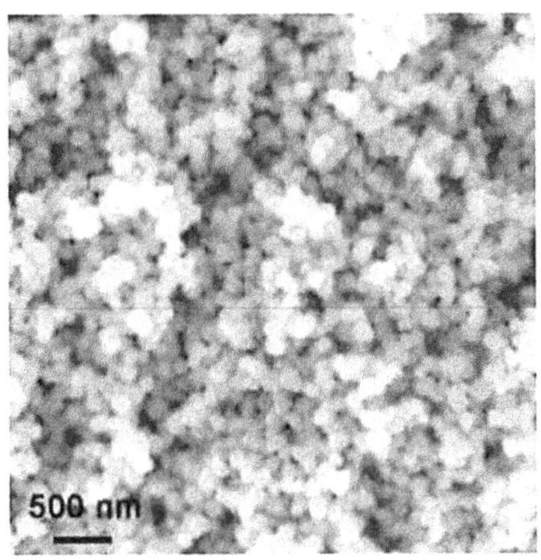

Important point from all these available research finding:

Very inadequate research work involves the change in solvent/surfactant in field of nanocomposite films. Also limited resources are available in switching studies of s-block/metal oxide elements and polar/non-polar polymers. Crystal structure is shown in Figure 3.

Structures of TiO2 and PMMA are shown in Figure 4 and 5.

Figure 3. Crystal of $BaTiO_3$

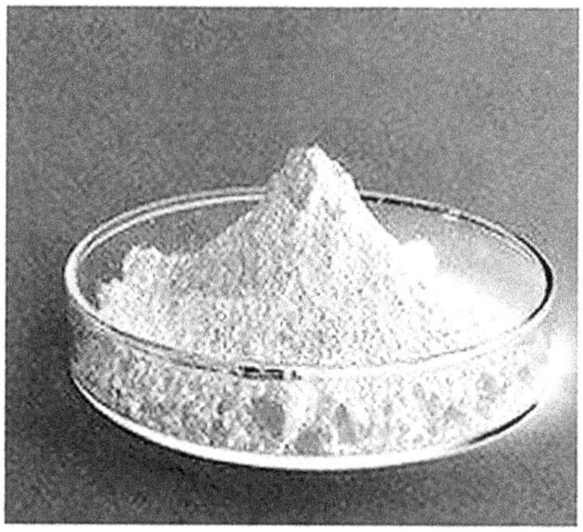

Figure 4. Structure of TiO_2

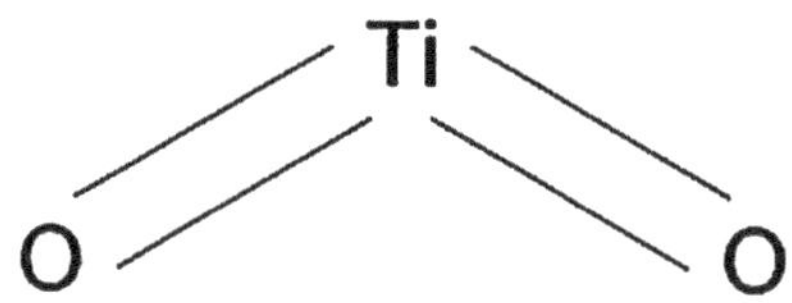

Figure 5. Structure of monomer of PMMA

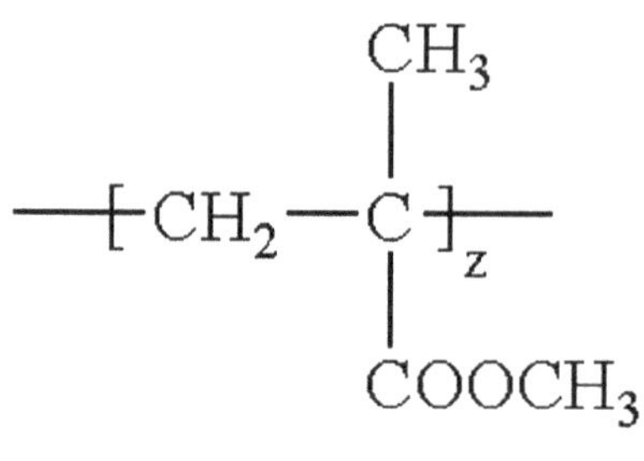

PREPARATION OF THIN FILM

Preparation Steps

- Preparation of the composite films based on layer deposition.
- Search the protocols to develop mixtures of polymer and dopants compounds.
- The composite structures changes due to the variation in solvent selection, cured time and temperature hence optimization of these variation would be studied.
- For preliminary establishment of the search strategy, a bench mark problem was chosen.
- Comparison of results with the previous work.

Implications

Having established basic framework, two implications were noticed:

1. Need of the best solvent, to put the successive development on the various substrates with a fixed temp and a fix time.
2. Need of various characterization and simulation software.

Approaches

The following approaches were adapted to form the thin films at higher flexibility.

- Avoiding expensive clean room technology and computational redundancy in calculations related to process.
- Zoning to exploit a prior knowledge about chemical method-inspired synthesis of thin films for cutting down overall time for optimization.
- These event lead to the evolution of the preparation strategy which is termed in this investigation as Design and synthesis of a composite thin films. 'Thinning Composite Films' useful for the design of the nano architecture structure.

CHARACTERIZATIONS

For design of various composites of polymeric material and elements & metal oxides:
For laboratory experiments:

- Especially some alkaline earth metals (i.e. Ba) and various metal oxide compound (ZnO, SnO, TiO2, PZT, $BaTiO_3$, and other 1 D & 2 D nano materials) are to be used.
- Characterization tools such as SEM (Scanning Electron microscopy), DSC (Differential Scanning Calorimetey), TEM (Transmission Electron Microscopy), TGA (Thermo Gravimetric Analysis), DLS (Dynamic Light Scattering), XRD (X-ray Diffraction), I – V (Current Voltage), Profilometer, FTIR (Fourier Transform Infrared) spectroscopy, PL (Photo Luminescence), HR-TEM-High Resolution-Transmission Electronic Microscopy, Rheology are helpful.
- XRD: Results are shown in Figure 6 and 7.

APPLICATION AND FUTURE ASPECTS

They have been used in various dielectric, ferroelectric, switching, pyroelectric, optoelectric and piezoelectric applications [Schmidt, H., 2000; May, Gary S., 2007; Lim, J. B., 2008; Morse, Daniel E., 2011; Bruley, John, 2013; Chocat, Noemie, 2012; Collins, David E., 1999).

Also, the nano composite film of $BaTiO_3$ found various applications in device fabrication such as super capacitor, Frequency Electro Mechanical System (FEMS), Micro Electro Mechanical System (MEMS),

Figure 6. XRD all peaks

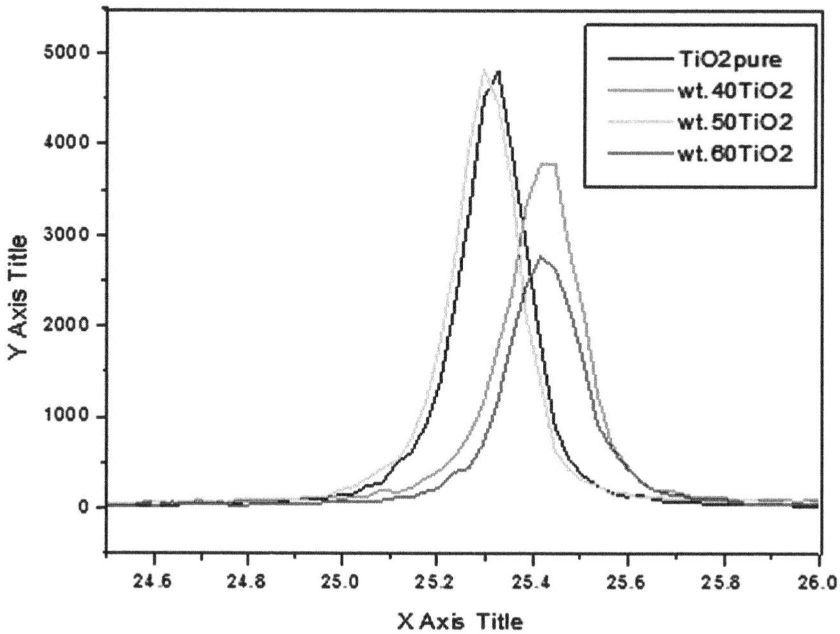

**For a more accurate representation see the electronic version.*

Figure 7. XRD first peaks

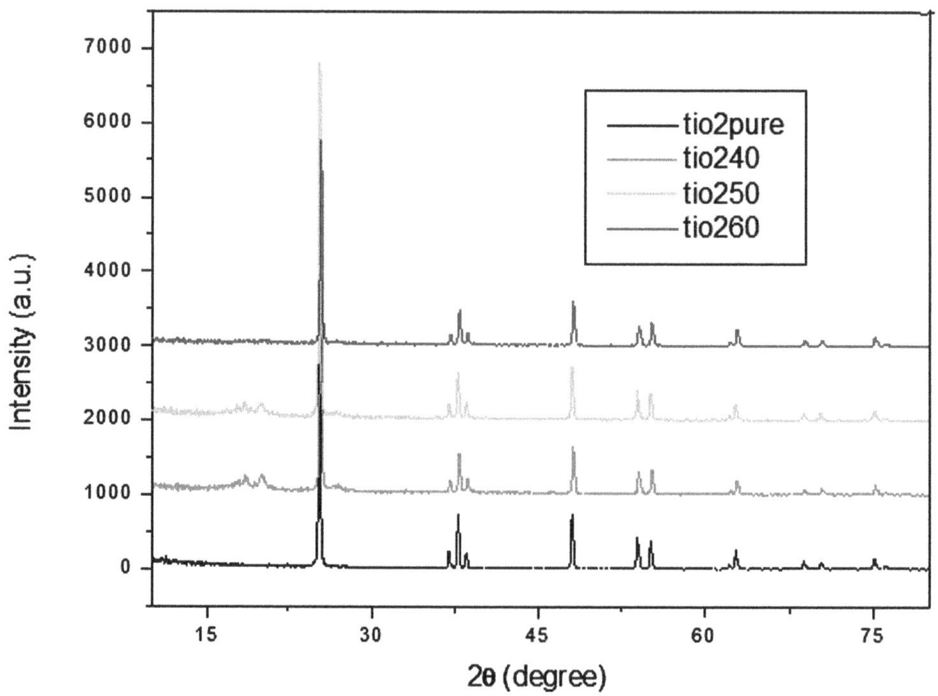

**For a more accurate representation see the electronic version.*

Nano Electro Mechanical System (NEMS), Actuators, Embedded capacitors etc (Zhang, Tianshui, 2014; Zhang, Jialiang, 2015; Cross, L. Eric, 1989).

Properly doped barium titanate has found wide application in semiconductors, positive temperature coefficient resistors, ultrasonic transducers, piezoelectric devices. Smart materials. Nature- inspired composite films (such as green nanocomposite film) are more suitable in field of the memory storage, micro electro mechanical system (MEMS), nano electro mechanical system (NEMS), FinFET, CCD (charge coupled devices), Acoustic Amplifier, Spintronics, MOSFET, Medical Imaging, and frequency electro mechanical system (FEMS) at various frequency [Murty, B. S., 2012; Bertacco, R., 2014;. E, Longo, 2013).

CONCLUSION

The average crystallite size of the $BaTiO_3$ particles in the composite films has been found to be lies in between ~ 20 – 30 n m. It has been found that the peak intensities increase with increasing the wt. % of $BaTiO_3$ in the composite films. The X R D analysis revealed that the addition of TiO_2 has played a crucial role to enhance the crystalline nature of the composite films at room temperature. Chemical based development can be an effective tool in solving thin films problems related to sensor arrays. Thinning in composite is a typical optimization problem, which can be solved by using a framework based on chemical approach. Techniques such as, physiochemical methods, and concept of acceptable solution are useful in reducing overall computational and preparation time. When operational requirements demand a much faster response time than is possible by real - time synthesis using the above concept.

REFERENCES

Abothu, I. R. (2007). Processing, Properties and Electrical Reliability of Embedded Ultra - Thin Film Ceramic Capacitors in Organic Packages. *Electronic Components and Technology Conference*, 1014–1018.

Bertacco, R. (2014). Electric control of magnetism at the Fe / BaTiO3 interface. *Nature Communications*, *5*(3404). PMID:24584546

Bhattacharya, S. (2007). Optimization of Epoxy - Barium Titanate Nanocomposite for High Performance Embedded Capacitor Components. *IEEE Transactions on Components and Packaging Technologies, 30*(2).

Bobic, J. D. (2008). History and Challenges of Barium Titanate: Part I I -. *Science of Sintering*, *40*(3), 235–244. doi:10.2298/SOS0803235V

Bruley, J. (2013). Switching of ferroelectric in without epitaxial conducting without bottom electrode a conducting BaTiO3 films on silicon bottom electrode. *Nature Nanotechnology*.

Chinchamalatpure & Ramkrishna. (2010). Synthesis and Electrical Characterization of BaTiO3 Thin Films on Si (100). *Materials Sciences and Applications, 1*, 187-190.

Chocat, N. (2012). *Multimaterial Acoustic Fibers* (PhD Thesis). Massachusetts Institute of Technology.

Collins, D. E., & Slamovich, E. B. (1999). Preparation of a Homogeneously Dispersed BaTiO3 Polymer Nanocomposite Thin Film. *Chemistry of Materials, 11*(9), 2319–2321. doi:10.1021/cm990349p

Eisenmenger, W. (1998). Internal Charge Generation in Polyvinylidene Fluoride Films during Poling Observed By Raman Spectroscopy. *Proceedings of International Symposium on Electrical Insulating Materials*, 399 – 401. 10.1109/ISEIM.1998.741767

Hegde, S. (2014). Effect of BaTiO3 Nanoparticle on Electro - Optical Properties of Polymer Dispersed Liquid Crystal Displays. *Journal of Crystallization Process and Technology, 4*, 60 - 63.

Komarneni, S. (1996). Nanophase and Nanocomposite Materials II. *Materials Research Society Symposium Proceedings, 457.*

Kotov, N. A. (2008). *Nanoscale Design of Ultra strong Materials by L B L Assembly - Biomedical Circuits and Systems Conference.* Baltimore, MD: IEEE.

Kumar, N. (2010). Ferroelectric properties of KNO3 - polymer composite films. *J. Pure Appl. & Ind. Phys., 1*, 21 – 35.

Lim, J. B. (2008). Dielectric Behavior in the BiSc03 - BaTi03 - (K1I2Bi1l2) Ti03 Ternary System. *IEEE Transactions.*

Longo, E. (2013). Fabrication and Characterization of PZT – Pani / PVDF Based Nano composite. *Joint UFFD, EFTF, and PFM Symposium.*

Malinovsky, V. K. (1990). The Prospects of ferroelectrics applications. *IEEE 7th International Symposium on Applications of Ferroelectrics*, 11 – 13.

May, G. S. (2007). Optimization of Nanocomposite Integral Capacitor Fabrication Using Neural Networks and Genetic Algorithms. *27th Annual IEEE/SEMI International Electronics Manufacturing Technology Symposium*, 123 – 129.

McQuaid, R. G. P., McGilly, L. J., Sharma, P., Gruverman, A., & Gregg, J. M. (2011). Mesoscale flux - closure domain formation in single - crystal BaTiO3. *Nature Communications, 2*, 404. doi:10.1038/ncomms1413 PMID:21792183

Morse, D. E. (2011). First Large - Scale Engineered Synthesis of BaTiO3 Nanoparticles Using Low Temperature Bioinspired Principles. *Nature Protocols, 6*(1), 97–104. doi:10.1038/nprot.2010.138 PMID:21212785

Rajanna, K. (2013). Packaging of Polyvinylidene fluoride nasal sensor for biomedical applications. *8th International Conference on Microsystems, Packaging, Assembly and Circuits Technology*, 356 – 358.

Schmidt, H. (2000). The Sol - Gel Process as a basic technology for nano particle - dispersed inorganic - organic composites. *Journal of Sol - Gel Science and Technology, 19*, 39–51.

Shi, T. (2015). Why Sn doping significantly enhances the dielectric properties of Ba (Ti 1 - x Sn x) O3. Nature Communications, 5(8606). doi:10.1038rep08606 PMID:25721479

Wang, H. (2015). Enhanced Dielectric Performance of BaTiO3 / PVDF Composites Prepared by Modified Process for Energy Storage Applications. *IEEE Transactions on Ultrasonics, Ferroelectrics, and Frequency Control, 62*(1).

Zhang, T. (2014). Low - Loss Composite NiCuZnCo – BaTiO3 With Matched Permeability and Permittivity in High Frequency Range. *IEEE Transactions on Magnetics, 50*(11).

Zhang, T. (2014). Low - Loss Composite NiCuZnCo – BaTiO3 with Matched Permeability and Permittivity in High Frequency Range. *IEEE Transactions on Magnetic, 50*(11).

Zhang, J. (2015). Unfolding grain size effects in barium titanate ferroelectric ceramics. *Nature Communications, 5*(9953).

Chapter 4
Innovative Strategies for Lipid-Based Drug Delivery

Navneet Sharma
Institute of Nuclear Medicine and Allied Sciences, India

Sabna Kotta
Buraydah Private Colleges, Saudi Arabia

Mohd Aleem
Institute of Nuclear Medicine and Allied Sciences, India

Shubham Singh
Institute of Nuclear Medicine and Allied Sciences, India

Rakesh Kumar
Defence Food Research Laboratory, India

ABSTRACT

In the last decade, there has been a mounting concern in lipid-based formulations to deliver water-soluble drugs. Lipid-based drug delivery systems are one of the budding and promising technologies designed to tackle the poor bioavailability problems. This chapter stresses the different mechanisms of lipophilic drug absorption along with its advantages and limitations. It points out the different mechanisms of how lipid-based excipients and the different formulations interact with the absorption process. This review provides a comprehensive summary about the lipid formulation classification scheme (LFCS), a guide for the selection of appropriate formulation and commonly used excipients for lipid-based formulations, along with the important factors to be considered in formulation design and excipient selection. This review also focuses on the formulation of solid lipid-based formulations, important evaluation aspects, and commercial formulations available for the purpose.

INTRODUCTION

Design and development of suitable drug delivery systems are necessary to localize and improve drug delivery. Targeting drugs to the specific sites with minimal side effects is not easy as specific carrier drug is needed to be get developed for the improved drug delivery. Different types of drugs as a carrier have

DOI: 10.4018/978-1-5225-4781-5.ch004

Copyright © 2018, IGI Global. Copying or distributing in print or electronic forms without written permission of IGI Global is prohibited.

been used depending on the routes of administration. The most commonly employed route owing to its safety as well as convenience and ease of administration to the patient is the oral administration of the drug (Umeyor, Kenechukwu, Uronnachi, Osonnwa, & Nwakile, 2012). Development of orally administered drug is challenging due to their stability or their absorption in the gastrointestinal tract (GIT) and it may be less effective at the target site (Nnamani, Attama, Ibezim, & Adikwu, 2010). To improve the absorption capacity of such drugs, lipid systems such as emulsions, micellar solutions, liposomes, lipid nanoparticles, structured lipid carriers, self-emulsifying lipid formulations, solid dispersions, dry emulsions, solid-liquid compacts, and drug-lipid conjugates are in use as drug carriers (Chime, Onyishi, Obito, Onunkwo, & Odo, 2013). Solid lipid microparticles (SLMs) have been developed, that have a lower risk of the reaction with the carrying substance in respect to the emulsion system. By altering either one or both the inner solid vesicle or the outer phospholipid layer the release rate of substance from the SLMs can be manipulated (Jaspart, S., Bertholet, P., Piel, G, Dogné, J.M., Delattre, L., & Evrard, B., 2007).

DIFFERENT TYPES OF ROUTES IN LIPID-BASED DRUG DELIVERY SYSTEM

Lipid-Based Drug Delivery Through the Skin

Among the different type of routes in lipid-based drug delivery system (Figure 1), skin is one of them. Routes like oral, parenteral, ocular, intranasal, dermal/transdermal, and vaginal can be preferred for the administration of the lipid based drug delivery systems (Gershkovich, P., Wasan, K.M., & Barta, C.A., 2008; Paveli, Z., Skalko-Basnet, N., Filipovi-Gr,ˇJ., Martinac, A., & Jalˇsenjak, I., 2005). Transdermal drug delivery has various advantages over conventional oral and intravenous routes. The amount of the drug may be reduced as a result of metabolism in the stomach when it is administered orally. Transdermal drug delivery has many other advantages over other routes of the drug administration such as minimization of pain, and possible controlled drug release (Subedi, Oh, Chun, & Choi, 2010). Drugs that have the capability to penetrate the skin may produce therapeutic effects at the target site inside the human body or in other animals. Drugs absorption through the skin may be affected by the stratum corneum, which has functioned as a first line of the defense in the skin (Bouwstra, J.A., Honeywell-Nguyen, P.L., & Gooris, G.M., 2006; Morgan, C.J., Renwick, A.G., & Friedmann, P.S., 2003). Penetration enhancers may be used to facilitate drug delivery through the skin. They may cause a temporary reversible reduction in the barrier function of the stratum corneum. Penetration enhancers are extensively used to increase percutaneous absorption (Bouwstra & Ponec, 2006). The important example of the penetration enhancer is terpenes (limonene or cineole) which are naturally occurring compounds consisting of isoprene (C_5H_8) units. They have been used in transdermal research as skin penetration enhancer. Food and Drug Administration (FDA) classified terpenes as an effective class of the penetration enhancers and its use is safe. Lipid nanoparticles composited in the terpene and evaluated for dermal delivery of All-*trans*-retinoic acids (ATRA) (Vikas, Seema, Gurpreet, Rana, & Baibhav, 2011).

Lipid based nanosystems that are colloidal nanocarriers are extensively used for transdermal drug delivery. Two types of lipid nanoparticles that have been shown to enhance transdermal permeation are solid lipid nanoparticles (SLNs) and nanostructured lipid carriers (NLCs). Lipid nanoparticles exhibit negligible skin irritation, higher stability, and more controlled release than other transdermal vehicle such as cream, tinctures, emulsions, and liposomes etc. (Manjunath, Reddy, & Venkateswarlu, 2005). NLCS represent the second generation of lipid nanoparticles based drug vehicles; consisting a mixture

Figure 1. Lipids based drug delivery through different routes

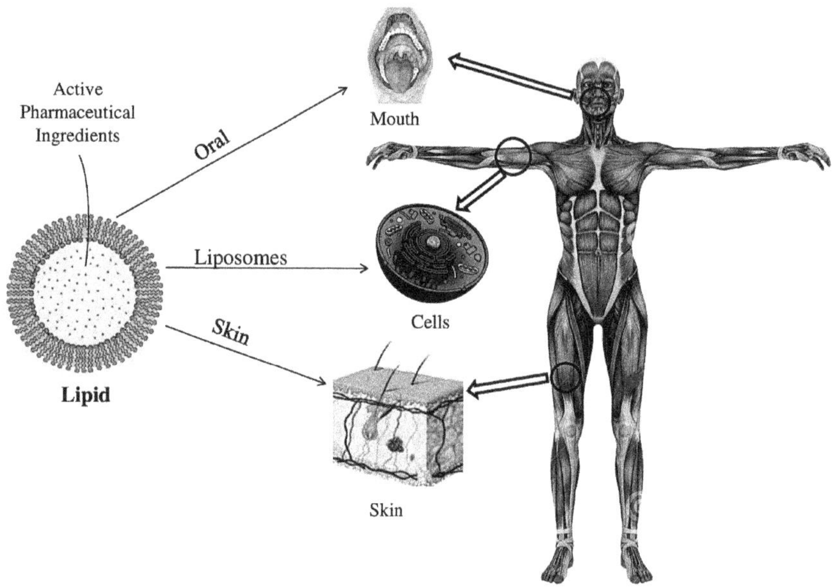

of solid and liquid lipids. The beneficial properties of NLCs have advantages over the SLNs because they produce efficient transdermal drug permeation (Gomes, Martins, Ferreira, Segundo, & Reis, 2014). NLCS overcome the limitations of SLNs including limited drug-loading capacity, drug leakage during storage, and risk of gelation (Müller, Radtke, & Wissing, 2002). Lipid-based nanosystems are in use for transdermal drug delivery in modern research. Alkaloids lappaconitine and ranaconitine isolated from *Aconitum sinomontanum* respectively are important examples of the NLCs that enhance the percutaneous permeation.

Lipid-Based Drug Delivery Through Oral Route

For well oral absorption, the drug should not be metabolized in the GI tract and it should be easily permeable in the GI membrane or in the intestine (Nagabandi, V., & Sambaraj, S., 2013; Wu, C.Y., & Benet, L.Z., 2005). Drugs with poor aqueous solubility, poor dissolution rate, and poor permeability are not suitable for oral delivery because the desirable amount of the drug do not reach the target site and produce less therapeutic effects at the target site (Hauss, 2007). The solubility, dissolution rate, permeability and the absorption of the drug can be enhanced by the suitable carrier of the drug delivery, for example, lipid based formulations have emerged as an effective and versatile technology that has been used as a carrier for lipid based drug delivery (Pouton & Porter, 2008).

The oral absorption of low soluble and low permeable of drugs can be enhanced by using a novel silica-lipid hybrid microparticulate system, these Silica-lipid hybrid microparticles increase drug solubilization, which leads to enhanced oral bioavailability, by producing the solubilizing effect of dispersed lipids and stabilizing the effect of hydrophilic silica (Sambaraj, 2013). The current review is focusing on the improvement of absorption of poorly water-soluble and poorly permeable drugs based on appropriately selected lipid excipients and the utilization of nanoparticle technology (Deshmukh, Nakhat, & Yeole, 2010).

Liposome Assisted Drug Delivery

Liposomes are an important example of the most common and well-investigated nanocarriers for targeted drug delivery. Liposomes have improved therapies in the area of biomedical because they enhance cellular and tissue uptake, and improving biodistribution of compounds to target sites *in vivo* (Koning, G.A., & Storm, G., 2003; Ding, B.S., Dziubla, T., Shuvaev, V.V., Muro, S., & Muzykantov, V. R., 2006; Hua, S., & Wu, S.Y., 2013). Liposomes are vesicles of phospholipid that have one or more concentric lipid bilayers enclosing discrete aqueous spaces. Liposomes are able to entrap both lipophilic and hydrophilic compounds enable a diverse range of drugs to be encapsulated by these vesicles. Drug into the liposomes can be loaded through the formation of the liposome in an aqueous solution saturated with soluble drug or pH gradient methods by using of organic solvents and solvent exchange methods. Drug loading into the liposome can occur by the use of lipophilic drugs. Liposomes can be used for oral (Rogers & Anderson 1998), ocular, pulmonary and transdermal delivery of drugs. Hydrophobic molecules are soluble in lipid and can be inserted into the bilayer membrane, and hydrophilic molecules are insoluble in lipid and can be located in the aqueous compartment. DNA, proteins and imaging agents can permeate across the lipid bilayer of the liposomes easily and the hydrophobic molecules get entrapped in the aqueous center of the liposome (Monteiro, Martins, Reis, & Neves, 2014). Conventional liposomes consist of a lipid bilayer that can be composed of cationic, anionic, or neutral (phospho) lipids and cholesterol, which enclose an aqueous compartment. Liposomal based drug delivery has been useful for improving the therapeutic index of encapsulated drugs (Koning, & Storm, 2003). The liposomes have a good permeability to both the cell and nuclear membrane of the tumor cell (Zhao, Y.Z., Dai, D.D., Lu, C.T., Chen, L.J., Lin, M., … Shen, X.T., 2013).

Drug Administration Through Lymphatic System

Another important system through which drug administered is the lymphatic system which may play a significant role in the transportation of drugs for a systemic circulation, from where the drug may be transported throughout the body (Figure 2). The major advantage of lymphatic administration of the drug is to avoid the first pass metabolism in the stomach that may lead to a reduction in the amount of the drug, thus, drug administration through the lymphatic system may provide an adequate amount of drug at the target sites. Drug administration through the lymphatic system may useful in lymphatic diseases; such as certain lymphomas and HIV. The transcellular absorption occurs due to increase in membrane fluidity that allows paracellular transport by the opening of tight junctions.

BARRIERS OF DRUG ABSORPTION AND IMPROVEMENTS IN PERMEABILITY

Skin Barrier and Permeability

Stratum corneum makes the first line of defense in the skin it consists of Corneocytes surrounded by lipids. This layer acts as a significant barrier to the penetration of most drugs (Wiechers, 1989). Topically applied drugs on the skin have to permeate through the lipid domain. The lipid domains in the skin are important for the skin barrier functions. The important components of this layer are generally long chain ceramides, free fatty acids, and *cholesterol* (Bouwstra, J.A., & Ponec, M., 2003). Stratum

Figure 2. Lipids based drug delivery through Lymphatic system

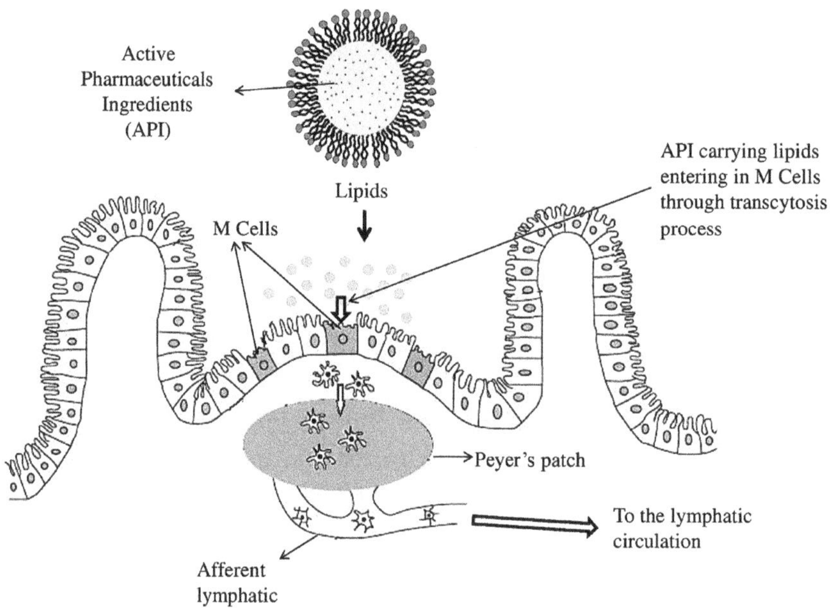

corneum have many defensive functions including negative influence on skin penetration, low pH, the presence of enzymes on the skin, and the transcutaneous concentration gradient (Geusens, B., Strobbe, T., Bracke, S., Dynoodt, P., Sanders, N., … VanGele, M., 2011). The two most important parameters determining the absorption and bioavailability of an active ingredient are solubility and permeability. The permeation of any agent or drug depends upon different factors such as agent's size, shape, superficial charges, lipophilicity, the presence of penetration enhancers, type of formulation, and physical state of the stratum corneum (D.D. Verma, S. Verma, Blume, & Fahr, 2003a).

Oral Route Barriers and Improvements in Drug Permeability

There are great challenges in innovative drug delivery system when given orally, such as poor solubility of drugs in water which leads to low solubility and bioavailability. Lipid-based drug delivery systems have been used to overcome this problem and improving the absorption and solubility of the drug. Encapsulating the drug or solubilization of the drug in lipid carrier can enhance drug absorption, resulting in greater bioavailability. The bioavailability of the drug can also be enhanced when it is co-administered along with food. The absorption of the drug in lipid-based drug delivery system may depend upon numerous factors, like particle size, the rate of dispersion, and degree of absorption (Porter, C.J., & Charman, W.N., 2001; Pouton, 2000). Absorption of the drug can be enhanced from the gastrointestinal tract when drug administered with the lipid excipients such as pure triglyceride oils, mixed glycerides, lipophilic surfactants, hydrophilic surfactants and water-soluble co-solvents. These lipid excipients may accelerate the dissolution process, facilitating the formation of solubilized phases by reduction of particle size to the molecular level that leads to the increase absorption of the drug through the gastrointestinal tract (Humberstone, A.J., & Charman, W.N., 1997; Porter, C.J., & Charman, W.N., 2001).

Gastric lipase initiates the digestion of exogenous excipients e.g., dietary triglyceride and formulation triglyceride after oral administration of lipid based formulations. Simultaneously, the mechanical mixing of the exogenous excipients and drug in the stomach facilitates the formation of a crude emulsion. Triglyceride is broken down to diglyceride, monoglyceride, and fatty acids by pancreatic lipase together in the small intestine. The secretion of endogenous biliary lipids from the gall bladder including bile salt, phospholipids and cholesterol, which are stimulated by exogenous lipids present in the small intestine. Monoglycerides, fatty acids, and products of lipid digestion lysophospholipid are subsequently incorporated into a series of colloidal structures, including micelles and unilamellar and multilamellar vesicles in the presence of bile salts that lead to the enhanced solubilization and absorption through the small intestine of lipid digestion products and drugs (Erlanson-Albertsson, 1992).

ADVANTAGES AND DISADVANTAGES OF LIPID-BASED DRUG DELIVERY

Advantages of Lipid-Based Drug Delivery

The principle objective of lipid-based drug delivery system is to enhance their bioavailability. Lipid-based drug delivery has been used to reduce the toxicity of various drugs by changing the biodistribution of the drug away from sensitive organs. Lipid-based carriers are safe to be used for the formulation in pharmaceutics, as well as vaccines, diagnostics, nutraceuticals, etc (Müller, R.H., Radtke M., & Wissing S.A., 2002; Prajapati, N.H., Patel, D.P., Patel, N.G., Dalrymple, D.M., & Serajuddin, A.T., 2011; Pouton, 2006).

Lipid-based drug delivery system has many unique advantages such as control and target drug release, encapsulate high drug content, improve the stability of pharmaceuticals, and have the capability to carrying both lipophilic and hydrophilic drugs etc. Lipid-based drug delivery system also is less expensive to prepare than polymeric/surfactant based carriers. Lipid-based drug delivery systems also have many advantages over polymer based systems which include enhanced drug absorption, reduce side effects, controlled drug release and site-specific targeting. For both the hydrophilic and hydrophobic substances, most of the lipid formulations have high stability, high carrier capacity, the feasibility of incorporation, and feasibility of variable routes of administration, including oral, topical, parenteral and pulmonary routes. Administration of some drugs with the food may increase their bioavailability (El Laithy, H.M., & El-Shaboury, K.M., 2002; Amidon, G.L., Lennernas, H., Shah V.P., & Crison, J.R., 1995; Charman, W.N., Porter, C.J., Mithani, S., & Dressman, J. B., 1997; Winstanley, P.A., & Orme, M.L.E., 1989). Lipid components of the food play important role in the absorption of lipophilic drugs and enhance their oral bioavailability. High-fat meals stimulate biliary and pancreatic secretions which decrease metabolism and efflux activity, to increase intestinal wall permeability and prolongation of gastrointestinal tract residence time (ElMaghraby, Barry, & Williams, 2008).

Advantages of Dermal Administration

The transdermal drug delivery technique is one of the highly successful alternative drug delivery methods. Skin of an average adult body covers a surface area of approximately $2m^2$ and come in contact of about one-third of the blood circulating through the body. Lipid-based nanosystems have been using for drug delivery and it has great potential for transdermal drug delivery. Transdermal drug delivery has various advantages over conventional oral and intravenous routes in the reduction of drug metabolism via first pass effect, minimization of pain, and possible controlled drug release (Subedi, Oh, Chun, & Choi, 2010). Transdermal drug delivery system is having an advantage over oral drug delivery system as it bypasses the first pass metabolism of the liver (Schäfer-Korting et al., 2007; ElMaghraby et al., 2008; Wang et al., 2008). The horny layer of the stratum corneum in the skin can impair penetration and absorption of drugs. Penetration of hydrophilic compounds is prevented by this layer more efficiently as compared to lipophilic compounds (Bouwstra, Honeywell-Nguyen, & Gooris, 2003).

Both lipids and excipients used in the formulation not only improve or enhance the bioavailability of the drug substance but also help in avoiding the erratic absorption. Lipids and its excipients keep the drugs in solubilized form which promote the lymphatic transport, altering the permeability of epithelia and also altering enterocyte-based drug transport (Jannin, Musakhanian, & Marchaud, 2008).

In particular, lipid based drug delivery system is avoided of reduction in the significant first-pass effect of the liver that can prematurely metabolize drugs. Transdermal drug delivery also has many advantages over hypodermic injections, which are painful, generate dangerous medical waste and pose the risk of disease transmission (Manjunath, Reddy, & Venkateswarlu, 2005). In addition, transdermal drug delivery systems are also non-invasive and can be self-administered. They provide control release of the drug, which also improve the patient compliance and the systems are generally inexpensive.

Only a limited number of drugs are amenable to administration by transdermal route and this is the greatest challenge for drug delivery. With current delivery methods, some drugs have molecular masses up to few hundred Daltons and exhibit octanol water partition coefficients. This favors lipid and require the doses of milligrams per day or less, which are successful in transdermal drug additives. One more great challenge in transdermal drug delivery is to exploit the transdermal route to deliver hydrophilic drugs (Guy, R.H., & Hadgraft, J., 2003; Prausnitz, M.R., Mitragotri, S., & Langer, R., 2004).

The transdermal delivery of vaccines is another area of great interest. In addition, transdermal vaccine delivery could improve immune responses by targeting delivery to immunogenic Langerhans cells in the skin to avoid from hypodermic needles (Glenn & Kenney, 2006).

Advantages of Oral Administration

The most convenient and noninvasive method of drug administration is the oral route of drug delivery which is having the highest degree of patient compliance. The solubility, dissolution rate, permeability and the absorption of the drug can be enhanced by the suitable carrier of the drug delivery. Low soluble and low permeable drugs absorption can be enhanced by the novel silica-lipid hybrid microparticulate system. Silica - lipid hybrid microparticulate system may increase drug solubilisation which leads to enhanced oral bioavailability (Sambaraj, 2013). Lipid-based formulations have emerged as an effective and versatile technology to improve the solubility and permeability of the drugs (Dening, Rao, Thomas, & Prestidge 2015). Silica-based materials enhance the oral absorption of drugs via increased wet ability in the aqueous medium, which leads to enhanced dissolution or release kinetics (Nagabandi, V., & Sambaraj, S., 2013; Bremmell, K.E., Tan, A., Martin, A., & Prestidge, C.A., 2013).

The ultimate goal of any oral lipid-based formulation is the efficient absorption of the drug by the intestinal mucosal cells. Absorption of the drug can be enhanced from the gastrointestinal tract when drug administered with the high-fat food or lipid excipients such as pure triglyceride oils, mixed glycerides, lipophilic surfactants, hydrophilic surfactants and water-soluble co-solvents. These lipid excipients may accelerate the dissolution process, facilitate the formation of solubilized phases by reduction of particle size to the molecular level that leads to the increase absorption of the drug through the gastrointestinal tract (Kalepu, Manthina, & Padavala, 2013). Administration of the drugs with the high fat containing food may elevate their intestinal absorption that leads to enhancing in the bioavailability of the drug. Triglycerides and long chain fatty acids in the food have an important role in prolonging the gastrointestinal residence time of the drug. High-fat meal may elevate the triglycerides rich lipoproteins which may react with drug molecules. The association of lipoproteins with drug molecules enhances intestinal lymphatic transport and leads to changes in drug disposition and finally changes the kinetics of the poorly soluble drugs in water (Gershkovich, Wasan, & Barta, 2008).

Lipid-based formulations can be used to reduce the dose of the drug while simultaneously enhancing its oral bioavailability. The bioavailability of food dependent drug can be significantly reduced by formulating the drug as a lipid-based formulation, which facilitates the formation of solubilized species and may increase the solubility, dissolution, and absorption of lipophilic drugs (Humberstone & Charman, 1997).

Advantages of Lymphatic System Administration

The lymphatic system is a part of the circulatory system and is comprised of a complex network of conduits that carry a clear fluid called lymph. The primary functions of the lymphatic system are to maintain the body's water balance by bringing back the extracellular fluid that has been leaked into the interstitial space to the systemic circulation and to transport immune cells to the lymph nodes (Miteva D.O., Rutkowski J.M., Dixon J.B., Kilarski W., Shields J.D., & Swartz M.A., 2010; Iqbal J., & Hussain M.M., 2009). Further, the lymphatic system has important roles in certain areas because of its non-uniform structure and function in our body. It plays a significant role in absorbing long chain fatty acids, triglycerides, cholesterol esters, lipid soluble vitamins, and xenobiotics (O'Driscol, 1992). Drug delivery via the lymphatic system has several major advantages, including circumventing the first-pass metabolism in the liver and targeting drugs to diseases that spread through the lymphatic system (e.g., certain types of cancer and human immunodeficiency virus). The lymphatic system also plays an active role in disseminating metastatic cancer cells and infectious agents throughout the body. Cancer cells use the lymph nodes as a reservoir to spread to other areas of the body (McCarter M.D., Clarke J.H., & Harken A.H., 2004; Pantel K., & Brakenhoff R.H., 2004; Sleeman, 2000, 2006).

Disadvantages of Lipid-Based Drug Delivery

Lipid-based drug formulations can also face challenges like maintaining their adequate chemical and physical stability of unsaturated lipid components which can undergo lipid per oxidation (Jyoti, Anroop, & Rachna, 2012). This can be minimized by use of saturated medium chain triglycerides and by use of appropriate antioxidants.

There are some major challenges for lipid excipients and drug delivery systems like the varying range of compounds they contain. Proper characterization and evaluation of these delivery systems, their stability, Solubility, dispersion, digestion, and absorption are essential.

Factors that can cause affect the oral administration of the drugs are its poor solubility, low permeability, instability, and rapid metabolism, all of which leads to the less oral bioavailability. The present significant challenge to the oral delivery of the lipophilic drug is their inherent low aqueous solubility, which generally leads to poor oral bioavailability, and lack of dose proportionality (Jyoti, Anroop, & Rachna, 2012).

Lipid components of the food play important role in the absorption of lipophilic drugs and enhance their oral bioavailability (Hunt, J.N., & Knox, M.T., 1968; Ravi, K., Shivjee, K., Shyam, S., Amit, K.J., 2011; Soumya, S., Doney, A.B., & Sabitha M., 2012; Attama, A.A., Momoh, M.A., & Builders, P.F., 2012). But the food and drug complex absorption lead to a serious concern about the sub-therapeutic plasma drug concentration when co-administered without food. Administration of the drug with food which has a narrow therapeutic index increased their bioavailability that may lead to serious opposite effects. Thus control or/and monitoring of food intake is required when such types of drugs administered.

However, a few limitations of the technology such as the stability of lipid-based formulations, manufacturing methods, the lack of a database considering the solubility of drugs in lipids, indicate that development of proper regulatory guidelines for lipid-based drug delivery system still need to be improvement in depth to advance the technology.

The Lipid Formulation Classification Scheme (LFCS)

LFCS working model was introduced in 2000, and revised in 2006 by adding an extra type of formulation. *In vivo* behavior of the formulation can be easily interpreted by this model. As per physicochemical nature of specific drugs, a most appropriate formulation can be selected by LFCS (Table 1) (Pouton, 2000).

Commonly Used Excipients for Lipid-Based Formulations

There are a wide range of lipid excipients (Figure 3) which are available from suppliers. The characteristics of this lipid should be carefully considered since they affect the absorption process (Wang, Ye, Zhoua, & Zhang, 2008). Miscibility, solvent capacity, digestibility, self-dispersibility and fate of digested products etc. are the important factors which affects the choice of excipient for a lipid-based formulation. The regulatory concerns like irritancy, toxicity, purity, melting point, compatibility with capsule shell chemical stability and cost should also be considered. Most of the lipids are amphiphilic in character which contain lipophilic and hydrophilic parts (Christie, 1987). As the chain length of fatty acid increases, the melting point also increases. The susceptibility to oxidation increases with increase in unsaturation of the fatty acid (Jannin, Musakhanian, & Marchaud, 2008). Lipid excipients are classified as triglycerides, mixed glycerides and polar oils, co-solvents, water-insoluble surfactants and water-soluble surfactants.

Triglycerides

Triglyceride vegetable oils are the most common excipient used in lipid-based drug delivery. Since they are completely digested and absorbed, they do not process any safety issue (Wang, Ye, Zhou, & Zhang, 2008). Triglycerides are mainly three types viz, long chain triglycerides, medium chain triglycerides and short chain triglycerides. The effective concentration of ester groups determines solvent capacity (Cao, Marra, & Anderson, 2004). Medium chain triglycerides show higher solvent capacity when compared to long chain and also they are less susceptible to oxidation (Kaukonen, Boyd, Porter, & Charman, 2004).

Figure 3. Commonly used excipients for lipid based formulations

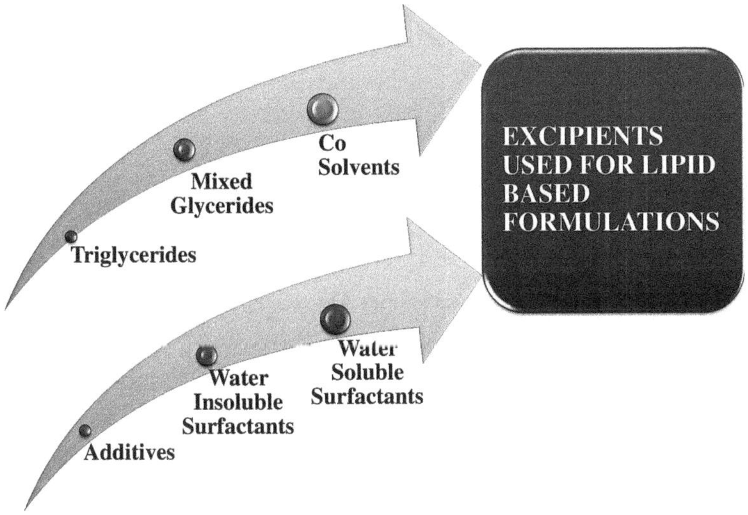

Mixedglycerides

These are obtained from partial hydrolysis of triglycerides, and its chemical composition is determined by the extent of hydrolysis. Medium chained glycerides have higher solvent capacity and dispersibility and also they are not susceptible to oxidation (Strickley, 2004, 2007).

Co Solvents

Co solvents are used in most of the products to enhance solubilization. Ethanol, poly ethylene glycols, glycerol and propylene glycol are the most commonly used co solvents. Precipitation of the solubilized drug from the solvent, incompatibility with the capsule shell, loss of the solvent capacity up on dilution and immiscibility with some oils are the limitations for the use of co-solvents (Yalkowsky, 2000; Cole, Cade, & Benameur, 2008).

Water-Insoluble Surfactants

These have an HLB (Hydrophilic - Lipophilic Balance) value of 8-12 and adsorb at oil–water interfaces. These have very limited solubility in water depending on the degree of ethoxylation. These do not process the property of self-emulsification due to their insufficient hydrophilic nature.

Water-Soluble Surfactants

These have an HLB value above 12 and are the most commonly used surfactant for self-emulsifying drug delivery system. They can form micellar solutions in low concentration by dissolving in water above their critical micellar concentration. These are produced by blending polyethylene glycols with hydrolyzed vegetable oils or by the reaction between alcohols and ethylene oxide to produce alkyl ether ethoxylate (Schick, M. J., 1987; Rowe, R.C., Sheskey, P.J., & Owen, S.C., 2006).

Additives

Mainly used additives are anti-oxidants to protect the formulation from oxidation. α-tocopherol, β-carotene, butylated hydroxyl toluene, or anisole are the most commonly used anti-oxidants in lipid-based systems (Gibson, 2007).

Factors to Be Considered in Formulation Design and Excipient Selection

Some factors like excipient Selection, the ability to self-emulsify in a large field of dilution with water, the droplet polarity, size and size distribution formed on dilution, significance of digestibility are very significant as far as formulation is considered. A clear understanding of the characteristics solvent capacity of the delivery system to solubilize the dose, loss of solvent capacity on dilution of lipid excipients, and how they influence performance *in vivo* is essential to guide formulation design strategies (O'Driscoll, 2002).

The low solvent capacity for some drugs and poor emulsification properties hamper the use of natural food grade oils even though they are safe and of natural origin. To overcome these issues polyglycolide glycerides and hydrolyzed oils are used. Non-ionic surfactants are the surfactants of choice due to their low oral toxicity. For absorption by lymphatic route oils with long chain fatty acids are preferred (Wenson, & Curtalo, 1992).

According to Craig et al self-emulsifying behavior was shown to be dependent on the polarity of the oils. Oils with high HLB value show a maximum tendency for self-emulsification to form O/W emulsions. The self-emulsification tendency is also dependent on the HLB of surfactant and nature of co-solvent (Craig, Agnes Chan, & Khan, 1995).

Due to a larger area to volume ratio, larger droplets are less stable than smaller droplets and so they grow by the expenditure of the smaller droplets. Droplet size can also affect the rate and extent of drug release. The polarity of the oil droplets is determined by the concentration of the emulsifier, ratio of oil and surfactant, it's HLB, fatty acid chain length and its degree of un saturation as well as the molecular weight of the hydrophilic portion (Yalkowsky, 2000).

Since the digested products of the oil phases show enhanced the solvent capacity good to choose oil phase which undergoes digestion of the final mixed micellar phases that forms *in vivo*. Mixed micelles having long chain fatty acids display a superior solvent capacity than the equivalent simple bile salts. Sometimes the surfactant also undergoes digestion, as a result, the solvent capacity will be altered. Therefore measurement in an *in vitro* lipolysis model is considered of supreme importance to assess the effect of digestion *in vivo* (Porter, C.J.H., Pouton, C.W., Cuine, J.F., & Charman, W.N., 2008; O' Driscoll, C.M., & Griffin, B.T., 2008).

Another important formulation design factor is the solvent capacity of the system to solubilize the required dose, as well as when contact with the intestinal media the drug should be properly solubilized inside the emulsion. If the solvent capacity is failed while intestinal transit, the drug will precipitate, and the precipitate must be dissolved take place the absorption. Usually, the chance of drug precipitation by dispersion or digestion is more for formulations which contain a relatively higher volume of water-soluble surfactants or co-solvent.

The appropriate excipient selection is an important formulation design factor to achieve desirable *in vivo* performance. Selecting formulation excipients should, therefore, involve a balance to ensure adequate solvent capacity for solubilizing the complete dose on initial dilution in the stomach, whereas also ensure that the lipids used in the formulation, during processing into the final micellar stage, should ensure the adequate solvent capacity of the drug (MacGregor, K.J., Embleton, J.K., Lacy, J. E., Perry, E. A., Solomon, L. J., Seager, H., & Pouton, C.W., 1997).

Formulation Aspects (Figure 4)

Oily Liquids

Highly lipophilic drugs like steroids show solubility only in oils, so these should be formulated in triglycerides only. So these should be formulated as oily liquids by incorporating the drug in oil. The main limitation is the amount of drug cannot be so high since the quantity of oil required to solubilize the entire dose will be very high (Larsen, D.B., Joergensen, S., Olsen, N.V., Hansen, S.H., & Larsen, C., 2002; Kalepun, S., Manthina, M., & Padavala, V., 2013).

Self-Emulsifying Systems

These systems consist of one or more surfactants apart from the oil phase. A microemulsion is formed in the GI fluid by self-emulsification due to the dispersion of oily vehicle by the surfactant. These systems may be SMEDDS (self - micro emulsifying drug delivery system) or SNEDD (self - nano emulsifying drug delivery system) depending up on the size of emulsion droplets (Kalepun, Manthina, & Padavala, 2013).

Figure 4. Formulation aspects of lipid based drug delivery systems

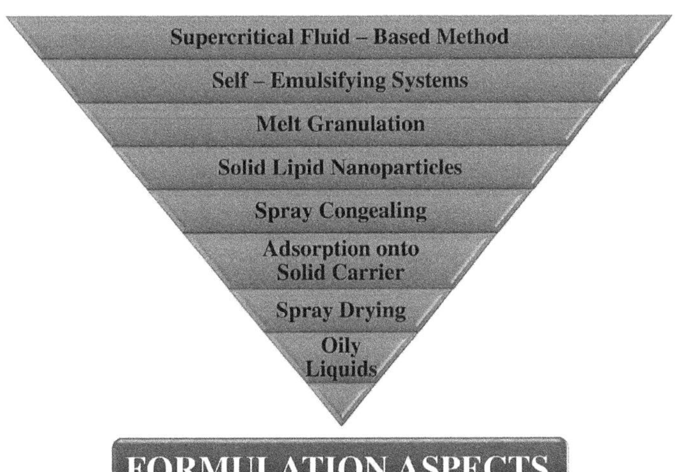

Melt Granulation

This method employs the conversion of a powder mixture containing the drug into pellets or granules. It is also called as pelletization. Here a molten binder is sprayed into the mixture of powder and then mixed using a high shear mixer. Due to the friction of particles the melted binder forms liquid bridges among powder particles and this leads to the formation of granules which convert into spheroid pellets in controlled conditions. Depending on the fineness of the powder, 15%–25% of the lipid-based binder can be used. The particle size of the binder, mixing time, the speed of impeller and binder solution viscosity is the important process parameters (Chambin, O., & Jannin, V., 2005; Evrard, B., Amighi, K., Beten, D., Delattre, L., & Moës A.J., 1999; Royce, A., Suryawanshi, J., Shah, J., & Vishnupad, K., 1996; Seo, A., & Schæfer, t., 2001).

Solid Lipid Nanoparticles

These are exploited as very good carriers for intestinal lymphatic delivery. They have gained much interest due to the bioavailability enhancement power apart from controlled and site-specific drug delivery. They have a solid lipid core matrix which is stabilized by surfactants and able to solubilize lipophilic molecules. They are spherical in shape with a size range of 10 to 1000nm. Mono, di and tri glycerides, fatty acids, waxes, and steroids are the commonly used lipids for the formulation of SLN (Kalepun, Manthina, & Padavala, 2013).

Spray Congealing

Here the molten lipid is sprayed into a cooling chamber, while contact with the cool air; it congeals into globular solid particles. These are collected from the bottom of the chamber. These solid particles can be compressed in to form tablets or filled into hard gelatin capsules. For spray cooling process ultrasonic atomizers are commonly used to produce solid particles. The Melting point of the excipient, temperature of the cooling air, the viscosity of the formulation is the important process parameters. This process is also called as spray cooling (Kalepun, Manthina, & Padavala, 2013).

Adsorption Onto Solid Carrier

Here a lipid formulation in a liquid state is adsorbed onto solid carriers like calcium silicate, silicon dioxide, or magnesium aluminum - metasilicate. A blender is used to mix the lipid and the carrier. The carrier should have good ability to adsorb the liquid formulation and must have good flow property after adsorption. Good content uniformity and high lipid contact are the main advantages of this method. This process is simple and economic as far as equipment investment is considered. (Venkatesan, N., Yoshimitsu, J., & Ohashi, Y., 2006; 2007; Ito, Y., Kusawake, T., Ishida, M., Tawa, R., Shibata, N., & Takada, K., 2005).

Spray Drying

This technique is to some extent similar to spray congealing but differs in the temperature of the air in the atomizing chamber. Here the drug solution in organic solution or water is sprayed into a hot air chamber so that the water or the organic solvent evaporates which results in the formation of solid microparticles of drug. During this process, solid carriers can also be used beside the lipid excipients. (Chauhan, Shimpi, & Paradkar, 2005a, 2005b).

Supercritical Fluid-Based Method

Here the drug and lipid-based excipients are solubilized in an organic solvent and then in a supercritical fluid by increasing the temperature and pressure. Here the lipid forms a coating around the drug particle to form a solid dispersion (Richard, T.C., Dos Santos, R., Rolland, V.H., & Benoit, J.P., 2003; Dos Santos, R., Thies, J., & Richard, T.C., 2003). The solubility of the coating material is reduced by decreasing the pressure and temperature in order to facilitate the coating process by precipitation of the coating particles on to drug. The important process parameters are solubility of the components in the supercritical fluid and its stability (Sethia, S., & Squillante, E., 2002; 2004).

Evaluation Aspects (Figure 5)

Organoleptic Properties

The appearance, color, odor and taste are important characteristics to be considered particularly in the orally administered formulation. Change in taste, mostly of active ingredient, may be due to changes in particle size, crystal habit, and subsequent particle dissolution. The difference in color, odor, and taste may also be due to chemical instability (Wei, Sun, Nie, & Pan, 2005).

Figure 5. Evaluation of lipid based drug delivery systems

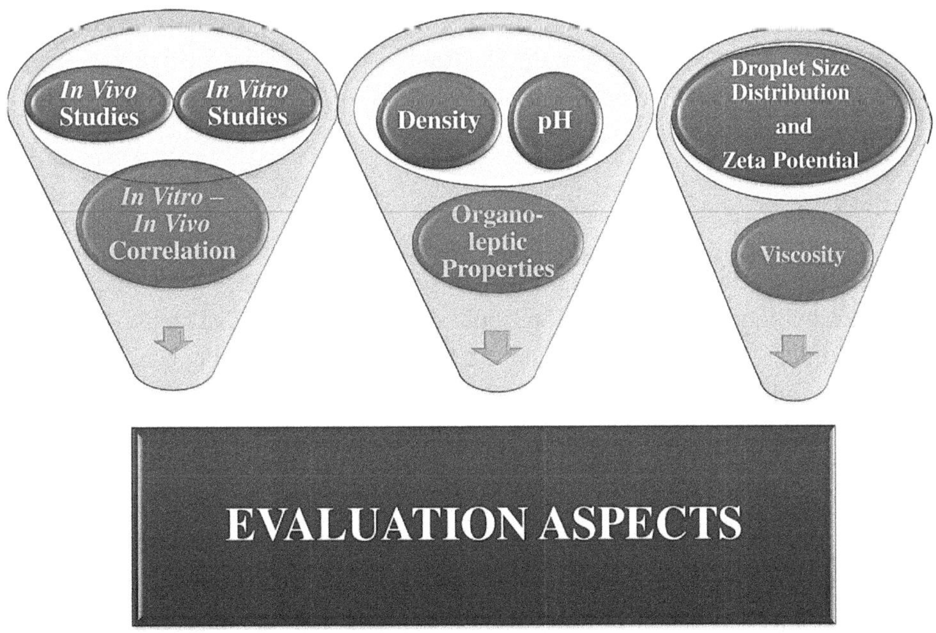

Density

The density of the formulation is a critical parameter since a decrease in density maybe due to air entrapment within the structure of the formulation. High precision hydrometers can be used to measure density (Wei, Sun, Nie, & Pan, 2005).

pH

The pH of the formulation can influence the overall stability. Changes in pH can be measured by a pH meter only after the system reaches equilibrium and also at given set of temperature conditions (Wei, L., Sun, P., Nie, S., & Pan, W., 2005; Shrestha, H., Bala, R., & Arora, S., 2014).

Droplet Size Distribution and Zeta Potential

The droplet size distribution of the system can be determined by both electron microscopy and light-scattering technique. Dynamic light scattering measurements are carried out at an angle of 90° in a dynamic light-scattering spectrophotometer. Recently, photon correlation spectroscopy (PCS) is also used to measure particle size distribution in terms of particle characterization and product physical stability.

Zeta potential analyzer measures the surface charge of the preparations. It gives information regarding repulsive forces among particles and droplets. To obtain stable nanoemulsions without flocculation and coalescence of the droplets, zeta potential should normally reach a value above 30 mV (Wei, Sun, Nie, & Pan, 2005).

Viscosity Measurement

The viscosity of the formulations of different compositions at different shear rates can be measured by Brookfield type rotary viscometer. The samples must be maintained at a temperature of 37°C. The instrument must be properly calibrated to measure the apparent viscosity of the formulation at equilibrium at a given temperature for establishing reproducibility Wei, L., Sun, P., Nie, S., & Pan, W., 2005; Shrestha, H., Bala, R., & Arora, S., 2014).

In Vitro Studies

A preface guideline for formulation development will be obtained from *in vitro* studies. It also gives a picture of *in vivo* evaluation of the formulation. Lipid digestion models can be used for *in vitro* assessment of the formulation. A method called simulated lipolysis release testing can be used to assess the performance of the excipient in formulation development and to forecast *in vivo* performance. The basic principle by which this system works is that if there is any change in pH, a constant pH is maintained by a reaction which releases or consumes hydrogen ions. If there is any deviation is found, it is compensated by the reagent addition. The model consists of a vessel maintained at constant temperature containing simulated intestinal fluid, composed of digestion buffer, phospholipids and also bile salts. The lipid-based formulation in a fluid state is added and to begin the digestion pancreatic lipase and colipase is also added. When the digestion process begins there will be the liberation of fatty acids, which cause a temporary fall in pH. This decrease in pH is measured by a pH electrode. This pH electrode is attached with a pH-stat meter controller and an automatic burette. An equimolar amount of base is added to titrate the liberated fatty acids for preventing the change in pH of the digestion medium. By quantifying the rate of base addition and taking into account the stoichiometric relationship among fatty acids and sodium hydroxide, the degree of digestion can be measured. During the process of digestion, samples are withdrawn and separated by a centrifuge into a poorly dispersed oil phase and dispersed aqueous phase, and also a precipitated pellet phase. Measurement of the drug in the dispersed aqueous phase designates that drug has not precipitated. So the *in vivo* performance can be assumed (Shrestha, H., Bala, R., & Arora, S., 2014; Prabhu, S., Ortega, M., & Ma, C., 2005).

In Vivo Studies

Since sufficient clinical data are not available and differences in methods in animal models used for the drug transport studies through the lymphatic system the *in vivo* studies are difficult. A thorough study of intestinal lymphatic absorption is required since the excipients play a major role in the bioavailability and pharmacokinetic profile of drugs (Shrestha, H., Bala, R., & Arora, S., 2014; Edwards, G.A., Porter, C.J.H., Caliph, S.M., Khoo, S., & Charman, W.N., 2001).

In Vitro-In Vivo Correlation

The drug development period can be shortened and product quality can be improved by the development of a suitable *in vitro - in vivo* correlation model. It will also assist to maximize the development potential and commercialization of the formulations. *In vitro* parameters like dissolution, lipolysis of the lipid excipient can be correlated with that of *in vivo* parameters like blood drug concentration, AUC etc. But these techniques give information about only some specific aspects of the formulation (Seeballuck, Ashford, & O'Driscoll, 2003).

Lipid-Based Formulations

Some important commercially available lipid-based formulations (Table 2) (Patel, M., Patel, S., & Patel, N., 2011; Sarpal, K., Pawar, Y.B., & Bansal, A.K., 2010).

Regulatory Framework

All excipients are not totally inert, and some may be toxic at higher concentrations. The FDA has published a list of substances that are commonly recognized as safe (GRAS) in the Code of Federal Regulations. A list of inactive ingredients for excipients permitted inactive ingredient guide that is approved and can be incorporated in marketed products are also available in it (Maincent, 2007). The maximum amount of allowed for excipients, allowed for a specific route of administration is also mentioned. For a new drug formulation by a particular route, an already approved excipient can be used without any review. The regulatory process is proper in a scientific standpoint since excipients have vital roles in formulation design. For launching a lipid-based dosage form into the market, quality and safety issues associated with preclinical and clinical studies are the main difficulties to be faced. Immunological safety and drug stability are the other key points to be addressed. Adequate details to address the type of dosage form and the mechanism of drug release also should be produced to the regulatory authorities for their acceptance. Safety assessment and the potential influence of biopharmaceutical factors on the drug or lipid excipients need to be explored. Based on *in vitro* details got by dissolution studies it will be difficult to assume the *in vivo* performance because of the complicated mechanism of lipid absorption through GIT.

For rationalizing the design of lipid formulation and to study the fate of a drug after oral administration of a lipid-based formulation, an association has been created by academics and industrial scientists. The consortium performs research for developing *in vitro* methods to review the performance of lipid-based formulation while dispersion and digestion since these are critical parameters. The most important objective is to build up guidelines for rationalizing and accelerating the development of drug candidates by identification of important performance criteria. They are also responsible for the validation and ultimate publication of worldwide standard tests and common operating procedures (Maincent, 2007; Chen, 2008).

CONCLUSION

Lipid-based delivery systems offer a new type of carrier system for drugs. Surface stabilization by emulsifying particles will lead to the increase in bioavailability of the less stable drugs. It is evident from the literature that, the bioavailability of the certain drugs increased by the sustained release of drug entrapped in lipid system. Use of lipid can be considered as new drug delivery approach for less stable drugs. However, some limitations of these carriers are poor physiochemical properties, lack of drug solubility database in lipids and unavailability of standard methodologies for in-vitro analysis. Lipid Fat environment is used to achieve the desired goal for controlled and safe delivery of drugs. It is important to maintain the structure of the formed colloidal species after passing the drug through GI tract. Further, it is important to achieve drug solubility in the formulation after digestion and dispersion. Medium chained triglycerides have greater drug solubility & stability whereas, for more bioavailability, we need long chained triglycerides which are responsible for the formation of bile salt lipid colloidal species. Type III B SMEDDS formulations depend upon the properties of surfactant used, so we can employ on – digestible surfactants for high bioavailability. Type IV formulation is more efficient and have high drug solubility if two surfactants are used in the formulation. But this needs to be designed very carefully, so that drug doesn't get precipitated.

REFERENCES

Amidon, G. L., Lennernas, H., Shah, V. P., & Crison, J. R. (1995). A theoretical basis for a biopharmaceutic drug classification: The correlation in vitro drug product dissolution and in vivo bioavailability. *Pharmaceutical Research, 12*(3), 413–420. doi:10.1023/A:1016212804288 PMID:7617530

Attama, A. A., Momoh, M. A., & Builders, P. F. (2012). *Lipid nanoparticulate drug delivery systems: a revolution in dosage form design and development in: recent advances in novel drug carrier systems* (A. D. Sezer, Ed.). InTech.

Bouwstra, J. A., Honeywell-Nguyen, P. L., & Gooris, G. M. (2003). Structure of the skin barrier and its modulation by vesicular formulations. *Progress in Lipid Research, 42*(1), 1–36. doi:10.1016/S0163-7827(02)00028-0 PMID:12467638

Bouwstra, J. A., & Ponec, M. (2006). The skin barrier in healthy and diseased state. *Biochimica et Biophysica Acta, 1758*(12), 2080–2095. doi:10.1016/j.bbamem.2006.06.021 PMID:16945325

Bremmell, K. E., Tan, A., Martin, A., & Prestidge, C. A. (2013). Tableting lipid-based formulations for oral drug delivery: A case study with silica nanoparticle-lipid-mannitol hybrid microparticles. *Journal of Pharmaceutical Sciences, 102*(2), 684–693. doi:10.1002/jps.23406 PMID:23242712

Cao, Y., Marra, M., & Anderson, B. D. (2004). Predictive relationships for the effects of triglyceride ester concentration and water uptake on solubility and partitioning of small molecules into lipid vehicles. *Journal of Pharmaceutical Sciences, 93*(11), 2768–2779. doi:10.1002/jps.20126 PMID:15389678

Chambin, O., & Jannin, V. (2005). Interest of multifunctional lipid excipients: Case of Gelucire 44/14. *Drug Development and Industrial Pharmacy, 31*(6), 527–534. doi:10.1080/03639040500215750 PMID:16109625

Charman, W. N., Porter, C. J., Mithani, S., & Dressman, J. B. (1997). Physiochemical and physiological mechanisms for the effects of food on drug absorption: The role of lipids and pH. *Journal of Pharmaceutical Sciences, 86*(3), 269–282. doi:10.1021/js960085v PMID:9050793

Chauhan, B., Shimpi, S., & Paradkar, A. (2005a). Preparation and evaluation of glibenclamidepolyglycolized glycerides solid dispersions with silicon dioxide by spray drying technique. *European Journal of Pharmaceutical Sciences, 26*(2), 219–230. doi:10.1016/j.ejps.2005.06.005 PMID:16087324

Chauhan, B., Shimpi, S., & Paradkar, A. (2005b). Preparation and characterization of etoricoxib solid dispersions using lipid carriers by spray drying technique. *AAPS PharmSciTech, 6*(3), E405–E409. doi:10.1208/pt060350 PMID:16353998

Chen, M. (2008). Lipid excipients and delivery systems for pharmaceutical development: A regulatory perspective. *Advanced Drug Delivery Reviews, 60*(6), 768–777. doi:10.1016/j.addr.2007.09.010 PMID:18077051

Chime, S. A., Onyishi, I. V., Obitte, N. C., Onunkwo, G. C., & Odo, G. I. (2013). Sustained release artemether-loaded solid lipid microparticles based on solidified reverse micellar solution (SRMS). *Innovare J Sci., 1*, 1–7.

Christie, W.W., (1987). *High-performance liquid chromatography and lipids: a practical guide.* Oxford, UK: Pergamon Press.

Cole, E. T., Cade, D., & Benameur, H. (2008). Challenges and opportunities in the encapsulation of liquid and semi-solid formulations into capsules for oral administration. *Advanced Drug Delivery Reviews, 60*(6), 747–756. doi:10.1016/j.addr.2007.09.009 PMID:18096270

Craig, D. Q. M., Agnes Chan, K. Y., & Khan, N. (1995). Article. *Pharmacy and Pharmacology Communications, 1*, 559.

Dening, T. J., Rao, S., Thomas, N., & Prestidge, A. (2016). Novel Nanostructured Solid Materials for Modulating Oral Drug Delivery from Solid-State Lipid-Based Drug Delivery Systems. *The AAPS Journal, 18*(1), 23–40. doi:10.120812248-015-9824-7 PMID:26354801

Deshmukh, A., Nakhat, P., & Yeole, P. (2010). Formulation and in-vitro evaluation of self microemulsifying drug delivery system (SMEDDS) of Furosemide. *Der Pharm Lett*, *2*(2), 94–106.

Ding, B. S., Dziubla, T., Shuvaev, V. V., Muro, S., & Muzykantov, V. R. (2006). Advanced drug delivery systems that target the vascular endothelium. *Molecular Interventions*, *6*(2), 98–112. doi:10.1124/mi.6.2.7 PMID:16565472

Dos Santos, R., Thies, J., Richard, T. C., Le Meurlay, D., Gajan, V., Vandevelde, V., & Benoit, J.-P. (2003). A supercritical fluid-based coating technology. 2: Solubility considerations. *Journal of Microencapsulation*, *20*(1), 97–109. doi:10.3109/02652040309178052 PMID:12519705

Edwards, G. A., Porter, C. J. H., Caliph, S. M., Khoo, S., & Charman, W. N. (2001). Animal models for the study of intestinal lymphatic drug transport. *Advanced Drug Delivery Reviews*, *50*(1-2), 45–60. doi:10.1016/S0169-409X(01)00148-X PMID:11489333

El Laithy, H. M., & El-Shaboury, K. M. (2002). The development of cutinalipogels and gel micromeulsion for topical administration of fluconazole. *AAPS PharmSciTech*, *3*, E35. PMID:12916929

ElMaghraby, G. M., Barry, B. W., & Williams, A. C. (2008). Liposomes and skin: From drug delivery to model membranes. *European Journal of Pharmaceutical Sciences*, *34*(4-5), 203–222. doi:10.1016/j.ejps.2008.05.002 PMID:18572392

Erlanson-Albertsson, C. (1992). Pancreatic colipase. Structural and physiological aspects. *Biochimica et Biophysica Acta*, *1125*(1), 1–7. doi:10.1016/0005-2760(92)90147-N PMID:1567900

Evrard, B., Amighi, K., Beten, D., Delattre, L., & Moës, A. J. (1999). Influence of melting and rheological properties of fatty binders on the melt granulation process in a high-shear mixer. *Drug Development and Industrial Pharmacy*, *25*(11), 1177–1184. doi:10.1081/DDC-100102285 PMID:10596355

Gershkovich, P., Wasan, K. M., & Barta, C. A. (2008). A review of the application of lipid-based systems in systemic, dermal/ transdermal, and ocular drug delivery. *Critical Reviews in Therapeutic Drug Carrier Systems*, *25*(6), 545–584. doi:10.1615/CritRevTherDrugCarrierSyst.v25.i6.20 PMID:19166393

Geusens, B., Strobbe, T., Bracke, S., Dynoodt, P., Sanders, N., ... VanGele, M. (2011). Lipid-mediated gene delivery to the skin. *European Journal of Pharmaceutical Sciences*, *43*(4), 199–211. doi:10.1016/j.ejps.2011.04.003 PMID:21515366

Gibson, L. (2007). Lipid-based excipients for oral drug delivery. In D. J. Hauss (Ed.), *Oral lipid-based formulations: enhancing the bioavailability of poorly water soluble drugs* (pp. 33–61). InformaHealthcare.

Glenn, G. M., & Kenney, R. T. (2006). Mass vaccination: Solutions in the skin. *Current Topics in Microbiology and Immunology*, *304*, 247–268. doi:10.1007/3-540-36583-4_14 PMID:16989274

Gomes, M. J., Martins, S., Ferreira, D., Segundo, M. A., & Reis, S. (2014). Lipid nanoparticles for topical and transdermal application for alopecia treatment: Development, physicochemical characterization, and in vitro release and penetration studies. *International Journal of Nanomedicine*, *9*, 1231–1242. PMID:24634584

Guy, R. H., & Hadgraft, J. (2003). *New York: Marcel Dekker, 2003. Transdermal Drug Delivery, Williams, A.* London: Pharmaceutical Press.

Hauss, D. J. (2007). *Oral lipid-based formulations: enhancing the bioavailability of poorly water soluble drugs*. New York, NY: Informa Healthcare.

Hua, S., & Wu, S. Y. (2013). The use of lipid-based nanocarriers for targeted pain therapies. *Frontiers in Pharmacology*, *4*, 143. doi:10.3389/fphar.2013.00143 PMID:24319430

Humberstone, A. J., & Charman, W. N. (1997). Lipid-based vehicles for the oral delivery of poorly water soluble drugs. *Advanced Drug Delivery Reviews*, *25*(1), 103–128. doi:10.1016/S0169-409X(96)00494-2

Hunt, J. N., & Knox, M. T. (1968). A relation between the chain length of fatty acids and the slowing of gastric emptying. *The Journal of Physiology*, *194*(2), 327–336. doi:10.1113/jphysiol.1968.sp008411 PMID:5639357

Iqbal, J., & Hussain, M. M. (2009). Intestinal lipid absorption. *American Journal of Physiology. Endocrinology and Metabolism*, *296*(6), E1183–E1194. doi:10.1152/ajpendo.90899.2008 PMID:19158321

Ito, Y., Kusawake, T., Ishida, M., Tawa, R., Shibata, N., & Takada, K. (2005). Oral solid gentamicin preparation using emulsifier and adsorbent. *Journal of Controlled Release*, *105*(1-2), 23–31. doi:10.1016/j.jconrel.2005.03.017 PMID:15908031

Jannin, V., Musakhanian, J., & Marchaud, D. (2008). Approaches for the development of solid and semi-solid lipid-based formulations. *Advanced Drug Delivery Reviews*, *60*(6), 734–746. doi:10.1016/j.addr.2007.09.006 PMID:18045728

Jannin, V., Musakhanian, J., & Marchaud, D. (2008). Approaches for the development of solid and semisolid lipid-based formulations. *Advanced Drug Delivery Reviews*, *60*(6), 734–746. doi:10.1016/j.addr.2007.09.006 PMID:18045728

Jaspart, S., Bertholet, P., Piel, G., Dogné, J. M., Delattre, L., & Evrard, B. (2007). Solid lipid microparticles as a sustained release system for pulmonary drug delivery. *European Journal of Pharmaceutics and Biopharmaceutics*, *65*(1), 47–56. doi:10.1016/j.ejpb.2006.07.006 PMID:16962749

Jyoti, W., Anroop, N., & Rachna, K. (2012). Emulsion forming drug delivery system for lipophilic drugs. *Acta Pol. Pharm. Drug Res.*, *69*(2), 179–191. PMID:22568032

Kalepu, S., Manthina, M., & Padavala, V. (2013). Oral lipid-based drug delivery systems – an overview. *Acta Pharmaceutica Sinica. B*, *3*(6), 361–372. doi:10.1016/j.apsb.2013.10.001

Kalepun, S., Manthina, M., & Padavala, V. (2013). Oral lipid-based drug delivery systems – an overview. *Acta Pharmaceutica Sinica. B*, *3*(6), 361–372. doi:10.1016/j.apsb.2013.10.001

Kaukonen, A. M., Boyd, B. J., Porter, C. J., & Charman, W. N. (2004). Drug solubilization behavior during *in vitro* digestion of simple triglyceride lipid solution formulations. *Pharmaceutical Research*, *21*(2), 245–253. doi:10.1023/B:PHAM.0000016282.77887.1f PMID:15032305

Koning, G. A., & Storm, G. (2003). Targeted drug delivery systems for the intracellular delivery of macromolecular drugs. *Drug Discovery Today*, *8*(11), 482–483. doi:10.1016/S1359-6446(03)02699-0 PMID:12818515

Koning, G. A., & Storm, G. (2003). Targeted drug delivery systems for the intracellular delivery of macromolecular drugs. *Drug Discovery Today*, *8*(11), 482–483. doi:10.1016/S1359-6446(03)02699-0 PMID:12818515

Larsen, D. B., Joergensen, S., Olsen, N. V., Hansen, S. H., & Larsen, C. (2002). *In vivo* release of bupivacaine from subcutaneously administered oily solution: Comparison with *in vitro* release. *Journal of Controlled Release*, *81*(1-2), 145–154. doi:10.1016/S0168-3659(02)00055-X PMID:11992687

MacGregor, K. J., Embleton, J. K., Lacy, J. E., Perry, E. A., Solomon, L. J., Seager, H., & Pouton, C. W. (1997). Influence of lipolysis on drug absorption from the gastro-intestinal tract. *Advanced Drug Delivery Reviews*, *25*(1), 33–46. doi:10.1016/S0169-409X(96)00489-9

Maincent, P. (2007). The regulatory environment: The challenges for lipid-based formulations. *Bulletin Technique Gattefossé*, *100*, 47–49.

Manjunath, K., Reddy, J., & Venkateswarlu, V. (2005). Solid lipid nanoparticles as drug delivery systems. *Methods and Findings in Experimental and Clinical Pharmacology*, *27*(2), 127–144. doi:10.1358/mf.2005.27.2.876286 PMID:15834465

McCarter, M. D., Clarke, J. H., & Harken, A. H. (2004). Lymphangiogenesis is pivotal to the trials of a successful cancer metastasis. *Surgery*, *135*(2), 121–124. doi:10.1016/S0039-6060(03)00342-8 PMID:14739845

Miteva, D. O., Rutkowski, J. M., Dixon, J. B., Kilarski, W., Shields, J. D., & Swartz, M. A. (2010). Transmural flow modulates cell and fluid transport functions of lymphatic endothelium. *Circulation Research*, *106*(5), 920–931. doi:10.1161/CIRCRESAHA.109.207274 PMID:20133901

Monteiro, N., Martins, A., Reis, R. L., & Neves, N. M. (2014). Liposomes in tissue engineering and regenerative medicine. *Journal of the Royal Society, Interface*, *11*(101), 1–23. doi:10.1098/rsif.2014.0459 PMID:25401172

Morgan, C. J., Renwick, A. G., & Friedmann, P. S. (2003). The role of stratum corneum and dermal microvascular perfusion in penetration and tissue levels of water-soluble drugs investigated by microdialysis. *British Journal of Dermatology*, *148*(3), 434–443. doi:10.1046/j.1365-2133.2003.05163.x PMID:12653734

Müller, R. H., Radtke, M., & Wissing, S. A. (2002). Solid lipid nanoparticles (SLN) and nanostructured lipid carriers (NLC) in cosmetic and dermatological preparations. *Advanced Drug Delivery Reviews*, *54*(Suppl 1), S131–S155. doi:10.1016/S0169-409X(02)00118-7 PMID:12460720

Nagabandi, V., & Sambaraj, S. (2013). Silica-Lipid Hybrid Microparticles for Improved Bioavailability of Bcs Class IV Drugs. *Am J Adv Drug Deliv*, *1*(5), 663–681.

Nnamani, P. O., Attama, A. A., Ibezim, E. C., & Adikwu, M. U. (2010). SRMS142-based solid lipid microparticles: Application in oral delivery of glibenclamide to diabetic rats. *European Journal of Pharmaceutics and Biopharmaceutics*, *76*(1), 68–74. doi:10.1016/j.ejpb.2010.06.002 PMID:20554020

O' Driscoll, C. M., & Griffin, B. T. (2008). Biopharmaceutical challenges associated with drugs with low aqueous solubility—The potential impact of lipid-based formulations. *Advanced Drug Delivery Reviews*, *60*(6), 617–624. doi:10.1016/j.addr.2007.10.012 PMID:18155800

O'Driscol, C. M. (1992). Anatomy and physiology of the lymphatics. In W. N. Charman & V. J. Stella (Eds.), *Lymphatic Transport of Drugs*. Boca Raton, FL: CRC Press Inc.

Pantel, K., & Brakenhoff, R. H. (2004). Dissecting the metastatic cascade. *Nature Reviews. Cancer*, *4*(6), 448–456. doi:10.1038/nrc1370 PMID:15170447

Patel, M., Patel, S., & Patel, N. (2011). A review: novel oral lipid based formulation for poorly soluble drugs. *International Journal of Pharmaceutical Sciences and Technology, 3*(4), 1181-1192.

Paveli, Z., & Skalko-Basnet, N. (2005). Development and in vitro evaluation of a liposomal vaginal delivery system for acyclovir. *Journal of Controlled Release*, *106*(1-2), 34–43. doi:10.1016/j.jconrel.2005.03.032 PMID:15979189

Porter, C. J., & Charman, W. N. (2001). In vitro assessment of oral lipid based formulations. *Advanced Drug Delivery Reviews*, *50*(Suppl. 1), 127–147. doi:10.1016/S0169-409X(01)00182-X PMID:11576699

Porter, C. J. H., Pouton, C. W., Cuine, J. F., & Charman, W. N. (2008). Enhancing intestinal drug solubilisation using lipid-based delivery systems. *Advanced Drug Delivery Reviews*, *60*(6), 673–691. doi:10.1016/j.addr.2007.10.014 PMID:18155801

Pouton, C. W. (2000). Lipid formulations for oral administration of drugs: Non emulsifying, self-emulsifying and 'self-microemulsifying' drug delivery systems. *European Journal of Pharmaceutical Sciences*, *11*(Suppl. 2), 93–98. doi:10.1016/S0928-0987(00)00167-6 PMID:11033431

Pouton, C. W. (2000). Lipid formulations for oral administration of drugs: Non emulsifying, self-emulsifying and 'self-microemulsifying' drug delivery systems. *European Journal of Pharmaceutical Sciences*, *11*, 93 98. doi:10.1016/S0928-0987(00)00167-6 PMID:11033431

Pouton, C. W. (2006). Formulation of poorly water-soluble drugs for oral administration: Physicochemical and physiological issues and the lipid formulation classification system. *European Journal of Pharmaceutical Sciences*, *29*(3-4), 278–287. doi:10.1016/j.ejps.2006.04.016 PMID:16815001

Prabhu, S., Ortega, M., & Ma, C. (2005). Novel lipid-based formulations enhancing the *in vitro* dissolution and permeability characteristics of a poorly water-soluble model drug, piroxicam. *International Journal of Pharmaceutics*, *301*(1-2), 209–216. doi:10.1016/j.ijpharm.2005.05.032 PMID:16046087

Prajapati, N. H., Patel, D. P., Patel, N. G., Dalrymple, D. M., & Serajuddin, A. T. (2011). Effect of difference in fatty acid chain lengths of medium chain lipids on lipid/surfactant/water phase diagrams and drug Solubility. *Journal of Excipients and Food Chemicals*, *2*, 73.

Prausnitz, M. R., Mitragotri, S., & Langer, R. (2004). Transdermal and Topical Drug Delivery, Current status and future potential of transdermal drug delivery. *Nature Reviews. Drug Discovery*, *3*(2), 115–124. doi:10.1038/nrd1304 PMID:15040576

Ravi, K., Shivjee, K., Shyam, S., & Amit, K. J. (2011). Vesicular system-carrier for drug delivery. Der. *Der Pharmacia Sinica*, *2*(4), 192–202.

Richard, T. C., Dos Santos, R., Rolland, V. H., & Benoit, J. P. (2003). A supercritical fluid-based coating technology 1: Process considerations. *Journal of Microencapsulation*, *20*(1), 87–96. doi:10.3109/02652040309178051 PMID:12519704

Rogers, J.A., & Anderson, K.E. (1998). The Potential of Liposomes in Oral Drug Delivery. *Critical Reviews™ in Therapeutic Drug Carrier Systems.*

Rowe, R. C., Sheskey, P. J., & Owen, S. C. (2006). Handbook of pharmaceutical excipients (5th ed.). Washington, DC: American Pharmaceutical Association.

Royce, A., Suryawanshi, J., Shah, J., & Vishnupad, K. (1996). Alternative granulation technique: Melt granulation. *Drug Development and Industrial Pharmacy*, *22*(9-10), 917–924. doi:10.3109/03639049609065921

Sambaraj, S. (2013). Silica-Lipid Hybrid Microparticles for Improved Bioavailability of Bcs Class IV Drugs. *Am J Adv Drug Deliv*, *1*(5), 663–681.

Sarpal, K., Pawar, Y.B., & Bansal, A.K. (2010). Self-emulsifying drug delivery systems: A strategy to improve oral bioavailablity. *Current Research and Information on Pharmaceutical Sciences, 11*(3), 42-49.

Schick, M. J. (1987). *Surfactant science series* (Vol. 23). NewYork: Marcel Dekker.

Seeballuck, F., Ashford, M. B., & O'Driscoll, C. M. (2003). The effects of Pluronic block copolymers and Cremophor EL on intestinal lipoprotein processing and the potential link with P-glycoprotein in Caco-2 cells. *Pharmaceutical Research*, *20*(7), 1085–1092. doi:10.1023/A:1024422625596 PMID:12880295

Seo, A., & Schæfer, T. (2001). Melt agglomeration with polyethylene glycol beads at a low impeller speed in a high shear mixer. *European Journal of Pharmaceutics and Biopharmaceutics*, *52*(3), 315–325. doi:10.1016/S0939-6411(01)00183-7 PMID:11677074

Sethia, S., & Squillante, E. (2002). Physicochemical characterization of solid dispersions of carbamazepine formulated by supercritical carbon dioxide and conventional solvent evaporation method. *Journal of Pharmaceutical Sciences*, *91*(9), 1948–1957. doi:10.1002/jps.10186 PMID:12210042

Sethia, S., & Squillante, E. (2004). *In vitro-in vivo* evaluation of supercritical processed solid dispersions: Permeability and viability assessment in Caco-2 cells. *Journal of Pharmaceutical Sciences*, *93*(12), 2985–2993. doi:10.1002/jps.20199 PMID:15468328

Shrestha, H., Bala, R., & Arora, S. (2014). Lipid-Based Drug Delivery Systems. *Journal of Pharmaceutics*, 1-10.

Sleeman, J. P. (2000). The lymph node as a bridgehead in the metastatic dissemination of tumors. *Recent Results in Cancer Research. Fortschritte der Krebsforschung. Progres Dans les Recherches Sur le Cancer*, *157*, 55–81. doi:10.1007/978-3-642-57151-0_6 PMID:10857162

Sleeman, J. P. (2006). The relationship between tumors and the lymphatics: What more is there to know. *Lymphology*, *39*, 62–68. PMID:16910096

Soumya, S., Doney, A. B., & Sabitha, M. (2012). Current trends in lipid based delivery systems and its applications in drug delivery. *Asian J. Pharm. Clin. Res.*, *5*(3), 4–9.

Strickley, R. G. (2004). Solubilizing excipients in oral and injectable formulations. *Pharmaceutical Research*, *21*(2), 201–230. doi:10.1023/B:PHAM.0000016235.32639.23 PMID:15032302

Strickley, R. G. (2007). Currently marketed oral lipid-based dosage forms: drugs products and excipients. In D. J. Hauss (Ed.), *Oral lipid-based formulations: enhancing the bioavailability of poorly water soluble drugs* (pp. 1–31). New York: Informa Healthcare.

Subedi, R. K., Oh, S. Y., Chun, M. K., & Choi, H. K. (2010). Recent advances in transdermal drug delivery. *Archives of Pharmacal Research*, *33*(3), 339–351. doi:10.100712272-010-0301-7 PMID:20361297

Umeyor, C. E., Kenechukwu, F. C., Uronnachi, E. M., Osonnwa, U. E., & Nwakile, C. D. (2012). Solid lipid microparticles (SLMs): An effective lipid based technology for controlled drug delivery. *Am J PharmTech Res.*, *2*, 1–18.

Venkatesan, N., Yoshimitsu, J., Ito, Y., Shibata, N., & Takada, K. (2005). Liquid filled nanoparticles as a drug delivery tool for protein therapeutics. *Biomaterials*, *26*(34), 7154–7163. doi:10.1016/j.biomaterials.2005.05.012 PMID:15967493

Venkatesan, N., Yoshimitsu, J., Ohashi, Y., Ito, Y., Sugioka, N., Shibata, N., & Takada, K. (2006). Pharmacokinetic and pharmacodynamic studies following oral administration of erythropoietin mucoadhesive tablets to beagle dogs. *International Journal of Pharmaceutics*, *310*(1-2), 46–52. doi:10.1016/j.ijpharm.2005.11.014 PMID:16439074

Verma, D. D., Verma, S., Blume, G., & Fahr, A. (2003a). Particle size of liposomes influences dermal delivery of substances into skin. *International Journal of Pharmaceutics*, *258*(1-2), 141–151. doi:10.1016/S0378-5173(03)00183-2 PMID:12753761

Vikas, S., Seema, S., Gurpreet, S., Rana, A. C., & Baibhav, J. (2011). Penetration enhancers: A novel strategy for enhancing transdermal drug delivery. *Int. Res. J. Pharm.*, *2*, 32–36.

Wagnera, D., Langguth, H. S., Hanafy, A., Koggela, A., & Langguth, P. (2001). Intestinal drug efflux: Formulation and food effects. *Advanced Drug Delivery Reviews*, *50*(Suppl. 1), 113–131. PMID:11576693

Wang, Q., Ye, J., Zhoua, X., & Zhang, N. (2008). Injectable loaded solid lipid nanoparticles as passive targeting therapeutic agents for rheumatoid arthritis. *International Journal of Pharmaceutics*, *352*(1-2), 273–279. doi:10.1016/j.ijpharm.2007.10.014 PMID:18054182

Wei, L., Sun, P., Nie, S., & Pan, W. (2005). Preparation and evaluation of SEDDS and SMEDDS containing carvedilol. *Drug Development and Industrial Pharmacy*, *31*(8), 785–794. doi:10.1080/03639040500216428 PMID:16221613

Wenson, E. S., & Curtalo, W. J. (1992). Article. *Advanced Drug Delivery Reviews*, *8*, 39. doi:10.1016/0169-409X(92)90015-I

Wiechers, J. W. (1989). The barrier functions of the skin in relation to percutaneous absorption of drugs. *Pharmaceutisch Weekblad. Scientific Edition*, *11*(6), 185–198. doi:10.1007/BF01959410 PMID:2694089

Winstanley, P. A., & Orme, M. L. E. (1989). The effects of food on drug bioavailability. *British Journal of Clinical Pharmacology*, *28*(6), 621–628. doi:10.1111/j.1365-2125.1989.tb03554.x PMID:2692684

Wu, C. Y., & Benet, L. Z. (2005). Predicting drug disposition via application of BCS: Transport/absorption/ elimination interplay and development of a biopharmaceutics drug disposition classification system. *Pharmaceutical Research*, *22*(1), 11–23. doi:10.100711095-004-9004-4 PMID:15771225

Yalkowsky, S.H. (2000). *Solubility and solubilization in aqueous media*. Washington, DC: American Chemical Society.

Zhao, Y.Z., Dai, D.D., Lu, C.T., Chen, L.J., Lin, M., … Shen, X.T. (2013). Epirubicin loaded with propyleneglycol liposomes significantly overcomes multidrug resistance in breast cancer. *Cancer Lett, 330*, 74–83.

Chapter 5
Lipid Nanocarriers for Advanced Therapeutic Applications

Vandana B. Patravale
Institute of Chemical Technology, India

Preshita P. Desai
Institute of Chemical Technology, India

Sanyat S. Mapara
Institute of Chemical Technology, India

ABSTRACT

Lipid nanocarriers are the mainstream of nanotechnology-based advanced healthcare systems. This field has reported extensive research activity, promising results, and market acceptability over the past few decades. This profound success of lipid nanocarriers as therapeutic delivery systems is a result of their unique properties, that is, biocompatibility and biodegradability, possible delivery by multiple routes of administration, ease of formulation and scale up, amicable dosage form development, enhanced stability, bioavailability, and possible drug targeting. The chapter aims to give a detailed overview of various types of lipid nanocarriers along with methods of fabrication and characterization. The chapter also describes multiple applications of lipid nanocarriers in advanced therapeutics and elaborates on the current market opportunities and future prospects.

INTRODUCTION

Nanotechnology has revolutionized the face of modern day pharmaceuticals. Among various types of nanocarriers, lipid nanocarriers have attracted remarkable attention and have become market reality in very short duration. This practical success of lipid nanocarriers has resulted from their unique properties like biodegradability, possible delivery by multiple routes of administration, amicable dosage form development, enhanced stability, bioavailability and possible drug targeting along with their commercial feasibility in terms of ease of formulation development, scale up and characterization. Through extensive research over the years, various types of novel and effective lipid nanocarrier systems have been

DOI: 10.4018/978-1-5225-4781-5.ch005

Copyright © 2018, IGI Global. Copying or distributing in print or electronic forms without written permission of IGI Global is prohibited.

invented and are extensively researched. A detailed overview of these multitude lipid nanocarriers along with their manufacturing methods, characterization techniques and applications in advanced healthcare system are discussed in subsequent sections.

TYPES OF LIPID NANOCARRIERS

Researchers have explored an extensive number of lipid nanocarriers over the last several decades as described below. Their broad classification is depicted in Figure 1.

Emulsion Based Lipid Nanocarriers

The pictorial representation of emulsion based lipid nanocarriers is shown in Figure 2.

Microemulsions, Nanoemulsions, and Multiple Emulsions

In 1943, Schulman and Hoar introduced the concept of the microemulsion (Pappinen & Urtti, 2016). Microemulsions are kinetically and thermodynamically stable, spontaneously formed colloidal dispersions of oil and water stabilized by an interfacial film of alternating surfactant and co-surfactant molecules. They are of 10-140 nm size, transparent, optically isotropic, self-preserving, sterilizable and have ultra-low interfacial tension (Agrawal & Agrawal, 2012). Their advantages include, low cost of production, good stability, easy scale-up, high drug solubilization capacity and drug protection (Prabhu & Patravale, 2014).

Winsor has classified microemulsion system based on their phase equilibrium as shown in Table 1 (Moulik & Kumar, 2008). Further, microemulsion type can be determined by surfactant critical packing ratio (CPP) which can be calculate using Equation 1 (Prabhu & Patravale, 2014).

$$\text{Critical Packing Ratio (CPP)} = \frac{Vo}{A \times l} \tag{1}$$

wherein 'Vo' is the volume of surfactant molecule, 'A' is the head group surface area and 'l' is the surfactant tail length.

For microemulsions, the oily phase is selected based on its biocompatibility, acceptability for the desired delivery route, drug solubilization capacity, ease of emulsification and additional benefits like P-GP efflux inhibition and oxidation stability etc. The surfactant is chosen on its biocompatibility, stabilization ability, chemical nature, acceptability for the desired delivery route, drug solubilization capacity and cloud point. Co-surfactant is selected based on its properties to decrease surface tension, increase interfacial fluidity and synergistically aid surfactant to stabilize microemulsion (Moulik & Kumar, 2008). Multiple mechanisms are involved in drug release from microemulsions and are depicted in Figure 3 (Pappinen & Urtti, 2016).

Nanoemulsions are kinetically stable colloidal dispersions of oil and water stabilized by an interfacial film of alternating surfactant and co-surfactant molecules with average size of 100nm and above. Unlike microemulsions, they are not thermodynamically stable and require energy intensive manufacturing techniques. On the contrary, nanoemulsions are relatively stable than microemulsions to changes in physical conditions like temperature and pressure etc. (Gupta, Eral, Hatton, & Doyle, 2016).

Multiple emulsions are polydispersed systems wherein both o/w and w/o emulsions exist simultaneously and are stabilized by hydrophilic and lipophilic surfactants respectively. Their types are water in oil in water (w/o/w) multiple emulsion and oil in water in oil (o/w/o) multiple emulsion. Here, an immiscible phase separates two miscible phases thereby acting as a semi-permeable membrane through which drug must diffuse to travel from one phase to another. The drug release through multiple emulsions can follow various mechanisms as described in Figure 4 (Sinha & Kumar, 2002).

Multiple emulsions possess advantages like biocompatibility, biodegradability, avoidance of undesired drug autoimmune response, possible drug targeting to reticuloendothelial system (RES), encapsulation of both hydrophilic and hydrophobic drugs, decrease in fluctuation in steady-state drug concentration and good taste masking (Prabhu & Patravale, 2014). However, multiple emulsion stabilization is the main issue and various strategies employed for their stabilization are shown in Figure 5 (Sinha & Kumar, 2002).

Self-Emulsifying Drug Delivery Systems (SEDDS), Self Micro-Emulsifying Drug Delivery Systems (SMEDDS), and Self Nano-Emulsifying Drug Delivery Systems (SNEDDS)

SEDDS, SMEDDS and SNEDDS are mixtures of oil and surfactants that can form o/w emulsion or microemulsion or nanoemulsion when introduced into an aqueous phase under mild conditions of gentle agitation. One of the main differences between them is size viz. SEDDS (200 nm-5 µ), SMEDDS (100 – 200nm) and SNEDDS (< 100nm) (Prabhu & Patravale, 2014).

They rapidly self-emulsify in the stomach with the help of gentle agitation received through gastrointestinal (GI) peristalsis. Their advantages include bioavailability enhancement of drugs thereby providing a window for dose and dosing frequency reduction, consistent drug absorption profiles, selective targeting inside GI tract, protection of drug from the hostile environment in GI tract, high drug loading, controlled drug release and flexibility to administer drug through various dosage forms (Kohli, Chopra, Dhar, Arora, & Khar, 2010; Venkata Ramana Rao & Shao, 2008).

Lipid Nanovesicular Systems

The various lipid nanovesicular drug delivery systems are shown in Figure 6.

Liposomes

British hematologist Alec Bangham first published his work on liposomes in 1964 (Bangham & Hornc, 1964) and were initially termed as 'bangosomes' (Sessa & Weissmann, 1968). Liposomes are bi-layered concentric spherical vesicles in which a membranous lipid bilayer encloses an aqueous volume.

The liposomal membrane consists of phospholipids, charge generating molecules and cholesterol. The phospholipid polar head groups of liposomes point outwards while the non-polar tail groups point inwards in the lamellar structure as shown in Figure 6. The hydrophilic drugs are incorporated in the core of liposomes while the lipophilic drugs are incorporated in the lipid bilayer (Crowley, 2013; Allen & Cullis, 2013; Siler-Marinkovic, 2016). Liposomes have a particle size ranging from 25nm to several micrometers. The thermodynamic properties and ability of lipids to self-assemble in an aqueous environment, influence the number and type of lipid bilayers that classifies various types of liposomes as depicted in Figure 7 (Prabhu & Patravale, 2014).

Liposomes gained importance owing to their advantages like similarity to biological membranes, biodegradability, biocompatibility, safety, versatility in entrapping both hydrophilic and hydrophobic drugs, increase in drug efficacy and therapeutic index, active targeting by coupling with site-specific ligands etc. However, their disadvantages include high production cost, probable drug leakage and the possibility of phospholipids to undergo oxidation and hydrolysis (Akbarzadeh, Rezaei-Sadabady, Davaran, Joo, Zarghami, Hanifehpour, … Nejati-Koshki, 2013).

The type of phospholipid used in the preparation of liposomes determines the rigidity of the lipid membrane. It is preferable to select lipids with glass transition temperature above the body temperature so that they maintain their rigidity The unsaturated phospholipids obtained from natural sources like Egg phosphatidylcholine are less rigid, more permeable and less stable than saturated phospholipids like hydrogenated synthetic glycerophospholipids. With conventional liposomes, entrapment efficiency was only ~30% depending upon the method of preparation and type of phospholipid used. Hence, poor drug loading and significant drug leakage were serious problems associated with classical liposomes. In this context, addition of cholesterol and other membrane tightening agents impart liposomal membrane rigidity especially in case of unsaturated phospholipids based liposomes thereby enhancing entrapment efficiency to a great extent. Moreover, it also inhibits lateral diffusion through the membrane preventing drug leakage (Akbarzadeh, Rezaei-Sadabady, Davaran, Joo, Zarghami, Hanifehpour, … Nejati-Koshki, 2013).

Surface charge plays a critical role in liposome-cell interactions and liposome-liposome interactions. Lack of surface charge can lead to aggregation of the liposomes (Siler-Marinkovic, 2016). The neutral liposome interacts with cells via simple adsorption due to non-specific hydrophobic interactions and is less significant. As a result, the drug can be released extracellularly prior to cell entry. The negative surface charge helps to increase liposome-cell interaction mainly via endocytosis and higher plasma clearance of liposomes is observed after systemic administration. The positively charged liposomes are taken up by fusion with cell membranes. Here, the lipid bilayer of liposomes fuses with the cell membrane and simultaneous drug release occurs. Cationic liposomes show enhanced cell interaction than anionic liposomes (Miller, Bondurant, McLean, McGovern, & O'Brien, 1998; Dan, 2002).

The RES rapidly removes the classical liposomes from the blood. Long-circulating liposomes were developed by polyethylene glycol modification of liposomes that prevents opsonization by RES. Smart liposomes like pH sensitive liposomes actively target solid tumors, inflamed regions and infarcts owing to the presence of slightly acidic pH. Moreover, temperature sensitive and magnetically sensitive liposomes are also explored in literature for targeted drug delivery (Sawant & Torchilin, 2010; Allen & Cullis, 2013). The classification of such smart and advanced liposomes based on their composition and properties is shown in Figure 8.

The development of liposomes has led to the invention of various other vesicular drug delivery systems which are discussed in the following sections.

Ethosomes

Liposomes have a poor skin penetration rendering practically no significance in transdermal or dermal drug delivery. There occurs accumulation of drug under skin layer due to poor skin penetration of liposomes. Ethosomes were developed with an aim to overcome this drawback and achieve efficient skin permeation (Liu, Wen, & Yang, 2012). They are highly malleable, vesicular carriers consisting of a phospholipid bilayer, high quantities of alcohol and water as shown in Figure 6. A typical ethosomal formulation consists of phospholipid (e.g. egg phosphatidylcholine), alcohol (e.g. ethanol, isopropyl alcohol), stabilizers (e.g. cholesterol), penetration enhancers (e.g. propylene glycol, transcutol), gel formers (e.g. carbopol) and water (Tyagi, Kumar, Maurya, & Kori, 2013).

The alcohol in ethosomes softens the skin lipid bilayer thereby enhancing the lipid membrane fluidity. As a result, these soft vesicles penetrate through the skin easily. Ethosomes are mainly used for transdermal and transcellular drug delivery. They enable delivery of hydrophilic as well as hydrophobic drugs and of large molecules like proteins, hormones and peptides through the skin. Besides, ethosomal drug delivery is non-toxic, user friendly and straightforward in comparison to techniques like iontophoresis. On the whole, ethosomes have paved their way into market owing to extensive applications in transdermal drug delivery (Ainbinder, Godin, & Touitou, 2016).

Transfersomes

Drug delivery through the skin is challenging owing to the outermost skin layer or stratum corneum, which acts as a barrier to any transport through it. Most of the drug carriers like liposomes, niosomes, SLNs, microemulsions and nanoemulsions face the similar problem of limited drug absorption through skin leading to deposition of drug on the skin surface. The pore size of stratum corneum is too small (<0.4 nm) to allow these drug carriers to pass through. To solve the problem of poor transdermal drug delivery, Gregor Cvec came up with Tranfersomes in the early 1990s (Cvec, 1992). Transfersomes (Figure 6), a trademark of IDEA AG, are highly deformable, flexible and elastic vesicles that consist of phospholipids like phosphatidylcholine, surfactants like Tween 80, sodium cholate, Span 80 and other additives like Myrj 45 and 49 or glycolipids or fatty oligoglycerol derivatives. These additives enhance the phospholipid bilayer adaptability and increase vesicle deformability (Benson, 2006).

Ethosomes have an ability to penetrate the skin membrane owing to significant alcohol content which softens the skin bilayer and allows the drug to penetrate through the skin. However, in the case of a non-occlusive application of ethosomes, the alcohol is lost via evaporation or transdermal diffusion rendering limited drug penetration. To achieve efficient drug delivery through skin, the vesicle carrier should remain intact while passing through the skin barrier and adapt according to the pore size. Transfersomes have a reversible ability to diminish their cross section unidirectionally to pass through a skin pore. These hydrophilic vesicles travel through the skin conduits along the natural hydration gradient present within the skin until they reach a well-hydrated point within the skin barrier. Therefore, it is advised that transfersomes must not be applied under occlusion as it blocks hydration. It has been proven that these elastic vesicles remain intact within stratum corneum but it is not substantiated that the vesicles retain their shape through the viable epidermis. A proper phospholipid-surfactant ratio is critical to achieve desired deformability and adaptability in transfersomes (Cevc & Chopra, 2016).

Transfersomes can deliver drugs into skin wherein the drug can directly diffuse in the bloodstream, deposit drug inside skin and transport drug via lymphatic drainage. The flexibility of transfersomes allows them to adapt to ambient stress and change its membrane composition reversibly and locally. The excess intra-vesicular water can flow out of the phospholipid bilayer and excess drug present on the outside of the vesicle can enter inside the deformed carrier (Benson, 2006). Transfersomes have shown a remarkable ability to deliver small molecules and large molecules like proteins and peptides through the skin. They have given an attractive alternative to iontophoresis, microneedle or electroporation methods for transdermal delivery. Transfersomes have a tremendous potential to deliver a variety of drugs efficiently through transdermal route in future.

Invasomes

After the development of ethosomes and transfersomes, a series of different vesicular drug carriers were developed. In 2002, Professor Alfred Fahr described invasomes (Figure 6), which consist of unsaturated phospholipids like soybean lecithin with high phosphatidylcholine, a mixture of terpenes like citral, d-limonene and a small amount of ethanol (Dragicevic, Verma, & Fahr, 2016). Terpenes act as permeation enhancers by enhancing the fluidity of stratum corneum lipid bilayer and impart deformability to vesicles. Lipophilic drugs display better skin penetration owing to their enhanced solubility in terpene treated stratum corneum. More the solubility in penetration enhancer better is the partition coefficient between stratum corneum/carrier and more is drug penetration. In case of hydrophilic drugs, the enhanced penetration through invasomes is due to increased diffusion coefficient caused by terpene mediated skin barrier disruption. On the whole, invasomes are believed to fragment on the upper stratum corneum layers thereby releasing its contents. The unsaturated phospholipids mix with lipid layers in the skin, modify them and thus increase penetration. Ethanol and terpenes act synergistically for permeation enhancement by fluidizing skin lipid bilayers, thereby forming microcavities, which facilitate diffusion (Dragicevic, N., Verma, D. D., & Fahr, 2016; Lakshmi, Kalpana, & Prasanthi, 2013).

Terpenes with low irritancy and Generally Regarded as Safe (GRAS) status are added in 1-5% concentration in invasomes. The presence of terpenes and ethanol make invasomes unique (Lakshmi, Kalpana, & Prasanthi, 2013). They have better penetration ability through the skin than liposomes and have facilitated delivery of a variety of drugs through the skin.

Pharmacosomes

Pharmacosomes (Figure 6) are amphiphilic, zwitterionic, colloidal bilayer vesicles wherein active hydrogen atom (-OH, -NH_2, -COOH) of drug is covalently complexed with the phosphate group of phospholipids (Ex. Phosphatidylcholine, Phosphatidylethanolamine) via esterification (Mueller-Goymann & Hamann, 1991). If the carboxylic group is not present in the drug but an active hydrogen atom like –OH, -NH_2 is present then spacers like succinic acid are used to carry out an esterification reaction (Semalty, Semalty, Rawat, Singh, & Rawat, 2009; Pandita & Sharma, 2013).

Both hydrophilic as well as lipophilic drugs can be incorporated into pharmacosomes. Unlike liposomes, there are no problems of drug leakage and removal of the unentrapped drug from the formulation as the drug is covalently bonded to the phospholipid in pharmacosomes. The drug release occurs via hydrolysis of the ester bond or by enzymatic degradation. The stability of the formulation depends on the melting point, phase transition temperature and solubility of drug-phospholipid complex. The membrane fluidity plays no role in drug release as the drug release occurs via hydrolysis. The drug release rate depends upon the rate of bond cleavage and crystallinity of drug (amorphous drugs release faster than crystalline). Further, the rate of bond cleavage can be tuned by optimizing the length of fatty acid chain in phospholipid and type of spacer (Semalty, Semalty, Rawat, Singh, & Rawat, 2009).

Since pharmacosomes are amphiphilic, they are quickly absorbed through GI tract and cell membrane, thereby rendering good bioavailability. The entrapment efficiency is quite high since it is predetermined based upon the drug-lipid complex. Pharmacosomes enable targeted drug delivery and reduction in toxicity. They tend to aggregate, fuse or hydrolyze on storage. On the whole, pharmacosomes are better drug delivery carriers for drugs with active hydrogen atoms over liposomes (Pandita & Sharma, 2013).

Phytosomes

Active constituents obtained from plants generally possess an inherent drawback of limited oral bioavailability and instability owing to their hydrophilic nature. These water-soluble phytoconstituents (e.g. flavonoids, tannins) have a large molecular size and poor lipophilicity, which hinders their entry through the cell membrane. To solve this problem, Indena® developed Phytosome® technology, which primarily conjugates a hydrophilic phytoconstituent to a phospholipid via hydrogen bonds (Indena, 2017). In phytosomes (Figure 6), phospholipid and phytoconstituent are present in a particular stoichiometric ratio of 1:2 or 2:1(Bhattacharya, 2009).

The phospholipids like phosphatidylcholine, phosphatidylserine phosphatidylethanolamine or phospholipids obtained from soy lecithin, swine or bovine are generally used for phytosome preparation. Phytosomes are lipophilic in nature, moderately soluble in fats and freely soluble in non-polar solvents. In an aqueous environment, they form micellar structure, which is similar to that of liposomes. Phytosomes enhance the oral as well as the topical bioavailability of hydrophilic phytoconstituents. This enables to reduce dose and thereby minimize toxicity. Phytosomes prevent degradation of active moiety in GI tract and enhance the stability of it. Since there is a bond formation between phytoconstituent and phospholipid, the entrapment efficiency is predetermined and good. Moreover, phytosomes are better than liposomes in transdermal and dermal drug delivery owing to their better skin penetration. Liver targeting is also possible using phytosomes. Thus, phytosomes have helped to solve many problems associated with herbal drug delivery and enabled to develop a plethora of marketed formulations of such drugs (Awasthi, Kulkarni, & Pawar, 2011;Bhattacharya, 2009).

Archaeosomes

Archaeosomes (Figure 6) are liposomes that consist of vesicles made from lipids or combination of lipids including archaeobacterial ether lipids in their composition. These archaeobacterial ether lipids have ether linkages at *sn*-2,3 glycerol carbons which attached regularly branched phytanyl chains. Their lipid membranes can be bilayer, monolayer or combination of both depending upon whether they are exclusively made from monopolar archaeol lipids, bipolar caldarchaeol lipids or their combination respectively (Patel & Sprott, 1999).

Archaeosomes are taken up by macrophages preferentially as compared to liposomes. Macrophages are of particular interest because the majority of antigen presenting cells responsible for an immune response against foreign bacteria and viruses are phagocytic in nature. Thus, archaesomes are useful carriers for the delivery of antigens or as an adjuvant responsible for immune stimulation. Archaeosomes have been found to stimulate CD8+ cytotoxic T lymphocyte response, which is an antigen-specific cell-mediated immune component. This response prevents the growth of tumor cells and tackles the growth of foreign bacteria or viruses inside the body. Archaeosomes have better resistance to phospholipase and bile salt-induced degradation and better acidic pH stability than liposomes. Besides, they are heat sterilizable. They have poor permeability than liposomes and owing to their negative charge they lack a potential for DNA antigen binding (Patel & Sprott, 1999; Prabhu & Patravale, 2014).

Cubosomes

In 1995, Larsson and his coworkers introduced the concept of cubosomes (Figure 6). Cubosomes are a colloidal dispersion of nanostructured, cubic, bicontinuous liquid crystalline particles of amphiphilic lipids (e.g. monoglyceride monoolein, phosphatidylethanolamine) in water stabilized using surfactants (e.g. poloxamer). Amphiphilic lipids self-assemble in thermodynamically stable, well-defined structures like lamellar (liposomes), hexagonal (hexosomes) and bicontinuous cubic phases (cubosomes). In case of cubosomes, a 3D honeycomb-like network is formed wherein lipid bilayer separates two distinct, continuous and non-intersecting hydrophilic sections (Karami & Hamidi, 2016).

Cubosomes have a size range of 10-300 nm and pore size of 5-10 nm. Cubosomes possess greater tolerance to rupture and higher area to particle volume ratios than liposomes. There occurs diffusion through cubosomes, which is responsible for the exchange of internal drug and water with external water. Excellent thermodynamic stability, biocompatibility and bioadhesiveness make cubosomes a great drug delivery system. The viscous nature of cubic phases enables sustained delivery of the drug through cubosomes. Hydrophobic drugs have an affinity for the lipophilic portions of cubosomes and therefore the drug release is slow. In case of hydrophilic drugs, problems like drug leakage can be prevented by incorporating surfactants which can interact with these drugs and retard their release. Moreover, incorporating charged molecules delay the release of oppositely charged drug through cubosomes. The bioadhesive nature of cubosomes has extensive applications in mucosal and topical drug delivery (Garg, Saraf, & Saraf, 2007) (Karami & Hamidi, 2016).

Cochleates

In 1975, Papahadjopoulos described cochleates for the first time. Cochleates (Figure 6) are crystalline structures consisting of spiral solid lipid bilayer sheets with little or no internal aqueous phase (Papahadjopoulos, Vail, Jacobson, & Poste, 1975). They are composed of negatively charged lipids like phosphatidylserine that fuse in the presence of a cation like calcium. Calcium has a tendency to displace water upon complex formation thereby dehydrating the membrane surface and bringing the bilayers of phosphatidylserine closer which leads to crosslinking of phosphatidylserine molecules. Therefore, little or no water is present inside the cochleates.

Cochleates form a stable spiral structure to minimize contact with external aqueous phase. This unique structure provides protection against degradation in GI tract. As a result, small molecules, large molecules and sensitive biopharmaceuticals can be delivered through cochleates via the oral route. Moreover, cochleates have been found to improve oral bioavailability of drugs. They can be easily freeze dried and reconstituted with liquid before administration (Zarif, Graybill, Perlin, & Manninoa, 2000).

Lipid Nanoparticulate Systems

Various types of lipid nanoparticulate systems are depicted in Figure 9.

Solid Lipid Nanoparticles (SLNs)

SLNs (Figure 9(a)) were developed in the early 1990s with an aim to combine the advantages of the existing colloidal drug carriers and overcome their drawbacks (R. H. Müller, Radtke, & Wissing, 2002)

. SLNs are lipid nanodispersions comprising solid lipids in an aqueous system stabilized with the help of emulsifiers. The lipids selected are solid at room and body temperature and are selected based on its biocompatibility, acceptability for the desired route of administration, solubilization capacity for the selected therapeutic agent, ease of stabilization, the rate of lipid crystallization, shape of lipid crystals and self-emulsifying ability. Few examples include mono, di and triglycerides (e.g. trilaurin, compritol), steroids (e.g. cholesterol), waxes (e.g. cetyl palmitate) and fatty acids (e.g. Palmitic acid) (Mäder & Mehnert, 2001). The emulsifier is chosen on its biocompatibility, ability to stabilize lipid dispersion, chemical nature, acceptability for the desired delivery route, drug solubilization capacity and cloud point. The SLN drug loading depends upon solubility of drug in the lipid and physical, chemical and polymorphic properties of lipid (Mäder & Mehnert, 2001). In general, the solubility of the drug must be considerably higher in solid lipid than in the emulsifier. There are three drug incorporation models in SLNs as shown in Figure 10. Their description is given in Table 2 (R. Müller, Mäder, & Gohla, 2000).

The SLNs have a highly ordered rigid lamellar crystal structure mainly due to the crystallinity of the solid lipid. Triglycerides that are commonly used in SLNs have many polymorphic forms with α and β form being the important ones. The recrystallization of lipid from the melt results into the transition from α, through a metastable β' to stable β form. The lamellar crystal lattice is the main structure for all the forms. The density and crystalline order increase from α to β form with the β form being the highest. As crystalline order increases, the ability to incorporate drugs and the rate of diffusion of drug decreases. Hence, poor drug loading is one of the major problems associated with SLNs. In general, long chain triglycerides undergo slower transformation to stable β form than short chain triglycerides. Therefore, if SLNs are produced in such a way that α form is preserved during the storage then using a trigger mechanism, natural transformation can be initiated inside the body to achieve a controlled release drug delivery system (Harms & Müller-Goymann, 2011).

The main advantages of SLNs are increased drug stability, possibility of drug targeting and controlled drug release, ease of scale-up, incorporation of both hydrophilic and lipophilic drugs, biocompatible carrier and easy sterilization.

Poor drug loading and complexity of lipid physical state are the serious drawbacks of SLNs and there was need to develop nanolipid carrier system retaining all advantages of SLNs but with higher drug loading (Naseri, Valizadeh, & Zakeri-Milani, 2015).

Nanostructured Lipid Carriers (NLCs)

In 1990s, R.H. Muller and his team realized that, a finite crystal order is responsible for molecular dispersion of drug between fatty chains of glycerides in SLNs and came with an idea to control the nanostructure of the lipid carrier to solve this problem. They observed that introduction of a liquid lipid in the solid lipid matrix increased its imperfections and flexibility leading to higher amount of drug loading. These imperfections are created due to the structural differences between liquid lipid and solid lipid thereby preventing the formation of a perfect crystal. Thus, NLCs, an unstructured solid lipid matrix consisting of a blend of liquid lipid and solid lipid dispersed in an aqueous phase using emulsifiers were developed. These modified SLNs were the first type of NLCS called as NLCs imperfect crystal type (Figure 9(b)) (Radtke & Müller, 2001). In the second type of NLCs, amorphous lipid particles are created (Figure 9(c)). As a result, the crystallinity and the resulting drug expulsion are avoided. Special precaution is needed to prevent transformation of the amorphous state into stable crystalline form during storage (Radtke & Müller, 2001). The third type of NLCs consist of lipid oil nano-compartments inside a solid lipid (Figure 9(d)). At times, drug has a higher solubility in liquid lipid than in the solid lipid. In case of SLNs, such drug solubilizes in melted lipid during the hot homogenization procedure but on cooling, the solubility of the drug reduces continuously leading to the expulsion of drug through the solid matrix. Hence in this type, melted solid lipid is mixed with liquid lipid at elevated temperatures. Using homogenization, the liquid lipid droplets are formed which are entrapped inside the solid lipid matrix upon cooling avoiding drug leakage (Radtke & Müller, 2001).

For NLCs, generally the solid lipids are mixed with liquid lipids in a ratio of 70:30 to as high as 99.9:0.1. On a whole, NLCs enable higher drug loading, enhanced stability of formulation, protection of drug from degradation and encapsulation of highly lipophilic drugs (Beloqui, Solinis, Rodriguez-Gascon, Almeida, & Preat, 2016).

Miscellaneous Nanolipid Systems

Lipid Drug Conjugates (LDCs)

Owing to their lipophilic nature, SLNs and NLCs have a poor affinity for hydrophilic drugs. As a result, the drug loading of such drugs is low. To overcome this disadvantage, LDCs were developed that consist of a drug molecule (generally hydrophilic drug molecule) conjugated to a lipid molecule (covalent linkage or salt formation). The drug can be conjugated with steroids, fatty acids, glycerides and phospholipids. The conjugation is typically in the form of ester bonds (easily cleaved), amide linkage (slow hydrolysis), disulfide bonds (cleavage in reductive environment), hydrazone bonds (pH sensitive, cleavage at acidic pH) (Figure 11) (Irby, Du, & Li, 2017). The miscellaneous bonds reported in literature include thioester linkage, carbamate bonds, phosphodiester bond etc. (Irby, Du, & Li, 2017). With LDCs, around 30-50% drug loading can be achieved but an efficient linker cleavage is essential for complete release of the drug.

LDCs make a hydrophilic drug, more lipophilic by conjugation with a lipid and thus have poor water solubility. Some LDCs can self-assemble into nanoparticles in aqueous solutions owing to their amphiphilic nature and they can be stabilized with or without using surfactants depending on the type of LDCs (e.g. squalene-based LDCs) (Prabhu & Patravale, 2014). On the contrary, most of the LDCs require specialized carriers like emulsions, micelles, lipid nanoparticles, liposomes, polymeric and inorganic nanoparticles and carbon nanotubes etc. for their delivery (Irby, Du, & Li, 2017).

LDCs provide advantages like increased drug stability, oral bioavailability, targeted drug delivery, improved drug loading, penetration into blood brain barrier, overcoming drug resistance, sustained drug release and better delivery of proteins and nucleic acids. Moreover, the research in the area is now focusing on developing stimuli sensitive LDCs to achieve site-specific drug release.

METHODS OF PREPARATION

Wide range of methods are reported in literature for formulation of lipid nanocarriers and are described below.

Emulsion Based Drug Delivery Systems

Microemulsion

Microemulsions are prepared using two techniques namely phase titration techniques and phase inversion method (Figure 12). In phase titration techniques, pseudo-ternary phase diagrams are drawn to determine the microemulsion region and find out ideal oil: water: surfactant-cosurfactant ratio for microemulsion formation (Agrawal & Agrawal, 2012). Phase Inversion occurs when the dispersed phase becomes the continuous phase. This can happen because of the addition of excess dispersed phase to a microemulsion. Moreover, heating of an o/w microemulsion above the phase inversion temperature and sudden cooling of it can result in formation of w/o microemulsion. This can occur in microemulsions prepared using non-ionic surfactants. The addition of electrolytes like sodium chloride to o/w microemulsion beyond a critical point can result into phase inversion (Moulik & Kumar, 2008).

Nanoemulsions

Initially, water soluble components are added to the aqueous phase and oil soluble components to the oily phase. Lipid phase is slowly added to the aqueous phase with continuous stirring. A homogeneous emulsion is formed. Depending upon the desired specifications, hydrophilic or lipophilic surfactant can be used to form o/w or w/o emulsion. This emulsion is then processed through energy intensive techniques like high-pressure homogenization, sonication or milling to form nanoemulsion (Gupta, Eral, Hatton, & Doyle, 2016)

Multiple Emulsions

Multiple Emulsions are prepared using double step emulsification technique and phase inversion technique. In the double step emulsification method, oil and water binary mixture is taken. An oil soluble surfactant is added to this mixture to form w/o emulsion. This is a primary emulsion generally formed using high shear techniques. Later, water and water-soluble surfactant are added to form w/o/w multiple emulsion. This secondary emulsion is formed using low shear techniques to prevent disruption of liquid membranes between inner and outer phases. Similarly, if the water-soluble surfactant is added first and oil and oil soluble surfactant later, o/w/o multiple emulsion can be obtained (Sinha & Kumar, 2002).

Phase inversion is another method wherein a multiple emulsion can be obtained by a one-step process. Here water and a hydrophilic surfactant solution are added to oil and lipophilic surfactant solution to form a w/o/w multiple emulsion. The volume fraction of aqueous phase must be above 0.7 to form a w/o/w multiple emulsion. It is essential to optimize the ratio of hydrophilic: lipophilic emulsifier (Sinha & Kumar, 2002).

SEDDS, SMEDDS and SNEDDS

The preparation method involved mixing of oil, surfactants, co-surfactants and drug to form homogenize one phase system that can be filled in solid unit dosage form as is or can be converted to solid formulations using various approached as summarized in Figure 13 (Prabhu & Patravale, 2014).

Lipid Nanovesicular Systems

Various techniques have been explored in literature for the preparation of vesicular drug delivery systems. Since ethosomes, transfersomes, pharmacosomes and invasomes are direct extensions of liposomes, their manufacturing methods are similar with minor changes depending upon the type of vesicular carrier. Table 3 summarizes the manufacturing methods for these vesicular carriers, special characteristics and their drawbacks. Besides, Figure 14 depicts the schematic outline of each of these production methods (Prabhu & Patravale, 2014).

Additionally, liposomes are also prepared using techniques like dried reconstituted vesicles (Dua, Rana, & Bhandari, 2012), double emulsion vesicles (Laouini, Sfar, Charcosset, Fessi, Jaafar-Maalej, & Limayem-Blouza, 2012), dialysis (Laouini, Sfar, Charcosset, Fessi, Jaafar-Maalej, & Limayem-Blouza, 2012) and micro-emulsification vesicles (Dua, Rana, & Bhandari, 2012) .

Phytosomes are prepared by reacting herbal extract dissolved in organic solvents like methylene chloride with phospholipid-like phosphatidylcholine. Later this solvent is evaporated under vacuum or by freeze drying (Awasthi, Kulkarni, & Pawar, 2011). In case of archeosomes, the archeal lipids are extracted from Archae biomass using solvents like methanol, chloroform or water. These lipids are then precipitated using cold acetone and resuspended in methanol/chloroform mixture. Hydration is carried out at around 35 °C to yield multilamellar archeosomes. The size of these archeosomes can be reduced using bath sonicator. Ultracentrifugation followed by washing is carried out to remove any unentrapped antigen. Finally, these archaesomes are resuspended in phosphate buffer saline or water and membrane filtration using 0.45μm filter is carried out (Krishnan & Sprott, 2008).

Cochleates are manufactured using techniques like hydrogel method, direct calcium dialysis method, trapping method, binary aqueous-aqueous emulsion system and liposomes before cochleates dialysis method. Figure 15 summarizes the schematic of each of these methods (Ravi Sankar & Dastagiri Reddy, 2010).

Cubosomes are manufactured using two techniques namely top-down approach and bottom-up approach. The top-down approach involves two steps. In the first step, lipids are mixed with a stabilizer to form viscous bulk cubic phase. In the second step, energy intensive techniques like high-pressure homogenization or sonication are used to disperse this cubic phase into the aqueous medium. Thus cubosomes are formed. The high-energy intensive process is the main drawback of this method which can also limit the incorporation of sensitive drugs like proteins and peptides.

In the bottom-up approach, a method known as solvent dilution method is used for the manufacturing of cubosomes. Here, a mixture of liquid crystal forming lipid, hydrotrope and polymer are dispersed in excess water to form nanosized cubosomes. The hydrotrope dissolves lipids, prevents the formation of viscous liquid crystal phase and creates liquid precursors. Lesser energy input, ability to incorporate sensitive materials, better efficiency in creating nanosized cubosomes, better long-term stability and easy scale-up are some of the advantages of bottom-up approach over top-down approach (Karami & Hamidi, 2016).

Lipid Nanoparticulate Systems

The manufacturing methods for various particulate drug delivery systems are quite similar with the minor changes tweaked to suit particular drug delivery system. In the following part, these techniques are discussed in detail.

High-Pressure Homogenization

This technique is commonly used for the manufacturing of SLNs and NLCs. Easy industrial scale up, improved drug loading and limited residual solvent content are some of the advantages of high pressure homogenization. There are two types of homogenization: cold homogenization and hot homogenization (Mäder & Mehnert, 2001).

Cold homogenization involves dispersion of the drug in solid lipid melt. Then the lipid melt is rapidly cooled using liquid nitrogen or dry ice and pulverized to form lipid microparticles (50-100 μm). A pre-suspension is formed by dispersing these particles into a cold surfactant solution. Later, SLNs are formed by homogenizing this pre-suspension at or below room temperature. Cold homogenization limits the melting of the lipid and thereby the loss of hydrophilic drugs to water is minimized. Thus, temperature sensitive compounds can be processed using this technique. However, it is essential that the difference between the melting point of lipid and homogenization temperature is high to prevent melting of lipid in a homogenizer (Müller, Mäder, & Gohla, 2000).

Hot homogenization involves heating above the melting point of the lipid. Here, a pre-emulsion of the drug, lipid melt and water is formed using a high shear mixer. This pre-emulsion is homogenized at 500 bar and 5-10°C temperature above the melting point of the lipid. The resulting nanoemulsion is cooled wherein solid lipid crystallizes out to form SLNs. In case of NLCs, specific changes to the homogenization method are made as mentioned in section to form the particular type of NLC (Mäder & Mehnert, 2001).

Solvent Emulsification/ Evaporation

Figure 16 depicts the schematic of this technique. There is no mechanical stress involved in this process. The presence of organic solvent is an issue in this technique (Naseri, Valizadeh, & Zakeri-Milani, 2015).

Microemulsion Template Technique

This technique involves slow addition of water, surfactant and co-surfactant solution to drug solid lipid melt mixture. Once the accurate ratio of water, lipid and surfactant: co-surfactant is fixed, a microemulsion is formed. This hot microemulsion is slowly added to cold water (2-3°C) and stirred gently to form SLNs (Müller, Mäder, & Gohla, 2000).

Supercritical Fluid Technique

Depending upon the solubility of drug in supercritical carbon dioxide, various techniques using supercritical carbon dioxide as solvent and anti-solvent can be used to manufacture particulate drug delivery systems. This technique is sustainable and no residual solvent is present. The technique is similar to solvent emulsification/evaporation technique wherein instead of an organic solvent, supercritical fluid is used (Naseri, Valizadeh, & Zakeri-Milani, 2015).

Spray Drying

In this technique, a solid drug product is produced from SLN dispersion. It is more economical than lyophilization. Owing to particle aggregation from high temperature and shear forces, this technique is not widely used for the manufacturing of SLNs (Naseri, Valizadeh, & Zakeri-Milani, 2015).

Double Emulsion Technique

In this technique, milli-Q water is inner aqueous phase which is added to dichloromethane containing lecithin and palmitin. Sonication is used to form w/o emulsion. Poloxamer solution is added to this w/o emulsion to form w/o/w double emulsion. Later, sonication is performed followed by dilution with poloxamer solution. Finally, solvent evaporation is carried out to form SLNs (Prabhu & Patravale, 2014).

High-Speed Homogenization

Hydrophilic surfactant and water mixture is heated 5-10°C above the melting point of lipid. The drug is added to solid lipid melt and heated to the same temperature. The lipid phase is slowing added to aqueous phase and stirred at high rpm to form a pre-emulsion. Sonication is used for size reduction. Subsequently, the nanoemulsion is cooled to form SLNs (Naseri, Valizadeh, & Zakeri-Milani, 2015).

CHARACTERIZATION TECHNIQUES

It is essential to analyze the formulations to understand whether they meet the desired specifications. The various lipid-based nanocarriers have similar characterization tests and are depicted in Table 4. Among these, particle size and zeta potential are very essential tests. It reveals an important information regarding size, surface charge, formulation stability, cellular interaction and permeability etc.

In addition to the tests mentioned in Table 4, there are several specific tests for different formulations. Conductivity test, Dye solubility test and fluorescence test are carried out to determine the type of microemulsion. Optical Birefringence test is used to ascertain the formation of a microemulsion. Dispersibility test is a crucial test to determine the self-emulsification ability of SEDDS, SMEDDS and SNEDDS. It helps to determine the type of emulsion and the rate of its formation in GI tract (Sachan, Khatri, & Kasture, 2010).

In case of vesicular drug delivery systems, lamellarity is an important test. It is determined using electron microscope or nuclear magnetic resonance. Degree of deformability test using extrusion method or by passing through microporous filters is carried out for vesicular drug delivery systems especially ethosomes, transfersomes and invasomes. The transition temperature for these carriers is measured using differential scanning calorimetry. The skin permeation studies are carried out for the carriers meant for transdermal delivery. Confocal laser scanning microscopy and fluorescence studies are used for this purpose. The occlusion effect is also checked for these carriers (Anwekar, Patel, & Singhai, 2011).

For particulate drug delivery systems, degree of crystallinity and lipid polymorphism are important tests (Harms & Müller-Goymann, 2011). On the whole, characterization techniques help to understand whether a formulation conforms to the specification and assures the quality of it.

APPLICATIONS OF LIPID NANOCARRIERS IN ADVANCED THERAPEUTICS

Lipid nanocarriers are the mainstream of nanotechnology based advanced healthcare systems and have been extensively explored for multiple radical therapeutic applications. An in-depth insight of these applications is given below with the help of few detailed examples along with an additional list of examples summarized in Table 5 .

Bioavailability, Permeability, and Efficacy Enhancement

Lipid nanocarriers are on the forefront for bioenhancement of poorly available drug and have proven to be effective for almost all routes of administration. This is possible because colloidal nature, lipophilicity, nanometric size and better interaction of lipid nanocarriers with biological membranes enable enhanced drug permeation and better drug solubility and/or loading.

Additionally, increased lymphatic uptake of certain lipid nanocarriers has gained an upper edge in increasing bioavailability of many drugs. This approach desires a careful selection of lipids that natively undergo lymphatic uptake and long chain lipids are considered good candidates for the same (Shete, Chatterjee, De, & Patravale, 2013). Some reported approaches include, Huperzine A SMEDDS that showed significant increase in oral bioavailability with 8 fold higher lymphatic uptake, SLNs of quetiapine fumarate that demonstrated 2.76 fold enhancement in bioavailability via lymphatic absorption and NLCs of tamoxifen with 2.71-fold bioavailability enhancement via selective intestinal lymphatic absorption pathway etc. (Li, Hu, Wang, Gui, Cheng, Gao, Ye, & Tang, 2017; Shete, Chatterjee, De, & Patravale, 2013; Yasir, Gaur, Puri, Shekar, & Kumar, 2017).

Micro and nanoemulsions of various drugs from BCS class II, III and IV have also shown promising results regarding bioavailability enhancement. Few examples include ampelopsin microemulsion, puerarin microemulsion, cyclosporine A microemulsion, baicalin nanoemulsion, silymarin nanoemulsion etc. (Hirunpanich, & Sato, 2009; Nagia, Iqbala, Kumara, Sharmaa, Alib, & Babootab, 2017; Solanki, Sarkar, & Dhanwani, 2012; Tang, Hu, Liao, Liu, & Xiang, 2013; Zhao, Wei, Huang, He, Zhou, & Fu, 2013).

Bilayered lipid vesicles have equally been investigated for bioenhancement. Yan et al. (2016), developed ethosomes of sinomenine hydrochloride (very short half-life) to enhance its bioavailability and in turn efficacy with reduced side effects for treatment of inflammatory conditions. The developed ethosomes demonstrated significant anti-inflammatory efficacy (~30.01%) in xylene-induced rodent ear edema model which can be attributed to increased skin penetration with the ethosomal carrier (Yan, Zhang, Sun, Wang, Dong, Dong, & Xing, 2016). In another investigation, phytosomes of quercetin (Size: ~70 nm) were developed that proved significant bioenhancement with the desired improvement in lipid profile, elevated calcium, inorganic phosphorus, glutathione content and reduced tumor necrosis factors and glucose level. Thus, the novel delivery platform herein presented a superior alternative for hormone replacement therapy instead of plain drug (Abd El-Fattah, Fathy, Ali, El-Garawany, & Mohamed, 2017).

In recent years, LDCs are emerging as novel adducts for bioenhancement by improving drug lipophilicity (Irby, Du & Li, 2017). In one study, LDCs of an anticancer drug, pemetrexed diacid salt with stearic acid were synthesized followed by the development of LDC nanoparticles (size: ~ 120nm). The developed system allowed oral delivery of the drug with almost 4.22-fold enhancement in bioavailability as compared to plain drug suspension. This can be attributed to enhanced GI permeation of complex which was also corroborated using ex vivo gut permeation studies (Soni Mujtaba, & Kohli, 2017). Interestingly, many LDCs have made it to early clinical studies which confirm their potential in future medicine. Some examples include gemcitabine LDC-CP4126 to overcome drug resistance with reduced drug toxicity in pancreatic cancer treatment (Venugopal, Awada, Evans, Dueland, Hendlisz, Rasch, … Aamdal, 2015), cytarabine 5′-monophosphate LDC with fatty alcohol (cytarabine ocfosfate) for better efficacy in hematological malignancies (as cited in Alexander, Kucera, & Pardee, 2016).

Controlled and Sustained Drug Delivery

Lipid nanocarriers play a key role in development of controlled release drug delivery systems as they offer advantages in terms of improved therapy and/ or patient compliance, efficacy, reduced drug dose and/or dosing frequency. Thus they are efficient in arresting associated drug toxicity, side-effects and resistance. For example, N-acetyl-L-carnosine is a prodrug of L-carnosine used for cataract treatment. L-carnosine is highly sensitive, degradable and hydrophilic dipeptide. Therefore, when it is given as eye drops, it cannot exhibit desired controlled or sustained release profile. For this, Abdelkader et al. (2016) developed L-carnosine phytosomes-hyaluronic acid systems (size: 380-450 nm) as controlled release ocular delivery platform. The phytosomal formulation controlled permeation across cornea significantly and retained human corneal cell viability. Additionally, the studies with ex vivo porcine lenses demonstrated higher efficacy in lens brunescence inhibition indicating a delay in cataractogenesis induced ill effects (Abdelkader, Longman, Alany, & Pierscionek, 2016).

In Hemophilia A, life-threatening bleeding occurs due to deficiency of factor VIII and first line treatment requires a replacement therapy with recombinant factor VIII. Currently, 15-30% patients develop neutralizing antibody against it thereby failing to respond to this treatment. As a solution, cochleates of recombinant factor VIII were developed (size: $\leq$ 500 nm) in which 75% of protein factor VIII was associated with cochleate complex lipid matrix followed by a slow and sustained release which inhibited high exposure of protein in the bloodstream and thus restricted the autoimmune response. Hence, the treatment efficacy restored and the hypothesis was further proven in mice model (Miclea, Varma, Peng, & Balu-Iyer, 2007).

In some cases, lipid nanocarriers can further be modified to achieve controlled release profiles. For example, Pham et al. (2017) developed mucoadhesive wafers comprising microemulsion of a model drug, mucoadhesive agent and mannitol for controlled buccal delivery. The wafer exhibited increased retention time in ex vivo studies with sustained drug release profile up to 6 hours (Pham, Van, Vo, Tran, Tran, & Tran, 2017). In another study, thermoresponsive microemulsion gel of 5-fluorouracil was developed for the treatment of colorectal cancer. The formulation exhibited tumor site-specific sustained and targeted drug release up to 10 hours owing to gel thermoresponsive properties. The formulation also demonstrated almost 5-fold higher intracellular uptake with reduced systemic and rectal side effects (Wang, Huang, Guo, Han, Zheng, & Jiang, 2016).

Stability Enhancement

Lipid nanocarriers allow stabilization of drugs by multiple pathways viz. entrapment in lipid matrix, restricting exposure to enzymatic and/or environmental degradation factors etc. Thus they form a premier option for stable formulation development of otherwise unstable drugs. For instance, pH and enzymatic stabilization of peptides are fundamental challenges. To address this, Boge et al. formulated cubosomes of antimicrobial peptides. The cubosomal formulation offered stability to antimicrobial peptide LL-37against proteolytic degradation and thereby resulted in superior antibacterial efficacy as compared to plain peptide (Boge, Umerska, Matougui, Bysell, Ringstad, Davoudi, … Andersson, 2017). However, as peptide size increases, effective delivery becomes an additional challenge. Consider the example of large peptide drug insulin. To impart stabilization with enhanced transdermal permeation, Malakar et al. (2017), developed transferosomal gel of insulin and delivered it via iontophoresis. The formulation proposed superior in vitro permeation flux and demonstrated sustained in vivo hypoglycemic effect in alloxan-induced diabetic rats. Additionally, the therapy could be considered more patient compliant considering its non-invasive nature and sustained delivery (Malakar, Sen, Nayak, & Sen, 2017).

Antioxidants are another sensitive class of drugs prone to degradation by auto-oxidation, pH, UV radiation etc. For their stabilization, a wide arena of lipid nanocarriers has been explored that includes resveratrol microemulsion for drug photostabilization, SNEDDS, phytosomes of curcumin etc. (Joshi, Negi, Kumar, Pawar, Munjal, Bansal, & Sharma, 2013; Juškaitė, Ramanauskienė, & Briedis, 2017; Mirzaei, Shakeri, Rashidi, Jalili, Banikazemi, & Sahebkar, 2017).

Toxicity Reduction

Drugs with low therapeutic index, side effects and non-site specific toxicities pose a great therapy challenge. Nanocarriers systems have been successfully designed to tackle these issues with lipid nanocarriers being at the forefront.

Docetaxel is prescribed as an adjuvant chemotherapeutic drug for the treatment of multiple solid tumors but causes severe myelosuppression toxicity. Yual et al. (2014) developed SLNs of docetaxel for the treatment of breast cancer. The studies confirmed a significant reduction in myelosuppression toxicity to mice bone marrow cells compared to commercial docetaxel (Taxotere®). They also demonstrated very effective tumor suppression in the human xenograft breast cancer mice model (Yuan, Han, Cong, Ge, Ma, Dai, … Bi, 2014). In another study, systemic toxicity of docetaxel SLNs was compared against Taxotere® in multiple animal models. In mice, docetaxel SLNs exhibited more than two fold higher maximum tolerated dose than marketed product. In Beagle dogs, weekly iv infusion of docetaxel SLNs at a dose of 4mg/kg for four weeks did not show any abnormal reactions whereas Taxotere® showed severe toxicity even at a dose of 1mg/kg. Thus, lipid nanocarrier system implied promising toxicity reduction (Gao, Yang, Zhang, Chen, Sun, & Li, 2010)

Another anticancer drug, cisplatin, is used in the treatment of peritoneal, testicle, ovarian, and lung carcinomas but associates itself with mucositis toxicity causing intestinal epithelium alterations. To overcome this, Araújo et al. developed long-circulating and pH-sensitive liposomes of cisplatin and experimentally proved lesser inflammatory infiltration, better histological parameters, reduced intestinal damage and possible recovery after 72 hours post treatment as compared to plain cisplatin treatment in mice model. This can be attributed to the reduced presentation of cisplatin directly at the intestinal epithelium using the modified liposomal system. (Araújo, Silveira, De Sales E Souza, Freire, De Souza, Reis, … Cardoso, 2017)

Targeted Drug Delivery

Achieving cell-specific targeting through nanocarriers is an extremely popular approach amongst scientist as it allows enhanced site-specific delivery and addresses issues related to non-site specific toxicities. Surface coating with a specific ligand, stimuli sensitization, modulation of size, shape, lipid composition, are amongst the most widely explored approaches to achieve the same. Some examples of surface modified target lipid nanocarrier include poly-ε-lysine (PεL)-coated cubosomes for endosomal uptake via energy-dependent pathways (Deshpande & Singh, 2017), chitosan coated microemulsion for efficient dermal delivery (Kumari, & Kesavan, 2017), chitosan stabilized camptothecin nanoemulsion for enhanced breast cancer targeting (Natesan, Sugumaran, Ponnusamy, Thiagarajan, Palanichamy, & Kandasamy, 2017), mucoadhesive nanoemulsion of quercetin for brain targeting using intranasal route (Ahmad, Ahmad, Naqvi, Alam, Ashafaq, Abdur Rub, & Ahmad, 2017) and surface modified SLNs using apolipoprotein E-derived peptide for brain targeting (Dal Magro, Ornaghi, Cambianica, Beretta, Re, Musicanti, … Sancini, 2017) etc.

In an interesting study, Ilbasmis-Tamer et al. developed a pH responsive doxorubicin lipid nanotubes comprising specially designed lipid molecule named AQUA [AQ-NH-$(CH_2)_{10}$COOH (AQ: anthraquinone group] for the treatment of colorectal cancer. The formulation exhibited an increase in drug loading with pH increase to reach maximum loading of 96% at pH 9 and showed drug release at lower pH value making it very suitable for accurate delivery at tumor sites exhibiting lower pH. The developed formulation was observed to be stable, non-toxic, biocompatible and biodegradable thus showing great potential in targeted colorectal carcinomas (Ilbasmis-Tamer, Unsal, Tugcu-Demiroz, Kalaycioglu, Degim,, & Aydogan, 2016)

Ethosomes, are comprehensively investigated to modulate the topical delivery of drugs. An antifungal drug, griseofulvin was incorporated in ethosomes (size: ~130nm) to overcome its low solubility and permeation resulting into poor deposition and bioavailability. Upon application, the nano size allowed localization of formulation in stratum corneum and the precise targeting to skin dermatophytes was proved through the skin diffusion assay (Marto, Vitor, Guerreiro, Severino, Eleutério, Ascenso, & Simões, 2016). For phytoconstituent delivery, Kumar et al. (2014) developed phytosomes of a hepatoprotective agent silymarine to achieve liver and inflammatory cell targeting. Upon oral administration, phytosomes exhibited enhanced selective hepatoprotection against paracetamol-induced hepatotoxicity in Wister rats. The formulation also demonstrated 3.5-fold higher bioavailability as compared to silymarine suspension (Kumar, Rai, Reddy, Raj, Jain, Deshpande, … Rao, 2014).

In another study, invasomes of Temoporfin were developed (size: <150nm) for photodynamic therapy of malignant or non-malignant cutaneous diseases. The invasomes exhibited significantly high deposition in stratum corneum as compared to liposomes and ethanolic solution. The formulation also showed significantly better efficacy in epidermoid tumor cell line A431 as compared to ethanoic solution, but the efficacy was observed to be similar in human colorectal tumor cell line HT29. Thus, the technology established its high potential in the treatment of superficial cutaneous malignancies with better and desired drug deposition properties (Dragicevic-Curic, Gräfe, Gitter, & Fahr, 2010; Dragicevic-Curic, Scheglmann, Albrecht, & Fahr, 2008). Scientists have also successfully developed invasomal gel of isotretenoin with an ability to specifically target the pilosebaceous follicular unit of the skin for treatment of Eosinophilic pustular folliculitis which is an HIV associated secondary symptom (Dwivedi, Sharma, & Pathak, 2017).

Specific lipid composition mediated cellular targeting is a unique approach and requires extremely meticulous selection of lipids. For example, Jain et al. reported NLCs comprising a lipid glyceryl-dilaurate with particular potential to target infected red blood cells (RBCs) only and have demonstrated proof of concept in malaria model using Plasmodium-infected RBCs (Jain, Garg, Kushwah, Thanki, Agrawal, & Dora, 2014).

Theranostics

Multifunctional nanocarriers are now revolutionizing the field of nanocarrier research and amongst those, nanocarriers allowing simultaneous therapy and diagnosis (theranostic) are of highest priority.

Lipid nanocarriers have made tremendous progress in this field (Charron, Chen, & Zhang, 2015). In one interesting study, transfersomal gel of vasodilator papaverine hydrochloride was developed for diagnosis and treatment of erectile dysfunction. Conventionally, a painful penile injection of the drug is used for this purpose. Development of tranferosomes not only presented an alternative to otherwise painful therapy but also showed significant result ($P<0.05$) in terms of dilating the desired cavernous artery allowing relief (Ali, Salem, Abdelmohsen, & Attia, 2015). Lozano et al. reported a novel targeted theranostic SLN system comprising dye indocyanine green (diagnosis) and drug doxorubicin (breast cancer therapeutic) which was functionalized with humanized antibody targeting Mucin 1 receptor (MUC-1) which is overexpressed in breast cancer. The strategy proved enhanced efficacy with breast cancer targeting in mice model (Lozano, Al-Ahmady, Beziere, Ntziachristos, & Kostarelos, 2015).

Thus, in a nutshell, lipid nanocarriers offer a wide range of therapeutic benefits and behold great future in clinical medicine.

MARKET STATUS, FUTURE PROSPECT, AND CONCLUSION

A significant number of lipid nanocarrier based formulations have already made their way in advanced clinical trials and many have become market reality (Table 6). This clearly portrays their market potential in near future. However, comparatively low drug loading and high formulation bulk is still an unmet challenge for some types of lipid nanocarriers and further breakthroughs in this area are desired.

Overall, pharmaceutical sector has witnessed the unprecedented growth in the field of lipid nanocarriers over the past few decades and their potential is widely accepted as advanced healthcare systems.

REFERENCES

Abd El-Fattah, A. I., Fathy, M. M., Ali, Z. Y., El-Garawany, A. E. A., & Mohamed, E. K. (2017). Enhanced therapeutic benefit of quercetin-loaded phytosome nanoparticles in ovariectomized rats. *Chemico-Biological Interactions*, *271*, 30–38. doi:10.1016/j.cbi.2017.04.026 PMID:28460884

Abdelkader, H., Longman, M. R., Alany, R. G., & Pierscionek, B. (2016). Phytosome-hyaluronic acid systems for ocular delivery of L-carnosine. *International Journal of Nanomedicine*, *11*, 2815–2827. doi:10.2147/IJN.S104774 PMID:27366062

Agrawal, O. P., & Agrawal, S. (2012). An overview of new drug delivery system: Microemulsions. *Asian Journal of Pharmaceutical Science & Technology*, *2*(1), 5–12.

Ahmad, N., Ahmad, R., Naqvi, A. A., Alam, M. A., Ashafaq, M., Abdur Rub, R., & Ahmad, F. J. (2017). Intranasal delivery of quercetin-loaded mucoadhesive nanoemulsion for treatment of cerebral ischaemia. *Artificial Cells, Nanomedicine, and Biotechnology*, *12*, 1–13. PMID:28604104

Ainbinder, D., Godin, B., & Touitou, E. (2016). Ethosomes: Enhanced Delivery of Drugs to and Across the Skin. In Percutaneous Penetration Enhancers Chemical Methods in Penetration Enhancement (pp. 61–75). Berlin: Springer Berlin Heidelberg. doi:10.1007/978-3-662-47862-2_4

Akbarzadeh, A., Rezaei-Sadabady, R., Davaran, S., Joo, S. W., Zarghami, N., Hanifehpour, Y., ... Nejati-Koshki, K. (2013). Liposome: Classification, preparation, and applications. *Nanoscale Research Letters*, *8*(1), 102. doi:10.1186/1556-276X-8-102 PMID:23432972

Al Shuwaili, A. H., Rasool, B. K., & Abdulrasool, A. A. (2016). Optimization of elastic transfersomes formulations for transdermal delivery of pentoxifylline. *European Journal of Pharmaceutics and Biopharmaceutics*, *102*, 101–114. doi:10.1016/j.ejpb.2016.02.013 PMID:26925505

Alavi, S. E., Mansouri, H., Esfahani, M. K., Movahedi, F., Akbarzadeh, A., & Chiani, M. (2014). Archaeosome: As new drug carrier for delivery of Paclitaxel to breast cancer. *Indian Journal of Clinical Biochemistry*, *29*(2), 150–153. doi:10.100712291-013-0305-4 PMID:24757295

Alexander, P., Kucera, G., & Pardee, T. S. (2016). Improving nucleoside analogs via lipid conjugation: Is fatter any better? *Critical Reviews in Oncology/Hematology*, *100*, 46–56. doi:10.1016/j.critrevonc.2016.01.015 PMID:26829896

Ali, M. F., Salem, H. F., Abdelmohsen, H. F., & Attia, S. K. (2015). Preparation and clinical evaluation of nano-transferosomes for treatment of erectile dysfunction. *Drug Design, Development and Therapy*, *9*, 2431–2447. doi:10.2147/DDDT.S81236 PMID:25995616

Allam, A. N., Komeil, I. A., & Abdallah, O. Y. (2015). Curcumin phytosomal softgel formulation: Development, optimization and physicochemical characterization. *Acta Pharmaceutica (Zagreb, Croatia)*, *65*(3), 285–297. doi:10.1515/acph-2015-0029 PMID:26431106

Allen, T. M., & Cullis, P. R. (2013). Liposomal drug delivery systems: From concept to clinical applications. *Advanced Drug Delivery Reviews*, *65*(1), 36–48. doi:10.1016/j.addr.2012.09.037 PMID:23036225

Anwekar, H., Patel, S., & Singhai, A. (2011). Liposome- as drug carriers. *International Journal of Pharmacy & Life Sciences*, *2*, 945–951.

Araújo, R. S., Silveira, A. L. M., De Sales, E., Souza, É. L., Freire, R. H., De Souza, C. M., ... Cardoso, V. N. (2017). Intestinal toxicity evaluation of long-circulating and pH sensitive liposomes loaded with cisplatin. *European Journal of Pharmaceutical Sciences*, *106*, 142–151. doi:10.1016/j.ejps.2017.05.046 PMID:28546107

Awasthi, R., Kulkarni, G. T., & Pawar, V. K. (2011). Phytosomes: An approach to increase the bioavailability of plant extracts. *International Journal of Pharmacy and Pharmaceutical Sciences*, *3*(2), 1–3.

Bangham, A. D., & Horne, R. W. (1964). Negative staining of phospholipids and their structural modification by surface-active agents as observed in the electron microscope. *Journal of Molecular Biology*, *8*(5), 660–IN10. doi:10.1016/S0022-2836(64)80115-7 PMID:14187392

Baowan, D., & Thamwattana, N. (2014). Modelling encapsulation of gold and silver nanoparticles inside lipid nanotubes. *Physica A*, *396*, 149–154. doi:10.1016/j.physa.2013.11.003

Batista-Duharte, A., Lastre, M., Romeu, B., Portuondo, D. L., Téllez-Martínez, D., & Manente, F. A. … Carlos, I. Z. (2016). Antifungal and immunomodulatory activity of a novel cochleate for amphotericin B delivery against Sporothrix schenckii. *International Immunopharmacology*. doi:10.1016/j.intimp.2016.09.008

Beloqui, A., Solinis, M. A., Rodriguez-Gascon, A., Almeida, A. J., & Preat, V. (2016). Nanostructured lipid carriers: Promising drug delivery systems for future clinics. *Nanomedicine; Nanotechnology, Biology, and Medicine*, *12*(1), 143–161. doi:10.1016/j.nano.2015.09.004 PMID:26410277

Benson, H. A. (2006). Transfersomes for transdermal drug delivery. *Expert Opinion on Drug Delivery*, *3*(6), 727–737. doi:10.1517/17425247.3.6.727 PMID:17076595

Bhattacharya, S. (2009). Phytosomes: The new technology for enhancement of bioavailability of botanicals and nutraceuticals. *International Journal of Health Research*, *2*(3), 225–232. doi:10.4314/ijhr.v2i3.47905

Boge, L., Umerska, A., Matougui, N., Bysell, H., Ringstad, L., Davoudi, M., ... Andersson, M. (2017). Cubosomes post-loaded with antimicrobial peptides: Characterization, bactericidal effect and proteolytic stability. *International Journal of Pharmaceutics*, *526*(1-2), 400–412. doi:10.1016/j.ijpharm.2017.04.082 PMID:28476579

Castilho-Fernandes, A., Lopes, T. G., Primo, F. L., Pinto, M. R., & Tedesco, A. C. (2017). Photodynamic process induced by chloro-aluminum phthalocyanine nanoemulsion in glioblastoma. *Photodiagnosis and Photodynamic Therapy,* S1572-1000(17)30195-3.

Cevc, G., & Chopra, A. (2016). Deformable (Transfersome®) vesicles for improved drug delivery into and through the skin. In Percutaneous Penetration Enhancers Chemical Methods in Penetration Enhancement (pp. 39–59). Berlin: Springer Berlin Heidelberg. doi:10.1007/978-3-662-47862-2_3

Chang, C. C., Liu, D. Z., Lin, S. Y., Liang, H. J., Hou, W. C., Huang, W. J., ... Liang, Y. C. (2008). Liposome encapsulation reduces cantharidin toxicity. *Food and Chemical Toxicology*, *46*(9), 3116–3121. doi:10.1016/j.fct.2008.06.084 PMID:18652872

Charron, D. M., Chen, J., & Zheng, G. (2015). Theranostic lipid nanoparticles for cancer medicine. *Cancer Treatment and Research*, *166*, 103–127. doi:10.1007/978-3-319-16555-4_5 PMID:25895866

Chourasia, M. K., Kang, L., & Chan, S. Y. (2011). Nanosized ethosomes bearing ketoprofen for improved transdermal delivery. *Results in Pharma Sciences*, *1*(1), 60–67. doi:10.1016/j.rinphs.2011.10.002 PMID:25755983

Crowley, M. (2013). Solutions, Emulsions, Suspensions, and Extracts. In L. Felton (Ed.), Remington: Essentials of Pharmaceutics (Vol. 1st, pp. 435–468). Pharmaceutical Press.

Cvec, G. (1992). *Preparation for drug application in minute droplet form*. European Patent Office.

Dal Magro, R., Ornaghi, F., Cambianica, I., Beretta, S., Re, F., Musicanti, C., ... Sancini, G. (2017). ApoE-modified solid lipid nanoparticles: A feasible strategy to cross the blood-brain barrier. *Journal of Controlled Release*, *249*, 103–110. doi:10.1016/j.jconrel.2017.01.039 PMID:28153761

Dan, N. (2002). Effect of liposome charge and PEG polymer layer thickness on cell? liposome electrostatic interactions. *Biochimica et Biophysica Acta (BBA) - Biomembranes*, *1564*(2), 343–348. doi:10.1016/S0005-2736(02)00468-6 PMID:12175916

Das, B., Sen, S. O., Maji, R., Nayak, A. K., & Sen, K. K. (2017). Transferosomal gel for transdermal delivery of risperidone: Formulation optimization and ex vivo permeation. *Journal of Drug Delivery Science and Technology*, *38*, 59–71. doi:10.1016/j.jddst.2017.01.006

Del Campo, J., Lindqvist, M., Cuello, M., Bäckström, M., Cabrerra, O., Persson, J., ... Harandi, A. M. (2010). Intranasal immunization with a proteoliposome-derived cochleate containing recombinant gD protein confers protective immunity against genital herpes in mice. *Vaccine*, *28*(5), 1193–1200. doi:10.1016/j.vaccine.2009.11.035 PMID:19945418

Deshpande, S., & Singh, N. (2017). Influence of cubosome surface architecture on its cellular uptake mechanism. *Langmuir*, *33*(14), 3509–3516. doi:10.1021/acs.langmuir.6b04423 PMID:28325047

Dragicevic, N., Verma, D. D., & Fahr, A. (2016). Invasomes: Vesicles for enhanced skin delivery of drugs. In Percutaneous Penetration Enhancers Chemical Methods in Penetration Enhancement (pp. 77–92). Berlin: Springer Berlin Heidelberg. doi:10.1007/978-3-662-47862-2_5

Dragicevic-Curic, N., Gräfe, S., Gitter, B., & Fahr, A. (2010). Efficacy of temoporfin-loaded invasomes in the photodynamic therapy in human epidermoid and colorectal tumour cell lines. *Journal of Photochemistry and Photobiology. B, Biology*, *101*(3), 238–250. doi:10.1016/j.jphotobiol.2010.07.009 PMID:20797872

Dragicevic-Curic, N., Scheglmann, D., Albrecht, V., & Fahr, A. (2008). Temoporfin-loaded invasomes: Development, characterization and in vitro skin penetration studies. *Journal of Controlled Release*, *127*(1), 59–69. doi:10.1016/j.jconrel.2007.12.013 PMID:18281119

Dua, J. S., Rana, A. C., & Bhandari, A. K. (2012). Liposome: Methods of preparation and applications. *International Journal of Pharmaceutical Studies and Research*, *3*(2), 14–20.

Duangjit, S., Nimcharoenwan, T., Chomya, N., Locharoenrat, N., & Ngawhirunpat, T. (2016). Design and development of optimal invasomes for transdermal drug delivery using computer program. *Asian Journal of Pharmaceutical Sciences*, *11*(1), 52–53. doi:10.1016/j.ajps.2015.10.039

Dwivedi, M., Sharma, V., & Pathak, K. (2017). Pilosebaceous targeting by isotretenoin-loaded invasomal gel for the treatment of eosinophilic pustular folliculitis: Optimization, efficacy and cellular analysis. *Drug Development and Industrial Pharmacy*, *43*(2), 293–304. doi:10.1080/03639045.2016.1239628 PMID:27649797

El-Komy, M., Shalaby, S., Hegazy, R., Abdel Hay, R., Sherif, S., & Bendas, E. (2016). Assessment of cubosomal alpha lipoic acid gel efficacy for the aging face: A single-blinded, placebo-controlled, right-left comparative clinical study. *Journal of Cosmetic Dermatology*. doi:10.1111/jocd.12298 PMID:27873449

Elitez, Y., Ekinci, M., Ilem-Ozdemir, D., Gundogdu, E., & Asikoglu, M. (2017). Tc-99m Radiolabeled Alendronate Sodium Microemulsion: Characterization and Permeability Studies across Caco-2 Cells. *Current Drug Delivery*. doi:10.2174/1567201814666170613082752 PMID:28606033

Gao, Y., Yang, R., Zhang, Z., Chen, L., Sun, Z., & Li, Y. (2011). Solid lipid nanoparticles reduce systemic toxicity of docetaxel: Performance and mechanism in animal. *Nanotoxicology*, *5*(4), 636–649. doi:10.3109/17435390.2010.551427 PMID:21306192

Garg, G., Saraf, S., & Saraf, S. (2007). Cubosomes: An Overview. *Biological & Pharmaceutical Bulletin*, *30*(2), 350–353. doi:10.1248/bpb.30.350 PMID:17268078

Ghanbarzadeh, S., & Arami, A. (2013). Formulation and evaluation of piroxicam transferosomal gel: An approach for penetration enhancement. *Journal of Drug Delivery Science and Technology*, *23*(6), 587–590. doi:10.1016/S1773-2247(13)50089-X

Ghanbarzadeh, S., Hariri, R., Kouhsoltani, M., Shokri, J., Javadzadeh, Y., & Hamishehkar, H. (2015). Enhanced stability and dermal delivery of hydroquinone using solid lipid nanoparticles. *Colloids and Surfaces. B, Biointerfaces*, *136*, 1004–1010. doi:10.1016/j.colsurfb.2015.10.041 PMID:26579567

Gupta, A., Eral, H. B., Hatton, T. A., & Doyle, P. S. (2016). Nanoemulsions: Formation, properties and applications. *Soft Matter*, *12*(11), 2826–2841. doi:10.1039/C5SM02958A PMID:26924445

Harms, M., & Müller-Goymann, C. C. (2011). Solid lipid nanoparticles for drug delivery. *Journal of Drug Delivery Science and Technology*, *21*(1), 89–99. doi:10.1016/S1773-2247(11)50008-5

He, R., Cui, D., & Gao, F. (2009). Preparation of fluorescence ethosomes based on quantum dots and their skin scar penetration properties. *Materials Letters*, *63*(20), 1662–1664. doi:10.1016/j.matlet.2009.05.003

Hirunpanich, V., & Sato, H. (2009). Improvement of cyclosporine A bioavailability by incorporating ethyl docosahexaenoate in the microemulsion as an oil excipient. *European Journal of Pharmaceutics and Biopharmaceutics*, *73*(2), 247–252. doi:10.1016/j.ejpb.2009.06.011 PMID:19560537

Huang, J., Peng, T., Li, Y., Zhan, Z., Zeng, Y., & Huang, Y., … Wu, C. (2017). Ocular cubosome drug delivery system for timolol maleate: Preparation, characterization, cytotoxicity, ex vivo, and in vivo evaluation. *AAPS PharmSciTech*. doi:10.120812249-017-0763-8

Ilbasmis-Tamer, S., Unsal, H., Tugcu-Demiroz, F., Kalaycioglu, G. D., Degim, I. T., & Aydogan, N. (2016). Stimuli-responsive lipid nanotubes in gel formulations for the delivery of doxorubicin. *Colloids and Surfaces. B, Biointerfaces*, *143*, 406–414. doi:10.1016/j.colsurfb.2016.03.070 PMID:27037777

Indena. (2017). *Phytosome*. Retrieved June 26, 2017, from https://www.phytosome.info/

Irby, D., Du, C., & Li, F. (2017). Lipid-drug conjugate for enhancing drug delivery. *Molecular Pharmaceutics*, *14*(5), 1325–1338. doi:10.1021/acs.molpharmaceut.6b01027 PMID:28080053

Jain, S., Garg, T., Kushwah, V., Thanki, K., Agrawal, A. K., & Dora, C. P. (2017). 1.α-Tocopherol as functional excipient for resveratrol and coenzyme Q10-loaded SNEDDS for improved bioavailability and prophylaxis of breast cancer. *Journal of Drug Targeting*, *25*(6), 554–565. doi:10.1080/1061186X.2017.1298603 PMID:28274130

Jain, S. A., Basu, H., Prabhu, P. S., Soni, U., Joshi, M. D., Mathur, D., ... Sharma, S. (2014). Parasite impairment by targeting Plasmodium-infected RBCs using glyceryl-dilaurate nanostructured lipid carriers. *Biomaterials*, *35*(24), 6636–6645. doi:10.1016/j.biomaterials.2014.04.058 PMID:24818881

Joshi, R. P., Negi, G., Kumar, A., Pawar, Y. B., Munjal, B., Bansal, A. K., & Sharma, S. S. (2013). SNEDDS curcumin formulation leads to enhanced protection from pain and functional deficits associated with diabetic neuropathy: An insight into its mechanism for neuroprotection. *Nanomedicine (London)*, *9*(6), 776–785. doi:10.1016/j.nano.2013.01.001 PMID:23347896

Juškaitė, V., Ramanauskienė, K., & Briedis, V. (2017). Testing of resveratrol microemulsion photostability and protective effect against UV induced oxidative stress. *Acta Pharmaceutica (Zagreb, Croatia)*, *67*(2), 247–256. doi:10.1515/acph-2017-0018 PMID:28590913

Karami, Z., & Hamidi, M. (2016). Cubosomes: Remarkable drug delivery potential. *Drug Discovery Today*, *21*(5), 789–801. doi:10.1016/j.drudis.2016.01.004 PMID:26780385

Kohli, K., Chopra, S., Dhar, D., Arora, S., & Khar, R. K. (2010). Self-emulsifying drug delivery systems: An approach to enhance oral bioavailability. *Drug Discovery Today*, *15*(21–22), 958–965. doi:10.1016/j.drudis.2010.08.007 PMID:20727418

Krishnan, L., & Sprott, G. D. (2008). Archaeosome adjuvants: Immunological capabilities and mechanism(s) of action. *Vaccine*, *26*(17), 2043–2055. doi:10.1016/j.vaccine.2008.02.026 PMID:18343538

Kumar, N., Rai, A., Reddy, N. D., Raj, P. V., Jain, P., Deshpande, P., ... Rao, C. M. (2014). Silymarin liposomes improves oral bioavailability of silybin besides targeting hepatocytes, and immune cells. *Pharmacological Reports*, *66*(5), 788–798. doi:10.1016/j.pharep.2014.04.007 PMID:25149982

Kumari, B., & Kesavan, K. (2017). Effect of chitosan coating on microemulsion for effective dermal clotrimazole delivery. *Pharmaceutical Development and Technology*, *22*(4), 617–626. doi:10.1080/10837450.2016.1230629 PMID:27574791

Lakshmi, P., Kalpana, B., & Prasanthi, D. (2013). Invasomes-novel vesicular carriers for enhanced skin permeation. *Systematic Reviews in Pharmacy*, *4*(1), 26. doi:10.4103/0975-8453.135837

Laouini, A., Sfar, S., Charcosset, C., Fessi, H., Jaafar-Maalej, C., & Limayem-Blouza, I. (2012). Preparation, characterization and applications of liposomes. *Journal of Colloid Science and Biotechnology*, *1*(2), 147–168. doi:10.1166/jcsb.2012.1020

Li, F., Hu, R., Wang, B., Gui, Y., Cheng, G., Gao, S., ... Tang, J. (2017). Self-microemulsifying drug delivery system for improving the bioavailability of huperzine A by lymphatic uptake. *Acta Pharmaceutica Sinica. B*, *7*(3), 353–360. doi:10.1016/j.apsb.2017.02.002 PMID:28540173

Li, G., Fan, Y., Fan, C., Li, X., Wang, X., Li, M., & Liu, Y. (2012). Tacrolimus-loaded ethosomes: Physicochemical characterization and in vivo evaluation. *European Journal of Pharmaceutics and Biopharmaceutics*, *82*(1), 49–57. doi:10.1016/j.ejpb.2012.05.011 PMID:22705640

Liu, Y. S., Wen, C. F., & Yang, Y. M. (2012). Development of ethosome-like catanionic vesicles for dermal drug delivery. *Journal of the Taiwan Institute of Chemical Engineers*, *43*(6), 830–838. doi:10.1016/j.jtice.2012.06.008

Lobovkina, T., Jacobson, G. B., Gonzalez-Gonzalez, E., Hickerson, R. P., Leake, D., Kaspar, R. L., ... Zare, R. N. (2011). In vivo sustained release of sirna from solid lipid nanoparticles. *ACS Nano*, *5*(12), 9977–9983. doi:10.1021/nn203745n PMID:22077198

Lozano, N., Al-Ahmady, Z. S., Beziere, N. S., Ntziachristos, V., & Kostarelos, K. (2015). Monoclonal antibody-targeted PEGylated liposome-ICG encapsulating doxorubicin as a potential theranostic agent. *International Journal of Pharmaceutics*, *484*(1-2), 2–10. doi:10.1016/j.ijpharm.2014.10.045 PMID:25445515

Lu, P. S., Inbaraj, B. S., & Chen, B. H. (2017). Determination of oral bioavailability of curcuminoid dispersions and nanoemulsions prepared from curcuma longa linnaeus. *Journal of the Science of Food and Agriculture*. doi:10.1002/jsfa.8437 PMID:28516478

Mäder, K., & Mehnert, W. (2001). Solid lipid nanoparticles: Production, characterization and applications. *Advanced Drug Delivery Reviews*, *47*(2–3), 165–196. doi:10.1016/S0169-409X(01)00105-3 PMID:11311991

Malakar, J., Sen, S., Nayak, A. K., & Sen, K. K. (2012). Formulation, optimization and evaluation of transferosomal gel for transdermal insulin delivery. *Saudi Pharmaceutical Journal*, *20*(4), 355–363. doi:10.1016/j.jsps.2012.02.001 PMID:23960810

Marto, J., Vitor, C., Guerreiro, A., Severino, C., Eleutério, C., Ascenso, A., & Simões, S. (2016). Ethosomes for enhanced skin delivery of griseofulvin. *Colloids and Surfaces. B, Biointerfaces*, *146*, 616–623. doi:10.1016/j.colsurfb.2016.07.021 PMID:27429295

Mazumder, A., Dwivedi, A., Du Preez, J. L., & Du Plessis, J. (2016). In vitro wound healing and cytotoxic effects of sinigrin–phytosome complex. *International Journal of Pharmaceutics*, *498*(1-2), 283–293. doi:10.1016/j.ijpharm.2015.12.027 PMID:26706438

Miclea, R. D., Varma, P. R., Peng, A., & Balu-Iyer, S. V. (2007). Development and characterization of lipidic cochleate containing recombinant factor VIII. *Biochimica et Biophysica Acta (BBA) -. Biomembranes*, *1768*(11), 2890–2898. doi:10.1016/j.bbamem.2007.08.001 PMID:17936245

Miller, C. R., Bondurant, B., McLean, S. D., McGovern, K. A., & O'Brien, D. F. (1998). Liposome-cell interactions in vitro: Effect of liposome surface charge on the binding and endocytosis of conventional and sterically stabilized liposomes. *Biochemistry*, *37*(37), 12875–12883. doi:10.1021/bi980096y PMID:9737866

Mirzaei, H., Shakeri, A., Rashidi, B., Jalili, A., Banikazemi, Z., & Sahebkar, A. (2017). Phytosomal curcumin: A review of pharmacokinetic, experimental and clinical studies. *Biomedicine and Pharmacotherapy*, *85*, 102–112. doi:10.1016/j.biopha.2016.11.098 PMID:27930973

Moreno, L. C., Cavalcanti, I. M., Satyal, P., Santos-Magalhães, N. S., Rolim, H. M., & Freitas, R. M. (2015). Acute toxicity and anticonvulsant activity of liposomes containing nimodipine on pilocarpine-induced seizures in mice. *Neuroscience Letters*, *585*, 38–42. doi:10.1016/j.neulet.2014.11.025 PMID:25445375

Morgado, L. F., Trávolo, A. R. F., Muehlmann, L. A., Narcizo, P. S., Nunes, R. B., Pereira, P. A. G., & Longo, J. P. F. (2017). Photodynamic Therapy treatment of onychomycosis with Aluminium-Phthalocyanine Chloride nanoemulsions: A proof of concept clinical trial. *Journal of Photochemistry and Photobiology. B, Biology*, *173*, 266–270. doi:10.1016/j.jphotobiol.2017.06.010 PMID:28622558

Moulik, P. S., & Kumar, R. A. (2008). Physicochemistry of W/O Microemulsions. In M. Fanun (Ed.), *Microemulsions: Properties and Applications* (pp. 17–40). Taylor and Francis Group, LLC; doi:10.1201/9781420089608.ch2

Mueller-Goymann, C., & Hamann, H. J. (1991). Pharmacosomes - multilamellar vesicles consisting of pure drug. *European Journal of Pharmaceutics and Biopharmaceutics*, *37*(2), 113–117.

Müller, R., Mäder, K., & Gohla, S. (2000). Solid lipid nanoparticles (SLN) for controlled drug delivery: A review of the state of the art. *European Journal of Pharmaceutics and Biopharmaceutics*, *50*(1), 161–177. doi:10.1016/S0939-6411(00)00087-4 PMID:10840199

Müller, R. H., Radtke, M., & Wissing, S. A. (2002). Solid lipid nanoparticles (SLN) and nanostructured lipid carriers (NLC) in cosmetic and dermatological preparations. *Advanced Drug Delivery Reviews*, *54*(SUPPL.), 131–155. doi:10.1016/S0169-409X(02)00118-7 PMID:12460720

Nagia, A., Iqbala, B., Kumara, S., Sharmaa, S., Alib, J., & Babootab, S. (2017). Quality by design based silymarin nanoemulsion for enhancement of oral bioavailability. *Journal of Drug Delivery Science and Technology*, *40*, 35–44. doi:10.1016/j.jddst.2017.05.019

Naseri, N., Valizadeh, H., & Zakeri-Milani, P. (2015). Solid lipid nanoparticles and nanostructured lipid carriers: Structure preparation and application. *Advanced Pharmaceutical Bulletin*, *5*(3), 305–313. doi:10.15171/apb.2015.043 PMID:26504751

Natesan, S., Sugumaran, A., Ponnusamy, C., Thiagarajan, V., Palanichamy, R., & Kandasamy, R. (2017). Chitosan stabilized camptothecin nanoemulsions: Development, evaluation and biodistribution in preclinical breast cancer animal mode. *International Journal of Biological Macromolecules,* S0141-8130(16)32673-3.

Paliwal, R., Rai, S., & Vyas, S. P. (2011). Lipid drug conjugate (LDC) nanoparticles as autolymphotrophs for oral delivery of methotrexate. *Journal of Biomedical Nanotechnology*, *7*(1), 130–131. doi:10.1166/jbn.2011.1235 PMID:21485837

Pandita, A., & Sharma, P. (2013). Pharmacosomes: An emerging novel vesicular drug delivery system for poorly soluble synthetic and herbal drugs. *ISRN Pharmaceutics*, *2013*(3), 1–10. doi:10.1155/2013/348186 PMID:24106615

Papahadjopoulos, D., Vail, W. J., Jacobson, K., & Poste, G. (1975). Cochleate lipid cylinders: Formation by fusion of unilamellar lipid vesicles. *Biochimica et Biophysica Acta*, *394*(3), 483–491. doi:10.1016/0005-2736(75)90299-0 PMID:805602

Pappinen, S., & Urtti, A. (2016). Microemulsions. In *Percutaneous Penetration Enhancers Chemical Methods in Penetration Enhancement* (pp. 253–262). Berlin: Springer Berlin Heidelberg; doi:10.1007/978-3-662-47862-2_16

Patel, G. B., & Sprott, G. D. (1999). Archaeobacterial ether lipid liposomes (archaeosomes) as novel vaccine and drug delivery systems. *Critical Reviews in Biotechnology*, *19*(4), 317–357. doi:10.1080/0738-859991229170 PMID:10723627

Pereira, S., Egbu, R., Jannati, G., & Al-Jamal, W. T. (2016). Docetaxel-loaded liposomes: The effect of lipid composition and purification on drug encapsulation and in vitro toxicity. *International Journal of Pharmaceutics*, *514*(1), 150–159. doi:10.1016/j.ijpharm.2016.06.057 PMID:27863659

Pérez, O., Bracho, G., Lastre, M., Zayas, C., González, D., Gil, D., & Solís, R. L. (2006). Proteliposome-derived Cochleate as an immunomodulator for nasal vaccine. *Vaccine*, *24*(2), S52–S53. doi:10.1016/j.vaccine.2005.01.127 PMID:16823925

Perinelli, D. R., Cespi, M., Pucciarelli, S., Vincenzetti, S., Casettari, L., & Lam, J. K. W. … Palmieri, G. F. (2017). Microemulsions for protein delivery: Loading optimization and stability. *Current Pharmaceutical Biotechnology*. doi:10.2174/1389201018666170508112947

Pham, M. N. Van, Vo, T., Tran, V. T., Tran, P. H., & Tran, T. T. (2017). Microemulsion-based mucoadhesive buccal wafers: wafer formation, in vitro release, and ex vivo evaluation. *AAPS PharmSciTech*. doi:10.120812249-017-0754-9

Prabhu, P., & Patravale, V. (2014). Lipid based drug delivery systems. In N. Udupa & S. Mutalik (Eds.), *Recent Trends in Novel Drug Delivery* (pp. 80–167). Prism Books Pvt. Ltd.

Prabhu, P., Suryavanshi, S., Pathak, S., Patra, A., Sharma, S., & Patravale, V. (2016). Nanostructured lipid carriers of artemether-lumefantrine combination for intravenous therapy of cerebral malaria. *International Journal of Pharmaceutics*, *513*(1-2), 504–517. doi:10.1016/j.ijpharm.2016.09.008 PMID:27596113

Prabhu, P., Suryavanshi, S., Pathak, S., Sharma, S., & Patravale, V. (2016). Artemether-lumefantrine nanostructured lipid carriers for oral malaria therapy: Enhanced efficacy at reduced dose and dosing frequency. *International Journal of Pharmaceutics*, *511*(1), 473–487. doi:10.1016/j.ijpharm.2016.07.021 PMID:27421912

Radtke, M., & Müller, R. (2001). Nanostructured lipid drug carriers. *New Drugs*, 1–4. Retrieved from http://www.pharmasol-berlin.de/files/nlc.pdf

Ravi Sankar, V., & Dastagiri Reddy, Y. (2010). Nanocochleate - A new approach in lipid drug delivery. *International Journal of Pharmacy and Pharmaceutical Sciences*, *2*(4), 3.

Ren, L. L., Chen, S. Z., Li, H. D., Zhang, Z. Y., Ye, C. H., Liu, M. L., & Zhou, X. (2015). MRI-visible liposome nanovehicles for potential tumor-targeted delivery of multimodal therapies. *Nanoscale*, *7*(30), 12843–12850. doi:10.1039/C5NR02144H PMID:26022345

Sachan, R., Khatri, K., & Kasture, S. (2010). Self-emulsifying drug delivery system a novel approach for enhancement of bioavailability. *International Journal of Pharm Tech Research*, *2*, 1738–1745.

Sawant, R. R., & Torchilin, V. P. (2010). Liposomes as "smart" pharmaceutical nanocarriers. *Soft Matter*, *6*(17), 4026. doi:10.1039/b923535n

Semalty, A., Semalty, M., Rawat, B. S., Singh, D., & Rawat, M. (2009). Pharmacosomes: The lipid-based new drug delivery system. *Expert Opinion on Drug Delivery*, *6*(6), 599–612. doi:10.1517/17425240902967607 PMID:19519287

Sessa, G., & Weissmann, G. (1968). Phospholipid spherules (liposomes) as a model for biological membranes. *Journal of Lipid Research*, *9*(3), 310–318. Retrieved from http://www.ncbi.nlm.nih.gov/pubmed/5646182 PMID:5646182

Sharma, P., Dube, B., & Sawant, K. (2012). Synthesis of cytarabine lipid drug conjugate for treatment of meningeal leukemia: Development, characterization and in vitro cell line studies. *Journal of Biomedical Nanotechnology*, *8*(6), 928–937. doi:10.1166/jbn.2012.1464 PMID:23030001

Shete, H., Chatterjee, S., De, A., & Patravale, V. (2013). Long chain lipid based tamoxifen NLC. Part II: Pharmacokinetic, biodistribution and in vitro anticancer efficacy studies. *International Journal of Pharmaceutics*, *454*(1), 584–592. doi:10.1016/j.ijpharm.2013.03.036 PMID:23535344

Siddiqui, R. A., Harvey, K. A., Xu, Z., Natarajan, S. K., & Davisson, V. J. (2014). Characterization of lovastatin-docosahexaenoate anticancer properties against breast cancer cells. *Bioorganic & Medicinal Chemistry*, *22*(6), 1899–1908. doi:10.1016/j.bmc.2014.01.051 PMID:24556504

Siler-Marinkovic, S. (2016). Liposomes as drug delivery systems in dermal and transdermal drug delivery. In *Percutaneous Penetration Enhancers Chemical Methods in Penetration Enhancement* (pp. 15–38). Berlin: Springer Berlin Heidelberg; doi:10.1007/978-3-662-47862-2_2

Sinha, V. R., & Kumar, A. (2002). Multiple emulsions: An overview of formulation, characterization-stability and applications. *Indian Journal of Pharmaceutical Sciences*, *64*(3), 191–199.

Solanki, S. S., Sarkar, B., & Dhanwani, R. K. (2012). Microemulsion drug delivery system: For bioavailability enhancement of ampelopsin. *ISRN Pharmaceutics*. PMID:22830055

Soni, K., Mujtaba, A., & Kohli, K. (2017). Lipid drug conjugate nanoparticle as a potential nanocarrier for the oral delivery of pemetrexeddiacid: Formulation design, characterization, ex vivo, and in vivo assessment. *International Journal of Biological Macromolecules*, *103*, 139–151. doi:10.1016/j.ijbiomac.2017.05.015 PMID:28499946

Sreekanth, V., Bansal, S., Motiani, R. K., Kundu, S., Muppu, S. K., Majumdar, T. D., ... Bajaj, A. (2013). Design, synthesis, and mechanistic investigations of bile acid-tamoxifen conjugates for breast cancer therapy. *Bioconjugate Chemistry*, *24*(9), 1468–1484. doi:10.1021/bc300664k PMID:23909664

Tang, T. T., Hu, X. B., Liao, D. H., Liu, X. Y., & Xiang, D. X. (2013). Mechanisms of microemulsion enhancing the oral bioavailability of puerarin: Comparison between oil-in-water and water-in-oil microemulsions using the single-pass intestinal perfusion method and a chylomicron flow blocking approach. *International Journal of Nanomedicine*, *8*, 4415–4426. doi:10.2147/IJN.S51469 PMID:24277986

Tyagi, L. K., Kumar, S., Maurya, S. S., & Kori, M. L. (2013). Ethosomes : Novel vesicular carrier for enhanced transdermal drug delivery system. *Bulletin of Pharmaceutical Research*, *3*(1), 6–13.

Venkata Ramana Rao, S., & Shao, J. (2008). Self-nanoemulsifying drug delivery systems (SNEDDS) for oral delivery of protein drugs. *International Journal of Pharmaceutics*, *362*(1–2), 2–9. doi:10.1016/j.ijpharm.2008.05.018 PMID:18650038

Venugopal, B., Awada, A., Evans, T. R., Dueland, S., Hendlisz, A., Rasch, W., ... Aamdal, S. (2015). A first-in-human phase I and pharmacokinetic study of CP-4126 (CO-101), a nucleoside analogue, in patients with advanced solid tumours. *Cancer Chemotherapy and Pharmacology*, *76*(4), 785–792. doi:10.100700280-015-2846-0 PMID:26289594

Wang, L. L., Huang, S., Guo, H. H., Han, Y. X., Zheng, W. S., & Jiang, J. D. (2016). In situ delivery of thermosensitive gel-mediated 5-fluorouracil microemulsion for the treatment of colorectal cancer. *Drug Design, Development and Therapy*, *10*, 2855–2867. doi:10.2147/DDDT.S111351 PMID:27660416

Yan, Y., Zhang, H., Sun, J., Wang, P., Dong, K., Dong, Y., & Xing, J. (2016). Enhanced transdermal delivery of sinomenine hydrochloride by ethosomes for anti-inflammatory treatment. *Journal of Drug Delivery Science and Technology*, *36*, 201 207. doi:10.1016/j.jddst.2016.10.013

Yasir, M., Gaur, P. K., Puri, D., Shekar, P., & Kumar, S. S. (2017). Solid lipid nanoparticles approach for lymphatic targeting through intraduodenal delivery of quetiapine fumarate. *Current Drug Delivery*, *14*(999), 1. doi:10.2174/1567201814666170525121049 PMID:28545354

Yu, X., Du, L., Li, Y., Fu, G., & Jin, Y. (2015). Improved anti-melanoma effect of a transdermal mitoxantrone ethosome gel. *Biomedicine and Pharmacotherapy*, *73*, 6–11. doi:10.1016/j.biopha.2015.05.002 PMID:26211575

Yuan, Q., Han, J., Cong, W., Ge, Y., Ma, D., Dai, Z., ... Bi, L. (2014). Docetaxel-loaded solid lipid nanoparticles suppress breast cancer cells growth with reduced myelosuppression toxicity. *International Journal of Nanomedicine*, *9*, 4829–4846. PMID:25378924

Zarif, L., Graybill, J. R., Perlin, D., & Manninoa, R. J. (2000). *Cochleates: New lipid-based drug delivery system*. Academic Press.

Zhang, Q., Li, J., Zhang, W., An, Q., Wen, J., Wang, A., ... Chen, S. (2015). Acute and sub-chronic toxicity studies of honokiol microemulsion. *Regulatory Toxicology and Pharmacology*, *71*(3), 428–436. doi:10.1016/j.yrtph.2014.11.007 PMID:25481277

Zhang, Q., Ye, X., Wang, L., Peng, B., Zhang, Y., Bao, J., ... Chen, S. (2016). Embryo-fetal development toxicity of honokiol microemulsion intravenously administered to pregnant rats. *Regulatory Toxicology and Pharmacology*, *74*, 117–122. doi:10.1016/j.yrtph.2015.11.012 PMID:26619782

Zhang, Y., He, L., Yue, S., Huang, Q., Zhang, Y., & Yang, J. (2017). Characterization and evaluation of a self-microemulsifying drug delivery system containing tectorigenin, an isoflavone with low aqueous solubility and poor permeability. *Drug Delivery*, *24*(1), 632–640. doi:10.1080/10717544.2017.1284946 PMID:28283000

Zhao, L., Wei, Y., Huang, Y., He, B., Zhou, Y., & Fu, J. (2013). Nanoemulsion improves the oral bioavailability of baicalin in rats: In vitro and in vivo evaluation. *International Journal of Nanomedicine*, *8*, 3769–3779. doi:10.2147/IJN.S51578 PMID:24124365

Zhao, Y., Chang, Y. X., Hu, X., Liu, C. Y., Quan, L. H., & Liao, Y. H. (2016). Solid Lipid Nanoparticles for Sustained Pulmonary Delivery of Yuxingcao Essential Oil: Preparation, Characterization and in Vivo Evaluation. *International Journal of Pharmaceutics*, *516*(1-2), 364–371. doi:10.1016/j.ijpharm.2016.11.046 PMID:27884712

ADDITIONAL READING

Charron, D. M., Chen, J., & Zheng, G. (2015). Theranostic lipid nanoparticles for cancer medicine. *Cancer Treatment and Research*, *166*, 103–127. doi:10.1007/978-3-319-16555-4_5 PMID:25895866

Irby, D., Du, C., & Li, F. (2017). Lipid-Drug Conjugate for Enhancing Drug Delivery. *Molecular Pharmaceutics*, *14*(5), 1325–1338. doi:10.1021/acs.molpharmaceut.6b01027 PMID:28080053

Prabhu, P., & Patravale, V. (2014). Lipid based drug delivery systems. In N. Udupa & S. Mutalik (Eds.), *Recent Trends in Novel Drug Delivery* (pp. 80–167). Prism Books Pvt. Ltd.

Puri, A., Loomis, K., Smith, B., Lee, J. H., Yavlovich, A., Heldman, E., Blumenthal, R. (2009). Lipid-based nanoparticles as pharmaceutical drug carriers: from concepts to clinic. *Critical Reviews™ in Therapeutic Drug Carrier Systems, 26*(6), 523-580.

KEY WORDS AND DEFINITIONS

Bioavailability: The rate and fraction of the administered dose which reaches the systemic circulation in unchanged form.

Controlled Drug Delivery Systems: The specially designed and optimized drug delivery systems in which the rate and extent of drug release from the delivery system (formulation) can be controlled/modified.

Drug Targeting: A smart drug delivery approach to deliver medication in such a manner that the drug concentration at the desired site inside the body is more than the other sites.

Lipid Nanocarriers: Particulate/vesicular systems comprising lipid, oils, modified lipids/oils alone or in combination which are suitably stabilized to achieve a nanoscale size (< 1000 nm).

Nanoparticles: The particulate systems with nanoscale size (< 1000 nm).

Nanovesicles: The vesicular systems with nanoscale size (< 1000 nm).

Permeation: The ability of drug to cross the biological membrane and transport across the cell.

Theranostics: A combination of diagnostic and therapeutic capabilities merged together to develop specific, individualized therapies for different diseases.

APPENDIX: TABLES AND FIGURES

Figure 1. Classification of lipid nanocarriers

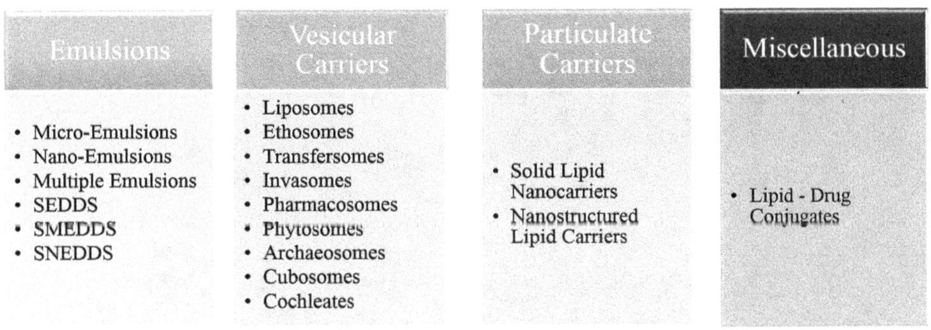

Figure 2. Pictorial representation of emulsion based lipid nanocarriers

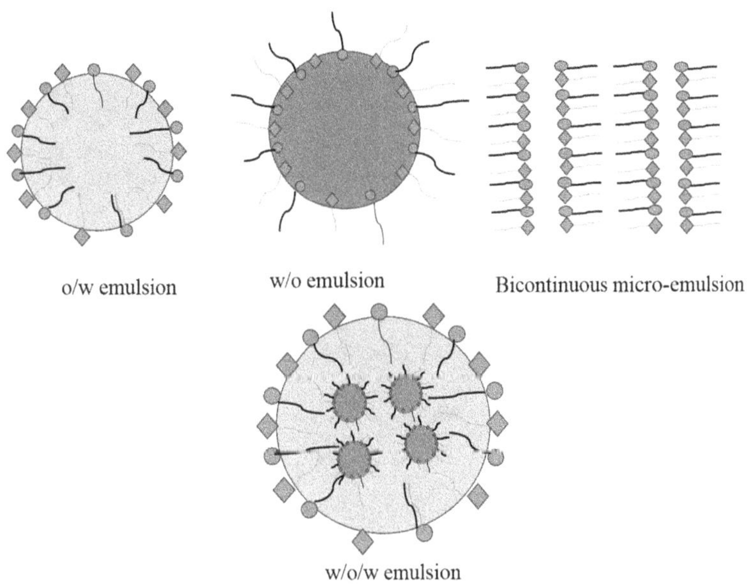

Figure 3. Drug release mechanism from microemulsion droplets. Drug distribution occurs based on its solubility in various phases of skin (1). Drug penetration into skin occurs from outer phase in the first mechanism (2). In the second mechanism, direct diffusion to the skin occurs from microemulsion droplets because of their high density in the microemulsion. (3). On contact with skin, droplets break down to release its content into the skin (4). Mixing occurs between microemulsion components and skin lipids.

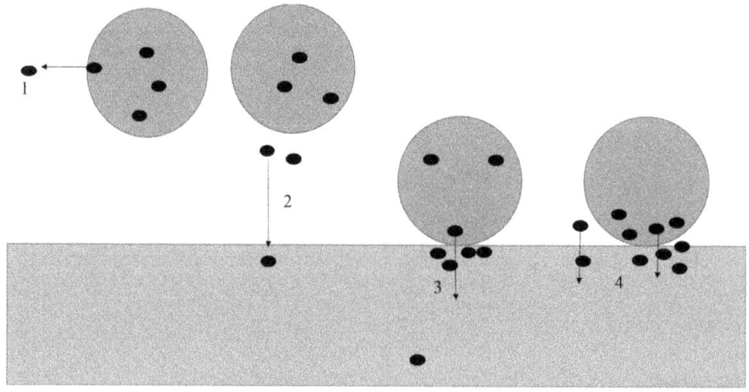

Figure 4. Mechanisms of drug release through multiple emulsions

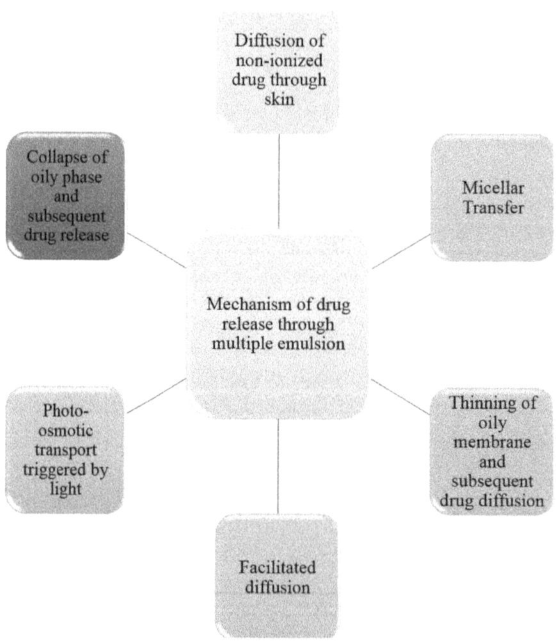

Figure 5. Stabilization strategies for multiple emulsions

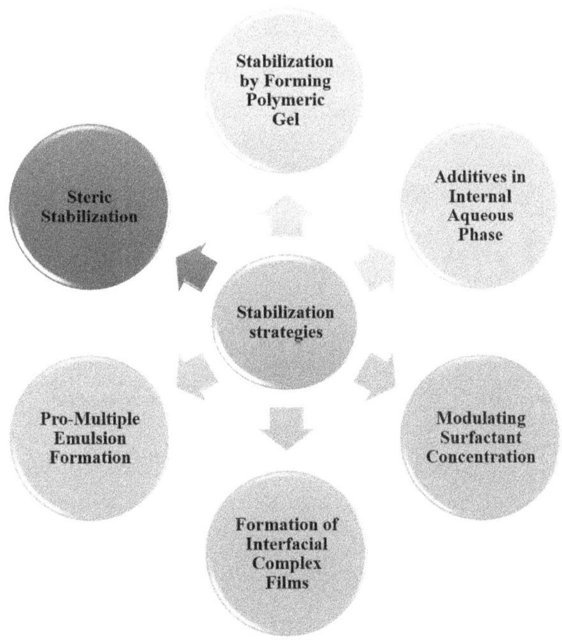

Figure 6. Pictorial description of vesicular drug delivery systems

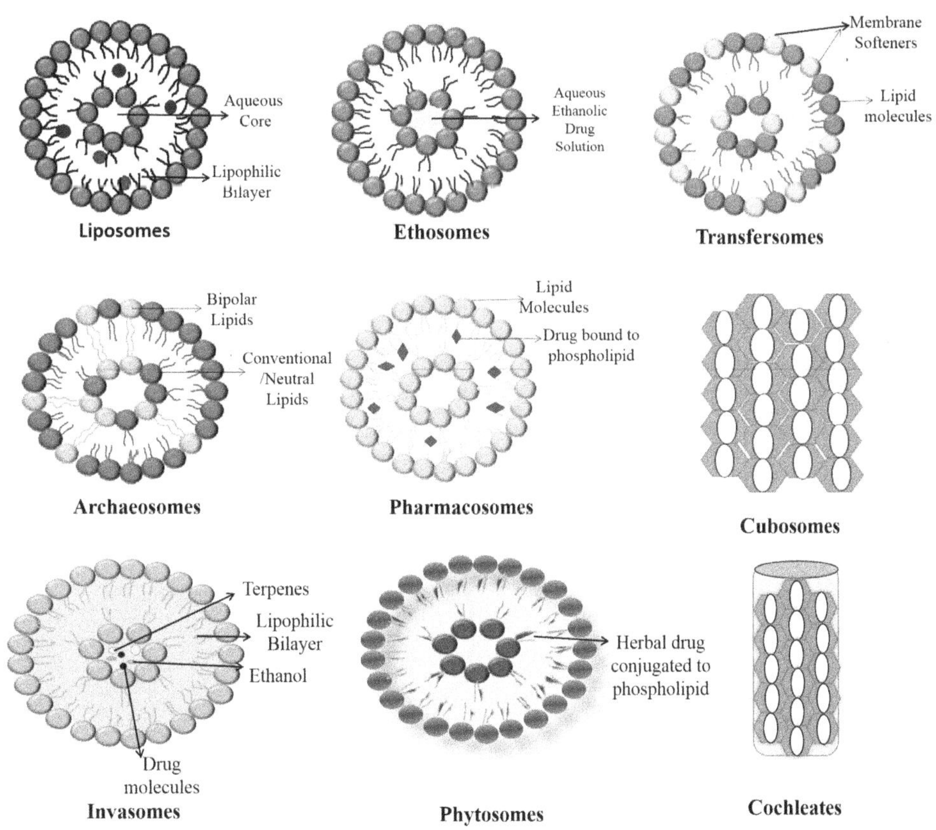

Figure 7. Classification of liposomes based on their structure

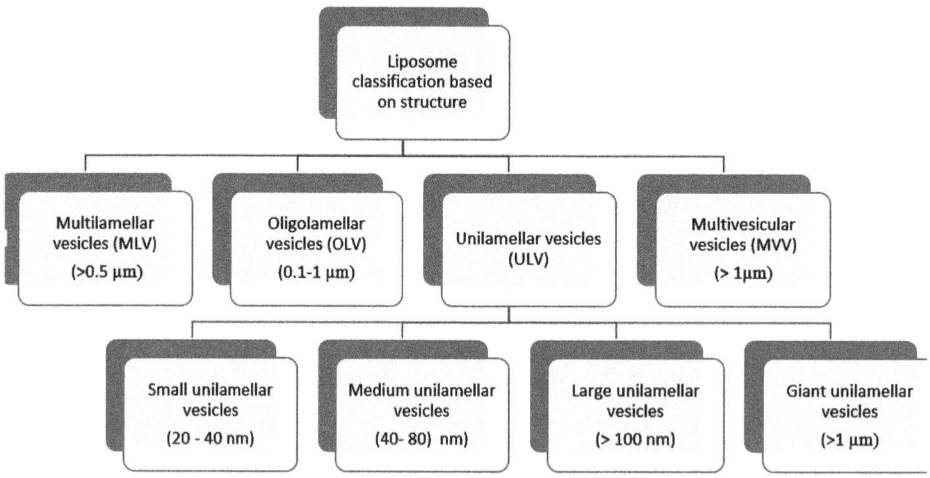

Figure 8. Classification of liposomes based on their composition

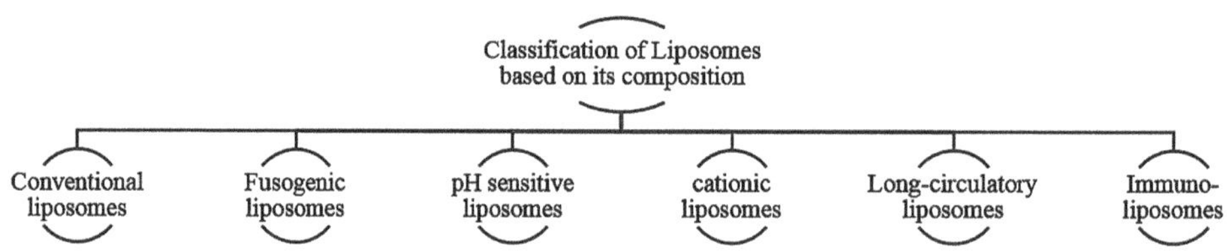

Figure 9. a) SLN pictorial representation b) NLC imperfect crystal c) NLC Amorphous Type d) NLC multiple type consisting of oil nano-compartments.

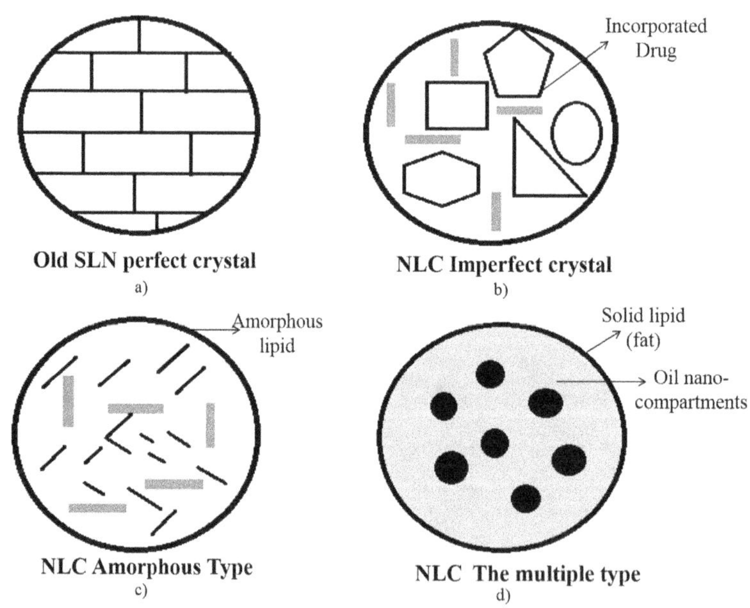

Figure 10. Drug incorporation models in SLNs. a) Solid solution model b) Core-shell method with drug enriched shell c) Core-shell model with drug enriched core.

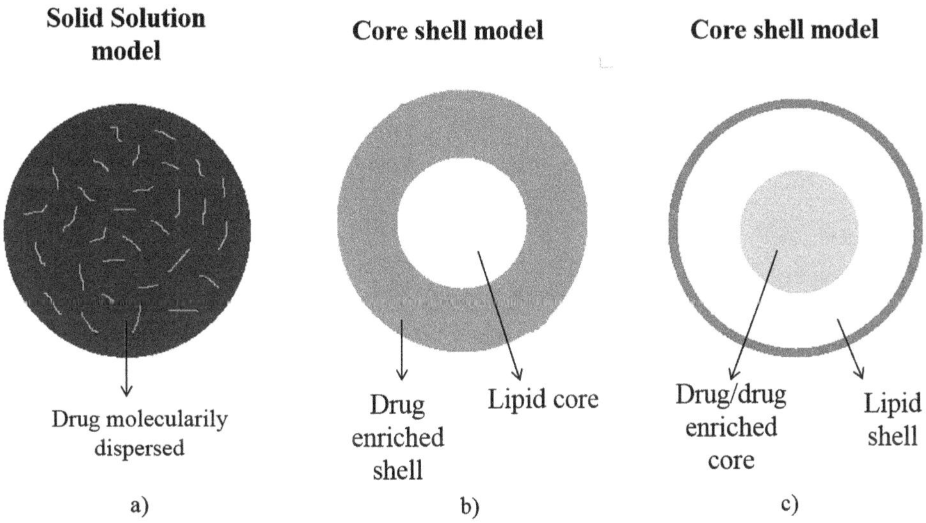

Figure 11. Types of lipid-drug linkage. a) Ester bond b) Amide bond c) Hydrazone bond d) Disulphide bond.

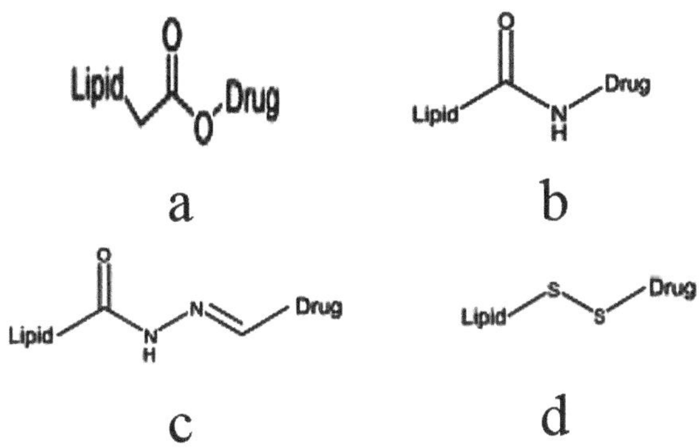

Figure 12. Schematic procedure for phase titration techniques

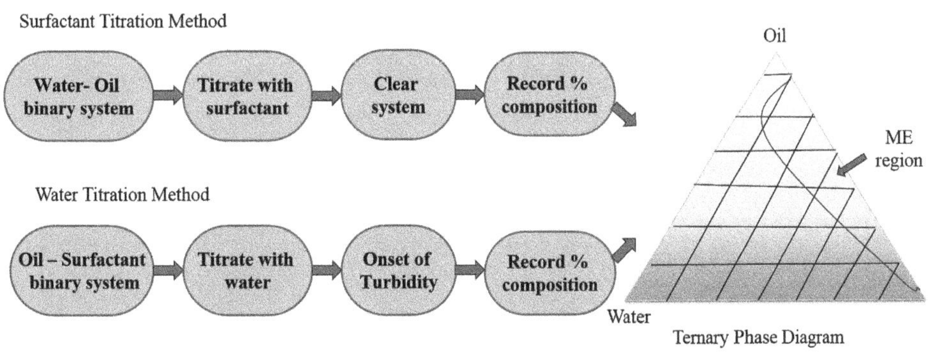

Figure 13. Manufacturing methods to form solid SEDDS, SMEDDS and SNEDDS

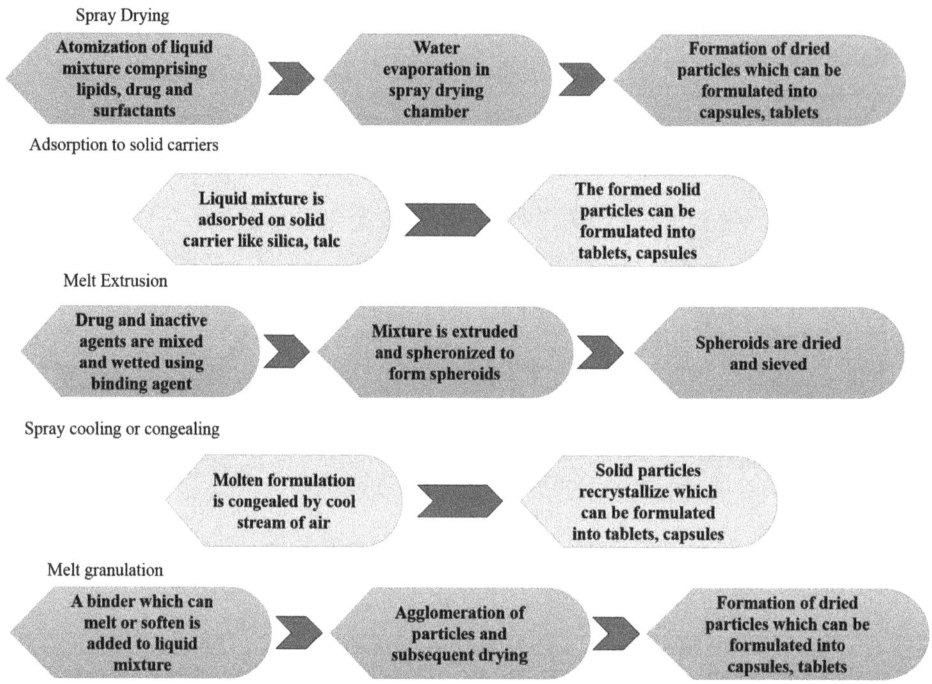

Figure 14. Schematic description of methods of preparation of various vesicular drug delivery systems

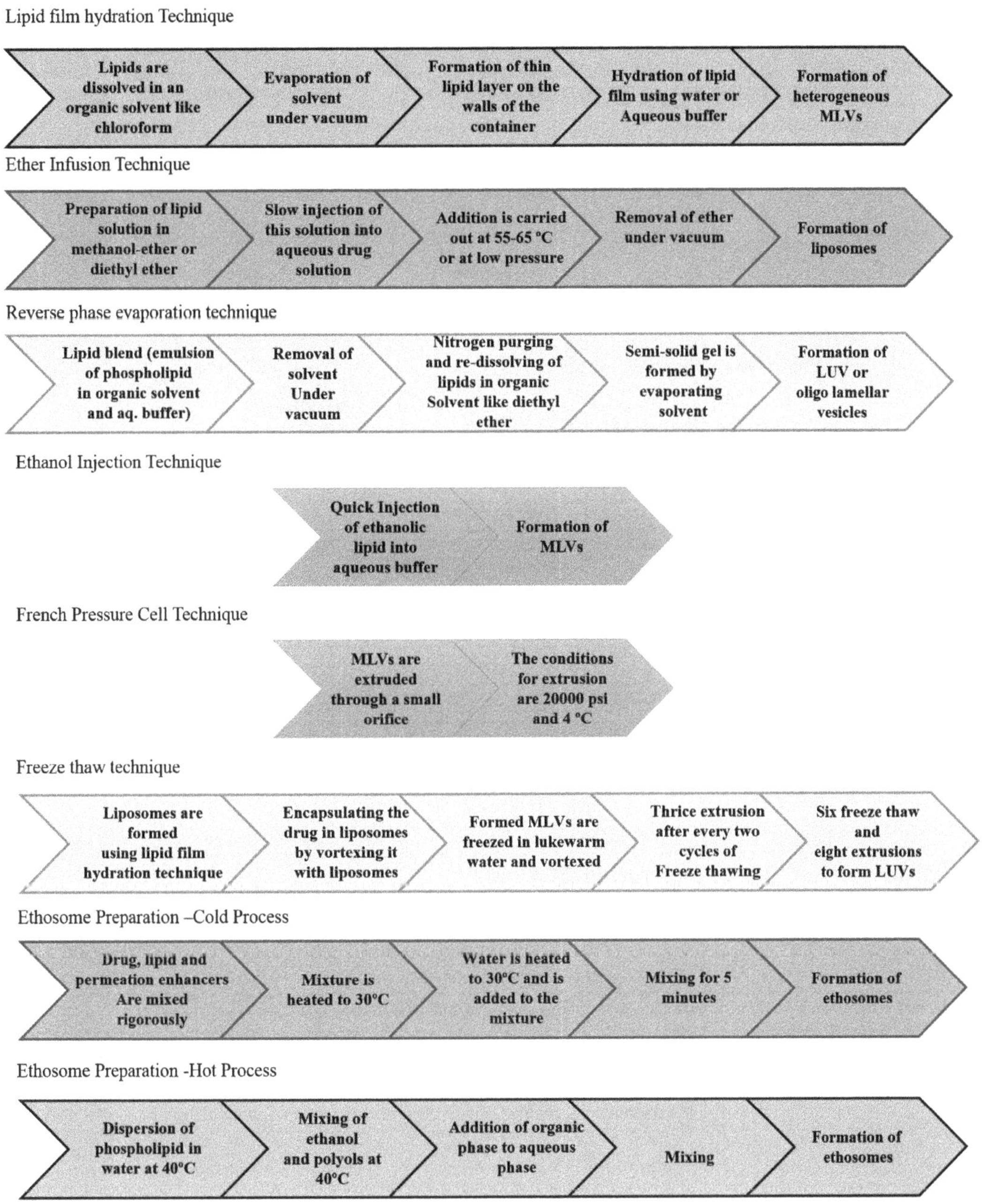

Figure 15. Schematic of methods of preparation of cochleates

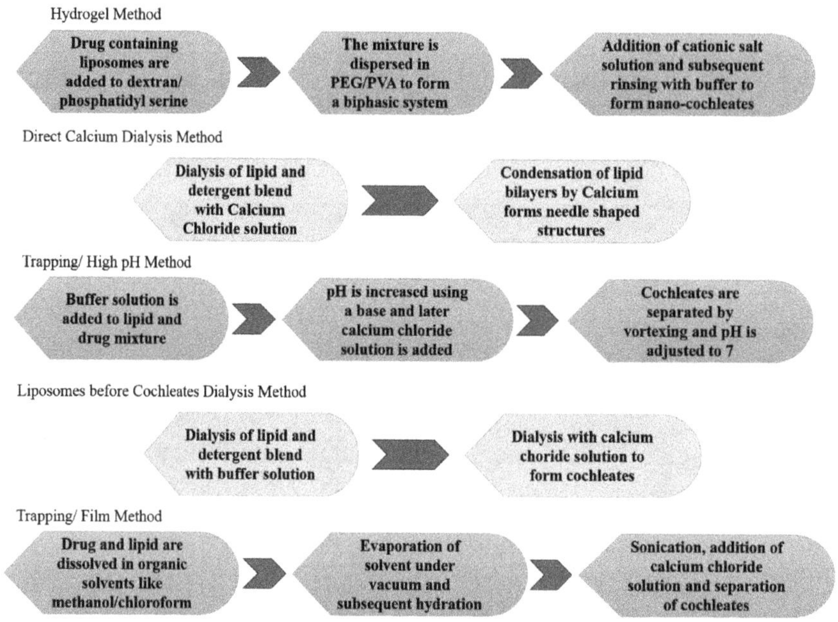

Figure 16. Schematic diagram of solvent emulsification/evaporation technique for the preparation of SLNs

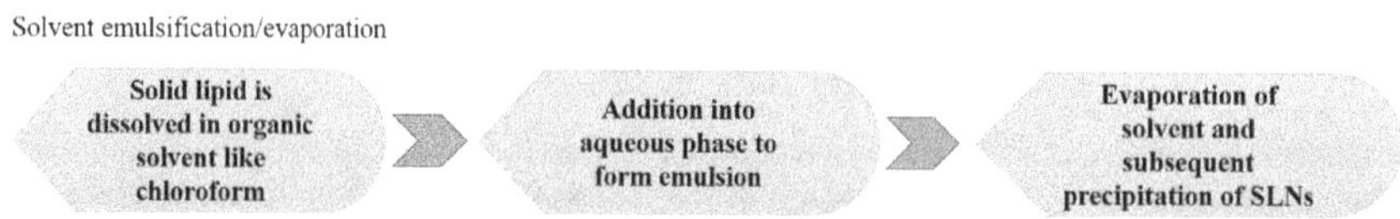

Table 1. Winson classification of microemulsion system

Type of Microemulsion	Description
Winsor I	Oil in water (o/w) microemulsion is in equilibrium with excess oil
Winsor II	Water in oil (w/o) microemulsion is in equilibrium with excess water
Winsor III	Bicontinuous microemulsion wherein both w/o and o/w microemulsion are present simultaneously
Winsor IV	Microemulsion is neither in equilibrium with water nor with oil

Table 2. Types of drug incorporation models in SLNs

Type of Drug Incorporation Model in SLN	Description
Solid solution model	Observed in case of cold homogenization wherein drug is homogeneously dispersed in the lipid matrix
Core-shell model with drug enriched shell	In case of hot homogenization, when the temperature increases beyond the melting point of lipid, the drug partitions from the lipid phase to water phase. On cooling, the lipid crystallizes out and the drug is repartitioned on the lipid shell to form a drug enriched shell.
Core-shell model with drug enriched core	When a nanoemulsion is cooled, supersaturation of drug occurs in melted lipid. The lipid crystallizes out on further cooling thereby surrounding the drug core giving drug enriched core

Table 3. Methods of preparation of vesicular drug delivery systems

Name of Method of Preparation	Type of Vesicular Nanocarrier	Special Characteristics	Drawbacks
	Liposome, ethosome, pharmacosome, transfersome, invasome	• Gel-liquid crystal transition temperature of the lipid should be lesser than the temperature of the hydrating medium • Water, saline solution, hydroalcoholic solution (for ethosomes) and buffer solution can be used as hydrating medium • Large multilamellar liposomes are formed • In case of transfersomes, surfactants are also dissolved in surfactants along with lipids in organic solvent • For invasome preparation, ethanol and terpene mixture are added after the hydrating solution • Ultrasonication or extrusion can be used for size reduction	Poor encapsulation efficiency of liposomes
Ether injection technique	Liposome, pharmacosome	• Ether solutions like diethyl ether or methanol-ether mixture are used • Reaction conditions are 55-65 °c and reduced pressure	• High particle dispersion index of liposomes (70-190 nm) • Exposure of drug to organic solvents.
Reverse phase evaporation technique	Liposome	• High encapsulation efficiency can be obtained upto 65% • Small and large macromolecules can be incorporated	Exposure of drug to organic solvents and sonication
Ethanol injection technique	Liposome	Multi-lamellar vesicles are formed using this technique	• Heterogeneous liposomes (30-110nm). • Difficulty in removal of ethanol
French pressure cell technique	Liposome	• Simple, reproducible, rapid and gentle handling of unstable materials. • Larger small unilamellar vesicles than those obtained from sonication	• Small working volume • Difficulty in achieving temperature
Sonication	All vesicular drug delivery systems	Aqueous phospholipid dispersions are sonicated to reduce the size of small unilamellar vesicles having initial size of 15-25 μ	Size variation between batches
Freeze thaw technique	Liposomes	This technique is used for the entrapment of proteins	• Costly method • Drugs unstable to freeze thawing cannot be entrapped using this method
Membrane extrusion	Liposomes, invasomes	• Liposomal dispersion is passed through a polycarbonate membrane with specific pore size for size reduction. • Uniformity and limited size variation are advantages	It is a slow process
Cold and hot method	Ethosomes	• In cold method, drug is dissolved in lipid mixture. • In hot method, drug is dissolved in aqueous or hydroalcoholic solution • The final size reduction can be carried out by sonication	Additional step of sonication or extrusion is required for size reduction

Dua, Rana, & Bhandari, 2012; Tyagi, Kumar, Maurya, & Kori, 2013; Benson, 2006; Semalty, Semalty, Rawat, Singh, & Rawat, 2009; Lakshmi, Kalpana, & Prasanthi, 2013; Prabhu& Patravale, 2014.

Table 4. Common characterization techniques for lipid nanocarriers

Characterization Test	Method of Analysis	Significance of the Test
Organoleptic test	• Visual appearance • Odour • Taste	These tests are essential to understand whether the formulation is visually acceptable and palatable
Particle/ droplet size and shape determination	• Scanning electron microscopy (SEM) • Transmission electron microscopy (TEM) • Small angle neutron scattering (SANS) • Small-angle x-ray scattering (SAXS) • Photon correlation spectroscopy (PCS)	Particle/droplet size determination is one of the most important techniques to determine whether the formulation is in nanodomain. Depending on the type of formulation the method of analysis varies. PCS can be used to measure the size of only particles in suspension or polymers in solution
Surface morphology	• SEM • TEM • Atom force microscopy (AFM) • Scanning tunneling microscope (STM)	These techniques are used to understand the surface morphology of the nanoparticle. Generally, these techniques are applicable for solid particles only. For liquid samples, special techniques like environmental scanning electron microscopy can be used.
Zeta potential/ surface charge	• Dynamic electrophoretic mobility • Electro acoustic mobility	Zeta potential is electric potential between interfacial double layer i.e. Between the stationery fluid layer attached to a particle and dispersion medium. The lower is the zeta potential, more is the tendency of particles to coagulate or flocculate in the system. It is influenced by factors like ionic strength, pH, amount of electrolytes and surfactants. Zeta potential above $\pm$ 25 mv renders good stability.
Rheological characteristics	• Brookfield viscometer • Plate viscometer	Optimum viscosity is essential for any formulation to pour/add them into a container. Depending upon desired rheological characteristics, viscosity should be modified using surfactants.
In vitro release	Dissolution apparatus	This test is essential to determine the rate of drug release through the formulation and correlate in vitro - in vivo drug release
pH	pH meter	Proper pH maintenance is crucial for the stability of a formulation. A fall in pH can affect zeta potential and destabilize a system.
Drug entrapment efficiency	Assay	This method enables to understand the amount of drug entrapped in the system thereby revealing the total amount of drug the system can release. Better the entrapment efficiency lesser is the requirement of the carrier
Stability testing	As per ICH guidelines	Stability testing is critical to ensure that the formulation adheres to the specifications throughout its shelf life. This testing also helps to determine the expiry date of the product
Related substances	Test to check presence of residual solvents, organometallic compounds and other colloidal compounds	This test ensures that the formulation contains materials within specifications.
Turbidity	Nephelometer	Microemulsions are transparent; nanoemulsions are translucent while liposomes are translucent to milky Exact turbidity analysis helps to determine the presence of other colloidal substances

Agrawal & Agrawal, 2012 ; Sinha & Kumar, 2002; Müller, Radtke, & Wissing, 2002; Prabhu & Patravale, 2014; Anwekar, Patel, & Singhai, 2011.

Table 5. Application summary of lipid nanocarriers for advanced therapeutics

Lipid Nanocarrier System	Drug	Indication	Delivery Route	Results and Key Features	Reference
Bioavailability, Permeability, and Efficacy Enhancement					
Nano emulsion	Curcumin	Antioxidant, neuroprotective	Oral	~5-fold increase in oral bioavailability	Lu, Inbaraj, & Chen, 2017
NLCs	Artemether-lumefantrine	Malaria	Oral	Enhanced efficacy with reduced dose and dosing frequency	Prabhu, Suryavanshi, Pathak, Sharma, & Patravale, 2016
SMEDDS	Tectorigenin	Osteosarcoma	Oral	Enhanced bioavailability	Zhang et al., 2017
Ethosome	Ketoprofen	Fungal infection	In vitro studies	Higher drug permeation and transdermal flux compared to *hydroethanolic drug solution*	Chourasia, Kang, & Chan, 2011
Ethosomes	Tacolimus	Atopic dermatitis	In vitro studies	Higher skin penetration compared to marketed ointment protopic®	Li et al., 2012
Phytosomess	Sinigrin	Wound healing	In vitro studies	Complete wound healing in 42h as compared to 71% healing with pain drug	Mazumdar, Dwivedi, Du Preez & Du Plessis, 2016
LDCs	Bile acid-tamoxifen conjugate	Breast cancer	Direct tumor invasion	Irreversible electrostatic membrane interactions due to LDC charge and hydrophobicity Enhanced in vivo anti-breast cancer efficacy	Sreekanth et al., 2013
LDCs	Lovastatin-docosahexaenoic acid conjugate	Breast cancer	In vitro studies	Synergistic increase in anticancer efficacy	Siddiqui, Harvey, Xu, Natarajan, & Davisson, 2014
Transferosomal transdermal gel	Risperidone	Schizophrenia	Ex vivo studies	Enhanced permeation	Das et al., 2017
Transferosomal transdermal gel	Piroxicam	Inflammation	Ex vivo studies	Enhanced permeation	Ghanbarzadeh, & Arami, 2013
Invasomes	Capsaicin	Pain relief	Transdermal	Enhanced permeation compared to liposomes and commercial product Attributed to size <100 nm	Duangjit, Nimcharoenwan, Chomya, Locharoenrat, & Ngawhirunpat, 2016
Cubosomal gel	Alpha lipoic acid	Ageing	Topical	Facial skin improvement with increased epidermal thickness compared to placebo group	El-komy et al., 2016
Cochleates	Proteoliposome	Vaccine	Nasal	Enhanced systemic igG and igA antibody responses	Perez et al., 2006
Cochleates	Proteoliposome with recombinant gD protein	Vaccine	Nasal	Strong immunity against genital herpes	Del Campo et al., 2010

continued on following page

Table 5. Continued

Lipid Nanocarrier System	Drug	Indication	Delivery Route	Results and Key Features	Reference
Controlled and Sustained Drug Delivery					
SLNs	Yuxingcao essential oil	Pulmonary abscess	In vitro studies	Sustained release upto 48h Ease of nebulization for pulmonary delivery	Zhao et al., 2016
SLNs	Sirna	Gene therapy	Intradermal	Sustained release upto10-13 hours	Lobovkina et al., 2011
LDC nanoparticles	Cytarabine-stearic acid conjugate	Meningeal leukemia	In vitro studies	Sustained drug release profile, enhanced stability and efficacy in leukemic cell line el-4	Sharma, Dube, & Sawant, 2012
Transferosomes	Pentoxifylline	Intermittent claudicatio, chronic occlusive arterial diseases	Transdermal	Sustained drug delivery with prolonged half life and enhanced drug permeation conventional sustained release tablets	Al Shuwaili, Rasool, & Abdulrasool, 2016
Cubosomes	Timolol maleate	Galucoma	Ocular deivery	Enhanced ex vivo permeation, in vivo efficacy and retention compared to marketed eye drops	Huang et al., 2017
Stability Enhancement					
SLNs	Hydroquinone	Hyperpigmentation	In vitro study	Increased drug stability against oxidative degradation with enhanced skin deposition	Ghanbarzadeh et al., (2015)
Microemulsion	Bovine serum albumin as model drug	-	In vitro study	Enhanced stability up to 6 months	Perinelli et al., (2017)
SNEDDS	α-tocopherol, resveratrol coenzyme Q10	Cancer	Parenetral	Enhanced stability with increased antioxidant and antitumor efficacy	Jain et al., (2017)
Phytosomal gel	Curcumin	Antioxidant, neuroprotective	In vitro study	Enhanced stability and drug solubility	Allam, Komeil, & Abdallah, 2015
Lipid nanotubes	Gold and silver nanoparticles	-	In vitro study	Stable incorporation of gold and silver nanospheres in lipid nanotube (radius: ~10.23nm	Baowan, & Thamwattana, 2014
Toxicity Reduction					
Microemulsion	Honokinol	Cancer, anxiety, digestive disorders	Intravenous	Non-toxicity up to 500µg/kg (acute and subacute toxicity study) 75 times higher embryo fetal toxicity than therapeutic dose.	Zhang et al., 2015, 2016
Nanoemulsion	Aluminium-phthalocyanine chloride-photodynamic therapy	Onychomycosis	Topical	Significantly high 60% cure with reduced systemic toxicity	Morgado et al., 2017

continued on following page

Table 5. Continued

Lipid Nanocarrier System	Drug	Indication	Delivery Route	Results and Key Features	Reference
Liposomes	Docetaxel	Cancer	In vitro study	Enhanced drug loading via steric stabilization leading to reduced toxicity and higher efficacy	Pereira, Egbu, Jannati, & Al-Jamal 2016
Liposomes	Nimodipine	Convulsions, Seizures	Intraperitoneal	Reduced central nervous system and systemic toxicity compared to plain drug	Moreno et al, (2015)
PEGylated liposomes	Cantharidin	Cancer	Intravenous	Significant reduction in systemic toxicity with higher antitumor efficacy	Chang et al., (2008)
Ethosomes	Mitoxantrone	Melanomas	Topical/ transdermal	Absence of significant side effects Non-invasive treatment	Yu, Du, Li, Fu, & Jin, 2015
Archeosomes	Paclitaxel	Breast cancer and other carcinomas	In vitro study	Improved therapeutic index with reduced toxicity and enhanced efficacy	Alavi et al ., (2014)
LDC nanoparticles	Methotrxate conjugate	Cancer	Oral	Reduced gastrointestinal toxicity with enhanced bioavailability	Paliwal, Rai & Vyas, 2011
Cochleates	Amphotericin b	Systemic fungal infections	Intraperitoneal	Reduced nephrotoxicity, improved immunomodulatory activity with enhanced antifungal efficacy	Batista-Duharte et al., (2016)
Targeted Drug Delivery					
NlCs	Artemether-lumefantrine	Cerebral malaria	intravenous	Enhanced brain permeation 100% survival in cerebral malaria mice model	Prabhu et al., (2016)
Nanoemulsion	Chloro-aluminum phthalocyanine	Glioblastoma multiforme	In vitro study	Targeted release using photoactivation	Castilho-Fernandes, Lopes, Primo, Pinto, & Tedesco, 2017
Liposome	Paclitaxel, MRI contrast agent (Gd-DOTA), and targeting agent (cyclic RGD peptide) and fluorophore	Cancer	Parenteral	Tumor targeting theranostic potential Enhanced efficacy	Ren et al., (2015)
Theranostics					
Ethosomes	Quantum dots	Scar labelling and healing	In vitro study	Fluorescence labelling property with skin scar therapy	He, Cui, & Gao, 2009
Microemulsion	Radiolabeled alendronate sodium	Osteaoporosis, Paget's disease	In vitro study	Bone disease diagnosis and therapy	Elitez et al., (2017)

Table 6. Market update of lipid nanocarriers for advanced therapeutic

Product	Lipid Nanocarrier System	Drug	Indication	Manufacturer
Marketed				
Mucosolvan® retard capsules	SLNs, lipid nanopellets	Ambroxol HCl	Acute and chronic bronchopulmonary diseases	Boehringer-Ingelheim Inc.
Doxil® (Caelyx)	PEGylated liposome	Doxorubicin	Ovarian/breast cancer	Orthobiotech Inc., Schering-Plough Inc.
Myocet®	Liposome	Doxorubicin	Breast cancer	Elan/Sopherion therapeutics Inc.
DaunoXome®	Liposome	Daunorubicin	Kaposi Sarcoma (HIV related)	Gilead Science Inc.
DepoCyt®	Liposomal	Cytarabine	Lymphomatous meningitis	Skye Pharma Inc., Enzon Inc.
Siliphos®	Phytosome	Silybin, silycristin, isosilbin, silydianin	hepatitis, cirrhosis and inflammation	Indena Inc.
Meriva®	Phytosomes	Curcumin	Antioxidant, neuroprotective	Thorne Research Inc.
Sandimun Neoral	Microemulsion	Cyclosporine	Immunosuppressant	Sandoz Inc.
Under Clinical Investigation				
Onco-TCS	Liposomal	Vincristine	Non-Hodgkin Lymphoma	Inex Inc.
Aroplatin	Liposome	Cispltin	Colorectal carcinoma	Antigenics Inc.
Rifamsolin	SLNs	Rifampicin	Tuberculosis	AlphaRx Inc.
Nektar -102	PEGylated lipodome	Irinotecan,	Breast /colorectal carcinoma	Nektar therapeutics Inc.

Chapter 6
Lipid Nanocarriers for Intracellular Delivery

Clara Bernard Fernandes
SVKM's NMIMS, India

Divya Suares
SVKM'S NMIMS, India

Vivek Dhawan
SVKM'S NMIMS, India

ABSTRACT

Recent trends in drug delivery indicate a growing trend to utilize nanotechnology to target diseased tissues with minimal adverse effects. However, in such cases, the biggest challenge encountered by the formulator is the intracellular delivery of the actives. Nevertheless, pharmaceutical nanocarriers have proven to possess distinct advantages for intracellular delivery of therapeutics over conventional approaches. They are versatile in terms of engineering and provide attractive options to deliver encapsulated or conjugated cargoes to cellular targets. In this chapter, the authors discuss important aspects of lipid-based nanocarriers for intracellular drug targeting. The chapter provides insight of different pathways to internalize lipid nanocarriers and the physicochemical factors affecting the intracellular fate of nanocarriers. Further, the chapter provides details of different types of lipid-based nanocarriers that have been explored for intracellular delivery in infectious diseases as well as cancer.

1. INTRODUCTION TO CHALLENGES OF INTERCELLULAR DRUG DELIVERY

Delivery of therapeutically active molecules to a desired target site still remains a daunting task. Although there are approaches being devised to address the issue, for intracellular targeting it's an uphill task to ensure that the drug reaches the cellular domain in the appropriate concentration (Hillaireau & Couvreur, 2009). To-date, nanotechnology has made successful ingress in this domain. There have been successful strides made in designing a variety of nanocarrier-based drug delivery and drug-targeting systems to minimize the drug loss through degradation and inactivation in biologic milieu, minimize side-effects,

DOI: 10.4018/978-1-5225-4781-5.ch006

Copyright © 2018, IGI Global. Copying or distributing in print or electronic forms without written permission of IGI Global is prohibited.

and increase drug bioavailability and targetability (Mozafari, M. R.; Pardakhty, A.; Azarmi, S.; Jazayeri, J. A.; Nokhodchi, A.; Omri, A., 2009). Numerous nanocarriers ranging from polymeric systems, lipidic systems, protein based nanoassemblies and inorganic systems have been explored for intracellular delivery. This chapter outlines the cellular pathways and factors affecting the cellular uptake of nanocarriers. Further, it gives insight about the variety of lipid based nanocarrier systems explored for intracellular delivery. Through this chapter, we intend to contribute to an understanding of these new technologies for the advancement of drug delivery systems with cell specificity, higher efficacy and lower toxicity.

2. MECHANISM OF CELLULAR UPTAKE OF NANOCARRIERS

It is believed that for small molecules, primary pathway for cellular entry is through passive diffusion or active transport. However, for nanomedicines the predominant route into cells is endocytosis (Kou, Sun, Zhai, & He, 2013). Endocytosis is broadly classified into phagocytosis and pinocytosis. Phagocytosis is generally associated with macrophages, monocytes and polymorphonuclear neutrophils (PMNs) while pinocytosis occurs in all cells (Wang, Byrne, Napier & DeSimone, 2011) (Figure 1).

2.1. Phagocytosis

This pathway predominantly relies on recognition and internalization of larger nanocarriers and pathogens. This pathway is characterized by three stepwise related events: 1) recognition of the nanocarriers by opsonization; 2) adhesion of opsonized nanocarriers onto the cell membrane; 3) ingestion of nanocarriers by the cells. For opsonization, various blood components such as proteins (immunoglubulins

Figure 1. Various mechanisms of cellular uptake of nanocarriers

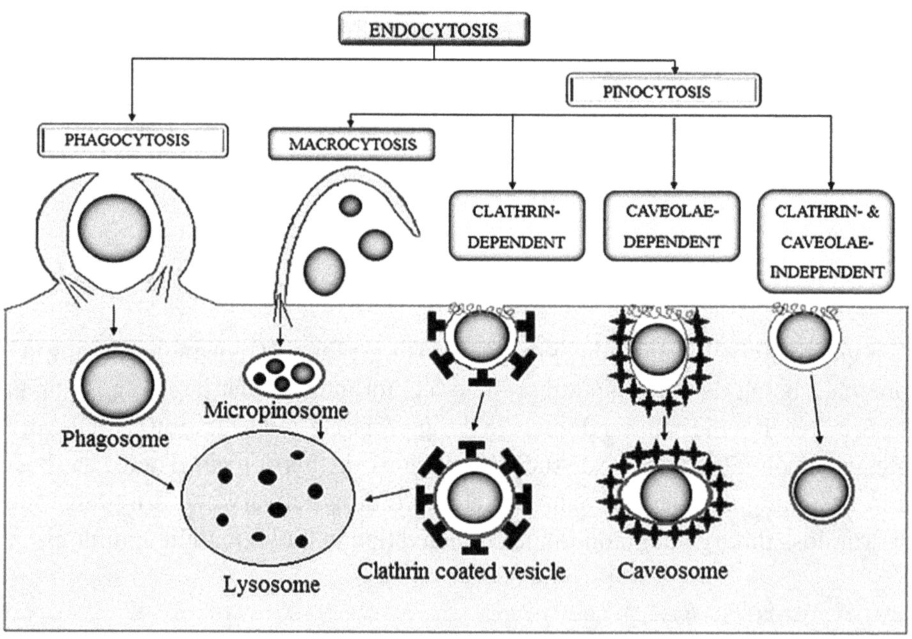

IgG, IgM), complement components (C3, C4, C5), blood serum proteins (including laminin, fibronectin, etc.) and others are adsorbed onto the nanocarrier surface. Post opsonization, the particles attach to the macrophage surface through Fc receptor (FcR) or complement receptors (CR) or other receptors such as mannose/ fructose and scavenger receptors (Sahay, Alakhova, & Kabanov, 2010). This receptor-ligand interaction results in actin rearrangement and formation of a phagosome (diameter of 0.5 µm-10 mm) which internalizes the nanocarriers in macrophages through attractive forces (i.e., van der Waals, electrostatic, ionic, hydrophobic/ hydrophilic) between the cells and nanoparticles surfaces (Yameen, Choi, Vilos, Swami, Shi, & Farokhzad, 2014). Thereafter, the phagosomes fuse with lysosomes, wherein the nanocarriers are destroyed by acidification and enzymolysis in the lysosomes (Kou, Sun, Zhai, & He, 2013). Although phagocytosis is a deterrent for site-specific targeting of intravenously administered nanocarriers, it has been exploited for targeting macrophages related infections e.g. liposomal and lipidic amphotericin B products (Ambisome, Abelcet and Amphocil) (Duncan & Richardson, 2012).

2.2. Pinocytosis

This pathway is characterized by internalization of fluid surrounding the cell, which clearly states that all nanocarriers dispersed in the fluid phase area of invagination are taken up simultaneously (Iversen, Skotland, & Sandvig, 2011). Based on the proteins involved in the endocytic pathways, pinocytosis is classified as clathrin-dependent endocytosis (also known as clathrin-mediated endocytosis (CME)) and clathrin-independent endocytosis. Further, the clathrin-independent pathways are classified as: 1) caveolae-mediated endocytosis; 2) clathrin- and caveolae-independent endocytosis and; 3) macropinocytosis (Sahay, Alakhova, & Kabanov, 2010).

2.2.1. Clathrin Mediated Endocytosis

This is a very well established route of cellular entry for nanocarriers present in all mammalian cells. It is associated with uptake of nutrients like cholesterol by low density lipoprotein (LDL) via the LDL receptor, or iron carried by transferrin (Tf) via the Tf receptor (Doherty & McMahon, 2009). The pathway is characterized by recruitment of clathrin protein from the cytosol to initiate clathrin-coating on the inner membrane of the cell in the presence of nanocarrier. Facilitating vesicle formation is an adaptor protein, Epsin, which aids the initial stages of membrane curvature and pit formation. In addition to this, there are accessory proteins such as dynamin (GTPase) which induce deformation of membrane and promote vesicle formation i.e. shallow to deep invagination by polymerization of the coat complex. Thereafter, with energy supplied by actin, clathrin-coated vesicle containing nanocarrier internally detaches from the donor membrane within the cell. Following this, clathrin and adaptor proteins uncoat the vesicle, thereby resulting in the fusion of vesicle within the cell and subsequent release of nanocarriers within the cell (Murugan, Choonara, Kumar, Bijukumar, du Toit, & Pillay, 2015).

2.2.2. Caveolae Mediated Endocytosis

This pathway bypasses lysosyme and relies on membrane cholesterol, dynamin, and cell receptor mediation. It is a preferred route of cellular entry by the pathogens including viruses and bacteria to avoid lysosomal degradation (Medina-Kauwe, 2007). Hence, it is often exploited to increase the cellular concentration and therapeutic efficacy of the cargo. The prominent protein governing endocytosis is a cluster of caveolin proteins (caveolin-1, -2, -3) that bind directly to membrane cholesterol. By binding to the receptors, nanocarriers induce, as observed in clathrin mediated endocytosis, actin reorganization and dynamin recruitment from the cytosol to stimulate a flask shaped membrane invagination (having a body diameter of 60–80 nm and a neck diameter of 10–15 nm) and subsequent, vesicle budding. Thereafter, the nanocarriers containing cell membrane get internalized and the caveolae membrane fuses into the acceptor compartment to release its contents (Kou, Sun, Zhai, & He, 2013). Unlike, clathrin-dependent endocytosis, this pathway is known to occur over relative longer time and have smaller vesicles in the process (Pelkmans, Kartenbeck, & Helenius, 2001).

2.2.3. Clathrin- and Caveolae-Independent Endocytosis

This is a distinct pathway, which is independent of clathrin and caveolae, occurring in cholesterol-rich microdomains on the plasma membrane, widely known as lipid rafts (Wang, Byrne, Napier, & DeSimone, 2011). This pathway also known as lipid raft mediated endocytosis is poorly understood. By definition, these lipid rafts are:

... small (10–200 nm), heterogeneous, highly dynamic sterol- and sphingolipid-enriched domains that compartmentalize cellular processes. (Pike, 2006)

There are reports that suggest these lipid rafts which play a role in cell signalling, membrane trafficking, endocytosis have been utilized by some viruses for budding (Simons & Gerl, 2010). Broadly, this pathway includes flotillin-dependent endocytosis, GTPase regulator associated with focal adhesion kinase-1 (GRAF1)-dependent endocytosis, adenosine diphosphate-ribosylation factor 6 (Arf6)-dependent endocytosis, and RhoA-dependent endocytosis (El-Sayed & Harashima, 2013). Although, it is unclear, it is believed that dynamins also play a dominant part in this pathway. Further, there are reports which suggest the role of clathrin-independent carrier (CLIC) or GPI-anchored protein-enriched early endosomal compartment (GEEC) (Benmerah & Lamaze, 2007). For detailed review, readers are referred to Canton & Battaglia, 2012.

2.2.4. Macropinocytosis

This pathway is a specialised clathrin-, caveolin-, and dynamin-independent process growth factor-induced, actin-driven endocytosis that leads to internalization of large volume of membrane together with extracellular fluid through irregularly formed vesicles called macropinosomes (Mercer & Helenius, 2009). These macropinosomes originating from coated vesicles, are significantly larger, thereby allowing for larger sized particles of sizes 0.5-10 µm to be internalized (Hansen & Nichols, 2009). This pathway is found in most of the cells with few exceptions, like brain microvessel endothelial cells (Kou, Sun, Zhai, & He, 2013). The endocytic pathway is initiated by activation of tyrosine kinases that signals the actin driven formation of protrusions from the cell membrane, which encapsulates the nanocarriers and subsequently fuses to the cell membrane. This generates an internalized macrosome vesicle following which the uncoated membrane of the macrosome eventually acidifies and fuses with the lysosomal compartment, consequently releasing the nanocarriers into the intracellular compartment (Hillaireau &

Couvreur, 2009). However, it is not generalized, in human A431 cells, the macropinosomes move to the cell surface and release the nanocarriers to the extracellular, making it cell specific (Mayor & Pagano, 2007).

3. FACTORS AFFECTING UPTAKE OF NANOCARRIERS

It is established that the endocytosis efficiency of nanocarriers is greatly governed by the physicochemical attributes, such as size, shape, charge and surface chemistry, as well as cell type (Figure 2). Hence, in this section, physicochemical attributes of lipid nanocarriers influencing the interaction of nanocarriers with cells is discussed in detail.

3.1. Nanocarrier Size

This is a critical parameter that governs the bodily responses to the nanocarriers i.e. uptake by the macrophage phagocyte system and at cellular level, the mechanism of cellular internalization (Jhaveri & Torchilin, 2016). Since most of the internalization process is receptor mediated, the size-dependent multiple interaction of nanocarriers with the receptor on the cell membrane becomes rate defining step (Albanese, Tang, & Chan, 2012). It is believed that in case of small nanocarrier, due to less ligand-

Figure 2. Overview of factors affecting cellular uptake of nanocarriers

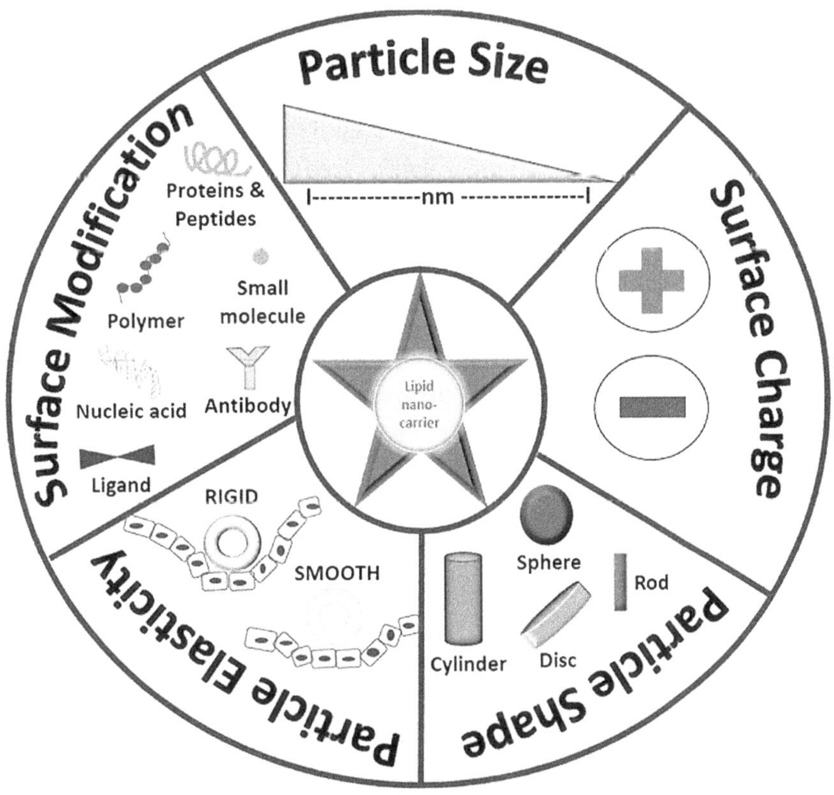

to-receptor interactions than large ones, to trigger membrane wrapping several small nanocarriers are required to interact simultaneously with receptors. Whereas, for large nanocarrier, an individual nanocarrier acts as a cross-linker to cluster receptors and facilitate its uptake (Shang, Nienhaus, & Nienhaus, 2014). Study conducted using gold nanocarriers suggest that nanocarriers in size range of 40- to 50-nm are preferable for receptor mediated internalization. The authors ascribe this to the possibility to balance between multivalent crosslinking of receptors and the membrane wrapping process occurring in receptor-mediated endocytosis (Jiang, Kim, Rutka, & Chan, 2008). Similar observations were made for lipid nanocarriers, wherein it was demonstrated that the nanocarriers with sizes of 20, 50, and 100 nm were taken up into the macrophages by complement receptor-mediated phagocytosis (Vonarbourg, Passirani, Saulnier, Simard, Leroux, & Benoit, 2006). However, in case of liposomes with sizes ranging from 100 to 2000 nm, the number of liposomes taken up by the macrophages showed proportional increase with size over the range 100–1000 nm, but the rate was found to remain constant with sizes over 1000 nm (Chono, Tanino, Seki, & Morimoto, 2007). Although the studies implicate the role of size in cellular uptake, it has to be noted that in biological milieu, the nanocarriers tend to aggregate, resulting in increase in their overall size. Thus, the particle size of nanocarrier should be considered only after thorough investigation whether the nanocarriers maintain their un-aggregated state in the biological media before they enter the cell (Oh & Park, 2014).

3.2. Nanocarrier Surface Charge

Surface charge of nanocarriers is governed by the chemical composition and it does influence the efficiency and the pathway of cellular uptake. This is based on the fact that biological interaction involves various forces i.e. ionic, electrostatic, van der Waals forces etc. between functionalized ligands of nanocarriers and lipid bilayer head groups. Owing to the negative charge of cell membranes (Yeung, Gilbert, Shi, Silvius, Kapus, & Grinstein, 2008), it is demonstrated that, positively charged nanocarriers are internalized to greater extent in comparison to negatively charged or neutral nanocarriers (Sun, Hu, Ji, Wright, & Gu, 2017). Literature states that cationic nanocarriers are internalized through clathrin-dependent pathway while anionic nanocarriers through caveolae-mediated pathway (Hammond, 2016, Harush-Frenkel, Debotton, Benita, & Altschuler, 2007). The charge also influences the nanocarrier interaction with serum proteins, where the positive charge on nanocarriers tend to attract serum proteins which results in protein corona, making it susceptible to clearance by immune cells. Further, this protein corona reduces the free energy of the nanocarrier surface. A prerequisite for internalization is cellular adhesion, for which nanocarriers with high surface energy is required, hence protein corona reduces the adhesion to the cell membrane as compared to bare nanocarriers, consequently uptake levels. Additionally, biomolecules in the corona may regulate the cellular uptake by inducing specific recognition by cell membrane receptors, further affecting rate of internalisation (Lesniak, Salvati, Santos-Martinez, Radomski, Dawson, & Åberg, 2013). Besides this, the cationic nanocarriers have tendency to disrupt platelets causing hemolysis, thrombogenicity and activation of complement system if positive charge density is high and eventually prove to be toxic (Arvizo, Miranda, Thompson, Pabelick, Bhattacharya, Robertson, & Mukherjee, 2010, Kumari & Yadav, 2011). The influence of surface charge was demonstrated by study carried out using R123-loaded solid lipid nanocarriers with mean size below 200 nm and slight negative surface charge (around −20 mV) demonstrated that the nanocarriers in four human glioma cell lines (A172, U251, U373 and U87) and a human macrophage cell line (THP1) were internalized in a higher amount than by macrophages through a clathrin-dependent endocytic pathway (Martins, Costa-Lima, Carneiro, Cordeiro-da-Silva, Souto, & Ferreira, 2012). Similarly, negatively charged nanoparticles, such as DOXIL® have shown preferential cellular uptake via caveolae-mediated pathway (Sahay, Kim, Kabanov, & Bronich, 2010).

3.3. Nanocarrier Shape

In recent times, diverse shapes of nanocarriers, nanospheres, nanodiscs, nanorods, and nanocylinders have been designed. The shape of nanocarrier has known to influence membrane wrapping time thereby affecting the cellular internalization. During the process of internalization, nanocarrier attachment and wrapping is influenced by two opposing energy factors; the adhesion-energy gained during contact between a nanocarrier and a membrane and the deformation-energy loss by the lipid bilayer. For favourable internalization, the adhesion strength is thought to be large enough to recompense the deformation-energy loss at the surface point of smallest curvature (Dasgupta, Auth, & Gompper, 2014). For internalization of any particle by the macrophage, the macrophage membrane undergoes structural changes to ensure that the membrane spreads around the geometry of the particle, starting from the initial contact site between particle and membrane. Thus, the progression of endocytic uptake of particles is dependent on this contact angle between particle and macrophage membrane. In case of an elliptical disk-shaped particle, if the particle attaches itself perpendicularly to the cell membrane, due to small contact angle, internalization is observed along its long axis. Consequently, particle gets engulfed because the membrane spreads symmetrically around the particle. Conversely, when the short axis is perpendicular to the membrane, due to increase in the angle of contact and the number of contact points with the membrane, the membrane spreads asymmetrically, thereby failing to engulf the particle (Champion & Mitragotri, 2006, Hirota & Terada, 2012). Literature cites that in comparison to rod-shaped particles, spherical particles of similar size were taken up 500% more, as elongated particles take longer membrane wrapping time owing to their elongated structure (Verma & Stellacci, 2010). Besides this, asymmetry in shape has shown to promote nanocarrier margination i.e. tumbling toward the wall of blood vessels under flow arising due to non-uniform distribution of hydrodynamic forces acting on the shape of nanocarrier. Owing to this, the asymmetry also contributes to enhancement of nanocarrier penetration and distribution inside solid tissues and tumors. This could be ascribed to the possibility that asymmetric nanocarriers approach the cell membrane at different contact angles resulting in variation of rates of internalization (Agarwal, Singh, Jurney, Shi, Sreenivasan, & Roy, 2015, Toy, Peiris, Ghaghada, & Karathanasis, 2014, Toy & Roy, 2016). From the perspective of circulation, cylindrical or disc-like shape versus spherical shape may demonstrate enhanced circulation half-time either by orienting the nanocarrier to follow blood flow or by tumbling in the blood vessels (Muro, Garnacho, Champion, Leferovich, Gajewski, Schuchman, Mitragotri, & Muzykantov, 2008). The study carried out in mammalian cells states that the cell uptake kinetics, efficiency, and mechanisms of uptake are governed by the shape of nanocarriers and cell type. The epithelial and immune cells were shown to preferentially internalize disc-shaped nanocarriers of high aspect ratios compared with nanorods and lower aspect-ratio nanodiscs while endothelial cells preferred nanodiscs with intermediate aspect ratio. In terms of efficiency, larger-sized hydrogel nanodiscs and nanorods were more efficiently internalized than their smallest counterparts. With regards to mechanism, macropinocytosis was found to be used by both epithelial and endothelial cells, while epithelial cells also exhibited caveolae-mediated pathway. On the other hand, human umbilical vein endothelial cells, preferentially used clathrin-mediated uptake for all shapes and had higher uptake efficiency compared with epithelial cells. The authors ascribed the behaviour to shape- and size-dependent parameters i.e. particle–cell adhesion, strain energy for membrane deformation, and sedimentation or local particle concentration at the cell membrane (Agarwal, Singh, Jurney, Shi, Sreenivasan, & Roy, 2013).

3.4. Nanocarrier Elasticity

This term accounts for the impact of interaction of rigid and soft nanocarriers with cellular membrane. It has been stated that, with increased stiffness of the nanocarrier, the energy expended by the cell membrane for wrapping a nanocarrier decreases, thereby making rigid nanoparticles easier for cellular uptake. It is assumed that for a rigid particle, the membrane deforms and wraps around the nanocarrier at a faster rate, in response to adhesive interaction between the particle and membrane. Whereas, for a soft particle, the deformation is slower and gradual. In case of soft nanocarrierrs, the particle initially spreads along the membrane without significantly deforming the membrane. Following this, at a later stage the membrane is compelled to bend and wrap around the particle. This causes an abrupt rise in elastic energy at the later stage of wrapping, as a result, greater adhesion energy is required to counterbalance the sudden inflection in elastic energy. In contrast, since the membrane deforms more easily for a rigid particle, the rise in elastic energy is gradual and consistent (Yi, Shi, & Gao, 2011). Further, since cellular internalization is difficult, it is believed soft nanocarriers undergo prolonged blood circulation residence time and increased organ deposition (Toy & Roy, 2016). The study revealed that the elasticity also influences choice of cellular internalization route. The soft nanocarriers are preferentially internalized by macropinocytosis, hard nanocarriers by clathrin-mediated routes and nanocarriers exhibiting intermediate elasticity are found to be internalized via multiple mechanisms giving rise to increased rate of cellular uptake (Banquy, Suarez, Argaw, Rabanel, Grutter, Bouchard, Hildgen, & Giasson, 2009). These observations were affirmed from the study involving polyethylene glycol (PEG)-based hydrogel nanoparticles of uniform size (200 nm) with elastic moduli ranging from 0.255 to 3000 kPa. The authors demonstrated that *in vivo* soft nanoparticles (10 kPa) exhibited longer circulation and subsequently enhanced targeting compared to hard nanoparticles (3000 kPa). Besides this, as discussed earlier, soft nanoparticles showed significantly reduced cellular uptake in immune cells (J774 macrophages), endothelial cells (bEnd.3), and cancer cells (Anselmo, Zhang, Kumar, Vogus, Menegatti, Helgeson, & Mitragotri, 2015).

3.5. Nanocarrier Surface Modification

It is well known that the type of ligand and ligand density on the surface of nanocarrier influences the biodistribution, cellular uptake and cellular association of nanocarrier as well as immune response to the nanocarrier. Further, ligand conjugation to a nanocarrier can be a tool to minimize cytotoxicity (Toy & Roy, 2016). However, the surface modification is a very critical step, as it is essential to note *in lieu* of conferring targetability to the nanocarrier, the healthy cells also share the receptors of the tumor cells albeit at a lower expression level (Sun, Hu, Ji, Wright, & Gu, 2017). The interaction between nanocarrier surface groups and membrane receptors is governed by the type of biomolecules/ chemicals (e.g., affinity) or by changing the density of surface biomolecules/ chemicals (e.g., avidity) (Zhu, Nie, Meng, Xia, Nel, & Zhao, 2012). One of the most common surface modification includes the use of polymers such as polyethylene glycol (PEG), predominantly to enhance particle hydrophilicity and reduce clearance by the reticuloendothelial system. Studies investigating the effect of PEG density have confirmed that the degree of PEG surface loading changes the particle biodistribution between hepatocytes and Kupffer cells (Liu, Hu, & Huang, 2014). Most commonly used ligands, include growth factors, folate receptors, transferrin receptors, epidermal growth factor receptors, antibodies, proteins, polypeptides, nucleic acids, and polysaccharides. This strategy has been prominently used to target tumor cells since the aforementioned receptors are overexpressed in cancerous cells (Ma, Ma, Li, Wang, Tang, Wang, Mou, Chen, & He, 2013).

4. ADVANTAGES OF LIPID-BASED NANOCARRIERS (MUKHERJEE, RAY, & THAKUR, 2009)

Although, both polymeric and lipid nanocarriers have been explored extensively for intracellular targeting, lipid nanocarriers have inherent advantages such as;

- Biodegradability and Biocompatibility.
- Ability to deliver both lipophilic and hydrophilic drugs.
- Amenable to improve targetability.
- Ability to modulate drug release.
- Confer stability of pharmaceuticals.
- Easily scalable.
- Economical.
- Products can be easily regulated for approvals.

5. TYPES OF LIPID-BASED PARTICULATE CARRIERS

In literature (Copland, Rades, Davies, & Baird, 2005; Fernandes, Prabhu, Guggulothu, & Patravale, 2011), lipid-based particulate systems have been broadly classified based on the structural alignment of lipid components contained in the formulation with the water i.e. at the air-liquid interface and in the bulk aqueous phase, using the categories of lipids proposed by Small (1969) (Figure 3).

5.1 Class I-Based Delivery Systems

This class constitutes insoluble non-swelling amphiphiles i.e. lipids which are insoluble in the bulk aqueous phase but spread at the air-liquid interface to form a stable monolayer. They comprise of the following types of delivery systems:

5.1.1 Microemulsions

Microemulsions are thermodynamically stable systems characterized by ultra-low interfacial tension between the immiscible phases stabilized by an interfacial film of surfactant or a mixture of surfactants, may include co-surfactant or co-solvent. Broadly, these systems may be classified based on their microstructure as water-in-oil, bicontinuous or oil-in-water type (Jain, Fernandes, & Patravale, 2010;

Figure 3. Different types of lipid-based particulate carriers

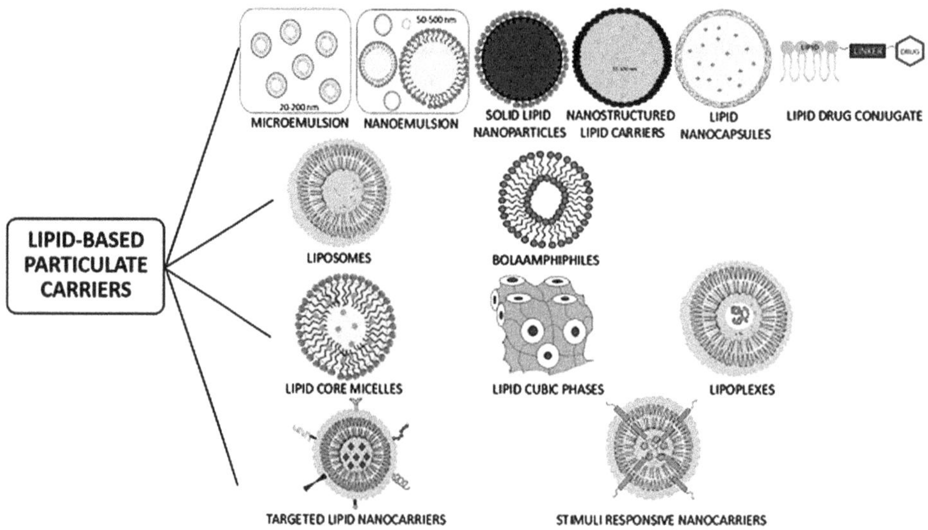

Fanun, 2012). They offer several benefits such as spontaneous formation, ease of manufacture, broad solubilisation capacity of lipophilic, hydrophilic and amphiphilic solutes, macroscopic homogeneity and microscopic heterogeneity (microdomains), large surface area per volume ratio for mass transfer, enormous interfacial area, and good shelf life (stability with time). By manipulating the components, they can be modified to protect labile drug, control drug release, increase bioavailability and in turn reduce patient variability (Lawrence & Rees, 2000).

Qu, et al. (2015) investigated anticancer effect of synergistic dual-drug; coix seed oil and etoposide in the form of microemulsion with globule size around 35 nm against A549 cells (human lung carcinoma). The study revealed that the microemulsion system promoted significant internalization of etoposide via clathrin-mediated endocytosis pathway. This enhanced uptake resulted 3.5-fold improvement in induction of cell apoptosis in A549 cells by microemulsion (20 μg/mL of etoposide) in comparison to free drug. Recently, study involving microemulsion of docetaxel (DTX) and Schizandrin A, a potent chemotherapeutic agent and a potential drug resistance modulator showed a 3.9-fold enhancement of DTX internalization in DTX-resistant EC109 (esophageal carcinoma) cells in comparison to that observed for EC109 cells at DTX (30 μg/mL) concentration. Likewise, the apoptotic rate of DTX-resistant EC109 increased up to 20-fold compared to free drug. Further, in nude mice bearing EC109/DDR tumor xenografts, drug loaded microemulsion had the highest survival rate (37.5%) during the observation period (Su, Gao, Shi, Feng, Liu, Qu, & Wang, 2017). Another study also established that the levamisole loaded microemulsion increased the phagocytosis rate, microbicidal activity and apoptosis index thereby increasing the functional activity of human mononuclear phagocytes against *G. lamblia* (Hernandes, Moraes, Ribeiro, Fagundes, Honorio-França, & França, 2017). Interestingly, a study demonstrated the negative effect of evodiamine and rutaecarpine loaded microemulsion which showed lower cellular uptake in mouse skin fibroblasts. The authors ascribed this to the fact that most of the drug loaded in microemulsion vehicle was transported via the intercellular space and did not exhibit endocytosed evodiamine and rutaecarpine (Zhang, Huang, Zhang, Zhao, Wang, Liu, & Feng, 2012).

5.1.2 Nanoemulsions

Nanoemulsions are colloidal dispersions of water and oil stabilised by an amphiphilic surfactant with mean droplet diameter smaller than ~500 nm (Singh, et al., 2017). In contrast to microemulsions, these systems are thermodynamically unstable and are only stable kinetically. Generally, unlike microemulsion which are spontaneously formed, these systems are prepared either by high-energy emulsification methods (e.g. high-pressure homogenizers) or ultrasound generators or by low energy methods or by phase-inversion temperature (PIT) method (Fernandes, Soni, & Patravale, 2010; Pidaparthi & Suares, 2016). They have been widely explored to solubilize and protect drugs against harsh environmental factors (oxidation, pH, hydrolysis), to target specific organs by exploiting enhanced permeability and retention effect, to evade reticuloendothelial system, to increase rate of drug dissolution and subsequently bioavailability (Singh, Meher, Raval, Khan, Chaurasia, Jain, & Chourasia, 2017).

The study carried out on paclitaxel nanoemulsion showed increased permeability through the Caco-2 cell monolayer and decreased efflux. Further, paclitaxel nanoemulsion in breast cancer cell line showed significant antiproliferation at lower IC50 values possibly due to enhanced uptake of paclitaxel through the oil core (Choudhury, et al., 2014). Similarly, another study combining paclitaxel and tocotrienol in nanoemulsion exhibited higher cytotoxicity in breast cancer cell line (MCF-7) when compared to free paclitaxel and marketed formulation (Taxol®). Cell cycle arrest study depicted that MCF-7 cells treated with paclitaxel loaded nanoemulsion showed high arrest in G2-M phase while blank nanoemulsion induced additional apoptosis in breast cancer cells through G1-S arrest by disrupting mitochondrial membrane potential. Further, both paclitaxel loaded nanoemulsion and blank nanoemulsion enhanced secretion of IL-12 and down-regulated secretion of IL-4 and IL-10 in macrophages (Pawar, Panchal, Singh, Meher, Sharma, Singh, Bora, Singh, Datta, & Chourasia, 2014).

5.1.3 Solid Lipid Nanoparticles

Solid lipid nanoparticles (SLNs) are sub-micron rigid colloidal carriers (50-1000 nm) which are composed of physiological lipid, dispersed in water or in an aqueous surfactant solution. (Fernandes, Mandawgade, & Patravale, 2013; Suares & Prabhakar, 2016). They comprise of lipids which are solid at room temperature as well as at body temperature. As a nanocarrier system, SLNs provide several advantages such as protection of photosensitive, moisture sensitive and chemically labile drugs, biocompatibility, biodegradability, controlled drug release and cost-effective scale-up process (Yoon, Park, & Yoon, 2013). However, the drug loading capacity is limited by the solubility of drug in lipid melt, structure of the lipid matrix and polymorphic state of the lipid matrix. It is assumed that if the lipid matrix consists of similar molecules (i.e. tristearin or tripalmitin), a highly ordered crystal lattice with few imperfections is formed. Since the drugs are located between fatty acid chains, between the lipid layers and also in crystal imperfections, large amounts of drug cannot be accommodated in nanoparticles (Mukherjee, Ray, & Thakur, 2009).

A study involving curcumin SLNs demonstrated that in comparison to solubilised solution, curcumin SLNs exhibited prolonged inhibitory activity in cancer cells, as well as time-dependent increase in intracellular uptake (Sun, Bi, Chan, Sun, Zhang, & Zheng, 2013). Using fluorescent dye, the cellular uptake ability of fluorescent SLNs with different lipid material was evaluated. The order of cellular uptake ability was found to be glycerol tristearate SLNs > monostearin SLNs > stearic acid SLNs >

Compritol 888 ATO SLNs (Yuan, Miao, Du, You, Hu, & Zeng, 2008). The study involving uptake of coumarin-6 (a drug model) in alveolar epithelial cells also demonstrated that there was enhancement in the drug uptake by 54.8% when SLNs of coumarin-6 was incorporated in the extracellular medium (Rivolta, Panariti, Lettiero, Sesana, Gasco, Gasco, Masserini, & Miserocchi, 2011).

5.1.4. Nanostructured Lipid Carriers

SLNs owing to the crystalline nature are plagued with issues such as drug expulsion, gelation and poor stability. To circumvent, nanostructured lipid carriers (NLCs) were explored. These systems are characterized by a solid lipid core consisting of a mixture of solid and liquid lipids. Based on the method of production and on the lipid blend composition, NLCs are broadly classified as: imperfect, amorphous and multiple type. In the imperfect type, lipid crystallization is altered by small amounts of oils. While in the amorphous type; the lipid matrix is solid and amorphous, achieved by mixing special lipids, for example, hydroxyoctacosanyl hydroxystearate with isopropyl myristate. Finally, in the multiple type, the solid lipid matrix contains tiny oil compartments obtained by including higher amount of oil (Battaglia & Gallarate, 2012; Beloqui, Solinís, Rodríguez-Gascón, Almeida, & Préat, 2016). The prominent advantage of NLCs is that the use of spatially different lipids creates spaces between the fatty acid chains of the glycerides and imperfections in the crystal lattice thereby generating space to accommodate drug molecules (Prabhu, Suryavanshi, Pathak, Sharma, & Patravale, 2016). The authors investigated the effect of glyceryl dilaurate NLCs in Plasmodium-infected red blood cells (iRBCs). The NLCs were found to be localized to the parasite mitochondrion, leading to mitochondrial-membrane polarization and Ca^{+2} ion accumulation, reactive oxygen species release, and stage-specific iRBC lysis. The treatment also resulted in externalization of iRBC-membrane phosphatidylserine and enhanced iRBC clearance by macrophages. Further, the NLCs disrupted the parasite-induced tubulovesicular network, a vital component for nutrient import by the parasite and restored iRBC flexibility (Jain, Basu, Prabhu, Soni, Joshi, Mathur, Patravale, Pathak, & Sharma, 2014).

5.1.5. Lipid-Drug Nanoconjugates

A prerequisite for SLNs is the drug should be lipophilic in nature. Hence, for hydrophilic drugs, the entrapment is generally low due to partitioning effects during the production process (Mukherjee, Ray, & Thakur, 2009). The lipid-drug conjugates (LDCs) are achieved either by salt formation (e.g., with a fatty acid) or by covalent linking (e.g., esters or ethers). Owing to the conjugation of lipids, the hydrophilic drug is rendered lipophilic, thereby resulting in diverse properties of drugs. Some LDCs have shown to form self-assembled nanoparticles, however, most LDCs are entrapped in nanocarriers. The lipid "tail" in the LDC, through a hydrophobic interaction, enables the loading of LDCs into delivery carriers and prevents the leakage of hydrophilic drugs, consequently increasing the formulation stability. This approach has several advantages, such as improved oral bioavailability, enhanced tumor targeting, reduced toxicity, and enhanced hydrophilic drug loading into delivery carriers (Irby, Du, & Li, 2017).

Researchers have investigated the influence of LDCs wherein the lipid-modified antisense oligonucleotides (LASOs) was shown to improve penetration and efficiency in inhibiting translationally controlled tumor protein (TCTP) expression in the absence of additional transfection agents, in androgen-independent prostatic cancer cell line PC-3. It was observed that transfection with TCTP-LASO resulted in rapid and prolonged internalization via macropinocytosis, TCTP down-regulation and significant decreased cell viability. Further, the lipid-modification led to delayed tumor progression in CRPC xenografts models, with no significant toxic effects (Karaki, Benizri, Mejías, Baylot, Branger, Nguyen, Vialet, Oumzil, Barthélémy, & Rocchi, 2017).

5.1.6. Lipid Nanocapsules

Lipid nanocapsules (LNCs), consisting of an oil-filled core with a surrounding polymer shell have special use for encapsulating and delivering hydrophobic drugs. They have similar particle size as SLNs and are prepared by a solvent free, soft-energy procedure. Generally, their oily core comprises of medium-chain triglycerides surrounded by a membrane made from a mixture of lecithin and a PEGylated surfactant. Mostly, they are formulated using phase inversion temperature phenomenon of an emulsion leading to lipid nanocapsule formation with good mono-dispersion (Huynh, Passirani, Saulnier, & Benoît, 2009; Heurtault, Saulnier, Pech, Proust, & Benoit, 2002).

A study carried out in rat glioma cells revealed that LNCs rapidly accumulated within cells (from 2 min exposure) through active and saturating mechanisms involving endogenous cholesterol with a major contribution of clathrin/ caveolae-independent pathways. The LNCs were found to bypass the endo-lysosomal compartment and only 10% of the cell-internalized fraction were found in isolated lysosomes after 2 h exposure. The LNCs were found to revert lysosome integrity in a size-dependent manner with small particle size showing maximum efficiency (Paillard, Hindré, Vignes-Colombeix, Benoit, & Garcion, 2010). Similarly, in glioma U251MG cells, the curcumin LNCs were found to be more cytotoxic than non-encapsulated curcumin after 24 h incubation via induction of G2/M arrest and autophagy (Zanotto-Filho, Coradini, Braganhol, Schröder, De Oliveira, Simões-Pires, Battastini, Pohlmann, Guterres, Forcelini, & Beck, 2013).

5.2 Class II-Based Delivery Systems

This class constitutes insoluble swelling amphiphiles which have a very low real aqueous solubility but swell to form well-defined liquid crystalline phases and stable monolayers.

5.2.1 Liposomes

This is the most widely known and well-investigated class of nanocarriers for targeted drug delivery. They are defined as phospholipid vesicles consisting of one or more concentric lipid bilayers enclosing discrete aqueous spaces. Overall the physical and chemical properties of a liposome are governed by the properties of the constituent phospholipids such as permeability, charge density and steric hindrance (Bawarski, Chidlowsky, Bharali, & Mousa, 2008). Owing to their morphology, they are able to encapsulate both lipophilic and hydrophilic compounds. It is believed that hydrophobic molecules are inserted into the bilayer membrane of liposomes, and hydrophilic molecules are contained in the aqueous spaces. Due to its versatility, they have been exploited for the delivery of small molecules and macromolecules, such as DNA, proteins. Prominent advantages of this includes biocompatibility, biodegradability, ability to encapsulate both hydrophobic and hydrophilic drugs, confer protection to drug, overcome obstacles to cellular and tissue uptake, and improve biodistribution of compounds to target sites *in vivo* (Sercombe, Veerati, Moheimani, Wu, Sood, & Hua, 2015; Malam, Loizidou, & Seifalian, 2009).

Most prominent example for liposomal formulation is Doxil®, a marketed formulation of the anthracycline drug doxorubicin used to treat cancer in AIDS-related Kaposi sarcoma and multiple myeloma. The formulation has well established greater efficacy and lower cardiotoxicity over free doxorubicin (Huwyler, Drewe, & Krähenbühl, 2008). Another study revealed that curcuminoid-loaded liposomes demonstrated high cellular uptake resulting in down-regulation of the expression of inflammatory markers on osteoblasts. In presence of interleukin (IL)-1β stimulation, the liposomal curcumin demonstrated a high osteoprotegerin (OPG)/ receptor activator of nuclear factor κB ligand (RANKL) ratio to prevent osteoclastogenesis compared to free drug (Yeh, Su, Lin, Chen, Shi, Chen, & Chang, 2015).

5.2.2. Bolaamphiphiles

They are also known as bolaform detergents or two-headed amphiphiles or bipolar amphiphiles. The characteristic of this type of amphiphiles is the presence of two hydrophilic head groups (ionic or non-ionic and they may be identical to or different from one another) which is separated by either one, two or three long hydrophobic spacers i.e. mostly alkyl chains, or steroids or porphyrins (Meister & Blume, 2007; Fariya, Jain, Dhawan, Shah, & Nagarsenker, 2014). Generally, bolaamphiphiles form less permeable and better durable monolayer with increased aqueous solubility. It is reported that the bolaamphiphiles have increased Critical Aggregation Concentration (CAC) in range of 10^{-4} to 10^{-6} M much higher in comparison to phospholipids (10^{-8} M). Basically, the chemical structure of bolaamphiphiles influence their arrangement into parallel or antiparallel sheets which contribute to the formation of either unsymmetrical or symmetrical monolayer membranes (MLMs). Typically, short-chain bolaamphiphiles form micelles, whereas long-chain bolaamphiphiles form vesicles (Puri, Loomis, Smith, Lee, Yavlovich, Heldman, & Blumenthal, 2009; Fuhrhop & Wang, 2004).

The study involving iron oxide nanoparticles demonstrated that iron oxide nanoparticles loaded bolavesicles enhanced internalization in b.End3 brain microvessel endothelial cells – an *in vitro* model of the blood–brain barrier (Philosof-Mazor, Dakwar, Popov, Kolusheva, Shames, Linder, Greenberg, Heldman, Stepensky, & Jelinek, 2013). Similar study was undertaken to investigate the ability of Bolaamphiphilic cationic vesicles decorated with acetylcholine (ACh) surface groups to deliver a model protein–bovine serum albumin conjugated to fluorescein isothiocyanate (BSA-FITC) across blood–brain barrier. Based on this study, it was confirmed that the vesicles were successfully internalized into brain endothelial b.End3 cells, at 37 °C, but not at 4 °C, indicating an active uptake process (Dakwar, Hammad, Popov, Linder, Grinberg, Heldman, & Stepensky, 2012).

5.3 Class III-Based Delivery Systems

This class constitutes soluble amphiphiles which form micellar solutions when added to an aqueous bulk phase. They are further sub classified as Class IIIa: Lipids which form micelles at a specific critical micelle-forming concentration of the amphiphile and form liquid crystal phases at high concentrations. Class IIIb: Lipids which do not exhibit lyotropic mesomorphism and form micelles in a stepwise fashion upon dissolution in the aqueous bulk.

5.3.1 Lipid Core Micelles

These micelles comprise of hydrophobic core made up of short and hydrophobic phospholipid residues containing two long-chain fatty acyls. The micelles are generally formed by conjugates of soluble co-polymers with lipids (such as polyethylene glycol-phosphatidyl ethanolamine conjugate, PEG-PE). The PEG block typically has a molecular weight range from 750 to 5000 Da. It is believed that use of lipid moieties as hydrophobic blocks confers superior particle stability when compared with conventional amphiphilic polymer micelles. Prominent advantages of these micelles include great solubilisation capacity of hydrophobic drugs, stealth property due to the outer PEG corona and amenability to target body areas with compromised vasculature (tumors, infarcts) via the enhanced permeability and retention (EPR) effect. In few cases, by modulating the charge of lipid-core mixed micelles with certain specific components (such as positively charged lipids), the micelles can be enabled to escape endosomes and release drug directly into the cell cytoplasm (Torchilin, 2005; Sawant & Torchilin, 2010; Gill, Kaddoumi, & Nazzal, 2015).

Recently, a stable mixed micelles made of 1,2-distearoyl-sn-glycero-3-phosphoethanolamine-N-[methoxy(polyethyleneglycol)-2000] (DSPE-PEG) mixed with d-α-tocopheryl polyethylene glycol 1000 succinate (TPGS) (PEG-succinate ester of vitamin E) formulation of berberine has been reported to induce significant enhanced apoptosis and overall cytotoxicity against monolayer and spheroid cultures of human prostate carcinomas (16- to 18-fold lower half-maximal inhibitory concentration values in PC3 and LNPaC, respectively), compared to free drug (Shen, Kim, Yao, & Elbayoumi, 2016). Similarly, due to enhanced cellular uptake, pro-apoptotic agent DM-PIT-1 loaded PEG–DSPE micelles were found to be effective against human U87MG glioblastoma cells at concentrations around 100 mM (Skidan, Miao, Thekkedath, Dholakia, Degterev, & Torchilin, 2009).

5.3.2 Lipid Cubic Phases

They are self-assembled mesophase system comprising of polar lipids and having features similar to crystalline solids and isotropic liquids. This ability to form various liquid-crystalline phases is governed by the molecular structure of polar lipid, packing parameter, water content, temperature and composition (Libster, Aserin, & Garti, 2015). Recently, non-lamellar liquid crystalline lipid systems, such as inverted bicontinuous cubic, hexagonal and sponge mesophases have been explored for drug delivery (Koynova & Tenchov, 2013). Among these, cubic and hexagonal are highly ordered internal structures making them suitable as a slow release matrix for active pharmaceutical ingredients with various sizes and polarities. The lipid based systems are formed when amphiphilic lipids exposed to aqueous environment, spontaneously form thermodynamically stable self-assembled structures and eventually convert into cubic and/or hexagonal liquid crystals by varying temperature and water content. Examples of lipid include glyceryl monooleate, phytantriol, monolinolein, monoelaidin, phosphatidylethanolamine, oleoylethanolamide, phospholipids, PEGylated phospholipids, alkyl glycerates, and glycolipids. The advantages of this system includes, biodegradability, biocompatibility, minimal toxicity, tunable nanoproperties, improved drug payload, and sustained release profile (Chen, Ma, & Gui, 2014). However, in recent times, phytantriol cubosomes have shown to be more toxic than glycerol monooleate cubosomes due to its greater ability to disrupt the cellular membrane (hemolytic activity) and induce oxidative stress (Hinton, Grusche, Acharya, Shukla, Bansal, Waddington, Monaghan, & Muir, 2014).

The anticancer effect of doxorubicn-loaded cubosome on the glioblastoma T98G cell line was found to be highly efficient and even at lower concentrations of drug, the cubosome was found to inhibit the proliferation of cancer cells than the effective concentrations of free drug (Nazaruk, Majkowska-Pilip, & Bilewicz, 2017). A study was carried out to investigate the intracellular uptake potential of Gambogenic acid loaded cubosomes in the human hepatic carcinoma (SMMC-7721) cells. The study revealed that increased cellular uptake of gambogenic acid from cubosomes and the possible mechanism of uptake for cubosome was ascribed to receptor-mediated endocytosis (Luo, Lin, Zhang, Zhu, Wang, Ji, Jia, Ge, Peng, & Chen, 2015).

5.3.3. Lipoplexes

This is a non-viral vector popular to deliver nucleic-acid-based drugs. The use of lipid nanocarriers is often preferred due to their ease of synthesis, low toxicity, low production cost, and the ability to deliver transgenes with different sizes. Generally, lipoplex nanocarriers incorporate amphiphilic lipids to encapsulate hydrophilic therapeutics (Boukany, Wu, Zhao, Kwak, Glazer, Leong, & Lee, 2014). They may exhibit different charges based on the ratio of the cationic charges of the lipid interacting with the anionic DNA phosphodiester bonds. As a result, anionic, neutral or cationic complexes are obtained, for higher transfection efficiency, lipoplexes with a slight excess of positive charge is acceptable (de Ilarduya, Sun, & Düzgüneş, 2010). Although it is well established that the carriers have to undergo endocytosis to ingress inside the cellular domain, post endocytosis, lipoplexes use a distinct mechanism to release their cargo into the cytosol. The mechanism relies on lipid interaction via fusion and/or formation of transient and local perturbations of the endosomal membrane through which nucleic acids may be released into the cytosol. For cationic lipids, the most widely used lipid, this is the inherent ability which aids in the formation of non-bilayer structures. Further, it is reported that the lipoplex-induced flip-flop of negatively charged phospholipids from the cytoplasm to the inner face of the endosome, thereby forming charged neutral ion pairs with the cationic lipids, resulting in destabilization of the lamellar membrane organization and simultaneous dissociation of the nucleic acids from the lipoplexes (Rehman, Hoekstra, & Zuhorn, 2013). Well-characterized cationic lipids such as N-[1-(2,3-dioleyloxy)propyl]-N,N,N-trimethylammonium chloride (DOTMA), 2,3-dioleyloxy-N-[2(sperminecarboxamido)ethyl]-N,N-dimethyl-l-propanaminium trifluoroacetate (DOSPA), [1,2-bis(oleoyloxy)-3-(trimethylammonio) propane] (DOTAP), 1,2-dimyristyloxypropyl-3dimethyl- hydoxyethylammonium (DMRIE) and 3β[N-(N′, N′-dimethylaminoethane)-carbamoyl] (DC) have been used for liposomal gene delivery to enhance transfection activity. However, their usefulness is limited by low efficacy owing to poor stability and rapid clearance, as well as the generation of inflammatory or anti-inflammatory responses (Yin, Kanasty, Eltoukhy, Vegas, Dorkin, & Anderson, 2014; Zhang, McIntosh, & Grinstaff, 2012).

A study reported the uptake of DOTAP/DNA lipoplexes by clathrin-mediated endocytosis and eventual degradation in lysosomes, which was proven by its inhibition by chlorpromazine and potassium depletion but were unaffected by filipin or genestein (Rejman, Bragonzi, & Conese, 2005). Similarly, another study also revealed that the uptake of SAINT/DOPE lipoplexes in the COS-7, CHO, and HepG2 cells was via cholesterol-dependent clathrin-mediated endocytosis pathway (Zuhorn, Kalicharan, & Hoekstra, 2002).

5.4. Targeted Lipid Nanocarriers

Targeting of lipid nanocarriers often exploits characteristics of disease tissues to selectively target their payloads, either by passive, active or physical targeting. Most commonly, passive targeting is employed wherein nanocarriers tend to localize into specific organs or site of disease via biological mechanisms, such as RES (reticuloendothelial system) or EPR (enhanced permeability and retention) effects. This targeting is non-selective process primarily governed by the leaky, underdeveloped tumour vasculature and inefficient drainage into the lymphatic system which permits size-dependent retention of macromolecules. Widely used in oncology, the advanced form targeting, i.e. active targeting, is an approach that involves use of ligands that bind to receptors that are overexpressed on the surface of rapidly dividing cancer cells. Example of receptors includes transferrin and folate receptors which conjugate with transferrin, folic acid or antibodies. However, these ligands are plagued with shortcomings as these receptors are native to other tissues too. Hence, there is a possibility that they may have non-specificity and could contribute to side effects. To overcome this drawback, new ligands rely on highly specific interactions of antibodies, aptamers (single-stranded oligonucleotides), peptides and oligonucleotides with cell surface receptors expressed only on target cells (Petros & DeSimone, 2010; Torchilin, V., 2014).

Recently, targeted lipid nanocarriers surface-functionalized with anti-CD4 monoclonal antibody were investigated to deliver siRNAs specifically to CD4+ T lymphocytes. The *ex vivo* study found this modality was specific only to primary CD4+ T lymphocytes and no other cell types. Further, *in vivo*, systemic intravenous administration of these nanocarriers was found to be selectively localized into CD4+ T lymphocytes in several anatomical sites including the spleen, inguinal lymph nodes, blood, and the bone marrow as well as in a subset of circulating CD4+ T lymphocytes (Ramishetti, Kedmi, Goldsmith, Leonard, Sprague, Godin, Gozin, Cullis, Dykxhoorn, & Peer, 2015). Another example demonstrated the targetability of fucose decorated SLNs of methotrexate in breast cancer cells. The authors revealed that ligand decorated nanocarries showed greater cellular uptake and better cytotoxicity at lower IC50 of methotrexate (MTX) in breast cancer cells. Further, *in vivo* studies affirmed the tumor targeting efficiency with minimum secondary drug distribution in various organs and sizeable reduction in tumor burden of anchored nanocarriers when compared with free drug (Garg, Singh, Jain, Nirbhavane, Sharma, Tyagi, Kushwah, Jain, & Katare, 2016). Similarly, cRGD peptides (ligand specific to $\alpha v\beta 3$ integrins expressed by tumour endothelium and cancer cells) surface grafted LNCs revealed superior internalization *in vitro* in U87MG glioma cells and superior *in vivo* tumor accumulation (Hirsjärvi, Belloche, Hindré, Garcion, & Benoit, 2014).

5.5. Stimuli Responsive Nanocarriers

For the stimuli responsive nanocarriers, stimuli can be endogenous i.e. intrinsic to the target tissue (such as changes in pH, temperature, redox condition or the activity of certain enzymes) or endogenous i.e. externally applied (such as a magnetic field, ultrasound and various types of irradiation) (Torchilin, 2014). For targeting at the cellular level, pH responsive system has shown to either trigger the release of the entrapped drug into late endosomes or lysosomes, or promote endosomal escape of the nanocarriers to the cell cytoplasm. Whereas for targeting at the tissue level, the targeted nanocarrier can be guided to the site of action in the body or for modulating release, for instance, using external magnetic stimuli based guiding of ultrasmall iron oxide-based nanoparticles (Arachchige, Reshetnyak, & Andreev, 2015). For detailed review, please refer (Mura, Nicolas, & Couvreur, 2013).

Based on this concept, there is concept of eliposomes. An emulsion liposomes (eLiposome) is a evolving concept which relies on ultrasound stimuli to release the content from the liposome. It is basically an emulsion nanodroplet encapsulated within the liposome which on the application of ultrasound causes the emulsion droplet to change from liquid to gas, thus causing the sudden increase in the internal volume resulting in rupture and release of the drug. This concept was explored to deliver doxorubicin in HeLa cells using perfluoropentane nanodroplet within the aqueous interior of a dipalmitoylphosphatidylcholine liposome, along with the anticancer drug doxorubicin (Dox). The eLiposome containing Dox (eLipoDox) was found to release Dox upon insonation with low intensity ultrasound at 20-kHz, 1.0-MHz and 3.0-MHz. The study demonstrated that the authors were successful in controlling the delivery of Dox by applying ultrasound to HeLa tumor cells *in vitro* (Lin, Javadi, Belnap, Barrow, & Pitt, 2014). Recently, pH-sensitive liposomes (HHG2C(18)-L and PEGHG2C(18)-L) based on zwitterionic oligopeptide lipids were evaluated for the multistage pH-response to tumor microenvironmental pH (pH(e), pH 6.0-7.0) and endosomal/ lysosomal pH (pH(i), pH 4.0-6.0) successively. Both these liposomes were shown to exhibit higher tumor cellular uptake due to electrostatic absorptive endocytosis at pH(e) (pH 6.5), producing proton sponge effect for endo-lysosomal escape, and subsequent accumulation inside mitochondria, based on stronger positive charge by the hydrolysis of a pH-sensitive linker at pH(i) (pH 5.5 and pH 4.5) (Mo, Sun, Li, & Zhang, 2013).

6. CONCLUSION AND PERSPECTIVES

The delivery of actives for infectious diseases and cancer has transformed with the advent of lipid nanocarriers. Nevertheless, these systems face incredulity from Pharma industry with respect to product manufacture and reproducibility. Such cynicism may be resolved by shifting the research focus from proof-of-concept to exhaustive fundamental studies and reliable manufacturing processes, followed by thorough preclinical ADME/ toxicology data and finally clinical studies. As depicted in the book chapter lipid nanocarriers are emerging as tools to target cells *in vivo*, promoting cellular uptake and increasing therapeutic efficacy.

REFERENCES

Agarwal, R., Jurney, P., Raythatha, M., Singh, V., Sreenivasan, S., Shi, L., & Roy, K. (2015). Effect of shape, size, and aspect ratio on nanoparticle penetration and distribution inside solid tissues using 3D spheroid models. *Advanced Healthcare Materials*, *4*(15), 2269–2280. doi:10.1002/adhm.201500441 PMID:26376024

Agarwal, R., Singh, V., Jurney, P., Shi, L., Sreenivasan, S. V., & Roy, K. (2013). Mammalian cells preferentially internalize hydrogel nanodiscs over nanorods and use shape-specific uptake mechanisms. *Proceedings of the National Academy of Sciences of the United States of America*, *110*(43), 17247–17252. doi:10.1073/pnas.1305000110 PMID:24101456

Albanese, A., Tang, P. S., & Chan, W. C. (2012). The effect of nanoparticle size, shape, and surface chemistry on biological systems. *Annual Review of Biomedical Engineering*, *14*(1), 1–16. doi:10.1146/annurev-bioeng-071811-150124 PMID:22524388

Anselmo, A. C., Zhang, M., Kumar, S., Vogus, D. R., Menegatti, S., Helgeson, M. E., & Mitragotri, S. (2015). Elasticity of nanoparticles influences their blood circulation, phagocytosis, endocytosis, and targeting. *ACS Nano*, *9*(3), 3169–3177. doi:10.1021/acsnano.5b00147 PMID:25715979

Arachchige, M. C. M., Reshetnyak, Y. K., & Andreev, O. A. (2015). Advanced Targeted Nanomedicine. *Journal of Biotechnology*, *202*, 88–97. doi:10.1016/j.jbiotec.2015.01.009 PMID:25615945

Arvizo, R. R., Miranda, O. R., Thompson, M. A., Pabelick, C. M., Bhattacharya, R., Robertson, J. D., & Mukherjee, P. (2010). Effect of nanoparticle surface charge at the plasma membrane and beyond. *Nano Letters*, *10*(7), 2543–2548. doi:10.1021/nl101140t PMID:20533851

Banquy, X., Suarez, F., Argaw, A., Rabanel, J. M., Grutter, P., Bouchard, J. F., ... Giasson, S. (2009). Effect of mechanical properties of hydrogel nanoparticles on macrophage cell uptake. *Soft Matter*, *5*(20), 3984–3991. doi:10.1039/b821583a

Battaglia, L., & Gallarate, M. (2012). Lipid nanoparticles: State of the art, new preparation methods and challenges in drug delivery. *Expert Opinion on Drug Delivery*, *9*(5), 497–508. doi:10.1517/17425247.2012.673278 PMID:22439808

Bawarski, W. E., Chidlowsky, E., Bharali, D. J., & Mousa, S. A. (2008). Emerging nanopharmaceuticals. *Nanomedicine; Nanotechnology, Biology, and Medicine*, *4*(4), 273–282. doi:10.1016/j.nano.2008.06.002 PMID:18640076

Beloqui, A., Solinís, M. Á., Rodríguez-Gascón, A., Almeida, A. J., & Préat, V. (2016). Nanostructured lipid carriers: Promising drug delivery systems for future clinics. *Nanomedicine; Nanotechnology, Biology, and Medicine*, *12*(1), 143–161. doi:10.1016/j.nano.2015.09.004 PMID:26410277

Benmerah, A., & Lamaze, C. (2007). Clathrin-Coated Pits: Vive La Différence? *Traffic (Copenhagen, Denmark)*, *8*(8), 970–982. doi:10.1111/j.1600-0854.2007.00585.x PMID:17547704

Boukany, P. E., Wu, Y., Zhao, X., Kwak, K. J., Glazer, P. J., Leong, K., & Lee, L. J. (2014). Nonendocytic delivery of lipoplex nanoparticles into living cells using nanochannel electroporation. *Advanced Healthcare Materials*, *3*(5), 682–689. doi:10.1002/adhm.201300213 PMID:23996973

Canton, I., & Battaglia, G. (2012). Endocytosis at the nanoscale. *Chemical Society Reviews*, *41*(7), 2718–2739. doi:10.1039/c2cs15309b PMID:22389111

Champion, J. A., & Mitragotri, S. (2006). Role of target geometry in phagocytosis. *Proceedings of the National Academy of Sciences of the United States of America*, *103*(13), 4930–4934. doi:10.1073/pnas.0600997103 PMID:16549762

Chen, Y., Ma, P., & Gui, S. (2014). *Cubic and hexagonal liquid crystals as drug delivery systems*. BioMed Research International.

Chono, S., Tanino, T., Seki, T., & Morimoto, K. (2007). Uptake characteristics of liposomes by rat alveolar macrophages: Influence of particle size and surface mannose modification. *The Journal of Pharmacy and Pharmacology*, *59*(1), 75–80. doi:10.1211/jpp.59.1.0010 PMID:17227623

Choudhury, H., Gorain, B., Karmakar, S., Biswas, E., Dey, G., Barik, R., & Pal, T. K. (2014). Improvement of cellular uptake, in vitro antitumor activity and sustained release profile with increased bioavailability from a nanoemulsion platform. *International Journal of Pharmaceutics*, *460*(1), 131–143. doi:10.1016/j.ijpharm.2013.10.055 PMID:24239580

Copland, M. J., Rades, T., Davies, N. M., & Baird, M. A. (2005). Lipid based particulate formulations for the delivery of antigen. *Immunology and Cell Biology*, *89*(2), 97–105. doi:10.1111/j.1440-1711.2005.01315.x PMID:15748206

Dakwar, G. R., Hammad, I. A., Popov, M., Linder, C., Grinberg, S., Heldman, E., & Stepensky, D. (2012). Delivery of proteins to the brain by bolaamphiphilic nano-sized vesicles. *Journal of Controlled Release*, *160*(2), 315–321. doi:10.1016/j.jconrel.2011.12.042 PMID:22261280

Dasgupta, S., Auth, T., & Gompper, G. (2014). Shape and orientation matter for the cellular uptake of nonspherical particles. *Nano Letters*, *14*(2), 687–693. doi:10.1021/nl403949h PMID:24383757

de Ilarduya, C. T., Sun, Y., & Düzgüneş, N. (2010). Gene delivery by lipoplexes and polyplexes. *European Journal of Pharmaceutical Sciences*, *40*(3), 159–170. doi:10.1016/j.ejps.2010.03.019 PMID:20359532

DM, S. (1969). Surface and bulk interactions of lipids and water with a classification of biologically active lipids based on these interactions. *Federation Proceedings*, *29*(4), 1320–1326. PMID:5459881

Doherty, G. J., & McMahon, H. T. (2009). Mechanisms of endocytosis. *Annual Review of Biochemistry*, *78*(1), 857–902. doi:10.1146/annurev.biochem.78.081307.110540 PMID:19317650

Duncan, R., & Richardson, S. C. (2012). Endocytosis and intracellular trafficking as gateways for nanomedicine delivery: Opportunities and challenges. *Molecular Pharmaceutics*, *9*(9), 2380–2402. doi:10.1021/mp300293n PMID:22844998

El-Sayed, A., & Harashima, H. (2013). Endocytosis of gene delivery vectors: From clathrin-dependent to lipid raft-mediated endocytosis. *Molecular Therapy*, *21*(6), 1118–1130. doi:10.1038/mt.2013.54 PMID:23587924

Fanun, M. (2012). Microemulsions as delivery systems. *Current Opinion in Colloid & Interface Science*, *17*(5), 306–313. doi:10.1016/j.cocis.2012.06.001

Fariya, M., Jain, A., Dhawan, V., Shah, S., & Nagarsenker, M. S. (2014). Bolaamphiphiles: A Pharmaceutical Review. *Advanced Pharmaceutical Bulletin*, *4*(Suppl 2), 483–491. PMID:25671179

Fernandes, C., Soni, U., & Patravale, V. (2010). Nano-interventions for neurodegenerative disorders. *Pharmacological Research*, *62*(2), 166–178. doi:10.1016/j.phrs.2010.02.004 PMID:20153429

Fernandes, C. B., Mandawgade, S., & Patravale, V. B. (2013). Solid lipid nanoparticles of etoposide using solvent emulsification diffusion technique for parenteral administration. *International Journal of Pharma Bioscience and Technology*, *1*(1), 27–33.

Fernandes, C. B., Prabhu, P. S., Guggulothu, D., & Patravale, V. B. (2011). Lipid Nanocarriers for Topical Anti-cancer Therapy: An Update. In E. B. Souto & E. B. Souto (Eds.), *Lipid Nanocarriers in Cancer Diagnosis and Therapy* (pp. 461–491). New York: Smithers Rapra Technology.

Fuhrhop, J. H., & Wang, T. (2004). Bolaamphiphiles. *Chemical Reviews*, *104*(6), 2901–2938. doi:10.1021/cr030602b PMID:15186184

Garg, N. K., Singh, B., Jain, A., Nirbhavane, P., Sharma, R., Tyagi, R. K., ... Katare, O. P. (2016). Fucose decorated solid-lipid nanocarriers mediate efficient delivery of methotrexate in breast cancer therapeutics. *Colloids and Surfaces. B, Biointerfaces*, *146*, 114–126. doi:10.1016/j.colsurfb.2016.05.051 PMID:27268228

Gill, K. K., Kaddoumi, A., & Nazzal, S. (2015). PEG–lipid micelles as drug carriers: Physiochemical attributes, formulation principles and biological implication. *Journal of Drug Targeting*, *23*(3), 222–231. doi:10.3109/1061186X.2014.997735 PMID:25547369

Hammond, P. T. (2016). Shooting for the moon: Nanoscale approaches to cancer. *ACS Nano*, *10*(2), 1711–1713. doi:10.1021/acsnano.6b01095 PMID:26902596

Hansen, C. G., & Nichols, B. J. (2009). Molecular mechanisms of clathrin-independent endocytosis. *Journal of Cell Science*, *122*(11), 1713–1721. doi:10.1242/jcs.033951 PMID:19461071

Harush-Frenkel, O., Debotton, N., Benita, S., & Altschuler, Y. (2007). Targeting of nanoparticles to the clathrin-mediated endocytic pathway. *Biochemical and Biophysical Research Communications*, *353*(1), 26–32. doi:10.1016/j.bbrc.2006.11.135 PMID:17184736

Hernandes, M. R. G., Moraes, L. C. A., Ribeiro, E. B., Fagundes, D. L. G., Honorio-França, A. C., & França, E. L. (2017). In vitro immunomodulatory effects of microemulsions with levamisole delivery systems on blood phagocytes interacting with Giardia lamblia. *Parasitology International*, *66*(3), 299–304. doi:10.1016/j.parint.2017.02.005 PMID:28257952

Heurtault, B., Saulnier, P., Pech, B., Proust, J. E., & Benoit, J. P. (2002). A novel phase inversion-based process for the preparation of lipid nanocarriers. *Pharmaceutical Research*, *19*(6), 875–880. doi:10.1023/A:1016121319668 PMID:12134960

Hillaireau, H., & Couvreur, P. (2009). Nanocarriers' entry into the cell: Relevance to drug delivery. *Cellular and Molecular Life Sciences*, *66*(17), 2873–2896. doi:10.100700018-009-0053-z PMID:19499185

Hinton, T. M., Grusche, F., Acharya, D., Shukla, R., Bansal, V., Waddington, L. J., ... Muir, B. W. (2014). Bicontinuous cubic phase nanoparticle lipid chemistry affects toxicity in cultured cells. *Toxicology Research*, *3*(1), 11–22. doi:10.1039/C3TX50075F

Hirota, K., & Terada, H. (2012). Endocytosis of particle formulations by macrophages and its application to clinical treatment. INTECH Open Access Publisher, 414-428.

Hirsjärvi, S., Belloche, C., Hindré, F., Garcion, E., & Benoit, J. P. (2014). Tumour targeting of lipid nanocapsules grafted with cRGD peptides. *European Journal of Pharmaceutics and Biopharmaceutics*, *87*(1), 152–159. doi:10.1016/j.ejpb.2013.12.006 PMID:24361535

Huwyler, J., Drewe, J., & Krähenbühl, S. (2008). Tumor targeting using liposomal antineoplastic drugs. *International Journal of Nanomedicine*, *3*(1), 21–29. doi:10.2147/IJN.S1253 PMID:18488413

Huynh, N. T., Passirani, C., Saulnier, P., & Benoît, J. P. (2009). Lipid nanocapsules: A new platform for nanomedicine. *International Journal of Pharmaceutics*, *379*(2), 201–209. doi:10.1016/j.ijpharm.2009.04.026 PMID:19409468

Irby, D., Du, C., & Li, F. (2017). Lipid-drug Conjugate for Enhancing Drug Delivery. *Molecular Pharmaceutics*, *14*(5), 1325–1338. doi:10.1021/acs.molpharmaceut.6b01027 PMID:28080053

Iversen, T. G., Skotland, T., & Sandvig, K. (2011). Endocytosis and intracellular transport of nanoparticles: Present knowledge and need for future studies. *Nano Today*, *6*(2), 176–185. doi:10.1016/j.nantod.2011.02.003

Jain, J., Fernandes, C., & Patravale, V. (2010). Formulation development of parenteral phospholipid-based microemulsion of etoposide. *AAPS PharmSciTech*, *11*(2), 826–831. doi:10.120812249-010-9440-x PMID:20464537

Jain, S. A., Basu, H., Prabhu, P. S., Soni, U., Joshi, M. D., Mathur, D., ... Sharma, S. (2014). Parasite impairment by targeting Plasmodium-infected RBCs using glyceryl-dilaurate nanostructured lipid carriers. *Biomaterials*, *35*(24), 6636–6645. doi:10.1016/j.biomaterials.2014.04.058 PMID:24818881

Javadi, M., Pitt, W. G., Belnap, D. M., Tsosie, N. H., & Hartley, J. M. (2012). Encapsulating nanoemulsions inside eLiposomes for ultrasonic drug delivery. *Langmuir*, *28*(41), 14720–14729. doi:10.1021/la303464v PMID:22989347

Jhaveri, A., & Torchilin, V. (2016). Intracellular delivery of nanocarriers and targeting to subcellular organelles. *Expert Opinion on Drug Delivery*, *13*(1), 49–70. doi:10.1517/17425247.2015.1086745 PMID:26358656

Jiang, W., Kim, B. Y., Rutka, J. T., & Chan, W. C. (2008). Nanoparticle-mediated cellular response is size-dependent. *Nature Nanotechnology*, *3*(3), 145–150. doi:10.1038/nnano.2008.30 PMID:18654486

Karaki, S., Benizri, S., Mejías, R., Baylot, V., Branger, N., Nguyen, T., ... Rocchi, P. (2017). Lipid-oligonucleotide conjugates improve cellular uptake and efficiency of TCTP-antisense in castration-resistant prostate cancer. *Journal of Controlled Release*, *258*, 1–9. doi:10.1016/j.jconrel.2017.04.042 PMID:28472637

Kou, L., Sun, J., Zhai, Y., & He, Z. (2013). The endocytosis and intracellular fate of nanomedicines: Implication for rational design. *Asian Journal of Pharmaceutical Sciences*, *8*(1), 1–10. doi:10.1016/j.ajps.2013.07.001

Koynova, R., & Tenchov, B. (2013). Recent patents on nonlamellar liquid crystalline lipid phases in drug delivery. *Recent Patents on Drug Delivery & Formulation*, *7*(3), 165–173. doi:10.2174/18722113113079990011 PMID:23829393

Kumari, A., & Yadav, S. K. (2011). Cellular interactions of therapeutically delivered nanoparticles. *Expert Opinion on Drug Delivery*, *8*(2), 141–151. doi:10.1517/17425247.2011.547934 PMID:21219249

Lawrence, M. J., & Rees, G. D. (2000). Microemulsion-based media as novel drug delivery systems. *Advanced Drug Delivery Reviews*, *45*(1), 89–121. doi:10.1016/S0169-409X(00)00103-4 PMID:11104900

Lesniak, A., Salvati, A., Santos-Martinez, M. J., Radomski, M. W., Dawson, K. A., & Åberg, C. (2013). Nanoparticle adhesion to the cell membrane and its effect on nanoparticle uptake efficiency. *Journal of the American Chemical Society*, *135*(4), 1438–1444. doi:10.1021/ja309812z PMID:23301582

Libster, D., Aserin, A., & Garti, N. (2015). Lipid Nano-Vehicles Based on Lyotropic Liquid crystals as drug delivery vehicles. *Lipids in Nanotechnology*, 191.

Lin, C. Y., Javadi, M., Belnap, D. M., Barrow, J. R., & Pitt, W. G. (2014). Ultrasound sensitive eLiposomes containing doxorubicin for drug targeting therapy. *Nanomedicine; Nanotechnology, Biology, and Medicine*, *10*(1), 67–76. doi:10.1016/j.nano.2013.06.011 PMID:23845926

Liu, Y., Hu, Y., & Huang, L. (2014). Influence of polyethylene glycol density and surface lipid on pharmacokinetics and biodistribution of lipid-calcium-phosphate nanoparticles. *Biomaterials*, *35*(9), 3027–3034. doi:10.1016/j.biomaterials.2013.12.022 PMID:24388798

Luo, Q., Lin, T., Zhang, C. Y., Zhu, T., Wang, L., Ji, Z., ... Chen, W. (2015). A novel glyceryl monoolein-bearing cubosomes for gambogenic acid: Preparation, cytotoxicity and intracellular uptake. *International Journal of Pharmaceutics*, *493*(1), 30–39. doi:10.1016/j.ijpharm.2015.07.036 PMID:26209071

Ma, N., Ma, C., Li, C., Wang, T., Tang, Y., Wang, H., ... He, N. (2013). Influence of nanoparticle shape, size, and surface functionalization on cellular uptake. *Journal of Nanoscience and Nanotechnology*, *13*(10), 6485–6498. doi:10.1166/jnn.2013.7525 PMID:24245105

Malam, Y., Loizidou, M., & Seifalian, A. M. (2009). Liposomes and nanoparticles: Nanosized vehicles for drug delivery in cancer. *Trends in Pharmacological Sciences*, *30*(11), 592–599. doi:10.1016/j.tips.2009.08.004 PMID:19837467

Martins, S., Costa-Lima, S., Carneiro, T., Cordeiro-da-Silva, A., Souto, E. B., & Ferreira, D. C. (2012). Solid lipid nanoparticles as intracellular drug transporters: An investigation of the uptake mechanism and pathway. *International Journal of Pharmaceutics*, *430*(1), 216–227. doi:10.1016/j.ijpharm.2012.03.032 PMID:22465548

Mayor, S., & Pagano, R. E. (2007). Pathways of clathrin independent endocytosis. *Nature Reviews. Molecular Cell Biology*, *8*(8), 603–612. doi:10.1038/nrm2216 PMID:17609668

Medina-Kauwe, L. K. (2007). "Alternative" endocytic mechanisms exploited by pathogens: New avenues for therapeutic delivery? *Advanced Drug Delivery Reviews*, *59*(8), 798–809. doi:10.1016/j.addr.2007.06.009 PMID:17707545

Meister, A., & Blume, A. (2007). Self-assembly of bipolar amphiphiles. *Current Opinion in Colloid & Interface Science*, *12*(3), 138–147. doi:10.1016/j.cocis.2007.05.003

Mercer, J., & Helenius, A. (2009). Virus entry by macropinocytosis. *Nature Cell Biology*, *11*(5), 510–520. doi:10.1038/ncb0509-510 PMID:19404330

Mo, R., Sun, Q., Li, N., & Zhang, C. (2013). Intracellular delivery and antitumor effects of pH-sensitive liposomes based on zwitterionic oligopeptide lipids. *Biomaterials*, *34*(11), 2773–2786. doi:10.1016/j.biomaterials.2013.01.030 PMID:23352118

Mozafari, M. R., Pardakhty, A., Azarmi, S., Jazayeri, J. A., Nokhodchi, A., & Omri, A. (2009). Role of nanocarrier systems in cancer nanotherapy. *Journal of Liposome Research*, *19*(4), 310–321. doi:10.3109/08982100902913204 PMID:19863166

Mukherjee, S., Ray, S., & Thakur, R. S. (2009). Solid Lipid Nanoparticles: A Modern Formulation Approach in Drug Delivery System. *Indian Journal of Pharmaceutical Sciences*, *71*(4), 349–358. doi:10.4103/0250-474X.57282 PMID:20502539

Mura, S., Nicolas, J., & Couvreur, P. (2013). Stimuli-responsive nanocarriers for drug delivery. *Nature Materials*, *12*(11), 991–1003. doi:10.1038/nmat3776 PMID:24150417

Muro, S., Garnacho, C., Champion, J. A., Leferovich, J., Gajewski, C., Schuchman, E. H., ... Muzykantov, V. R. (2008). Control of endothelial targeting and intracellular delivery of therapeutic enzymes by modulating the size and shape of ICAM-1-targeted carriers. *Molecular Therapy*, *16*(8), 1450–1458. doi:10.1038/mt.2008.127 PMID:18560419

Murugan, K., Choonara, Y. E., Kumar, P., Bijukumar, D., du Toit, L. C., & Pillay, V. (2015). Parameters and characteristics governing cellular internalization and trans-barrier trafficking of nanostructures. *International Journal of Nanomedicine*, *10*, 2191. PMID:25834433

Nazaruk, E., Majkowska-Pilip, A., & Bilewicz, R. (2017). Lipidic Cubic-Phase Nanoparticles—Cubosomes for Efficient Drug Delivery to Cancer Cells. *ChemPlusChem*, *82*(4), 570–575. doi:10.1002/cplu.201600534

Oh, N., & Park, J.-H. (2014). Endocytosis and exocytosis of nanoparticles in mammalian cells. *International Journal of Nanomedicine*, *9*(Suppl 1), 51–63. PMID:24872703

Paillard, A., Hindré, F., Vignes-Colombeix, C., Benoit, J. P., & Garcion, E. (2010). The importance of endo-lysosomal escape with lipid nanocapsules for drug subcellular bioavailability. *Biomaterials*, *31*(29), 7542–7554. doi:10.1016/j.biomaterials.2010.06.024 PMID:20630585

Pawar, V. K., Panchal, S. B., Singh, Y., Meher, J. G., Sharma, K., Singh, P., ... Chourasia, M. K. (2014). Immunotherapeutic vitamin E nanoemulsion synergies the antiproliferative activity of paclitaxel in breast cancer cells via modulating Th1 and Th2 immune response. *Journal of Controlled Release*, *196*, 295–306. doi:10.1016/j.jconrel.2014.10.010 PMID:25459427

Pelkmans, L., Kartenbeck, J., & Helenius, A. (2001). Caveolar endocytosis of simian virus 40 reveals a new two-step vesicular-transport pathway to the ER. *Nature Cell Biology*, *3*(5), 473–483. doi:10.1038/35074539 PMID:11331875

Petros, R. A., & DeSimone, J. M. (2010). Strategies in the design of nanoparticles for therapeutic applications. *Nature Reviews. Drug Discovery*, *9*(8), 615–627. doi:10.1038/nrd2591 PMID:20616808

Philosof-Mazor, L., Dakwar, G. R., Popov, M., Kolusheva, S., Shames, A., Linder, C., ... Jelinek, R. (2013). Bolaamphiphilic vesicles encapsulating iron oxide nanoparticles: New vehicles for magnetically targeted drug delivery. *International Journal of Pharmaceutics*, *450*(1), 241–249. doi:10.1016/j.ijpharm.2013.04.017 PMID:23623794

Pidaparthi, K., & Suares, D. (2016). Comparison of Nanoemulsion and Aqueous Micelle Systems of Paliperidone for Intranasal Delivery. *AAPS PharmSciTech*, 1–10. PMID:27714701

Pike, L. J. (2006). Rafts defined: A report on the Keystone Symposium on Lipid Rafts and Cell Function. *Journal of Lipid Research*, *47*(7), 1597–1598. doi:10.1194/jlr.E600002-JLR200 PMID:16645198

Prabhu, P., Suryavanshi, S., Pathak, S., Sharma, S., & Patravale, V. (2016). Artemether-lumefantrine nanostructured lipid carriers for oral malaria therapy: Enhanced efficacy at reduced dose and dosing frequency. *International Journal of Pharmaceutics*, *511*(1), 473–487. doi:10.1016/j.ijpharm.2016.07.021 PMID:27421912

Puri, A., Loomis, K., Smith, B., Lee, J. H., Yavlovich, A., Heldman, E., & Blumenthal, R. (2009). Lipid-based nanoparticles as pharmaceutical drug carriers: from concepts to clinic. *Critical Reviews™ in Therapeutic Drug Carrier Systems*, *26*(6),523-580.

Qu, D., Ma, Y., Sun, W., Chen, Y., Zhou, J., Liu, C., & Huang, M. (2015). Microemulsion-based synergistic dual-drug codelivery system for enhanced apoptosis of tumor cells. *International Journal of Nanomedicine*, *10*, 1173–1187. PMID:25709440

Ramishetti, S., Kedmi, R., Goldsmith, M., Leonard, F., Sprague, A. G., Godin, B., ... Peer, D. (2015). Systemic gene silencing in primary T lymphocytes using targeted lipid nanoparticles. *ACS Nano*, *9*(7), 6706–6716. doi:10.1021/acsnano.5b02796 PMID:26042619

Rehman, Z. U., Hoekstra, D., & Zuhorn, I. S. (2013). Mechanism of polyplex-and lipoplex-mediated delivery of nucleic acids: Real-time visualization of transient membrane destabilization without endosomal lysis. *ACS Nano*, *7*(5), 3767–3777. doi:10.1021/nn3049494 PMID:23597090

Rejman, J., Bragonzi, A., & Conese, M. (2005). Role of clathrin-and caveolae-mediated endocytosis in gene transfer mediated by lipo-and polyplexes. *Molecular Therapy*, *12*(3), 468–474. doi:10.1016/j.ymthe.2005.03.038 PMID:15963763

Rivolta, I., Panariti, A., Lettiero, B., Sesana, S., Gasco, P., Gasco, M. R., ... Miserocchi, G. (2011). Cellular uptake of coumarin-6 as a model drug loaded in solid lipid nanoparticles. *Journal of Physiology and Pharmacology*, *62*(1), 45–53. PMID:21451209

Sahay, G., Alakhova, D. Y., & Kabanov, A. V. (2010). Endocytosis of Nanomedicines. *Journal of Controlled Release*, *145*(3), 182–195. doi:10.1016/j.jconrel.2010.01.036 PMID:20226220

Sahay, G., Kim, J. O., Kabanov, A. V., & Bronich, T. K. (2010). The exploitation of differential endocytic pathways in normal and tumor cells in the selective targeting of nanoparticulate chemotherapeutic agents. *Biomaterials*, *31*(5), 923–933. doi:10.1016/j.biomaterials.2009.09.101 PMID:19853293

Sawant, R. R., & Torchilin, V. P. (2010). Multifunctionality of lipid-core micelles for drug delivery and tumour targeting. *Molecular Membrane Biology*, *27*(7), 232–246. doi:10.3109/09687688.2010.516276 PMID:20929339

Sercombe, L., Veerati, T., Moheimani, F., Wu, S. Y., Sood, A. K., & Hua, S. (2015). Advances and challenges of liposome assisted drug delivery. *Frontiers in Pharmacology*, *6*, 286. doi:10.3389/fphar.2015.00286 PMID:26648870

Shang, L., Nienhaus, K., & Nienhaus, G. U. (2014). Engineered nanoparticles interacting with cells: Size matters. *Journal of Nanobiotechnology*, *12*(1), 5. doi:10.1186/1477-3155-12-5 PMID:24491160

Shen, R., Kim, J. J., Yao, M., & Elbayoumi, T. A. (2016). Development and evaluation of vitamin E d-α-tocopheryl polyethylene glycol 1000 succinate-mixed polymeric phospholipid micelles of berberine as an anticancer nanopharmaceutical. *International Journal of Nanomedicine*, *11*, 1687–1700. PMID:27217747

Simons, K., & Gerl, M. J. (2010). Revitalizing membrane rafts: New tools and insights. *Nature Reviews. Molecular Cell Biology*, *11*(10), 688–699. doi:10.1038/nrm2977 PMID:20861879

Singh, Y., Meher, J. G., Raval, K., Khan, F. A., Chaurasia, M., Jain, N. K., & Chourasia, M. K. (2017). Nanoemulsion: Concepts, development and applications in drug delivery. *Journal of Controlled Release*, *252*, 28–49. doi:10.1016/j.jconrel.2017.03.008 PMID:28279798

Skidan, I., Miao, B., Thekkedath, R. V., Dholakia, P., Degterev, A., & Torchilin, V. (2009). In vitro cytotoxicity of novel pro-apoptotic agent DM-PIT-1 in PEG-PE-based micelles alone and in combination with TRAIL. *Drug Delivery*, *16*(1), 45–51. doi:10.1080/10717540802517951 PMID:19555308

Su, X., Gao, C., Shi, F., Feng, X., Liu, L., Qu, D., & Wang, C. (2017). A microemulsion co-loaded with Schizandrin A–docetaxel enhances esophageal carcinoma treatment through overcoming multidrug resistance. *Drug Delivery*, *24*(1), 10–19. doi:10.1080/10717544.2016.1225854 PMID:28155336

Suares, D., & Prabhakar, B. (2016). Oral delivery of rosuvastatin lipid nanocarriers: Investigation of *in vitro* and *in vivo* profile. *International Journal of Pharmaceutical Sciences and Research*, *7*(12), 4856.

Sun, J., Bi, C., Chan, H. M., Sun, S., Zhang, Q., & Zheng, Y. (2013). Curcumin-loaded solid lipid nanoparticles have prolonged in vitro antitumour activity, cellular uptake and improved in vivo bioavailability. *Colloids and Surfaces. B, Biointerfaces*, *111*, 367–375. doi:10.1016/j.colsurfb.2013.06.032 PMID:23856543

Sun, W., Hu, Q., Ji, W., Wright, G., & Gu, Z. (2017). Leveraging Physiology for Precision Drug Delivery. *Physiological Reviews*, *97*(1), 189–225. doi:10.1152/physrev.00015.2016

Torchilin, V. P. (2005). Lipid-core micelles for targeted drug delivery. *Current Drug Delivery*, *2*(4), 319–327. doi:10.2174/156720105774370221 PMID:16305435

Torchilin, V. P. (2014). Multifunctional, stimuli-sensitive nanoparticulate systems for drug delivery. *Nature Reviews. Drug Discovery*, *13*(11), 813–827. doi:10.1038/nrd4333 PMID:25287120

Toy, R., Peiris, P. M., Ghaghada, K. B., & Karathanasis, E. (2014). Shaping cancer nanomedicine: The effect of particle shape on the in vivo journey of nanoparticles. *Nanomedicine (London)*, *9*(1), 121–134. doi:10.2217/nnm.13.191 PMID:24354814

Toy, R., & Roy, K. (2016). Engineering nanoparticles to overcome barriers to immunotherapy. *Bioengineering & Translational Medicine*, *1*(1), 47–62. doi:10.1002/btm2.10005 PMID:29313006

Verma, A., & Stellacci, F. (2010). Effect of surface properties on nanoparticle–cell interactions. *Small*, *6*(1), 12–21. doi:10.1002mll.200901158 PMID:19844908

Vonarbourg, A., Passirani, C., Saulnier, P., Simard, P., Leroux, J. C., & Benoit, J. P. (2006). Evaluation of pegylated lipid nanocapsules versus complement system activation and macrophage uptake. *Journal of Biomedical Materials Research. Part A*, *78*(3), 620–628. doi:10.1002/jbm.a.30711 PMID:16779767

Wang, J., Byrne, J. D., Napier, M. E., & DeSimone, J. M. (2011). More Effective Nanomedicines through Particle Design. *Small (Weinheim an Der Bergstrasse, Germany)*, *7*(14), 1919–1931.

Yameen, B., Choi, W. I., Vilos, C., Swami, A., Shi, J., & Farokhzad, O. C. (2014). Insight into nanoparticle cellular uptake and intracellular targeting. *Journal of Controlled Release*, *190*, 485–499. doi:10.1016/j.jconrel.2014.06.038 PMID:24984011

Yeh, C.-C., Su, Y.-H., Lin, Y.-J., Chen, P.-J., Shi, C.-S., Chen, C.-N., & Chang, H.-I. (2015). Evaluation of the protective effects of curcuminoid (curcumin and bisdemethoxycurcumin)-loaded liposomes against bone turnover in a cell-based model of osteoarthritis. *Drug Design, Development and Therapy*, *9*, 2285–2300. PMID:25945040

Yeung, T., Gilbert, G. E., Shi, J., Silvius, J., Kapus, A., & Grinstein, S. (2008). Membrane phosphatidylserine regulates surface charge and protein localization. *Science*, *319*(5860), 210–213. doi:10.1126cience.1152066 PMID:18187657

Yi, X., Shi, X., & Gao, H. (2011). Cellular uptake of elastic nanoparticles. *Physical Review Letters*, *107*(9), 098101. doi:10.1103/PhysRevLett.107.098101 PMID:21929271

Yin, H., Kanasty, R. L., Eltoukhy, A. A., Vegas, A. J., Dorkin, J. R., & Anderson, D. G. (2014). Non-viral vectors for gene-based therapy. *Nature Reviews. Genetics*, *15*(8), 541–555. doi:10.1038/nrg3763 PMID:25022906

Yoon, G., Park, J. W., & Yoon, I. S. (2013). Solid lipid nanoparticles (SLNs) and nanostructured lipid carriers (NLCs): Recent advances in drug delivery. *Journal of Pharmaceutical Investigation*, *43*(5), 353–362. doi:10.100740005-013-0087-y

Yuan, H., Miao, J., Du, Y. Z., You, J., Hu, F. Q., & Zeng, S. (2008). Cellular uptake of solid lipid nanoparticles and cytotoxicity of encapsulated paclitaxel in A549 cancer cells. *International Journal of Pharmaceutics*, *348*(1), 137–145. doi:10.1016/j.ijpharm.2007.07.012 PMID:17714896

Zanotto-Filho, A., Coradini, K., Braganhol, E., Schröder, R., De Oliveira, C. M., Simões-Pires, A., ... Beck, R. C. R. (2013). Curcumin-loaded lipid-core nanocapsules as a strategy to improve pharmacological efficacy of curcumin in glioma treatment. *European Journal of Pharmaceutics and Biopharmaceutics*, *83*(2), 156–167. doi:10.1016/j.ejpb.2012.10.019 PMID:23219677

Zhang, X.-X., McIntosh, T. J., & Grinstaff, M. W. (2012). Functional lipids and lipoplexes for improved gene delivery. *Biochimie*, *94*(1), 42–58. doi:10.1016/j.biochi.2011.05.005 PMID:21621581

Zhang, Y. T., Huang, Z. B., Zhang, S. J., Zhao, J. H., Wang, Z., Liu, Y., & Feng, N. P. (2012). In vitro cellular uptake of evodiamine and rutaecarpine using a microemulsion. *International Journal of Nanomedicine*, *7*, 2465–2472. PMID:22679361

Zhu, M., Nie, G., Meng, H., Xia, T., Nel, A., & Zhao, Y. (2012). Physicochemical properties determine nanomaterial cellular uptake, transport, and fate. *Accounts of Chemical Research*, *46*(3), 622–631. doi:10.1021/ar300031y PMID:22891796

Zuhorn, I. S., Kalicharan, R., & Hoekstra, D. (2002). Lipoplex-mediated transfection of mammalian cells occurs through the cholesterol-dependent clathrin-mediated pathway of endocytosis. *The Journal of Biological Chemistry*, *277*(20), 18021–18028. doi:10.1074/jbc.M111257200 PMID:11875062

Chapter 7
Magnetic Nano-Systems in Drug Delivery and Biomedical Applications

Saritha R. Shetty
SKVM's NMIMS, India

Archana Upadhya
SKVM's NMIMS, India

ABSTRACT

Nanotechnology is that sphere of technology that involves the participation of biology, chemistry, physics, and engineering sciences. Nanoscale science defines the chemistry and physics of structures lying in the range of 1-100 nm. Among the nanosystems researched, magnetic nanosystems are highlighted due their unique ability, which enables their targeting to specific locations on application of an external magnetic field. The exhibited property of these magnetic nanosystems being super-paramagnetism, there is no retention of magnetic property on removal of the magnetic field, thus enabling a reversion of the targeting process. For effective utilization of these nanosystems, they should be reduced to nanosizes, layered with biocompatible entities, stabilized, and functionalized. In the chapter, synthesis and functionalization and stabilization are elucidated. The biomedical applications such as targeted delivery, MRI, magnetic hyperthermia, tissue engineering, gene delivery, magnetic immunotherapy, magnetic detoxification, and nanomagnetic actuation are discussed.

INTRODUCTION

Novel technologies with innovative ideas that modify drug attributes and therapeutic strategies for increased efficacy and cost-effective products to patients is the need of the hour. Nanotechnology in combination with novel delivery systems opens up possibilities for effective treatment regimens (Lyer, Singh, Tietze & Alexiou, 2015). Nanotechnology is a multifaceted area in research and development that brings together the various facets of science viz. chemistry, biology, engineering, and medicine (Banerjee, Katsenovich, Lagos, McIintosh, Zhang, & Li, 2010). Nanoscale science defines the chemistry and physics of struc-

DOI: 10.4018/978-1-5225-4781-5.ch007

Copyright © 2018, IGI Global. Copying or distributing in print or electronic forms without written permission of IGI Global is prohibited.

tures lying in the range of 1-100 nm, or < 100 nm (Nikalje, 2015) (Figure 1 is adapted from Nikalje, 2015). Magnetic nanoparticles (MNPs) principally comprise of metals (iron and cobalt), alloys (spinel type ferromagnetic substances viz. magnesium ferrite ($MgFe_2O_4$), manganese ferrite ($MnFe_2O_4$), cobalt ferrite ($CoFe_2O_4$) and oxides such as iron oxide magnetite (Fe_3O_4) and maghemite (γ-Fe_2O_3). Magnetic materials can be classified based on magnetic susceptibility, which is defined as magnetism induced on application of an external magnetic field (Barakat, 2009). Based on the response of the intrinsic MNP magnetic dipole and the net magnetization in the presence and absence of an applied magnetic field, commonly there are five types of magnetic materials (Issa, Obaidat, Albiss & Haik, 2013) (Kolhatkar, Jamison, Litvinov, Wilson & Lee, 2013).

- Ferromagnetic materials (such as iron, nickel, and cobalt) are atoms having a net magnetic moment due to unpaired electrons. When this material is placed in a magnetic field, the magnetic moments of the domains align themselves along the direction of the applied magnetic field forming a large net magnetic moment. However, it is observed that a residual magnetic moment does exist even after the removal of the magnetic field.
- Paramagnetic materials (such as gadolinium, magnesium, lithium, and tantalum) are characterized by unpaired electrons and the absence of magnetic domain. Due to this, in a magnetic field, the material produces a weak net magnetic moment and fails to retain magnetic moment in the absence of magnetic field.
- Diamagnetic materials (such as copper, silver, and gold) are atoms with no unpaired electrons and zero net magnetic moment. These materials repel the applied magnetic field and orient themselves in a direction opposite to the applied field.

Figure 1. Size of particles in nanoscale
Adapted from Nikalje, 2015

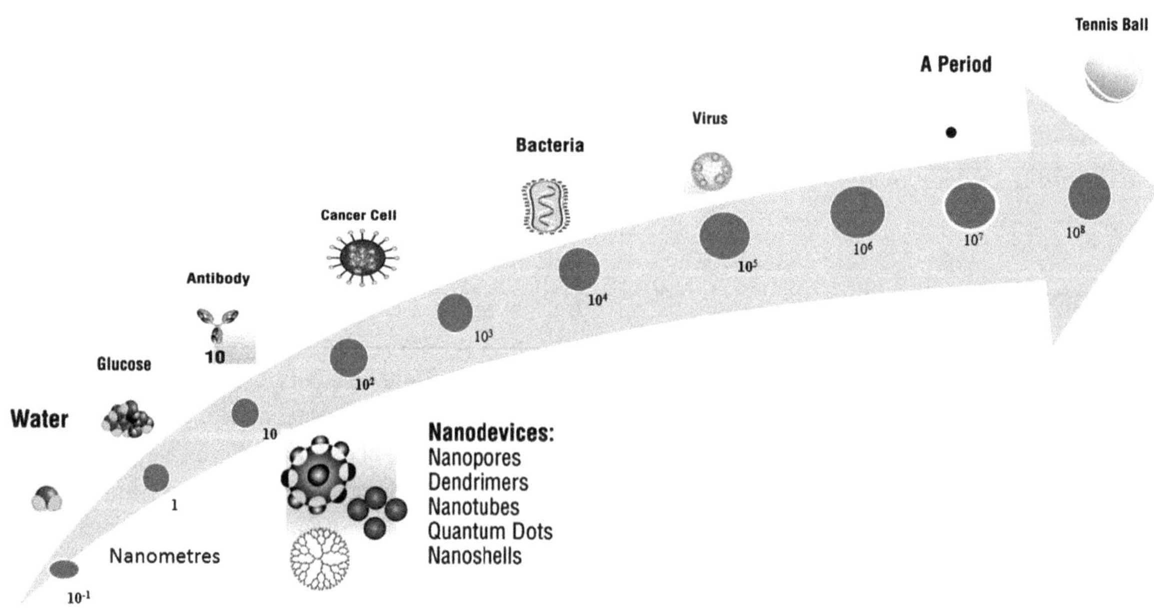

- Antiferromagnetic materials (such as manganese oxide (MnO), Cobalt oxide (CoO), and nickel oxide (NiO), copper chloride ($CuCl_2$) are compounds of two different atoms that occupy different lattice positions. The two atoms have magnetic moments that are equal in magnitude and opposite in direction which result in zero net magnetic moment.
- Ferrimagnetic materials (such as Fe_3O_4 and γ-Fe_2O_3) are compounds of different atoms residing on different lattice sites with anti-parallel magnetic moments. However, due to different magnitude, these materials do not cancel each other's magnetic moments resulting in a net spontaneous magnetic moment.

Superparamagnetism is a property occurring principally in small, single-domain magnetic particles without magnetic memory. The property is more related to ferromagnetism than paramagnetism. When a ferrimagnetic, multidomain sample is reduced in size to less than 40 nm, a single domain magnetic particle will be formed. Because only a single domain is involved, the susceptibility of a superparamagnetic substance is not as great as a ferromagnetic substance. Additionally, since each domain is a separate particle, there can be no interactions or ordering of domains within a sample (Issa, Obaidat, Albiss & Haik, 2013) Thus super paramagnetic substances do not retain any net magnetization once the external field has been removed. Magnetic nanoparticles usually exhibit superparamagnetism. Magnetic nanoparticles which are used in biomedical applications are mainly iron oxide particles such as magnetite (Fe_3O_4) and its two oxidized products tetragonal maghemite (γ-Fe_2O_3) and hexagonal hematite (α-Fe_2O_3). These natural materials are found in biological materials.

Body's defense system that serve to protect the body against foreign entities including injected therapeutics, contrast agents prevent them from reaching their target site are known as 'biological barriers' (Veiseh, Gunn & Zhang, 2010). Nanoparticle functions are restricted by these barriers either by blocking their movement, causing physical changes to them or by inducing a negative host response using biochemical signalling (Kagadis, Ford, Karnabatidis & Loudos, 2016). In addition to this, nanoparticles must overcome anatomical size restrictions to access the target site. E.g., Brain and kidney. Obstacles from the barriers illustrates the requirements for the formulator to manipulate the core and the surface functionalization of magnetic nanoparticles and to tailor the physicochemical properties like size, shape, surface charges for its ideal requisite properties E.g. Target drug delivery. Magnetic nanodelivery acts as a promising targeting drug delivery system to evade reticuloendothelial system (RES) with the aid of magnetic field. This ensures efficient drug accumulation in smaller blood vessels with lower blood flow rate than in central vessels with a faster blood flow. This chapter focuses on different aspects of magnetic nanoparticles and their diverse biomedical applications in healthcare sciences.

Preparation of Magnetic Nanosystems

Design strategies for development of magnetic nanoparticles (MNPs) need to be considered before the synthesis of magnetic nanoparticles. The fundamental pre-requisites for tailoring the nanosystems are(Kolhatkar, Jamison, Litvinov, Willson & Lee, 2013):

1. Fundamental concepts of nanomagnetism.
2. Nature of nanostructure material.
3. Selection of biocompatible, non-toxic entity.

4. Formulation strategies to develop the pharmaceutical product that can surpass the physiological barriers and gain access to its cellular target.
5. Physical characteristics that can promote the functionality *in vivo.*

Synthesis of Magnetic Nanoparticles

Past a decade, significant research on efficient synthesis and coating of magnetic nanoparticles have shown to produce highly stable monodispersed, well controlled shape, and low toxic and biocompatible product. In order to develop product uniformity, reproducibility and good characteristic properties, few process parameters need to be considered during synthetic process. Due to low toxicity and biocompatibility, the ferrite colloids, magnetite (Fe_3O_4) and maghemite (γFe_2O_3) represent magnetic nanoparticles. There are various means of synthesis process like physical, chemical and microbial route (Reddy, Arias, Nicolas& Couvreur, 2012). In this chapter emphasis is given on most commonly chosen synthetic process by the researchers in the area of magnetic nanosystems.

Microemulsion/Reverse Micelle System

Microemulsion is a dispersion made of water, oil, and surfactant(s) that is an isotropic and thermodynamically stable system with dispersed domain diameter varying approximately from 1 to 100 nm, usually 10 to 50 nm. At the interface between the oil and water, surfactant molecules may form a monolayer with the hydrophobic tails of the surfactant molecules dissolved in the oil phase and the hydrophilic head in the aqueous phase (Tang, Qiu & Zhao, 2013). In a non-polar solvent, it is the exposure of the hydrophilic head groups to the surrounding solvent that is energetically unfavourable, giving rise to a water-in-oil system. In this case, the hydrophilic groups are sequestered in the micelle core and the hydrophobic groups extend away from the centre. These reverse micelles are proportionally less likely to form on increasing head group charge, since hydrophilic sequestration would create highly unfavourable electrostatic interactions (Lu, Salabas & Schüth, 2007). Spirin and co-workers (Spirin, Brichkin & Razumov, 2005) revealed that the synthesized mean size of gold nanoparticles in Triton X-100 reverse micelles in the presence of sodium sulfite was markedly smaller than that of particles prepared in sodium bis (2-ethylhexyl) sulfosuccinate (AOT) reverse micelles. $MnFe_2O_4$ nanoparticles are synthesised through formation of water-in-toulene inverse micelles with sodium dodecylbenzenesulfonate (NaDBS) as surfactant that gave controllable sizes from about 4–15 nm (Liu, Zou, Rondinone & Zhang, 2000). In this method, the reactants, Manganese nitrate [Mn $(NO_3)_2$] and Iron nitrate [Fe $(NO_3)_3$] are taken. To this metal salt solution, NaDBS aqueous solution is added, subsequent to this addition of toluene forms reverse micelles. The volume ratio of water and toluene determines the size of the resulting $MnFe_2O_4$ nanoparticles. The main advantage of the reverse micelle or emulsion technology is the diversity of nanoparticles that can be obtained by varying the nature and amount of surfactant and co-surfactant, the oil phase, or the reacting conditions (Hasany, Ahmed, Rajan, & Rehman, 2012). However, the main disadvantage of microemulsion method is consumption of large quantities of solvents, low yield, difficulty in scale up technology, reporting the adverse effects of residual surfactants as per regulatory norms.

Co-Precipitation

Two methods are followed for the synthesis of magnetite spherical particles in solution. One method consists of partially oxidizing ferrous hydroxide suspensions with different oxidizing agents (Lu, Salabas, & Schüth, 2007) while the other method consists of aging stoichiometric mixtures of ferrous and ferric hydroxides in aqueous media, yielding spherical magnetite particles homogeneous in size. This technique is the most efficient chemical pathway to obtain magnetic particles. By an aging stoichiometric mixture of ferrous and ferric salts in aqueous medium magnetic particles of iron oxides (either Fe_3O_4 or γFe_2O_3) are usually synthesised (Laurent, Forge, Port, Roch, Robic, Vander Elst & Muller, 2008). The chemical reaction of Fe_3O_4 formation may be written as Equation 1.

$$Fe^{2+} + 2Fe^{3+} + 8OH^{-} \rightarrow Fe_3O_4 + 4H_2O \quad (1)$$

As per the thermodynamics of this reaction, complete precipitation of Fe_3O_4 should be expected at a pH between 8 and 14, with a stoichiometric ratio of 2:1 (Fe^{3+}/Fe^{2+}) in a non-oxidizing oxygen environment. However, magnetite (Fe_3O_4) is not very stable and is sensitive to oxidation. Magnetite is transformed into maghemite (γFe_2O_3) in the presence of oxygen. (Equation 2)

$$Fe_3O_4 + 2H^{+} \rightarrow \gamma Fe_2O_3 + Fe^{2+} + H_2O \quad (2)$$

Under acidic and anaerobic conditions, surface Fe^{2+} ions are desorbed as hexa-aqua complexes in solution, whereas, under basic conditions, the oxidation of magnetite involves the oxidation-reduction of the surface of magnetite. The oxidation of ferrous ions is always correlated with migration of cations through the lattice framework, creating cationic vacancies to maintain the charge balance, explaining the structure of maghemite (Laurent, Forge, Port, Roch, Robic, Vander Elst, & Muller, 2008). However, the control of particle size distribution is limited, because only kinetic factors are controlling the growth of the crystal. Key factors such as the type of salts used, the Fe^{2+}/Fe^{3+} ratio, the reaction temperature, the pH value and ionic strength of the media decides the size, shape, and composition of the magnetic nanoparticles. Use of stabilizers and/ or reducing agents can be used to produce monodisperse particles. Freitas and co-workers (2015) studied the effect of ultrasonic cavitation on changing the reaction environment by using homogeneous co-precipitation method i.e. sonochemically assisted reaction between ferrous chloride solution as precursor and urea with different ultrasound power to prepare magnetic nanoparticles The higher the energy dissipated in the reaction medium higher is the number of nuclei formed, leading to formation of precipitates with a smaller particle size. This behavior suggests that the ultrasonic energy accelerates the reactions (Freitas, Branco, Lisboa, Costa, Campos, Jafelicci Júnior & Marques, 2015).

Hydrothermal Synthesis

Autoclaves or aqueous media in reactors at pressure higher than 2000 psi and temperature above 200°C (Hasany, Ahmed, Rajan, & Rehman, 2012) are used in hydrothermal synthesis. This method rely on the ability of water to hydrolyze and dehydrate metal salts on elevated conditions. At these conditions, the very low solubility of the resulting metal oxides in water generates supersaturation (Hao & Teja, 2003). By hydrothermal synthesis, Xu, et al., (2008) investigated various process parameters like effect of precursor concentration, temperature and residence time that affects the particle size and morphology of nanoparticles. Xu et al., co-workers studied that the presence of polyvinyl alcohol (PVA) during synthesis prevents the aggregation of particles and nanoparticle size can be controlled. With increase in PVA concentration, narrow particle size distributions are obtained. The average particle size is shown to increase with temperature and residence time, and may change its morphology. In this method, the residence time shows significant impact on the average particle size than feed concentration (Xu & Teja, 2008). The main advantage of this method is that it gives controllable reproducible narrow range of nanostructured materials. The multi-component reaction mixtures like ethylene glycol, sodium acetate, and polyethylene glycol were used as a high boiling point reducing agent to produce metal/metal oxide nanoparticles, electrostatic stabilizer and surfactant to prevent particle agglomeration. Thus, this method uses a multi-component approach to obtain a number of different materials like monodisperse, hydrophilic, crystalline ferrite microspheres (Banerjee, Katsenovich, Lagos, McIintosh, Zhang, & Li, 2010).

Thermal Decomposition

Considerable interest is observed in thermal decomposition of organometallic compounds. This method derives the synthesis of high-quality semiconductor nanocrystals used to produce magnetic nanoparticles of controlled shapes and sizes (Hyeon, 2003). This occurs in high boiling organic solvents with stabilizing surfactants such as oleic acid or hexadecylamine (Lu, Salabas, & Schüth, 2007). The decomposition of iron precursors in the presence of hot organic surfactants has yielded markedly improved samples with good size control, narrow size distribution and good crystallinity of individual and dispersible magnetic iron oxide nanoparticles. Biomedical applications like magnetic resonance imaging, magnetic cell separation or magneto relaxometry strongly depend on particle size and thus magnetic nanoparticles produced by this method could be potentially used for these applications. E.g. Sun and Zeng co-worker (2002) prepared monodispersed magnetite nanoparticles ranging from 3 to 20nm. The reaction of iron (III) acetylacetonate ($Fe(acac)_3$) in phenyl ether in the presence of alcohol, oleic acid, and oleylamine was performed at high-temperature (265°C). By effectively controlling the varied synthetic parameters like the ratio of the organometallic compounds, surfactants, and solvents apart from parameters like reaction temperature, reaction time, and aging period stable well defined magnetic nanoparticles are formed (Sun & Zeng, 2002). Metallic iron nanoparticles that have larger magnetization compared to metal oxides, are synthesized by thermal decomposition of $[Fe(CO)_5]$ in the presence of polyisobutene in decalin under nitrogen atmosphere at 170°C (Lu, Salabas, & Schüth, 2007). For biotechnological applications, water soluble magnetite magnetic nanoparticles, are desirable and synthesized under reflux (245 °C) using $FeCl_3{\cdot}6H_2O$ as the iron source and 2-pyrrolidone as a coordinating solvent. Thermal decomposition represents a complicated synthesis method requiring an inert atmosphere carried out at high temperatures for prolonged periods. Though this method allows precise control over shape and size along with high crystalinity and narrow size distribution, they are unsuitable for biological or medical applications due to the use of nonpolar solvents and non-biocompatible surfactants (Banerjee, Katsenovich, Lagos, McIintosh, Zhang, & Li, 2010).

Aerosol/Vapour Method

Aerosol technologies like spray and laser pyrolysis have shown to be potential techniques for the direct and continuous production of well-defined magnetic nanoparticles differing only in the final state (based on aggregation). In spray pyrolysis technique, solution is sprayed into a series of reactors where the aerosol droplets undergo condensation and solvent evaporates. Condensation within the droplet is followed by drying and thermolysis of the precipitated particle at higher temperature to obtain nanoparticles. The resulting dried residue consists of particles whose size depends upon the initial size of the original droplets (Laurent, Forge, Port, Roch, Robic, Vander Elst, & Muller, 2008). This technique is used to produce maghemite nanoparticles start with a Fe^{3+} salt and a certain organic compound that acts as the reducing agent. In this procedure, Fe^{3+} is partially reduced to a mixture of Fe^{2+} and Fe^{3+} in the presence of organic compounds with the formation of magnetite, which is finally oxidized to maghemite. Without the presence of a reducing agent, hematite is found to be formed instead of maghemite (Lu, Fan, Stump, Ward, Rieker & Brinker, 1999). Maghemite particles with size ranging from 5 to 60 nm with different shapes have been obtained using different iron precursor salts in alcoholic solution (Ali, Hira Zafar, ul Haq, Phull, Ali & Hussain, 2016).

Laser pyrolysis technique involves heating a flowing mixture of gases with a continuous wave CO_2 laser, which initiates and sustains a chemical reaction. Above a certain pressure and laser power, a critical concentration of nuclei is reached in the reaction zone, which leads to homogeneous nucleation of particles that are further transported to a filter by an inert gas. Small particle size, narrow particle size distribution, and near absence of aggregation are amongst the salient features of this technique. The CO_2 laser pyrolysis device is used to produce pure, well-crystallized and uniform γ-Fe_2O_3 nanoparticles in a single step. In this device, a small reaction zone is defined by the overlap between vertical reactant gas stream and horizontal laser beam. The reaction zone is safely separated from the chamber walls. This provides an ideal environment for the nucleation of small particles (3.5-5 nm range), with less contamination and narrower size distribution (Tartaj, Veintemillas-Verdaguer, & Serna, 2003).

Polyols

Polyols is a very promising technique for preparation of well-defined shape and size controlled nanoparticles that could be used in biomedical applications (Ali, Hira Zafar, ul Haq, Phull, Ali, & Hussain, 2016) which is achieved by controlling the kinetic of the precipitation. A better control of the average size of the metal particles can be obtained by seeding the reactive medium with foreign particles (heterogeneous nucleation). In this way, nucleation and growth steps can be completely separated and uniform particles result. Iron particles around 100 nm can be obtained by dis-proportionation of ferrous hydroxide in organic media (Hasany, Ahmed, Rajan, & Rehman, 2012). The solvents as polyols for example, polyethylene glycol, offer interesting properties: owing to their high dielectric constants, they act as solvents able to dissolve inorganic compounds, and owing to their relatively high boiling points, they offer a wide operating-temperature range (from 25°C to the boiling point) for preparing inorganic compounds (Joseyphus, Kodama, Matsumoto, Sato, Jeyadevan & Tohji, 2007). Polyols also serve as reducing agents as well as stabilizers to control particle growth and prevent inter particle aggregation (Liu, Ko, Wu, Jung, Min, Lee, & Kim, 2007) evaluated several factors governing the production yield of Fe particles like type of polyols, ferrous salts, ferrous ion concentration, hydroxyl ion concentration, and reaction temperature. The yield and size of Fe particles varied depending upon the reduction potential of the polyols (Liu, Ko, Wu, Jung, Min, Lee, ... & Kim, 2007). Other examples for polyols are ethylene glycol (EG), diethyleneglycol (DEG), triethylene glycol (TREG), and tetraethylene glycol (TEG). The influence of the nature of the polyol, on the production and the morphological characteristics of Fe particles were studied by Joseyphus and co-workers (2007). The yield and size of Fe particles varied depending upon the reduction potential of the polyols.

Multisynthesis Processing Method

The combination and variation of polyol method and thermal decomposition routes (Hong, Leroueil, Majoros, Orr, Baker & Holl, 2007) wherein high temperature organic or solution phase synthesis is followed by a size selective separation technique to obtain relatively monodisperse (<5%) nanoparticles is known as multisynthesis process (MSP). Nucleation is observed immediately when rapid injection of the organometallic precursor into a hot solution containing the stabilizing agents is performed. Physicochemical characteristics like size and morphology can be controlled by adjusting reaction parameters like time, temperature, precursor concentration, surfactant type, and surfactant concentration (Banerjee, Katsenovich, Lagos, McIintosh, Zhang, & Li, 2010). High temperature reduction of platinum acetylacetonate and thermal decomposition of iron carbonyl in the presence of stabilizing agents, oleic acid and oleyl amine produced monodisperse FePt nanoparticles and self-assembled superlattices (Teng, Black, Watkins, Gao & Yang, 2003). The composition was controlled by the ratio of iron precursor to that of platinum precursor to obtain the controlled magnetic nanoparticles.

Coating of Magnetic Nanoparticles

One of the major criteria dominating the choice of materials used for coating magnetic nanoparticles is that they should enable formation of conjugates with any given biological entity (Barakat, 2009). The role of coating polymers is to inhibit opsonisation, thereby permitting longer circulation time. Since they are used for biomedical purposes the coating materials ought to be safe, less toxic, stable and biocompatible. Cationic excipients for coating are favoured for entry of magnetic nanoparticles into negatively charged cells. When polymeric materials are employed as stabilizers, the adsorption of polymers onto the MNPs confer protective steric repulsion and act as a barrier against the interaction between the particles, thereby stabilizing the particles and preventing them from agglomeration. Such protection is most efficient when using amphiphilic copolymers bearing a hydrophilic segment with a tendency to spread into the aqueous medium and a hydrophobic segment anchoring onto the particle surface. If the polymer chains are charged, an additional electrostatic repulsion may occur, thus conferring a combined ionic and steric (electrosteric) stabilization effect. In other words, polymeric coatings can be designed with surface properties (chemical functionality and surface charge) on the MNPs and constitute an excellent barrier for preventing aggregation, leading to physicochemically stable magnetic nanoformulations. Regarding, the vascular administration [intravenous (i.v.) or intra-arterial] of MNPs, the gravitational settling in the blood flow can be considered as negligible, thanks to these polymer coatings that generally decrease the mean density of the magnetic cores. After particles are injected into the blood stream they are rapidly coated by components such as plasma proteins, by a mechanism known as Opsonization and this formation will dictate the circumstances of injected particles. However the macrophages cells of RES will uptake these opsonised particles. Hence to avoid this, surface coatings with biodegradable polymers or non-biodegradable organic and inorganic coatings are used to retard the uptake by macrophages cells of liver, spleen etc to name few. Key characteristics of the polymer such as length and molecular weight, chemical structure (biodegradability and hydrophobic/hydrophilic character), conformation, degree of surface coverage, and attachment mechanism to the particle surface (covalent, hydrophobic, or ionic binding) must be taken into consideration. Common coatings used on magnetic nanoparticles are derivatives of dextran, Polyethylene glycol, polyethyleneime, poloxamers, polyoxamines (Barakat, 2009). Co-polymerization with polymeric acidic amino acids such as poly (L-glutamate) or poly (L-aspartate) provide additional functional groups to interact and form conjugates with the biological entity. Two most commonly used coating techniques are discussed below:

- **Emulsion Polymerization Method:** In this technique polymer coating is carried at a high surfactant to monomer ratio in a given microemulsion system. Magnetite nanoparticles are prepared by co-precipitation and further coated these nanoparticles using emulsion polymerization method. Here methyl methacrylate (MMA) and acrylic acid are used as comonomers with a weight ratio of 9/1 with high surfactant to monomer ratio conducted in microemulsion system. The sodium dodecyl sulphate acts as surfactant and potassium persulphate as initiator (Sayar, Güven, & Pişkin, 2006; Businova, Chomoucka, Prasek, Hrdy, Drbohlavova, Sedlacek & Hubalek, 2011).
- **Co-Precipitation Method:** In this method, polyethylene glycol (PEG) is most commonly used. PEG, a linear neutral polyether acts at the surface by providing a stealth shielding effect, delaying the action of RES from protein resistant character of PEGylated surfaces. This contributes to lower the interfacial energy in water and steric stabilization effect (Meng, Engbers & Feijen, 2004). However, hydrophobic surfaces on the particles are effectively coated with plasma components and rapidly excreted, whereas particles that are more hydrophilic can resist this coating process and are cleared slowly (Gaur, Sahoo, De Tapas. Ghosh, Maitra & Ghosh, 2000).

Characterization of Magnetic Nanosystems

For effective and stable magnetic nanosystems its structural and physicochemical characterization plays a critical role in product development. Magnetic properties of nanoparticles depend upon their physical structure i.e. size and shape of the particles, microstructure, and chemical phases in which they are embodied in the nanosystems. Properties such as size distribution, average particle diameter, particle charge also affect the physical stability and the *in vivo* distribution of the nanoparticles. Size and shape with polydispersity, charge, and nature of the coating are crucial parameters for exhibiting biological or pharmacological activities.

Various techniques (Table 1) that are used to investigate the surface properties of coated iron oxide nanoparticles, the nature and strength of the bonds between the iron core and coatings, their influence on the magnetic nanoparticle are (Di Marco, Guilbert, Port, Robic, Couvreur & Dubernet, 2007):

1. Atomic and chemical force microscopy (AFM and CFM),
2. Thermogravimetric analysis (TGA),
3. Differential scanning calorimetry (DSC),
4. X-ray photoelectron spectroscopy,
5. Thermally programmed desorption,
6. Infrared spectroscopy (IR),
7. Fourier transform infrared spectroscopy (FTIR),
8. Secondary ion mass spectra (SSIMS and TOF-SIMS),
9. Conductimetry, potentiometry, and
10. Solid-state NMR.

"Size" is an ambiguous concept. Characterization of nanoparticles based on the size, morphology and surface charge, can be done using advanced microscopic techniques such as atomic force microscopy (AFM), scanning electron microscopy (SEM) and transmission electron microscopy (TEM). However, in magnetic nanoparticles the different parts of the nanoparticle are crystalline parts of the core, whole iron core (crystalline and amorphous), the core, the shell, and the hydrated layer, or even a size with no geometrical meaning on the particle but just a physical meaning. Since nanoparticles are polydisperse and have heterogeneity of sizes it gives rise to different values. This depends upon whether the technique gives access to a number, volume, or even intensity (volume to the power of two)-weighted mean size (Laurent et al., 2007). TEM reports the total particle size of the core crystalline or amorphous parts and gives access to a number-weighted mean value. Furthermore, it provides details on the size distribution and the shape. Atomic arrangement can be interpreted by High-resolution transmission electron microscopy (HRTEM). It can be used to study local microstructures (such as lattice vacancies and defects, lattice fringe, glide plane, or screw axes) and surface atomic arrangement of crystalline nanoparticles. Properties like surface morphology, size and overall shape are determined by electron microscopy techniques. X-ray diffraction method can be performed to obtain the crystalline structure of the particles. By comparing the intensities of experimental peak and reference peak in a diffraction pattern, the intensity can be used to quantify the proportion of iron oxide formed in a mixture. Using the Scherrer formula, crystal size can be calculated from the line broadening observed in the XRD pattern (Rao & Houska, 1986). Extended X-ray absorption fine structure (EXAFS) gives information on the particle size, especially for small sizes (Calvin, Miller, Goswami, Cheng, Mulvaney, Whitman & Harris, 2003). For characterization of suspension and to improve the characterization of fine structure details, Energy dispersive X-ray diffraction (EDXD) is used as advanced tool. Small-angle neutron scattering (SANS) is a powerful technique to obtain information on the size, polydispersity, shape (form factor), and even the structure of nanoparticles (Lindner, 2002). The singularity of neutrons is that they interact with the nuclei of the atoms present in the sample. The technique of contrast variation (or contrast matching) relies on the differential scatter of hydrogen versus deuterium (Laurent, 2007). This can be used to study independently the size of the core and the shell of the nanoparticles. Photon correlation spectroscopy (PCS), also called dynamic light scattering (DLS) or quasi-elastic light scattering (QELS), is a common technique to obtain a nanoparticle size. The determination of the diffusion co-efficient of the nanoparticles in solution gives access to the hydrodynamic radius of a corresponding sphere and the polydispersity of colloidal solution (Faraji, Yamini & Rezaee, 2010). Determination of the mean crystal size and various other parameters can be calculated from the magnetometry and relaxivity profiles recorded in the magnetic field. Different characterization tools and methods for nanoparticles are mentioned in Table 1 (Bhatia, 2016).

Stabilization of Magnetic Nanosystems

In the production of the magnetic colloidal nanosystems, stabilization is the crucial step. The nanosystem should be stable against aggregation in both a biological medium and a magnetic field. This stability results from the equilibrium between attractive and repulsive forces. Theoretically, four kinds of forces can contribute to the interparticle potential in the system, namely Van der Waals forces, electrostatic forces, steric forces and dipole magnetic interactions. Van der Waals forces induce strong short-range isotropic attractions. The electrostatic repulsive forces can be partially screened by adding salt to the

Table 1. Various characterization tools and methods for nanoparticles

Characterization Parameter	Technology Used
Carrier-Drug Interaction	Differential Scanning Calorimetry (DSC)
Charge Determination	• Laser Doppler Anemometry • Zeta potentiometer
Chemical Analysis of Surface	Static secondary ion mass spectrometry Sorptometer
Drug Stability	• Bioassay of drug extracted from nanoparticles • Chemical analysis of drug
Nanoparticle Dispersion Stability	• Critical Flocculation Temperature (CFT) • Atomic Force Microscopy (AFM)
Particle Size and Distribution	• Laser Defractometry • Photon Correlation Spectroscopy (PCS) • Scanning Electron Microscopy (SEM) • Transmission Electron Microscopy (TEM)
Release Profile	*In vitro* release characteristics under physiologic and sink conditions (Dissolution and / or Diffusion studies).
Surface Hydrophobicity	• Rose Bengal (dye) binding • Water contact angle measurement • X-ray photoelectron spectroscopy

suspension (Laurent, Forge, Port, Roch, Robic, Vander Elst, & Muller, 2008). Derjaguin-Landau-Verwey-Overbeek (DLVO) theory explains about these forces and particle-particle interactions (Derjaguin, 1941; Verwey, Overbeek & Overbeek, 1999). For magnetic suspensions, magnetic dipolar forces between two particles must be added. These forces induce anisotropic interactions, which are found to be globally attractive if the anisotropic interparticle potential is integrated over all directions. Dependent upon the pH of the solution, the surface of the magnetite will be positive or negative. The isoelectric point is observed at pH 6.8 (Bacri, Perzynski, Salin,Cabuil & Massart, 1990) and around this point [point of zero charge (PZC)], the surface charge density (Σ) is too small and the particles are no longer stable in water and flocculate. Either one or both of the two repulsive forces: electrostatic and steric repulsion are required for stabilizing the magnetic particles. The force strength among these particles dictate the stability of the nanosystem. The steric force is difficult to predict and quantify (Napper, 1970; Fritz, Schädler, Willenbacher & Wagner, 2002). Stability factor (W) is measured for the effectiveness of the potential barrier in preventing the particles from aggregation. W is defined as the ratio of the number of collisions between particles and the number of collisions resulting in aggregation (Laurent, Forge, Port, Roch, Robic, Vander Elst, & Muller, 2008). Stability factor is expressed as $W = k_{fast}/k$, where k_{fast} is the rate constant describing rapid aggregation (every collision leads to an aggregation) and k is the aggregation rate constant at the salt concentration used (Baudry, Bertrand, Rouzeau, Greffier, Koenig, Dreyfus, & Lequeux, 2004; Mylon, Chen & Elimelech, 2004). Techniques that are used for the measurement of stability factor are light scattering (static or dynamic) or turbidimetric measurements. The stabilization of magnetic particles can be classified as detailed in the Table 2 and Figure 2 is the schematic representation of surface coating stabilization in magnetic nanoparticle: a.) With Inorganic stabilization; b.) Organic or Poymeric Stabilization; c.) Nanoencapsulation as nanospheres using polymers; d.) Nanocapsules (Figure 2 is adapted from Reddy, Arias, Nicolas, & Couvreur, 2012).

Table 2. Classification of stabilizers used in magnetic nanoparticles

Strategies	Examples	Few References
Monomeric Stabilizers	Carboxylates, Phosphates and sulphates	LiNianqiang, 2013; Ballesteros-Gómez, & Rubio, 2009.
In-Organic Materials	Silica, Metal(Gold) or Non metal Metal oxides/Sulfides	Lin, Zhou, Kumbhar, Wiemann, Fang, Carpenter & O'Connor, 2001; Li, Liu & He, 2010.
Polymer Stabilizers	Dextran, Polyethylene glycol (PEG), Polyvinyl Alcohol (PVA), Alginate, Chitosan, Polyethyleneimine (PEI), Co-polymers, Liposomes/ micelles, Other Polymers: PEO, PVP, PAA etc.	Chen, Yang, Ma, & Wu, 2011; Tang,Li, He, Zhang, Ma, Li & He, 2013; Pradhan, Giri, Rieken, Koch, Mykhaylyk, Döblinger,, ... & Plank, 2010.
Surface Modification Chemistry	Covalent linkages and Physical Interactions	Lu,Yin, Mayers& Xia, 2002; Wang, Wang,He, Zhang & Chen, 2009; Lin & Samia, 2006; Akbarzadeh, Samiei & Davaran, 2012.
Target Strategies	Small organic molecules, Peptides, Aptamers, Antibodies and Proteins	Guven, Basaran-Akgul, Temur, Tamer & Boyacı, 2011; Bamrungsap, Chen, Shukoor, Chen, Sefah, Chen, & Tan, 2012.

Figure 2. Different surface coatings in magnetic nanoparticles
Adapted from Reddy et al., 2012

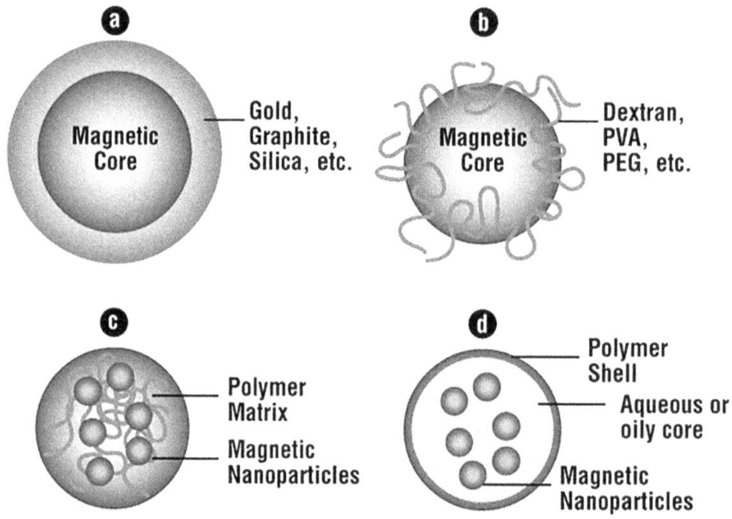

- **Monomeric Stabilizers:** Monomeric stabilizers can be tailored for dispersibility into oil/hydrocarbon carrier fluids or aqueous media. E.g. Carboxylates, phosphates and sulphates. By co-ordinating via one or two of the carboxylate functionalities, depending upon steric necessity and the curvature of the surface, citric acid may be adsorbed on the surface of the magnetite nanoparticles (Sahoo, Goodarzi, Swihart, Ohulchanskyy, Kaur, Furlani & Prasad, 2005). By this method one of the carboxylic acid group gets exposed to the solvent and makes the surface negatively charged and hydrophilic.
- **Inorganic Materials:** Inorganic coatings not only provide stability to the nanoparticles in solution but also help in binding various biological ligands to the nanoparticle surface. These nanopar-

ticles have an inner iron oxide core with an outer metallic shell of inorganic materials (Laurent, Forge, Port, Roch, Robic, Vander Elst, & Muller, 2008). An inert silica coating on the surface of magnetite nanoparticles prevents their aggregation in liquid, improves their chemical stability, and provides better protection against toxicity (Hosseini, Memari, Ganjali,, Khoobi, Faridbod, Shafiee, ... & Hajinezhad, 2014). Silica shields the magnetic dipole interaction with the silica shell and the silica nanoparticles are negatively charged, hence the silica coating enhances the coulomb repulsion of the magnetic nanoparticles. Tartaj and co-workers (2003) prepared submicronic silica coated magnetic sphere aerosol by the pyrolysis method. The presence of surface silanol groups reacts easily with various coupling agents to covalently attach specific ligands to these magnetic particles, and stability is enhanced. (Ulman, 1996; Liu, Xu, Finch, & Egerton, 1998).

- **Gold Coating:** Two methods used in gold coating nanoparticles are direct and indirect methods. In direct coating for nanoparticles (Silva, Tavallaie, Sandiford, Tilley & Gooding, 2016), gold shell can be formed directly or indirectly onto the magnetic core. The Au shell is formed directly on the core surface, while in the indirect methods, a ''glue material'' is used between core and Au shell. Direct gold coating onto cores can be achieved using magnetite particles that are in aqueous or organic phase. For particles that are in aqueous solution the most common procedures reduce Au^{3+} by using reducing agents such as sodium citrate and sodium borohydride. A shell is made by attaching the gold atoms by using the sodium citrate reduction of gold chloride (Ahmad,Bae, Rhee, Chang, Jin & Hong, 2012; Chen, Qi, Zhou, Jia, Gao, Koh, & Yin, 2015; Ghorbani, Hamishehkar, Arsalani & Entezami, 2015). Under vigorous stirring, boiling gold chloride aqueous solution is mixed with synthesized magnetic nanoparticles and sodium citrate is added wherein Au layer is formed. Sodium citrate also confers stability against aggregations by coating the gold magnetic nanoparticles by citrate moieties. Colour change from brownish to burgundy is observed as Au shell is formed around magnetic nanoparticles (Zhou, Lee, Park, Lee, Park& Lee, 2012). Gold MNPs obtained by indirect gold coating are characterized by having a ''glue layer''. The glue layer ensures the stability of the product and has the ability to chelate metal ions that binds the magnetic core inorder to promote gold shell growth. Hence the choice and preparation of the glue layer is the keyfactor to obtain multifunctional properties of gold magnetic nanoparticles. (Hu, Meng, Niu & Lu, 2013)
- **Polymer Stabilizers:** Polymers functionalised iron oxide nanoparticles are gaining lots of demand in biomedical applications. Polymer coating increases repulsive forces to balance the magnetic and the van der Waals attractive forces acting on the NPs. Moreover, polymer functionalized iron oxide NPs have been extensively investigated due to interest in their unique physicochemical properties. The saturation magnetization value of iron oxide NPs will decrease after polymers functionalization. Monomer polymerization method or synthesis in the microporous of polymeric microsphere gives uniform magnetic composite NPs with high content of iron oxide NPs (Guin & Manorama, 2008). List of various polymers used in stabilization of magnetic nanosystems are detailed in Table 3. (Wu, He, & Jiang, 2008).

Surface Modification Chemistry

Chemical approaches are categorised as covalent linkages (Direct nanoparticle conjugation, click chemistry and covalent linker chemistry) and physical interactions (Electrostatic, hydrophilic/hydrophobic, affinity interactions). Covalent linkages are strong and stable covalent bonds specifically formed with

Table 3. List of various polymers used in stabilization of magnetic nanosystems

Type of Polymer	Examples	Mechanism
Natural Polymers	Dextran	Enables optimum polar interactions with iron oxides surfaces and improves the blood circulation time, stability and biocompatibility
	Starch	Improves biocompatibility, good for MRI and drug target delivery
	Gelatin	Used as gelling agent, hydrophilic emulsifier and biocompatible
	Chitosan	Non-toxic, alkaline, hydrophilic, non-viral gene delivery biocompatible and hydrophilic
Synthetic Polymers	Polyethylene glycol (PEG)	Enhances the hydrophilicity and water solubility, improves blood circulation and biocompatible.
	Polyvinyl Alcohol (PVA)	Prevents agglomeration
	Poly Lactic Acid (PLA)	Improves biocompatibility, biodegradable and low toxic
	Alginate	Improves stability and biocompatibility
	Polymethylmethacrylate (PMMA)	Thermosensitive drug delivery and cell separation
	Poly Acrylic Acid(PAA)	Improves stability, biocompatibility and bioconjugation.

functional groups like carboxylic acid, amino and thiol groups on the nanoparticle surfaces and ligands. E.g. Polymer coatings (Chitosan, dextran) dictated the type and number of functional group on each nanoparticle or terminal ends (PEG).

- **Direct Nanoparticle Conjugation:** Here functional groups are directly bonded to reactive ligands or linkage reactions and are facilitated by the aid of catalysts. Eg: Amine, sulphide, aldehyde etc.
- **Click Chemistry:** Sharpless and co-workers developed a new approach of direct conjugation known as Click chemistry (Kolb, Finn & Sharpless, 2001). These reactions are fast, efficient and require mild reaction conditions and create water soluble biocompatible ligands. E.g. Azide and alkyne reactive groups are highly specific and unreactive functional groups ensuring specific conjugation at the desired locations on the reactive moiety (Hein, Liu & Wang, 2008). Disadvantage: Since copper is most commonly used catalyst in the reaction, the use of Cu or consumptions may be linked to few disorders like neurological disorder, kidney disorder, hepatitis etc.
- **Linker Chemistry:** Linker molecule offers control over the molecular orientation of bound ligand, critical when protecting ligand functionality. Additionally linkers are selectively cleaved for the use of ligand quantification, controlled release and other applications (Veiseh, Gunn& Zhang, 2010).
- **Physical Interactions:** Have unique advantages like rapid speed of binding, high efficiencies and no need for intermediate modification steps. Many scientists have worked with magnetic nanoparticles coated with cationic polymers like PEI, which is then complexed with negatively charged plasmid DNA molecules (Chorny, Polyak, Alferiev, Walsh, Friedman & Levy, 2007 ; Park, Ng, Wang, Chu, Yuan, Zhang, & Pun, 2008). Hydrophobic/hydrophilic interactions are highly useful for adsorbing hydrophobic drugs on magnetic nanosystems. Affinity interactions have shown effective for bioconjugation of targeting ligands to nanosystems. The linkages formed are highly stable and the strongest of all non-covalent linkages. Unlike hydrophobic and electrostatic inter-

actions, affinity binding is not sensitive to the environment conditions like change in pH, salinity and hydrophilicity (Gunn, Wallen, Veiseh, Sun, Fang, Cao, ... & Zhang, 2008) hence used in immunotherapy applications.

Target Strategies

Targeting agents are used in nanosystems against specific surface markers on target cells. Few target agents play a dual role as therapeutics as well as target agents. They also initiate endocytosis of nanoparticles to which they are bound, making it particularly attractive for drug delivery applications. The following parameters need to be considered while designing the nanosystem for targeting capabilities (Veiseh, Gunn, & Zhang, 2010):

1. Nanosystem binding specificity,
2. Type of ligand,
3. Method of nanoparticle attachment.

Figure 3 is adapted from Veiseh et al., (2010), represents the various molecules that are organised on to the nanoparticle surfaces and depicts some of the advantages and disadvantages of each ligand. E.g. Bulkier molecules like proteins and antibodies are difficult to assemble on to the surface due to lack of covalent bonding and orientation of proteins or may be due to non specific physical interactions by protein's charged, hydrophobic or hydrophilic regions with the nanoparticle surface. Alternatively the smaller molecules, aptamer or peptides are designed for one active molecular handle per molecule to ensure consistent linking on to the surface of nanoparticle and hence no loss of binding activity (Hong, Leroueil, Majoros, Orr, Baker, & Holl, 2007).

Biomedical Applications

Magnetic nanoparticles may be utilized for various biomedical applications only if they possess the desirable characteristics (Polyak & Friedman, 2009) as explained below:

Figure 3. Organisation of various molecules on surface of magnetic nanoparticles
Adapted from Veiseh et al., 2010

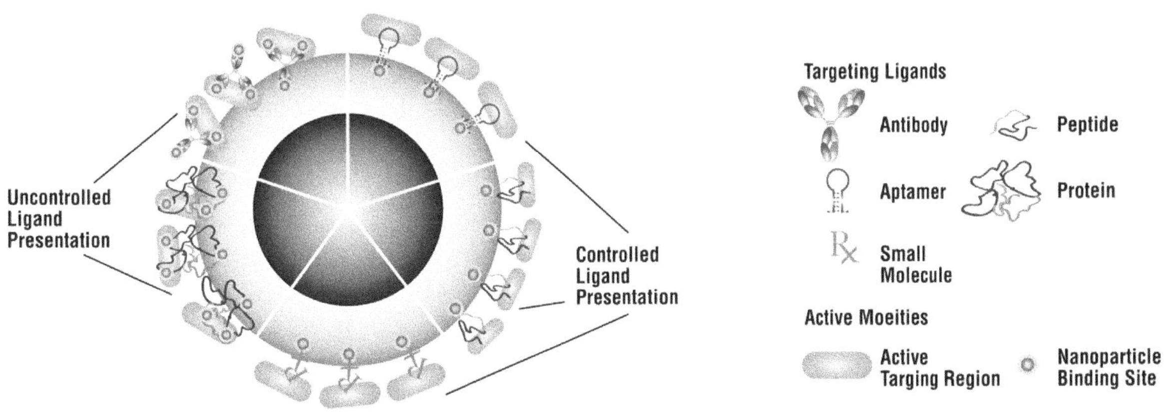

1. Nanoparticles should possess sufficient magnetic moment to overcome drag effects in the circulation, thereby permitting their localization in specific tissues on application of an external or implanted magnetic field.
2. Magnetic particles should exhibit super-paramagnetism, i.e there should be no remnants of magnetization in particles on removal of the magnetic field. The property is essential to prevent uncontrolled aggregation of particles *in vivo*. Aggregation may lead to formation of emboli in the vasculature which could be lethal.
3. Formulation of magnetic nanoparticles should be biocompatible to minimize occurrence of inflammatory responses and to prevent toxicity.
4. Nanoparticle formulation should be biodegradable so that they can be effectively shunted out of the body.
5. Magnetic nanoparticles should be layered with appropriate coating polymers to enable the loading of moieties aimed at targeting specific tissues. The coatings should also confer stealth to the nanoparticles, prolong their half-life in circulation by avoiding opsonisation, and prevent particulate aggregation under physiological conditions.
6. The formulated magnetic nanoparticles should be structurally stable to survive the magnetization applied through an external magnetic field for targeted delivery. Figure 4 represents the biomedical applications of magnetic nanoparticles.

Targeted Drug Delivery Systems

The delivery of a given drug to its target organ through nanoparticles may be achieved by active or passive targeting. The efficient active targeting of magnetic nanoparticulate formulations is primarily determined by the nature of ligands on its surface to enable interlocking with appropriate receptors

Figure 4. Biomedical Applications of MNPs

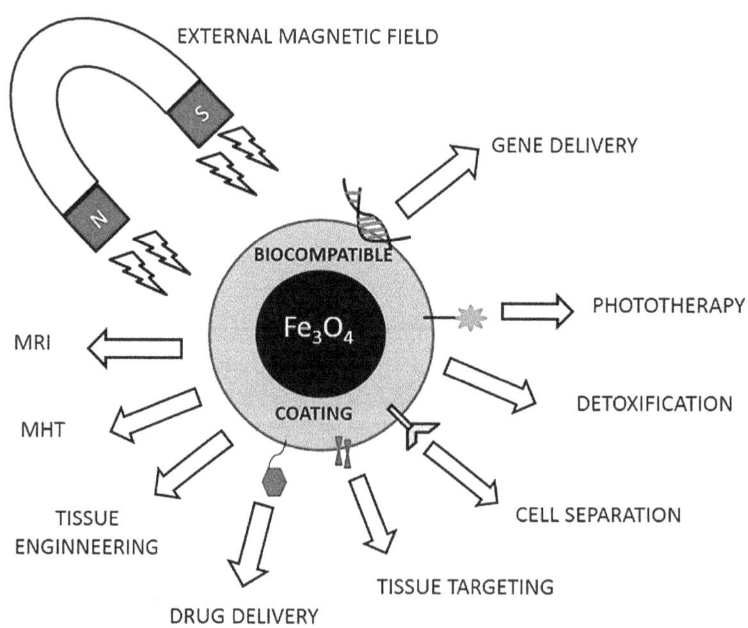

on the target tissue. For passive targeting, important characteristics that need to be addressed are the hydrodynamic size and shape of the nanoparticles. These features influence the bioavailability, elimination, and vascular permeability of the nanoparticles. For instance, though permeation through most endothelial vessels is facilitated when the size of the nanoparticles is <150 nm, the requirements of the blood brain barrier are more stringent due to presence of tight junctions at the blood brain interface and may be facilitated at sizes ≤50 nm. Size of the nanoparticles also determine their destination in the body with reports indicating that nanoparticles of size (30-150nm) accumulate in the bone marrow, heart, kidney and stomach; larger nanoparticles (150-300nm) tend to reach the liver and spleen, while smaller nanoparticles (<20nm) are efficiently excreted by the kidney. Apart from size, anisotropy also plays a role in bioavailiability, with spherical particles being removed from circulation faster than rod shaped nanoparticles (Veisch, Gunn, & Zhang, 2010).

Site Specific Drug Delivery for Cancer Therapy

Iron oxide nanoparticles are usually decorated with ligands targeting related receptors that are highly expressed in cancerous cells. The ligands could be antibodies (not usually preferred due to their large size), peptides and small molecules (Peng, Qian, Mao, & Wang, 2008). For E.g. Methotrexate (MTX) which is an analogue of folic acid and a therapeutic was conjugated to iron oxide nanoparticles. The iron-oxide nanoparticles were found to accumulate to a greater extent in cancerous tissues that overexpress the folate receptor compared to their normal counterparts (Kohler, Sun, Wang & Zhang, 2005).

Site Specific Drug Delivery Systems of Skeletal Muscles

The skeletal system comprises of bone matrix, bone tissue and bone cells. The common diseases that affect the bone are osteoarthritis, bone cancer and osteoporosis. Targeted delivery to bone is essential to reduce unwanted side-effects and increase the therapeutic window at the diseased site. Targeting moieties to the bone can be classified into bone tissue targeting moieties and bone cell targeting moieties. The readers are referred to the review by Dang and his colleagues for a detailed description of the bone targeting ligands (Dang, Liu, Li, Wang, Li, Guo, ... & Badshah, 2016). Although there are no reports of magnetic nanoparticles being used *in vivo* for bone targeting, magnetic nanoparticles have been investigated for bone repair in *ex vivo* conditions (Wang, Yan, Yang & Li, 2016). The utility of magnetic iron oxide nanoparticles (IONPs) for targeting the skeletal tissue in the treatment of the above mentioned maladies could be the answer for effective drug localization in the bone but the treatment modality needs to be further developed (Barakat, 2009).

Site Specific Drug Delivery Systems for Lung Delivery

Lung specific delivery can be accomplished by use of magnetized aerosols (Babu, Templeton, Munshi & Ramesh, 2013) In the case of a specific lung cancer called non-small-cell lung carcinoma (NSCLC), the magnetized particles may be equipped with ligands that target receptors that are overexpressed in the tumour tissue. Sadhuka and colleagues., (Sadhuka, Wiedmann & Panvam, 2013) targeted super paramagnetic iron oxide inhalable nanoparticles to the lung via a ligand that targeted the epidermal growth factor receptor (EGFR/Her1) receptor over expressed in NSCLC. Enhanced tumour retention of the particles was observed and on application of magnetic hyperthermia treatment, improved tumour cell kill was observed.

Site Specific Drug Delivery Systems for Topical Delivery

Cell labeling and targeting via magnetic nanoparticles may aid in diagnosis of skin diseases. Alternatively they can be exploited for wound healing applications (Baroli, Ennas, Loffredo, Isola, Pinna, & López-Quintela, 2007). The factors that determine interaction of nanoparticles with skin include the physicochemical properties of nanoparticles such as size, surface charge, properties of nanomaterial used, drug-loading efficiency, lamellarity and mode of application (Desai, Patlolla & Singh, 2010). Baroli et al. (2007) showed that the rigid magnetic nanoparticles <10 nm can passively penetrate the skin through the SC lipid matrix and hair follicle orifices, and can reach up to the stratum granulosum. The application of the nanoparticles for treatment of skin disorders however requires further investigation.

Magnetic Hyperthermia

Introduction to Hyperthermia (HT)

Hyperthermia (HT) refers to a kind of therapy used especially in oncology, wherein the temperature of the target region is increased to a temperature between 41 - 45°C for the period of a few minutes to several hours (Dahl & Overgaard, 1995), through an external agent. The main purpose of using HT is to kill cancerous cells and the form of therapy may be used as an adjuvant to radiotherapy, chemotherapy, gene therapy and immunotherapy. The extent of cancerous cell kill depends on the temperature achieved and the duration of HT. Denaturation of critical proteins involved in maintenance of cellular morphology, signaling, cellular communication, DNA repair is affected on application of HT leading to apoptosis or necrosis. Cancerous tissue is more susceptible to HT than normal tissue due to abnormal conditions within the cell such as hypoxia, low pH, deprivation of nutrients and high metabolic activity. Cancer cells that are in S-phase (the phase which is refractory to radiation) are found to be more susceptible to HT treatments (Chicheł, Skowronek, Kubaszewska & Kanikowski, 2007). There are three types of treatment modalities used in hyperthermia; local hyperthermia, partial or regional hyperthermia and whole body hyperthermia. Whole body hyperthermia utilizes thermal chambers, hot water blankets, infra-red radiation and may be used to treat metastatic disease. Partial hyperthermia applied to treat locally advanced cancer is achieved by perfusion or microwaves. Local hyperthermia is specified for small tumours (≤ 3 cm upto 5-6 cm in diameter) (Chicheł, Skowronek, Kubaszewska, & Kanikowski, 2007) located superficially or within an accessible body cavity such as rectum or oesophagus and is accomplished by utilizing ultrasound, microwave or near –infrared radiation (Moros, 2012).

Magnetic Hyperthermia (MHT)

Magnetic hyperthermia involves the use of an external magnetic field to generate heat in the tissue impregnated with magnetic iron oxide nanoparticles (IONPs). MHT was initially introduced by Gilchrist and his fellow researchers (Gilchrist, Medal, Shorey, Hanselman, Parrott, & Taylor, 1957). Heat generation in the tissue can be controlled by modulating the external magnetic field and by developing IONPs with high specific absorption rate (SAR) so that low concentrations of IONPs can be employed thereby reducing toxicity (Shetake, Balla, Kumar & Pandey, 2016). Local HT can be achieved by injecting the tumour with the IONPs and subjecting the area to alternating magnetic fields. The method is superior to other techniques used for heat generation for the following reasons; 1) Alternating magnetic field can penetrate tissues to a greater depth than light or acoustic methods (Perigo, Hemery, Sandre, Ortega, Garaio, Plazaola, & Teran, 2015); 2) Heat generation can be coupled with MRI imaging of the tissue combining therapy and diagnosis (Tran & Webster, 2010); 3) Magnetic nanoparticles may be manipulated to increase residence time in the tissue to avoid repeated injections; 4) Magnetic nanoparticles may be loaded with chemotherapeutic agents, radionuclides or immunotherapy agents to achieve a combinatorial therapy and; 5) The technique is minimally invasive. Heat generated due to application of oscillating magnetic fields (~kHz-MHz) to magnetic iron oxide nanoparticles embedded in the target region are primarily due to two mechanisms which are size dependent (nanoparticles <100nm); one being Brown relaxation (due to occurrence of friction arising from total particle oscillations) and the other being Neél relaxation (heat generated due to rotation of the magnetic moment with each field oscillation) (Cherukuri, Glazer & Curly, 2010). The parameters which affect heat efficiency of magnetic hyperthermia are: 1) magnitude of the applied magnetic field; 2) iron oxide nanoparticle diameter; 3) iron oxide nanoparticle anisotropy and; 4) collective behavior of the nanoparticles (Deatsch & Evans, 2014). Reports of application of MHT in preclinical settings are several for example; treatment of head and neck cancers with magnetic hyperthermia in mouse showed an elevated temperature in the tumour centre from body temperature of 37°C to 40°C in a matter of 5-10 seconds causing necrosis in the tumour tissue (Zhou, Lee, Park, Lee, Park, & Lee, 2012). In another study, Shetake and colleagues administered oleic acid coated IONPs to tumours of murine fibrosarcoma and subjected the tumours to MHT. The treatment resulted in the induction of apoptosis by influencing the heat shock protein 90 (Hsp 90/AKT) pathway (Shetake, Kumar, Gaikwad, Ray, Desai, Ningthoujam, Vatsa, & Pandey, 2015).

Bioimaging: Magnetic Resonance Imaging (MRI)

Introduction

Bioimaging techniques are diagnostic tools involving live-cell/tissue imaging by non-invasive methods. Bio-imaging encompasses various imaging platforms; computed X-ray tomography (CT), optical imaging, magnetic resonance imaging (MRI), positron emission tomography (PET), single photon emission computed tomography (SPECT) and ultrasound. Among the imaging modalities mentioned above, MRI technology enables acquisition of 3-D tomographical information of tissues, including soft tissues with high resolution without use of ionizing radiation (CT) or administration of radioactive tracers (PET and SPECT). MRI scanners reconstruct images from electromagnetic signals generated by the stimulation and relaxation of protons in the tissue environment. Contrast agents are used to selectively change the longitudinal and transverse relaxation times (T1 and T2 respectively) of the protons in the biological tissues. They are involved in transfer of energies which occur between magnetic elements and the spins of the protons. T1 weighted images produce superior anatomical images of tissues while T2 weighted images provide pathological information (Stephen, Kievit & Zhang, 2011). The use of MRI contrast agents thus allows differentiation between normal and diseased cells of the tissues. These agents enhance the contrast of the images obtained by the MRI scanner; increase in signals are caused by positive contrast agents while negative contrast agents decrease the signals. Based on their composition, MRI contrast agents can be divided into gadolinium based contrast agents, manganese based contrast agents and iron oxide based contrast agents.

MARKERS USED FOR MRI

Gadolinium (Gd^{+3}) MRI Contrast Agents

Gd^{+3}, a lanthanide metal ion, has 7 unpaired electrons in its 4f orbitals and has a magnetic moment of 7.94. The properties of Gd provide slow electronic relaxation and thus increase the longitudinal (T1) relaxation times. Small molecules like Gd-DTPA (Gd-diethyltriaminepentaacetic acid) and Gd-DOTA (Gd-N,N',N'',N'''-tetracarboxymethyl-1, 4,7, 10-tetraazacyclododecane) are therefore used as T1 weighted or positive contrast MRI agents (Zhu, Liu, Ma, Liu & Wang, 2013). Commercial preparations containing Gd-based chelates include Magnevist™, Dotarem™, Omniscan™, Prohance™, Optimark™ and Gadovist™ (Rohrer, Bauer, Mintorovitch, Requardt & Weinmann, 2005). These agents, though widely used, have short blood circulation times and poor detection sensitivity.

Manganese (Mn^{+2}) MRI Contrast Agents

The transition metal ion, Mn^{+2} has 5 unpaired electrons in its 3f orbitals and has a lower magnetic moment of 5.92. The element (Mn) could be used in the preparation of MRI contrast agents. These agents would also be categorized as T1 weighted/positive contrast agents (Zhu, Liu, Ma, Liu, & Wang, 2013).

Iron Oxide MRI Contrast Agents

Superparamagnetic iron oxide nanoparticles (SPIONs) are preferred agents for MRI imaging. Iron oxide nanoparticles are divided into two classes; SPIONs and ultra-small SPIONs. SPIONs are typically made of magnetite (Fe_3O_4) or maghemite (γ-Fe_2O_4). SPIONs have a hydrodynamic radius of > 50 nm while USPIONs possess hydrodynamic radius of < 50 nm. The difference in hydrodynamic radii confers different relaxometric properties on the iron oxide particles. SPIONs are preferentially used in cell labeling, liver cancer diagnosis (since they are captured by macrophages and end up in the liver) while USPIONs are used in molecular targeted images and blood pool/angiography procedures since they tend to stay in the circulation for longer times (Fortin, 2017). SPIONs produce T2-weighted /negative contrast images while USPIONs are used in T1-weighted imaging. Several formulations of SPIONs have been approved by the Food and Drug Administration, which include Lumiren® for bowel imaging (Wang, Hussain & Krestin, 2001), Feridex IV ® (hydrodynamic radius 160nm) (Bliasak, van Veggel & Tomanek, 2013) for liver and spleen imaging (Bonnemain et al., 1998) and Combidex® (hydrodynamic radius 30nm) (Blasiak, van Veggel, & Tomanek, 2013) for lymph node and metastasis imaging (Harisinghani, Barentsz, Hahn, Deserno, Tabatabaei, van de Kaa, ... & Weissleder, 2003).

Photoablation Therapy: Photodynamic and Photothermal Therapy

Photodynamic Therapy With Magnetic Nanosystems

Photodynamic therapy (PDT) involves administration of a photosensitizer (PS) which on exposure to light (600-800nm) results in a photochemical reaction leading to production of singlet oxygen species. The highly reactive singlet oxygen when produced in cells causes tissue damage in the form of apoptosis, necrosis and autophagy. Photodynamic therapy against cancer is a minimally invasive method and is viewed as an adjunct to the conventional modes of cancer therapy; chemotherapy, radiotherapy and surgery (Agostinis, Berg, Cengel, Foster, Girotti, Gollnick ... & Korbelik, 2011). To improve the tissue targetability of the PSs in PDT, they could be coupled with magnetic nanoparticles. The approach not only enables their accumulation at the desired site under the influence of an external magnetic field but enables MRI of the tissue as well. In a research study, a photosensitizer chlorine e6 (Ce6) was coated on magnetic nanoparticles (Ce6-MNP) and administered to nude mice implanted subcutaneously with human gastric cancer (MGC083) cells. Tumour targeting under the influence of a magnetic field with simultaneous PDT and imaging was achieved, which resulted in tumour regression and procurement of superior images of the tumour tissue (Huang, Li, Lin, Yang, Gao, Xu, ... & Hu, 2011). In another study iron oxide (IO) nanoparticles were coated with (Fmp) fibronectin-mimetic peptide (for tumour targeting) and a new generation photosensitizer; silicon phthalocyanine photosensitizer Pc 4 to generate Fmp-IO-Pc4 magnetic nanoparticles which on administration to nude mice achieved regression of xeno graft tumours after localized PDT under influence of a magnetic field (Wang, Fei, Halig, Qin, Hu, Xu, ... & Chen, 2014).

Photothermal Therapy (PTT) Using Magnetic Nanosystems

Temperature is one of the most critical parameters determining the dynamics and viability of biological systems (Jaque, Maestro, Del Rosal, Haro-Gonzalez, Benayas, Plaza, ... & Sole, 2014). Photothermal therapy (PTT) employs near infrared (NIR) (650-1000nm) laser photoabsorbers to generate heat when exposed to NIR laser irradiation. When such optical nanoparticles are implanted in cancer tissue and NIR light irradiated, the intense heat produced causes destruction of the cancer cells. Some of the photothermal nanotherapeutics (PTNs) explored include Au nanostructures, nanocarbons, transition metal sulfides/oxides nanomaterials and organic nanomaterials (Shanmugam, Selvakumar & Yen, 2014). PTT is being considered as an approach to treat the menace of cancer metastasis (Zou, Wang, He, Zeng, Tan, Cao, ... & Li, 2016). Hybrid magnetic nanosystems employing iron oxide nanoparticles and NIR absorbing substances are suitable for achieving cancer tissue specific accumulation of the hybrid PTNs on application of an external magnetic field and tumour destruction following subsequent PTT. The technique enables imaging (MRI) of the concerned tissue as well providing advantage of treatment monitoring. In one of the reports, the metastasis of 4T1 murine breast cancer cells to sentinel lymph nodes (SLN) were treated by hybrid nanoparticulate systems consisting of gold (Au) shelled and polyethylene glycol coated (PEG) iron oxide nanoclusters (IONC). The nanoparticles IONC@Au-PEG were administered to mice 12 days post 4T1 implantation. After magnetic targeting for 4 hours, primary tumours and SLN of mice were irradiated with an 808 nm NIR light for photothermal ablation. The mice that were treated in this fashion showed greater survival than those without the magnetic field treatment (Liang, Song, Chen, Liu,

Song, Peng, & Liu, 2015). Biocompatible polymer coated specific iron oxide particles have also shown to have NIR absorbing properties. Sun and fellow researchers from the University of Michigan have prepared and patented the use of highly crystallized iron-oxide nanoparticles (HCIONP) surrounded by polysiloxane-containing copolymer for photothermal treatment of cancer (Chen, Burnett, Zhang, Zhang, Paholak, & Sun, 2014; Chen & Sun, 2017).

Tissue Engineering Using Magnetic Nanosystems

The concept of tissue engineering was introduced by Langer and Vacanti in 1993 (Langer & Vacanti, 1993). This multidisciplinary science utilizes bioengineering principles towards development of a biological substitute that restores, maintains or improves tissue or whole organ function. Magnetic force assisted tissue engineering is often referred to as "Mag-TE" (Ito & Honda, 2006). Mag-TE involves remote controlling of cells in the tissue scaffold through magnetic force. Thus the primary step in Mag-TE would be the transfection of target cells by magnetite nanoparticles coated by cationic/neutral lipid moieties to which various cell specific or organelle specific ligands may be attached (Ito & Honda, 2007). The coated magnetic nano particles are allowed to bind to their receptors on the cell membrane or in the intracellular compartment. Magnetic fields may then be applied to these cells in the scaffold to: 1) influence cellular function; 2) cause the cells to secrete extracellular matrix components; 3) guide adherence of cells to the scaffold and; 4) seed cells in the scaffold. The level of magnetic force applied can be varied in different regions of the tissue scaffold by changing the magnetic field geometry, type of particle attached to each region or the number of particles attached to each region (Cartmell & Dobson, 2009). In one example of Mag-TE; for creation of 3-D tissues of tightly connected cardio myocytes, positively charged magnetic particles were attached to primary rat cardio myocytes at 100 pg/ cell with no toxicity observed after 24 hours. Multi-layered sheets of cardio myocytes were then constructed by seeding the cell suspension in a tissue culture plate and applying a magnetic field to draw all cells to the bottom of the dish. The cells later stained positive for connexin 43 within the cardio-myocyte sheets confirming the presence of gap junctions required for effective cardiac function (Shimizu, Ito, Lee, Yoshida, Miwa, Ishiguro, ... & Honda, 2007). For further examples of Mag-TE, the reader is requested to refer the excellent review by Cartmell and Dobson (Cartmell & Dobson, 2009).

Magnetic Particle Based Immunotherapy

Immunotherapy or biologic therapy is a type of cancer therapy wherein the body's immune defenses are boosted to fight cancer. There are several types of immunotherapeutics comprising of monoclonal antibodies, cytokines (interferons and interleukins), oncolytic viruses, T-cells and cancer vaccines (www.cancer.net). The tumour site specific location may be increased on tagging these therapeutics with magnetic nanaoparticles and applying an external magnetic force near the desired area. To prove the concept, researchers initially induced a tumour in female C57BL/6 mice by injecting a chemical carcinogen 3-methylcholalnthrene in the right leg. IFN-γ (interferon gamma) was adsorbed on magnetite nanoparticles coated with dimercaptosuccinic acid (DMSA) to generate IFN-γ-DMSA-NP and injected into the mice twice a week after the tumour size reached 300 mm^3. On application of an external magnet (0.4T) near the tumour site they observed an increase in IFN-γ concentration in the tumour and reduction in tumour growth compared to the controls of phosphate buffered saline and IFN-γ-DMSA-NP without application of an external magnetic field (Gutiérrez et al., 2012). Other researchers made supermagnetic iron-oxide nanoparticles conjugated to with anti-VEGF-R2 (vascular epithelial growth factor receptor 2) and used them as probes to monitor the angiogenesis of gliomas in mice by MRI techniques (Towner, Smith, Asano, He, Doblas, Saunders, ... & Seeney, 2010).

Detoxification of Biological Fluid by Magnetic Nanosystems

Detoxification of biological fluids is based on magnetic dialysis techniques wherein a magnetic separator eliminates toxin-loaded magnetic spheres from blood. In a proposed method, a suspension of magnetic adsorbent (ferro-carbon) particles may be injected into an extracorporeal system. During movement with the blood stream, it would then adsorb low, medium and high molecular weight toxic compounds from blood. A high gradient magnetic separator could be then used to remove magnetic particles and the purified blood returned to the organism. This process is known as haemosorption (Bahadur & Giri, 2003). Key components of such magnetic dialysis system would include: 1) externally applied magnetic fields; 2) use of hemostatically inert materials and physiological flow conditions to avoid blood clotting during procedure; 3) a biocompatible insertion tube; 4) small ferromagnetic wires; 5) high separation capacity and; 6) first pass capture efficiency (Chen, 2007).

Magnetic Cell Separation

Magnetic particles have an important application in the process of isolation and separation of specific biomolecules/cells in crude samples such as blood, bone marrow, tissue homogenates, stool, cultivation media, food, water and soil. The procedure for magnetic biomolecule/cell separation comprise of the following steps: 1) preparation of magnetic particles coupled to specific ligands (antibodies/antigens/receptors), 2) Incubation of mixtures with the magnetic labels, 3) Application of an external magnetic field for sedimentation of the magnetic label-cells/biomolecules, 4) Collection or discard of supernatant, 5) Washing of magnetic label-cell/biomolecules and 6) Elution of the desired cell/biomolecule from the magnetic particles. (Barakat, 2009). One application demonstrated is the separation of $CD4^+$ T cells from human blood containing a population of different cell types using iron oxide nanoparticles coupled to anti-$CD4^+$ antibody (Mandal, Ghosh & Mandal, 2009). Some commercial available systems for cell separation are Dynabeads™ and MagniSort™ (ThermoFisher Scientific).

Magnetic Nanosystems in Nucleic Acid Delivery

The generic term used for magnetically driven intracellular delivery of nucleic acids is magnetofection (Planck, Scherer, Schillinger & Anton, 2000). Magnetofection is defined as nuclear acid delivery under the influence of a magnetic field acting on nucleic acid vectors associated with magnetic (nano) particles. In cell cultures the vector-conjugated magnetic particles are sedimented on the target cells with the help of static or oscillating magnets placed below the plated cells. The diffusion barrier to nuclear delivery is thus surmounted and the introduction of genetic material is synchronized as a large percentage of cells get transfected (Plank & Rosenecker, 2009). The method enables a greater number of transfected viable cells since there is no disruption of cell membranes and the non-toxic, biodegradable magnetic particles enter the cell by endocytosis or pinocytosis (Arora, Gupta, Singh & Singh, 2013). More than 15 years have passed since the employment of the magnetic nanosystems for nucleic acid delivery. Since its inception many commercially available magnetofection agents are available. One class of magneto nanosystems for gene delivery, based on affinity interactions of streptavidin (coated on magnetic nanoparticles) and biotin (on the delivery vector) are Streptavidin MagneSphere® (Promega), Dynabeads™ MyOne™ Streptavidin C1(Thermo Fisher Scientific), and Sphero™ Avidin coated magnetic particles (Spherotech). Polycation and polyanion coated magnetic nanoparticles are also available such as CombiMAG, PolyMAG and SilenceMAG (OZBiosciences) which permit non-specific electrostatic/hydrophobic interactions between the magnetic nanoparticles and the vector, thus obliterating the step of having to introduce biotin/streptavidin groups on the nucleic acid carrier. For more information on characterization, design of these systems the reader is directed to excellent reviews by Plank and associates on the topic (Plank, Zelphati & Mykhalylyk, 2011; Plank, Vlaskou, Sanchez-Antequera & Mykhaylyk, 2015).

Nanomagnetic Actuation

Mechanical stimulation of cells within three dimensional constructs are essential for appropriate tissue regeneration/formation. *In vitro* mechanical stimulation may be applied within bioreactors equipped with piston/compression systems, substrate bending technology, hydrodynamic compression and fluid shear. Magnetically mediated mechanical stimulation or nanomagnetic actuation allows manipulation of cellular functions at a distance (Sesenig, Sapir, MacDonald, Cohen & Polyak, 2012) unlike the conventional methods. An external magnetic field can be applied to magnetic nanoparticles bound to specific cellular receptors to actuate processes such as activation of ion channels (Hughes, El Haj & Dobson, 2005) within the target cell despite the presence of intervening tissues. The technique thus enables *in vitro* and *in vivo* manipulation of target cells. In one example of *in vitro* actuation, RBL-2H3 mast cells were pre-incubated with IgE directed against the dinitrophenyl (DNP) antigen resulting in exposure of the IgE on the surface of the cells. Superparamagnetic nanobeads of size 30 nm were covalently conjugated to DNP through a lysine linker (DNP-Lys), (1DNP/bead) and incubated with the pre-treated cells. The beads were bound to the cells via the IgE-FcεR1 receptor. In absence of an external magnetic field there was no signal activation i.e. no increase in intracellular calcium was observed. However when an external magnetic field through an electromagnetic needle was applied, the beads aggregated due to bead-bead attraction causing clustering of the associated receptors and subsequent signaling path activation leading to an increase in intracellular calcium. The calcium signaling was proportional to the proximity of the electromagnetic needle tip and could be manipulated (Mannix, Kumar, Cassiola, Montoya-Zavala, Feinstein, Prentiss, & Ingber, 2008).

CONCLUSION AND FUTURE PERSPECTIVES

This chapter basically reviews the basic principles of magnetic nanoparticles, chemical synthetic pathways, its characterization and stabilization methods. The design strategies, its performance and biomedical applications are discussed. Magnetically responsive nanodevices have a crucial role in *In-vivo* applications like MRI, imaging of transplanted cells or tissue reconstruction, stem cell labeling and tracking *in vivo*, imaging-assisted drug and gene delivery, molecular targeting of chronic diseases such as atherosclerosis and cancer, disease therapy, safety and biocompatibility to name few. Toxicity of MNPs is multifactorial and depends upon their composition, physicochemical properties such as size and surface characteristics, route of administration, and dose. Knowledge about the complex issues involving physiological, physicochemical and molecular processes of magnetic nanosystems need to be considered for understanding the clinical toxicity These magnetic nanosystems are of great advantage for nonsurgical removable neoplasia (i.e., brain cancers or hemorrhagic tumors) but limited to accessible tumor nodules. Hence surface functionalization is important for target delivery because of specificity toward the target cells overexpressing unique surface receptors. The biocompatibility of nanoparticles must be assessed *in vitro*, prior to measuring their magnetic and relaxometric properties. Finally, the biological kinetics (blood retention, organ uptake, clearance) and contrast-enhancement effects of each new nanoparticulate system, must be carefully studied *in vivo*. Nano carrier systems have demonstrated to induce cytotoxicity and /or genotoxicity whereas their antigenicity remains poorly characterized. Identification of best magnetic and irradiation technologies is the requirement for the efficient delivery of magnetic nanosystems. Emitters of magnetic fields are potentially expensive and hence remain the major challenge for daily clinical practice. Finally, the expansion of hybrid imaging modalities (MRI/PET, MRI/luminescence, MRI/SPECT, MRI/echography), call for the development of multifunctional and increasingly complex imaging tracers. Huge progress has been observed in this area of magnetic nanosystem, but various challenges need to be addressed with respect to clinical medicine and ensure the smooth transition of these concepts from labs to market. Regulatory guidance enforce very strict requirements over the design, manufacturing, reproducibility, potential toxicity and pharmacokinetic performance of such magnetic nanosystems. In this context, the 2020 nanomedicine research outlook as viewed by the European Commission, is to establish a stronger and faster transition of nanomedical R&D from a laboratory to clinical development and approval (www.etp-nanomedicine.eu).

REFERENCES

Agostinis, P., Berg, K., Cengel, K. A., Foster, T. H., Girotti, A. W., Gollnick, S. O., ... Korbelik, M. (2011). Photodynamic therapy of cancer: An update. *CA: a Cancer Journal for Clinicians*, *61*(4), 250–281. doi:10.3322/caac.20114 PMID:21617154

Ahmad, T., Bae, H., Rhee, I., Chang, Y., Jin, S. U., & Hong, S. (2012). Gold-coated iron oxide nanoparticles as a T 2 contrast agent in magnetic resonance imaging. *Journal of Nanoscience and Nanotechnology*, *12*(7), 5132–5137. doi:10.1166/jnn.2012.6368 PMID:22966533

Akbarzadeh, A., Samiei, M., & Davaran, S. (2012). Magnetic nanoparticles: Preparation, physical properties, and applications in biomedicine. *Nanoscale Research Letters*, *7*(1), 144. doi:10.1186/1556-276X-7-144 PMID:22348683

Ali, A., & Hira Zafar, M. Z. (2016). Synthesis, characterization, applications, and challenges of iron oxide nanoparticles. *Nanotechnology, Science and Applications*, *9*, 49–67. doi:10.2147/NSA.S99986 PMID:27578966

Babu, A., Templeton, A. K., Munshi, A., & Ramesh, R. (2013). Nanoparticle-based drug delivery for therapy of lung cancer: Progress and challenges. *Journal of Nanomaterials*, *2013*, 14. doi:10.1155/2013/863951

Bacri, J. C., Perzynski, R., Salin, D., Cabuil, V., & Massart, R. (1990). Ionic ferrofluids: A crossing of chemistry and physics. *Journal of Magnetism and Magnetic Materials*, *85*(1-3), 27–32. doi:10.1016/0304-8853(90)90010-N

Bahadur, D., & Giri, J. (2003). Biomaterials and magnetism. *Sadhana*, *28*(3-4), 639–656. doi:10.1007/BF02706451

Ballesteros-Gómez, A., & Rubio, S. (2009). Hemimicelles of alkyl carboxylates chemisorbed onto magnetic nanoparticles: Study and application to the extraction of carcinogenic polycyclic aromatic hydrocarbons in environmental water samples. *Analytical Chemistry*, *81*(21), 9012–9020. doi:10.1021/ac9016264 PMID:19785448

Bamrungsap, S., Chen, T., Shukoor, M. I., Chen, Z., Sefah, K., Chen, Y., & Tan, W. (2012). Pattern recognition of cancer cells using aptamer-conjugated magnetic nanoparticles. *ACS Nano*, *6*(5), 3974–3981. doi:10.1021/nn3002328 PMID:22424140

Banerjee, R., Katsenovich, Y., Lagos, L., McIintosh, M., Zhang, X., & Li, C. Z. (2010). Nanomedicine: Magnetic nanoparticles and their biomedical applications. *Current Medicinal Chemistry*, *17*(27), 3120–3141. doi:10.2174/092986710791959765 PMID:20629620

Barakat, N. S. (2009). Magnetically modulated nanosystems: A unique drug-delivery platform. *Nanomedicine (London)*, *4*(7), 799–812. doi:10.2217/nnm.09.66 PMID:19839815

Baroli, B., Ennas, M. G., Loffredo, F., Isola, M., Pinna, R., & López-Quintela, M. A. (2007). Penetration of metallic nanoparticles in human full-thickness skin. *The Journal of Investigative Dermatology*, *127*(7), 1701–1712. doi:10.1038j.jid.5700733 PMID:17380118

Baudry, J., Bertrand, E., Rouzeau, C., Greffier, O., Koenig, A., Dreyfus, R., ... Lequeux, N. (2004). Colloids for studying molecular recognition. [). Lavoisier.]. *Annales de chimie*, *29*(1), 97–106. doi:10.3166/acsm.29.97-106

Bhatia, S. (2016). Nanoparticles Types, Classification, Characterization, Fabrication Methods and Drug Delivery Applications. In *Natural Polymer Drug Delivery Systems* (pp. 33–93). Springer International Publishing. doi:10.1007/978-3-319-41129-3_2

Blasiak, B., van Veggel, F. C., & Tomanek, B. (2013). Applications of nanoparticles for MRI cancer diagnosis and therapy. *Journal of Nanomaterials*, *2013*, 12. doi:10.1155/2013/148578

Bonnemain, B. (1998). Superparamagnetic agents in magnetic resonance imaging: Physicochemical characteristics and clinical applications a review. *Journal of Drug Targeting*, *6*(3), 167–174. doi:10.3109/10611869808997890 PMID:9888302

Businova, P., Chomoucka, J., Prasek, J., Hrdy, R., Drbohlavova, J., Sedlacek, P., & Hubalek, J. (2011). Polymer coated iron oxide magnetic nanoparticles: Preparation and characterization. *Nanocon*, *9*, 21–23.

Calvin, S., Miller, M. M., Goswami, R., Cheng, S. F., Mulvaney, S. P., Whitman, L. J., & Harris, V. G. (2003). Determination of crystallite size in a magnetic nanocomposite using extended x-ray absorption fine structure. *Journal of Applied Physics*, *94*(1), 778–783. doi:10.1063/1.1581344

Cartmell, S. H., & Dobson, J. (2009) The use of magnetic particles in tissue engineering. In Nanomaterials for Life Sciences: Magnetic Nanomaterials (pp. 293-308). Wiley-VCH.

Chen, H., Burnett, J., Zhang, F., Zhang, J., Paholak, H., & Sun, D. (2014). Highly crystallized iron oxide nanoparticles as effective and biodegradable mediators for photothermal cancer therapy. *Journal of Materials Chemistry. B, Materials for Biology and Medicine*, *2*(7), 757–765. doi:10.1039/C3TB21338B

Chen, H., Ebner, A. D., Bockenfeld, D., Ritter, J. A., Kaminski, M. D., Liu, X., ... Rosengart, A. J. (2007). A comprehensive in vitro investigation of a portable magnetic separator device for human blood detoxification. *Physics in Medicine and Biology*, *52*(19), 6053–6072. doi:10.1088/0031-9155/52/19/023 PMID:17881819

Chen, H., Qi, F., Zhou, H., Jia, S., Gao, Y., Koh, K., & Yin, Y. (2015). Fe 3 O 4@ Au nanoparticles as a means of signal enhancement in surface plasmon resonance spectroscopy for thrombin detection. *Sensors and Actuators. B, Chemical*, *212*, 505–511. doi:10.1016/j.snb.2015.02.062

Chen, H., & Sun, D. (2017). U.*S. Patent No. 9,533,045*. Washington, DC: U.S. Patent and Trademark Office.

Chen, J. P., Yang, P. C., Ma, Y. H., & Wu, T. (2011). Characterization of chitosan magnetic nanoparticles for in situ delivery of tissue plasminogen activator. *Carbohydrate Polymers*, *84*(1), 364–372. doi:10.1016/j.carbpol.2010.11.052

Cherukuri, P., Glazer, E. S., & Curley, S. A. (2010). Targeted hyperthermia using metal nanoparticles. *Advanced Drug Delivery Reviews*, *62*(3), 339–345. doi:10.1016/j.addr.2009.11.006 PMID:19909777

Chicheł, A., Skowronek, J., Kubaszewska, M., & Kanikowski, M. (2007). Hyperthermia–description of a method and a review of clinical applications. *Reports of Practical Oncology and Radiotherapy: Journal of Greatpoland Cancer Center in Poznan and Polish Society of Radiation Oncology*, *12*(5), 267–275. doi:10.1016/S1507-1367(10)60065-X

Chorny, M., Polyak, B., Alferiev, I. S., Walsh, K., Friedman, G., & Levy, R. J. (2007). Magnetically driven plasmid DNA delivery with biodegradable polymeric nanoparticles. *The FASEB Journal*, *21*(10), 2510–2519. doi:10.1096/fj.06-8070com PMID:17403937

Dahl, O., & Overgaard, J. (1995). A century with hyperthermic oncology in Scandinavia. *Acta Oncologica*, *34*(8), 1075–1083. doi:10.3109/02841869509127234 PMID:8608032

Dang, L., Liu, J., Li, F., Wang, L., Li, D., Guo, B., ... Badshah, S. A. (2016). Targeted delivery systems for molecular therapy in skeletal disorders. *International Journal of Molecular Sciences*, *17*(3), 428. doi:10.3390/ijms17030428 PMID:27011176

Deatsch, A. E., & Evans, B. A. (2014). Heating efficiency in magnetic nanoparticle hyperthermia. *Journal of Magnetism and Magnetic Materials*, *354*, 163–172. doi:10.1016/j.jmmm.2013.11.006

Derjaguin, B. V. (1941). Theory of the stability of strongly charged lyophobic sols and the adhesion of strongly charged particles in solutions of electrolytes. *Acta Physicochim. USSR*, *14*, 633–662.

Desai, P., Patlolla, R. R., & Singh, M. (2010). Interaction of nanoparticles and cell-penetrating peptides with skin for transdermal drug delivery. *Molecular Membrane Biology*, *27*(7), 247–259. doi:10.3109/09687688.2010.522203 PMID:21028936

Di Marco, M., Guilbert, I., Port, M., Robic, C., Couvreur, P., & Dubernet, C. (2007). Colloidal stability of ultrasmall superparamagnetic iron oxide (USPIO) particles with different coatings. *International Journal of Pharmaceutics*, *331*(2), 197–203. doi:10.1016/j.ijpharm.2006.11.002 PMID:17141984

Faraji, M., Yamini, Y., & Rezaee, M. (2010). Magnetic nanoparticles: Synthesis, stabilization, functionalization, characterization, and applications. *Journal of the Indian Chemical Society*, *7*(1), 1–37.

Fortin, M. (n.d.). *Magnetic nanoparticles for MRI applications in medicine*. Retrieved from http://www.cqmfscience.com/wpcontent/uploads/2013/05/Fortin_Chapter.pdf

Freitas, J. C. D., Branco, R. M., Lisboa, I. G. O., Costa, T. P. D., Campos, M. G. N., Jafelicci Júnior, M., & Marques, R. F. C. (2015). Magnetic Nanoparticles Obtained by Homogeneous Coprecipitation Sonochemically Assisted. *Materials Research*, *18*(suppl 2), 220–224. doi:10.1590/1516-1439.366114

Fritz, G., Schädler, V., Willenbacher, N., & Wagner, N. J. (2002). Electrosteric stabilization of colloidal dispersions. *Langmuir*, *18*(16), 6381–6390. doi:10.1021/la015734j

Gaur, U., Sahoo, S. K., De Tapas, K., Ghosh, P. C., Maitra, A., & Ghosh, P. K. (2000). Biodistribution of fluoresceinated dextran using novel nanoparticles evading reticuloendothelial system. *International Journal of Pharmaceutics*, *202*(1), 1–10. doi:10.1016/S0378-5173(99)00447-0 PMID:10915921

Ghorbani, M., Hamishehkar, H., Arsalani, N., & Entezami, A. A. (2015). Preparation of thermo and pH-responsive polymer@ Au/Fe3O4 core/shell nanoparticles as a carrier for delivery of anticancer agent. *Journal of Nanoparticle Research*, *17*(7), 305. doi:10.100711051-015-3097-z

Gilchrist, R. K., Medal, R., Shorey, W. D., Hanselman, R. C., Parrott, J. C., & Taylor, C. B. (1957). Selective inductive heating of lymph nodes. *Annals of Surgery*, *146*(4), 596–606. doi:10.1097/00000658-195710000-00007 PMID:13470751

Guin, D., & Manorama, S. V. (2008). Room temperature synthesis of monodispersed iron oxide nanoparticles. *Materials Letters*, *62*(17), 3139–3142. doi:10.1016/j.matlet.2008.02.005

Gunn, J., Wallen, H., Veiseh, O., Sun, C., Fang, C., Cao, J., ... Zhang, M. (2008). A multimodal targeting nanoparticle for selectively labeling T cells. *Small*, *4*(6), 712–715. doi:10.1002mll.200701103 PMID:18528851

Gupta, G., Arora, S., Singh, S., & Singh, N. (2014). Advances in magnetofection magnetically guided nucleic acid delivery: A review. *Journal of Pharmaceutical Technology. Research Management*, *1*, 19–29.

Gutiérrez, L., Mejías, R., Barber, D. F., Veintemillas-Verdaguer, S., Serna, C. J., Lázaro, F. J., & Morales, M. P. (2012, February). Fighting cancer with magnetic nanoparticles and immunotherapy. In *SPIE BiOS* (pp. 82320X–82320X). International Society for Optics and Photonics. doi:10.1117/12.905890

Guven, B., Basaran-Akgul, N., Temur, E., Tamer, U., & Boyacı, İ. H. (2011). SERS-based sandwich immunoassay using antibody coated magnetic nanoparticles for Escherichia coli enumeration. *Analyst (London)*, *136*(4), 740–748. doi:10.1039/C0AN00473A PMID:21125089

Hao, Y., & Teja, A. S. (2003). Continuous hydrothermal crystallization of α–Fe_2O_3 and Co_3O_4 nanoparticles. *Journal of Materials Research*, *18*(02), 415–422. doi:10.1557/JMR.2003.0053

Harisinghani, M. G., Barentsz, J., Hahn, P. F., Deserno, W. M., Tabatabaei, S., van de Kaa, C. H., ... Weissleder, R. (2003). Noninvasive detection of clinically occult lymph-node metastases in prostate cancer. *The New England Journal of Medicine*, *348*(25), 2491–2499. doi:10.1056/NEJMoa022749 PMID:12815134

Hasany, S. F., Ahmed, I., Rajan, J., & Rehman, A. (2012). Systematic review of the preparation techniques of iron oxide magnetic nanoparticles. *Nanoscience and Nanotechnology*, *2*(6), 148–158. doi:10.5923/j.nn.20120206.01

Hein, C. D., Liu, X. M., & Wang, D. (2008). Click chemistry, a powerful tool for pharmaceutical sciences. *Pharmaceutical Research*, *25*(10), 2216–2230. doi:10.100711095-008-9616-1 PMID:18509602

Hong, S., Leroueil, P. R., Majoros, I. J., Orr, B. G., Baker, J. R., & Holl, M. M. B. (2007). The binding avidity of a nanoparticle-based multivalent targeted drug delivery platform. *Chemistry & Biology*, *14*(1), 107–115. doi:10.1016/j.chembiol.2006.11.015 PMID:17254956

Hosseini, M., Memari, Z., Ganjali, M. R., Khoobi, M., Faridbod, F., Shafiee, A., ... Hajinezhad, A. (2014). A novel mercury-sensitive fluorescent nano-chemosensor using new functionalized magnetic core-shell Fe3O4@ SiO2 nanoparticles. *International Journal of Environmental of Research*, *8*(4), 861–870.

Hu, Y., Meng, L., Niu, L., & Lu, Q. (2013). Facile synthesis of superparamagnetic Fe3O4@ polyphosphazene@ Au shells for magnetic resonance imaging and photothermal therapy. *ACS Applied Materials & Interfaces*, *5*(11), 4586–4591. doi:10.1021/am400843d PMID:23659588

Huang, P., Li, Z., Lin, J., Yang, D., Gao, G., Xu, C., ... Hu, H. (2011). Photosensitizer-conjugated magnetic nanoparticles for in vivo simultaneous magnetofluorescent imaging and targeting therapy. *Biomaterials*, *32*(13), 3447–3458. doi:10.1016/j.biomaterials.2011.01.032 PMID:21303717

Hughes, S., El Haj, A. J., & Dobson, J. (2005). Magnetic micro-and nanoparticle mediated activation of mechanosensitive ion channels. *Medical Engineering & Physics*, *27*(9), 754–762. doi:10.1016/j.medengphy.2005.04.006 PMID:15985383

Hussain, S. M., & Krestin, G. P. (2001). Superparamagnetic iron oxide contrast agents: Physicochemical characteristics and application in MR imaging. *European Journal of Radiology*, *11*(11), 2319–2331. doi:10.1007003300100908

Hyeon, T. (2003). Chemical synthesis of magnetic nanoparticles. *Chemical Communications*, (8): 927–934. doi:10.1039/b207789b PMID:12744306

Issa, B., Obaidat, I. M., Albiss, B. A., & Haik, Y. (2013). Magnetic nanoparticles: Surface effects and properties related to biomedicine applications. *International Journal of Molecular Sciences*, *14*(11), 21266–21305. doi:10.3390/ijms141121266 PMID:24232575

Ito, A., & Honda, H. (2006). Magnetic nanoparticles for tissue engineering. In *Nanotechnologies for the Life Sciences*. Wiley-VCH Verlag GmbH & Co. KGaA.

Jaque, D., Maestro, L. M., Del Rosal, B., Haro-Gonzalez, P., Benayas, A., Plaza, J. L., ... Sole, J. G. (2014). Nanoparticles for photothermal therapies. *Nanoscale*, *6*(16), 9494–9530. doi:10.1039/C4NR00708E PMID:25030381

Joseyphus, R. J., Kodama, D., Matsumoto, T., Sato, Y., Jeyadevan, B., & Tohji, K. (2007). Role of polyol in the synthesis of Fe particles. *Journal of Magnetism and Magnetic Materials*, *310*(2), 2393–2395. doi:10.1016/j.jmmm.2006.10.1132

Kagadis, G. C., Ford, N. L., Karnabatidis, D. N., & Loudos, G. K. (Eds.). (2016). *Handbook of Small Animal Imaging: Preclinical Imaging, Therapy, and Applications*. CRC Press. doi:10.1201/b19052

Kohler, N., Sun, C., Wang, J., & Zhang, M. (2005). Methotrexate-modified superparamagnetic nanoparticles and their intracellular uptake into human cancer cells. *Langmuir*, *21*(19), 8858–8864. doi:10.1021/la0503451 PMID:16142971

Kolb, H. C., Finn, M. G., & Sharpless, K. B. (2001). Click chemistry: Diverse chemical function from a few good reactions. *Angewandte Chemie International Edition*, *40*(11), 2004–2021. doi: PMID:11433435

Kolhatkar, A. G., Jamison, A. C., Litvinov, D., Willson, R. C., & Lee, T. R. (2013). Tuning the magnetic properties of nanoparticles. *International Journal of Molecular Sciences*, *14*(8), 15977–16009. doi:10.3390/ijms140815977 PMID:23912237

Langer, R., & Vancanti, J. P. (1993). Tissue engineering. *Science*, *260*(5110), 920–926. doi:10.1126cience.8493529 PMID:8493529

Laurent, S., Forge, D., Port, M., Roch, A., Robic, C., Vander Elst, L., & Muller, R. N. (2008). Magnetic iron oxide nanoparticles: Synthesis, stabilization, vectorization, physicochemical characterizations, and biological applications. *Chemical Reviews*, *108*(6), 2064–2110. doi:10.1021/cr068445e PMID:18543879

Li, N. J. (Ed.). (2013). Biosensors based on nanomaterials and nanodevices. CRC Press.

Li, S., Liu, H., & He, N. (2010). Covalent binding of streptavidin on gold magnetic nanoparticles for bead array fabrication. *Journal of Nanoscience and Nanotechnology*, *10*(8), 4875–4882. doi:10.1166/jnn.2010.2385 PMID:21125822

Liang, C., Song, X., Chen, Q., Liu, T., Song, G., Peng, R., & Liu, Z. (2015). Magnetic Field-Enhanced Photothermal Ablation of Tumor Sentinel Lymph Nodes to Inhibit Cancer Metastasis. *Small*, *11*(37), 4856–4863. doi:10.1002mll.201501197 PMID:26179806

Lin, J., Zhou, W., Kumbhar, A., Wiemann, J., Fang, J., Carpenter, E. E., & O'Connor, C. J. (2001). Gold-coated iron (Fe@ Au) nanoparticles: Synthesis, characterization, and magnetic field-induced self-assembly. *Journal of Solid State Chemistry*, *159*(1), 26–31. doi:10.1006/jssc.2001.9117

Lin, X. M., & Samia, A. C. (2006). Synthesis, assembly and physical properties of magnetic nanoparticles. *Journal of Magnetism and Magnetic Materials*, *305*(1), 100–109. doi:10.1016/j.jmmm.2005.11.042

Lindner, P. (2002). Scattering experiments: experimental aspects, initial data reduction and absolute calibration. *Neutrons, X-Rays and Light: Scattering methods applied to soft condensed matter*, 23-48.

Liu, C., Zou, B., Rondinone, A. J., & Zhang, Z. J. (2000). Reverse micelle synthesis and characterization of superparamagnetic MnFe2O4 spinel ferrite nanocrystallites. *The Journal of Physical Chemistry B*, *104*(6), 1141–1145. doi:10.1021/jp993552g

Liu, H. L., Ko, S. P., Wu, J. H., Jung, M. H., Min, J. H., Lee, J. H., ... Kim, Y. K. (2007). One-pot polyol synthesis of monosize PVP-coated sub-5nm Fe 3 O 4 nanoparticles for biomedical applications. *Journal of Magnetism and Magnetic Materials*, *310*(2), e815–e817. doi:10.1016/j.jmmm.2006.10.776

Liu, Q., Xu, Z., Finch, J. A., & Egerton, R. (1998). A novel two-step silica-coating process for engineering magnetic nanocomposites. *Chemistry of Materials*, *10*(12), 3936–3940. doi:10.1021/cm980370a

Lu, A. H., Salabas, E. E., & Schüth, F. (2007). Magnetic nanoparticles: Synthesis, protection, functionalization, and application. *Angewandte Chemie International Edition*, *46*(8), 1222–1244. doi:10.1002/anie.200602866 PMID:17278160

Lu, Y., Fan, H., Stump, A., Ward, T. L., Rieker, T., & Brinker, C. J. (1999). Aerosol-assisted self-assembly of mesostructured spherical nanoparticles. *Nature*, *398*(6724), 223–226. doi:10.1038/18410

Lu, Y., Yin, Y., Mayers, B. T., & Xia, Y. (2002). Modifying the surface properties of superparamagnetic iron oxide nanoparticles through a sol– gel approach. *Nano Letters*, *2*(3), 183–186. doi:10.1021/nl015681q

Lyer, S., Singh, R., Tietze, R., & Alexiou, C. (2015). Magnetic nanoparticles for magnetic drug targeting. *Biomedical Engineering/Biomedizinische Technik, 60*(5), 465-475.

Mandal, S. M., Ghosh, A. K., & Mandal, M. (2008). Iron oxide nanoparticle assisted purification and mass spectrometry based proteolytic mapping of intact CD4+ T cells from human blood. *Preparative Biochemistry & Biotechnology*, *39*(1), 20–31. doi:10.1080/10826060802589510 PMID:19090418

Mannix, R. J., Kumar, S., Cassiola, F., Montoya-Zavala, M., Feinstein, E., Prentiss, M., & Ingber, D. E. (2008). Nanomagnetic actuation of receptor-mediated signal transduction. *Nature Nanotechnology*, *3*(1), 36–40. doi:10.1038/nnano.2007.418 PMID:18654448

Meng, F., Engbers, G. H., & Feijen, J. (2004). Polyethylene glycol–grafted polystyrene particles. *Journal of Biomedical Materials Research. Part A*, *70*(1), 49–58. doi:10.1002/jbm.a.30056 PMID:15174108

Moros, E. (2012). *Physics of thermal therapy: fundamentals and clinical applications*. Taylor & Francis.

Mylon, S. E., Chen, K. L., & Elimelech, M. (2004). Influence of natural organic matter and ionic composition on the kinetics and structure of hematite colloid aggregation: Implications to iron depletion in estuaries. *Langmuir*, *20*(21), 9000–9006. doi:10.1021/la049153g PMID:15461479

Napper, D. H. (1970). Flocculation studies of sterically stabilized dispersions. *Journal of Colloid and Interface Science*, *32*(1), 106–114. doi:10.1016/0021-9797(70)90107-4

Nikalje, A. P. (2015). Nanotechnology and its Applications in Medicine. *Medicinal Chemistry (Shariqah, United Arab Emirates)*, *5*(2), 81–89.

Park, I. K., Ng, C. P., Wang, J., Chu, B., Yuan, C., Zhang, S., & Pun, S. H. (2008). Determination of nanoparticle vehicle unpackaging by MR imaging of a T 2 magnetic relaxation switch. *Biomaterials*, *29*(6), 724–732. doi:10.1016/j.biomaterials.2007.10.018 PMID:18006052

Peng, X. H., Qian, X., Mao, H., & Wang, A. Y. (2008). Targeted magnetic iron oxide nanoparticles for tumor imaging and therapy. *International Journal of Nanomedicine*, *3*(3), 311. PMID:18990940

Perigo, E. A., Hemery, G., Sandre, O., Ortega, D., Garaio, E., Plazaola, F., & Teran, F. J. (2015). Fundamentals and advances in magnetic hyperthermia. *Applied Physics Reviews*, *2*(4), 041302. doi:10.1063/1.4935688

Plank, C., & Rosenecker, J. (2009). Magnetofection: the use of magnetic nanoparticles for nucleic acid delivery. *Cold Spring Harbor Protocols, 2009*(6), pdb-prot5230.

Plank, C., Scherer, F., Schillinger, U., & Anton, M. (2000). Magnetofection: enhancement and localization of gene delivery with magnetic particles under the influence of a magnetic field. *J Gene Med, 2*(5), S24.

Plank, C., Vlaskou, D., Sanchez-Antequera, Y., & Mykhaylyk, O. (2015). Magnetofection: Using Magnetic Particles and Magnetic Force to Enhance and Target Nucleic Acid Delivery. In Gene and Cell Therapy: Therapeutic Mechanisms and Strategies, Fourth Edition (pp. 347-420). CRC Press.

Plank, C., Zelphati, O., & Mykhaylyk, O. (2011). Magnetically enhanced nucleic acid delivery. Ten years of magnetofection—Progress and prospects. *Advanced Drug Delivery Reviews*, *63*(14), 1300–1331. doi:10.1016/j.addr.2011.08.002 PMID:21893135

Polyak, B., & Friedman, G. (2009). Magnetic targeting for site-specific drug delivery: Applications and clinical potential. *Expert Opinion on Drug Delivery*, *6*(1), 53–70. doi:10.1517/17425240802662795 PMID:19236208

Pradhan, P., Giri, J., Rieken, F., Koch, C., Mykhaylyk, O., Döblinger, M., ... Plank, C. (2010). Targeted temperature sensitive magnetic liposomes for thermo-chemotherapy. *Journal of Controlled Release*, *142*(1), 108–121. doi:10.1016/j.jconrel.2009.10.002 PMID:19819275

Rao, S., & Houska, C. R. (1986). X-ray particle-size broadening. *Acta Crystallographica. Section A, Foundations of Crystallography*, *42*(1), 6–13. doi:10.1107/S0108767386099981

Reddy, L. H., Arias, J. L., Nicolas, J., & Couvreur, P. (2012). Magnetic nanoparticles: Design and characterization, toxicity and biocompatibility, pharmaceutical and biomedical applications. *Chemical Reviews*, *112*(11), 5818–5878. doi:10.1021/cr300068p PMID:23043508

Rohrer, M., Bauer, H., Mintorovitch, J., Requardt, M., & Weinmann, H. J. (2005). Comparison of magnetic properties of MRI contrast media solutions at different magnetic field strengths. *Investigative Radiology*, *40*(11), 715–724. doi:10.1097/01.rli.0000184756.66360.d3 PMID:16230904

Sadhukha, T., Wiedmann, T. S., & Panyam, J. (2013). Inhalable magnetic nanoparticles for targeted hyperthermia in lung cancer therapy. *Biomaterials*, *34*(21), 5163–5171. doi:10.1016/j.biomaterials.2013.03.061 PMID:23591395

Sahoo, Y., Goodarzi, A., Swihart, M. T., Ohulchanskyy, T. Y., Kaur, N., Furlani, E. P., & Prasad, P. N. (2005). Aqueous ferrofluid of magnetite nanoparticles: Fluorescence labeling and magnetophoretic control. *The Journal of Physical Chemistry B*, *109*(9), 3879–3885. doi:10.1021/jp045402y PMID:16851439

Sayar, F., Güven, G., & Pişkin, E. (2006). Magnetically loaded poly (methyl methacrylate-co-acrylic acid) nano-particles. *Colloid & Polymer Science*, *284*(9), 965–978. doi:10.100700396-005-1383-5

Sensenig, R., Sapir, Y., MacDonald, C., Cohen, S., & Polyak, B. (2012). Magnetic nanoparticle-based approaches to locally target therapy and enhance tissue regeneration in vivo. *Nanomedicine (London)*, *7*(9), 1425–1442. doi:10.2217/nnm.12.109 PMID:22994959

Shanmugam, V., Selvakumar, S., & Yeh, C. S. (2014). Near-infrared light-responsive nanomaterials in cancer therapeutics. *Chemical Society Reviews*, *43*(17), 6254–6287. doi:10.1039/C4CS00011K PMID:24811160

Shetake, N. G., Balla, M. M., Kumar, A., & Pandey, B. N. (2016). Magnetic hyperthermia therapy: An emerging modality of cancer treatment in combination with radiotherapy. *Journal of Radiation and Cancer Research*, *7*(1), 13. doi:10.4103/0973-0168.184606

Shetake, N. G., Kumar, A., Gaikwad, S., Ray, P., Desai, S., Ningthoujam, R. S., ... Pandey, B. N. (2015). Magnetic nanoparticle-mediated hyperthermia therapy induces tumour growth inhibition by apoptosis and Hsp90/AKT modulation. *International Journal of Hyperthermia*, *31*(8), 909–919. doi:10.3109/02656736.2015.1075072 PMID:26416812

Shimizu, K., Ito, A., Lee, J. K., Yoshida, T., Miwa, K., Ishiguro, H., ... Honda, H. (2007). Construction of multi-layered cardiomyocyte sheets using magnetite nanoparticles and magnetic force. *Biotechnology and Bioengineering*, *96*(4), 803–809. doi:10.1002/bit.21094 PMID:16865728

Silva, S. M., Tavallaie, R., Sandiford, L., Tilley, R. D., & Gooding, J. J. (2016). Gold coated magnetic nanoparticles: From preparation to surface modification for analytical and biomedical applications. *Chemical Communications*, *52*(48), 7528–7540. doi:10.1039/C6CC03225G PMID:27182032

Spirin, M. G., Brichkin, S. B., & Razumov, V. F. (2005). Synthesis and stabilization of gold nanoparticles in reverse micelles of aerosol OT and Triton X-100. *Colloid Journal*, *67*(4), 485–490. doi:10.100710595-005-0122-4

Stephen, Z. R., Kievit, F. M., & Zhang, M. (2011). Magnetite nanoparticles for medical MR imaging. *Materials Today*, *14*(7), 330–338. doi:10.1016/S1369-7021(11)70163-8 PMID:22389583

Sun, S., & Zeng, H. (2002). Size controlled synthesis of magnetite nanoparticles. *Journal of the American Chemical Society*, *124*(28), 8204–8205. doi:10.1021/ja026501x PMID:12105897

Tang, C., Qiu, F., & Zhao, X. (2013). Molecular design and applications of self-assembling surfactant-like peptides. *Journal of Nanomaterials*, *2013*, 15. doi:10.1155/2013/469261

Tang, Y., Li, Z., He, N., Zhang, L., Ma, C., Li, X., ... He, L. (2013). Preparation of functional magnetic nanoparticles mediated with PEG-4000 and application in Pseudomonas Aeruginosa rapid detection. *Journal of Biomedical Nanotechnology*, *9*(2), 312–317. doi:10.1166/jbn.2013.1493 PMID:23627062

Tartaj, P., Veintemillas-Verdaguer, S., & Serna, C. J. (2003). The preparation of magnetic nanoparticles for applications in biomedicine. *Journal of Physics. D, Applied Physics*, *36*(13), R182–R197. doi:10.1088/0022-3727/36/13/202

Teng, X., Black, D., Watkins, N. J., Gao, Y., & Yang, H. (2003). Platinum-maghemite core– shell nanoparticles using a sequential synthesis. *Nano Letters*, *3*(2), 261–264. doi:10.1021/nl025918y

Towner, R. A., Smith, N., Asano, Y., He, T., Doblas, S., Saunders, D., ... Seeney, C. E. (2009). Molecular magnetic resonance imaging approaches used to aid in the understanding of angiogenesis in vivo: Implications for tissue engineering. *Tissue Engineering. Part A*, *16*(2), 357–364. doi:10.1089/ten.tea.2009.0233 PMID:19663584

Tran, N., & Webster, T. J. (2010). Magnetic nanoparticles: Biomedical applications and challenges. *Journal of Materials Chemistry*, *20*(40), 8760–8767. doi:10.1039/c0jm00994f

Ulman, A. (1996). Formation and structure of self-assembled monolayers. *Chemical Reviews*, *96*(4), 1533–1554. doi:10.1021/cr9502357 PMID:11848802

Veiseh, O., Gunn, J. W., & Zhang, M. (2010). Design and fabrication of magnetic nanoparticles for targeted drug delivery and imaging. *Advanced Drug Delivery Reviews*, *62*(3), 284–304. doi:10.1016/j.addr.2009.11.002 PMID:19909778

Verwey, E. J. W., Overbeek, J. T. G., & Overbeek, J. T. G. (1999). *Theory of the stability of lyophobic colloids*. Courier Corporation.

Wang, D., Fei, B., Halig, L. V., Qin, X., Hu, Z., Xu, H., ... Chen, Z. (2014). Targeted iron-oxide nanoparticle for photodynamic therapy and imaging of head and neck cancer. *ACS Nano*, *8*(7), 6620–6632. doi:10.1021/nn501652j PMID:24923902

Wang, Q., Yan, J., Yang, J., & Li, B. (2016). Nanomaterials promise better bone repair. *Materials Today*, *19*(8), 451–463. doi:10.1016/j.mattod.2015.12.003

Wang, X., Wang, L., He, X., Zhang, Y., & Chen, L. (2009). A molecularly imprinted polymer-coated nanocomposite of magnetic nanoparticles for estrone recognition. *Talanta*, *78*(2), 327–332. doi:10.1016/j.talanta.2008.11.024 PMID:19203590

Wu, W., He, Q., & Jiang, C. (2008). Magnetic iron oxide nanoparticles: Synthesis and surface functionalization strategies. *Nanoscale Research Letters*, *3*(11), 397–415. doi:10.100711671-008-9174-9 PMID:21749733

Xu, C., & Teja, A. S. (2008). Continuous hydrothermal synthesis of iron oxide and PVA-protected iron oxide nanoparticles. *The Journal of Supercritical Fluids*, *44*(1), 85–91. doi:10.1016/j.supflu.2007.09.033

Zhao, Q., Wang, L., Cheng, R., Mao, L., Arnold, R. D., Howerth, E. W., ... Platt, S. (2012). Magnetic nanoparticle-based hyperthermia for head & neck cancer in mouse models. *Theranostics*, *2*(1), 113–121. doi:10.7150/thno.3854 PMID:22287991

Zhou, H., Lee, J., Park, T. J., Lee, S. J., Park, J. Y., & Lee, J. (2012). Ultrasensitive DNA monitoring by Au–Fe 3 O 4 nanocomplex. *Sensors and Actuators. B, Chemical*, *163*(1), 224–232. doi:10.1016/j.snb.2012.01.040

Zhu, D., Liu, F., Ma, L., Liu, D., & Wang, Z. (2013). Nanoparticle-based systems for t1-weighted magnetic resonance imaging contrast agents. *International Journal of Molecular Sciences*, *14*(5), 10591–10607. doi:10.3390/ijms140510591 PMID:23698781

Zou, L., Wang, H., He, B., Zeng, L., Tan, T., Cao, H., ... Li, Y. (2016). Current approaches of photothermal therapy in treating cancer metastasis with nanotherapeutics. *Theranostics*, *6*(6), 762–772. doi:10.7150/thno.14988 PMID:27162548

Chapter 8
Mesoporous Silica Nanoparticles:
A Multifunctional Nanocarrier for Therapeutic Applications

Viney Lather
JCDM College of Pharmacy, India

Neelam Poonia
JCDM College of Pharmacy, India

Deepti Pandita
JCDM College of Pharmacy, India

ABSTRACT

Integration of nanotechnology and biomedicine has offered great opportunities for the development of nanoscaled therapeutic platforms. Amongst various nanocarriers, mesoporous silica nanoparticles (MSNs) is one of the most developed and promising inorganic materials-based drug delivery system for clinical translations due to their simple composition and nanoporous structure. MSNs possess unique structural features, for example, well-defined morphology, large surface areas, uniform size, controllable structure, flexible pore volume, tunable pore sizes, extraordinarily high loading efficiency, and excellent biocompatibility. Progress in structure control and functionalization may endow MSNs with functionalities that enable medical applications of these integrated nanoparticles such as molecularly targeted drug delivery, multicomponent synergistic therapy, in vivo imaging and therapeutic capability, on-demand/stimuli-responsive drug release, etc. In this chapter, the authors overview MSNs' characteristics and the scientific efforts developed till date involving drug delivery and biomedical applications.

DOI: 10.4018/978-1-5225-4781-5.ch008

Copyright © 2018, IGI Global. Copying or distributing in print or electronic forms without written permission of IGI Global is prohibited.

INTRODUCTION

Magic Bullet, a term coined by Nobel laureate Paul Ehrlich in the late 19th century, as a scientific concept to improve the efficacy of therapeutic drugs has been made into reality with the advances in nanotechnology. Nanotechnology, especially nanoparticles, offers an excellent opportunity to enhance our ability to treat various diseases including cancer, cardiovascular and inflammatory diseases. The prerequisites for an effective delivery of therapeutic moieties are to increase its target selectivity and endow it with the means to overcome the biological barriers that prevent it from reaching its target. Nanoparticle-based medicines have evolved with time to maximize therapeutic efficacy, facilitate targeting to tumors and across complex biological barriers, and offer multifunctionality while carrying multiple diagnostic/therapeutic payloads (Bobo, Robinson, Islam, Thurecht, & Corrie, 2016).

Various forms of nanoparticles, organic/inorganic, *viz.* liposomes, micelles, polymeric particles, dendrimers, quantum dots, carbon nanotubes and gold nanoparticles have been synthesized and investigated for therapeutic applications (Jeevanandam, Chan, & Danquah, 2016). Their current expectations and clinical achievements in overcoming the shortcomings of conventional therapeutic modalities have offered multiple possibilities in pharmaceutical and medical research.

NANOCARRIERS AND THEIR ONGOING CHALLENGES

Development of nanoparticle based therapeutics has come a long way since polymer-drug conjugate and first liposomal-drug formulation were reported in 1955 and 1973 respectively (Petros & DeSimone, 2010, Bobo, Robinson, Islam, Thurecht, & Corrie, 2016). Figure 1 presents the nanoparticle based medicines which are approved by the US FDA. Nanoparticles have provided a universal platform for drug delivery owing to their unique characteristics like use of different types of material in their design (e.g. polymer, metal oxides, silica, carbon and metals), accommodation of wide range of bioactive components (e.g. small molecules, proteins, nucleic acids, diagnostics etc.), functionalization with multiple functional groups for drug and gene targeting. Despite several advantages, there are several limitations associated with the nanoparticle based delivery systems like poor drug loading or limited carrying capacity, burst release, inadequate tissue distribution, scale up issues, rapid clearance via reticuloendothelial system, toxicity, and regulatory issues etc (Couvreur, 2013; Cho, Wang, Nie, Chen, & Shin, 2008). Table 1 lists the advantages and disadvantages of the different nanotherapeutic carriers and eventually cites the needs for developing new nanosystem overcoming these cons. (Wicki, Witzigmann, Balasubramanian, & Huwyler, 2015).

Inorganic nanoparticles have shown a promising potential in drug delivery owing to their versatile physicochemical properties like easy and diverse availability, rich functionality, biocompatibility, controlled and targeted drug delivery, zero premature release and dual-drug delivery etc (Kim & Hyeon, 2014). Last decade has seen several type of inorganic nanoparticles including gold, silver, platinum, iron oxide, cerium oxide, zinc oxide and carbon derivatives.

Silica (SiO_2), a natural abundantly available inorganic material classified as "Generally Recognized as Safe" (GRAS) by FDA has been utilized widely as a carrier for therapeutic and diagnostic applications (Feng, Panwar, Tng, Tjin, Wang, & Yong, 2016). Silica based nanomaterials, mesoporous silica nanoparticles (MSNs) have attracted wide attention in the field of nanomedicine due to their unique characteristics such as easy synthesis, uniform and tunable particle size/pore size, high surface area and

Figure 1. An overview of FDA approved nanomedicines stratified by material category

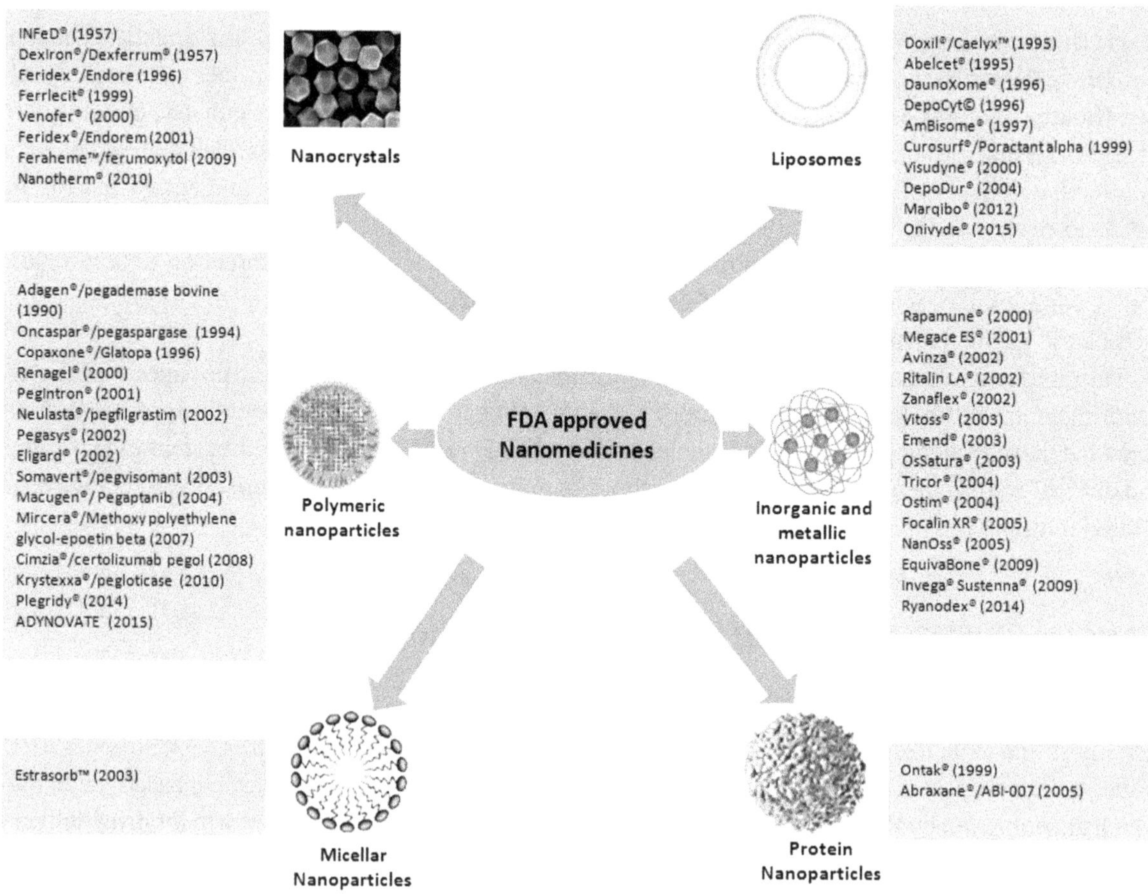

Table 1. Advantages and disadvantages of different nanoplatforms in drug delivery

Nanoplatform	Advantages	Disadvantages
Lipid-Based Nanocarriers • Conventional liposomes • PEGylated liposomes	Clinically used Biocompatible/biodegradable, Reduced adverse drug effects Passive targeting, reduced toxicity	Rapid clearance via RES Dependent on EPR effect, No improved efficacy
Protein-Based Nanosystems	Clinically used	Immunogenic, metabolic instability
Polymeric Nanoparticles	Chemically versatile	No clinically approved product, Degradation products of the nanocarrier
Drug Conjugates • Antibody drug conjugates • Polymer drug conjugates	Clinically used, small size Active targeting Tailored biodistribution of drug	Limited carrying capacity Coupling strategies, necessitates specific target Mostly passive targeting
Viral Nanoparticles	Gene therapy approach	Immunogenic, viral spread to other organs
Inorganic Nanoparticles	May improve imaging	No drug delivery Degradation products of the nanoparticles

RES: reticuloendothelial system
EPR: enhanced permeability and retention effect

pore volume, prominent biocompatibility, facile surface functionalization, capacity to carry disparate payloads of various size, shapes and functionalities such as drugs, genes, DNAs, and proteins within the porous core and effective protection for the payloads ((Feng, Panwar, Tng, Tjin, Wang, & Yong, 2016). One of the unique features of MSNs functionalization with different organic groups through grafting procedures has led to its high potential for selective adsorption and release of diverse drug molecules.

MSNs AND THEIR CHARACTERISTICS

Structure and Properties

MSNs are featured as solid materials with an ordered array of 2D hexagonal micro- or mesopore structure, uniform particle sizes (50-300 nm), high surface areas (> 1000 m^2/g), large pore volume (0.5-2.5 cm^3/g), tunable pore diameter (1.3-30 nm), controllable particle morphology, good chemical and thermal stability and tunable exterior and interior surfaces which could be modified with different functional groups (Slowing, Vivero-Escoto, Wu, & Lin, 2008).

The first mesoporous silica materials were discovered by Kresge and his team at Mobil Oil Corporation (Kresge, Leonowicz, Roth, Vartuli, & Beck, 1992) and Kuroda group at Waseda University, Japan (Yanagisawa, 1990) while aiming to discover materials with pores larger than the zeolites. Broadly, MSNs are classified as M41S type MSN family, organically modified silica (ORMOSIL) nanoparticles and hollow type MSNs (Figure 2) ((Feng, Panwar, Tng, Tjin, Wang, & Yong, 2016).

M41S Type MSN Family

Mobile Crystalline Material-41 (MCM-41) is the earliest and widely known representative of M41S family with a 2D hexagonal mesoporous structure and has been used widely for biomedical applications (Vallet-Regi, Rámila, del Real, & Pérez-Pariente, 2001). Figure 3a shows different structures of the M41S family. With a controllable synthesis using Stöber method (known as sol-gel technique) (Stöber, Fink, & Bohn, 1968), MCM-41 nanomaterials possess large surface area, high thermal stability and narrow size distribution. The structural parameters could be easily tuned by varying the solutions composition and concentrations. Another commonly used M41S MSNs for drug delivery applications include Santa Barbara Amorphous (SBA-15), which is synthesized using amphiphilic triblock copolymers having

Figure 2. Schematic representation of different type of MSNs

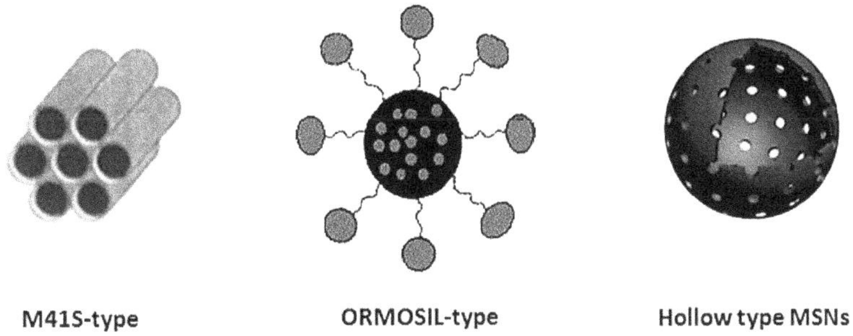

Figure 3. (a) Structural arrangements of M41S family: (top) surfactant supramolecular assemblies and (bottom) TEM images of the final materials. Reproduced with permission from ref. (Linares, Silvestre-Albero, Serrano, Silvestre-Albero, & Garcia-Martinez, 2014). Copyright © 2014, Royal Society of Chemistry. (b) Schematic representation for fabrication of MCM-41 with CTAB surfactant micelles as template. Reproduced with permission from ref. (Yang, Gai, & Lin, 2012). Copyright © 2012, Royal Society of Chemistry.

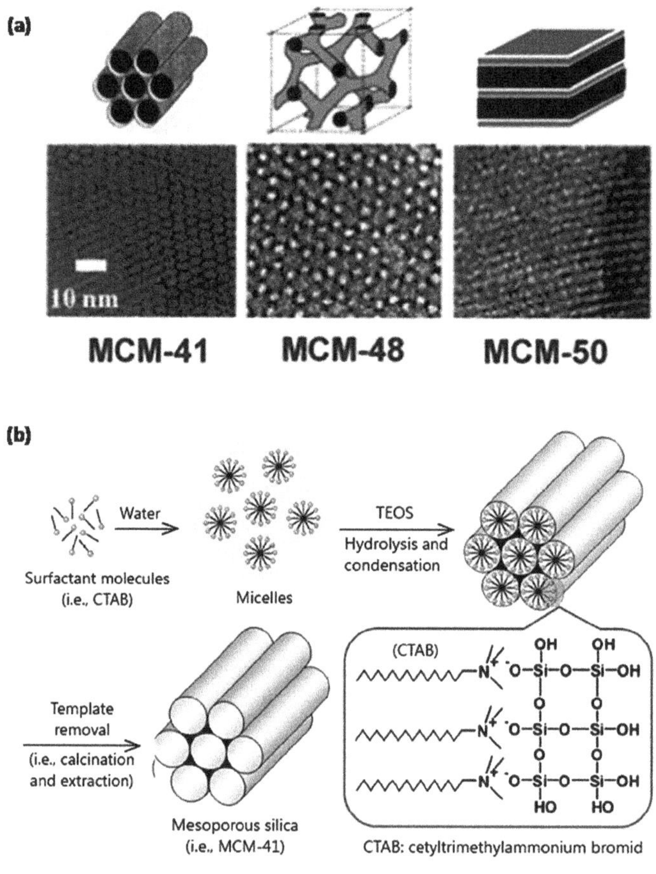

mesostructural ordering properties (Zhao, Feng, Huo, Melosh, Fredrickson, Chmelka, & Stucky, 1998). Though sharing a 2D hexagonal structure, SBA-15 nanomateirals bears a wider, tunable pore size and greater hydrothermal stability than MCM-41. The basic principle of synthesis of these MSNs includes the condensation of silica precursors directed by self-assembled liquid-crystal arrays of surfactants (Figure 3b) (Hoffmann, Cornelius, Morell, & Fröba, 2006).

ORMOSIL Nanoparticles

Despite the fact that M41S type MSNs display interesting structural properties as discussed earlier, their large size (>200 nm), structural and colloidal instabilities need to be defined for more applications and ORMOSIL nanoparticles have evolved as interesting hybrid materials for biomedical applications (Roy, Kumar, Kumar, Ohulchanskyy, Yong, & Prasad, 2014). A condensation of tetraethyl orthosilicate

(TEOS)/vinyltriethoxysilane (VTES) as inorganic silica precursors, and hydrophobic organoaloxysilane such as (3-aminopropyl) triethoxysilane (APTES)/ mercaptopropyltrimethoxysilane (MPTMS)/ diethylenetriamine (DETA) in presence of weak alkali solutions as catalyst can easily form o/w microemulsion at room temperature (Figure 4). ORMOSIL nanoparticles display several advantages for biomedical applications like:

1. Surface functionalization with different groups like hydroxyl, amino, thiol and carboxyl groups which can be used for fluorescence and targeting.
2. The morphology and particle size (from 10 to 100 nm) can be easily controlled by varying the amount of added organoalkoxysilanes.
3. Self assembly of nanoparticles due to the presence of hydrophobic and hydrophilic groups on the precursors.

Hollow Type MSNs

Hollow MSNs with a hollow core and shell with mesopores possess the characteristics of macroporous and mesoporous structures in a single system and thus improves the drug loading efficiency. Extending

Figure 4. (a) One-pot synthesis of doped, PEGylated and functional ORMOSIL nanoparticles. Reproduced with permission from ref. (Selvestrel et al., 2013). Copyright © 2013, Royal Society of Chemistry. (b) TEM images of ORMOSIL nanoparticles of sized (A) 30 nm, (B) 50 nm and (C) 80 nm. Reproduced with permission from ref. (Roy, Kumar, Kumar, Ohulchanskyy, Yong, & Prasad, 2014). Copyright © 2014, Royal Society of Chemistry.

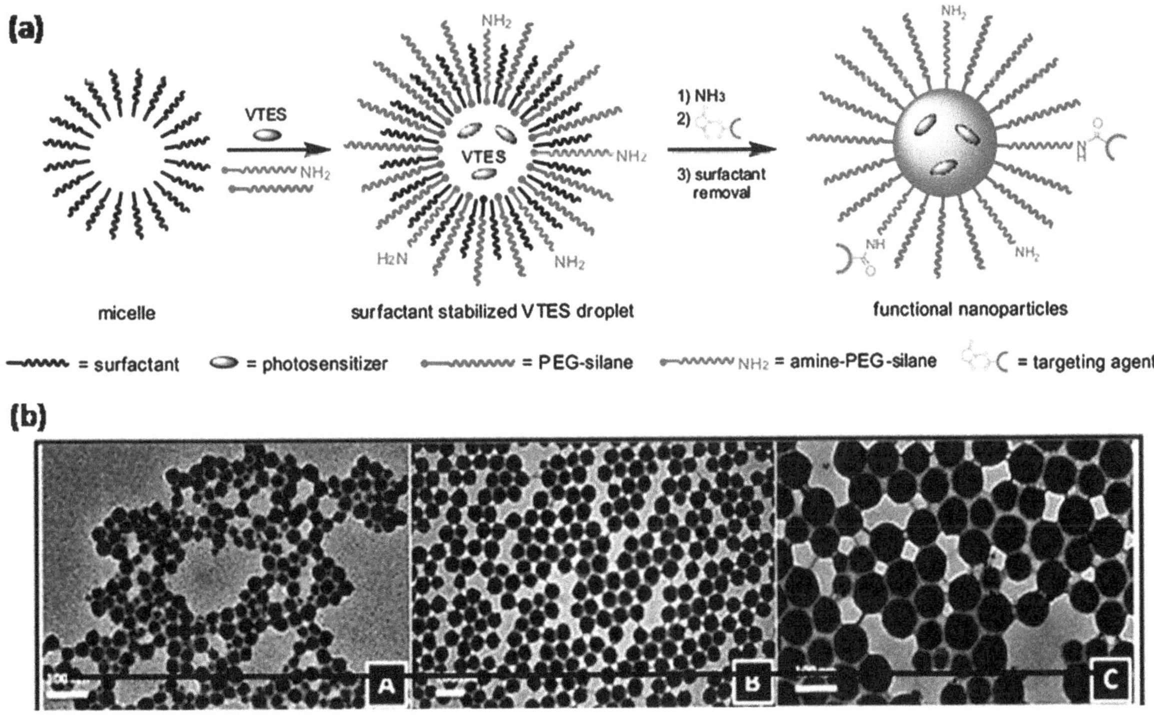

a high drug loading capacity and abundant surface chemistry hollow MSNs are being widely explored as ideal drug delivery system particularly in the treatment and diagnosis of cancer. The well-defined mesopores in the shell create the diffusion path for guest molecules. The commonly used method for the synthesis of hollow MSNs is based on "templating method", wherein different soft or hard templates are used as substrates and shells with desirable characteristics are coated on their surface (Lou, Archer, & Yang, 2008). Removal of templates leads to the formation of hollow spheres. Commonly, hollow MSNs are synthesized by three approaches including hard-template, soft-template and self-template.

- **Hard-Template Method:** Non-siliceous materials like metal or metal-oxide nanoparticles, polymer beads and semiconductor nanoparticles are used as templates. The common strategy involves the synthesis of core template followed by surface activation of polymer latexes and then silicification to form shell layer. Selective removal of templates by calcination or in alkaline/acidic conditions leads to the formation of hollow MSNs (Figure 5a). The shell thickness can be easily tuned by adjusting the ratio of nanoparticle and surfactant and the amount of silica source. Multi-functional MSNs can be synthesized using this method by incorporating capping agents or metallic nanoparticles as theranostics. Kim et al. (2008) synthesized Fe_3O_4@MSNs using cetyltrimethylammonium bromide (CTAB) acting both as a stabilizer and mesostructural directing agent, which after polyethylene glycol (PEG) surface modification could be used as a T_2-weighting magnetic resonance imaging (MRI) agent as well as a therapeutic agent (Kim, Kim, Lee, Kim, Kim, Yu, Song, Moon, & Hyeon, 2008).
- **Soft-Template Method:** Soft template method involves the use of dual or multi-surfactants to fabricate a complex template for preparing mesoporous shell and hollow interior at the same time. The soft templates being used include micelles, micremulsion droplets, vesicular structures etc (Pal & Bhaumik, 2013). One of the attractive features of the soft-template method is their ability to encapsulate multifunctional modalities during the synthetic process itself resulting in the versatility as compared to hard template. For example, Li et al. (2017) fabricated Au@HMSNs having high catalytic activity using a ternary w/o microemulsion system (Li, Xu, Gong, Wang, Liu, & Guo, 2017). Although this method is quiet simple and facile, however a precise control on particle size and thickness remains a challenge and also use of huge amount of surfactants is troublesome due to toxicity issues (Shi, Chen, & Cai, 2013).
- **Self-Template Method:** Self-templating method does not employ an additional template structure. Figure 5 (b-c) illustrates self-template method for synthesizing hollow MSNs. It involves the structural transformation by surface dissolution of the precursor followed by nucleation of the second phase on the surface of preformed particles. Hollow MSNs were fabricated by alkaline treatment of poly(dimethydiallylammonium chloride) coated mesoporous silica spheres (Tang, Li, & Chen, 2012). Self-templating involves a simple, cost-effective and self-driven technique with no additional requirement of templates or protective surfactants.

Control of Structural Properties

MSNs used in the field of nanomedicine have evolved from mesoporous silicas having amorphous chunks and particles with different shapes and sizes used for the applications like catalysis, separation, and sensors. However with advancements in surface-templated synthesis, the key structural features of

Figure 5. (a) Scheme of hard-templating methodology for hollow MSNs by using surfactant or polymer. Reproduced with permission from ref. (Wu, Mou, & Lin, 2013). Copyright © 2013, Royal Society of Chemistry. (b) Fabrication process of hollow type MSNs with silica shell in the presence of ammonia solution. TEM images show the poly(dimethydiallylammonium chloride) pre-coated mesoporous silica spheres during different instants of 1M ammonia solution treatment. Reproduced with permission from ref. (Ren, Wang, Yang, Zhang, Yang, Yue, Gao, & Tang, 2005). Copyright © 2005, American Chemical Society. (c) Formation schematics of hollow/rattle-type mesoporous silica spheres (left) and the microscopic structure schematics (right). Route A represents the selective-etching procedure in Na solution and route B for that in ammonia solution under hydrothermal treatment. The local microscopic structure (right) shows the existence of long carbon chains of C_{18}TMS that constitutes the hydrophobic cores. Reproduced with permission from ref. (Chen, Chen, Guo, He, Chen, Zhou, Feng, & Shi, 2010). Copyright © 2010, American Chemical Society.

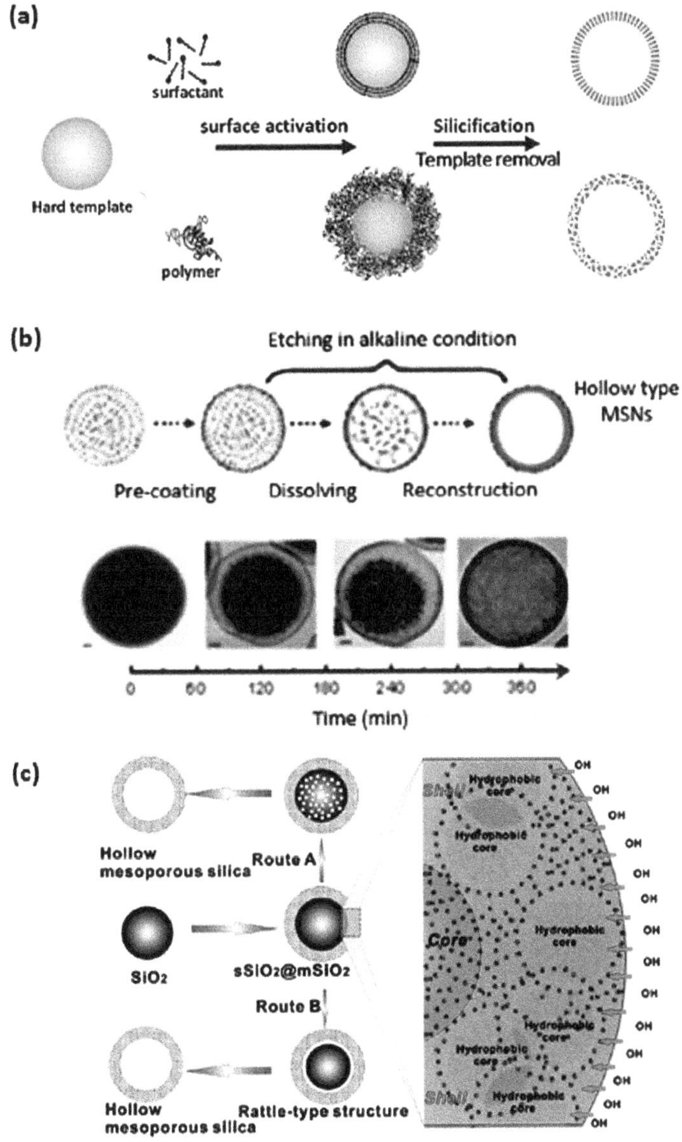

MSNs including size and shape of the particles and pores, surface chemistry and structural characteristics can be precisely controlled and modified making them a versatile carrier for payloads of different drug molecules for diverse therapeutic and diagnostic applications.

Size Control

Particle and Pore Size

MSNs owing to their unique properties have attracted a lot of attention in the field of nanomedicine. The unique properties include (Slowing, Vivero-Escoto, Wu, & Lin, 2008):

1. **Tunable Particle Size:** The particle size can be easily tuned from 30-300 nm which facilitates endocytosis by living cells with no significant toxicity.
2. **Stable and Rigid Framework:** The chemical and physical stability of MSNs in comparison to other polymer-based nanosystems gives a significant edge in their use as drug delivery carriers.
3. **Uniform and Tunable Pore Size:** A narrow pore size distribution having a diameter of 2-10 nm can be used to precisely control the drug loading and its release kinetics.
4. **High Surface Area and Large Pore Volume:** Higher values of both total surface area (>900 m^2/g) and pore volume (>0.9 cm^3/g) account for high drug payload.
5. **Two Functional Surfaces:** Both the internal and external surfaces of MSNs can be functionalized with different moieties.
6. **Unique Porous Structure:** With cylindrical porous channels running from one end to other in MSNs, a zero premature release effect can be easily achieved as long as both ends of the channels are capped.

Horcajada et al. (2004) synthesized MCM-41 MSNs of different pore sizes by using surfactants of different alky chain lengths and studied them for ibuprofen loading. It was observed that MSNs with pore size of 3.6 nm and 2.5 nm were able to load 19 wt % and 11 wt % of drug respectively (Horcajada, Rámila, Pérez-Pariente, & Vallet, 2004). Similarly, Zhang et al. (2010) observed that drug loading of telmisartan, a poorly water-soluble drug was found to increase from 48.9 to 59.7% when the pore size changed from 3.6 to 12.9 nm. The drug release was also controlled efficiently by using aminopropyl modified MSNs as compared to unmodified MSNs (Zhang, Zhi, Jiang, Zhang, Wang, & Wang, 2010). A similar result was also observed by Jia and co-workers who synthesized MSNs with different pore sizes by using $NaBH_4$ etching method. MSNs with pore size of 9.68 nm, 5.63 nm, and 3.03 nm had paclitaxel loading efficiencies of 21.6%, 16.7% and 12.1%, respectively. The anti-tumor activity against breast cancer cell lines MCF-7 was found to improve significantly with increase in the pore size (Jia, Shen, Li, Zhang, Zhang, Liu, Zheng, & Tian, 2013). MCM-41 nanoparticles loaded with tetracycline were studied for the treatment of *Escherichia coli* (Koneru, Shi, Wang, Chavala, Miller, Holbert, Conson, Ni, & Di Pasqua, 2015). Tetracycline (TC) content measured using UV-vis spectroscopy was 18.6% and 17.7% w/w for the two different sizes of MSNs prepared: MCM-41A (~41 nm) and MCM-41B (~406 nm), respectively. The efficacies of the nanoparticles were of the order: TC-MCM-41A>TC-MCM-41B> free TC, *in vivo*, against *Escherichia coli* in culture over a 24 h period, while blank nanoparticles had no effect (Figure 6a-b).

Figure 6. (a) TEM images of tetracycline-containing MCM-41 nanoparticles of size (A) 41 ± 4 nm and (B) 406 ± 55 nm. (b) Survival (%) of E. coli treated by TC, MCM-41A, MCM-41B, TC-MCM-41A and TC-MCM-41B, determined using UV-vis spectroscopy. (A) TC concentration: 0.5 µg/ml and (B) TC concentration: 1.0 µg/ml. Reproduced with permission from ref. (Koneru, Shi, Wang, Chavala, Miller, Holbert, Conson, Ni, & Di Pasqua, 2015). Copyright © 2015, MDPI. (c) (A) TEM image of sample S-MSNs illustrating the porous structure, (B) SEM image of samples S-MSN$_1$ (C) S-MSP$_2$ and (D) NR-MSNs. (d) Cellular uptake of uncoated MSNs in two different cancer cell lines after 4-h incubation. (A) HeLa 10 µg/ml, (B) HeLa 2 µg/ml, (C) Caco-2 10 µg/ml and (D) Caco-2 2 µg/ml; NR-MSNs (green), S-MSN$_1$(pink) and S-MSN$_2$ (blue). The shaded area is the control (no particles). Reproduced with permission from ref. (Karaman, Desai, Senthilkumar, Johansson, Ratts, Oden, Eriksson, Sahlgren, Toivola, & Rosenholm, 2012). Copyright © 2012, licensee Springer.

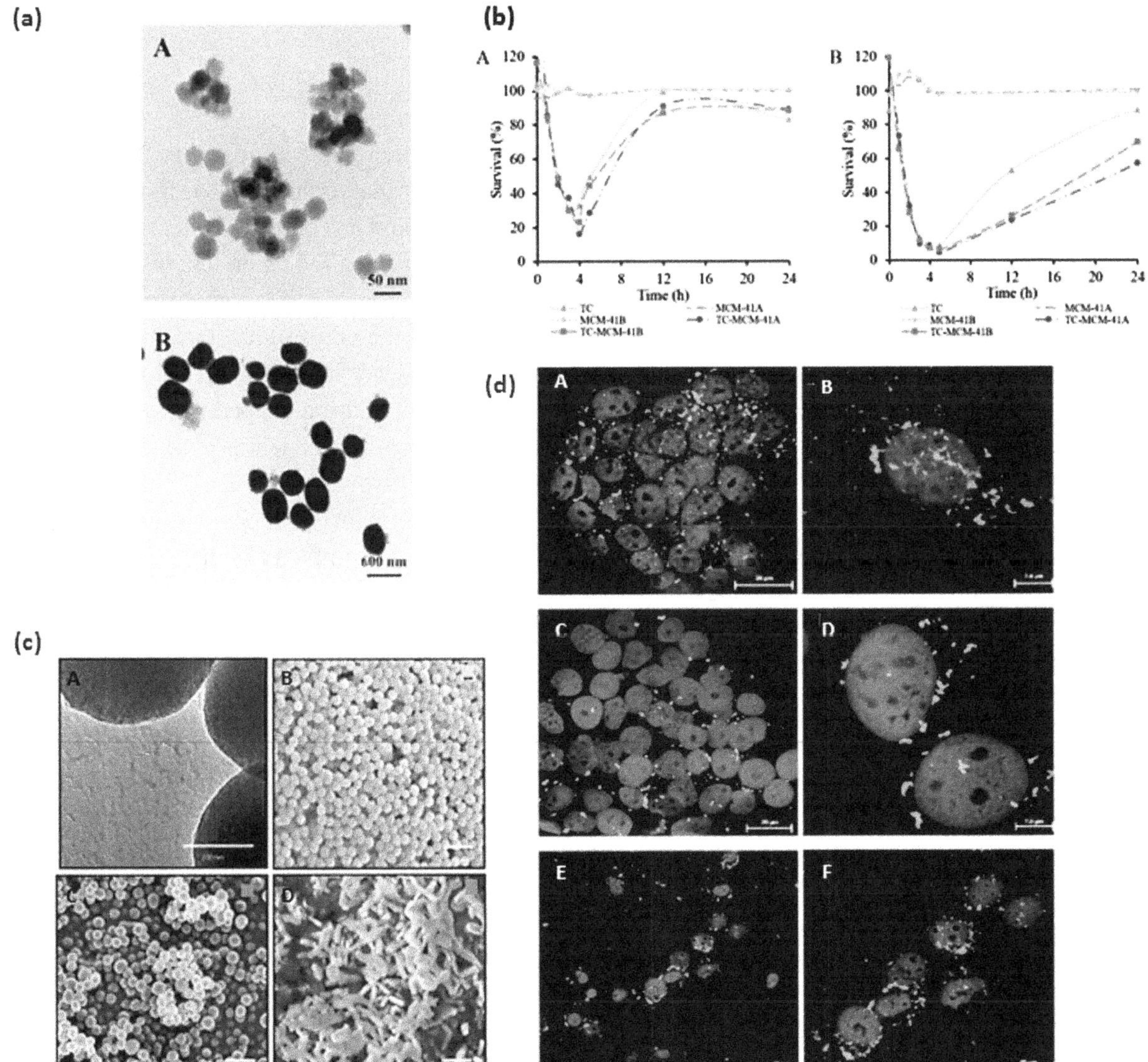

Surface Area and Pore Volume

MSNs carry different surface areas and pore volumes (MCM-41 type MSNs possess surface area of 1000 m^2/g and pore volume of 0.61 cm^3/g; SBA-15 possess surface area of 750 m^2/g and pore volume of 0.7 cm^3/g) and can adsorb or encapsulate large amount of drug molecules. The molecules which are adsorbed on the surface of MSNs either form a monolayer or multilayers. The drug loading capacity of MSNs increases with increase in surface area in case of monolayers, whereas in case of multilayers it becomes dependent on both surface area as well as the pore volume (Xu, Riikonen, & Lehto, 2013). Xu et al. (2009) studied the effect of MSNs surface area on ibuprofen adsorption and found that MSNs with largest surface area of 1283 cm^3/g had a drug loading capacity of 24.3 wt %. Surface capping by trimethylsilyl groups both on the external and internal surface had a delayed drug release profile (Xu, Gao, Xu, Wu, Sun, Shen, & Deng, 2009).

Shape Control

The shape of nanoparticles remains a major factor in determining their behaviour *in vitro* or *in vivo*, as the shape affects the agglomeration and circulation (phagocytosis by macrophages). The morphology of pores and particles of MSNs plays a key role in the drug adsorption and its controlled release properties. The shape of MSNs can be tuned by different methods like varying the alkyl chain lengths of the templates used (Trewyn, Whitman, & Lin, 2004), co-condensation reaction of TEOS and different organoalkoxysilanes (Huh, Wiench, Yoo, Pruski, & Lin, 2003b), changing the ratios of reactants like doubling the concentrations of TEOS, CTAB and NaOH (Huh, Wiench, Trewyn, Song, Pruski, & Lin, 2003a).

Karaman et al. (2012) synthesized MSNs of spherical (S-MSNs) and rod-shaped (NR-MSNs) morphologies and tested the cellular uptake efficiency in HeLa and Caco-2 cells. It was observed that both rod-like and spherical particles were internalized by HeLa cells readily, whereas Caco-2 cells were able to internalize rod-shaped particles more efficiently (Figure 6c-d) (Karaman, Desai, Senthilkumar, Johansson, Ratts, Oden, Eriksson, Sahlgren, Toivola, & Rosenholm, 2012). The impact of sphere shaped MSNs with different pore sizes on serum proteins and red blood cells was studied (Ma, Bai, Wang, & Jiang, 2014). The authors observed that the conformation of absorbed human serum albumin and fibrinogen was affected by the pore size and surface morphology of the MSNs and the hemolytic activity of MSNs was pore size dependent.

Surface Functionalization

The surface of the unmodified MSNs is largely covered with –OH groups and thus hydrogen bonding remains the major force of intermolecular interaction. However with surface functionalization, thc electrostatic and hydrophobic interactions can be introduced and could be used as a multifunctional platform for targeted drug delivery, stimuli-responsive drug delivery and increase/decrease of drug loading capacity etc. MSNs surface can be functionalized commonly by three methods: co-condensation, grafting and imprint coating method.

Co-condensation involves the synthesis of MSNs by the co-condensation of tetraalkoxysilanes (TEOS or TMOS) and terminal trialkoxyorganosilanes in the presence of structure directing agents leading to particles with organic residues attached covalently to the pore walls (Hoffmann, Cornelius, Morell, & Fröba, 2006). Grafting involves the silylation on free (Si-OH) and germinal silanol ($Si(OH)_2$) groups.

Both the internal and external (pore) surfaces can be functionalized by this method. Lu et al. (2007) functionalized the external surface of MSNs with trihydroxysilylpropyl methylphosphonate using grafting to reduce the aggregation and increase the stability of particles in aqueous solution (Lu, Liong, Zink, & Tamanoi, 2007). Imprint coating involves coating of MSNs surface with ligands already bound to metal ions rather than the free ligands. On removal of metal ions, ligands were positioned for complexation with metal ions of same type (Burleigh, Dai, Hagaman, Barnes, & Xue, 2000).

FUNCTIONALIZATION OF MSNs FOR VARIOUS THERAPEUTIC APPLICATIONS

Various nanocarriers have been employed in drug delivery for improving the bioavailability of poorly water-soluble drugs, prolonging the half-life of drug systemic circulation, release of drugs at a sustained rate, deliver drugs in a targeted manner and thus, minimize side effects. Extensive amount of work has been done worldwide in last decade on MSNs as multifunctional platforms for nanomedicine applications.

Drug Delivery

MSNs are competitive carriers and have hosted a variety of therapeutic agents e.g. drugs and genes (Table 2). Literature revealed applications of MSNs extends to treatment of various diseases including respiratory disorders, diabetes, infectious diseases, inflammation, cancer etc. The large amount of payloads (e.g. paclitaxel, doxorubicin [DOX], ibuprofen, small interfering RNA [siRNA], DNA plasmids etc.) are favourably adsorbed by electrostatic/van der Waals forces of attraction or hydrogen bonding between drug molecules and internal surface of MSNs (Jia, Shen, Li, Zhang, Zhang, Liu, Zheng, & Tian, 2013; Kamarudin, Jalil, Triwahyono, Salleh, Karim, Mukti, Hameed, & Ahmad, 2013; Minati, Antonini, Dalla Serra, Speranza, Enrichi, & Riello, 2013; Roberts, Shahin, Wen, Finlay, Dong, Wang, Dellinger Zink, Tamanoi, & Glackin, 2017). Investigations on MSNs to improve the efficacy of drug and gene delivery have grown exponentially since the first report by Vallet-Regi (Vallet-Regi, Rámila, del Real, & Pérez-Pariente, 2001). These systems have shown promising potential for various routes of administration (oral, topical, intravenous etc.) as well. Figure 7 gives an overview of the versatility of drug delivery applications of MSNs.

In a study, loading and release profile of three anti-epileptic model drugs carbamazepine, oxcarbazepine and rufinamide within ordered MSNs was investigated to boost the *in vitro* dissolution profile of these hydrophobic drugs which otherwise depict poor oral bioavailability issues limiting their clinical applications (Thomas, Slipper, Walunj, Jain, Favretto, Kallinteri, & Douroumis, 2010). Formerly, encapsulation of itraconazole, a BCS class II drug within SBA-15 type MSNs had shown *in vivo* oral bioavailability enhancement in rabbits and dogs *via* enhanced transepithelial intestinal transport (Mellaerts, Mols, Jammaer, Aerts, Annaert, Van Humbeeck, Van den Mooter, Augustijns, & Martens, 2008). Amine functionalized MSNs were examined of lately for improving the solubility and oral bioavailability of curcumin in mice (Hartono, Hadisoewignyo, Yang, Meka, Antaresti, & Yu, 2016). Further, Tao and co-workers conjugated cytosine-phosphate-guanosine oligodeoxynucleotides to amine functionalized MSNs of 60 nm size via electrostatic attraction to enhance the cellular uptake of bonded nucleotide which is otherwise susceptible to degradation by nucleases. Superior immunostimulatory action was observed in case of developed system compared to free nucleotide (Tao, Zhu, Li, & Hanagata, 2015). DOX loaded in carboxylic acid modified MSNs showed high passive accumulation within liver cells.

Table 2a. Various bioactives investigated on mesoporous silica nanoparticles for drug delivery applications: Drug delivery

Drug	Silicon Source	Surfactant	Functional Group	Particle Size (nm)	Drug Loading (% w)	Research Highlights	Refs.
Drug Delivery							
Ampicillin	TEOS	Pluronic copolymer 123, CTAB	Amino	n.d.	23.7	The chemical nature of the matrix's surface plays a role for sustaining the release of drug from it and amine functionalized MSNs was found to be suitable candidate for local sustained release of antibiotic drugs.	(Nairi, Medda, Monduzzi, & Salis, 2017)
Ascorbic Acid	TEOS, aminopropyltri-ethoxysilane	CTAB	-	94.9	n.d.	Developed MSNs exhibited more significant induction efficiency of stem cell differentiation than the treatment by ascorbic acid alone.	(Ren, Han, Li, Feng, & Ouyang, 2015)
Budesonide	TEOS	N-hexadecyltri-methylammonium-bromide	Amino	100	49	Amino-functionalized MSN provided sustained release of budesonide. Cytoprotective effect of budesonide loaded in the MSNs was more pronounced on damaged HT-29 cells compared to pure budesonide.	Yoncheva et al., (2014)
Curcumin	TEOS	Pluronic P123	β-Cyclodextrin	n.d.	88.55	Maximum loading efficiency 88.55% was obtained at 43 h of loading time and 1.22 of the weight ratio using response surface methodology. Maximum drug release was obtained at 5.16 of pH and 107 h of release time.	(Abdous, Sajjadi, & Mamani, 2017)
Curcumin	TEOS	Tergitol® NP-9	Amino	n.d.	MSU-2 type: 4.3 MCM-41 type: 3.6	Two silica materials (MSU-2 and MCM-41) were found to be biocompatible in non-cancerous CHO cell line. Curcumin loaded amine functionalized MSNs obtained from both materials exhibited significant cytotoxicity in different cancer cells (A549, MCF-7, B16F10) compared to pristine curcumin.	Bollu et al., (2016)
Cytosine-Phosphate-Guanosine Oligodeoxynu-Cleotides	TEOS	Hexadecyltri-methyl-ammonium p-toluenesulfonate	Amino	75	5	Developed MSNs exhibited superior immunostimulatory action of drug.	(Tao, Zhu, Li, & Hanagata, 2015)
Doxorubicin	TEOS	CTAB	Carboxylic	55	21.6	*In vivo* study suggested the ability of drug loaded MSNs to inhibit the tumor growth and prolong the survival time of mice bearing hepatocellular carcinoma in situ.	M. Xie et al., (2014)
Doxorubicin	TEOS	CTAB	Phosphonate	175	6.9	Modification of MSNs with hydrophilic phosphonate groups resulted in increased stability and dispersibility of the carrier in aqueous solution even after drying process. Drug loading capacity of phosphonate modified MSNs was found to be higher (6.9 wt %) compared to unmodified MSNs (2.8 wt %).	Che et al., (2014)
Doxorubicin	TEOS	Hexadecyl trimethyl ammonium chloride	PEG	72	9.3	The pharmacokinetic study in healthy rats demonstrated that drug loaded in functionalized MSNs presented the longer circulation time and lower plasma clearance rate compared with free drug solution.	(Zhang, Zhao, Li, Liu, & Du, 2017)
Doxorubicin	TEOS and 3-aminopropyltri-ethoxysilane	CTAB	Aminopropyl	130	34.52	Doxorubicin loaded amino-functionalized MSNs showed higher drug loading capacity (34.52%) than bare MSNs (17.6%), which was attributed to the stronger hydrogen bond formed between the amino group of MSNs and drug molecules.	X. Wang et al., (2017)
Doxorubicin	TEOS	Hexadecyl-trimethyl ammonium bromide	Polyelectrolyte complex layer	83	27.2	The functionalization of the MSNs with polyelectrolytes increased the colloidal stability of the nanoparticles in high ionic strength solution and in biological medium used for the *in vitro* tests.	Minati et al., (2013)
Griseofulvin	TEOS, (3-aminopropyl) triethoxysilane, chlorotrimethylsilane	CTAB, sodium lauryl sulfate	Amino, methyl	100-200	15.76-19.92	The surface functionalization on MSNs showed enhancement in solubility and drug release of griseofulvin. The hydrophobic modification (methyl group) led to a retarded drug release, which is caused by the poor wetting effect.	Jambhrunkar et al., (2014)

continued on following page

Table 2a. Continued

Drug	Silicon Source	Surfactant	Functional Group	Particle Size (nm)	Drug Loading (% w)	Research Highlights	Refs.
Drug Delivery							
Ibuprofen	TEOS	Pluronic P123	Lanthanum	n.d.	n.d.	The storage capacity of the modified silicas obtained increased with increasing their average pore diameter and percentage content of lanthanum. The amount of ibuprofen adsorbed onto KIT-6 silica modified with lanthanum was higher than that adsorbed onto SBA-15 materials.	(Goscianska, Olejnik, Nowak, Marciniak, & Pietrzak, 2015)
Ibuprofen	TEOS	CTAB	Amino	n.d.	n.d.	Functionalization of MSNs provided sustained release of drug.	Kamarudin et al., (2013)
Indomethacin	Tetramethoxysilane 3-aminopropyltri-ethoxysilane	n.d.	Amino	>100	18.7	Amine modified MSNs provided higher drug loading and enhanced dissolution release compared to bare MSNs.	J. Li et al., (2016)
Irinotecan	TEOS	CTAB	Pluronic P123 grafted 1,2-dioleoyl-sn-glycero-3-phosphoethanolamine	112	2.9	Drug loaded MSNs showed high therapeutic performance and low toxicity in BALB/c nude mice bearing drug resistant breast tumors, with an inhibition rate of 81.2% compared to free drug treatment group.	X. Zhang et al., (2014)
Paclitaxel	TEOS	CTAB	n.d.	232.4-243.4	9.6	The *in vitro* anti-tumor studies on MCF-7 cells demonstrated that paclitaxel loaded MSNs produced higher cytotoxicity than free drug.	L. Jia et al., (2012)
Phyto-Chemicals	TEOS	CTAB	-	220	11-14	Confocal microscopy demonstrated nanoparticles of <500 nm were able to accumulate within cells with FITC-loaded MSNs showing membrane localised and cytoplasmic accumulation following a 2 h incubation.	(Lungare, Hallam, & Badhan, 2016)
Quercetin	TEOS, 3-aminopropyl triethoxysilane	CTAB	Aminopropyl	250	3.2-9.5	The grafting of aminopropyl groups over surface of MSNs resulted in increase in quercetin penetration into the skin as suggested by the *ex vivo* porcine skin experiments.	Sapino et al., (2015)
Resveratrol	TEOS	CTAB	-	150-300	23	The therapeutic efficacy of resveratrol was increased by 13 times in CHO cells.	Tsai et al., (2011)
Salidroside	TEOS	CTAB	Poly(acrylic acid)	442.7	2.1	Poly(acrylic acid) layer over the surface of MSNs regulated in higher uptake and release of salidroside.	Peng et al., (2013)
siRNA	TEOS	CTAB	Polyethylene imine	120	-	Mice treated with cisplatin plus gene loaded MSNs exhibited lower tumor burden than mice treated with cisplatin alone.	Roberts et al., (2017)
Telmisartan	TEOS	Hexadecyltrimethyl ammonium bromide	Amino propyl	20-90	50.7-60.3	The release rate of drug from the functionalized MSNs was effectively controlled due to the presence of an ionic interaction between the carboxyl groups of drug and the amine groups on the surface of MSNs.	Y. Zhang et al., (2010)
Ursolic Acid	3-[2-(2-aminoethylamino) ethylamino] propyltri-methoxysilane	Hexadecyltri-methylammonium bromid	-	102-219	22	*In vitro* cytotoxicity testing demonstrated that developed MSNs exhibited higher proliferation inhibition, cell cycle arrest at the G2/M phase and significantly caused the early and late apoptosis in HepG2 cells, which would be contributed to high loading capacity, high cellular uptake and sustained release of ursolic acid.	T. Li et al., (2017)
Vitamin B_{12}	TEOS, octadecyltri-methoxysilane	n.d.	-	25	1	Developed nanocomposite of mesoporous-silica-coated NaYF4:Yb/Er composite nanoparticles incorporated with photosensitizer (Vitamin B_{12}) exhibited a better performance for the photodynamic therapy of cancer cells under NIR-irradiation.	F. Xu et al., (2016)

n.d.: not defined
FITC: fluorescein isothiocyanate

Table 2b. Various bioactives investigated on mesoporous silica nanoparticles for drug delivery applications: Dual drug delivery

Therapeutic Agents	Silicon Source	Surfactant	Functional Group	Particle Size (nm)	Drug Loading (% w)	Research Highlights	Refs.
Dual-Drug Delivery							
Campothecin, Fluoresceine (Photosensitizer Agent)	TEOS, aminopropyltri-ethoxysilane	CTAB	Galactose	n.d.	n.d.	MSN combining drug delivery and photodynamic therapy showed a dramatic enhancement of cancer cell death compared to separate treatments tested on three cancer cell lines (HCT-116, MDA-MB-231, Capan-1).	Gary-Bobo et al., (2012a)
Campothecin, Porphyrin (Photosensitizer Agent)	TEOS	CTAB	α-d-mannose	n.d.	n.d.	Treatment studies on retinoblastoma cell lines (RB Y-79) demonstrated the active endocytosis of the MSNs through carbohydrate receptors with strong cell death after only a short irradiation at a low fluence.	Gary-Bobo et al., (2012b)
Chlorin e6 (Photodynamic Therapy) Gold Nano Rods (Photothermal Therapy)	TEOS	CTAB	Gold nano rods	193.5	n.d.	Synergistic anti-tumor effects were observed both *in vitro* and *in vivo* due to photothermal and photodynamic therapy provided by gold nano rods and chlorine e6, respectively.	Q. Sun et al., (2017)
Copper Ions, Silver Nanoparticles and Curcumin	[3-(2-Amino-ethylamino) propyl] trimethoxysilane, TEOS	CTAB	-	200	Copper: 2.78 Silver: 0.09 Curcumin: 12	Multifunctional nanohybrid showed excellent photodynamic inactivation against E. coli due to the synergistic antibacterial effects of silver, copper ions and curcumin compared to sole curcumin.	Kuthati et al., (2017)
Doxorubicin Hydrochloride, Indocyanine Green, C60 Fullerene	TEOS	Triton X-100	Hyaluronan	60	48.5	*In vitro* cytotoxicity study of the system on MDA-MB-231 triple-negative human breast cells showed synergistic cytotoxic profile on near infrared irradiation compared to free drug and MSNs encapsulating only doxorubicin only due to synergistic photothermal and photodynamic effect in conjunction with chemotherapy. Multifunctional delivery system also showed superior *in vivo* anti-tumor efficacy in orthotopic tumor model in mice.	H. Wang et al., (2016)
Doxorubicin, Tumor-Targeting Cellular Membrane-Penetrating Peptide and a Mitochondria-Targeting Therapeutic Peptide	Piperidine tetraethyl-orthosilicate	CTAB	Tumor-targeting cellular membrane-penetrating peptide and a mitochondria-targeting therapeutic peptide	120	Peptides: 8.1 Drug: 5.3	Developed system showed synergistic anti-cancer effect on Hela cells.	Cheng et al., (2016)
Doxorubicin, siRNA	TEOS	CTAB	Polyethylenimine	241-1201	-	The dual delivery of drug and siRNA in KB-V1 cells was capable of increasing the intracellular as well as intranuclear drug concentration to levels exceeding that of free doxorubicin or the drug being delivered by MSNs in the absence of siRNA co-delivery	H. Meng et al., (2010)
HydrochlorotHiazide, Amlodipine, Losartan and Simvastatin	TEOS	CTAB	-	150	Hydrochloro-thiazide: 12.5 Amlodipine: 2.5 Losartan: 25 Simvastatin: 40	Amlodipine, losartan and simvastatin were released from the polypill-MSN-41 system in a controlled way and diuretic hydrochlorothiazide was quickly released from the system.	(Doadrio, Sánchez-Montero, Doadrio, Salinas, & Vallet-Regí, 2017)
Paclitaxel, Doxorubicin	(3-Aminopropyl) triethoxysilane	CTAB	Lipid coating	202-235	Paclitaxel: 4.5 Doxorubicin: 40	Dual loaded MSNs exhibited a marked synergistic effect in inhibiting the proliferation of A549 cells. The pharmacokinetic study demonstrated that MSNs could significantly improve the relative bioavailability of both drugs.	Qiu et al., (2017)
Paclitaxel and Tetrandrine	TEOS	CTAB	-	125.4	Paclitaxel: 7.23 Tetrandrine: 1.21	Co-delivery of paclitaxel with the multidrug resistance reversal agent completely reversed the resistance of MCF-7/ADR cells to paclitaxel and the resistance reversion index was 72.3.	L. Jia et al., (2015)
Tirapazamine, Supramolecular Photosensitizers	TEOS	Cetyl-trimethyl-ammonium chloride	Hyaluronic acid	49.6	Tirapazamine: 3.9 Photosensitizer: 2.8	*In vivo* studies carried out in SCC-7 tumor-bearing mice showed preferential accumulation of developed system in tumor site and significantly inhibited the tumor progression by the collaboration of photodynamic therapy and bioreductive chemotherapy under NIR fluorescence/MRI guidance.	W. Chen et al., (2017)
Topotecan, TriphenylphoSphonium and Antibiotic Peptide (KLAKLAK)2	TEOS	CTAB	Poly(ethylene glycol)-blocked-2,3-dimethylmaleic anhydride-modified poly(L-lysine)	120	9.6	*In vitro* results demonstrated a significant enhancement of tumor cellular uptake, excellent mitochondria damage ability, and improved anti-tumor efficiency of the multifunctional enveloped MSNs.	J. Zhang et al., (2013)

n.d.: not defined

Table 2c. Various bioactives investigated on mesoporous silica nanoparticles for drug delivery applications: Targeted delivery

Drug	Silica Precursors	Surfactant	Targeting Moiety	Particle Size (nm)	Drug Loading (% in Weight)	Research Highlights	Refs.
Targeted Delivery							
Bevacizumab	TEOS, 2-cyanopropyltri-ethoxysilane	CTAB	Tumor endothelial marker 1 (TEM1)/ endosialin (Ab-/scFv)	166	n.d.	Developed MSNs increased the intracellular concentration of drug and enhanced the anti-cancer effect of active therapeutic agent in ovarian cancer cells.	Y. Zhang et al., (2015b)
Camptothecin	TEOS	CTAB	Folic acid	100 - 130	n.d.	Folate modification dramatically increased tumor-suppressing effects of drug loaded MSNs in murine models with pancreatic cancers.	(Lu, Li, Zink, & Tamanoi, 2012)
Camptothecin	TEOS	Hexadecyltri-methyl-ammonium bromide	Folic acid	120	-	Targeted MSNs depicted specific detection of folate receptors present on HeLa cells.	(Chan & Lin, 2015)
Carboplatin	TEOS	CTAB	EpCAM antibody	148.5	n.d.	Developed MSNs exhibited a superior anti-cancer effect in retinoblastoma cells (Y79).	(Qu, Meng, Yu, & Wang, 2017)
Celastrol	Tetramethoxysilane	Cetyltri-methylammonium-chloride	Glucose	250-300	2.16	Anti-apoptotic studies showed superior anti-tumor effect of drug loaded targeted MSNs on A 549 and HeLa cells.	(Niemela, Desai, Nkizinkiko, Eriksson, & Rosenholm, 2015)
Docetaxel	3-aminopropyl triethoxysilane	CTAB	Folic acid	50	18.19	Developed system showed targeted delivery of docetaxel in breast cancer cells expressing folate receptor.	Khosravian et al., (2016)
Doxorubicin	TEOS	Cetyltri-methylammonium-chloride	Folic acid, N-acetyl glucosamine	60	28.9-58.51	Cytotoxicity results showed that drug loaded N-acetyl glucosaminegrafted MSNs exerted significant higher cytotoxicity effect on both the cell lines (MCF-7 and MDA-MB-231) than folate tareted MSNs.	(Kumar, Tambe, Paknikar, & Gajbhiye, 2017)
Doxorubicin	TEOS	Cetyltri-methylammonium-chloride	CD44 monoclonal antibody	60	8.9	CD44-engineered MSNs provided active target, which promoted more cellular uptake and retention of doxorubicin in the resistant cells compared to unengineered counterpart.	Y. Wang et al., (2015b)
Doxorubicin	TEOS	Hexadecyl trimethyl -ammonium chloride	EpCAM aptamer	181	20.7	Results demonstrated that EpCAM conjugation increased binding of MSNs to EpCAM receptor overexpressing SW620 colon cancer cells but not EpCAM-negative Ramos cells, resulting in enhanced cellular uptake and increased cytotoxicity of the drug in SW620 cells when compared to non-modified nanoparticles.	X. Xie et al., (2016)
Doxorubicin	TEOS	CTAB	Folic acid	203.3	4.3	Targeted MSNs were efficiently trapped by folate-receptor-rich HeLa cancer cells through receptor mediated endocytosis, while folate-receptor-poor human embryonic kidney 293 normal cells showed much lower endocytosis towards nanoparticles under the same conditions.	Q. Zhang et al., (2012)
Doxorubicin	TEOS	Cetyltri-methyl-ammonium-chloride	Hyaluronic acid	40	14.1	Developed MSNs exhibited higher cellular uptake efficacy via CD44-mediated endocytosis by HeLa cells (CD44 over-expressed cells) than by LO2 cells (CD44 deficient cells).	J. Zhang et al., (2016)
5-fluorouracil	TEOS	Triton X-100	Epidermal growth factor	120	19.45	The high specificity and excellent targeting performance of epidermal growth factor grafted MSNs was observed on SW480 cells.	She et al., (2015)
Gemcetabine	TEOS	CTAB	Urokinase plasminogen activator	115	n.d.	*In vivo*, targeted MSNs demonstrated orthotopic pancreatic tumor specific accumulation compared to liver or kidney as identified using multispectral optoacoustic tomography (p b 0.05) and confirmed by *ex vivo* analysis.	Gurka et al., (2016)

n.d.: not defined

Figure 7. Overview of the versatility of drug delivery applications of MSNs

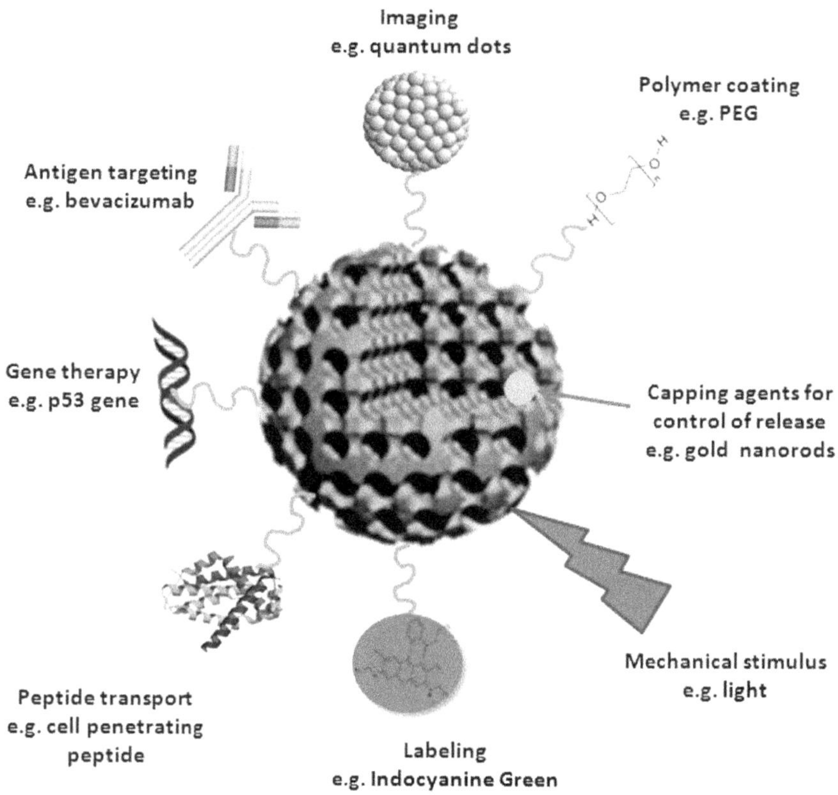

Carboxylic acid modification provided high dispersity to MSNs along with pH-sensitive release of loaded cargo. *In vivo* studies carried out in hepatocellular carcinoma bearing mice showed superior inhibition of the tumor growth compared to free DOX. The side effects of free drug on liver and heart cells were also surmounted after encapsulation within MSNs as suggested by histological examination of both organs post treatment (Xie, Xu, Shen, Shen, Ge, & Xie, 2014). In addition, Li et al. developed MSNs coupled with aerosol technology for treatment of respiratory diseases *via* inhalation route. Polyethyleneimine-PEG coated MSNs reached bronchial tree and gas exchange regions of respiratory tract suggested by necropsies of mice done at 1st and 7th day of post inhalation (Xu, Lü, Gao,Wang, Bai, Gao, & Liu, 2015).

Furthermore, controlled drug delivery of various categories of drugs has been accomplished till date by decorating the pore as well as MSNs surface with different functional groups and has provided several exciting results *via* precise control over the release kinetics of the therapeutics packed within these nanomaterials. Such as, PAA was grafted on MSNs employing acid cleavable linker for intracellular controlled DOX release and tumor therapy *in vivo* (Figure 8) (Chen, He, Wang, He, Yang, Qiu, & Chen, 2014). Bollu et al. (2016) formulated different silica based MSU-2 and MCM-41 mesoporous materials for delivery of curcumin. Results of release kinetic studies revealed slow and sustained release of curcumin from these materials at physiological conditions (pH 7.4). Formulations also showed inhibition of different cancer cells proliferation (CHO cell lines). The formation of intracellular reactive oxygen species and down regulation of anti-apoptotic proteins (EGFR and BCL-2) leading to the induction of an apoptotic pathway have been found to be the underlying mechanisms behind the anti-cancer proper-

Figure 8. Schematic illustration of an acid cleavable linker involved mesoporous silica–polymer hybrid nano-container for anti-cancer drug controlled release: synthesis of the particle, loading of the cargo, capping of the pore, and the delivery of anti-cancer drug to the tumor. Reproduced with permission from ref. (Chen, He, Wang, He, Yang, Qiu, & Chen, 2014). Copyright © 2014, Royal Society of Chemistry.

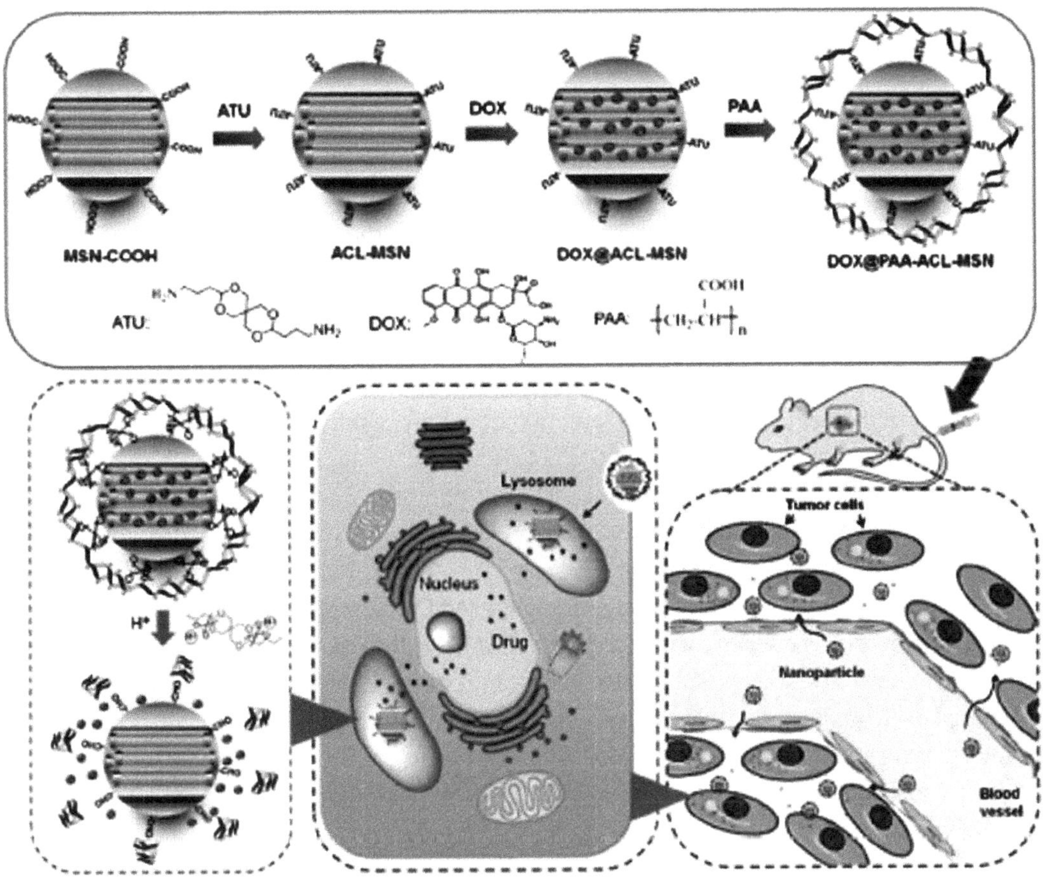

ties of developed formulations (Bollu, Barui, Mondal, Prashar, Fajardo, Briones, Rodriguez-Dieguez, Patra, & Gomez-Ruiz, 2016).

Multidrug resistance (MDR) has been one of the biggest hurdles to the success of cancer chemotherapy and MSNs have been exploited extensively in overcoming MDR. For instance, polymer-lipid (Pluronic P123 grafted 1,2-dioleoyl-sn-glycero-3-phosphoethanolamine) coated MSNs showed high intracellular uptake of irinotecan to drug resistant MCF-7/BCRP cancer cells owing to pH-responsive release facilitated by coated membrane. Also, surface coated dual polymer-lipid inhibited breast cancer resistance protein mediated drug efflux in tested cancer cells (Zhang, Luo, Liu, Ding, Li, & Cai, 2014).

Dual-Drug Delivery

Dual-drug delivery platforms have been proposed owing to their several benefits over single drug loaded systems i.e. they provide synergistic therapeutic action, combat MDR issues and helps in minimization of side effects (Boissenot, Bordat, Fattal, & Tsapis, 2016). MSNs possess capability of loading a wide variety of bioactive combinations owing to their large surface area (>1000 m^2/g), and tunable pore size and surface chemistry (Tarn, Ashley, Xue, Carnes, Zink, & Brinker, 2013). Multicomponent MSNs was fabricated for multi-drug delivery with the perspective of improvising the therapeutic efficacy by dose and toxicity reduction of each anti-cancer drug. Herein, DOX was entrapped within mesopores and cisplatin was conjugated to the mesoporous shells (Figure 9a). The developed system showed increased cytotoxicity of dual loaded MSNs compared to free individual drugs or single drug loaded MSNs at the same dose tested (Li, Wu, Pan, & Shi, 2016). In an interesting study, co-delivery of insulin and cyclic adenosine monophosphate (cAMP) encapsulated within glucose-responsive MSNs was investigated (Figure 9b). Delivery of insulin alone within this system suffered from typical decrease in levels of insulin release on repeated glucose treatment. This problem was overcome with the co-delivery of cAMP which could facilitate the secretion of insulin from pancreatic β cells during the shortage of insulin (Zhao, Trewyn, Slowing, & Lin, 2009).

MSNs co-loaded with camptothecin and a photosensitizer (fluoresceine) showed superior cytotoxic effects on colorectal tumor cells compared to single therapy owing to synergistic effect (Zhao, Huang, Shi, Tang, Li, & Chen, 2014). Wang et al. (2015) also reported enhanced cell death of SK-BR-3 cells due to collegial effect of the heat generated on irradiation of semi-graphitized carbon and chemotherapeutic effect of DOX, with a combination index of 0.253 (Wang, Liu, Wang, Shi, Zhou, Wang, Wu, Zeng, Li, Sun, Wang, Zhang, Teng, & Lu, 2015). In a recent study, photosensitizing agent (chlorine e6) and photo thermal agents (gold nanorods) co-loaded within rod shaped MSNs demonstrated superior anti-tumor effect in breast tumor bearing mice (Sun, You, Pang, Tan, Wang, Liu, Guo, Tan, & Li, 2017). Double delivery of combretastatin A4, an anti-angiogenic agent and DOX in MSNs for achieving improved anti-tumor efficacy at low doses of drug owing to their combined action that facilitated disruption of vascular structure has also been investigated lately (Li, Xu, Wang, Yang, Liu, Pan, & Li, 2016).

Co-delivery of therapeutics with molecules/inhibitors targeting anti-apoptotic or other mechanisms of resistance have been attempted to overcome MDR issues in cancer. For example, co-delivery MSNs based system encapsulating siRNA to silence the expression of efflux transporter and an anti-cancer drug i.e. DOX was developed. This dual drug delivery system provided superior inhibition of tumor growth compared to free DOX and MSNs loaded with single therapeutics in MCF-7/MDR xenograft murine model resolving MDR issues (Meng, Mai, Zhang, Xue, Xia, Lin, Wang, Zhao, Ji, Zink, & Nel, 2013). Also, co-delivery of tetrandrine (P-glycoprotein inhibitor) along with paclitaxel reversed the resistance of MCF-7/ADR cancer cells to paclitaxel with the resistance reversion index of 72.3 (Jia, Li, Shen, Zheng, Tian, Guo, & Chang, 2015).

Targeted Delivery

MSNs offer the possibility of construction of functional supramolecular assemblies for targeted drug delivery capable of overcoming various biological, biophysical, and biomedical barriers that the body stages against a standard intervention. MSNs are functionalized using different pathways *viz.* grafting (post-synthetic modification of the pore surface of a purely inorganic silica material), co-condensation (one-pot synthesis), imprint coating method, or production of periodic mesoporous organosilicas (PMOs) (incorporation of organic groups as bridging components directly into the pore walls) to render them targeting capability (Pandita et al., 2015). Various targeting moieties have been attempted on MSNs including ligands, peptides, antibodies etc. till date (Zhang, Liu, Nguyen, Ma, Wang, Xing, & Zhao, 2012; Niemela, Desai, Nkizinkiko, Eriksson, & Rosenholm, 2015). For instance, anti-tumor endothelial

Figure 9. Schematic illustration of the (a) synthesis and drug release behavior of Pt@PAA-MSN$_{DOX}$. Reproduced with permission from ref. (Li, Xu, Wang, Yang, Liu, Pan, & Li, 2016). Copyright © 2016, Royal Society of Chemistry. (b) glucose-responsive MSNs based delivery system for controlled release of bioactive gluconic acid-modified insulin (G-Ins) and cAMP. Reproduced with permission from ref. (Zhao, Trewyn, Slowing, & Lin, 2009). Copyright © 2009, American Chemical Society.

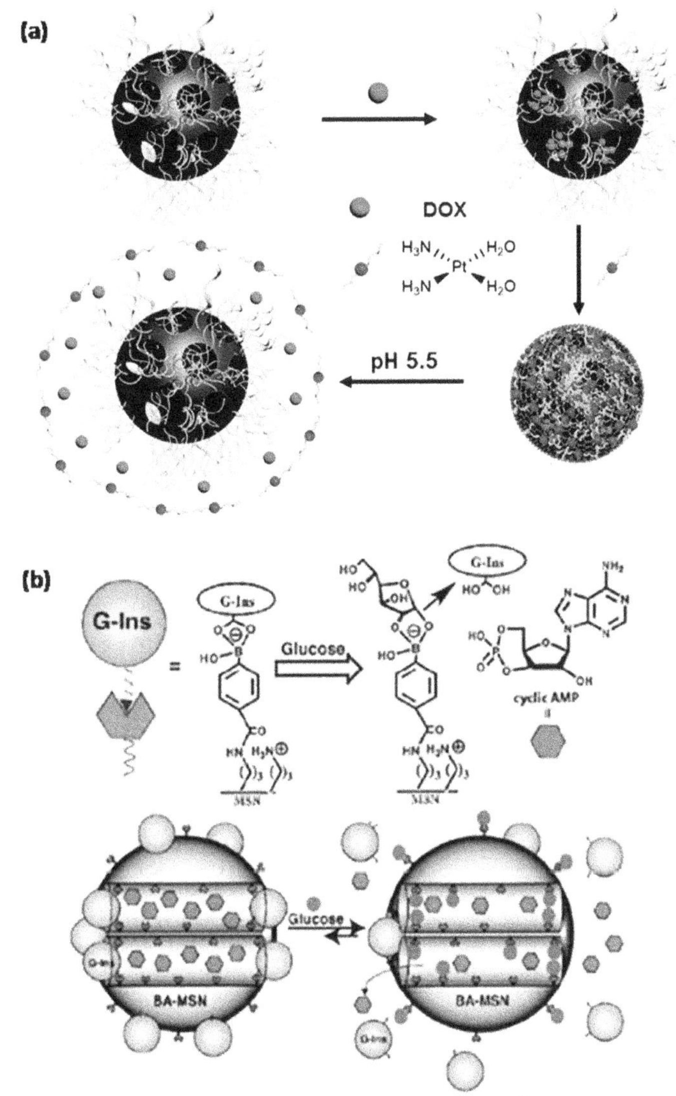

marker 1 [TEM1] antibody [Ab]/single-chain variable fragment conjugated MSNs were synthesized for achieving enhanced concentration of bevacizumab in the ovarian tumor tissues. The targeted system showed high intracellular uptake of drug in OVCAR-5 cell lines with overexpressed receptors along with pronounced anti-cancer effect (Zhang, Guo, Zhang, Li, Zhang, Gao, Liu, & Sheng, 2015c). Epidermal growth factor ligand binding to surface of hollow MSNs also rendered them high specificity to colorectal cancers due to high ligand receptor binding (She, Chen, Velleman, Li, Zhu, He, Wang, Shigdar, Duan, &

Kong, 2015). The system also allowed loading of large amount of 5-fluorouracil (194.5 mg/g) due to its large surface area. Similarly, hollow MSNs were modified with PEG and tLyp-1 peptide to achieve dual targeted drug delivery to tumor cells and tumor vessels (Li, Xue, Raabe, Aaron, Eisen, Evans, Hayes, Inaga, Tagmount, Takeuchi, Vulpe, Zink, Risbud, & Pinkerton, 2015). Wu et al. (2016) studied RGD peptide targeted arsenic trioxide loaded MSNs to treat MDA-MB-231 breast tumors. The results exhibited efficient tumor targeting thus enhanced therapeutic efficacy in a murine model of MDA-MB-231 breast tumor (Figure 10a) (Wu, Han, Schur, & Lu, 2016). Tumor bearing mice were treated every five days with MSNs, drug loaded MSNs, targeted MSNs and pure drug. Highest tumor reduction in case of mice treated with targeted MSNs was observed after 20th day. Lately, different ideas to design MSNs to explore its wide potential in drug delivery have been laid down by researchers. Likewise, transferrin decorated and stimuli-responsive MSNs were prepared through a facile approach for targeted and controlled drug delivery. Transferrin caped the mesopores, endowed MSNs' with targeting capacity, and also achieved redox-reponsive drug release while conjugated on MSNs through disulfide linkage (Chen, Luo, Qiu, Lei, Liu, Wang, & Zhang, 2017). Ligand targeted and pH-responsive MSNs have also been attempted for theranostic delivery to pancreatic tumors *in vivo* (Gurka, Pender, Chuong, Fouts, Sobelov, McNally, Mezera, Woo, & McNally, 2016).

Epithelial cell adhesion molecule (EpCAM), a transmembrane glycoprotein is reported to overexpress in many kind of carcinomas. The targeting capacity of aptamer, a kind of single-stranded DNA recognizing specific target molecule was employed and evaluated against EpCAM over expressed in colon cancer cells after its conjugation to surface of DOX loaded MSNs (Xie, Li, Zhang, Lu, Lian, Lin, Gao, & Jia, 2016). Recently, EpCAM modified MSNs were targeted to retinoblastoma cancer to increase the therapeutic efficacy of carboplatin. The apoptosis assay of drug loaded antibody conjugated MSNs depicted around 65% of apoptosis of retinoblastoma cells with over expressed EpCAM whereas, only 15% and 40% of apoptosis of cells was observed when cells were treated with free drug and drug loaded MSNs demonstrated receptor mediated interaction as major factor in high cytotoxic behavior of targeted MSNs (Qu, Meng, Yu, & Wang, 2017). Further, a comparative study of two different targeting moieties showed higher cellular uptake of N-acetyl glucosamine conjugated MSNs compared to folic acid grafted MSNs in breast cancer cells suggesting higher potential of N-acetyl glucosamine in targeted delivery to breast tissues

(Kumar, Kulanthaivel, Mondal, Mishra, Banerjee, Bhaumik, Banerjee, & Giri, 2017). Correspondingly, a detailed study investigating the prospect of polydopamine (PDA) and peptide modified DOX loaded MSNs for bladder targeted cancer therapy has been presented (Wei, Gao, Wang, Shi, Wei, Zhou, Zhou, & Ge, 2017). Cell cytotoxicity experiments carried out on HT-1376 cells showed higher cytotoxic effect of DOX loaded targeted MSNs (MSNs@PDA-PEP) compared to polydopamine modified MSNs (MSNs@PDA), drug loaded MSNs and free drug owing to the high ligand–receptor recognition facilitated by grafted peptide (Figure 10b).

Stimuli-Responsive Drug Delivery

The design and production of smart nanoplatform with a capacity to perform in response to a specific stimulus also needs to be accounted. Stimulus responsive behaviour can be imprinted on MSNs through surface modification such that the burst or premature release of the encapsulated therapeutic agents, which significantly limits its efficacy, may be surmounted before reaching the site of action. MSNs are developed with the on/off strategies of releasing the drug molecules by attaching capping agent. The

*Figure 10. (a) (A) RGD peptide targeted MSNs-based drug delivery system of arsenic trioxide (ATO) (ATO-MSNs-RGD) for treating MDA-MB-231 breast cancer model. In vivo treatment of MDA-MB-231 breast tumors with MSNs, ATO-MSNs, ATO-MSNs-RGD, and ATO every five days: (B) Tumor volume change with treatment days at the ATO dosage of 0.75 mg/kg. Error bars indicate SD of the means (n = 5). (C) Tumor weights treated with different drugs at day 20. Error bars indicate SD of the means (n = 5). (D) Digital camera images of tumors treated with different drugs at day 20. Reproduced with permission from ref. (Wu, Han, Schur, & Lu, 2016). Copyright © 2016, American Chemical Society. (b) (A) Schematic representation of the preparation techniques of DOX-loaded MSNs@PDA-PEP. Viability of HT-1376 cells incubated with free DOX, DOX-loaded MSNs, DOX-loaded MSNs@PDA and DOX-loaded MSNs@PDA-PEP at the same drug concentrations: (B) 24 h; (C) 48 h (n =3). *p<0.05; **p<0.01; ***p<0.001. Reproduced with permission from ref. (Wei, Gao, Wang, Shi, Wei, Zhou, Zhou, & Ge, 2017). Copyright © 2017, The Author(s). Published by Informa UK Limited, trading as Taylor & Francis Group.*

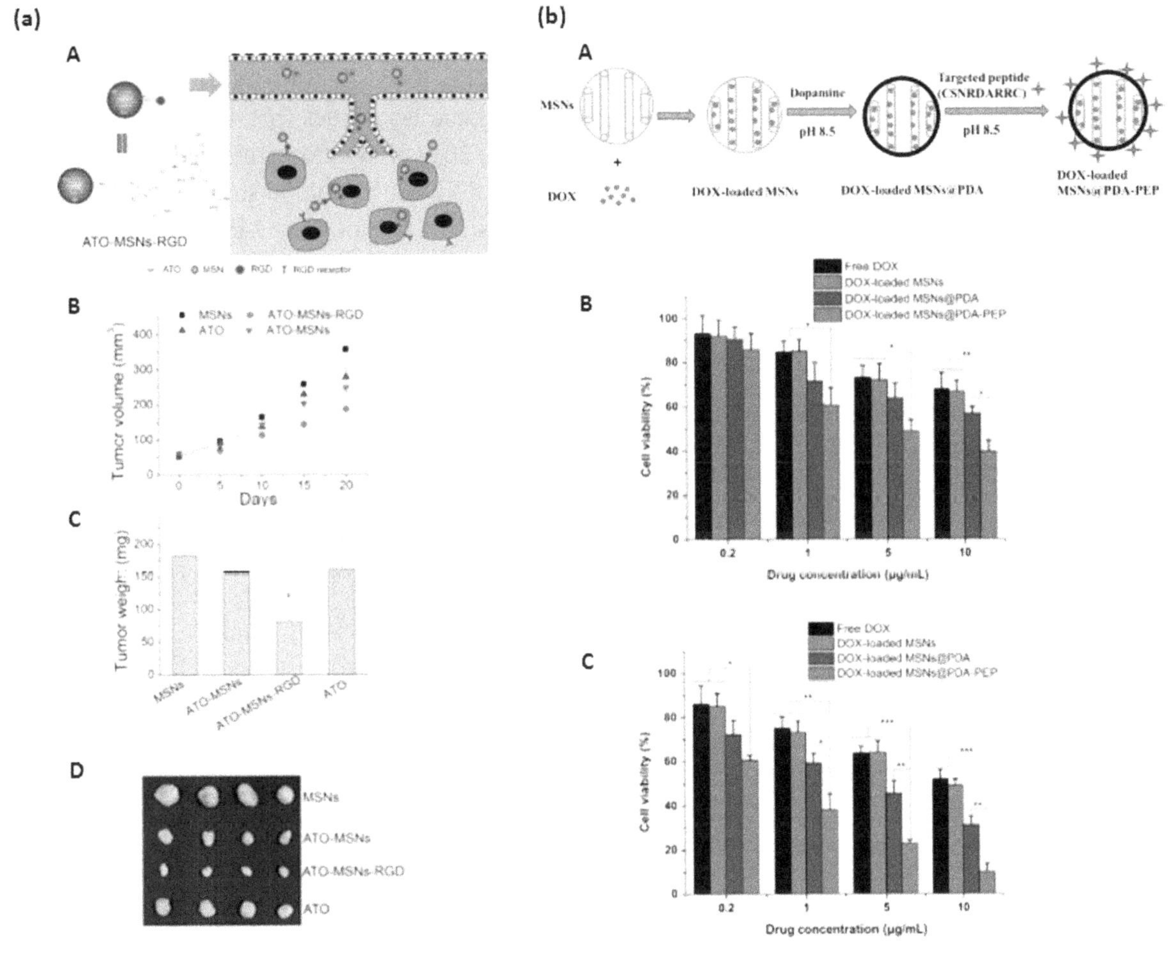

general strategy to cap the pores can be classified into three different types of gatekeepers i.e. molecules/particle pore gating, coating of the external particle surface and internal pore binding. Due to the blockage of mesopores, drug molecules are unable to leach out and premature release is prevented. Up to now, different types of gatekeepers *viz.* organic and inorganic nanoparticles, polymers, linear and macrocyclic molecules, cyclodextrin-based supramolecular systems, other supramolecular systems, peptide, biomacromolecules etc. have been investigated (Zhang, Ang, Li, Tan, Qu, Luo, & Zhao, 2015; Croissant, Chaix, Mongin, Wang, Clément, Raehm… & Zink, 2014, Ma, Wang, Chen, Wang, Wang, Wang, Zhu, Cheng, & Zhang, 2015; Li, Liu, Wang, Liu, Hu, Luo, Chen, Rong, & Zhang, 2013; Li, Liu, Hu, Xu, Liu, Jia, Chen, Lei, Rong, & Zhang, 2014; Huang, Bao, Lin, Chen, Liu, & Zhu, 2013; Zhang, Balogh, Wang, Sung, Nechushtai, & Willner, 2013). The gatekeepers are removed under exposure to the respective stimuli, triggering the release of loaded therapeutic molecules. Several stimuli-responsive based MSNs have been developed *viz.* pH, redox potential, temperature, magnetic field responsive (Figure 11). Table 3 enlists different types of stimuli-responsive MSNs investigated for drug delivery.

pH-Responsive MSNs

Biological pH-sensitive activation of MSNs is of special interest since delivery can be autonomously activated *in vitro* and *in vivo*. Human body exhibits different pH along the gastrointestinal tract, i.e., pH= 1.0-3.0 in stomach, to pH= 6.5-7.0 in the small intestine and then to pH= 7.0-8.0 in colon. In addition, the pH value of tumor microenvironment (pH 6.5-7.2) is lower than the normal tissues (pH ~ 7.4). Intracellular organelles such as endosomes (pH 5.5-6.0) and lysosomes (pH 4.5-5.0) have mildly acidic pH than normal tissues (Zhu, Wang, Lin, Xie, & Wang, 2014). Therefore, this pH gradient offers an effective way to control the specific drug profiles from MSNs into the blood stream or the targeted tumor tissues. Many methods have been developed to synthesize pH-responsive MSNs based systems.

Chang and co-workers developed pH-responsive MSNs, poly(4-vinylphenybronic acid-co-2(dimethylamino)ethyl [P(VPBA-DMAEA)] acted as the pH-sensitive nanovalve. The drug release

Figure 11. Schematic representation of cargo loading and its stimuli-responsive release from MSNs

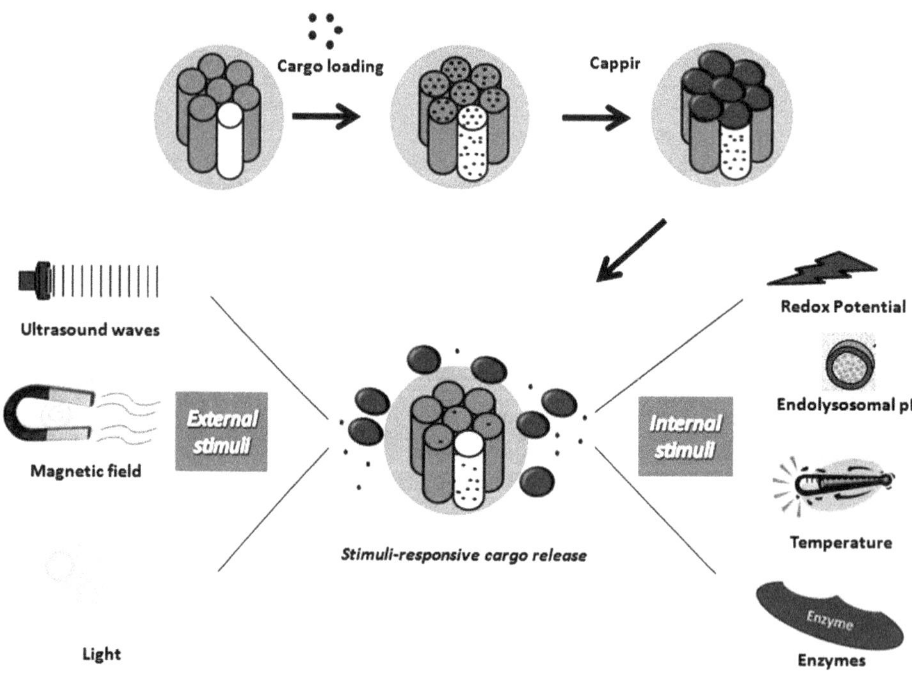

Table 3. Different types of stimuli-responsive mesoporous silica nanoparticles investigated for drug delivery

Stimulus/ Stimuli	Guest Molecule(s)	Capping Agent	Release Triggering Mechanism	Refs.
pH	Curcumin	Polyamidoamine dendrimers	Dendrimers expand in a great extent at low pH, owing to electrostatic repulsion between the primary and tertiary amine, which brings about a consequence that the dendrimer structure become very open and there is significant penetration of water molecules, leading to the channels open and the drug release.	X. Xu et al., (2015)
pH	Doxorubicin	Polydopamine	Polydopamine coating gets partially peeled off from the surface of MSNs in the acid media and releases drug.	Q. Zheng et al., (2014)
pH	Doxorubicin hydrochloride	Chitosan/poly (methacrylic acid)	Weaker electrostatic interaction between drug and polymer shell at low pH.	H. Tang et al., (2011)
pH	Doxorubicin	poly(PDM-b- poly(ethylene glycol) methyl ether methacrylate)	Under weakly acidic condition, the hydrophobic segments hydrolyzed into hydrophilic segments, resulting in the changes of hydrophobic–hydrophilic property, which is favorable for controlled drug release.	Mei et al., (2012)
pH	Doxorubicin	Dextrin dialdehyde, cross-linked by tetraethylenepentamine through a pH-sensitive Schiff's base	Schiff's base hydrolyzes in acidic pH and releases the drug.	H. Chen et al., (2016)
pH	Doxorubicin	Poly(l-glutamic acid) grafted MSNs by the surface-initiated N-carboxyanhydride polymerization	N-carboxyanhydride ring-opening polymerization of γ-benzyl-l-glutamate N-carboxyanhydride present on the surface of MSNs at acidic pH.	(Zheng, Tian, Sun, Lu, & Yang, 2013)
pH	Gemcetabine	Chitosan	Chitosan is insoluble in neutral and basic pH, but in acidic environments it is protonated to a water soluble form.	Gurka et al., (2016)
Redox	Doxorubicin	Hyaluronic acid linked to MSNs with disulphide bonds	Disulfide bonds are removed by the intracellular glutathione, which would also lead to the drug release.	J. Zhang et al., (2016)
Redox	Doxorubicin, p53 gene	Dendronized chitosan derivative attached to MSNs surface *via* disulfide bonds	Disulfide bonds are removed by the intracellular glutathione, which would also lead to the drug release.	J. Lin et al., (2017)
Temperature	Bovine hemoglobin	poly(n-isopropylacrylamide)	N-isopropylacrylamide exhibits a lower critical solution temperature at 33 °C and releases drug.	E. Yu et al., (2017)
Temperature	Cytochrome C	*In situ* co-polymerization of a vinyl group-functionalized MSNs with 1-butyl-3-vinyl imidazolium bromide and N-isopropylacrylamide monomers	Drug release when polymer expands at low temperature.	Eltohamy et al., (2016)
Temperature	Quercetin	Copolymerization of N-isopropylacrylamide and 3-(methacryloxypropyl) trimethoxysi-lane inside the mesopores	N-isopropylacrylamide exhibits a lower critical solution temperature at 33 °C and releases drug.	Ugazio et al., (2016)
Enzyme	5-flurouracil	Guar gum	Selective and irreversible degradation of guar gum 'capping' layer in presence of colonic enzymes.	B. Kumar et al., (2017)
pH and Redox	Rhodamine B	Poly(acrylic acid) grafted on the outlets of MSNs via the cleavable disulfide bonds	Poly(acrylic acid) chains possess an abundance of carboxyl groups which can effectively load and block drugs within the pore channels of MSNs by the electrostatic interactions. At acidic pH, the polymer gets protonized, which would cause the dissociation of the electrostatic interaction and the release of the drug. Also, disulfide bonds can be removed by the intracellular glutathione, which would also lead to the drug release.	Y. Wang et al., (2015a)
pH and Redox	Doxorubicin	Chitosan grafted on the surface of hollow MSNs via the cleavable disulfide bonds	Amino groups of chitosan get protonated in the acidic condition and provide pH-responsive drug release. Disulfide bond are removed in presence of glutathione and provides redox-responsive release.	Jiao et al., (2016a)

behaviour from the system could be altered by changing the molar ratio of vinylphenybronic acid and dimethylamino)ethyl, and the valve could be switched 'on' from pH 4.0 to 8.0 and 'off' vice-versa (Chang, Liu, Zhao, Yang, Wang, Wang, Lin, & Yang, 2015). In a study, intracellularly intelligent MSNs were designed based on the host–guest recognition between β-cyclodextrin and adamantine. This system exhibited faster drug release behavior compared to pH insensitive system as studied in two cancer cell lines (Chen, Zhang, Yao, Chen, & Chen, 2015).

Polymers can undergo structural changes in response to pH variations and thus facilitate controlled drug delivery. For example, poly(acrylic acid) (PAA) and poly (methacrylic acid) (PMAA) chains when grafted onto the surface of MSNs serves as pH-sensitive gatekeeper, i.e., at high pH value, the polymer chains extend whereas compact at acidic pH, thus releasing and blocking the loaded drug respectively (Hong, Li, & Pan, 2009; Gao, Xu, Wu, Sun, & Li, 2009). In an interesting study, pH-responsive property of poly(l-glutamic acid), PLGA, a synthetic polypeptide attracted Zheng and co-workers to design PLGA grafted MSNs, by the surface-initiated N-carboxyanhydride polymerization method, having superior properties and potentially more effective as anti-cancer drug delivery carrier when compared to unmodified MSNs (Zheng, Tian, Sun, Lu, & Yang, 2013). More recently, MSNs based nanocomposite was developed having a smart double-shell composed of green fluorescent marked transferrin (Tf) and diblock copolymer (mPEG45-PDPAn) layers facilitating targeting capability and pH-controlled protective cover, respectively. The copolymer layers could dissolve at acidic pH as investigated by UV spectrophotometry i.e. 100% transmittance of the copolymer solutions was observed at pH 5.0. Also, the drug release from developed MSNs was found to increase with reduction in pH (Figure 12) (Hao, Shen, Liu, Shang, Zhang, Xu, & Liu, 2017).

Polysaccharides and their derivatives *viz.* chitosan, starch, dextrin etc. are attractive gatekeepers owing to their properties like biocompatibility, biodegradability and facile surface modification. These may be grafted on the MSNs surface via layer-by-layer adsorption technique, free radical and surface-initiated polymerizations. Chitosan undergoes protonation (of amino acids) in acidic medium, as a gatekeeper and opens the gate to release the cargo. MSNs- chitosan-PMAA composite was prepared via *in situ* polymerization and the microspheres apparently showed pH-sensitive drug release and were effectively taken up by HeLa cells (Tang, Guo, Sun, Chang, Ren, & Yang, 2011). Chen et al. (2016) developed a pH-responsive MSNs-based system by using a dextrin dialdehyde (DDA)/tetraethylenepentamine (TEPA) modified coating to perform drug delivery to HeLa cancer cells. In this study, DOX was used as a model drug and modified dextrin layered were assembled *via* cross linking of DDA and TEPA on MSNs surface. The *in vitro* assays showed that an increased amount of drug was released, 28% to 94% in 24 h, when the pH was reduced from 7.4 to 6.0. Such results can be explained by the cross linking of DDA and TEPA on MSNs surface that could block the pores of MSNs and prevent premature release. Further, *in vivo* results showed that drug loaded modified MSNs have longer retention time and can passively target at tumor area rather than pure drug suspension (Chen, Zhang, Yu, Zhang, & He, 2016). More recently, the same group further observed controlled intracellular drug release, the hydrazone bond between MSNs and modified DDAs ruptured in the weakly acidic intracellular environment i.e. pH ~ 5.5 resulting in drug release. MSNs complexes were fabricated by capping on its surface three types of DDAs obtained by oxidation of dextran using varying concentration of sodium periodate which in turn accounted in controlling the drug loading capacity, entrapment efficiency and release rates (Zhang, Liu, Kuang, Li, Zheng, Song, Chen, Chen, Xu, Li, & Jiang, 2017).

Further, PDA as novel pH-sensitive gatekeeper has been proposed for MSNs owing to the oxidative self-polymerization of dopamine in neutral pH (Zheng, Li, Wu, Guo, Ye, Hao, Guo, Jiang, Fu, & Chen,

Figure 12. (a) Schematic of the intracellular drug delivery and release of the pH-sensitive MSN@Tf@Polymer. (b) DOX release from the various MSN@Tf@Polymers at pH 7.4, pH 6.5 and pH 5.0 (37°C). Drug release of (A) bare MSNs (3 mg/ml) at various pH values; (B) MSN@Tf@Polymer covered by different types of copolymers at pH 7.4; and (C), (D), (E) and (F) MSN@Tf@Polymer prepared using Tf concentrations of 0.1, 0.5, 1.0 and 2.0 mg/ml, respectively. Reproduced with permission from ref. (Hao, Shen, Liu, Shang, Zhang, Xu, & Liu, 2017). Copyright © 2017, Royal Society of Chemistry.

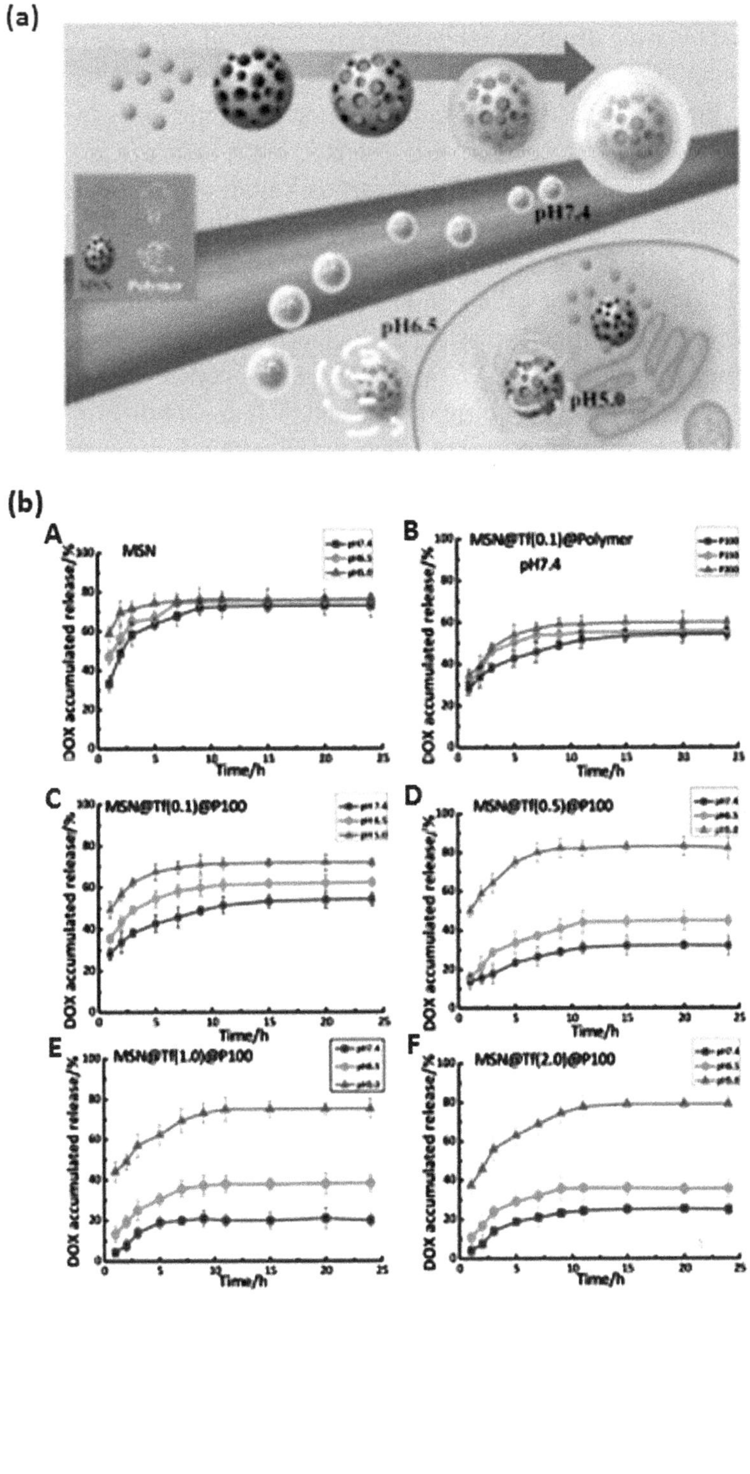

2014). MSNs with large pore size were synthesized by using 1,3,5-trimethylbenzene as pore expanding agent and further modified with PDA coating which controlled the release of DOX in acidic media whereas blocked it in neutral media.

Redox-Responsive MSNs

Redox-stimuli are an efficient strategy for attaining a controlled cargo release from MSNs. MSNs framework can be modified by using disulfide bonds. In human body, glutathione (GSH) is found in significant different concentrations, ~ 2-10 μM and ~ 2-10 mM in extracellular and intracellular environment, respectively, also, in the cancer tissues GSH concentration is several times higher than normal tissues (Saito, Swanson, & Lee, 2003). Intracellular GSH triggered redox breakage of the disulfide bonds inside cells can achieve intracellular degradation of nanoparticles along with drug release, and thus acts as a gatekeeper that works as an on-off switch in response to redox signals. Various studies have focused on the GSH mediated drug delivery for designing MSNs (Liu, Zhao, Wu, & Feng, 2008; Cui, Dong, Cai, Wang, & Li, 2012). PEG linked to the MSNs through disulfide bonds could be removed by GSH (Chen, Zheng, Wang, & Wang, 2014). Formerly researchers had focused only on designing various gatekeepers (Zhang, Li, Guo, Chen, Wang, Li, & Gan, 2014), Wang and co-workers, advance studied the influence of grafting density of gatekeepers on the drug release and biocompatibility of MSNs. The authors prepared PEG modified MSNs and documented an increase in MSNs' biocompatibility with the increase of PEG grafting density. Also, MSNs with PEG modification had the best capping efficiency (Wang, Han, Zhao, Bai, Li, Jiang, & Wang, 2015b).

Redox-responsive MSNs for dual delivery of DOX and p53 gene were recently designed. MSNs were modified using biocleavable poly(amidoamine) conjugated chitosan via a disulfide linker, which released the drug and gene under GSH conditions and depicted better inhibitory activity studied on HeLa cells (Lin, Liu, Zhu, Rong, Liang, Wang, Ma, Sun, & Wang, 2017). In addition, other redox-responsive systems have also been developed. It was reported that Mn_3O_4 nanoparticles are redox-responsive and can be reduced to Mn^{2+} (Wang, Guo, Wang, Zhao, Qi, Muhammad, Chen, Guo, Nguyen, & Zhu, 2014). The authors utilized Mn_3O_4 nanoparticles as a capping agent on the surface of MSNs (Figure 13). These Mn_3O_4 nanoparticles not only induced redox triggered drug release, but also allowed both *in vitro* and *in vivo* magnetic resonance imaging owing to their magnetic properties.

Lately, Jiao et al. (2016) developed a smart redox-responsive MSN system for controlled drug delivery and *in vivo* bioimaging by linking fluorescent carbon dots on the particle surface through disulfide bond. The carboxyl-abundant carbon dots were prepared by hydrothermal polymerization of PAA. In this study MSNs were initially incubated at pH 7.4, in the absence and presence of GSH, DOX release was found to be 15% and 35% respectively for a period of 24 h. Further increase in the drug release rate was observed at pH 5.0 in the presence of GSH. Moreover, cellular studies and imaging results showed that modified MSNs had excellent therapeutic effect towards A549 cancer cells. Such results suggest that polymer coated redox-responsive MSNs had great potential in real-time imaging to track the behaviour of nanoparticles during tumor therapy (Jiao, Liu, Li, Liu, Di, Zhang, Zhao, & Wang, 2016b).

Thermo-Responsive MSNs

Temperature stimuli have emerged as an appealing trigger used for controlled drug delivery systems. Thermo-responsive polymers used as gatekeepers remain in solid state at normal body temperature

Figure 13. (a) Schematic illustration of the synthesis of Mn_3O_4 paramagnetic nanocrystals capped MSNs and intracellular redox trigger release of camptothecin from MSNs. (b) (A) SEM and (B) TEM micrographs of Mn_3O_4 capped MSNs. (C) and (D) TEM micrographs of the sample obtained after incubation in 0.5 mM and 1.0 mM GSH solutions, showing the dissolution of the Mn_3O_4 nanolid. Reproduced with permission from ref. (Wang, Guo, Wang, Zhao, Qi, Muhammad, Chen, Guo, Nguyen, & Zhu, 2014). Copyright © 2014, Royal Society of Chemistry.

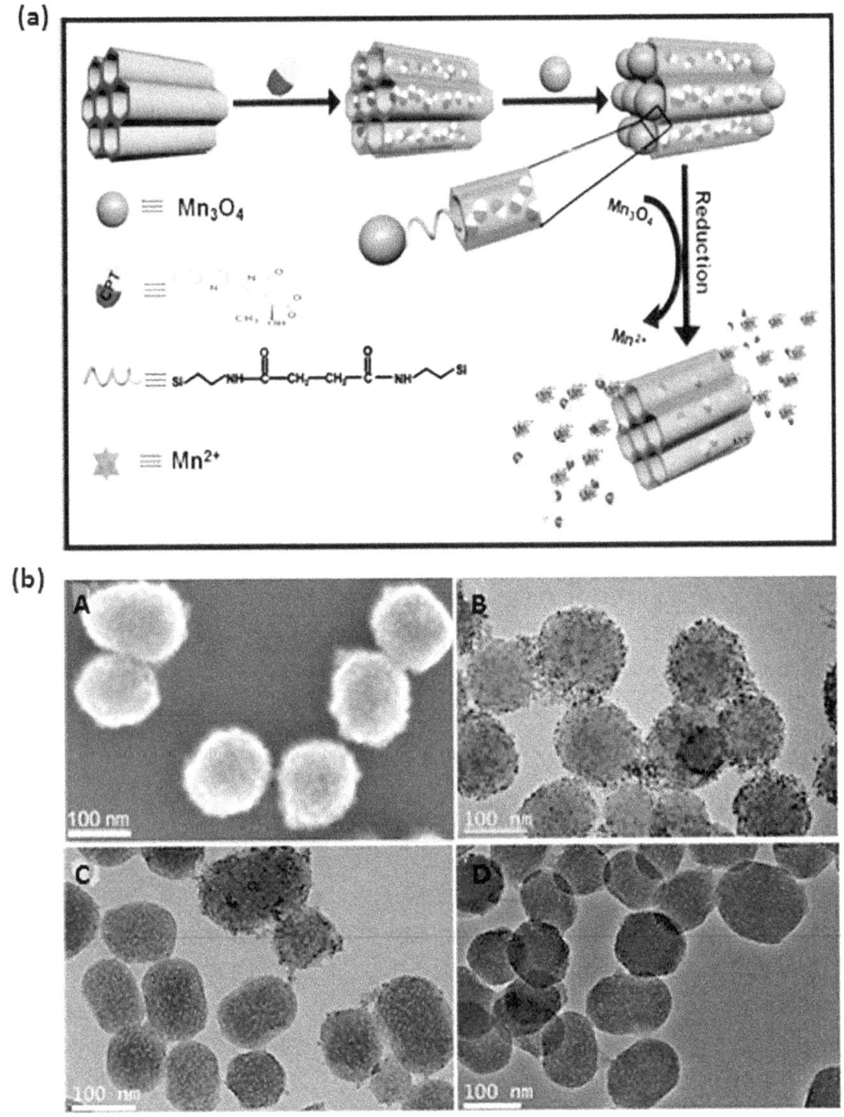

(37°C) but convert to liquid phase when temperature is raised above 37°C. Poly(Nisopropylacrylamide) (PNIPAM) polymer is widely used in thermo-responsive systems as it undergoes phase transition from a hydrophilic water-swollen state to a hydrophobic globular state when heated above its lower critical solution temperature (LCST) i.e. 30-35°C in aqueous solution (Ward & Georgiou, 2011). Recently, various approaches have been proposed to synthesize thermo-responsive MSNs. For example, a simple, efficient and convenient strategy has been proposed to fabricate hybrid MSNs with thermo-responsive on-off drug release (Brunella, Jadhav, Miletto, Berlier, Ugazio, Sapino, & Scalarone, 2016). The nanoparticles were prepared through single-step polymer grafting strategy by simultaneous polymerization and grafting of NIPAM and 3- methacryloxypropyltrimethoxysilane. The process was reproducible and further demonstrated stability and thermo-responsive property when tested at temperatures below and above the LCST of the copolymer. A proof-of-concept study of thermo-responsive MSNs for advanced dermal delivery was documented recently (Ugazio, Gastaldi, Brunella, Scalarone, Jadhav, Oliaro-Bosso, Zonari, Berlier, Miletto, & Sapino, 2016). MSNs of two different pore sizes i.e. 3.5 and 5.0 nm were prepared and evaluated to verify their capability of triggering the flavonoid release upon skin contact. The permeation and accumulation of antioxidant (quercetin) through the skin from the formulation were studied *ex vivo*. The effect of pore size in the design of thermo-responsive hybrid multimodal porous silica nanoparticles was studied. The authors reported that the selection of MSNs and pore diameter were important parameters to be considered in synthesizing thermo-responsive systems (Jadhav, Brunella, Ugazio E., Sapino, & Berlier, 2017a). More recently, the same group further studied the thermo-responsive porous silica systems for the stimuli-responsive rutin delivery. As mentioned previously, the thermo-sensitive property of NIPAM-based polymers (due to a coil-to-globule transition of the polymer chains in aqueous solution) was utilized. The copolymer with highest molecular weight and LCST was grafted on MSNs and further assessed for temperature triggered delivery (Jadhav, Brunella, Scalarone, & Berlier, 2017b).

Furthermore, a novel magnetic MSNs designed by coating a thermo-sensitive copolymer shell able to perform remotely controlled release of small molecules and proteins in response to an alternating magnetic field has been presented. In this study, iron oxide nanocrystals were encapsulated inside MSNs while the surface was decorated with poly(ethyleneimine)-b-NIPAM. The smart nanodevice was able to release different therapeutic agents in response to external stimuli i.e. magnetic field or temperature. Figure 14 show the effect of the external stimuli on the protein and fluorescein release. The system has the potential for the development of next generation of nanotherapeutics toward efficient cancer therapy (Baeza, Guisasola, Ruiz-Hernández, & Vallet-Regí, 2012).

Others

Enzyme-responsive MSNs for targeted delivery have also been presented. In one such example Yun and co-workers designed matrix metalloproteinases (MMPs) responsive MSNs for tumor targeting (Yun, Xingwei, Jinghua, Zhong, Yan, Junjie, Liangliang, Jun, Changjun, & Kaiyong, 2015). MMPs overexpressed in liver tumor's microenvironment triggered the release of DOX from peptide functionalized MSNs. Bovine serum albumin, a macromolecular protein was used as end-cap and lactobionic acid was the targeting ligand. The similar stimuli-responsive strategy was utilized for potential application as an oral medicine carrier for treating intestinal disease. The authors used a simple and green method to fabricate β-mannanase responsive mesoporous silica with high specificity and excellent biocompatibility, coated with Konjac oligosaccharide to seal the nanopores till it reached the colon i.e. the target site. Figure 15a illustrates the preparation and controlled release of oligosaccharide decorated MSNs. The release profile could be manipulated using varying amounts of oligosaccharide and enzyme (Guo, Yang, Cui, Lin, & Qu, 2014).

In addition, glucose-responsive nanosystems have been fabricated using glucose oxidase, glucose binding proteins and phenylboronic acid as the glucose-sensing moieties (Yu, Zhang, Bomba, & Gu, 2016). Novel glucose triggered mesoporous silica particles were prepared for insulin delivery (Zhao,

Figure 14. (a) Schematic presentation of preparation of magnetic MSN-NIPAM. (b) Time dependent (A) protein and (B) fluorescein release at 20°C, 45°C, and under alternating magnetic field exposition, as determined by HPLC and fluorescence spectroscopy respectively. Reproduced with permission from ref. (Baeza, Guisasola, Ruiz-Hernández, & Vallet-Regí, 2012). Copyright © 2012, American Chemical Society.

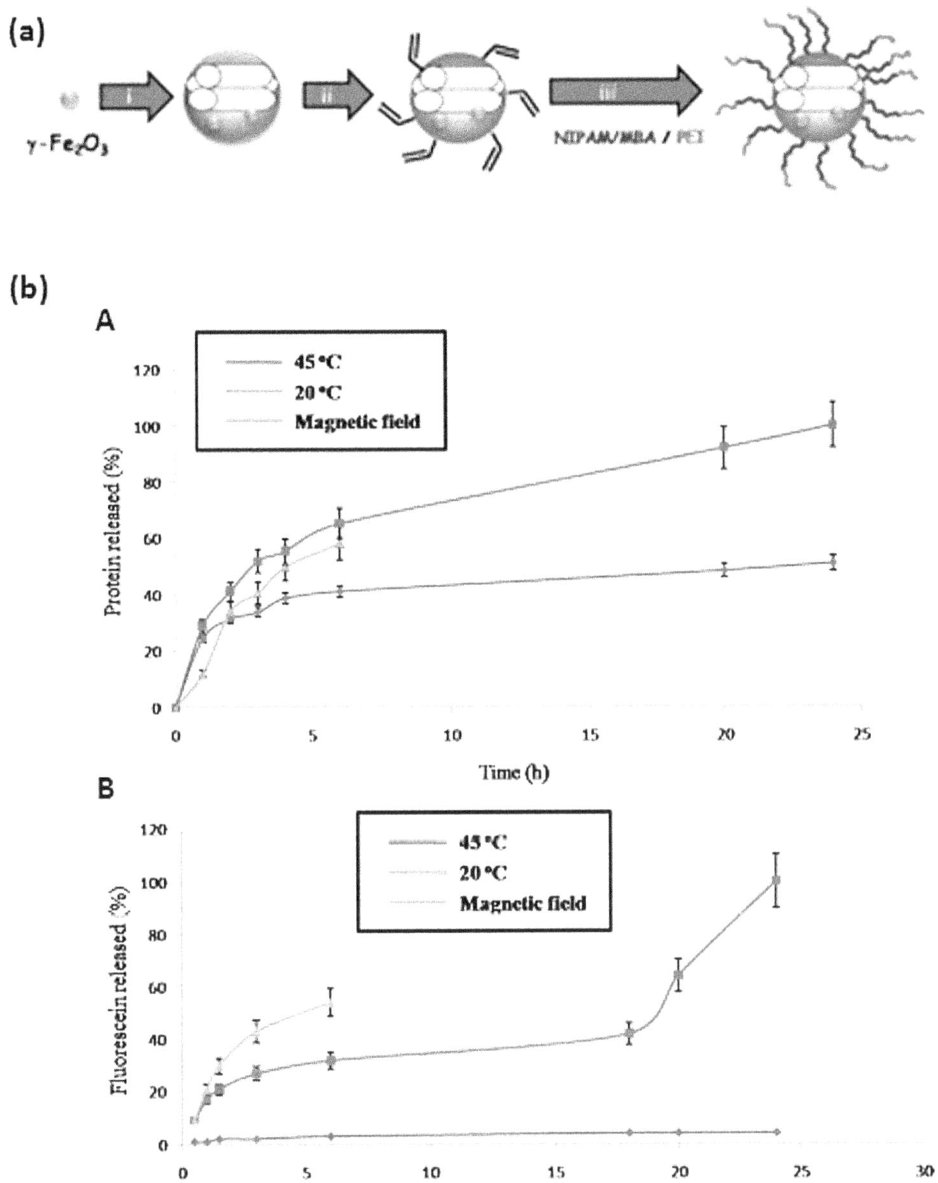

**For a more accurate representation see the electronic version.*

Zhang, He, Li, Gu, Li, Li, & Shi, 2011). Boronic acid-functionalized MSNs for glucose-responsive double delivery of insulin and cyclic adenosine monophosphate has also been attempted (Zhao, Trewyn, Slowing, & Lin, 2009).

It is highly desirable to seek smart strategies to explore MSNs' potential in drug delivery, this has paved the way for dual-responsive multifunctional hybrid MSNs. In the same line, redox and pH dual-responsive multifunctional hybrid hollow MSNs were studied for controlled drug release (Jiao, Li, Zhang, Liu, Di, Zhang, Zhao, & Wang, 2016a). Chitosan was grafted on the surface of hollow MSNs through disulfide bonds as the gatekeeper. Subsequently, PEG was grafted on the surface of chitosan in order to increase the stability of system under physiological conditions. In the release experiments, authors verified that in the presence of 10mM GSH there was an increase in DOX release. Further, the modified hollow MSNs incubated at pH 5.0 in the absence of 10mM GSH resulted in small release of DOX, while at pH 7.4 drug release was blocked. The nanocarrier's redox-responsive behaviour (in the presence of GSH) was justified by cleavage of disulfide bond formed between polymer and hollow MSNs. In an important study, redox and pH dual-responsive MSNs based co-delivery system for targeted treatment of breast cancer was synthesized (Zhou, Chen, Nie, Wang, Qin, Mo, Wang, & He, 2016). The system composed of polyethylenimine-polylysine copolymers (PEI-PLL) modification via cleavable disulfide bonds and further folate-linked PEG conjugation for targeting folate receptor that are overexpressed in breast cancer cells (Figure 15b). The cell viability and apoptosis assays presented an increased therapeutic efficacy by simultaneous delivery of DOX and Bcl-2 siRNA. The nanocarrier's redox-responsive behaviour (in the presence of GSH) was justified by cleavage of disulfide bond formed between the caps of PEI-PLL copolymer and MSNs. Also, the drug release followed pH-responsive trend, as it was significantly promoted (three times higher) at pH 5.0 compared to pH 7.4. Quite recently, pH and light dual responsive MSNs were developed depicting AND logic (Zhao, He, Li, Cheng, & Liu, 2017). The system was designed so as to control the drug release in small amounts.

Theranostics

The term theranostics implies the fusion of therapeutic and diagnostic modalities into a single smart platform, combining the therapeutic and diagnostic capabilities to enable more specific and individualized therapies for diseases like cancer. Nanotechnology has revolutionized the field of medicine in ways how the diseases are detected and treated and carries an answer to bring together the diagnosis and therapy by designing such nanosystems wherein the diagnostic modality is allowed to run throughout the disease treatment coining a new term called "Nanotheranostics". The nanotheranostics enabling the monitoring of circulation and biodistribution of drug delivery carrier will allow delivery of drug molecules to target tissues and simultaneous real-time non-invasive monitoring of biological responses to the treatment. The current imaging modalities are optical imaging, positron emission tomography (PET), single photon emission tomography (SPECT), MRI, computer tomography (CT), and ultrasound (US) imaging (Debbage & Jaschke, 2008; Janib, Moses, & MacKay, 2010). These modalities make use of contrast agents like iodine and barium in CT, gadolinium or iron oxide nanoparticles for MRI, 18F-fluorodeoxyglucose for PET, and 111In and 99mTc for SPECT (Sun, 2010). Clinically gadolinium complexes and anti-cancer drug molecules face limitations like short blood circulation time, nonspecific distribution, and lack of water solubility. Nanotheranostics have emerged as potential candidates offering functionalized surface, increased blood circulation time and encapsulation of contrast agents and drug molecules (Janib, Moses, & MacKay, 2010; Singh, Patel, Leong, & Kim, 2017).

Several types of nanoparticles like colloidal gold nanoparticles (Chen, Zhang, Yu, Zhang, & He, 2016; Kim, Chung, Lee, Kim, & Lee, 2016), semiconducting quantum dots (Kilina, Tamukong, & Kilin, 2016), superparamagnetic iron oxide nanoparticles (Kim, Chung, Lee, Kim, & Lee, 2016; Chen, Zhang, Yu, Zhang, & He, 2016; Lin, Hyeon, Lanza, Zhang, & Meade, 2009; Kwon, Singh, Perez, Abou Neel, Kim, & Chrzanowski, 2013; Singh & Kim, 2013), carbon nanotubes (Kam, Liu, & Dai, 2005), metal-organic

Figure 15. (a) Schematic presentation of preparation and controlled release process of $mSiO_2$@KOGC. Reproduced with permission from ref. (Guo, Yang, Cui, Lin, & Qu, 2014). Copyright © 2014, American Chemical Society. (b) (A) Construction of the dual-responsive DOX@MSNs-PPPFA/Bcl-2 siRNA complexes for targeted co-delivery of drug and siRNA into cancer cells, (B) In vitro release of DOX from DOX@MSNs-PPPFA with/without GSH at pH 5.0 and 7.4., and (C) pH-responsive release of DOX from DOX@MSNs-PPPFA. Reproduced with permission from ref. (Zhou, Chen, Nie, Wang, Qin, Mo, Wang, & He, 2016). Copyright © 2016, American Chemical Society.

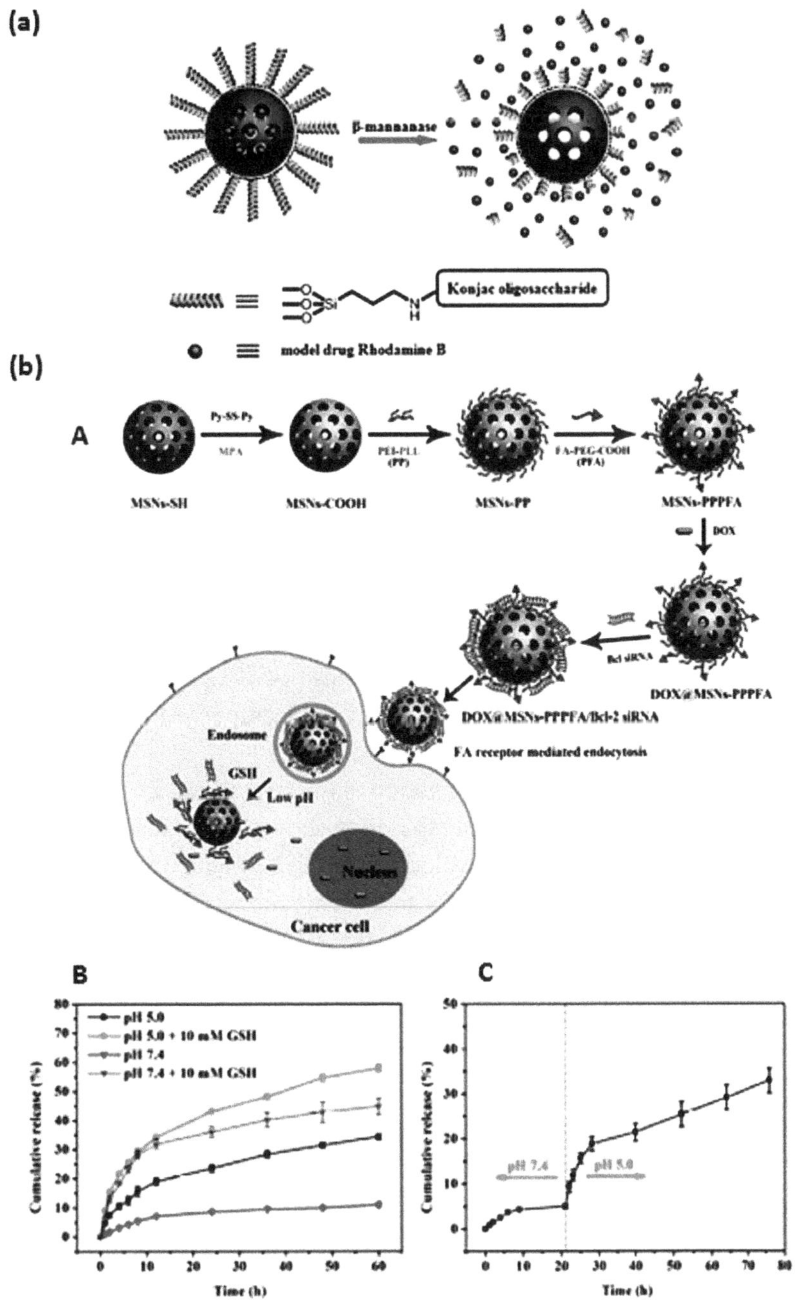

frameworks (Liu, Lu, Poon, & Lin, 2014) etc. have been explored for different theranostic applications like MRI, CT imaging and optical imaging. However, limitations such as toxicity in quantum dots and carbon nanotubes, high production cost in gold nanoparticles, etc. pose restrictions in their applications in medicine (Xie, Lee, & Chen, 2010).

The attributes of MSNs like the mesoporous structure, surface functionalization characteristics, and biocompatible nature make them a fascinating platform for theranostic applications (Pandita, & Lather, 2015). The smart incorporation of both therapeutic and diagnostic modalities into MSNs further potentiated by targeting capability offers an ideal system for medicine. The imaging modalities can be incorporated into MSNs by two approaches i.e. intrinsic and extrinsic as described in Figure 16a. The intrinsic approach involves the development of MSNs exhibiting self-activating fluorescence properties enabled by the control of intrinsic defect chemistry. For instance, MSNs with intrinsic luminescence capability were synthesized capable of carrying and monitoring accumulation and degradation profile of encapsulated. Also, MSNs showed no evidence of toxicity in mice and were cleared in short period of time via renal route (Park, Gu, Von Maltzahn, Ruoslahti, Bhatia, & Sailor, 2009). In a study, oxygen defects-induced luminescence property in MSNs was employed for tracking the cellular internalization of loaded DOX into breast cancer cells (MCF-7 and BT-474) (He, Shi, Cui, Wei, Zhang, Wu, Bu, Chen, & Wu, 2011). It has also been reported that calcination of MSNs at 400 °C can grant them luminescence property due to generation of carbon dots without influencing their drug loading capacity (Figure 16b). These label-free luminescent MSNs provided effective delivery of loaded DOX to cancerous cells in U87MG subcutaneous tumor models (Chen, Zhen, Tang, Todd, Chuang, Wang, Pan, & Xie, 2013). Recently, defect-related luminescent MSNs of 100 nm size were fabricated which exhibited bright white-blue luminescence under UV excitation. Developed MSNs acted as potential luminescent probe for monitoring release of DOX within cancer cells (Ge, Zhang, Jia, Ren, Wang, Tan, Liang, Zang, & Zhang, 2015). Lately, carbon-defect related MSNs were created for effective delivery of anti-cancer drug and optical imaging simultaneously. The treatment of cancer cells with these MSNs enabled multicolor visualization, signifying the possibility of cell tracing. Results of *in vivo* studies were also consistent with these depicting strong optical signals along with marked suppression of the tumor growth (Kang, Singh, Kim, Kim, Patel, & Kim, 2017).

The extrinsic method involves either the conjugation of imaging agents i.e. nanoparticles or chemicals onto the MSNs surface or their incorporation into the silica networks. For instance, MSNs functionalized with fluorescein isothiocyanate-conjugated β-cyclodextrin were fabricated for effectively delivering DOX into tumor site and tracking the pathway during the treatment process (Chen, Yao, Wang, Chen, & Chen, 2015). The researchers coupled ultra small lanthanide doped upconverting nanoparticles to the surface of MSNs via pH-sensitive linker for the delivery of anti-cancer agent and effective MRI. In another study, MSNs based nanocomposite was synthesized encapsulating superparamagnetic manganese ferrite nanoparticles with mesoporous silica shell. Surface of MSNs was modified with folic acid for targeting purpose and DOX was loaded within mesopores. Various mechanistic studies such as cytotoxicity assay, fluorescence microscopy, and apoptosis studies showed superior anti-cancer effects of MSNs based system. Also, this system acted as superior MRI contrast agent for facilitating simultaneous imaging (Sahoo, Devi, Dutta, Maiti, Pramanik, & Dhara, 2014). In an interesting study, MSNs based theranostic system based on MMP-2 responsive fluorescence imaging and cyclo[Arg-Gly-Asp-Phe(D)-Lys(N3)] peptide facilitated targeting capability demonstrating effective camptothecin delivery to SCC-7 cells was developed (Figure 16c). Fluorescence dye 5(6)-carboxytetramethylrhodamine hydrochloride and quencher 4,4-dimethylamino-azobenzene-4'-carboxylic acid were conjugated on the terminal of enzyme

Figure 16. Schematic illustrations of (a) Intrinsic and extrinsic approaches used to provide imaging modalities to MSNs for theranostic purposes. Reproduced with permission from ref. (Singh, Patel, Leong, & Kim, 2017). Copyright © 2017, American Chemical Society. (b) The particle formation and drug loading. After being calcinated at 400 °C, MSNs are rendered fluorescent due to the generation of carbon dots in the matrix. These fluorescent MSNs can be loaded with drug molecules (e.g. DOX) and coupled with targeting motifs (e.g. RGD peptide) for simultaneous imaging and drug delivery. Reproduced with permission from ref. (Chen, Zhen, Tang, Todd, Chuang, Wang, Pan, & Xie 2013). Copyright © 2013, Ivyspring International Publisher. (c) (A) Cell uptake via cRGD-mediated interaction; (B) MMP-2-activated fluorescence imaging with triggering the drug release; (C) drug diffusing into the nucleus and apoptosis of tumor cells. Reproduced with permission from ref. (Hu, Liu, Li, Zhuo, & Zhang, 2016). Copyright © 2016, Royal Society of Chemistry.

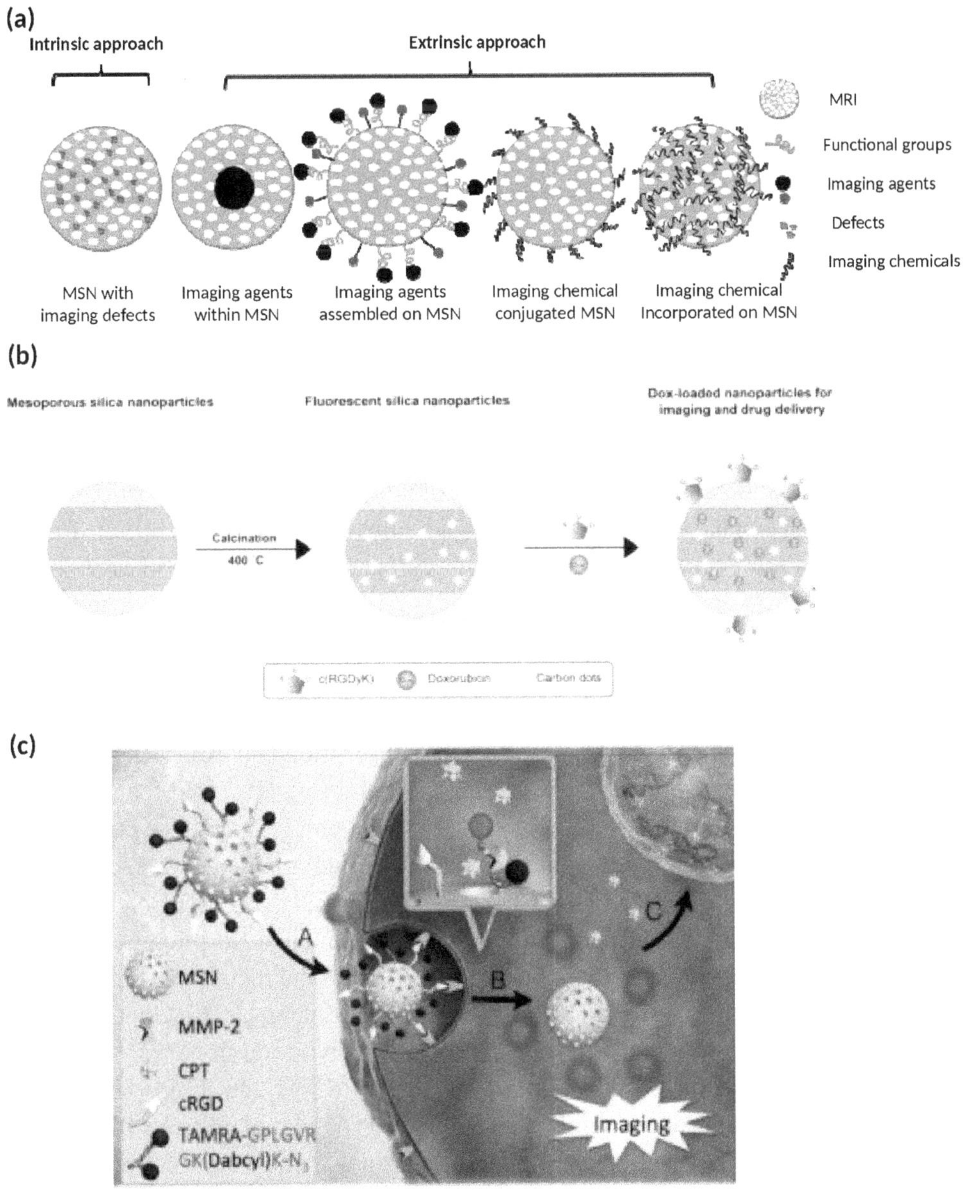

sensitive substrate peptide. No fluorescence was observed in absence of enzyme and the fluorescence of dye was recuperated efficiently when the drug loaded MSNs reached tumor site with over expressed enzyme, thus realizing the tumor imaging and triggering drug release (Hu, Liu, Li, Zhuo, & Zhang, 2016). Lately, multifunctional targeted MSNs specific for CD44 receptors were synthesized with dual treatment modalities and diagnostic properties. Herein, triapazamine was loaded within MSNs, and photosensitizer and targeting moiety were deposited by layer-by- layer assembly over the surface and thereafter, MRI contrast agent (gadolinium-III) was conjugated to the photosensitizing agent. The system showed superior accumulation in tumor site and significant suppression of tumor progression in SCC-7 tumor-bearing mice (Chen, Sun, Hu, Han, Liu, & Hu, 2017). Table 4 lists literature references on MSNs for theranostic applications. MSNs are eyeing for further improvement in bioimaging sensitivity and targeting specificity conjointly with the development in nanomaterials, drug and imaging technologies.

BIOCOMPATIBILITY, SAFETY, AND BIODEGRADABILITY

MSNs have been considered as possible protagonists in bringing revolution in field of biomedicine due to their unique properties. These have been widely explored for therapeutic applications over the last decade and shown potential benefits, but toxicity studies on these systems are limited till date. It is well known that silanol groups over MSNs can ionize and interact with phosphatidylcholine groups of RBCs leading to their hemolysis (Paula, Martinez, Araujo Júnior, Souza Filho, & Alves, 2012). Therefore, evaluation of their safety profile both *in vitro* and *in vivo* is crucially needed to bring them to clinics. Among the various ongoing studies to evaluate toxicity of MSNs, it has been reported that biocompatibility/biodegradation of MSNs is related to their physio-chemical properties such as size, morphology, porosity, surface charge and surface functionalization etc. (Asefa & Tao, 2012). For instance, the degradation rate of MSNs was found to be higher than that of nonporous silica nanoparticles because of the presence of mesopores (Yamada, Urata, Aoyama, Osada, Yamauchi, & Kuroda, 2012). The aggregation of MSNs also hampers their degradation rate and non-aggregated MSNs degrade easily because of the colloidal dispersity.

Further, it was observed that rod shaped MSNs with high aspect ratio were more cytotoxic compared to spherical shaped MSNs with lesser aspect ratio (Huang, Li, Liu, Hao, Liu, Chen, & Tang, 2011). In an acute toxicity and biodistribution study, orally administered MSNs with different aspect ratio (1, 1.75 and 5) showed different *in vivo* biodegradation, systematic absorption and excretion profile. MSNs with lowest aspect ratio have been found to be more biocompatible (Li, Liu, Fu, Tan, Meng, & Liu, 2015). Lin et al. reported negative co-relation between size of MSNs and hemolytic activity i.e. smaller sized (25 nm) MSNs caused higher hemolysis compared to MSNs of 225 nm diameter (Lin & Haynes, 2010). In contrary to this, the study on the interactions of different sized MSNs with RBC membranes suggested that MCM-41-type MSNs (~100 nm) did not cause any disruption but adsorption of large SBA-15 type MSNs (~600 nm) on their surface led to hemolysis due to strong local membrane deformation of RBCs resulting in particle internalization followed by hemolysis (Zhao, Zhang, He, Li, Gu, Li, Li, & Shi, 2011).

In addition, various comparative studies on evaluation of hemolytic activity of bare and functionalized MSNs have suggested that functionalization on the surface of MSNs with lipids, amine groups, PEG etc. reduces their hemolytic effect due to diminished interaction of silanol groups with RBCs membrane (Roggers, Joglekar, Valenstein, & Trewyn, 2014; Paula, Martinez, Araujo Júnior, Souza Filho, & Alves, 2012; Lin and Haynes, 2010). For example, only 10% haemolysis was observed when soybean lecithin,

Table 4. Literature references on mesoporous silica nanoparticles for theranostic applications

Therapeutic Agent	Type of Probe	Imaging Modalities	Research Highlights	Refs.
Camptothecin	Silica nanocrystals	Near-infrared fluorescence imaging	Developed theranostic system showed high cytotxicity on breast cancer cells and fluorescently images them simultaneously on near infrared irradiation.	(He, Ma, Wei, & Shi, 2012)
Campothecin	Europium and gadolinium ions	MRI and fluorescence imaging	Folate targeted nano-platform impeded tumor growth *in vitro* and *in vivo* and simultaneously provided photoluminescence imaging and MRI.	(Chan & Lin, 2015)
Chlorin e6 Gold Nano Rods	Chlorin e6 Gold nano rods	Photoacoustic and fluorescence imaging	Synergistic anti-tumor effects were observed both *in vitro* and *in vivo* due to photothermal and photodynamic therapy provided by gold nano rods and chlorine e6, respectively. Both agents also facilitated dual-imaging *in vivo*.	Q. Sun et al., (2017)
Curcumin	PAMAM dendrimers	Fluorescent imaging	The drug loading ratio was found to be increased due to the introduction of the PAMAM dendrimers, which possess lots of primary amine groups as further reaction site for drug molecules. PAMAM dendrimers served as pH-sensitive capping and self-fluorescent agents.	X. Xu et al., (2015)
Doxorubicin	NaYF4:Yb,Er nanoparticles	Luminescence imaging	Doxorubicin loaded folate targeted nanoparticles exhibited greater cytotoxicity to KB cells than free drug due to the specific cell uptake by KB cells *via* folate receptor-mediate endocytosis.	Liang et al., (2017)
Doxorubicin	Manganese oxide nanoparticles	MRI	The release of manganese in acidic condition from nanoparticles dispersed within mesostructure significantly enhances MRI-T_1 performance of manganese-based contrast agents. Nanocarrier also improved the intracellular uptake of drug.	Y. Chen et al., (2012)
Doxorubicin	Fluorescein isothiocyanate	Optical fluorescence imaging	MSNs were coated with fluorescein isothiocyanate modified chitosan and sodium alginate using layer-by-layer assembly technology for effective delivery of doxorubicin.	(Du, Zhao, Zeng, Guo, & Liu, 2015)
Doxorubicin	Near-infrared Fluorescent dye (Cy 5)	Fluorescent imaging	Nanocarrier was able to locate in the cytoplasm of MCF-7 cells and exhibited enhanced intracellular uptake efficacy and stronger effect on killing tumor cells.	M. Xie et al., (2013)
Doxorubicin	Polymer-coated carbonaceous nanodots	Fluorescence imaging	MSNs simultaneously delivered drug into cancer cells with pH-responsive release and facilitated efficient fluorescence imaging with high resolution.	Y. Wang et al., (2016)
Gemcetabine	Indocyanine Green	Multispectral optoacoustic tomography	Accumulation and biodistribution of tumor targeted nanoparticles was easily monitored in an orthotopic pancreatic tumor without the requirement for euthanasia and high-resolution images were obtained in real-time and to quantify nanoparticle biodistributions, *in vivo* at depths >1 cm.	Gurka et al., (2016)
Ibuprofen	Poly(p-phenylenevinylene)	Confocal fluorescent imaging	Developed system provided sustained release of drug and facilitated imaging as investigated on human cervical cancer cells.	(Qu, Feng, Tong, Liu, & Lü, 2013)
L-Cysteine	Gadolinium, Europium	MRI, fluorescence imaging	Confocal laser scanning microscopy confirmed that the targeting specificity and the cell uptake efficiency of folic acid grafted on the surface of developed MSNs lead to more nanomedicine particles in the HeLa cells than the L929 cells.	Hsiao et al., (2017)
Pro-Apoptotic Peptide i.e. KLA (HGGKLAKLAKKLAKLAK)	Gadolinium	MRI	The pro-apoptotic peptide encapsulated into the MSNs enters into the cells successfully to induce mitochondrial swelling and apoptosis.	Jin et al., (2017)
Salvianolic Acid B	Fluorescent dye rhodamine B	Optical fluorescence imaging	Enhanced cellular drug uptake, drug bioaccessability and efficacy for anti- ROS/hepatic fibrosis.	Q. He et al., (2010)
Sodium Nitroprusside	Fluorescein dye	Fluorescence imaging	MSNs loaded with drug led to a rapid relaxation of aortic vessels that was sustained over the 3 h period.	(Farooq, Tosheva, Azzawi, & Whitehead, 2016)
Tirapazamine, Supramolecular Photosensitizers	Gadolinium-III	MRI	*In vivo* studies carried out in SCC-7 tumor-bearing mice showed preferential accumulation of developed system in tumor site and significantly inhibited the tumor progression by the collaboration of photodynamic therapy and bioreductive chemotherapy under NIR fluorescence/MRI guidance.	W. Chen et al., (2017)

PAMAM: Polyamidoamine

1,2-Distearoyl-sn-glycero-3-phosphoethanolamine-N-[methoxy(PEG)-2000 was coated over the surface of MSNs whereas, it was 65.8% in case of bare MSNs suggesting suitability of surface functionalization (Han, Wang, Bai, Liu, Wang, Gao, Jiang, Kang, & Wang, 2016). Trimethyl silyl ether and triethyl silyl ether modified MSNs showed negligible toxicity to HeLa cells (Yan, Fu, Wang, & Lu, 2017). Also, methionine and amine conjugated MSNs showed no significant cytotoxicity on MCF-7 cells after 24 h of treatment suggesting their biocompatible nature (Khosravian, Shafiee Ardestani, Khoobi, Ostad, Dorkoosh, Akbari Javar, & Amanlou, 2016). Increase in density of PEG over surface of MSNs simultaneously reduced hemolytic activity and cytotoxic effect of MSNs paving pathway for development of safe MSNs.

Different routes of administration have presented different toxicity profile of MSNs i.e. MSNs were reported to be non-toxic when administered via subcutaneous route in mice whereas, the same doses of MSNs led to death of mice when administrated via intraperitoneal and intravenous route (Hudson, Padera, Langer, & Kohane, 2008).

Overall, by tuning the physico-chemical properties of MSNs a safe carrier system can be developed for drug delivery.

FUTURE OUTLOOK

The development of MSNs is increasing exponentially with various types of modifications satisfying diverse requirements of physico-chemical properties, specific therapeutic functions etc. by employing facile/innovative synthetic approaches and fine tuning the mesopore structure (pore size, shape and porosity) and chemistry of MSNs (internal and external surface). Multifunctional MSNs can efficiently provide high loading of diverse bioactives, controlled and stimuli-responsive release; and moreover can accomplish drug delivery and bioimaging simultaneously. C-dots (Cornell dots), the first dye-doped silica-based nanoparticles approved by FDA for stage I human clinical trial for targeted molecular imaging of cancer, were deemed safe for humans. Recently, it has been reported that the particles have shown intrinsic therapeutic properties, this makes an important and hopeful step towards realizing the treatment of tumors.

Advances in MSNs for therapeutics have indeed increased with an increased understanding of interaction between these nanomaterials and biological systems. Even so, more studies are needed with respect to long-term efficacy and stability, and nuclear targeted drug delivery to form optimized nanoplatforms for clinical translation in disease treatments.

REFERENCES

Abdous, B., Sajjadi, S. M., & Mamani, L. (2017). β-Cyclodextrin modified mesoporous silica nanoparticles as a nano-carrier: Response surface methodology to investigate and optimize loading and release processes for curcumin delivery. *Journal of Applied Biomedicine*, *133*, 1–9.

Asefa, T., & Tao, Z. (2012). Biocompatibility of Mesoporous Silica Nanoparticles. *Chemical Research in Toxicology*, *25*(11), 2265–2284. doi:10.1021/tx300166u PMID:22823891

Baeza, A., Guisasola, E., Ruiz-Hernández, E., & Vallet-Regí, M. (2012). Magnetically Triggered Multidrug Release by Hybrid Mesoporous Silica Nanoparticles. *Chemistry of Materials*, *24*(3), 517–524. doi:10.1021/cm203000u

Bobo, D., Robinson, K. J., Islam, J., Thurecht, K. J., & Corrie, S. R. (2016). Nanoparticle-Based Medicines: A Review of FDA-Approved Materials and Clinical Trials to Date. *Pharmaceutical Research*, *33*(10), 2373–2387. doi:10.100711095-016-1958-5 PMID:27299311

Boissenot, T., Bordat, A., Fattal, E., & Tsapis, N. (2016). Ultrasound-triggered drug delivery for cancer treatment using drug delivery systems: From theoretical considerations to practical applications. *Journal of Controlled Release*, *241*, 144–163. doi:10.1016/j.jconrel.2016.09.026 PMID:27667179

Bollu, V. S., Barui, A. K., Mondal, S. K., Prashar, S., Fajardo, M., Briones, D., ... Gomez-Ruiz, S. (2016). Curcumin-loaded silica-based mesoporous materials: Synthesis, characterization and cytotoxic properties against cancer cells. *Materials Science and Engineering C*, *63*, 393–410. doi:10.1016/j.mscc.2016.03.011 PMID:27040234

Brunella, V., Jadhav, S. A., Miletto, I., Berlier, G., Ugazio, E., Sapino, S., & Scalarone, D. (2016). Hybrid drug carriers with temperature-controlled on–off release: A simple and reliable synthesis of PNIPAM-functionalized mesoporous silica nanoparticles. *Reactive & Functional Polymers*, *98*, 31–37. doi:10.1016/j.reactfunctpolym.2015.11.006

Burleigh, M. C., Dai, S., Hagaman, E. W., Barnes, C. E., & Xue, Z. L. (2000). *Stepwise Assembly of Surface Imprint Sites on MCM-41 for Selective Metal Ion Separations. In Nuclear Site Remediation* (pp. 146–158). American Chemical Society.

Chan, M. H., & Lin, H. M. (2015). Preparation and identification of multifunctional mesoporous silica nanoparticles for in vitro and in vivo dual-mode imaging, theranostics, and targeted tracking. *Biomaterials*, *46*, 149–158. doi:10.1016/j.biomaterials.2014.12.034 PMID:25678124

Chang, Y. J., Liu, X. Z., Zhao, Q., Yang, X. H., Wang, K. M., Wang, Q., ... Yang, M. (2015). P(VPBA-DMAEA) as a pH-sensitive nanovalve for mesoporous silica nanoparticles based controlled release. *Chinese Chemical Letters*, *26*(10), 1203–1208. doi:10.1016/j.cclet.2015.08.005

Che, E., Wan, L., Zhang, Y., Zhao, Q., Han, X., Li, J., ... Wang, S. (2014). Development of phosphonate-terminated magnetic mesoporous silica nanoparticles for pH-controlled release of doxorubicin and improved tumor accumulation. *Asian Journal of Pharmaceutical Sciences*, *9*(6), 317–323. doi:10.1016/j.ajps.2014.07.003

Chen, H., Zhen, Z., Tang, W., Todd, T., Chuang, Y. J., Wang, L., ... Xie, J. (2013). Label-free luminescent mesoporous silica nanoparticles for imaging and drug delivery. *Theranostics*, *3*(9), 650–657. doi:10.7150/thno.6668 PMID:24052805

Chen, H., Zheng, D., Liu, J., Kuang, Y., Li, Q., Zhang, M., ... Jiang, B. (2016). pH-Sensitive drug delivery system based on modified dextrin coated mesoporous silica nanoparticles. *International Journal of Biological Macromolecules*, *85*, 596–603. doi:10.1016/j.ijbiomac.2016.01.038 PMID:26776872

Chen, L., Zhang, Z., Yao, X., Chen, X., & Chen, X. (2015). Intracellular pH-operated mechanized mesoporous silica nanoparticles as potential drug carries. *Microporous and Mesoporous Materials*, *201*, 169–175. doi:10.1016/j.micromeso.2014.09.023

Chen, L., Zheng, Z., Wang, J., & Wang, X. (2014). Mesoporous SBA-15 end-capped by PEG via l-cystine based linker for redox responsive controlled release. *Microporous and Mesoporous Materials, 185*, 7–15. doi:10.1016/j.micromeso.2013.10.025

Chen, M., He, X., Wang, K., He, D., Yang, S., Qiu, P., & Chen, S. (2014). A pH-responsive polymer/mesoporous silica nano-container linked through an acid cleavable linker for intracellular controlled release and tumor therapy in vivo. *Journal of Materials Chemistry. B, Materials for Biology and Medicine, 2*(4), 428–436. doi:10.1039/C3TB21268H

Chen, W., Zhang, S., Yu, Y., Zhang, H., & He, Q. (2016). Structural-Engineering Rationales of Gold Nanoparticles for Cancer Theranostics. *Advanced Materials, 28*(39), 8567–8585. doi:10.1002/adma.201602080 PMID:27461909

Chen, W. H., Luo, G. F., Qiu, W. X., Lei, Q., Liu, L. H., Wang, S. B., & Zhang, X. Z. (2017). Mesoporous silica-based versatile theranostic nanoplatform constructed by layer-by-layer assembly for excellent photodynamic/chemo therapy. *Biomaterials, 117*, 54–65. doi:10.1016/j.biomaterials.2016.11.057 PMID:27936417

Chen, X., Sun, H., Hu, J., Han, X., Liu, H., & Hu, Y. (2017). Transferrin gated mesoporous silica nanoparticles for redox-responsive and targeted drug delivery. *Colloids and Surfaces. B, Biointerfaces, 152*, 77–84. doi:10.1016/j.colsurfb.2017.01.010 PMID:28088015

Chen, X., Yao, X., Wang, C., Chen, L., & Chen, X. (2015). Mesoporous silica nanoparticles capped with fluorescence-conjugated cyclodextrin for pH-activated controlled drug delivery and imaging. *Microporous and Mesoporous Materials, 217*, 46–53. doi:10.1016/j.micromeso.2015.06.012

Chen, Y., Chen, H., Guo, L., He, Q., Chen, F., Zhou, J., ... Shi, J. (2010). Hollow/Rattle-Type Mesoporous Nanostructures by a Structural Difference-Based Selective Etching Strategy. *ACS Nano, 4*(1), 529–539. doi:10.1021/nn901398j PMID:20041633

Chen, Y., Yin, Q., Ji, X., Zhang, S., Chen, H., Zheng, Y., ... Shi, J. (2012). Manganese oxide-based multifunctionalized mesoporous silica nanoparticles for pH-responsive MRI, ultrasonography and circumvention of MDR in cancer cells. *Biomaterials, 33*(29), 7126–7137. doi:10.1016/j.biomaterials.2012.06.059 PMID:22789722

Cheng, Y. J., Zeng, X., Cheng, D. B., Xu, X. D., Zhang, X. Z., Zhuo, R. X., & He, F. (2016). Functional mesoporous silica nanoparticles (MSNs) for highly controllable drug release and synergistic therapy. *Colloids and Surfaces. B, Biointerfaces, 145*, 217–225. doi:10.1016/j.colsurfb.2016.04.051 PMID:27182657

Cho, K., Wang, X., Nie, S., Chen, Z. G., & Shin, D. M. (2008). Therapeutic nanoparticles for drug delivery in cancer. *Clinical Cancer Research, 14*(5), 1310–1316. doi:10.1158/1078-0432.CCR-07-1441 PMID:18316549

Couvreur, P. (2013). Nanoparticles in drug delivery: Past, present and future. *Advanced Drug Delivery Reviews, 65*(1), 21–23. doi:10.1016/j.addr.2012.04.010 PMID:22580334

Croissant, J., Chaix, A., Mongin, O., Wang, M., Clément, S., Raehm, L., ... Zink, J. I. (2014). Two-Photon-Triggered Drug Delivery via Fluorescent Nanovalves. *Small, 10*(9), 1752–1755. doi:10.1002mll.201400042 PMID:24678053

Cui, Y., Dong, H., Cai, X., Wang, D., & Li, Y. (2012). Mesoporous silica nanoparticles capped with disulfide-linked PEG gatekeepers for glutathione-mediated controlled release. *ACS Applied Materials & Interfaces*, *4*(6), 3177–3183. doi:10.1021/am3005225 PMID:22646097

Debbage, P., & Jaschke, W. (2008). Molecular imaging with nanoparticles: Giant roles for dwarf actors. *Histochemistry and Cell Biology*, *130*(5), 845–875. doi:10.100700418-008-0511-y PMID:18825403

Doadrio, A. L., Sánchez-Montero, J. M., Doadrio, J. C., Salinas, A. J., & Vallet-Regí, M. (2017). Mesoporous silica nanoparticles as a new carrier methodology in the controlled release of the active components in a polypill. *European Journal of Pharmaceutical Sciences*, *97*, 1–8. doi:10.1016/j.ejps.2016.11.002 PMID:27818251

Du, P., Zhao, X., Zeng, J., Guo, J., & Liu, P. (2015). Layer-by-layer engineering fluorescent polyelectrolyte coated mesoporous silica nanoparticles as pH-sensitive nanocarriers for controlled release. *Applied Surface Science*, *345*, 90–98. doi:10.1016/j.apsusc.2015.03.151

Eltohamy, M., Seo, J. W., Hwang, J. Y., Jang, W. C., Kim, H. W., & Shin, U. S. (2016). Ionic and thermo-switchable polymer-masked mesoporous silica drug-nanocarrier: High drug loading capacity at 10 degrees C and fast drug release completion at 40 degrees C. *Colloids and Surfaces. B, Biointerfaces*, *144*, 229–237. doi:10.1016/j.colsurfb.2016.04.023 PMID:27092438

Farooq, A., Tosheva, L., Azzawi, M., & Whitehead, D. (2016). Real-time observation of aortic vessel dilation through delivery of sodium nitroprusside via slow release mesoporous nanoparticles. *Journal of Colloid and Interface Science*, *478*, 127–135. doi:10.1016/j.jcis.2016.06.004 PMID:27288578

Feng, Y., Panwar, N., Tng, D. J. H., Tjin, S. C., Wang, K., & Yong, K. T. (2016). The application of mesoporous silica nanoparticle family in cancer theranostics. *Coordination Chemistry Reviews*, *319*, 86–109. doi:10.1016/j.ccr.2016.04.019

Gao, Q., Xu, Y., Wu, D., Sun, Y., & Li, X. (2009). pH-Responsive Drug Release from Polymer-Coated Mesoporous Silica Spheres. *The Journal of Physical Chemistry C*, *113*(29), 12753–12758. doi:10.1021/jp9043978

Gary-Bobo, M., Hocine, O., Brevet, D., Maynadier, M., Raehm, L., Richeter, S., ... Durand, J. O. (2012a). Cancer therapy improvement with mesoporous silica nanoparticles combining targeting, drug delivery and PDT. *International Journal of Pharmaceutics*, *423*(2), 509–515. doi:10.1016/j.ijpharm.2011.11.045 PMID:22178618

Gary-Bobo, M., Mir, Y., Rouxel, C., Brevet, D., Hocine, O., Maynadier, M., ... Durand, J. O. (2012b). Multifunctionalized mesoporous silica nanoparticles for the in vitro treatment of retinoblastoma: Drug delivery, one and two-photon photodynamic therapy. *International Journal of Pharmaceutics*, *432*(1-2), 99–104. doi:10.1016/j.ijpharm.2012.04.056 PMID:22569231

Ge, K., Zhang, C., Jia, G., Ren, H., Wang, J., Tan, A., ... Zhang, J. (2015). Defect-Related Luminescent Mesoporous Silica Nanoparticles Employed for Novel Detectable Nanocarrier. *ACS Applied Materials & Interfaces*, *7*(20), 10905–10914. doi:10.1021/acsami.5b02146 PMID:25943277

Goscianska, J., Olejnik, A., Nowak, I., Marciniak, M., & Pietrzak, R. (2015). Ordered mesoporous silica modified with lanthanum for ibuprofen loading and release behaviour. *European Journal of Pharmaceutics and Biopharmaceutics*, *94*, 550–558. doi:10.1016/j.ejpb.2015.07.003 PMID:26170160

Guo, W., Yang, C., Cui, L., Lin, H., & Qu, F. (2014). An Enzyme-Responsive Controlled Release System of Mesoporous Silica Coated with Konjac Oligosaccharide. *Langmuir*, *30*(1), 243–249. doi:10.1021/la403494q PMID:24380643

Gurka, M. K., Pender, D., Chuong, P., Fouts, B. L., Sobelov, A., McNally, M. W., ... McNally, L. R. (2016). Identification of pancreatic tumors in vivo with ligand-targeted, pH responsive mesoporous silica nanoparticles by multispectral optoacoustic tomography. *Journal of Controlled Release*, *231*, 60–67. doi:10.1016/j.jconrel.2015.12.055 PMID:26763377

Han, N., Wang, Y., Bai, J., Liu, J., Wang, Y., Gao, Y., ... Wang, S. (2016). Facile synthesis of the lipid bilayer coated mesoporous silica nanocomposites and their application in drug delivery. *Microporous and Mesoporous Materials*, *219*, 209–218. doi:10.1016/j.micromeso.2015.08.006

Hao, W., Shen, Y., Liu, D., Shang, Y., Zhang, J., Xu, S., & Liu, H. (2017). Dual-pH-sensitivity and tumour targeting core-shell particles for intracellular drug delivery. *RSC Advances*, *7*(2), 851–860. doi:10.1039/C6RA25224A

Hartono, S. B., Hadisoewignyo, L., Yang, Y., Meka, A. K., Antaresti, & Yu, C. (2016). Amine functionalized cubic mesoporous silica nanoparticles as an oral delivery system for curcumin bioavailability enhancement. *Nanotechnology*, *27*(50), 505–605. doi:10.1088/0957-4484/27/50/505605 PMID:27875331

He, Q., Ma, M., Wei, C., & Shi, J. (2012). Mesoporous carbon@silicon-silica nanotheranostics for synchronous delivery of insoluble drugs and luminescence imaging. *Biomaterials*, *33*(17), 4392–4402. doi:10.1016/j.biomaterials.2012.02.056 PMID:22425026

He, Q., Shi, J., Cui, X., Wei, C., Zhang, L., Wu, W., ... Wu, H. (2011). Synthesis of oxygen-deficient luminescent mesoporous silica nanoparticles for synchronous drug delivery and imaging. *Chemical Communications*, *47*(28), 7947–7949. doi:10.1039/c1cc11479d PMID:21499640

He, Q., Zhang, J., Chen, F., Guo, L., Zhu, Z., & Shi, J. (2010). An anti-ROS/hepatic fibrosis drug delivery system based on salvianolic acid B loaded mesoporous silica nanoparticles. *Biomaterials*, *31*(30), 7785–7796. doi:10.1016/j.biomaterials.2010.07.008 PMID:20674009

Hoffmann, F., Cornelius, M., Morell, J., & Fröba, M. (2006). Silica-Based Mesoporous Organic–Inorganic Hybrid Materials. *Angewandte Chemie International Edition*, *45*(20), 3216–3251. doi:10.1002/anie.200503075 PMID:16676373

Hong, C. Y., Li, X., & Pan, C. Y. (2009). Fabrication of smart nanocontainers with a mesoporous core and a pH-responsive shell for controlled uptake and release. *Journal of Materials Chemistry*, *19*(29), 5155–5160. doi:10.1039/b820534e

Horcajada, P., Rámila, A., Pérez-Pariente, J., & Vallet, M. (2004). Influence of pore size of MCM-41 matrices on drug delivery rate. *Microporous and Mesoporous Materials*, *68*(1-3), 105–109. doi:10.1016/j.micromeso.2003.12.012

Hsiao, S. M., Peng, B. Y., Tseng, Y. S., Liu, H. T., Chen, C. H., & Lin, H. M. (2017). Preparation and characterization of multifunctional mesoporous silica nanoparticles for dual magnetic resonance and fluorescence imaging in targeted cancer therapy. *Microporous and Mesoporous Materials*, *250*, 210–220. doi:10.1016/j.micromeso.2017.04.050

Hu, J. J., Liu, L. H., Li, Z. Y., Zhuo, R. X., & Zhang, X. Z. (2016). MMP-responsive theranostic nanoplatform based on mesoporous silica nanoparticles for tumor imaging and targeted drug delivery. *Journal of Materials Chemistry. B, Materials for Biology and Medicine*, *4*(11), 1932–1940. doi:10.1039/C5TB02490K

Huang, Q., Bao, C., Lin, Y., Chen, J., Liu, Z., & Zhu, L. (2013). Disulfide-phenylazide: A reductively cleavable photoreactive linker for facile modification of nanoparticle surfaces. *Journal of Materials Chemistry. B, Materials for Biology and Medicine*, *1*(8), 1125–1132. doi:10.1039/c2tb00420h

Huang, X., Li, L., Liu, T., Hao, N., Liu, H., Chen, D., & Tang, F. (2011). The Shape Effect of Mesoporous Silica Nanoparticles on Biodistribution, Clearance, and Biocompatibility in Vivo. *ACS Nano*, *5*(7), 5390–5399. doi:10.1021/nn200365a PMID:21634407

Hudson, S. P., Padera, R. F., Langer, R., & Kohane, D. S. (2008). The biocompatibility of mesoporous silicates. *Biomaterials*, *29*(30), 4045–4055. doi:10.1016/j.biomaterials.2008.07.007 PMID:18675454

Huh, S., Wiench, J. W., Trewyn, B. G., Song, S., Pruski, M., & Lin, V. S. Y. (2003a). Tuning of particle morphology and pore properties in mesoporous silicas with multiple organic functional groups. *Chemical Communications*, (18), 2364–2365. doi:10.1039/b306255d PMID:14518916

Huh, S., Wiench, J. W., Yoo, J. C., Pruski, M., & Lin, V. S. Y. (2003b). Organic Functionalization and Morphology Control of Mesoporous Silicas via a Co-Condensation Synthesis Method. *Chemistry of Materials*, *15*(22), 4247–4256. doi:10.1021/cm0210041

Jadhav, S. A., Brunella, D. S. V., Ugazio, E., Sapino, S., & Berlier, G. (2017a). Thermoresponsive copolymer-grafted SBA-15 porous silica particles for temperature-triggered topical delivery systems. *Express Polymer Letters*, *11*(2), 96–105. doi:10.3144/expresspolymlett.2017.11

Jadhav, S. A., Brunella, V., Scalarone, D., & Berlier, G. (2017b). Poly(NIPAM-co-MPS)-grafted multimodal porous silica nanoparticles as reverse thermoresponsive drug delivery system. *Asian Journal of Pharmaceutical Sciences*, *12*(3), 279–284. doi:10.1016/j.ajps.2017.02.002

Jambhrunkar, S., Qu, Z., Popat, A., Karmakar, S., Xu, C., & Yu, C. (2014). Modulating in vitro release and solubility of griseofulvin using functionalized mesoporous silica nanoparticles. *Journal of Colloid and Interface Science*, *434*, 218–225. doi:10.1016/j.jcis.2014.08.019 PMID:25203914

Janib, S. M., Moses, A. S., & MacKay, J. A. (2010). Imaging and drug delivery using theranostic nanoparticles. *Advanced Drug Delivery Reviews*, *62*(11), 1052–1063. doi:10.1016/j.addr.2010.08.004 PMID:20709124

Jeevanandam, J., Chan, Y. S., & Danquah, M. K. (2016). Nano-formulations of drugs: Recent developments, impact and challenges. *Biochimie*, *128-129*, 99–112. doi:10.1016/j.biochi.2016.07.008 PMID:27436182

Jia, L., Li, Z., Shen, J., Zheng, D., Tian, X., Guo, H., & Chang, P. (2015). Multifunctional mesoporous silica nanoparticles mediated co-delivery of paclitaxel and tetrandrine for overcoming multidrug resistance. *International Journal of Pharmaceutics*, *489*(1-2), 318–330. doi:10.1016/j.ijpharm.2015.05.010 PMID:25956050

Jia, L., Shen, J., Li, Z., Zhang, D., Zhang, Q., Duan, C., ... Tian, X. (2012). Successfully tailoring the pore size of mesoporous silica nanoparticles: Exploitation of delivery systems for poorly water-soluble drugs. *International Journal of Pharmaceutics*, *439*(1-2), 81–91. doi:10.1016/j.ijpharm.2012.10.011 PMID:23078857

Jia, L., Shen, J., Li, Z., Zhang, D., Zhang, Q., Liu, G., ... Tian, X. (2013). In vitro and in vivo evaluation of paclitaxel-loaded mesoporous silica nanoparticles with three pore sizes. *International Journal of Pharmaceutics*, *445*(1-2), 12–19. doi:10.1016/j.ijpharm.2013.01.058 PMID:23384728

Jiao, J., Li, X., Zhang, S., Liu, J., Di, D., Zhang, Y., ... Wang, S. (2016a). Redox and pH dual-responsive PEG and chitosan-conjugated hollow mesoporous silica for controlled drug release. *Materials Science and Engineering C*, *67*, 26–33. doi:10.1016/j.msec.2016.04.091 PMID:27287095

Jiao, J., Liu, C., Li, X., Liu, J., Di, D., Zhang, Y., ... Wang, S. (2016b). Fluorescent carbon dot modified mesoporous silica nanocarriers for redox-responsive controlled drug delivery and bioimaging. *Journal of Colloid and Interface Science*, *483*, 343–352. doi:10.1016/j.jcis.2016.08.033 PMID:27569517

Jin, Y., Zhang, N., Li, C., Pu, K., Ding, C., & Zhu, Y. (2017). Nanosystem composed with MSNs, gadolinium, liposome and cytotoxic peptides for tumor theranostics. *Colloids and Surfaces. B, Biointerfaces*, *151*, 240–248. doi:10.1016/j.colsurfb.2016.12.024 PMID:28024200

Kam, N. W. S., Liu, Z., & Dai, H. (2005). Functionalization of Carbon Nanotubes via Cleavable Disulfide Bonds for Efficient Intracellular Delivery of siRNA and Potent Gene Silencing. *Journal of the American Chemical Society*, *127*(36), 12492–12493. doi:10.1021/ja053962k PMID:16144388

Kamarudin, N. H. N., Jalil, A. A., Triwahyono, S., Salleh, N. F. M., Karim, A. H., Mukti, R. R., ... Ahmad, A. (2013). Role of 3-aminopropyltriethoxysilane in the preparation of mesoporous silica nanoparticles for ibuprofen delivery: Effect on physicochemical properties. *Microporous and Mesoporous Materials*, *180*, 235–241. doi:10.1016/j.micromeso.2013.06.041

Kang, M. S., Singh, R. K., Kim, T. H., Kim, J. H., Patel, K. D., & Kim, H. W. (2017). Optical imaging and anticancer chemotherapy through carbon dot created hollow mesoporous silica nanoparticles. *Acta Biomaterialia*, *55*, 466–480. doi:10.1016/j.actbio.2017.03.054 PMID:28373086

Karaman, D. S., Desai, D., Senthilkumar, R., Johansson, E. M., Ratts, N., Oden, M., ... Rosenholm, J. M. (2012). Shape engineering vs organic modification of inorganic nanoparticles as a tool for enhancing cellular internalization. *Nanoscale Research Letters*, *7*(1), 358. doi:10.1186/1556-276X-7-358 PMID:22747910

Khosravian, P., Shafiee Ardestani, M., Khoobi, M., Ostad, S. N., Dorkoosh, F. A., Akbari Javar, H., & Amanlou, M. (2016). Mesoporous silica nanoparticles functionalized with folic acid/methionine for active targeted delivery of docetaxel. *OncoTargets and Therapy*, *9*, 7315–7330. doi:10.2147/OTT.S113815 PMID:27980423

Kilina, S. V., Tamukong, P. K., & Kilin, D. S. (2016). Surface Chemistry of Semiconducting Quantum Dots: Theoretical Perspectives. *Accounts of Chemical Research*, *49*(10), 2127–2135. doi:10.1021/acs.accounts.6b00196 PMID:27669357

Kim, H., Chung, K., Lee, S., Kim, D. H., & Lee, H. (2016). Near-infrared light-responsive nanomaterials for cancer theranostics. *Wiley Interdisciplinary Reviews. Nanomedicine and Nanobiotechnology*, *8*(1), 23–45. doi:10.1002/wnan.1347 PMID:25903643

Kim, J., Kim, H. S., Lee, N., Kim, T., Kim, H., Yu, T., ... Hyeon, T. (2008). Multifunctional uniform nanoparticles composed of a magnetite nanocrystal core and a mesoporous silica shell for magnetic resonance and fluorescence imaging and for drug delivery. *Angewandte Chemie International Edition in English*, *47*(44), 8438–8441. doi:10.1002/anic.200802469 PMID:18726979

Kim, T., & Hyeon, T. (2014). Applications of inorganic nanoparticles as therapeutic agents. *Nanotechnology*, *25*(1), 012001. doi:10.1088/0957-4484/25/1/012001 PMID:24334327

Koneru, B., Shi, Y., Wang, Y. C., Chavala, S. H., Miller, M. L., Holbert, B., ... Di Pasqua, A. J. (2015). Tetracycline-Containing MCM-41 Mesoporous Silica Nanoparticles for the Treatment of Escherichia coli. *Molecules (Basel, Switzerland)*, *20*(11), 19690–19698. doi:10.3390/molecules201119650 PMID:26528964

Kresge, C. T., Leonowicz, M. E., Roth, W. J., Vartuli, J. C., & Beck, J. S. (1992). Ordered mesoporous molecular sieves synthesized by a liquid-crystal template mechanism. *Nature*, *359*(6397), 710–712. doi:10.1038/359710a0

Kumar, B., Kulanthaivel, S., Mondal, A., Mishra, S., Banerjee, B., Bhaumik, A., ... Giri, S. (2017). Mesoporous silica nanoparticle based enzyme responsive system for colon specific drug delivery through guar gum capping. *Colloids and Surfaces. B, Biointerfaces*, *150*, 352–361. doi:10.1016/j.colsurfb.2016.10.049 PMID:27847225

Kumar, P., Tambe, P., Paknikar, K. M., & Gajbhiye, V. (2017). Folate/N-acetyl glucosamine conjugated mesoporous silica nanoparticles for targeting breast cancer cells: A comparative study. *Colloids and Surfaces. B, Biointerfaces*, *156*, 203–212. doi:10.1016/j.colsurfb.2017.05.032 PMID:28531877

Kuthati, Y., Kankala, R. K., Busa, P., Lin, S. X., Deng, J. P., Mou, C. Y., & Lee, C. H. (2017). Phototherapeutic spectrum expansion through synergistic effect of mesoporous silica trio-nanohybrids against antibiotic-resistant gram-negative bacterium. *Journal of Photochemistry and Photobiology. B, Biology*, *169*, 124–133. doi:10.1016/j.jphotobiol.2017.03.003 PMID:28319867

Kwon, S., Singh, R. K., Perez, R. A., Abou Neel, E. A., Kim, H. W., & Chrzanowski, W. (2013). Silica-based mesoporous nanoparticles for controlled drug delivery. *Journal of Tissue Engineering*, *4*, 204–211. doi:10.1177/2041731413503357 PMID:24020012

Li, H., Yu, H., Zhu, C., Hu, J., Du, M., Zhang, F., & Yang, D. (2016). Cisplatin and doxorubicin dual-loaded mesoporous silica nanoparticles for controlled drug delivery. *RSC Advances*, *6*(96), 94160–94169. doi:10.1039/C6RA17213J

Li, J., Xu, L., Wang, H., Yang, B., Liu, H., Pan, W., & Li, S. (2016). Comparison of bare and amino modified mesoporous silica@poly(ethyleneimine)s xerogel as indomethacin carrier: Superiority of amino modification. *Materials Science and Engineering C, 59*, 710–716. doi:10.1016/j.msec.2015.10.072 PMID:26652425

Li, L., Liu, T., Fu, C., Tan, L., Meng, X., & Liu, H. (2015). Biodistribution, excretion, and toxicity of mesoporous silica nanoparticles after oral administration depend on their shape. *Nanomedicine; Nanotechnology, Biology, and Medicine, 11*(8), 1915–1924. doi:10.1016/j.nano.2015.07.004 PMID:26238077

Li, M., Xu, G., Gong, Y., Wang, W., Liu, Y., & Guo, J. (2017). Green preparation of hollow mesoporous silica nanosphere inside-loaded gold nanoparticles and the catalytic activity. *Journal of Macromolecular Science, Part A., 54*(6), 376–381. doi:10.1080/10601325.2017.1313128

Li, T., Chen, X., Liu, Y., Fan, L., Lin, L., Xu, Y., ... Shao, J. (2017). pH-Sensitive mesoporous silica nanoparticles anticancer prodrugs for sustained release of ursolic acid and the enhanced anti-cancer efficacy for hepatocellular carcinoma cancer. *European Journal of Pharmaceutical Sciences, 96*, 456–463. doi:10.1016/j.ejps.2016.10.019 PMID:27771513

Li, X., Wu, M., Pan, L., & Shi, J. (2016). Tumor vascular-targeted co-delivery of anti-angiogenesis and chemotherapeutic agents by mesoporous silica nanoparticle-based drug delivery system for synergetic therapy of tumor. *International Journal of Nanomedicine, 11*, 93–105. PMID:26766908

Li, X., Xue, M., Raabe, O. G., Aaron, H. L., Eisen, E. A., Evans, J. E., ... Pinkerton, K. E. (2015). Aerosol droplet delivery of mesoporous silica nanoparticles: A strategy for respiratory-based therapeutics. *Nanomedicine (London), 11*(6), 1377–1385. doi:10.1016/j.nano.2015.03.007 PMID:25819886

Li, Z. Y., Liu, Y., Hu, J. J., Xu, Q., Liu, L. H., Jia, H. Z., ... Zhang, X. Z. (2014). Stepwise-Acid-Active Multifunctional Mesoporous Silica Nanoparticles for Tumor-Specific Nucleus-Targeted Drug Delivery. *ACS Applied Materials & Interfaces, 6*(16), 14568–14575. doi:10.1021/am503846p PMID:25103086

Li, Z.-Y., Liu, Y., Wang, X. Q., Liu, L. H., Hu, J. J., Luo, G. F., ... Zhang, X. Z. (2013). One-Pot Construction of Functional Mesoporous Silica Nanoparticles for the Tumor-Acidity-Activated Synergistic Chemotherapy of Glioblastoma. *ACS Applied Materials & Interfaces, 5*(16), 7995–8001. doi:10.1021/am402082d PMID:23869943

Liang, X., Fan, J., Wang, Y., Zhao, Y., Jin, R., Sun, T., ... Wang, X. (2017). Synthesis of hollow and mesoporous structured NaYF4:Yb,Er upconversion luminescent nanoparticles for targeted drug delivery. *Journal of Rare Earths, 35*(5), 419–429. doi:10.1016/S1002-0721(17)60929-3

Lin, J. T., Liu, Z. K., Zhu, Q. L., Rong, X. H., Liang, C. L., Wang, J., ... Wang, G. H. (2017). Redox-responsive nanocarriers for drug and gene co-delivery based on chitosan derivatives modified mesoporous silica nanoparticles. *Colloids and Surfaces. B, Biointerfaces, 155*, 41–50. doi:10.1016/j.colsurfb.2017.04.002 PMID:28407530

Lin, W., Hyeon, T., Lanza, G. M., Zhang, M., & Meade, T. J. (2009). Magnetic Nanoparticles for Early Detection of Cancer by Magnetic Resonance Imaging. *MRS Bulletin, 34*(06), 441–448. doi:10.1557/mrs2009.120 PMID:26166945

Lin, Y. S., & Haynes, C. L. (2010). Impacts of Mesoporous Silica Nanoparticle Size, Pore Ordering, and Pore Integrity on Hemolytic Activity. *Journal of the American Chemical Society*, *132*(13), 4834–4842. doi:10.1021/ja910846q PMID:20230032

Linares, N., Silvestre-Albero, A. M., Serrano, E., Silvestre-Albero, J., & Garcia-Martinez, J. (2014). Mesoporous materials for clean energy technologies. *Chemical Society Reviews*, *43*(22), 7681–7717. doi:10.1039/C3CS60435G PMID:24699503

Liu, D., Lu, K., Poon, C., & Lin, W. (2014). Metal–Organic Frameworks as Sensory Materials and Imaging Agents. *Inorganic Chemistry*, *53*(4), 1916–1924. doi:10.1021/ic402194c PMID:24251853

Liu, R., Zhao, X., Wu, T., & Feng, P. (2008). Tunable Redox-Responsive Hybrid Nanogated Ensembles. *Journal of the American Chemical Society*, *130*(44), 14418–14419. doi:10.1021/ja8060886 PMID:18841893

Liu, Y., Chen, Q., Xu, M., Guan, G., Hu, W., Liang, Y., ... Liu, H. (2015). Single peptide ligand-functionalized uniform hollow mesoporous silica nanoparticles achieving dual-targeting drug delivery to tumor cells and angiogenic blood vessel cells. *International Journal of Nanomedicine*, *10*, 1855–1867. doi:10.2147/IJN.S75098 PMID:25834425

Lou, X. W., Archer, L. A., & Yang, Z. (2008). Hollow Micro-/Nanostructures: Synthesis and Applications. *Advanced Materials*, *20*(21), 3987–4019. doi:10.1002/adma.200800854

Lu, J., Li, Z., Zink, J. I., & Tamanoi, F. (2012). In vivo tumor suppression efficacy of mesoporous silica nanoparticles-based drug-delivery system: Enhanced efficacy by folate modification. *Nanomedicine; Nanotechnology, Biology, and Medicine*, *8*(2), 212–220. doi:10.1016/j.nano.2011.06.002 PMID:21703996

Lu, J., Liong, M., Zink, J. I., & Tamanoi, F. (2007). Mesoporous silica nanoparticles as a delivery system for hydrophobic anticancer drugs. *Small*, *3*(8), 1341–1346. doi:10.1002mll.200700005 PMID:17566138

Lungare, S., Hallam, K., & Badhan, R. K. (2016). Phytochemical loaded mesoporous silica nanoparticles for nose-to-brain olfactory drug delivery. *International Journal of Pharmaceutics*, *513*(1-2), 280–293. doi:10.1016/j.ijpharm.2016.09.042 PMID:27633279

Ma, N., Wang, W. J., Chen, S., Wang, X. S., Wang, X. Q., Wang, S. B., ... Zhang, X. Z. (2015). Cucurbit[8]uril-mediated supramolecular photoswitching for self-preservation of mesoporous silica nanoparticle delivery system. *Chemical Communications*, *51*(65), 12970–12973. doi:10.1039/C5CC04631A PMID:26176026

Ma, Z., Bai, J., Wang, Y., & Jiang, X. (2014). Impact of Shape and Pore Size of Mesoporous Silica Nanoparticles on Serum Protein Adsorption and RBCs Hemolysis. *ACS Applied Materials & Interfaces*, *6*(4), 2431–2438. doi:10.1021/am404860q PMID:24460090

Mei, X., Chen, D., Li, N., Xu, Q., Ge, J., Li, H., & Lu, J. (2012). Hollow mesoporous silica nanoparticles conjugated with pH-sensitive amphiphilic diblock polymer for controlled drug release. *Microporous and Mesoporous Materials*, *152*, 16–24. doi:10.1016/j.micromeso.2011.12.015

Mellaerts, R., Mols, R., Jammaer, J. A., Aerts, C. A., Annaert, P., Van Humbeeck, J., ... Martens, J. A. (2008). Increasing the oral bioavailability of the poorly water soluble drug itraconazole with ordered mesoporous silica. *European Journal of Pharmaceutics and Biopharmaceutics*, *69*(1), 223–230. doi:10.1016/j.ejpb.2007.11.006 PMID:18164930

Meng, H., Liong, M., Xia, T., Li, Z., Ji, Z., Zink, J. I., & Nel, A. E. (2010). Engineered Design of Mesoporous Silica Nanoparticles to Deliver Doxorubicin and P-Glycoprotein siRNA to Overcome Drug Resistance in a Cancer Cell Line. *ACS Nano*, *4*(8), 4539–4550. doi:10.1021/nn100690m PMID:20731437

Meng, H., Mai, W. X., Zhang, H., Xue, M., Xia, T., Lin, S., ... Nel, A. E. (2013). Codelivery of an optimal drug/siRNA combination using mesoporous silica nanoparticles to overcome drug resistance in breast cancer in vitro and in vivo. *ACS Nano*, *7*(2), 994–1005. doi:10.1021/nn3044066 PMID:23289892

Minati, L., Antonini, V., Dalla Serra, M., Speranza, G., Enrichi, F., & Riello, P. (2013). pH-activated doxorubicin release from polyelectrolyte complex layer coated mesoporous silica nanoparticles. *Microporous and Mesoporous Materials*, *180*, 86–91. doi:10.1016/j.micromeso.2013.06.016

Nairi, V., Medda, L., Monduzzi, M., & Salis, A. (2017). Adsorption and release of ampicillin antibiotic from ordered mesoporous silica. *Journal of Colloid and Interface Science*, *497*, 217–225. doi:10.1016/j.jcis.2017.03.021 PMID:28285049

Niemela, E., Desai, D., Nkizinkiko, Y., Eriksson, J. E., & Rosenholm, J. M. (2015). Sugar-decorated mesoporous silica nanoparticles as delivery vehicles for the poorly soluble drug celastrol enables targeted induction of apoptosis in cancer cells. *European Journal of Pharmaceutics and Biopharmaceutics*, *96*, 11–21. doi:10.1016/j.ejpb.2015.07.009 PMID:26184689

Pal, N., & Bhaumik, A. (2013). Soft templating strategies for the synthesis of mesoporous materials: Inorganic, organic-inorganic hybrid and purely organic solids. *Advances in Colloid and Interface Science*, *189-190*, 21–41. doi:10.1016/j.cis.2012.12.002 PMID:23337774

Pandita, D., & Lather, V. (2015). Silica-Based Nanoparticles for Theranostic Applications. In B. Singh, M. S. Sachdeva, & A. Liopo (Eds.), *NanoBioMedicine* (Vol. 3, pp. 383–422). Houston, TX: Studium Press, LLC.

Pandita, D., Poonia, N., & Lather, V. (2015). Mesoporous Silica Nanoparticles in Drug Delivery and Targeting. In B. Singh, J. R. Kanwar, & O. P. Katare (Eds.), *NanoBioMedicine* (Vol. 1, pp. 267–336). Houston, TX: Studium Press, LLC.

Park, J. H., Gu, L., Von Maltzahn, G., Ruoslahti, E., Bhatia, S. N., & Sailor, M. J. (2009). Biodegradable luminescent porous silicon nanoparticles for in vivo applications. *Nature Materials*, *8*(4), 331–336. doi:10.1038/nmat2398 PMID:19234444

Paula, A. J., Martinez, D. S. T., Araujo Júnior, R. T., Souza Filho, A. G., & Alves, O. L. (2012). Suppression of the hemolytic effect of mesoporous silica nanoparticles after protein corona interaction: Independence of the surface microchemical environment. *Journal of the Brazilian Chemical Society*, *23*(10), 1807–1814. doi:10.1590/S0103-50532012005000048

Peng, H., Dong, R., Wang, S., Zhang, Z., Luo, M., Bai, C., ... Xiong, H. (2013). A pH-responsive nanocarrier with mesoporous silica nanoparticles cores and poly(acrylic acid) shell-layers: Fabrication, characterization and properties for controlled release of salidroside. *International Journal of Pharmaceutics*, *446*(1-2), 153–159. doi:10.1016/j.ijpharm.2013.01.071 PMID:23395877

Petros, R. A., & DeSimone, J. M. (2010). Strategies in the design of nanoparticles for therapeutic applications. *Nature Reviews. Drug Discovery*, *9*(8), 615–627. doi:10.1038/nrd2591 PMID:20616808

Qiu, Y., Wu, C., Jiang, J., Hao, Y., Zhao, Y., Xu, J., ... Ji, P. (2017). Lipid-coated hollow mesoporous silica nanospheres for co-delivery of doxorubicin and paclitaxel: Preparation, sustained release, cellular uptake and pharmacokinetics. *Materials Science and Engineering C*, *71*, 835–843. doi:10.1016/j.msec.2016.10.081 PMID:27987779

Qu, W., Meng, B., Yu, Y., & Wang, S. (2017). EpCAM antibody-conjugated mesoporous silica nanoparticles to enhance the anticancer efficacy of carboplatin in retinoblastoma. *Materials Science and Engineering C*, *76*, 646–651. doi:10.1016/j.msec.2017.03.036 PMID:28482574

Qu, Y., Feng, L., Tong, C., Liu, B., & Lü, C. (2013). Poly(p-phenylenevinylene) functionalized fluorescent mesoporous silica nanoparticles for drug release and cell imaging. *Microporous and Mesoporous Materials*, *182*, 155–164. doi:10.1016/j.micromeso.2013.08.045

Ren, M., Han, Z., Li, J., Feng, G., & Ouyang, S. (2015). Ascorbic acid delivered by mesoporous silica nanoparticles induces the differentiation of human embryonic stem cells into cardiomyocytes. *Materials Science and Engineering C*, *56*, 348–355. doi:10.1016/j.msec.2015.06.048 PMID:26249600

Ren, N., Wang, B., Yang, Y. H., Zhang, Y. H., Yang, W. L., Yue, Y. H., ... Tang, Y. (2005). General Method for the Fabrication of Hollow Microcapsules with Adjustable Shell Compositions. *Chemistry of Materials*, *17*(10), 2582–2587. doi:10.1021/cm0502828

Roberts, C. M., Shahin, S. A., Wen, W., Finlay, J. B., Dong, J., Wang, R., ... Glackin, C. A. (2017). Nanoparticle delivery of siRNA against TWIST to reduce drug resistance and tumor growth in ovarian cancer models. *Nanomedicine; Nanotechnology, Biology, and Medicine*, *13*(3), 965–976. doi:10.1016/j.nano.2016.11.010 PMID:27890656

Roggers, R. A., Joglekar, M., Valenstein, J. S., & Trewyn, B. G. (2014). Mimicking Red Blood Cell Lipid Membrane To Enhance the Hemocompatibility of Large-Pore Mesoporous Silica. *ACS Applied Materials & Interfaces*, *6*(3), 1675–1681. doi:10.1021/am4045713 PMID:24417657

Roy, I., Kumar, P., Kumar, R., Ohulchanskyy, T. Y., Yong, K. T., & Prasad, P. N. (2014). Ormosil nanoparticles as a sustained-release drug delivery vehicle. *RSC Advances*, *4*(96), 53498–53504. doi:10.1039/C4RA10293B

Sahoo, B., Devi, K. S. P., Dutta, S., Maiti, T. K., Pramanik, P., & Dhara, D. (2014). Biocompatible mesoporous silica-coated superparamagnetic manganese ferrite nanoparticles for targeted drug delivery and MR imaging applications. *Journal of Colloid and Interface Science*, *431*, 31–41. doi:10.1016/j.jcis.2014.06.003 PMID:24980623

Saito, G., Swanson, J. A., & Lee, K. D. (2003). Drug delivery strategy utilizing conjugation via reversible disulfide linkages: Role and site of cellular reducing activities. *Advanced Drug Delivery Reviews*, *55*(2), 199–215. doi:10.1016/S0169-409X(02)00179-5 PMID:12564977

Sapino, S., Ugazio, E., Gastaldi, L., Miletto, I., Berlier, G., Zonari, D., & Oliaro-Bosso, S. (2015). Mesoporous silica as topical nanocarriers for quercetin: Characterization and in vitro studies. *European Journal of Pharmaceutics and Biopharmaceutics*, *89*, 116–125. doi:10.1016/j.ejpb.2014.11.022 PMID:25478737

Selvestrel, F., Moret, F., Segat, D., Woodhams, J. H., Fracasso, G., Echevarria, I. M., ... Mancin, F. (2013). Targeted delivery of photosensitizers: Efficacy and selectivity issues revealed by multifunctional ORMOSIL nanovectors in cellular systems. *Nanoscale*, *5*(13), 6106–6116. doi:10.1039/c3nr00402c PMID:23728482

She, X., Chen, L., Velleman, L., Li, C., Zhu, H., He, C., ... Kong, L. (2015). Fabrication of high specificity hollow mesoporous silica nanoparticles assisted by Eudragit for targeted drug delivery. *Journal of Colloid and Interface Science*, *445*, 151–160. doi:10.1016/j.jcis.2014.12.053 PMID:25617610

Shi, S., Chen, F., & Cai, W. (2013). Biomedical applications of functionalized hollow mesoporous silica nanoparticles: Focusing on molecular imaging. *Nanomedicine (London)*, *8*(12), 2027–2039. doi:10.2217/nnm.13.177 PMID:24279491

Singh, R. K., & Kim, H. W. (2013). Inorganic nanobiomaterial drug carriers for medicine. *Tissue Engineering and Regenerative Medicine*, *10*(6), 296–309. doi:10.100713770-013-1092-y

Singh, R. K., Patel, K. D., Leong, K. W., & Kim, H. W. (2017). Progress in Nanotheranostics Based on Mesoporous Silica Nanomaterial Platforms. *ACS Applied Materials & Interfaces*, *9*(12), 10309–10337. doi:10.1021/acsami.6b16505 PMID:28274115

Slowing, I. I., Vivero-Escoto, J. L., Wu, C. W., & Lin, V. S. Y. (2008). Mesoporous silica nanoparticles as controlled release drug delivery and gene transfection carriers. *Advanced Drug Delivery Reviews*, *60*(11), 1278–1288. doi:10.1016/j.addr.2008.03.012 PMID:18514969

Stöber, W., Fink, A., & Bohn, E. (1968). Controlled growth of monodisperse silica spheres in the micron size range. *Journal of Colloid and Interface Science*, *26*(1), 62–69. doi:10.1016/0021-9797(68)90272-5

Sun, D. (2010). Nanotheranostics: Integration of Imaging and Targeted Drug Delivery. *Molecular Pharmaceutics*, *7*(6), 1879–1879. doi:10.1021/mp1003652 PMID:21128687

Sun, Q., You, Q., Pang, X., Tan, X., Wang, J., Liu, L., ... Li, N. (2017). A photoresponsive and rod-shape nanocarrier: Single wavelength of light triggered photothermal and photodynamic therapy based on AuNRs-capped & Ce6-doped mesoporous silica nanorods. *Biomaterials*, *122*, 188–200. doi:10.1016/j.biomaterials.2017.01.021 PMID:28131043

Tang, F., Li, L., & Chen, D. (2012). Mesoporous Silica Nanoparticles: Synthesis, Biocompatibility and Drug Delivery. *Advanced Materials*, *24*(12), 1504–1534. doi:10.1002/adma.201104763 PMID:22378538

Tang, H., Guo, J., Sun, Y., Chang, B., Ren, Q., & Yang, W. (2011). Facile synthesis of pH sensitive polymer-coated mesoporous silica nanoparticles and their application in drug delivery. *International Journal of Pharmaceutics*, *421*(2), 388–396. doi:10.1016/j.ijpharm.2011.10.013 PMID:22001840

Tao, C., Zhu, Y., Li, X., & Hanagata, N. (2015). Binding of CpG oligodeoxynucleotides to mesoporous silica nanoparticles for enhancing delivery efficiency. *Microporous and Mesoporous Materials, 204*, 91–98. doi:10.1016/j.micromeso.2014.11.007

Tarn, D., Ashley, C. E., Xue, M., Carnes, E. C., Zink, J. I., & Brinker, C. J. (2013). Mesoporous Silica Nanoparticle Nanocarriers: Biofunctionality and Biocompatibility. *Accounts of Chemical Research, 46*(3), 792–801. doi:10.1021/ar3000986 PMID:23387478

Thomas, M. J., Slipper, I., Walunj, A., Jain, A., Favretto, M. E., Kallinteri, P., & Douroumis, D. (2010). Inclusion of poorly soluble drugs in highly ordered mesoporous silica nanoparticles. *International Journal of Pharmaceutics, 387*(1-2), 272–277. doi:10.1016/j.ijpharm.2009.12.023 PMID:20025947

Trewyn, B. G., Whitman, C. M., & Lin, V. S. Y. (2004). Morphological Control of Room-Temperature Ionic Liquid Templated Mesoporous Silica Nanoparticles for Controlled Release of Antibacterial Agents. *Nano Letters, 4*(11), 2139–2143. doi:10.1021/nl048774r

Tsai, C. H., Vivero-Escoto, J. L., Slowing, I. I., Fang, I. J., Trewyn, B. G., & Lin, V. S. Y. (2011). Surfactant-assisted controlled release of hydrophobic drugs using anionic surfactant templated mesoporous silica nanoparticles. *Biomaterials, 32*(26), 6234–6244. doi:10.1016/j.biomaterials.2011.04.077 PMID:21684000

Ugazio, E., Gastaldi, L., Brunella, V., Scalarone, D., Jadhav, S. A., Oliaro-Bosso, S., ... Sapino, S. (2016). Thermoresponsive mesoporous silica nanoparticles as a carrier for skin delivery of quercetin. *International Journal of Pharmaceutics, 511*(1), 446–454. doi:10.1016/j.ijpharm.2016.07.024 PMID:27421910

Vallet-Regi, M., Rámila, A., del Real, R. P., & Pérez-Pariente, J. (2001). A New Property of MCM-41: Drug Delivery System. *Chemistry of Materials, 13*(2), 308–311. doi:10.1021/cm0011559

Wang, A., Guo, M., Wang, N., Zhao, J., Qi, W., Muhammad, F., ... Zhu, G. (2014). Redox-mediated dissolution of paramagnetic nanolids to achieve a smart theranostic system. *Nanoscale, 6*(10), 5270–5278. doi:10.1039/C3NR05687B PMID:24695417

Wang, H., Agarwal, P., Zhao, S., Yu, J., Lu, X., & He, X. (2016). Combined cancer therapy with hyaluronan-decorated fullerene-silica multifunctional nanoparticles to target cancer stem-like cells. *Biomaterials, 97*, 62–73. doi:10.1016/j.biomaterials.2016.04.030 PMID:27162075

Wang, K., Yao, H., Meng, Y., Wang, Y., Yan, X., & Huang, R. (2015). Specific aptamer-conjugated mesoporous silica-carbon nanoparticles for HER2-targeted chemo-photothermal combined therapy. *Acta Biomaterialia, 16*, 196–205. doi:10.1016/j.actbio.2015.01.002 PMID:25596325

Wang, X., Li, C., Fan, N., Li, J., He, Z., & Sun, J. (2017). Multimodal nanoporous silica nanoparticles functionalized with aminopropyl groups for improving loading and controlled release of doxorubicin hydrochloride. *Materials Science and Engineering C, 78*, 370–375. doi:10.1016/j.msec.2017.04.060 PMID:28575997

Wang, X., Liu, Y., Wang, S., Shi, D., Zhou, X., Wang, C., ... Lu, G. (2015). CD44-engineered mesoporous silica nanoparticles for overcoming multidrug resistance in breast cancer. *Applied Surface Science, 332*, 308–317. doi:10.1016/j.apsusc.2015.01.204

Wang, Y., Cui, Y., Huang, J., Di, D., Dong, Y., Zhang, X., ... Wang, S. (2015a). Redox and pH dual-responsive mesoporous silica nanoparticles for site-specific drug delivery. *Applied Surface Science*, *356*, 1282–1288. doi:10.1016/j.apsusc.2015.07.151

Wang, Y., Han, N., Zhao, Q., Bai, L., Li, J., Jiang, T., & Wang, S. (2015b). Redox-responsive mesoporous silica as carriers for controlled drug delivery: A comparative study based on silica and PEG gatekeepers. *European Journal of Pharmaceutical Sciences*, *72*, 12–20. doi:10.1016/j.ejps.2015.02.008 PMID:25701727

Wang, Y., Shi, W., Wang, S., Li, C., Qian, M., Chen, J., & Huang, R. (2016). Facile incorporation of dispersed fluorescent carbon nanodots into mesoporous silica nanosphere for pH-triggered drug delivery and imaging. *Carbon*, *108*, 146–153. doi:10.1016/j.carbon.2016.07.009

Ward, M. A., & Georgiou, T. K. (2011). Thermoresponsive Polymers for Biomedical Applications. *Polymers*, *3*(4), 1215–1242. doi:10.3390/polym3031215

Wei, Y., Gao, L., Wang, L., Shi, L., Wei, E., Zhou, B., ... Ge, B. (2017). Polydopamine and peptide decorated doxorubicin-loaded mesoporous silica nanoparticles as a targeted drug delivery system for bladder cancer therapy. *Drug Delivery*, *24*(1), 681–691. doi:10.1080/10717544.2017.1309475 PMID:28414557

Wicki, A., Witzigmann, D., Balasubramanian, V., & Huwyler, J. (2015). Nanomedicine in cancer therapy: Challenges, opportunities, and clinical applications. *Journal of Controlled Release*, *200*, 138–157. doi:10.1016/j.jconrel.2014.12.030 PMID:25545217

Wu, S. H., Mou, C. Y., & Lin, H. P. (2013). Synthesis of mesoporous silica nanoparticles. *Chemical Society Reviews*, *42*(9), 3862–3875. doi:10.1039/c3cs35405a PMID:23403864

Wu, X., Han, Z., Schur, R. M., & Lu, Z. R. (2016). Targeted Mesoporous Silica Nanoparticles Delivering Arsenic Trioxide with Environment Sensitive Drug Release for Effective Treatment of Triple Negative Breast Cancer. *ACS Biomaterials Science & Engineering*, *2*(4), 501–507. doi:10.1021/acsbiomaterials.5b00398

Xie, J., Lee, S., & Chen, X. (2010). Nanoparticle-based theranostic agents. *Advanced Drug Delivery Reviews*, *62*(11), 1064–1079. doi:10.1016/j.addr.2010.07.009 PMID:20691229

Xie, M., Shi, H., Ma, K., Shen, H., Li, B., Shen, S., ... Jin, Y. (2013). Hybrid nanoparticles for drug delivery and bioimaging: Mesoporous silica nanoparticles functionalized with carboxyl groups and a near-infrared fluorescent dye. *Journal of Colloid and Interface Science*, *395*, 306–314. doi:10.1016/j.jcis.2013.01.001 PMID:23394807

Xie, M., Xu, Y., Shen, H., Shen, S., Ge, Y., & Xie, J. (2014). Negative-charge-functionalized mesoporous silica nanoparticles as drug vehicles targeting hepatocellular carcinoma. *International Journal of Pharmaceutics*, *474*, 223–231. PMID:25149125

Xie, X., Li, F., Zhang, H., Lu, Y., Lian, S., Lin, H., ... Jia, L. (2016). EpCAM aptamer-functionalized mesoporous silica nanoparticles for efficient colon cancer cell-targeted drug delivery. *European Journal of Pharmaceutical Sciences*, *83*, 28–35. doi:10.1016/j.ejps.2015.12.014 PMID:26690044

Xu, F., Ding, L., Tao, W., Yang, X. Z., Qian, H. S., & Yao, R. S. (2016). Mesoporous-silica-coated upconversion nanoparticles loaded with vitamin B12 for near-infrared-light mediated photodynamic therapy. *Materials Letters*, *167*, 205–208. doi:10.1016/j.matlet.2015.12.105

Xu, W., Gao, Q., Xu, Y., Wu, D., Sun, Y., Shen, W., & Deng, F. (2009). Controllable release of ibuprofen from size-adjustable and surface hydrophobic mesoporous silica spheres. *Powder Technology*, *191*(1-2), 13–20. doi:10.1016/j.powtec.2008.09.001

Xu, W., Riikonen, J., & Lehto, V. P. (2013). Mesoporous systems for poorly soluble drugs. *International Journal of Pharmaceutics*, *453*(1), 181–197. doi:10.1016/j.ijpharm.2012.09.008 PMID:22990124

Xu, X., Lü, S., Gao, C., Wang, X., Bai, X., Gao, N., & Liu, M. (2015). Facile preparation of pH-sensitive and self-fluorescent mesoporous silica nanoparticles modified with PAMAM dendrimers for label-free imaging and drug delivery. *Chemical Engineering Journal*, *266*, 171–178. doi:10.1016/j.cej.2014.12.075

Yamada, H., Urata, C., Aoyama, Y., Osada, S., Yamauchi, Y., & Kuroda, K. (2012). Preparation of Colloidal Mesoporous Silica Nanoparticles with Different Diameters and Their Unique Degradation Behavior in Static Aqueous Systems. *Chemistry of Materials*, *24*(8), 1462–1471. doi:10.1021/cm3001688

Yan, Y., Fu, J., Wang, T., & Lu, X. (2017). Controlled release of silyl ether camptothecin from thiol-ene click chemistry-functionalized mesoporous silica nanoparticles. *Acta Biomaterialia*, *51*, 471–478. doi:10.1016/j.actbio.2017.01.062 PMID:28131940

Yanagisawa, T., Shimizu, T., Kuroda, K., & Kato, C. (1990). The Preparation of Alkyltrimethylammonium-Kanemite Complexes and Their Conversion to Microporous Materials. *Bulletin of the Chemical Society of Japan*, *63*(4), 988–992. doi:10.1246/bcsj.63.988

Yang, P., Gai, S., & Lin, J. (2012). Functionalized mesoporous silica materials for controlled drug delivery. *Chemical Society Reviews*, *41*(9), 3679–3698. doi:10.1039/c2cs15308d PMID:22441299

Yoncheva, K., Popova, M., Szegedi, A., Mihaly, J., Tzankov, B., Lambov, N., ... Valoti, M. (2014). Functionalized mesoporous silica nanoparticles for oral delivery of budesonide. *Journal of Solid State Chemistry*, *211*, 154–161. doi:10.1016/j.jssc.2013.12.020

Yu, E., Lo, A., Jiang, L., Petkus, B., Ileri Ercan, N., & Stroeve, P. (2017). Improved controlled release of protein from expanded-pore mesoporous silica nanoparticles modified with co-functionalized poly(n-isopropylacrylamide) and poly(ethylene glycol) (PNIPAM-PEG). *Colloids and Surfaces. B, Biointerfaces*, *149*, 297–300. doi:10.1016/j.colsurfb.2016.10.033 PMID:27776334

Yu, J., Zhang, Y., Bomba, H., & Gu, Z. (2016). Stimuli-responsive delivery of therapeutics for diabetes treatment. *Bioengineering & Translational Medicine*, *1*(3), 323–337. doi:10.1002/btm2.10036 PMID:29147685

Yun, L., Xingwei, D., Jinghua, L., Zhong, L., Yan, H., Junjie, L., ... Kaiyong, C. (2015). Enzyme responsive drug delivery system based on mesoporous silica nanoparticles for tumor therapy in vivo. *Nanotechnology*, *26*(14), 145102. doi:10.1088/0957-4484/26/14/145102 PMID:25789511

Zhang, B., Luo, Z., Liu, J., Ding, X., Li, J., & Cai, K. (2014). Cytochrome c end-capped mesoporous silica nanoparticles as redox-responsive drug delivery vehicles for liver tumor-targeted triplex therapy in vitro and in vivo. *Journal of Controlled Release*, *192*, 192–201. doi:10.1016/j.jconrel.2014.06.037 PMID:25034575

Zhang, J., Sun, Y., Tian, B., Li, K., Wang, L., Liang, Y., & Han, J. (2016). Multifunctional mesoporous silica nanoparticles modified with tumor-shedable hyaluronic acid as carriers for doxorubicin. *Colloids and Surfaces. B, Biointerfaces*, *144*, 293–302. doi:10.1016/j.colsurfb.2016.04.015 PMID:27107383

Zhang, J., Yuan, Z. F., Wang, Y., Chen, W. H., Luo, G. F., Cheng, S. X., ... Zhang, X. Z. (2013). Multifunctional Envelope-Type Mesoporous Silica Nanoparticles for Tumor-Triggered Targeting Drug Delivery. *Journal of the American Chemical Society*, *135*(13), 5068–5073. doi:10.1021/ja312004m PMID:23464924

Zhang, M., Liu, J., Kuang, Y., Li, Q., Zheng, D. W., Song, Q., ... Jiang, B. (2017). Ingenious pH-sensitive dextran/mesoporous silica nanoparticles based drug delivery systems for controlled intracellular drug release. *International Journal of Biological Macromolecules*, *98*, 691–700. doi:10.1016/j.ijbiomac.2017.01.136 PMID:28174081

Zhang, Q., Liu, F., Nguyen, K. T., Ma, X., Wang, X., Xing, B., & Zhao, Y. (2012). Multifunctional Mesoporous Silica Nanoparticles for Cancer-Targeted and Controlled Drug Delivery. *Advanced Functional Materials*, *22*(24), 5144–5156. doi:10.1002/adfm.201201316

Zhang, Q., Zhao, H., Li, D., Liu, L., & Du, S. (2017). A surface-grafted ligand functionalization strategy for coordinate binding of doxorubicin at surface of PEGylated mesoporous silica nanoparticles: Toward pH-responsive drug delivery. *Colloids and Surfaces. B, Biointerfaces*, *149*, 138–145. doi:10.1016/j.colsurfb.2016.10.018 PMID:27750088

Zhang, X., Li, F., Guo, S., Chen, X., Wang, X., Li, J., & Gan, Y. (2014). Biofunctionalized polymer-lipid supported mesoporous silica nanoparticles for release of chemotherapeutics in multidrug resistant cancer cells. *Biomaterials*, *35*(11), 3650–3665. doi:10.1016/j.biomaterials.2014.01.013 PMID:24462359

Zhang, Y., Ang, C. Y., Li, M., Tan, S. Y., Qu, Q., Luo, Z., & Zhao, Y. (2015a). Polymer-Coated Hollow Mesoporous Silica Nanoparticles for Triple-Responsive Drug Delivery. *ACS Applied Materials & Interfaces*, *7*(32), 18179–18187. doi:10.1021/acsami.5b05893 PMID:26221866

Zhang, Y., Guo, J., Zhang, X. L., Li, D. P., Zhang, T. T., Gao, F. F., ... Sheng, X. G. (2015b). Antibody fragment-armed mesoporous silica nanoparticles for the targeted delivery of bevacizumab in ovarian cancer cells. *International Journal of Pharmaceutics*, *496*(2), 1026–1033. doi:10.1016/j.ijpharm.2015.10.080 PMID:26541303

Zhang, Y., Guo, J., Zhang, X. L., Li, D. P., Zhang, T. T., Gao, F. F., ... Sheng, X. G. (2015c). Antibody fragment-armed mesoporous silica nanoparticles for the targeted delivery of bevacizumab in ovarian cancer cells. *International Journal of Pharmaceutics*, *496*(2), 1026–1033. doi:10.1016/j.ijpharm.2015.10.080 PMID:26541303

Zhang, Y., Zhi, Z., Jiang, T., Zhang, J., Wang, Z., & Wang, S. (2010). Spherical mesoporous silica nanoparticles for loading and release of the poorly water-soluble drug telmisartan. *Journal of Controlled Release*, *145*(3), 257–263. doi:10.1016/j.jconrel.2010.04.029 PMID:20450945

Zhang, Z., Balogh, D., Wang, F., Sung, S. Y., Nechushtai, R., & Willner, I. (2013). Biocatalytic Release of an Anticancer Drug from Nucleic-Acids-Capped Mesoporous SiO2 Using DNA or Molecular Biomarkers as Triggering Stimuli. *ACS Nano*, *7*(10), 8455–8468. doi:10.1021/nn403772j PMID:23985013

Zhao, D., Feng, J., Huo, Q., Melosh, N., Fredrickson, G. H., Chmelka, B. F., & Stucky, G. D. (1998). Triblock Copolymer Syntheses of Mesoporous Silica with Periodic 50 to 300 Angstrom Pores. *Science*, *279*(5350), 548–552. doi:10.1126cience.279.5350.548 PMID:9438845

Zhao, J., He, Z., Li, B., Cheng, T., & Liu, G. (2017). AND logic-like pH- and light-dual controlled drug delivery by surface modified mesoporous silica nanoparticles. *Materials Science and Engineering C*, *73*, 1–7. doi:10.1016/j.msec.2016.12.056 PMID:28183586

Zhao, W., Zhang, H., He, Q., Li, Y., Gu, J., Li, L., ... Shi, J. (2011). A glucose-responsive controlled release of insulin system based on enzyme multilayers-coated mesoporous silica particles. *Chemical Communications*, *47*(33), 9459–9461. doi:10.1039/c1cc12740c PMID:21779606

Zhao, Y., Sun, X., Zhang, G., Trewyn, B. G., Slowing, I. I., & Lin, V. S. Y. (2011). Interaction of Mesoporous Silica Nanoparticles with Human Red Blood Cell Membranes: Size and Surface Effects. *ACS Nano*, *5*(2), 1366–1375. doi:10.1021/nn103077k PMID:21294526

Zhao, Y., Trewyn, B. G., Slowing, I. I., & Lin, V. S. Y. (2009). Mesoporous Silica Nanoparticle-Based Double Drug Delivery System for Glucose-Responsive Controlled Release of Insulin and Cyclic AMP. *Journal of the American Chemical Society*, *131*(24), 8398–8400. doi:10.1021/ja901831u PMID:19476380

Zhao, Z. X., Huang, Y. Z., Shi, S. G., Tang, S. H., Li, D. H., & Chen, X. L. (2014). Cancer therapy improvement with mesoporous silica nanoparticles combining photodynamic and photothermal therapy. *Nanotechnology*, *25*(28), 285701. doi:10.1088/0957-4484/25/28/285701 PMID:24971525

Zheng, J., Tian, X., Sun, Y., Lu, D., & Yang, W. (2013). pH sensitive poly(glutamic acid) grafted mesoporous silica nanoparticles for drug delivery. *International Journal of Pharmaceutics*, *450*(1-2), 296–303. doi:10.1016/j.ijpharm.2013.04.014 PMID:23598077

Zheng, Q., Lin, T., Wu, H., Guo, L., Ye, P., Hao, Y., ... Chen, G. (2014). Mussel-inspired polydopamine coated mesoporous silica nanoparticles as pH-sensitive nanocarriers for controlled release. *International Journal of Pharmaceutics*, *463*(1), 22–26. doi:10.1016/j.ijpharm.2013.12.045 PMID:24393764

Zhou, X., Chen, L., Nie, W., Wang, W., Qin, M., Mo, X., ... He, C. (2016). Dual-Responsive Mesoporous Silica Nanoparticles Mediated Codelivery of Doxorubicin and Bcl-2 SiRNA for Targeted Treatment of Breast Cancer. *The Journal of Physical Chemistry C*, *120*(39), 22375–22387. doi:10.1021/acs.jpcc.6b06759

Zhu, C. L., Wang, X. W., Lin, Z. Z., Xie, Z. H., & Wang, X. R. (2014). Cell microenvironment stimuli-responsive controlled-release delivery systems based on mesoporous silica nanoparticles. *Journal of Food and Drug Analysis*, *22*(1), 18–28. doi:10.1016/j.jfda.2014.01.002 PMID:24673901

KEY TERMS AND DEFINITIONS

Drug Delivery: Transporting bioactives safely to the site of action for desired therapeutic effect.

Dual-Drug Delivery: Delivery of drug combinations in a single system owing to their several benefits over single drug loaded systems.

Functionalization: Modification in properties of the carrier system by incorporation/adsorption/attachment of moieties like polymers, ligands, or antibodies to their surface.

Mesoporous Silica Nanoparticles: Nanosized mesoporous form of silica particles in shape of spheres or rods.

Nanomedicine: Submicron size (<0.1 μm or 100 nm) modules, used for treatment, diagnosis, monitoring, and control of biological system.

Photodynamic Therapy: Treatment with light using a particular type of drug called photosensitizers.

Stimuli-Responsive Drug Delivery: Delivery of drug at desired site in response to external/internal stimuli (e.g., light, heat, enzyme, etc.).

Targeted Drug Delivery: Delivery of drug to the desired site with the assistance of smart carriers.

Theranostics: A term coined to combine diagnostic and therapeutic capabilities for therapy.

Chapter 9
Micro- and Nanosponges-Based Carriers in Advanced Drug Delivery Applications

Kamla Pathak
Uttar Pradesh University of Medical Sciences, India

Ankur Vaidya
Uttar Pradesh University of Medical Sciences, India

ABSTRACT

Microsponges, a patented technology for chronotherapeutic topical drug delivery, has evolved for oral, pulmonary, and parenteral drug delivery. Various advances have been made with this carrier particle resulting in the development of novel carrier particles, namely nanosponges, nanoferrosponges, and porous microbeads. This chapter deals with the application for topical delivery of pharmaceuticals and for cosmetic purpose; potential of the delivery system for oral drug delivery, pulmonary, and parenteral purpose; and also provides an insight on the recent advances made in this field and future prospect. While many commercial products are available for topical purpose, the use of the technology for sustained/controlled/targeted delivery of pharmaceuticals/biopharmaceuticals via alternative routes is still in infancy. Extensive research inputs are required to resolve preclinical and clinical intricacies before the technology can be put into use for alternative administrative routes and for tissue engineering.

INTRODUCTION

Multiparticulate systems can control the drug release via temporal control or spatial control or both. These offer the advantages of ease of fabrication, high degree of dispersion in gastrointestinal tract (Asghar & Chandran 2006), reduced risk of dose dumping (Solanki, Patel, Barot, Parijiya, & Shelat, 2012), leading to less inter- and intra-subject variability (Goyel, Prajapati, Purohit, & Mehta, 2010), and efficient drug loading. Due to their advantages these have been widely explored as drug carriers and sequentially this has led to the development of microsponges in 1988. These porous microspheres were exclusively designed for chronotherapeutic topical drug delivery but attempts to utilize them for oral, pulmonary

DOI: 10.4018/978-1-5225-4781-5.ch009

Copyright © 2018, IGI Global. Copying or distributing in print or electronic forms without written permission of IGI Global is prohibited.

and parenteral drug delivery were also made (Smith, Morhenn, & Webster, 2006). Various advances have been made with this carrier particle resulting in the development of various novel developments.

The microsponge technology was introduced for topical delivery of drug products to facilitate the controlled release of active drug into the skin in order to reduce systemic exposure and minimize local cutaneous reactions to active drugs. Also known as solid phase porous microsphere (Figure 1); is a patented microparticulate system, comprising of highly cross-linked, polymeric porous microspheres having numerous interconnected voids in the particle, loaded with active agent within a collapsible structure (Embil & Nacht 1996) with large porous surface to entrap wide range of active agents with varying pharmacological activities administered in different doses that can be released at the desired site of absorption (Sharma & Pathak 2006).

The pores in the microparticle form a continuous arrangement open to the exterior surface of particles which permits the outward diffusion of the entrapped drug molecule at a controlled rate depending on the pore size (Nacht & Kantz, 1992). High degree of polymeric cross-linking results in insoluble, inert microparticles with satisfactory strength to withstand high shear. These microparticles were once visualized to consist of several nanoparticles enclosed in a porous polymeric outer surface (Katz, Cheng, & Nacht, 1999). A microsponge of size approximating 25 μm can have up to 3000 mm/g of pore length with a pore volume of about 1 ml/g (Gans, 1999). In addition to efficient entrapment of active ingredients, the technology is predicted to minimize side effects, improve stability, increase elegance and enhance formulation flexibility (Srivastava & Pathak 2012).

Primarily the products lined up for commercial purpose include those intended for topical applications due to the favourable features namely- The microsponge system can prevent excessive accumulation of ingredients within the epidermis and the dermis. It can absorb oil up to 6 times its weight without drying and extends drug release for up to 12 h. The microsponge system can significantly reduce the irritation of effective drugs without reducing their efficacy. The microsponges are then washed away with the next cleansing (Kaity, Maiti, Ghosh, Pal, Ghosh, & Banerjee, 2010). The characteristics of microsponges and the active pharmaceutical ingredient to be incorporated therein are listed in Table 1.

The microsponges may be prepared using any one of the following methods (1) Liquid-liquid suspension polymerization [Bottom-up approach] (Tansel et al 1992) ; (2) Quasi-Emulsion Solvent diffusion[Top down approach] (Kawashima, Niwa, Handa, Takeuchi, Iwamoto, & Itoh, 1989); (3) Water in oil in water (w/o/w) emulsion solvent diffusion (Rawat, Majumder, & Ahsan, 2008); Oil in oil emulsion solvent diffusion (Mandal, Bostanian, Graves, Chapman, & Idodo, 2001); (4) Addition of porogen (Bae, Son, Park, & Han, 2009); Lyophilization (Liu, Liu, Ng, Froix, Ohno, & Heller, 1997) and Electrohydrodynamic atomization (Pancholi, Ahras, Stride, Edirisinghe, & Samarasinghe, 2009). Table 2 lists the evaluation parameters of microsponges along with the determination method/equipment.

Advantages and Limitations

In addition to those listed in preceding text, microsponges depict improved thermal, physical and chemical stability over other microparticulate systems (Aritomi, Yamasaki, Yamada, Honda, & Koshi, 1996). Using these carrier systems liquids can be converted into powders leading to improved material processing. In this context microsponges present amenability to their development as novel dosage forms (Srivastava, Kumar, & Pathak, 2010). Microsponges are readily compressible when compared to other microparticulate systems or to the physical mixture of the drug and the polymer (Comoglu, Gonul, & Baykara, 2002). In addition, the entrapment of actives in the microsponge allows for both co-loading and coatings. Physiologically, the time required to traverse the small and large intestine is significantly increased via microsponge system thus maximizing the amount of drug that can be absorbed. Drugs that are not soluble in water can be entrapped in microsponge pores, which are extremely small; thus, the drug functions as microscopic particles, producing a greater surface area and increasing the rate of solubilization (Chadawar & Shaji, 2007)

Irrespective of the listed advantages, the system is subject to limitations. These include non-reproducibility the production techniques and almost no efforts for pilot plant on commercial level. Though research has demonstrated the efficacy of microsponges for protein delivery; but post release, microsponges do not offer protection against microbial flora at the site of release. Although smaller pores of microsponges limit the entry of microorganisms to the bulk but the microbes can grow on the surface of microsponges (Giovagnoli, Blasi, Schoubben, Rossi, & Ricci, 2007). Similarly, the use of biodegradable polymers for the delivery of amino acids and proteins has lead to generation of monomers at the site which may cause harm to the physiology of the human body. Another aspect relates to it colon targeting ability. Microsponges can be suitably converted to a colon-targeted tablet by using pectin for compression coating (Orlu, Cevher, & Araman, 2006) or calcium pectinate as matrix former (Srivastava, Kumar, & Pathak, 2010) but the microsponges on their own, cannot protect the active ingredient from being released in upper part of GIT.

Applications

Microsponges are primarily used for topical delivery of actives and recently for oral administration as well as biopharmaceutical delivery. It offers the formulator a range of alternatives to develop drug and cosmetic products. These are developed to deliver an active ingredient efficiently at the low dose and also to enhance stability, reduce side effects and modify drug release. Various categories of actives that can be delivered via microsponges for specific application (s) are shown in Table 3.

Topical Drug Delivery

Microsponges are frequently used for topical delivery and due to their elegance these carrier systems also applications in cosmetics. Benzoyl peroxide is used for the treatment of acne and athletes foot. Skin irritation is a common side effect, and it has been predicted that controlled release of benzoyl peroxide from the microsponge on to the skin could reduce the side effect while reducing percutaneous absorption (Jelvehgari, Siahi-Shadbad, & Azarmi, 2006; Nokhodchi, Jelvehgari, & Mozafari, 2007; Wester, Patel, Natch, Leyden, Melendres, & Maibach, 1991). Benzoyl peroxide microsponges appear to reduce sebum accumulation and associated facial shine. In one split-face trial, subjects cleansed the face with a gentle skin cleanser, then applied BPO microsphere cream 5.5% to one half of the face and no product to the control side. Measurements were taken with a sebumeter at baseline and 30 minutes, two hours, four hours, and six hours after the regimen. Actively treated sides had greater surface sebum reduction at all time points (Del Rosso, 2009). Hydroquinone bleaching creams are considered the gold standard for treating hyperpigmentation. A new formulation of hydroquinone (4%) with retinol (0.15%) entrapped in microsponges was developed for gradual release of hydroquinone to prolong treatment and to minimize skin irritation (Grimes 2004).

Tretinoin is used for the treatment of photodamage and acne, that contribute to premature aging of skin and has been implicated in skin cancer. A topical formulation containing 0.1 and 0.04% tretinoin entrapped in microsponges was formulated for treatment of acne vulgaris. The formulation uses patented methyl methacrylate/glycol dimethacrylate cross polymer porous microspheres to enable inclusion of the active ingredient, tretinoin, in an aqueous gel; marketed as Retin-A-Micro® by Ortho-McNeil pharmaceuticals (www.accessdata.FDA.com).

Topical retinoids are a mainstay in acne treatment since 1962. All-trans retinoic acid was the first and is still in use. Its irritation potential has led to the new galenics, i.e. incorporation in microsponges and in propolyomers, which increase the tolerability significantly. The isomer of tretinoin, isotretinoin, has the same clinical efficacy, but also a lower irritancy (Gollnick HPM & Krautheim 2003) is a potential candidate for MDS. In a multicenter, double-blind, randomized, parallel-group study conducted by Leyden et al. (2002) in patients with mild-to-moderate inflammatory facial acne vulgaris; the efficacy and tolerability of tazarotene 0.1% gel and tretinoin 0.1% microsponge gel were evaluated. A total of 169 patients were randomized to once-daily applications of one of these topical retinoids for 12 weeks. Both agents were associated with significant reductions from baseline in the non-inflammatory and inflammatory lesion counts. Tazarotene treatment was associated with a significantly greater incidence of treatment success (defined as > or = 50% global improvement [67 versus 49%; P = 0.03]) and significantly greater reductions in overall disease severity (36 versus 26%; P = 0.02) and non-inflammatory lesion count (60 versus 38% at week 12; P = 0.02) than tretinoin microsponge treatment. Both drugs were well tolerated, with mean levels of dryness, burning, pruritus, erythema, and peeling generally being no more than trace throughout the study. Clinically, no significant between-group differences were observed in measures of tolerability. The mean amount of medication applied was 0.28 g per application with tazarotene and 0.41 g per application with tretinoin microsponge, resulting in cost-effectiveness ratios of $81.45 per treatment success with tazarotene and $108.24 per treatment success with tretinoin microsponge. Tazarotene was observed to have greater efficacy and comparable tolerability and to be a cost-effective alternative to tretinoin 0.1% microsponge gel.

Hydroxyzine HCl loaded microsponges prepared using solvent diffusion method depicted nearly 98% encapsulation efficiency and 60-70% porosity. The pharmacodynamic effect of the optimized formulation was tested on the shaved back of histamine-sensitized rabbits. After topical application of the optimized microsponge preparations (plain or medicated) on the inflamed back of rabbits, the mean wheal areas were recorded at various time intervals in each group of rabbit. The wheal disappeared completely in the group treated with medicated microsponges (optimized formulation); whereas, the group receiving plain microsponges showed 21.2% reduction in the inflamed area at corresponding time interval. In comparison with the initial wheal areas, all the medicated preparations showed wheal area suppression after 4 h. The wheal suppression was about 80% after the first 2 h in the case of the rabbits treated with F2, while its maximum suppression (99.46%) was reached after 4 h (Rizkalla, 2011).

In an attempt to determine the influence of microsponge formulation on the flux for percutaneous drug delivery, Maiti et al. (2011) developed diclofenac sodium loaded ethyl cellulose microsponges loaded gel through w/o/w emulsion technique. The authors reported reduced flux of drug via microsponges across the skin thus suggested drug retention at the delivery site. These formulations reduced the drug permeation through skin and maintained the required concentration of drug at the desired site.

Drug Release Mechanism

As the microsponges have an open structure and the active ingredient is free to move in and out from the particle and into the vehicle until equilibrium is reached. Once the finished product is applied to the skin, the drug that is already in the vehicle will be absorbed into the skin, depleting the vehicle, which will become unsaturated, therefore, disturbing the equilibrium. This will start a flow of the drug from the microsponge particle into the vehicle, and from it to the skin, until the vehicle is either dried or absorbed. Even after that the microsponge particles retained on the surface of the stratum corneum will continue to gradually release the drug to the skin, providing prolonged release over time. Release can also be controlled through diffusion or other external triggers such as pressure, temperature and solubility (Khopade, Jain, & Jain, 1996; Shah 1989).

- **Pressure:** Applied pressure / rubbing can release active ingredient from microsponge on to skin.
- **Temperature Change:** At room temperature, few entrapped active ingredients can be too viscous to flow suddenly from microsponges onto the skin. With increase in skin temperature, flow rate is also increased and therefore release is also enhanced.
- **Solubility:** The microsponge loaded with water-soluble ingredients like antiperspirants and antiseptics will release the ingredient(s) in the presence of water. Thus release may be achieved based on the ability of external medium to dissolve the active ingredient, the concentration gradient varies or the ability to swell the microsponge network (Embil & Nacht, 1996).

Marketed Formulations

Microsponge delivery systems are used for topical prescription, over-the-counter and personal care products. Products under development or in the marketplace utilize the microsponge system in three primary ways: (1) As reservoirs releasing active ingredients over an extended period of time; (2) As receptacles for adsorbing undesirable substances, such as excess skin oils; (3) As closed containers holding ingredients away from the skin for superficial action (Embil 2000). Table 4 highlights some of the marketed formulations of microsponges.

Oral Drug Delivery

A microsponge system offers the potential to hold active ingredients in a protected environment and provide controlled delivery of oral medication to the lower gastrointestinal tract, where it will be released upon exposure to specific enzymes in the colon. This approach opened up entirely new opportunities for MDS. In oral applications, the microsponge system has been shown to increase the rate of solubilization of poorly water-soluble drugs by entrapping such drugs in the microsponge system pores. As the pores are very small, the drug is in effect reduced to microscopic particles and the significantly increased surface area thus greatly increases the rate of solubilization (Kaity, Maiti, Ghosh, Pal, Ghosh, & Banerjee, 2010). Furthermore, as explained in the earlier text the transit time across the small and large intestine is considerably increased with MDS resulting in maximization of drug absorption.

Kawashima et al (1992) reported controlled oral delivery of ibuprofen via microsponges made with an acrylic polymer, Eudragit RS. The authors achieved controlled delivery by modulating its intra-particle density. Sustained release formulation of chlorpheniramine maleate, using powder coated microsponges, was prepared by the dry impact blending method. Preparation of powder coated microsponges by dry impact blending method was first reported by Ukita et al (1989) . The same was utilized for fabricating chlorpheniramine maleate loaded microsponges. The researchers observed that the powder-coated microsponges demonstrated lower C_{max} and longer T_{max} than powder chlorpheniramine maleate, following oral administration in dogs.

In a study by Comoglu et al (2003) the effects of different mixing speeds, drug-polymer ratios, solvent-polymer ratios on the physical characteristics of the microsponges as well as the in vitro release rate of the drug from the microsponges were investigated. All the factors investigated had an influence on the physical characteristics of the microsponges. The in vitro dissolution results depicted that the release rate of ketoprofen was modified in all formulations. The same research group reported tablets of microsponges prepared by direct compression method. Different pressure values were applied to the tablet powder mass in order to determine the optimum pressure value for compression of the tablets. Results indicated that microsponge compressibility was much improved over the physical mixture of the drug and polymer and owing to the plastic deformation of sponge-like structure, microsponges produce mechanically strong tablets (Comoglu, Gonul, & Baykara, 2002)

The purpose of this study was to design novel colon specific drug delivery system containing flurbiprofen (FLB) microsponges. Microsponges containing FLB and Eudragit RS 100 were prepared by quasi-emulsion solvent diffusion method. Additionally, FLB was entrapped into a commercial Microsponge 5640 system using entrapment method. Afterwards, the effects of drug:polymer ratio, inner phase solvent amount, stirring time and speed and stirrer type on the physical characteristics of microsponges were investigated. The thermal behaviour, surface morphology, particle size and pore structure of microsponges were examined. The colon specific formulations were prepared by compression coating and also pore plugging of microsponges with pectin: hydroxypropylmethyl cellulose (HPMC) mixture followed by tabletting. In vitro dissolution studies were done on all formulations and the results were kinetically and statistically evaluated. The microsponges were spherical in shape, between 30.7 and 94.5 μ in diameter and showed high porosity values (61-72%). The pore shapes of microsponges prepared by quasi-emulsion solvent diffusion method and entrapment method were found as spherical cylindrical holes, respectively. Mechanically strong tablets were obtained owing to the plastic deformation of microsponges. In vitro studies exhibited that the drug release from compression coated colon specific tablet was initiated at the 8th hour corresponding to the proximal colon arrival time due to the addition of enzyme, following a modified release pattern while the drug release from the colon specific formulations prepared by pore plugging the microsponges showed an increase at the 8th hour which was the time point that the enzyme addition made. The study presented a new approach based on microsponges for colon specific drug delivery (Orlu, Cevher, & Araman, 2006).

A study by Jain and Singh (2010) reported dicyclomine loaded, Eudragit RS 100 based microsponges with potential for colonic delivery. The delivery system depicted biphasic drug release with an initial burst effect of 16-30% of drug release in the first hour. Cumulative release from microsponges over 8 hours ranged from 59-86%. Kinetic analysis revealed Higuchi matrix controlled diffusion as the main mechanism of drug release. Lack of in vivo studies did not provide proof of concept. Same authors attempted colon targeting of paracetamol by employing microsponges coated with natural polysaccharides like citrus pectin. *In vitro* release studies exhibited that compression coated colon specific tablet formulations started releasing the drug at 6th hour corresponding to the arrival time at proximal colon (Jain & Singh 2010) on addition of enzyme pectinase in the release media. This study also affirmed capability of the microsponges to load the drugs required to be used in the high dose, thus proving that the microsponges have better loading efficiency than other microparticulate (microballoons, microcapsules and microspheres) system. The utility of Eudragit RS 100 for fabricaton of microsponges has also been reported by Devrim and Canefe (2006). The researchers prepared microsponges for the delivery of ibuprofen and also studied the effect of polymers (Eudragit RS100, Eudragit RS PM and Eudragit RL 100) on various characteristics of the microsponges including rheological properties along with the particle size and release characteristics and concluded that all the microsponges possessed good flow properties, required for the maintenance of the dose and weight uniformity during tablet compression or capsule filling. They also observed that smaller particles that offered better control over drug release were obtained with Eudragit RS100 when compared to those fabricated using other grades of Eudragit. Jain et al. (2010) reaffirmed the capability of Eudragit S 100 for colon targeting. The authors designed microsponge-based novel colon-specific drug delivery system bearing dicyclomine. Eudragit S-100-based microsponges containing the drug in varying amount were prepared using quasi-emulsion solvent diffusion method. In vitro release data showed a biphasic pattern with an initial burst effect. In the first hour, drug release from microsponges was found to be between 17% and 31%. The cumulative percent release at the end of eighth hour was between 53 and 83%. The colon-specific tablets were prepared by compressing the microsponges followed by coating with pectin: hydroxypropyl methylcellulose mixture. In vitro release studies exhibited that compression-coated colon-specific formulations started releasing the drug at the sixth hour corresponding to the arrival time at colon.

In the same year, Dhawale et al. (2010) prepared fluorouracil-loaded porous microspheres for colonic delivery using pH - sensitive polymers Eudragit S 100 and L 100 by a simple oil /water emulsification process. Eudragit S100, pure or in mixture, was found to retain drug release at pH 4.5 less than 41% within 6 h. At pH 7.4, nearly immediate release (within 30 min) was observed for pure S100, while mixtures enabled to prolong the release slightly. However, the formulation proved its applicability in-vitro, as a promising device for pH-dependent colon delivery of 5-fluorouracil. The authors concluded development of porous microspheres, which can control the drug release up to 6 h and hence can prevent the acid decomposition in stomach. Later on, a report by our research group featured the development of colon specific microsponge based calcium-pectinate matrix tablet of meloxicam. The optimized colon-targeted tablet shielded meloxicam loaded microsponges in gastrointestinal region and selectively delivered them to colon, as visualized by vivo fluoroscopy in rabbits. The pharmacokinetic evaluation of the tablet (MS5T2) in rabbits, revealed appearance of drug appeared in plasma after a lag time of 7 h; a t_{max} of 30 h with Fr = 61.047%, thus presenting a formulation suitable for targeted colonic delivery. CLSM studies provided an evidence for colonic luminal retentive ability of microsponges at the end of 8 h upon oral administration of MS5T2. Thus a promising system for the colon-specific delivery of meloxicam was developed that has potential for use as an adjuvant therapy for colorectal cancer (Srivastava, Kumar, & Pathak, 2012).

Sareen et al developed and optimized the microsponges of curcumin for colon specific drug delivery in a view to bypass the upper GIT for enhanced therapeutic effect. The optimized formulation revealed that microsponges prevented the premature release of curcumin in upper GIT and specifically released the drug at colonic pH. Pharmacodynamic study of curcumin loaded microsponges caused a significant decrease in edema, necrosis, and hemorrhage of colon as compared to free curcumin in acetic acid induced colitis model in rats. The study proved that curcumin loaded microsponges may act as a promising drug delivery system for treatment of ulcerative colitis.

Another report on curcumin microsponges was published by our research group wherein the gastroretentive potential of microsponges was validated via optimization of targeted floating of curcumin microsponges for improved site specific absorption for gastric cancer. The in vitro permeation of curcumin through gastric mucin gel layer affirmed the capability of microsponges to deliver the drug across mucin and reach the target site to treat gastric cancer. Anticancer oral dose of microsponges was calculated as

50 mg by cytotoxicity assay in human cancer cell line KB. The pharmacokinetic evaluation of MS5 in rabbits revealed 10-fold increase in bioavailability as compared to native curcumin, and demonstrated the superiority of microsponges over native curcumin (Figure 2). The study presented a new approach based on floating ability of microsponges for treatment of gastric cancer.

Other research reports from our lab that validate the gastroretentive ability of microsponges include those on cinnarizine (Raghuvanshi & Pathak, 2016) and loratadine (Singh & Pathak, 2016). The interesting element of the publications was utilization of Acconon MC8-2 EP/NF as a bioadhesive material for developing modulated release bioadhesive gastroretentive microsponges of the actives. Bioadhesivity was also conferred by coating the microsponges with capmul GMO-50 and compared to bioadhesive microsponges prepared using Acconon MC8-2 EP/NF as bioadhesive raw material. Chemically, acconon MC 8-2 EP/NF is known as PEG-8 caprylic/capric glycerides. It is a mixture of monoesters, diesters, triesters of glycerol and monoesters, and diesters of polyoxyethylene glycol (Hansen, Neilsen, & Norling, 1999). The composition contains free macrogols as well. Both caprylic acid and polyethylene glycol/macrogol have been assessed to impart bioadhesive character (Gizurarson, 2004). The acconon MC 8-2 based microsponges displayed optimal in vitro buoyancy and bioadhesivity comparable to microsponges of cinnarizine made with EC (coated /uncoated) in dynamic in vitro bioadhesion test.

Delivery System for Biopharmaceuticals

The MDS is used for the delivery of biopharmaceuticals and in tissue engineering also. Sun et al.(2009) also investigated the potential of porous microspheres as injectable drug delivery system for controlled protein delivery. A new approach for protein delivery based on biodegradable porous PLGA microspheres blocked with calcium alginate hydrogel was introduced. Porous microspheres of three-dimensional network structure with interconnecting pores were prepared by solvent evaporation method using sodium oleate as an extractable porogen. Human serum albumin was adsorbed into micropores of porous microspheres by solution immersing method. The calcium alginate hydrogel was fabricated to block micropores of protein-loaded porous microspheres to achieve sustained protein release, in vitro. The authors claimed retention of protein's structural integrity and claimed potential application of porous microspheres for proteins, vaccines and gene delivery.

Three-dimensional scaffolds play an important role in tissue engineering as an adhesive substrate for implanted cells and a physical support to guide the formation of new organs. The scaffolds should facilitate cell adhesion, promote cell growth, allow the retention of differentiated cell functions, and be biocompatible, biodegradable, highly porous with a large surface-to-volume ratio, mechanically strong, and malleable. A cross section of applications of microsponges in tissue engineering is detailed in the preceding text. Bone substitute compounds were obtained by mixing pre-polymerized powders of polymethylmethacrylate and liquid methylmethacrylate monomer with two aqueous dispersions of a-tri calcium phosphate grains and calcium deficient hydroxyapatite powders. The final composites appeared to be porous and acted as microsponges (Berutoa, Bottera, & Milena, 2002). A biodegradable hybrid sponge of PLGA and collagen was fabricated by forming microsponges of collagen in the pores of PLGA sponge. The mechanical strength of the hybrid sponge was higher than that of either PLGA or collagen sponges, in both dry and wet states. The wettability with water was improved by hybridization with collagen, which facilitated cell seeding in the hybrid sponge. Mouse fibroblast L929 cells attached well and spread uniformly on the surfaces of the microsponges of collagen in the hybrid sponge. Use of the PLGA sponge as a skeleton facilitated formation of the hybrid sponge into desired shapes with high mechanical strength while collagen microsponges contributed good cell interaction and hydrophilicity; a useful tissue engineering application (Cheng, Ushida, & Tateishi, 2001).

Storage and release of endogenous growth factors by the extracellular matrix (ECM) are important biological events that control tissue homeostasis and regeneration. Kanematsu et al. (2004) in their investigation revealed that bFGF spontaneously interacts with type I collagen solution and sponges under *in vitro* and *in vivo* physiological conditions, and is protected from the proteolytic environment by the collagen. bFGF incorporated in a collagen sponge sheet was sustainedly released in the mouse subcutis corresponding to the biodegradation of the sponge matrix (Figure 4), and exhibited local angiogenic activity in a dose-dependent manner. Intramuscular injection of collagen microsponges incorporating bFGF induced a significant increase in the blood flow in the murine ischemic hindlimb, which could never have been attained by bolus injection of bFGF. These results suggest the significance and therapeutic utility of type I collagen as a reservoir of bFGF.

Biodegradable materials with autologous cell seeding have attracted much interest as potential cardiovascular grafts. However, pretreatment of these materials requires a complicated and invasive procedure that carries the risk of infection. A biodegradable graft material containing the collagen microsponge was developed for cardiovascular tissue grafting, as it would permit the regeneration of the autologous vessel tissue. The poly(lactic-co-glycolic acid)-collagen microsponge patch with and without precellularization showed good histologic findings and durability. This patch shows promise as a bioengineered material for promoting in situ cellularization and the regeneration of autologous tissue in cardiovascular surgery. (Iwai, Sawa, Ichikawa Taketani, Uchimura, Chen, Hara, Miyake, & Matsuda, 2004).

A thin biodegradable hybrid mesh synthetic PLGA and naturally derived collagen was for a three-dimensional culture of human skin fibroblasts. The hybrid mesh was constructed by forming web like collagen microsponges in the openings of a PLGA-knitted mesh. The results indicated that the web-like collagen microsponges formed in the openings of the PLGA knitted mesh increased the efficiency of cell seeding, improved cell distribution, and therefore facilitated rapid formation of dermal tissue having a uniform thickness. PLGA-collagen hybrid mesh may be useful for skin tissue engineering.

Advances in Microsponge Drug Delivery System

Various advances were made by modifying the methods to form nanosponges, nanoferrosponges and porous microbeads.

Nanosponges

Nanosponges are hyper-cross-linked cyclodextrins that can be synthesized using α, β and γ cyclodextrins, either alone or as mixtures, cross-linked with a suitable cross-linking agent. Interesting results have already been obtained as drug carriers by using an active carbonyl compound, e.g., carbonyldimiidazole, triphosgene, diphenyl carbonate, or organic dianhydrides.

Using ultrasound-assisted synthesis and an appropriate cross-linker molar ratio, spherical nanosponges (Figure 5a) of submicron size are obtained (Trotta, Cavalli, Tumiatti, Zerbinati, Roggero, & Vallero, 2006). The cross-linking produces a powder consisting of cyclodextrin connected by nanochannels to form a cage-like structure (Trotta & Tumiatti, 2003).

Nanosponges can be obtained by cross-linking different types of cyclodextrins (CD) with a carbonyl or a dicarboxylate compound as cross-linker (Trotta & Cavalli, 2009). The porous microparticles of cross-linked β -CD can serve as carrier for efficient loading of drugs. Obtained synthetically, these could be either in poorly crystalline (paracrystalline) or in crystalline form. These nano-structured materials can form inclusion and non-inclusion complexes with different compounds and forms a nanosuspension of rather uniform spherical shaped nanoparticles after dispersion in water under stirring. Structural characterization of nanosponges showed that the carbonate linkage is added to the primary hydroxyl groups of the parent β-CD unit. Thus, the drug molecules could be included inside the nanocavities of β-CD and due to the cross-linking further interactions of the guest molecules with more β-CD units might be thought. Moreover, the presence of the cross-linked network might also form nanochannels in the nanosponges structure for the polymer mesh (Cavalli et al. 2009). This peculiar structural organization might be responsible for the increased solubilization and protection capacities of nanosponges in comparison with the parent cyclodextrin. β-CD nanosponges can be used for hydropobic as well as hydrophilic drugs, in contrast to polymeric micro- or nanosponges.

By using different amounts of cross-linking agent, or by changing the type of cyclodextrin, it is possible to modulate the channels between the cyclodextrin molecules, thereby tuning the formation of the porous network and consequently affecting both the inclusion capacity and the solublizing ability of the nanosponges. Acid nanosponges carrying free carboxylic groups can be obtained using pyromellitic anhydride or other dianhydrides as a cross-linker, forming true cation exchange sites. The presence of free hydroxy groups in the nanosponges network allows further surface modification. For example carboxylated nanosponges can be obtained by reacting pristine carbonate nanosponges with succinic anhydride. The zeta potential of carbonate nanosponges is about −25 mV, which is sufficiently high to produce stable water suspension that does not undergo aggregation over time (Trotta, Zanetti, & Cavalli, 2012). For parenteral application it is possible to synthesize nanosponges with a mean diameter in the range of 200–300 nm with narrow size distribution.

Applications

The nanoporous structure of cyclodextrin nanosponges can be visualized as peculiar and versatile structure suitable for a broad range of potential and actual applications like water treatment, catalysis applications and in agriculture. By virtue of their biocompatibility and versatility, nanosponges have many potential applications in the pharmaceutical field. They can be used as excipients in preparing tablets, capsules, pellets, granules, suspensions, solid dispersions, or topical dosage forms (Ortega, Lorenzo, Concheiro, & Loftsson, 2012) or as new nanotechnological, multifunctional carriers. In particular, the design of new nanodelivery systems to improve drug administration is currently being studied. Many drugs show poor solubility, low permeability, a short half-life, low stability, and/or high molecular weight, and as a consequence their formulation is challenging.

Nanosponges have the capacity to incorporate drugs within their structure, either as inclusion complexes or as non-inclusion complexes. There are far more interaction sites available for incorporation within a nanosponge structure than in β-CD molecules, and they also show different mesh polarities (hydrophobic cyclodextrin cavities surrounded by hydrophilic nanochannels of the polymeric network) thereby enabling significant interactions between molecules with different lipophilicities and structures.

The ability of CD nanosponges to encapsulate drugs has been studied widely for both hydrophilic and lipophilic molecules, as shown in Table 5. When administered systemically, the nanosponges circulate around the body to reach the specific target site and adhere to it and initiate drug release a controlled and predictable manner. Another important character of these sponges is their aqueous solubility; this allows the use of these systems effectively for drugs with poor solubility (Selvamuthukumar, Anandam, Krishnamoorthy, & Rajappan, 2012). Poorly water soluble drugs, those belonging to BCS Class II (e.g. antihypertensives, immunosuppressants, cardiovascular drugs, antineoplastic agents etc) can be successfully delivered via nanosponges. The nanosponges may be formulated as oral, parenteral, topical or inhalation dosage forms. For the oral administration, the nanosponges may be dispersed in a matrix of excipients for the preparation of capsules or tablets. For the parenteral, administration they may be simply carried in sterile water, saline or other aqueous solutions and for topical administration they can be effectively incorporated into topical hydrogel.

The major limitation of these nanosponges is their ability to include only small molecules. The nanosponges could be either paracrystalline or in crystalline form. The loading capacity of nanosponges depends primarily on the degree of crystallization. Accordingly, paracrystalline nanosponges can show different loading capacities. By definition, paracrystalline materials are defined as having short and medium range ordering in their lattice (similar to the liquid crystal phases) but lacking crystal like long-range ordering at least in one direction (Voyles, Zotov, Nakhmanson, Drabold, Gibson, Treacy, & Keblinski, 2001).

Shankar et al. (2013) synthesized nanosponges by crosslinking of β- cyclodextrins (CDs) with diphenyl carbonate. It is a hyper-branched polymer with an ultra high encapsulation efficiency leading to formation of colloidal systems. Complexes of dexamethasone with three types of β –CD nanosponges were achieved with different cross-linking ratio. Nano-encapsulation was done by incubation-lyophilization technique to yield various formulations of nanosponges. Corneal permeability of dexamethasone from optimized formulation on excised bovine cornea in corneal holders showed that the nanosponge formulation showed higher permeability than the marketed formulation. Same research group fabricated β–CD nanosponges of resveratrol by reacting CD with a cross-linker such as carbonyldiimidazole. Resveratrol loaded nanosponges were in the size range between 400 to 500 nm with low polydispersity indices and high zeta potential. Cytotoxic studies on HCPC-I cell showed that resveratrol formulations were more cytotoxic than plain resveratrol. The permeation study indicates that the resveratrol nanosponge formulation showed good permeation in pigskin. The accumulation study in rabbit mucosa showed better accumulation of resveratrol nanosponge formulation than plain drug. These results signify that resveratrol nanosponge formulation can be used for buccal delivery and topical application (Ansari, Vavia, Trotta, & Cavalli, 2011).

Later on the research group proposed the application of nanosponges for protection of camptothecin from physicochemical degradation and for sustained release. In the study, the authors reported camptothecin loaded β-CD-based nanosponges obtained by the reaction of β-cyclodextrin with diphenylcarbonate. TEM measurements revealed mean particle size of about 400 nm and 900 nm for plain crystalline and paracrystalline nanosponges, respectively, and a size increase for the drug loaded crystalline nanosponges (450 nm). The nanosponges showed prolonged release profiles for 24 h. An initial burst effect due to non-complexed drug (3h), was followed by nearly linear and sustained release profiles of the drug (inclusion complexed drug) was observed. Camptothecin rapidly converts to the pharmacologically less active carboxylate form. The hydrolysis of camptothecin was slower when the drug was formulated in nanosponges compared to the plain drug. The complexation favoured the carboxylate/lactone-equilibrium towards the more hydrophobic active lactone form of the drug. Moreover, camptothecin loaded formulations showed negligible haemolytic activity and a strong cytotoxicity against HT-29 cells. The latter was correlated to the increased stability of the complexed drug. The lactone ring, as stated by the authors, is essential for passive diffusion of the drug into cancer cells (Swaminathan, Pastero, Serpe, Trotta, Vavia, Aquilano, Trotta, Zara, & Cavalli, 2010).

Swellable nanosponges of cyclodextrin-based poly(amidoamine) nanosponges were developed by cross linking β-CD with either 2,2-bis(acrylamidoacetic acid) or a short polyamido-amine chain deriving from 2,2-bis(acrylamidoacetic acid) and 2-methylpiperazine, respectively. The pH sensitive swellable nanosponges designed for protein delivery were used for encapsulating bovine serum albumin. High protein-complexation capacity (> 90%) was achieved for both the nanosponges and *in vitro* release depicted prolonged release of albumin (Ranucci, Ferruti, Manfredi, & Cavalli, 2012) from the two swellable β-CD-nanosponges over a period of 24 h. The researchers have also utilized the system to incorporate lysozyme that showed a high loading capacity. These lysozyme-loaded nanosponges released the enzyme at a pH-dependent rate with prolonged kinetics, whilst maintaining its biological activity

Nanoferrosponges

Nanoferrosponge is, a novel approach constituting self-pore forming carriers having better penetration to the targeted site due to the external magnetic trigger which enforces the carriers

to penetrate to the deeper tissue and then causing the removal of magnetic material from the particle leaving a porous system. Drug delivery from the magnetic sensitive ferrogels can be triggered by a non-contact force (an external magnetic field), which is superior to the traditional stimuli response polymers, such as pH or temperature sensitive polymer. By this concept, Magnetic Targeted Carriers have been designed which could adsorb pharmaceutical agents through application of an externally magnetic field for site specific targeting and sustained release of drugs (Fricker & Writer, 2001). A direct current magnetic field can be used to manipulate the drug release behaviors from a smart magnetic hydrogel through an on off switch of a magnetic field (Liu, Hu, Liu, Liu, & Chen, 2006). Magnetic-sensitive sponge hydrogel (ferrosponges) was developed by Hu et al. (2007). Two fundamentals were applied: Firstly, applying a "non-contact" external magnetic field to manipulate the drug release is considered robustic. Secondly, the porous structures (sponge) can improve the magnetic sensitivity because the magnetic nanoparticles are localized in a higher concentrate within thin polymeric walls (sponge's walls) than those spreading over the entire volume of the bulk or non-porous form. Furthermore, magnetic sensitive walls of ferrosponges constructed by magnetic nanoparticles can effectively reduce their wall permeability and decrease the drug release via a given magnetic field as shown in Figure 7.

Nano-ferrosponges with tunable magnetic sensitive behavior were successfully prepared by an in-situ synthesis of magnetic nanoparticles in the presence of gelatin. Nanopores with size ranging from 2 to 100 nm in diameter were synthesized within the magnetic nanoparticulate network. The nanopores were then manipulated to a reduced size by externally controlled magnetic field that allowed controlled release of active agent from ferrosponges. Release kinetics of a model drug, (vitamin B12) showed a series of tunable kinetic parameters under magnetization, and this finding allowed a slow release of drug molecules achievable for practical uses. The peculiar magnetic sensitive behaviors of the ferrosponges, can be used to design novel drug delivery system for medical uses.

Self Assembled Microsponge System

Lee et al. (2012) developed a self-assembled microsponge system for the delivery of short interfering RNA (siRNA). They reported the synthesis of a delivery vehicle that combines carrier and cargo: RNA interference (RNAi) polymers that self assemble into nanoscale pleated sheets of hairpin RNA, which in turn form sponge-like microspheres. The RNAi-microsponges consist entirely of cleavable RNA strands, and are processed by the cell's RNA machinery to convert the stable hairpin RNA to siRNA only after cellular uptake, thus inherently providing protection for siRNA during delivery and transport to the cytoplasm. More than half a million copies of siRNA can be delivered to a cell with the uptake of a single RNAi-microsponge. They also observed an improved stability of RNA and relatively effective encapsulation process of siRNA. The approach could lead to novel therapeutic routes for siRNA delivery. According to Grabow and Jaeger (2012) Self-assembled microsponges of hairpin RNA polymers achieve, with one thousand times lower concentration, the same degree of gene silencing in tumour-carrying mice as conventional nanoparticle-based siRNA delivery vehicles. However, when developing silencing therapeutics, the strength and duration of gene silencing needed for treatment may vary.

Porous Microbeads

Porous spherical beads, are classified on the basis of their pore size as macro-(>50 nm), meso- (50–2 nm) and microporous (< 20 nm). The porous nature and higher crosslinking degree differentiate them from gel-type polymer particles and confer them characteristics such as high surface area, ability to uptake various solvents with different polarity and increased brittleness. Various synthetic approaches have been reported for preparation of porous microbeads. Lindh et al (2016) utilized reductive amination technique to produce micrometer sized beads. The reductive amination of 2,3-dialdehyde cellulose beads with diaminaes produced micrometer-sized beads with porosity and increased specific surface area. Both aliphatic and aromatic diamines were found to be capable of producing porous micro beads with pores in the range of 10 to 100 nm.

El-Aassar et al., (2016) reported porous alginate microbeads containing silver nanoparticles (300µm) with strong antimicrobial activity compared to alginate/silver nanoparticles. Porous microbeads serve as scaffold to culture cells *in vitro* for improved implants and are thus utilized in tissue engineering. For the same PLGA porous microbeads were fabricated by introducing a phase separated emulsion into a simple fluidic device seeded with fibroblast. The fibroblast loaded PLGA microbeads were cultured into molds to desired shape. These fibroblast loaded PLGA microbeads were connected to neighboring beads by a network of cells and extracellular matrices to form the beginnings of a tissue construct inside the mold (Wang, 2011).

Future Prospects

Microsponge drug delivery system is a promising carrier that finds application pharmaceutical arena in terms of enhanced product performance and elegancy, extended release, improved drug release profile, reduced irritation, and improved physical, chemical and thermal stability. Controlled drug delivery systems comprising microsponges hold immense potential to reduce the dosing frequency, enable site-specific delivery, and increase the efficacy of the active compound and improving its safety. These microparticulate porous systems with a collapsible structure enable the improved drug entrapment; form a carrier system for chronotherapeutic drug delivery.

The real challenge lies in its development for the oral peptide delivery. New classes of pharmaceuticals, biopharmaceuticals (peptides, proteins and DNA-based therapeutics) are fueling the rapid evolution of drug delivery technology. The use of bioerodible and biodegradable polymers for the drug delivery is enabling safe delivery of the active(s).

As these porous systems have been explored for pulmonary drug delivery which indicates that these system effectively release drug even in the scarce dissolution fluid; thus colon could be an interesting site for targeted drug release. These carriers are also required to be developed for alternative drug administration routes like parenteral and pulmonary route. The particles can also be used as the cell culture media and thus can also be employed for stem cell culture and cellular regeneration in the body. These characteristic features of porous microspheres motivated the researchers to develop other such particles including nanosponges, nanoferrosponges and porous microbeads. These developments open new ways for drug delivery.

CONCLUSION

Microsponge delivery system that was developed for topical drug delivery has emerged as a carrier for controlled oral drug delivery. Various researchers have explained the potential of microsponges for targeting the drug molecule to the various parts of gastrointestinal tract including ascending colon and stomach. The carrier system also helped in increasing the stability of drug in formulation. The real challenge of microsponge delivery system is its utilization for the delivery of biopharmaceuticals. The system has also evolved as variants namely nanosponges, nanoferrosponges and porous microbeads that have widened the characteristics and applications of the delivery system. The research arena of micro-/nanosponges holds promise for extensive research for further development of technology for pharmaceutical and cosmetic applications.

REFERENCES

Anderson, D. L., Cheng, C. H., & Nacht, S. (1994). Flow characteristics of loosely compacted macroporous microsponge polymeric systems. *Powder Technology*, *78*(1), 15–18. doi:10.1016/0032-5910(93)02764-2

Ansari, K. A., Vavia, P. R., Trotta, F., & Cavalli, R. (2011). Cyclodextrin-based nanosponges for delivery of resveratrol: In vitro characterization, stability, cytotoxicity and permeation study. *AAPS PharmSciTech*, *12*(1), 279–286. doi:10.120812249-011-9584-3 PMID:21240574

Aritomi, H., Yamasaki, Y., Yamada, K., Honda, H., & Koshi, M. (1996). Development of sustained release formulation of chlorpheniramine maleate using powder coated microsponges prepared by dry impact blending method. *Journal of Pharmaceutical Science and Technology*, *56*(1), 49–56.

Arya, P., & Pathak, K. (n.d.). Assessing the viability of microsponges as gastro retentive drug delivery system of curcumin: Optimization and pharmacokinetics. *International Journal of Pharmaceutics*, *2*, 1–12. PMID:24184218

Asghar, L. F. A., & Chandran, S. (2006). Multiparticulate formulation approach to colon specific drug delivery: Current perspectives. *Journal of Pharmacy & Pharmaceutical Sciences*, *9*(3), 327–338. PMID:17207416

Bae, S. E., Son, J. S., Park, K., & Han, D. K. (2009). Fabrication of covered porous PLGA microspheres using hydrogen peroxide for controlled drug delivery and regenerative medicine. *Journal of Controlled Release*, *133*(1), 37–43. doi:10.1016/j.jconrel.2008.09.006 PMID:18838089

Berutoa, D. T., Bottera, R., & Milena, M. (2002). The effect of water in inorganic microsponges of calcium phosphates on the porosity and permeability of composites made with polymethylmethacrylate. *Biomaterials*, *23*(12), 2509–2517. doi:10.1016/S0142-9612(01)00385-4 PMID:12033598

Cavalli, R., Trotta, F., & Tumiatti, W. (2006). Cyclodextrin-based nanosponges for drug delivery. *Journal of Inclusion Phenomena and Macrocyclic Chemistry*, *56*(1-2), 209–213. doi:10.100710847-006-9085-2

Cavalli, R., Trotta, F., Tumiatti, W., Serpe, L., & Zara, G. P. (2006). 5-Fluorouracile loaded β-cyclodextrin nanosponges: invitro characterization and cytotoxicity. *International Cyclodextrin Symposium*, *13*, 207.

Chadawar, V., & Shaji, J. (2007). Microsponge delivery system. *Current Drug Delivery*, *4*(2), 123–129. doi:10.2174/156720107780362320 PMID:17456031

Chen, G., Sato, T., Ohgusi, H., Ushida, T., Tateishi, T., & Tanaka, J. (2005). Culturing of skin fibroblasts in a thin PLGA_collagen hybrid mesh. *Biomaterials*, *26*(15), 2559–2566. doi:10.1016/j.biomaterials.2004.07.034 PMID:15585258

Cheng, G., Ushida, T., & Tateishi, T. (2000, August). A Biodegradable Hybrid Sponge Nested with collagen microsponges. *Journal of Biomedical Materials Research*, *51*(2), 273–279. doi: PMID:10825227

Comoglu, C. T., Gonul, N., & Baykara, T. Preparation and *in vitro* evaluation of modified release ketoprofen microsponges. *ILFarmaco, 58,* 101–106.

Comoglu, T., Gonul, N., & Baykara, T. (2002). The effects of pressure and direct compression on tabletting of microsponges. *International Journal of Pharmaceutics*, *242*(1-2), 191–195. doi:10.1016/S0378-5173(02)00155-2 PMID:12176245

Del, R. J. Q. (2009). Benzoyl peroxide formulations: What is the science supporting microsphere vehicle technology and clinical use. *The Journal of Clinical and Aesthetic Dermatology*, *2*(9), 46–54. PMID:20729960

Devrim, B., & Canefe, K. (2006). Preparation and evaluation of modified release ibuprofen microspheres with acrylic polymers (Eudragit) by quasi-emulsion solvent diffusion method: Effect of variables. *Acta Poloniae Pharmaceutica*, *63*(6), 521–534. PMID:17438870

Dhawale, S. C., Bankar, A. S., & Patro, M. N. (2010). Formulation and evaluation porous microspheres of 5- Fluorouracil for colon targeting. *International Journal of Pharm Tech Research*, *2*(2), 1112–1118.

El-Aassar, M. R., & Mo, X. (2016). Development of porous alginate microbeads containing silver nanoparticles and their antibacterial efficacy. *Advances in Polymer Technology*, *35*(3), 298–306. doi:10.1002/adv.21555

Embil, K., & Nacht, S. (1996). The microsponge delivery system (MDS) a Topical Delivery System with reduced irritancy incorporating multiple triggering Mechanisms for the release of actives. *Journal of Microencapsulation*, *13*(5), 575–588. doi:10.3109/02652049609026042 PMID:8864994

Embil, V. P. (2000). OTC external analgesic cream/topical analgesic anti-inflammatory, counter irritant utilizing the microsponge delivery system for controlled release of actives. *UK Patent 01010586.*

Fricker, J., & Writer, F. (2001). Drugs with a magnetic attraction to tumours. *Drug Discovery Today, 6*(8), 387–389. doi:10.1016/S1359-6446(01)01771-8 PMID:11301276

Gans, E. H. (1999). Polymer developments of cosmetic interest. *Cosmetics & Toiletries, 114*, 53–60.

Giovagnoli, S., Blasi, P., Schoubben, A., Rossi, C., & Ricci, M. (2007). Preparation of large porous biodegradable microspheres by using a simple double-emulsion method for capreomycin sulfate pulmonary delivery. *International Journal of Pharmaceutics, 333*(1-2), 103–111. doi:10.1016/j.ijpharm.2006.10.005 PMID:17079101

Gizurarson, S. (2004). A bioadhesive agent. *European Patent 1480673A1.*

Gollnick, H. P. M., & Krautheim, A. (2003). Topical Treatment in Acne: Current Status and Future Aspects. *Dermatology (Basel, Switzerland), 206*(1), 29–36. doi:10.1159/000067820 PMID:12566803

Goyel, M., Prajapati, R., Purohit, K. K., & Mehta, S. C. (2010). Floating drug delivery system. *Journal of Current Pharma Research, 5*, 7–18.

Grabow, W. W., & Jaeger, L. (2012). siRNA delivery: Loaded-up microsponges. *Nature Materials, 11*(4), 268–269. doi:10.1038/nmat3286 PMID:22437781

Grimes, P. E. (2004). A microsponge formulation of hydroquinone 4% and retinol 0.15% in the treatment of melasma and post inflammatory hyperpigmentation. *Cutis, 74*(6), 362–368. PMID:15663072

Hansen, J., Neilsen, L. S., & Norling, T. (1999). Use of fatty acid esters as bioadhesive substances. *U.S. Patent 5955502A.*

Hu, S. H., Liu, T. Y., Liu, D. M., & Chen, S. Y. (2007). Nanoferrosponges for controlled drug release. *Journal of Controlled Release, 121*(3), 181–189. doi:10.1016/j.jconrel.2007.06.002 PMID:17644206

Iwai, S., Sawa, Y., Ichikawa, H., Taketani, S., Uchimura, E., Chen, G., ... Matsuda, H. (2004). Biodegradable polymer with collagen microsponge serves as a new bioengineered cardiovascular prosthesis. *The Journal of Thoracic and Cardiovascular Surgery, 128*(3), 472–479. doi:10.1016/j.jtcvs.2004.04.013 PMID:15354111

Jain, V., Jain, D., & Singh, R. (2010). Factors affecting the morphology of Eudragit RS100 based microsponges bearing dicyclomine for colonic delivery. *Journal of Pharmaceutical Sciences, 100*(4), 1–8. PMID:20960455

Jain, V., & Singh, R. (2010). Development and characterization of Eudragit RS 100 loaded microsponges and its colonic delivery using natural polysaccharides. *Acta Poloniae Pharma-Drug Research, 67*, 407–415. PMID:20635537

Jain, V., & Singh, R. (2010). Dicyclomine loaded Eudragit based microsponge with potential for colonic delivery: Preparation and characterization. *Tropical Journal of Pharmaceutical Research, 9*(1), 67–72. doi:10.4314/tjpr.v9i1.52039

Jelvehgari, M., Siahi-Shadbad, M. R., Azarmi, S., Martin, G. P., & Nokhodchi, A. (2006). The microsponge delivery system of benzoyl peroxide: Preparation, characterization and release studies. *International Journal of Pharmaceutics*, *308*(1-2), 124–132. doi:10.1016/j.ijpharm.2005.11.001 PMID:16359833

Kaity, S., Maiti, S., Ghosh, A. K., Pal, D., Ghosh, A., & Banerjee, S. (2010). Microsponges: A novel strategy for drug delivery system. *Journal of Advanced Pharmaceutical Technology & Research*, *1*(3), 283–290. doi:10.4103/0110-5558.72416 PMID:22247859

Kanematsu, A., Marui, A., Yamamoto, S., Ozeki, K., Hirano, Y., Yamamoto, M., ... Tabata, Y. (2004, September). Type 1 collagen can function as a reservoir of basic fibroblast growth factor. *Journal of Controlled Release*, *99*(2), 281–292. doi:10.1016/j.jconrel.2004.07.008 PMID:15380637

Katz, M. A., Cheng, C. H., & Nacht, S. (1999). Methods and composition for topical delivery of benzoyl peroxide. US5879716.

Kawashima, Y., Niwa, T., Handa, T., Takeuchi, H., Iwamoto, T., & Itoh, K. (n.d.). Preparation of controlled-release microspheres of ibuprofen with acrylic polymers by a novel quasi-emulsion solvent diffusion method. Journal of Pharmaceutical Sciences, 78, 68–72.

Kawashima, Y., Niwa, T., Takeuchi, H., Hino, T., & Itoh, Y. (1992). Control of prolonged drug release and compression properties of ibuprofen microsponges with acrylic polymer, Eudragit RS, by changing their intraparticle density. *Chemical & Pharmaceutical Bulletin*, *40*(1), 196–201. doi:10.1248/cpb.40.196 PMID:1576674

Khopade, A. J., Jain, S., & Jain, N. K. (1996). The microsponge. *Eastern Pharmacist*, *39*, 49–53.

Lee, J. B., Hong, J., Bonner, D. K., Poon, Z., & Hammond, P. T. (2012). Self-assembled RNA interference microsponges for efficient siRNA delivery. *Nature Materials*, *11*(4), 316–322. doi:10.1038/nmat3253 PMID:22367004

Leyden, J. J., Tanghetti, E. A., Miller, B., Ung, M., Berson, D., & Lee, J. (2002). Once daily tazarotene 0.1% gel versus once-daily tretinoin 0.1% microsponge gel for the treatment of facial acne vulgaris: A double-blind randomized trial. *Cutis*, *69*, 12–19. PMID:12095064

Lindh, J., Ruan, C., Strømme, M., & Mihranyan, A. (2016). Preparation of porous cellulose beads via introduction of diamine spacers. *Langmuir*, *32*(22), 5600–5607. doi:10.1021/acs.langmuir.6b01288 PMID:27181427

Liu, L. S., Liu, S. Q., Ng, S. Y., Froix, M., Ohno, T., & Heller, J. (1997). Controlled release of interleukin-2 for tumour immunotherapy using alginate/chitosan porous microspheres. *Journal of Controlled Release*, *43*(1), 65–74. doi:10.1016/S0168-3659(96)01471-X

Liu, T. Y., Hu, S. H., Liu, K. H., Liu, D. M., & Chen, S. Y. (2006). Preparation and characterization of smart magnetic hydrogels and its use for drug release. *Journal of Magnetism and Magnetic Materials*, *304*(1), e397–e399. doi:10.1016/j.jmmm.2006.01.203

Maiti, S., Kaity, S., Ray, S., & Sa, B. (2011). Development and evaluation of xanthan gum-facilitated ethyl cellulose microsponges for controlled percutaneous delivery of diclofenac sodium. *Acta Pharmaceutica (Zagreb, Croatia)*, *61*(3), 257–270. doi:10.2478/v10007-011-0022-6 PMID:21945905

Mandal, T. K., Bostanian, L. A., Graves, R. A., Chapman, S. R., & Idodo, T. U. (2001). Porous biodegradable microparticles for delivery of pentamidine. *European Journal of Pharmaceutics and Biopharmaceutics*, *52*(1), 91–96. doi:10.1016/S0939-6411(01)00150-3 PMID:11438428

Mognetti, B., Barberis, A., Marino, S., Berta, G., Francia, D. S., Trotta, F., & Cavalli, R. J. (2012). *In vitro* enhancement of anticancer activity of paclitaxel by a Cremophor free cyclodextrin-based nanosponge formulation. *Journal of Inclusion Phenomena and Macrocyclic Chemistry*, *74*(1-4), 201–210. doi:10.100710847-011-0101-9

Nacht, S., & Kantz, M. (1992). The microsponge: A novel topical programmable delivery system. *Topical Drug Delivery Systems*, *42*, 299–325.

Nokhodchi, A., Jelvehgari, M., & Mozafari, M. (2007). Factors affecting the morphology of benzoyl peroxide microsponges. *Micron (Oxford, England)*, *38*(8), 834–840. doi:10.1016/j.micron.2007.06.012 PMID:17692528

Orlu, M., Cevher, E., & Araman, A. (2006). Design and evaluation of colon specific drug delivery system containing flurbiprofen microsponges. *International Journal of Pharmaceutics*, *318*(1-2), 103–117. doi:10.1016/j.ijpharm.2006.03.025 PMID:16687222

Ortega, M. M. D., Lorenzo, A. C., Concheiro, A., & Loftsson, T. (2012, May). Cyclodextrin-based nanogels for pharmaceutical and biomedical applications. *International Journal of Pharmaceutics*, *428*(1-2), 152–163. doi:10.1016/j.ijpharm.2012.02.038 PMID:22388054

Pancholi, K., Ahras, N., Stride, E., Edirisinghe, M. J., & Samarasinghe, S. (2009). Novel electrohydrodynamic preparation of porous chitosan particles for drug delivery. *Journal of Materials Science. Materials in Medicine*, *20*(4), 917–923. doi:10.100710856-008-3638-4 PMID:19034624

Raghuvanshi, S., & Pathak, K. (2016). Bioadhesive floating microsponges of cinnarizine as novel gastroretentive delivery: Capmul GMO bioadhesive coating and acconon MC 8-2 EP/NF as bioadhesive raw material. *International Journal of Pharmaceutical Investigation*, *6*(4), 181–193. doi:10.4103/2230-973X.195923 PMID:28123987

Ranucci, E., Ferruti, P., Manfredi, A., & Cavalli, R. (2012). Cross-linked resins by stepwise polyaddition of β-cyclodextrin with bisacrylamides and assessment of their potential as ph-sensitive NPs for site-specific protein delivery. *Proceedings CRS 2012*, 99.

Rao, M., Bajaj, A., Khole, I., Mumjapara, G., & Trotta, F. (2013). In vitro and in vivo evaluation of β-cyclodextrin based nanosponges of telmisartan. *Journal of Inclusion Phenomena and Macrocyclic Chemistry*, *77*(1-4), 135–145. doi:10.100710847-012-0224-7

Rawat, A., Majumder, Q. H., & Ahsan, F. (2008). Inhalable large porous microspheres of low molecular weight heparin: In vitro and in vivo evaluation. *Journal of Controlled Release*, *128*(3), 224–232. doi:10.1016/j.jconrel.2008.03.013 PMID:18471921

Rizkalla, C. M. Z., Aziz, R. L., & Soliman, I. I. (2011). In vitro and in vivo evaluation of hydroxyzine hydrochloride microsponges for topical delivery. *AAPS PharmaScitech*, *12*(3), 989–1001. doi:10.120812249-011-9663-5 PMID:21800216

Sapino, S., Carlotti, M. E., Cavalli, R., Ugazio, E., Berlier, G., Gastaldi, L., & Morel, S. (2013). Photochemical and antioxidant properties of gamma-oryzanol in beta-cyclodextrin-based nanosponges. *Journal of Inclusion Phenomena and Macrocyclic Chemistry*, *75*(1-2), 69–76. doi:10.100710847-012-0147-3

Sareen, R., Nath, K., Jain, N., & Dhar, K. L. (2014). Curcumin loaded microsponges for colon targeting in inflammatory bowel disease: Fabrication, optimization, and *in vitro* and pharmacodynamic evaluation. *BioMed Research International*, *2014*, 1–8. doi:10.1155/2014/340701 PMID:25093165

Selvamuthukumar, S., Anandam, S., Krishnamoorthy, K., & Rajappan, M. (2012). Nanosponges: A novel class of drug delivery system—review. *Journal of Pharmacy & Pharmaceutical Sciences*, *15*(1), 103–111. doi:10.18433/J3K308 PMID:22365092

Shah, V. P., Elkins, J., Lam, S.-Y., & Skelly, J. P. (1989). Determination of *in-vitro* release from hydrocortisone creams. *International Journal of Pharmaceutics*, *53*(1), 53–59. doi:10.1016/0378-5173(89)90361-X

Sharma, R., & Pathak, K. (2011). Polymeric nanosponges as an alternative carrier for improved retention of econazole nitrate on to the skin through topical hydrogel formulation. *Pharmaceutical Development and Technology*, *16*(4), 367–376. doi:10.3109/10837451003739289 PMID:20367024

Singh, S., & Pathak, K. (2016). Assessing the bioadhesivity of Acconon MC 8-2 EP/NF for gastroretention of floating microsponges of loratadine and achieving controlled drug delivery. *Pharmaceutical and Biomedical Research*, *2*(2), 58–74. doi:10.18869/acadpub.pbr.2.2.58

Smith, S., Morhenn, V., & Webster, G. (2006). The characteristics and utility of solid phase porous microspheres: A review. *Journal of Drugs in Dermatology*, *5*(10), 969–974. PMID:17373146

Solanki, B., Patel, R., Barot, B., Parijiya, P., & Shelat, P. (2012). Multiple unit dosage form: A review. *Ph Tech Med*, *1*, 11–21.

Srivastava, R., Kumar, D., & Pathak, K. (2010). Colonic luminal surface retention of meloxicam microsponges delivered by erosion based colon targeted matrix tablet. *International Journal of Pharmaceutics*, *427*(2), 153–162. doi:10.1016/j.ijpharm.2012.01.036 PMID:22306039

Srivastava, R., & Pathak, K. (2012). Microsponges: A futuristic approach for drug delivery. *Expert Opinion on Drug Delivery*, *9*(7), 863–878. doi:10.1517/17425247.2012.693072 PMID:22663167

Summary Basis of Approval Retin-A Micro 0.1%. (n.d.). Available at: www.accessdata.FDA.com

Sun, L., Zhou, S., Wang, W., Li, X., Wang, J., & Weng, J. (2009). Preparation and characterization of porous biodegradable microspheres used for controlled protein delivery. *Colloids and Surfaces. A, Physicochemical and Engineering Aspects*, *345*(1-3), 173–181. doi:10.1016/j.colsurfa.2009.04.053

Swaminathan, S., Pastero, L., Serpe, L., Trotta, F., Vavia, P., Aquilano, D., ... Cavalli, R. (2010). Cyclodextrin-based nanosponges encapsulating camptothecin: Physicochemical characterization, stability and cytotoxicity. *European Journal of Pharmaceutics and Biopharmaceutics*, *74*(2), 193–201. doi:10.1016/j.ejpb.2009.11.003 PMID:19900544

Swaminathan, S., Vavia, P. R., Trotta, F., & Roberta, C. (2013, June 01). Nanosponges encapsulating dexamethasone for ocular delivery: Formulation design, physicochemical characterization, safety and corneal permeability assessment. *Journal of Biomedical Nanotechnology*, *9*(6), 998–1007. doi:10.1166/jbn.2013.1594 PMID:23858964

Swaminathan, S., Vavia, P. R., Trotta, F., & Torne, S. (2007). Formulation of betacyclodextrin based nanosponges of itraconazole. *Journal of Inclusion Phenomena and Macrocyclic Chemistry*, *57*(1-4), 89–94. doi:10.100710847-006-9216-9

Torne, S., Darandale, S., Vavia, P., Trotta, F., & Cavalli, R. (2013). Cyclodextrin-based nanosponges: Effective nanocarrier for tamoxifen delivery. *Pharmaceutical Development and Technology*, *18*(3), 619–625. doi:10.3109/10837450.2011.649855 PMID:22235935

Torne, S. J., Ansari, K. A., Vavia, P. R., Trotta, F., & Cavalli, R. (2010). Enhanced oral paclitaxel bioavailability after administration of paclitaxel-loaded nanosponges. *Drug Delivery*, *17*(6), 419–425. doi:10.3109/10717541003777233 PMID:20429848

Trotta, F., & Cavalli, R. (2009). Characterization and application of new hyper-cross-linked cyclodextrins. *Composite Interfaces*, *16*(1), 39–48. doi:10.1163/156855408X379388

Trotta, F., Cavalli, R., Tumiatti, W., Zerbinati, O., Roggero, C., & Vallero, R. (2006). Ultrasound assisted synthesis of cyclodextrin based nanosponges. *WO 0002814 A1*.

Trotta, F., & Tumiatti, W. (2003). Cross-linked polymers based on cyclodextrins for removing polluting agents. *WO 03/085002 A1*.

Trotta, F., Zanetti, M., & Cavalli, R. (2012). Cyclodextrin-based nanosponges as drug carriers. *Beilstein Journal of Organic Chemistry*, *8*, 2091–2099. doi:10.3762/bjoc.8.235 PMID:23243470

Ukita, K., Kuroda, M., Honda, H., & Koishi, M. (1989). Characterization of powder coated microsponge prepared by dry impact blending method. *Chemical & Pharmaceutical Bulletin*, *37*(12), 3367–3371. doi:10.1248/cpb.37.3367

Vavia, P. R., Swaminathan, S., Trotta, F., & Cavalli, R. (2006). Applications of nanosponges in drug delivery. *Proceedings XIII International Cyclodextrin Symposium*, p. 207.

Voyles, P. M., Zotov, N., Nakhmanson, S. M., Drabold, D. A., Gibson, J. M., Treacy, M. M. J., & Keblinski, P. (2001). Structure and physical properties of paracrystalline atomistic models of amorphous silicon. *Journal of Applied Physics*, *90*(9), 4437–4451. doi:10.1063/1.1407319

Wang, J. (2011). Porous microbeads as three-dimensional scaffold for tissue engineering. *NNIN Reu Research Accomplished*, 32-33.

Wester, R., Patel, R., Natch, S., Leyden, J., Melendres, J., & Maibach, H. (1991). Controlled release of benzoyl peroxide from a porous microsphere polymeric system can reduce topical irritancy. *Journal of the American Academy of Dermatology*, *24*(5), 720–726. doi:10.1016/0190-9622(91)70109-F PMID:1869643

APPENDIX: FIGURES AND TABLES

Table 1. Characteristics of microsponges and the active pharmaceutical ingredient to be incorporated therein

Characteristics of Microsponges Aritomi et al. (1996)	Characteristics of Active Ingredients Kawashima et al. (1992)
• Stable over a pH range of 1 to 11 • Stable up to 130° C temperature • Compatible with the many of the vehicles and active ingredients • Self-sterilizing as their average pore size is 0.25μm where bacteria cannot penetrate • Higher pay load (50 to 60%) • Free flowing and cost effective	• It should be miscible in monomer. • Miscible by addition of small amount of a water immiscible solvent. • It should be water immiscible or at most only slightly soluble. • It should be inert to monomers. • It should be stable in contact with polymerization catalyst and conditions of polymerization.

Table 2. Evaluation parameters for microsponges

Parameter	Method/ Equipment
Particle Size	Laser light diffractometry
Morphology and Surface Topography	SEM/TEM
True density	Pycnometer
Pore structure	Mercury intrusion porosimetry
Compatibility	TLC and FTIR
Effect of polymerization on crystallinity of the drug	XRD and DSC
Polymer / Monomer Composition	Assessment of release profiles
Resiliency (viscoelastic properties)	Monitoring drug release
Drug release	Dissolution test apparatus/ Franz diffusion cell
Safety Considerations	• Skin/ eye irritation studies in rabbits • Oral toxicity studies in rats • Mutagenicity in bacteria • Allergenicity in guinea pigs

Table 3. Therapeutic category wise applications of microsponges

Category	Applications
Sunscreens	Long lasting product efficacy, improved protection against sunburns and sun related injuries even at elevated concentration, reduced irritancy and sensitization.
Anti-acne agents	Enhanced efficacy with decreased skin irritation and sensitization.
Antiinflammatory	Long lasting activity with reduction of skin allergic response and dermatoses.
Antifungals	Sustained release of actives.
Antidandruff agents	Reduced unpleasant odour. lower irritation, extended safety and efficacy.
Antipruritics	Extended and improved activity.
Skin depigmenting agents	Improved stabilization against oxidation with improved efficacy.
Rubefacients	Prolonged activity, reduced irritancy greasiness and odour.

Table 4. A cross section of marketed formulations of microsponges

Product Name	Description	Manufacturer
Retin-A-Micro	0.1 and 0.04% tretinoin entrapped in MDS, for topical treatment of acne vulgaris. Uses patented methyl methacrylate/glycol+ dimethacrylate cross-polymer porous microspheres.	Ortho-McNeil Pharmaceutical, Inc., Raritan, New Jersey, United States.
Carac Cream	Contains 0.5% fluorouracil, with 0.35% being incorporated into microsponge composed of methyl methacrylate/glycol dimethacrylate cross-polymer and dimethicone.	Dermik Laboratories, Inc. Berwyn,PA19312 USA
Biomedic Retinol Cream	The retinol the microsponge system helps to maximize the retinol dosage, while reducing the possibility of irritation.	La Roche Posay, Singapore
Retinol 15 Nightcream	The cream with microsponge system contains pure retinol for diminishment of fine lines and wrinkles, and improvement in skin discoloration.	Sothys, Paris, France
EpiQuin™ Micro and EpiQuin™ Micro XD	Contains hydroquinone 4% and retinol incorporated into MDS composed of methyl methacrylate/glycol dimethacrylate crosspolymer.	Skin Medica Inc, Inc. Carlsbad, CA 9200,
Sports Cream RS and XS	Topical analgesic-anti-inflammatory and counterirritant actives in a MDS for management of musculoskeletal conditions	Embil Pharmaceutical Co, Ltd,Turkey.
Salicylic Peel 20 and 30	Salicylic acid 20% and 30%, Microsponge Technology. Excellent exfoliation	Biophora, Toronto, Canada
Micro Peel Plus	The Micro peel® Plus, stimulates cell turnover through the application of salicylic acid in the form of microcrystals using Microsponge® technology.	Southeastern Oral Maxillofacial & Facial Cosmetic Surgery center, P. C. Alabama
Solar Defense Oil Free Matte Block Spf-20	Ultra-sheer, weightless lotion that provides UVA and UVB protection. Microsponge technology absorbs and controls oil, maintaining an all day matte finish and preventing shine.	Dermalogica, California US
Dermalogica Oil Control Lotion	A feather-light lotion, formulated with oil absorbing Microsponge® technology and hydrating botanicals. The naturally antiseptic skin response complex helps soothe the skin.	Dermalogica, California US
Aramis Fragrances	A 24 h high performance antiperspirant spray sustained release of fragrance in the microsponge. The microsponge comes in the form of an ultra light powder, it can absorb fragrant oil easily, while maintaining a free-flowing powder characteristic where release is controlled due to moisture and temperature.	Aramis Inc, NY, US
Shine Stopper	This oil-absorbing primer gives a soft, powder-like finish. The unique Microsponge® technology keeps oily skin shine-free for up to 6 hours, whilc minimising thc appearance of pores.	Paula's Choice, Seattle, WA 98104, USA.

Table 5. A cross section of drugs formulated as cyclodextrin nanosponges

Drug	Therapeutic Category	Route of Administration	Reference
Doxorubicin	Antineoplastic	Parenteral	Trotta and Cavalli (2009)
Itraconazole	Antifungal	Topical	Swaminathan et al. 2010)
Flurbiprofen	Antiinflammatory	Oral	Trotta and Cavalli (2009)
Progesterone	Hormonal	Oral	Trotta and Cavalli (2009)
Paclitaxel	Antineoplastic	Oral	Torne et al. (2010)
5-flurouracil	Antineoplastic	Parenteral, topical	Dhawale et al (2010) Cavalli et al, (2006)
Tamoxifen	Antiestrogenoral	Oral	Torne et al. (2013)
Omeprazole	Antiulcerative	Oral	Vavia et al, (2006)
γ- oryizanol	Antioxidant	Topical	Sapino et al (2013)
Dexamethasone	Antiinflammatory	Parenteral	Trotta and Cavalli (2009)
Temisartan	Antihypertensive	Oral	Rao et al (2013)
Econazole nitrate	Antifungal	topical	Sharma and Pathak (2011)

Figure 1. Scanning electron micrographs of microsponges. The magnified view shows the porous surface of the microsponge.

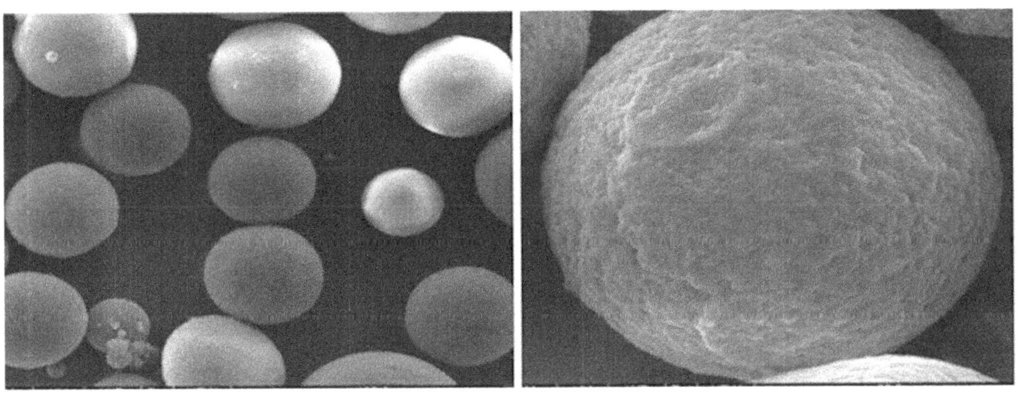

Figure 2. Plasma concentration versus time plot of curcumin in rabbits following oral administration of curcumin (suspension) and optimized microsponge formulation in fed state of stomach.

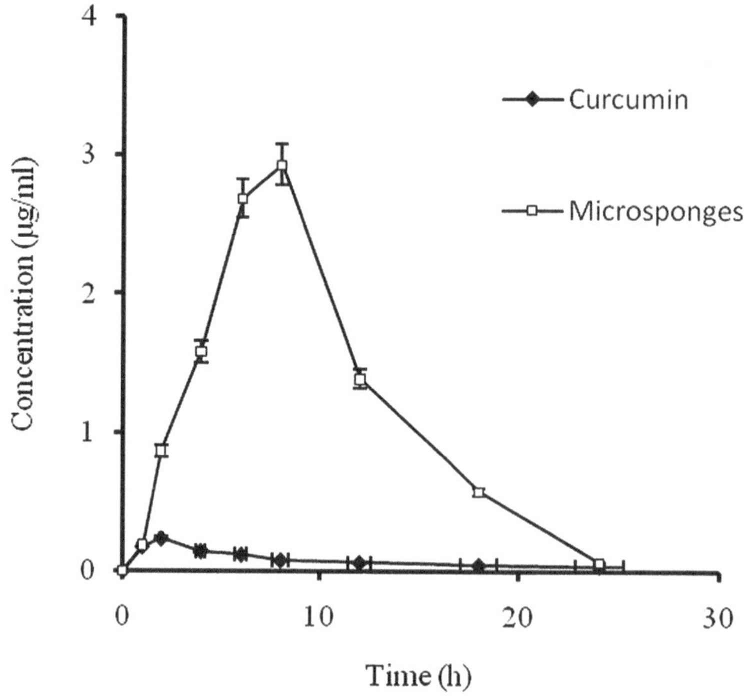

Figure 3. (A) Uncoated microsponges; (B) Capmul GMO coated bioadhesive microsponges of cinnarazine

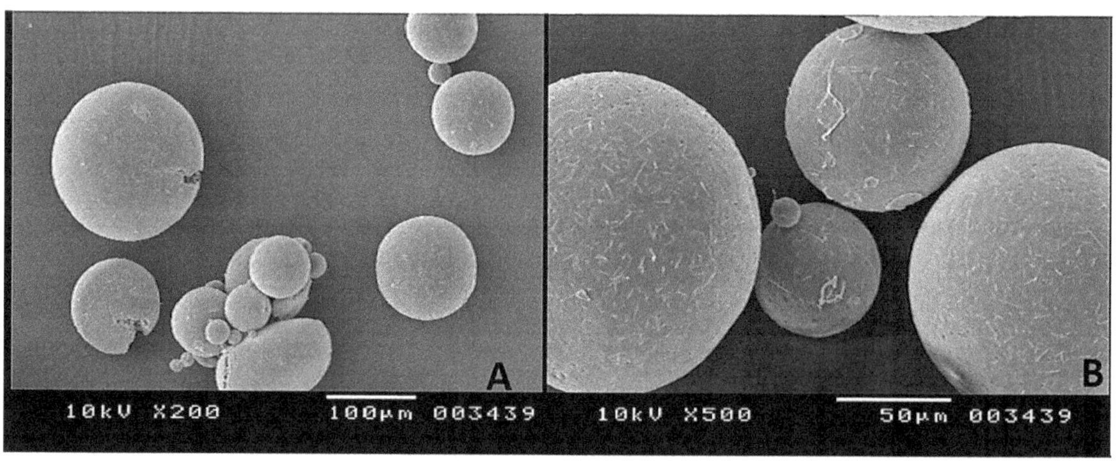

Figure 4. Schematic representation of bFGF incorporated in a collagen sponge sheet for sustained release in the mouse subcutis corresponding to the biodegradation of the sponge matrix.

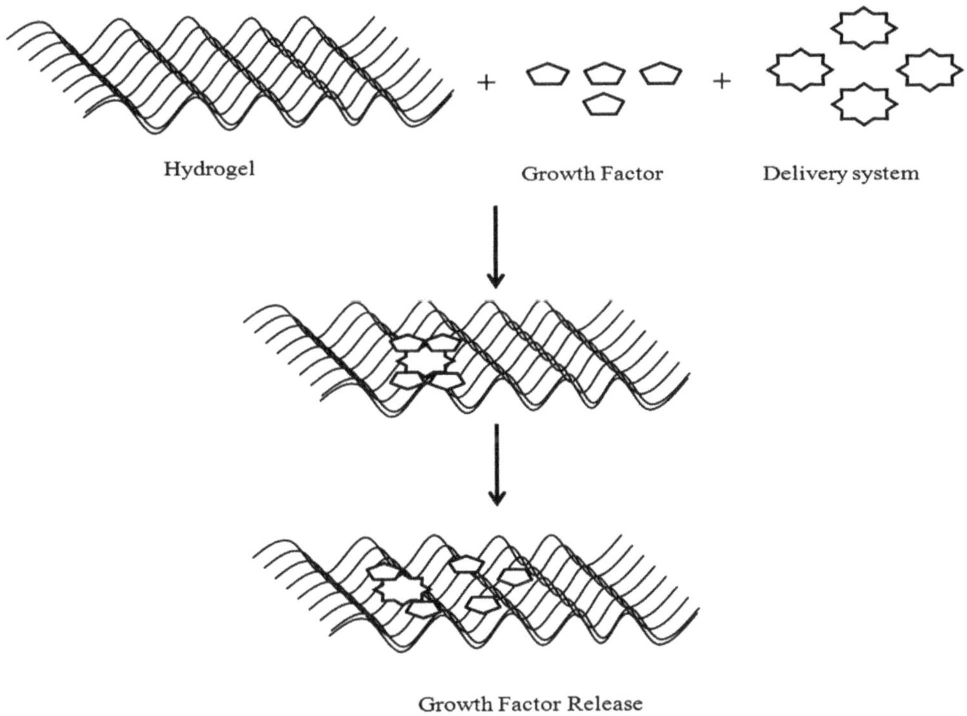

Figure 5. (A) SEM of nanosponges; (B) Diagrammatic representation of inclusion complexation of drug in nanocavity of cyclodextrin molecule.

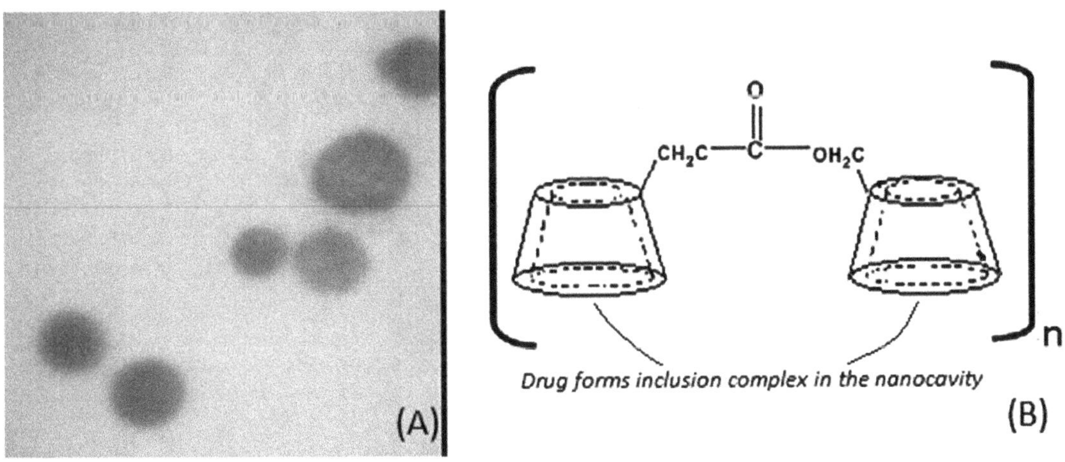

Figure 6. Synthetic routes to cyclodextrin nanosponges (A) Cyclodextrin carbonate nanosponges (B) Cyclodextrin carboxylate nanosponges.

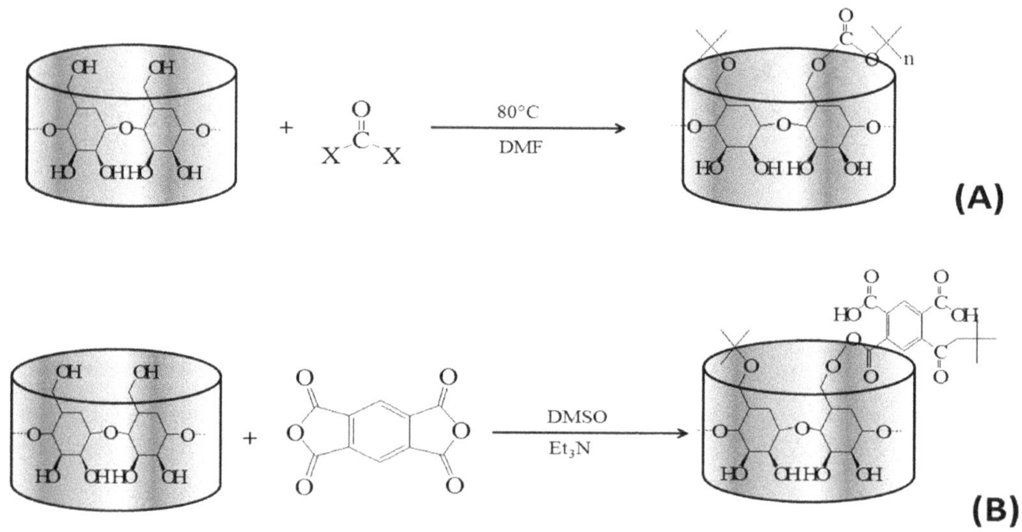

Figure 7. Diagrammatic representation of decrease in the drug release from magnetically sensitive walls of ferrosponges constructed by magnetic nanoparticles can effectively reduce their wall permeability and decrease the drug release via a given magnetic field.

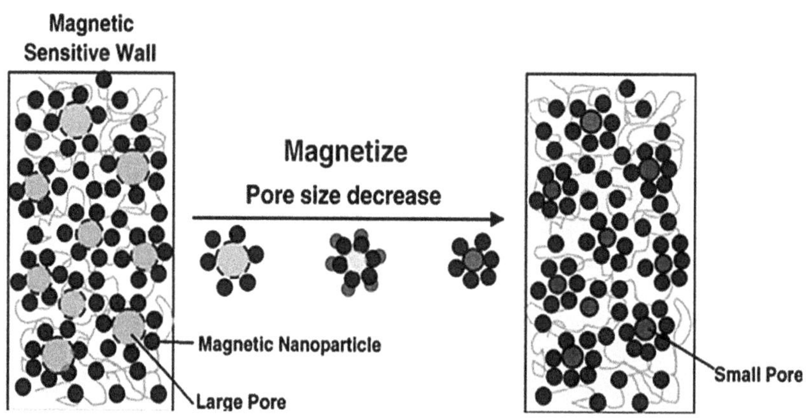

Chapter 10
Multicomponent Solid Forms: A New Boost to Pharmaceuticals

Rahul B. Chavan
NIPER Hyderabad, India

Balvant Yadav
NIPER Hyderabad, India

Anurag Lodagekar
NIPER Hyderabad, India

Nalini R. Shastri
NIPER Hyderabad, India

ABSTRACT

Multicomponent systems provide the option of combining drugs at the supramolecular level. Among these, co-crystals have gained a widespread interest in pharmaceutical industry as US Food and Drug Administration (FDA) recently introduced new regulatory guidelines regarding this solid form that is anticipated to expand patent portfolios. Apart from co-crystals, other multi-component adducts such as co-amorphous system and eutectics are also a topic of interest for pharmaceutical researchers as they provide therapeutic advantages along with improved the aqueous solubility, dissolution, and bioavailability of poorly soluble drugs. This chapter provides a brief overview of multicomponent solid forms, their preparation methodologies, characterization, evaluation, biopharmaceutical aspects, scale up issues, and regulatory perspectives related to these solid forms. In addition, a section on future perspectives that sheds light on new therapeutic hybrids deploying drug-drug and drug-neutraceuticals combinations with improved pharmaceutical and biopharmaceutical attributes is also included.

1. INTRODUCTION

Concurrent administration of two or more therapeutic agents which have similar or different mechanisms of action are termed as *multi drug therapy* and can be used to combat various ailments (Shin, Alani, Rao, Rockich, & Kwon, 2009). In comparison to single drug therapy, this approach help in targeting different key signal transduction pathways which can be more efficacious in management of diseases, since they

DOI: 10.4018/978-1-5225-4781-5.ch010

Copyright © 2018, IGI Global. Copying or distributing in print or electronic forms without written permission of IGI Global is prohibited.

can evade cellular resistance mechanisms. The advantages offered by multi-drug therapy are schematically depicted in Figure 1. To date, this approach has been successfully implemented for management of diseases such as HIV/AIDS, cancer, multiple sclerosis, malaria, infectious diseases, cardiovascular and metabolic diseases, hypertension, auto immune disorders and many psychiatric maladies (Conway, & Cohen, 2010; Thipparaboina, Chavan, Kumar, Modugula, & Shastri , 2015). Multi drug therapy when administered in fixed dose combinations (FDC) are cost-effective which help in reducing pill load without any additional risk of adverse events or drug resistance and hence improve the patient compliance. FDC also facilitate the reduction of managerial and manufacturing costs by reducing the outflow related to packaging and drug prescriptions. FDC products contain simple drug–drug combinations or drug–device combinations, such as drug-eluting stents or drug-biological products for use in cancer therapy. The benefits offered by FDC are often overshadowed because of its severe disadvantages such as stability issues, and solubility differences and incompatibility between the parent drugs (Thipparaboina, Chavan, Kumar, Modugula, & Shastri , 2015). Hence, there is a need to develop alternative approach which will facilitate the development of therapeutic hybrids to counter such problems. Multicomponent solids such as cocrystals, co amorphous system (CAM) and eutectics may provide solution required for delivering the drug-drug combinations with improved benefits in terms of stability, improved solubility and dissolution when compared to FDC.

Clinical success of Novartis product Entrestot a multi drug cocrystal which was approved in 2015 for effective management of chronic heart pain, is comprised of monosodium sacubitril, disodium valsartan

Figure 1. Advantages offered by multi drug therapy: MDR- multi drug resistance

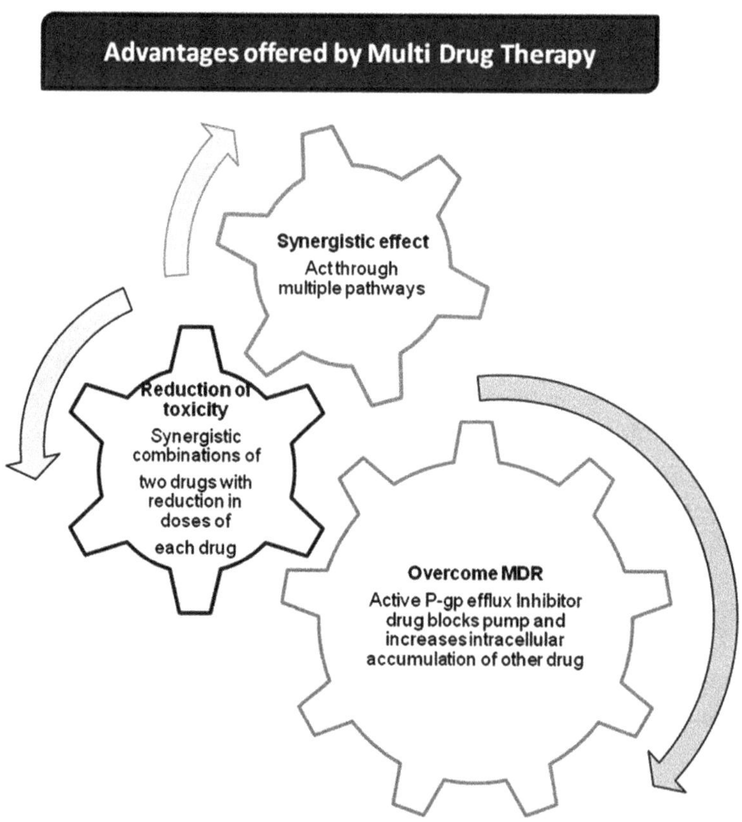

and water, and has given a boost to pharmaceutical industry to improve the pharmaceutical attributes using multi component systems. However, developments of such multi component solid system need careful attention as it require supportive evidence on its pharmacological action and safety such as synergistic or additive effect of two drugs in addition to stability and formulation related attributes. This book chapter aims to provide a brief overview on multi component solid forms (cocrystals, co amorphous system, eutectics) and furnish information ranging from preparation, characterization, scale up and regulatory concerns related to these systems.

2. MULTI DRUG COCRYSTALS

As per FDA, co-crystals are dissociable multicomponent solid crystalline supramolecular complexes which contain two or more components within the same crystal lattice where in the components are in neutral state and interact via nonionic interactions' (Aitipamula, Banerjee, Bansal, Biradha, Cheney, Choudhury, . . . Duggirala, 2012). First report on cocrystal came in 1844 for quinhydrone complex by Wholer, which was later found to be a 1:1 co-crystal of quinone and hydroquinone (Nangia, 2010). In 1995, Gautam Desiraju introduced the concept of the supramolecular synthon, or hydrogen bonded building units in crystal structures with leads from the field of supramolecular chemistry and crystal engineering (Desiraju, 1995). This concept led to a spurt of research that was responsible for the extensive growth in the field of cocrystals.

Drug-drug cocrystals are a subset of pharmaceutical cocrystals wherein the conformer is a bioactive molecule which possess independent drug activity instead of being an inert coformer. Multidrug cocrystals (MDC) offer numerous advantages from enhanced bioavailability to reduction of multidrug resistance, synergistic and/or additive effects, enhanced solubility and dissolution of at least one component, possible stabilization of unstable components through intermolecular interactions, lifecycle management of existing products, and finally combination therapies (Thipparaboina, Kumar, Chavan, & Shastri, 2016). The authors research group was the first one to propose the definition of co-crystals to MDC systems, and defined it as 'dissociable solid crystalline supramolecular complexes comprising two or more therapeutically effective components in a stoichiometric ratio within the same crystal lattice, wherein the components may predominantly interact via nonionic interactions and rarely through hybrid interactions (a combination of ionic and nonionic interactions involving partial proton transfer and hydrogen bonding) with or without the presence of solvate molecules' (Thipparaboina, Kumar, Chavan, & Shastri, 2016). Approval of Entresto a drug-drug cocrystal appeared just after the EMA reflection paper and FDA guidance stimulated the interest of the pharmaceutical industry in drug-drug cocrystals as materials for drug products. Interestingly, the first drug-drug cocrystal was reported by Nakao, S., *et al.*, way back in 1977 who developed theophylline: phenobarbital MDC (Nakao, FuJII, Sakaki, & Tomita, 1977). A partial list of some of the reported MDC along with their preparation methods and applications are depicted in Table 1.

2.1 Prediction of Formation of MDC

Before preparation of MDC, prediction of MDC formation is found to be crucial. To date, there are no confirmed systematic computational approaches for prediction the MDC formation. However, due to the similarity in the bond formation, the well developed prediction models of co-crystal formation

Table 1. Reported drug-drug/ drug-neutraceutical cocrystal

Drug Combination	Preparation Method	Pharmaceutical Attributes	Therapeutic Category	Reference
Theophylline–Phenobarbital	Distillation	Dissolution	Antiasthmatic and sedative hypnotic	Nakao et al., (1977)
Sulfadimidine–Aspirin	Solvent evaporation	-	Antibacterial and NSAID	(Caira, 1992)
Sulfadimidine–4-ASA				
Theophylline–5-FU	Solvent evaporation	-	Antiasthmatic and Anticancer	Zaitu et al., (1995)
Trimethoprim–Sulfadimidine	Solvent evaporation	-	Antibacterial	Sardone et al., (1997)
Trimethoprim–Sulfamethoxy Pyridazine	Heating at boiling point followed by instant cooling	-	Antibacterial	Bettinetti et al., (2000)
Piracetam–Gentisic Acid	Co-grinding, slurrying in water and solvent evaporation	-	Nootropic agent and NSAID	Vishweshwar et al., (2005)
Carbamazepine–Salicylic Acid	In situ cocrystallization mediated by water released by dibasic calcium phosphate dihydrate	-	Antiepileptic and anti-inflammatory	E. Lu et al., (2008)
Lamivudine–Zidovudine	Solvent evaporation	-	Antiviral	Bhatt et al., (2008)
Theophylline–Gentisic Acid	Thermally assisted solvent evaporation	-	Antiasthmatic and NSAID	Aitipamula et al., (2009)
p-Coumaric Acid-Caffeine and Theophylline	-	-	Antiasthmatic	Schultheiss et al., (2011)
Sulfamethazine–theophylline	Solvent evaporation	Hygroscopicity	Antibacterial and antiasthmatic	J. Lu et al., (2010)
Meloxicam–Aspirin	Solution crystallization, slurry and solvent drop grinding methods	Solubility, bioavailability (AUC, MRT, C_{max} and MAT)	NSAID	Cheney et al., (2011)
Isoniazid–4-ASA Pyrazinamide–4-ASA	Solvent drop grinding	-	Antitubercular drugs	Grobelny et al., (2011)
Pyrazinamide–Diflunisal	Ball mill grinding	-	Antitubercular and NSAID	Évora et al., (2011)
Curcumin–Pyrogallol	Liquid-assisted manual grinding	Dissolution	Anticancer	Sanphui et al., (2011)
Aceclofenac–Paracetamol	Various methods	Solubility	NSAID	Chandel et al.,(2011)
Piracetam–Lithium Chloride	Solvent evaporation and grinding	IDR	Nootropic agent and mood-stabilizing agent	(Braga et al., 2012)
Furosemide–Pentoxifylline	Solvent evaporation	-	Loop diuretic; the latter drug is used to treat intermittent claudication	Stepanovs et al., (2012)
Isoniazid–2-Chloro-4-Nitro Benzoic Acid	Solvent evaporation	-	Antitubercular and antiviral compounds	(Lemmerer, 2012)
Pyrimethamine–Carbamazepine	Solvent evaporation	-	Antimalarial and antiepileptic	Delori et al., (2013)
Pyrimethamine–Theophylline			Antimalarial and antiasthmatic	

continued on following page

Table 1. Continued

Drug Combination	Preparation Method	Pharmaceutical Attributes	Therapeutic Category	Reference
Ciprofloxacin–Norfloxacin	Solvent evaporation	-	Antibacterial	Pinto Vitorino et al., (2013)
Isoniazid- p-Coumaric Acid	Slow solvent evaporation	Log P	Antitubercular, anti cancer, antioxidant and anti inflammatory	Ravikumar et al., (2013)
Paracetamol–Indomethacin and Mefenamic Acid	Solvent evaporation	-	NSAIDs	Pathak et al., (2013)
Sildenafil–aspirin	Solvent evaporation	IDR	Antihypertensive and NSAID	Žegarac et al.,(2014)
Diclofenac and Diflunisal–Theophylline	Solvent drop grinding and solvent evaporation	Stability and dissolution	Antiasthmatic and NSAID	Surov et al., (2014)
Dapsone–Sulfanilamide Flavone, Luteolin, Caffeine and Benzothiazolone	Solution crystallization	Stability and solubility	Antileprotic, antibacterial and antioxidants	Jiang et al., (2014)
Sinapic Acid-ij6-Propyl-2-Thiouracil (PTU)	Solution crystallization	Stability	Anti-oxidant, anti-microbial, anti-inflammatory, anti-cancer, and anti-anxiety	Sinha et al., (2015)
Glicalzide and Metformin	Solvent evaporation	Solubility, dissolution and hygroscopicity	Antidiabetic	Putra et al., (2016)
Vitamin D2 and D3	Solvent evaporation	Chemical stability	Hormonal therapy	Wang et al., (2016)
Norfloxacin and Sulfathiazole	Liquid assisted grinding	Solubility, diffusion and antimicrobial activity	Antibacterial and antimicrobial	Gopi et al., (2016)
Telmisartan-atenolol	Liquid assisted grinding	Solubility, IDR, stability and in vivo pharmacodynamic activity	Antihypertensive	Haneef et al., (2017)
4-aminosalicylic acid-caffein	Solvent evaporation	Solubility and thermo chemical stability	Antituberculous and antiasthmatic	Drozd et al., (2017)
Flufenamic acid, ethenzamide	Solvent evaporation	Solubility, stability	NSAID	Nechipadappu et al., (2017)
Ethenzamide- gentisic acid	Solid state grinding	Compressibility, stability and solubility	NSAID, analgesic and antipyretic activity	Sokal et al., (2017)

between drugs and coformers can be successfully extrapolated for the prediction of MDC formation. These approaches may be based on knowledge or experimental screening (Figure 2). pKa based models, use of molecular descriptors, hydrogen-bonding propensity and synthonic engineering are promising knowledge based methods (Duggirala, Perry, Almarsson, & Zaworotko , 2016). These methods can be successfully applied to any two molecule systems and, thus, can be used for drug–drug systems. Synthon based approach is most widely used strategies to understand molecular interactions. Structural units of

Figure 2. Different approaches for prediction of MDC formation

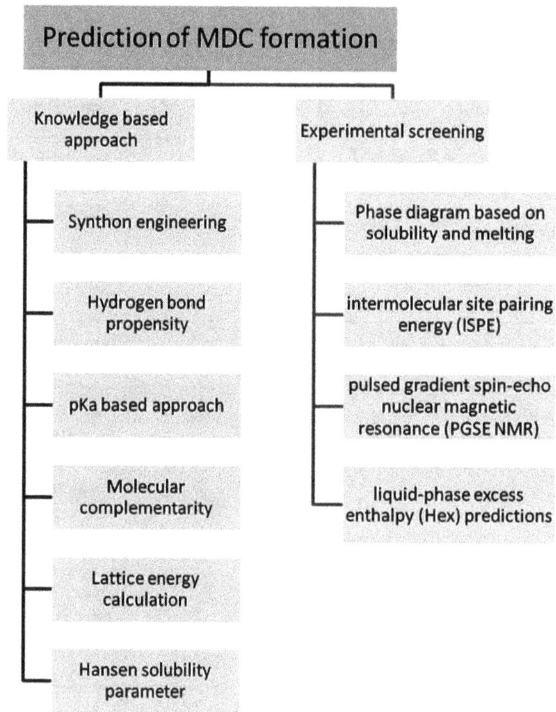

supermolecules are identified that can be assembled to form intermolecular interactions. Use of this synthon-based retrosynthetic strategy for the development of lamivudine and zidovudine MDC was reported by Prashant *et al* (Bhatt, Azim, Thakur, & Desiraju , 2008). This approach can predict with reasonable degree of success using simple molecules, but become complex in molecules with multiple hydrogen-bond donors and acceptors. Numerous attempts have been made to develop new prediction model for coformer selection. Delori et al.(2017), implemented hydrogen bonding propensity calculations for predicting the formation of a MDC of pyrimethamine with theophylline and carbamazepine (Delori, Galek, Pidcock, Patni, & Jones, 2013). Etter, M. C. et al (1990), developed a set of empirical rules to determine the tendency for hydrogen bonding of various donor/acceptor combinations. These rules are based on the fact that the best proton donors will form a hydrogen bond with the best proton acceptor (Etter, MacDonald, & Bernstein, 1990). Apart from these approaches, Childs et al. (2007), proposed ΔpKa based method which involves pKa values of drug and coformers. In their work on theophylline–acid complexes, they categorized a $0 < \triangle pKa < 2.5$ region as a salt/co-crystal continuum zone (Childs, Stahly, & Park , 2007). Cruz Cabeza et al.(2012) after studying the 6465 crystalline complexes in the CSD, and validating and quantifying the △pKa rule, stated that △pKa would be one of the most prominent and simplest methods to use in predicting co-crystal formation. They concluded that $\triangle pKa < -1$ would exclusively result in a non-ionized complex; $\triangle pKa < 4$ would result in an ionized complex; and between $1 \leq \triangle pKa \leq 4$, a 1 △pKa difference would increase the probability of proton transfer by 17% from 10% at $\triangle pKa = -1$ to 95% at $\triangle pKa = 4$ (Cruz-Cabeza, 2012). Use of Hansen solubility parameters (Mohammad, M. A., Alhalaweh, A., & Velaga, 2011), lattice energy calculations (Issa, Karamertzanis, Welch, & Price, 2008) and many other knowledge based methods are also available for prediction of cocrystal preparation which can be extrapolated to MDC (Duggirala, Perry, Almarsson, & Zaworotko, 2016).

Similar to these knowledge based prediction methods, literature also lacks in experimental screening methods for MDC formation. However, methods such as Ternary phase diagrams based on solubility and melting, liquid-phase excess enthalpy predictions, pulsed gradient spin-echo nuclear magnetic resonance (PGSE NMR), and intermolecular site pairing energy which were investigated for cocrystals can be extrapolated for MDC preparation but require proper validation before developing robust prediction model for screening of MDC.

2.2 Preparation and Characterization

Once the prediction of MDC formation is completed, then the next step is preparation or synthesis of MDC. The conventional cocrystal preparation methods and methods used for MDC preparation are similar. As depicted in Table 1, conventional cocrystal preparation methods such as mechanical grinding (both neat and solvent-drop or liquid assisted), slow solvent evaporation and slurry mediated transformation can be used for MDC preparation. Apart from these conventional methods, other methods that are reported for formation of MDC include microfluidic approach, high-throughput screening, supercritical fluid technologies and ultrasound assisted solution cocrystallization. Figure 3 outlines the general preparation methods of MDC. For more details on co-crystals preparation methods and their applications in the synthesis of MDC, interested readers may refer to previously published studies (Duggirala, Perry, Almarsson, & Zaworotko, 2016).

Prepared novel crystals are primarily characterized using techniques such as differential scanning calorimetry (DSC), powder X- ray diffraction (PXRD), single crystal X- ray diffraction, spectroscopic techniques (infrared spectroscopy, near infrared spectroscopy, Raman spectroscopy and tetra hertz spectroscopy), solid state nuclear magnetic resonance (ssMNR) and thermogravimetric analysis (TGA). As single crystals are not always available during initial stages of discovery, application of advanced spectroscopic techniques may help in determining the structure from the powder samples. Raman spectroscopy finds application in identifying cocrystal formation during high-throughput slurry screening (Kojima, Tsutsumi, Yamamoto, Ikeda, & Moriwaki , 2010), discriminating a cocrystal and a physical mixture in formulated tablets (Burley, Alkhalil, Bloomfield, & Matousek, 2012) and also in quantifying the cocrystals from binary or ternary mixtures (Allesø, Velaga, Alhalaweh, Cornett, Rasmussen, Berg, . . . Rantanen , 2008). Near infrared spectroscopy has been reported for identification and quantification of cocrystals in binary or ternary mixtures and final finished dosage form (Mukherjee, Tothadi, Chakraborty, Ganguly, & Desiraju, 2013). Terahertz time-domain-spectroscopy has also been employed to differentiate among the chiral and racemic of cocrystals of theophylline with malic acid and tartaric acid. Use of ssNMR for characterization of cocrystals was explained by Vogt et al., who diagnosed hydrogen bonding and local conformational changes by ^{1}H–^{1}H, ^{1}H–^{13}C and ^{19}F–^{13}C coupling (Vogt, Clawson, Strohmeier, Edwards, Pham, & Watson, 2008). Brief overview of various characterization techniques has been provided in Figure 4.

2.3 Evaluation of MDC

Major objective behind the development of MDC is to improve the therapeutic efficacy through synergistic or additive effect of second drug component of MDC, in addition to other pharmaceutical at-

Figure 3. Preparation methods of cocrystals
Reprinted from Thipparaboina R., et al.(2016), after minor modifications and with permission from Elsevier.

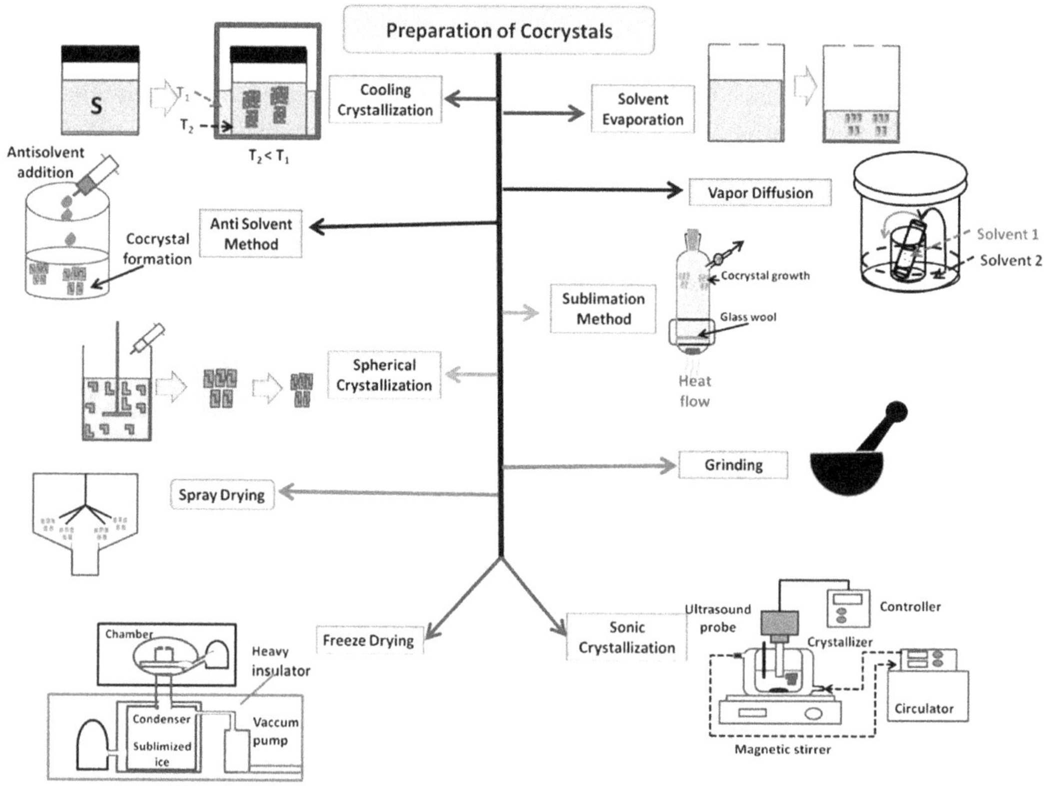

tributes (solubility, dissolution, stability and mechanical properties). Currently more than 15 articles on MDC have demonstrated improvement of solubility, stability and dissolution. However, fewer reports are available on MDC that address the biopharmaceutical aspects of MDC (Table 1). Analysis of the reported pharmacokinetic data generated from the MDC suggests that an improvement in area under curve (AUC) can be mainly attributed to the solubility advantage of MDC. Impact of MDC on other pharmacokinetic parameters was also found to be significant by few authors. Cheney et al (2011)., developed meloxicam: aspirin MDC which showed significant improvement in bioavailability (4 fold) as compared to plain drug. Five and four fold enhancement in C_{max} and AUC was reported by the authors (Cheney, Weyna, Shan, Hanna, Wojtas, & Zaworotko, 2011). However, an extensive literature search has revealed an absence of reports on pharmacodynamic or efficacy studies of MDC, which is more crucial, as combination of two drugs in MDC can only prove beneficial once their pharmacological potential is evaluated and proven experimentally.

2.4 Scale Up

Scale up of MDC is a major challenge in pharmaceutical industry. However, recent publications on scale up of cocrystals are expected to boost the scale up process for MDC as the preparation techniques for both cocrystals and MDC are similar. Methods like solution crystallization, hot melt extrusion, spray

Figure 4. Characterization tools used for MDC
Reprinted from Thipparaboina R., et al., (Thipparaboina et al., 2016) after minor modifications and with permission from Elsevier.

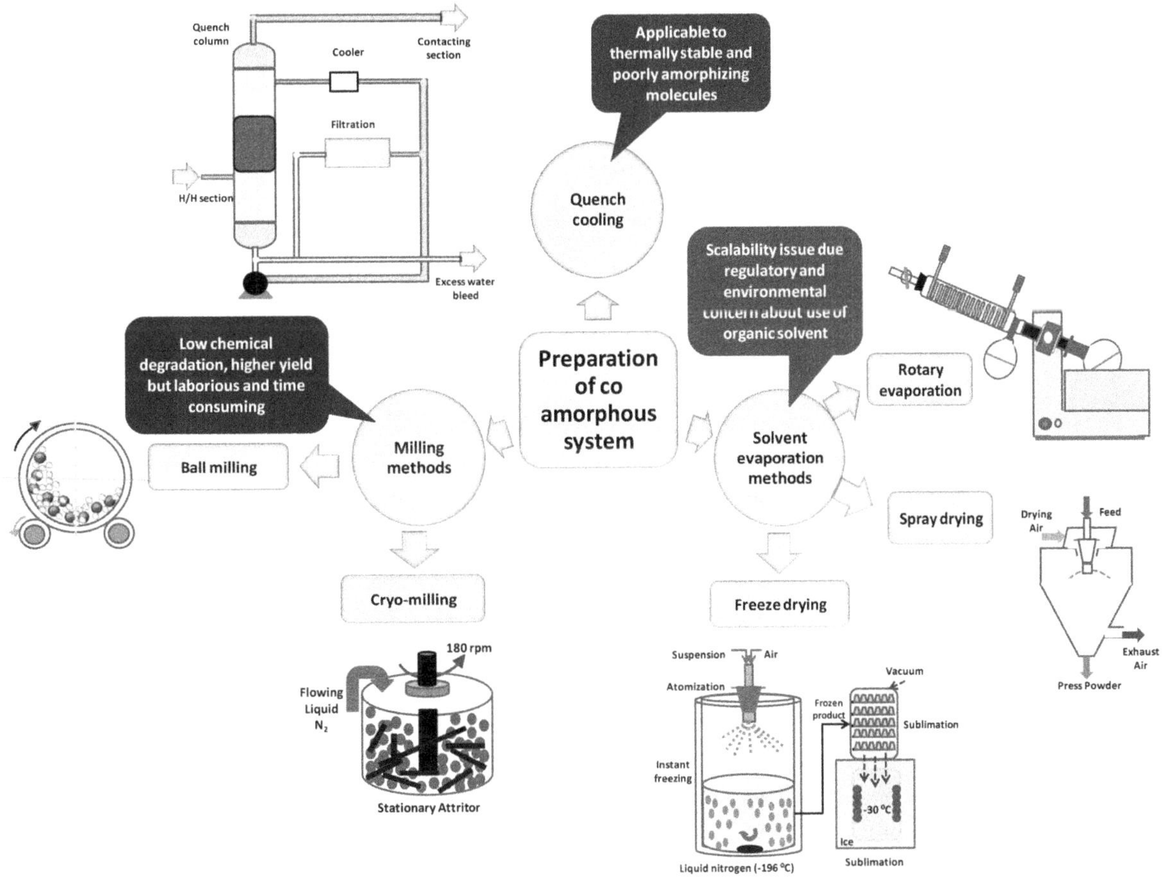

drying, high shear granulation are scalable for cocrystals. Solution crystallization is preferred for scale up of cocrystals. However, a challenge of difference in solubility of drug and coformer in the selected solvent that may result in preferential crystallization of individual substances has to be addressed. In this scale up process, ternary phase diagram of drug, coformer and solvent was found to be critical as it give a cocrystal region to produce cocrystals. Dennis H. Leung et al (2012), reported cocrystal of anti diabetic molecule with benzoic acid and scaled up to 2 gm using solution crystallization (Leung, Lohani, Ball, Canfield, Wang, Rhodes, & Bak, 2012). Apart from solution crystallization, other scalable techniques that are attempted by researchers include hot melt extrusion, spray drying, resonant acoustic mixing, high shear granulation etc. Nagaudi et al.(2017), reported scale up theophylline oxalic acid cocrystals up to 80 gm with 94% yield in resonant acoustic mixing by using design of experiment approach (Nagapudi, Umanzor, & Masui, 2017).

Large scale production of MDC requires study of process parameters and their interactions. Bulk production of MDC can be achieved successfully by using existing techniques, mainly spray-drying technologies, solvent assisted crystallization methodologies and spherical co-crystallization. However, solvent-free processes like hot melt extrusion or twin screw extrusion systems may also serve as eco-friendly alternatives for the production of MDC at large-scale.

3. CO AMORPHOUS SYSTEM

Last few years has evidenced rapid growth of binary amorphous systems. This binary system referred as co amorphous systems (CAM) are systems where drug is incorporated with small molecules instead polymers (Dengale, Grohganz, Rades, & Löbmann , 2016). Co amorphous term was coined by Chieng *et al.* with an intention to differentiate amorphous mixture containing two small molecules from the term polymeric amorphous solid dispersion (PASD) (Chieng, Aaltonen, Saville, & Rades , 2009). CAM is defined as:

... multi-component single phase amorphous solid system which lacks periodicity in lattice and is associated by weak and discrete intermolecular interactions between the components (Suresh, Mannava, & Nangia, 2014).

They possess short-range interactions such as hydrogen bonding of carboxylic acids, phenols/alcohols and carboxamides similar to amorphous system of single component systems. However, this system differs from cocrystal, salt or eutectic primarily by its amorphous nature which is characterized by presence of broad hump ('amorphous halo') in the X-ray diffractogram. Two types of co-amorphous systems have been proposed so far, namely drug–drug combinations and drug–excipient mixtures. Among these, drug-drug CAM have gained importance as two pharmacologically relevant drugs intended for multidrug therapies are combined to stabilize both the drugs in amorphous form. Both drugs thus act as an active component and a stabilizing excipient at the same time. As a result of the stable amorphous system, both drugs if poorly soluble achieve higher solubility and dissolution rate. Several drug-drug CAMs were reported in last few years (Table 2). These systems are developed with an intention to improve solubility, dissolution rate and physical stability of amorphous form of drug. Apart from the advantage of stabilization, solubility and dissolution, CAM also offers a platform for the development of new combinational therapy. Combination of drugs from two different therapeutic categories helps in more efficient therapy. Generally CAM are produced in a molar ratio of 1:1, which may show improvement in stability as it is assumed that both components of CAM interact at molecular level through hydrogen bonds (Alleso, Chieng, Rehder, Rantanen, Rades, & Aaltonen, 2009; Löbmann, Laitinen, Grohganz, Gordon, Strachan, & Rades , 2011; Suresh, Mannava, & Nangia, 2014). In addition to the potential therapeutic advantage, co amorphous approach offers bioavailability enhancement as one of the drugs may act as dissolution-enhancing and amorphous stabilizing agent for the second drug (Dengale, Ranjan, Hussen, Krishna, Musmade, Shenoy, & Bhat , 2014). To date, more than 20 drug-drug CAMs are reported, probably due to the limited availability of pharmacologically relevant drug pairs with glass forming ability that can be used in combination therapy.

3.1 Screening of Coformer for Co Amorphous System Preparation

Selection of right coformer is the biggest challenge in the development of CAM, since coformer decides the fate of the final product in terms of stability and pharmaceutical performance. Screening process involves systematic investigation of crystallization tendency of co-former. To make these processes easy and predictable, quantum mechanics can be used for assigning various molecular interactions in FTIR and Raman spectra to provide insights into the near range order of amorphous systems and help in identification of CAM formation via molecular interactions. Lobmann et al. (2013), investigated the

Table 2. Reported drug-drug/ drug-neutraceutical CAM, PK- Pharmacokinetic

Sr. No.	CAM	Preparation Method	Solubility	Dissolution	Stability	PK	Ref.
1	Cimetidine: indomethacin	Solvent evaporation method	✓	✓			Yamamura et al., (2000)
2	Cimetidine: diflunisal		✓	✓			Yamamura et al., (2002)
3	Cimetidine: naproxen	Ball milling		✓	✓		Allesø et al., (2009)
4	Indomethacin: ranitidine hydrochloride						Chieng et al., (2009)
5	Indomethacin: naproxen	Quench cooling		✓	✓		Löbmann et al., (2011)
6	Simvastatin: glipizide	Cryo milling and ball milling			✓		Löbmann et al., (2012)
7	Atorvastatin: carvedilol: glibenclamide	Solvent evaporation method			✓	✓	Shayanfar et al., (2013)
8	Indomethacin: naproxen	Quench cooling		✓	✓		Löbmann et al.,(2013)
9	Curcumin: artemisinin	Solvent evaporation method	✓			✓	Suresh et al., (2014)
10	Ritonavir: indomethacin		✓	✓			Swapnil J Dengale et al., (2014)
11	Ritonavir: quercetin		✓			✓	Swapnil J Dengale et al., (2015)
12	Ezetimibe: indapamide	Quench cooling			✓		Knapik et al., (2015)
13	Nateglinide: metformin hydrochloride	Ball milling	✓	✓			Wairkar et al., (2015)
14	Talinolol: naringin	Quench cooling	✓			✓	Teja et al., (2015)
15	Glipizide: atorvastatin	Cryo milling		✓	✓		Renuka et al., (2015)
16	indomethacin–cimetidine and naproxen–cimetidine	Quench cooling, co-evaporation and ball milling	-	-	✓	-	Lim et al., (2016)
17	Tranilast and Diphenhydramine Hydrochloride	Quench cooling			✓		Ueda et al., (2017)
18	Glipizide and atorvastatin	Cryomilling	-	✓	✓		Renuka et al., (2017)
19	Naproxen–indomethacin		-	-	-		Beyer, Radi, et al., (2016)
20	Naproxen/indomethacin	Melt-quenching	-	-	-		Beyer, Grohganz, et al., (2016)
21	Naproxen/indomethacin		-	-	-		Beyer et al., (2017)

formation of heterodimer in indomethacin and naproxen CAM through analysis of molecular interaction by quantum mechanics (Löbmann, Laitinen, Grohganz, Strachan, Rades, & Gordon , 2013). Russo et al (2016), further explored the applicability of quantum mechanics in evaluating intermolecular interactions between drug and co-former of CAM by studying the hydrogen bonding interactions between omeprazole and amoxicillin (Russo, Sancho, Silva, Baldoni, Venancio, Ellena, & Narda, 2016). Multivariate analysis (partial least squares discriminative analysis, PLS-DA) was also explored by Ueda et al.(2016), to study the contribution of physicochemical properties of co-former in the formation and stabilization of CAM (Ueda,Muranushi, Sakuma, Ida, Endoh, Kadota, & Tozuka, 2016). Use of parameters like Flory-Huggins interaction parameter (Pajula, Wittoek, Lehto, Ketolainen, & Korhonen , 2014) and solubility parameter to predict the miscibility of the components is well documented. However, mere understanding of stabilization potential of coformer is not sufficient to develop drug-drug CAM, because such combination might not provide any therapeutic benefits unless and until justifiable evidence about practical application of such combination in therapy or synergism or drug-drug interactions has not been provided. The scarcity of such reports can be attributed to the requirement of detailed clinical investigation.

3.2 Preparation and Scale Up of Co Amorphous System

Preparation techniques reported for CAM are still in infancy as most of the reported techniques are only applicable for lab scale production. These techniques are ideal for screening purpose but for large or industrial scale manufacturing, extensive research is required for checking their feasibility. Summary of the preparation techniques utilized for CAM are depicted in Figure 5. Scale up of CAM poses major challenge as existing preparation methods are suitable for making few milligrams to grams of CAM products.

Ball milling has already proven its scalability for single component amorphous systems. However, it faces few challenges such as high mechanical stress and difficulty in achieving a homogeneous mix of drug and coformer for large scale processes. Additionally, product obtained from milling possesses charge which cause aggregation and may aggravate the recrystallization tendency in the product. Such milled product due to charge development may stick to the wall of the milling chamber and create problem in product recovery from chamber. Milling temperature is one of the key operational parameter that has direct impact on the product. Heat generated during milling affects the stability of the product (Qi, McAuley, Yang, & Tipduangta, 2014). Hence, application of this method should be restricted to thermally stable drugs and co-formers with higher T_g.

Scale up is not expected for melting methods which is widely used for screening or optimization of CAM. Use of jacketed vessels and heat transfer coil systems only improve efficacy of this method marginally as such methods face risk of non homogeneity of the final product. In addition to this, in-line degradation and uneven mixing limit the melt methods for CAM preparation (Qi, McAuley, Yang, & Tipduangta, 2014). However, on the other hand, newer techniques such as hot melt extrusion (HME) which work on the same principle of melting of components has proved its efficacy in manufacturing of PASD products, with several PASDs available in market that are manufactured by HME process. HME may be extrapolated for CAM preparation due to the physical similarity of the end product desired. Advantages offered by HME includes continuous and solvent free processing with ease of scale-up due to availability of different equipment capacities to develop and optimize at bench and pilot plant level. To reach a commercial viable scale, various process variables of HME and their impact on the performance of the final product need to be extensively studied (Qi, McAuley, Yang, & Tipduangta, 2014; Vasconcelos, Marques, das Neves, & Sarmento , 2016).

Figure 5. Techniques available for preparation of co amorphous system
Reprinted from Chavan et al., (Chavan et al., 2016) with permission from Elsevier.

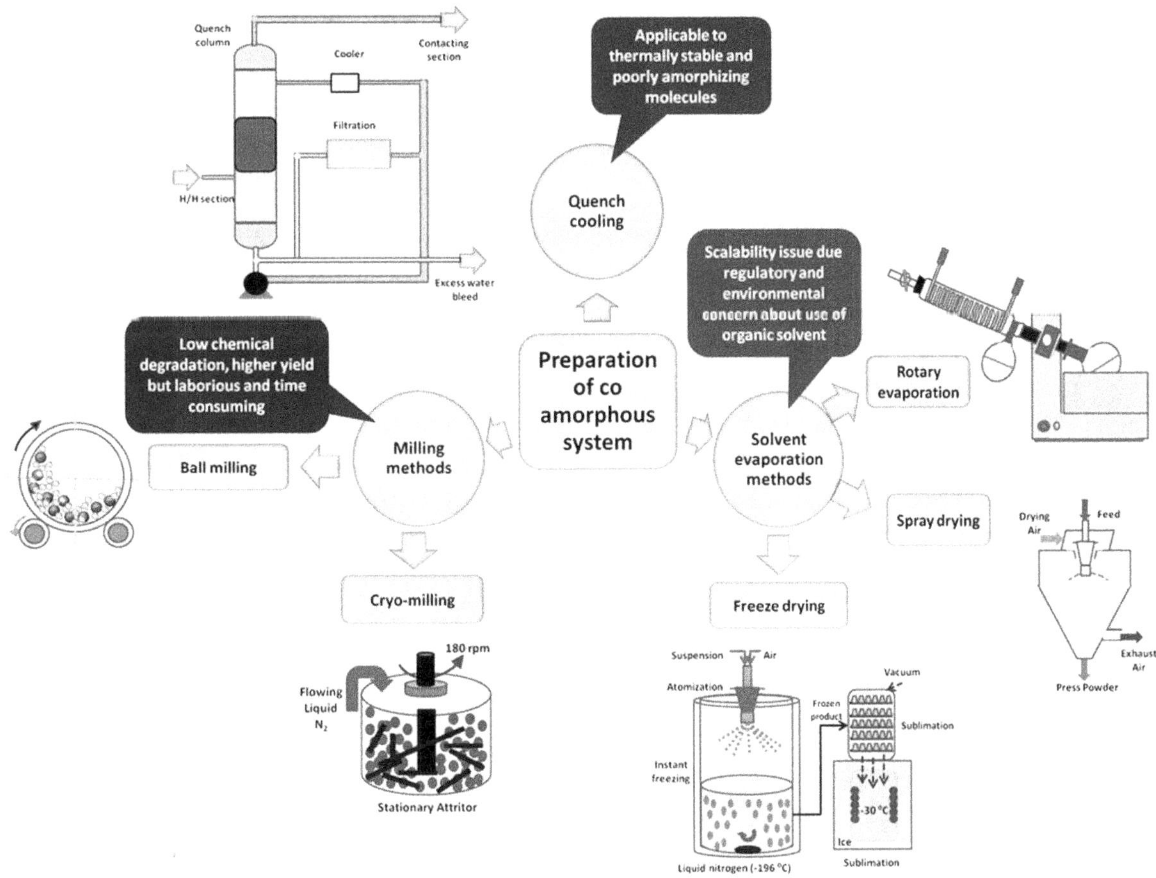

Solvent evaporation is third most widely used technique for CAM preparation. Spray-drying is already an established technique for the production of stable amorphous glass solutions, as its robustness during scale up of solid dispersions is well documented (Qi, McAuley, Yang, & Tipduangta, 2014). Recently, few reports have emerged where CAM products were produced by spray drying (Jensen, Blaabjerg, Lenz, Bohr, Grohganz, Kleinebudde, . . . Lobmann, 2016) which were subsequently formulated into final dosage forms (Lenz, Jensen, Blaabjerg, Knop, Grohganz, Lobmann, . . . Kleinebudde, 2015). Factors which are important for large scale production by using this technique involve thermal stability of drugs/excipients, molecular mixing, phase separation, temperature, solvent induced recrystallization, solvent toxicity, and amorphous to crystalline ratio in final product, need careful deliberation and study. Solvent evaporation technique in addition may pose environmental challenges (Paudel, Worku, Meeus, Guns, & Van den Mooter , 2013).

3.3 Characterization of Co Amorphous System

To understand the stability and performance of CAM, different advanced characterization tools are utilized. These analytical tools help in determination of molecular interactions, crystallinity, miscibility, molecular mobility, phase separation, moisture or solvent residue, surface chemistry and morphology of CAM at qualitative or quantitative level. However, use of simultaneous estimation tools or hyphenated techniques has increased for collecting the integrated information with a spatiotemporal resolution. Analytical tools utilized for CAM characterization are categorized based on the application in CAM and depicted in Figure 6.

3.4 Biopharmaceutical Aspects

As discussed earlier, CAM is a newer approach to solve the stability and dissolution related issues of amorphous system. However, limited studies have been published on *in vivo* performance of these systems. Results of reported pharmacokinetic studies of co amorphous system provide a general conclusion that enhanced AUC is likely due to improved solubility. Most of the CAM showed significant improvement in C_{max} and AUC. Improvement in C_{max} ranged from around 1.3 to 30 fold increase (Suresh, Mannava, & Nangia, 2014) while AUC showed enhancements of nearly 1 to 5 folds. In addition, significant reduction in T_{max} of CAM was documented in literature which was mainly attributed to the solubility advantage of these systems (Dengale, Hussen, Krishna, Musmade, Shenoy, & Bhat, 2015).

Apart from poor solubility, poor intestinal permeability is also a significant contributor to poor bioavailability of drugs. Physicochemical properties of the drug molecule (size and polarity) are found to be responsible for poor permeability of drug. Similarly, intestinal efflux pumps also contribute to poor permeability of drug across the intestine. This factor is found to be crucial for drugs which are P-gp substrate because permeation of such drugs across GI membrane might have been compromised due to poor solubility of drug, which limits the concentration of drug penetrating into the enterocyte by preventing

Figure 6. Analytical tools used for characterization of co amorphous system

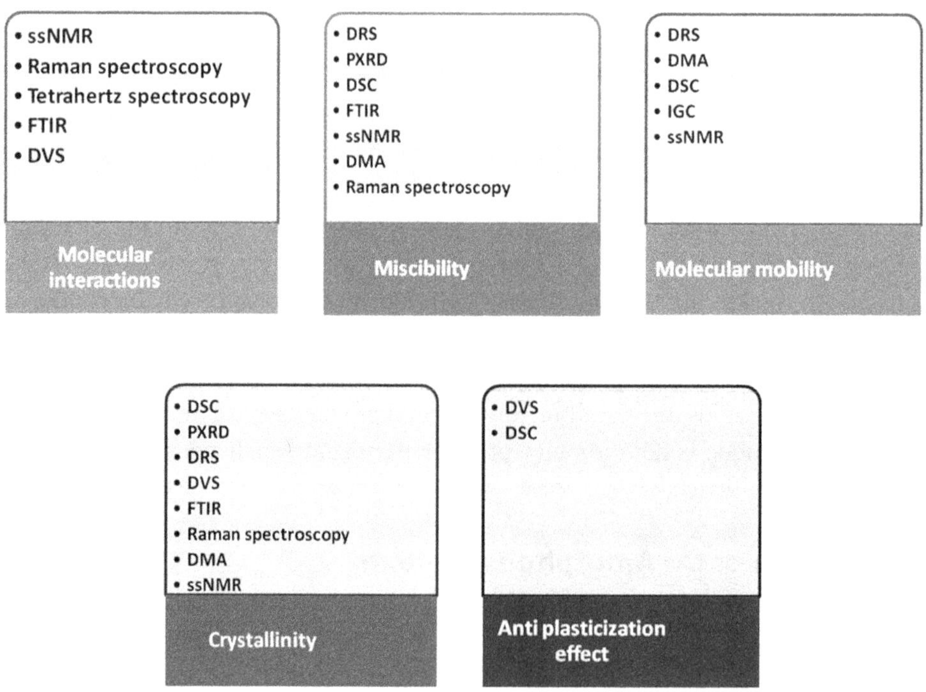

the saturation of efflux transporters. It is well known that these P-gp efflux transporters are amenable to saturation; hence solubility advantage of CAM might solve the problem by maintaining the higher luminal concentration of drug which will result into saturation of transporters thus leading to enhanced absorption of drug across GIT. Additionally, use of P-gp inhibitors in combination with the P-gp substrate drug may help in overcoming such permeability issues due to efflux transporters and multiply the effect of CAM for improving the bioavailability of such poorly soluble and permeable drugs. Teja et al.(2015) applied a similar hypothesis for improving the bioavailability issue of P-gp substrate drug talinolol by combining it with P-gp inhibitor drug naringin for development of co amorphous formulation. Using this approach, they were able to improve the dissolution rate with simultaneous enhancement in absorption of talinolol through efflux pump inhibition by the co-administered naringin. The bioavailability study of talinolol in Wister rat showed nearly 5.4 fold enhancement in AUC of talinolol. In order to evaluate the role of naringin on improvement of permeability of talinolol, permeability study was conducted using *in situ* intestinal closed loop method. Outcome of this permeability studies confirmed the effect of naringin on P-gp inhibition wherein the permeability of talinolol was increased to 3.16×10^{-5} cm/s in contrast to 2.48×10^{-5} cm/s in absence of naringin (Teja, Musmade, Khade, & Dengale, 2015). Conversely, Dengale et al. (2015), reported that increased permeation of ritonavir through enterocyte after oral administration of ritonavir- quercetin co amorphous system to rats might be due to solubility advantage of co amorphous system and not because of P-gp inhibition (Dengale, Hussen, Krishna, Musmade, Shenoy, & Bhat, 2015).

3.5 Regulatory Issues

Few patents have been granted to CAM in last few decades. These patents satisfy all three preliminary requisite (novelty, non obviousness and utility) for issuing of patents. Such intellectual property protection helps in life cycle management of drug products. CAM is comprised of amorphous form of drug, hence face similar regulatory challenges as that of PASD wherein the key risk factor is to prove the stability of amorphous form during manufacturing and shelf life, in order to fulfill quality requirement (Rahman, Siddiqui, Gupta, & Khan , 2014). Hence, during the final product development, monitoring and controlling the stability of amorphous based system is a crucial regulatory challenge. This is due to the fact that such products normally meets the quality specifications at the time of release but fails in quality control testing such as dissolution on aging of the product during storage. Recrystallization of amorphous drug during storage may lead to similar type of discrepancy in quality control testing. However, market existence of numerous PASD based products may help in clearing a path for commercialization of CAM as both CAM and PASD are conceptual similar. This will also assist a formulator in applying the same principles for regulatory documentation. However, multifold concern has been raised for drug-drug CAM since pharmacological relevancy creates big challenge for patient safety. This highlights major regulatory constraint of administering more than one drug in a fixed ratio between the two drugs which need to be addressed.

4. MULTI DRUG EUTECTICS

The Greek term eutectics means easy melting (eu=easy and teksis= melting). Well known definition of eutectic state that these are the solid materials which possess low melting point in comparison to their individual counterparts. Examples of eutectic solid ranges from ceramics, to glass, energy storage devices, traditional refrigeration, as an anti-freeze purpose in vehicles, snow removal and to limited extent in pharmaceutical industries. Eutectics are distinguishable from co crystal, based on their unit cell integrity (cocrystal shows the different x ray diffraction pattern whereas eutectics shows similar diffraction pattern of their parent molecules). As per IUPAC Gold Book, eutectic formation is defined as

... an isothermal, reversible reaction between two (or more) solid phases during the heating of a system, as a result of which a single liquid phase is produced (Cherukuvada, & Nangia , 2014).

However, Cherukuvada and Nangia recently redefined the eutectics as conglomerates of solid solution (Cherukuvada, & Nangia , 2014). As per the solid dispersion classification, eutectic can be defined as 1st generation crystalline solid dispersion system which consist of two crystalline phases (biphasic system) and differ from solid solution which is a single phase system (Dengale, Grohganz, Rades, & Löbmann, 2016; Vo, Park, & Lee, 2013). Comparison of eutectics, solid solution and cocrystals has been provided in Table 3.

Literature suggest that eutectics are the undesired/desired fruits during the screening of cocrystals which can be ascribed to a straight tussle between the molecules to reach the stable supramolecular assembly through various non covalent interaction (Thipparaboina, Thumuri, Chavan, Naidu, & Shastri, 2017). Drug eutectics were reported long back in 17th century and their inbuilt potential to improve the pharmaceutical attributes was well recognized when the Sekiguchi et al.(1961:1964), developed eutectic formulation of antimicrobial sulfathiazole and antibiotic chloramphenicol with urea to improve the physicochemical and biopharmaceutical properties (dissolution and bioavailability) of both drugs (Sekiguchi, & Obi , 1961; Sekiguchi, K., Obi, & Ueda , 1964). Later, Goldberg has given the experimental evidence for urea-acetaminophen eutectic system for improving the dissolution rate (Goldberg, Gibaldi, & Kanig , 1966). However, these systems are less explored in pharmaceutical field when compared to other systems such as solid solution and cocrystals; this might be due to its mysterious or partially explored mechanism of formation and lack of specific analytical tools for characterization.

Eutectic systems are classified into three classes based upon volume fraction of each phase involved, viz. rounded rod (the interphase surface energy for phases of eutectic isotropic and volume fraction of second phase less than 0.28), lamellar rod (surface energy for phases of eutectic anisotropic, volume of second phase more than 0.28) and faceted rod (conjugation of the several planes of eutectic phase with low energy). Recently Hemant Jain et al.(2014), further classified the eutectic system based on entropy

Table 3. Difference between eutectics, solid solution, and cocrystal

Solid Form	Phases Involved	Nature of Component	Lattice Structure	Nature of Interaction	Example
Eutectic	2	Can be similar or dissimilar	Similar to components	Predominantly cohesive	Curcumin–hydroquinone
Solid Solution	1	Isomorphous	Similar to components ensemble of solid solutions(Cherukuvada et al., 2014)	Cohesive	Benzoic acid–4-fluorobenzoic acid
Cocrystal	1	Can be similar or dissimilar	Different from components	Predominantly adhesive	Curcumin–resorcinol

Cherukuvada, S., & Nangia, 2014.

of fusion of component into three classes mainly lamellar or rod shape with coupled growth, irregular or regular complex structure and irregular structure without coupled growth (Table 4) (Jain, Khomane, & Bansal , 2014).

Apart from drug excipient eutectics system, researchers have explored drug-drug eutectic systems for improving pharmaceutical attributes to achieve the therapeutic benefits. First report on drug-drug eutectics emerged in 1985, where eutectic systems of local anesthetics were prepared for improving the permeation of drug. Recently, the authors group has reported eutectics of etodolac with paracetamol and propranolol hydrochloride for improving the pharmaceutical attributes such as dissolution, compressibility and biopharmaceutical properties (Thipparaboina, Thumuri, Chavan, Naidu, & Shastri, 2017). Repurposed activity of etodolac was improved due to synergistic action of paracetamol. To date less than 12 drug-drug eutectic systems are reported, among them only few were focused towards improving the therapeutic efficacy of the drugs (Table 5).

Methods for preparation of eutectics are similar to cocrystal preparation, ranging from solution crystallization to co grinding and slow solvent evaporation. However, major challenge in development of eutectic is its characterization, as they share some of the properties with solid solution (similar lattice structure) and cocrystal (similar or dissimilar nature of component). Various conventional characterization tools such as thermal (DSC, hot stage microscopy), microscopic (confocal laser scanning microscopy, optical and polarized microscopy and scanning electron microscopy) and spectroscopic techniques (IR, FT-Raman and ssNMR) along with PXRD are used for identification of eutectic systems, but have limited capacity to distinguish between the eutectics and cocrystal. Novel characterization techniques such as atomic pair distribution function (atomic arrangement measurement and local structural ordering determination), structure determination from powder diffraction (determine the microstructure based on solid-solid solubility) and total scattering PDF (differentiation of internal structural of eutectics) are promising approach for thorough characterization of the eutectic system in addition to conventional characterization tools.

As discussed under MDC, motivation behind drug-drug or drug- neutraceutical MDC or eutectics is to improve the pharmaceutical or biopharmaceuticals attributes. Apart from solubility and dissolution improvement, drug-drug eutectics have shown significant enhancement in pharmacokinetic and pharmacodynamic parameters. Among the reported eutectics (Table 5), simvastatin: aspirin and etodolac: paracetamol/ propranolol hydrochloride demonstrated synergistic/ additive effect when evaluated for their respective pharmacological action. In addition to improved fast dissolving capability, etodolac paracetamol eutectics showed improvement in hardness values thus making them suitable for tableting. This system has shown significant reduction of inflammatory markers such as TNF-α, IL-6 and COX-2 in cell culture analysis. Etodolac propranolol hydrochloride eutectic system decreased the IC_{50} value

Table 4. Classification of eutectics proposed by Hemant Jain et al, (2014)

Entropy of Fusion	Eutectic Mixture
Both components have low entropies of fusion (<2 J/gK)	Lamellar or rod shape, couple growth
One component has low entropy of fusion (<2 J/gK)	Irregular or regular complex structure
Both components have high entropies of fusion (>2 J/gK)	Irregular structure no couple growth, grow near each other

Table 5. Reported drug-drug eutectics

Drug Components	Pharmaceutical Attributes Addresses	Preparation Methods	Therapeutic Indication	Ref.
Aspirin and Paracetamol	Compressibility	Solvent evaporation	NSAIDs	Jain et al., (2014)
Simvastatin: Aspirin	Dissolution	Co grinding	Lipid lowering agent and NSAID	Górniak et al., (2013)
Curcumin: Hydroquinone	IDR	Co grinding	Anti cancer	Goud et al., (2012)
Pyrazinamide and Isoniazid	IDR	Co grinding	Anti tubercular	Cherukuvada et al., (2012)
Fenofibrate: Acetylsalicylic Acid	Dissolution	Co grinding	Lipid lowering agent and NSAID	Górniak et al., (2011)
Acetaminophen: Caffeine and Acetaminophen: Propylphenazone	Mechanical strength	In situ Melting / fusion	NSAID and antipyretic	Bi et al., (2003)
Prilocaine:Lidocaine (w/w), and their combinations with, etidocaine, mupivacaine, etc.	Permeation	Heat melted	Local anesthesia	Broberg et al., (1985)
Pyrodoxin and Isoniazid	-	Co grinding	Vitamin and anti tubercular activity	Ganduri et al., (2015)
Hydrochlorothiazide-Atenolol	Solubility, dissolution and stability	Co grinding	Anti hypertensive	Haneef et al., (2017)
Posaconazole and Benznidazole	Solubility and dissolution	Evaporative crystallization, hot melt and cooling	In Chagas disease treatment and anti fungal activity	Figueirêdo et al., (2017)
Etodolac:Paracetamol and Etodolac:Propranolol Hydrochloride	Solubility, dissolution and mechanical properties In vitro cytotoxicity study	Co grinding	Prostate cancer and inflammatory conditions osteoarthritis	Thipparaboina et al., (2017)

by 4.8 folds when compared to plain etodolac, which was recently repurposed for treatment of prostate cancer. Efficacy of this combination during in vitro experiment was analyzed by using Chou-Talalay method where different plots Fa-CI plot (combination index plot or Chou-Talalay plot) and Fa-DRI plot (dose reduction index plot or Chou-Martin plot) were determined (Figure 7). Output of these plots clearly indicated that etodolac propranolol hydrochloride eutectic system showed enhanced cytotoxic effects with synergistic combination index and favorable dose reduction index.

Although reported drug eutectics fulfill the desired goal such as enhanced physico-chemical properties, the design of these systems are still semi-empirical or by trial-and-error instead of chemical and deliberate. Eutectics are not popular as that of cocrystals or solid dispersions in spite their proven efficiency for improving various pharmaceutical and biopharmaceutical attributes. There will be always a few down-side issues with any technology, and eutectics are no exception. The concern with eutectics in the pharmaceutical industry might be due to the lack of proper understanding of their microstructures and difficulties in their complete characterization.

Figure 7. Combination index (CI) and dose reduction index (DRI) plots (E-etodolac and PHC-propranolol hydrochloride)
Reprinted from Thipparaboina R., et al., (2017), with permission from Elsevier.

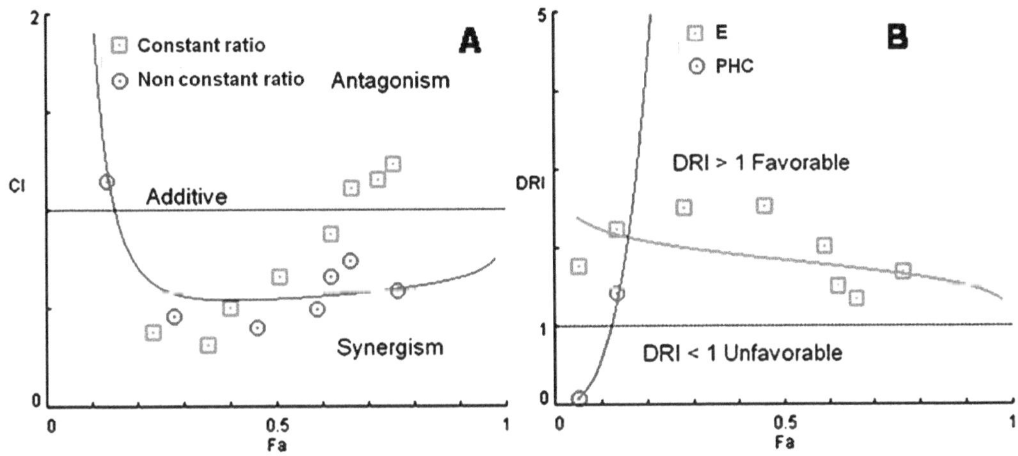

5. FUTURE PERSPECTIVES AND CONCLUDING REMARKS

Novel solid forms such as cocrystals, CAM and eutectics can modulate various pharmaceutical attributes (solubility, permeability, dissolution and pharmacokinetic parameters such as T_{max}, C_{max} and AUC for drugs with poor solubility) and tackle many challenges involved in delivery of therapeutic agents. Progress in the field of multi component solid forms is growing by leaps and bounds and is found promising, as numerous reports on drug-drug/ drug-neutraceutical cocrystals, CAM and eutectics have emerged in recent past with demonstrated potential to provide alternative to existing FDC or multi drug therapy. These multi component solid forms by enhancing the therapeutic activity may prove to be singularly advantageous over existing therapy by improving various pharmaceutical attributes. For successful development of multi component solid forms, selection of appropriate drug combination is a challenging task which requires careful consideration of key factors such as therapeutic applications, differential solubility, and drug–drug interactions. Drug-neutraceutical based combinations may tackle the bioavailability and stability issues of the neutraceuticals with an added advantage of providing new therapeutic hybrids with a unique combination of pharmaceuticals and therapeutically effective neutraceuticals for synergistic benefits and reduced adverse effects. From regulatory point of view, these solid forms are considered novel, non-obvious with potential utility and hence can be protected by composition of matter patents. To date, the existing work in this field is more focused towards coformer screening, preparation and characterization of multi component solid form, formation mechanism, stability and evaluation of pharmaceutical attributes. However, pharmacokinetics and pharmacodynamic of multi component solid forms are largely unexplored and represent a potential avenue for further studies. Similarly, the scale up related challenges needs to be addressed to ensure successful commercialization. Meanwhile, with marketing approval granted for Entresto and Ertugliflozin cocrystal in clinical development stage, one might be justified in expecting a bright future for multi component solid forms.

REFERENCES

Aitipamula, S., Banerjee, R., Bansal, A. K., Biradha, K., Cheney, M. L., Choudhury, A. R., ... Duggirala, N. (2012). Polymorphs, salts, and cocrystals: What's in a name? *Crystal Growth & Design*, *12*(5), 2147–2152. doi:10.1021/cg3002948

Aitipamula, S., Chow, P. S., & Tan, R. B. (2009). Theophylline–gentisic acid (1/1). *Acta Crystallogr. E: Struct. Rep. Online*, *65*(9), o2126–o2127. doi:10.1107/S1600536809031031 PMID:21577539

Alleso, M., Chieng, N., Rehder, S., Rantanen, J., Rades, T., & Aaltonen, J. (2009). Enhanced dissolution rate and synchronized release of drugs in binary systems through formulation: Amorphous naproxen–cimetidine mixtures prepared by mechanical activation. *Journal of Controlled Release*, *136*(1), 45–53. doi:10.1016/j.jconrel.2009.01.027 PMID:19331842

Allesø, M., Chieng, N., Rehder, S., Rantanen, J., Rades, T., & Aaltonen, J. (2009). Enhanced dissolution rate and synchronized release of drugs in binary systems through formulation: Amorphous naproxen–cimetidine mixtures prepared by mechanical activation. *Journal of Controlled Release*, *136*(1), 45–53. doi:10.1016/j.jconrel.2009.01.027 PMID:19331842

Allesø, M., Velaga, S., Alhalaweh, A., Cornett, C., Rasmussen, M. A., Berg, F., ... Rantanen, J. (2008). Near-infrared spectroscopy for cocrystal screening. A comparative study with Raman spectroscopy. *Analytical Chemistry*, *80*(20), 7755–7764. doi:10.1021/ac8011329 PMID:18798651

Bettinetti, G., Caira, M. R., Callegari, A., Merli, M., Sorrenti, M., & Tadini, C. (2000). Structure and solid-state chemistry of anhydrous and hydrated crystal forms of the trimethoprim-sulfamethoxypyridazine 1: 1 molecular complex. *Journal of Pharmaceutical Sciences*, *89*(4), 478–489. doi: PMID:10737909

Beyer, A., Grohganz, H., Löbmann, K., Rades, T., & Leopold, C. S. (2016). Influence of the cooling rate and the blend ratio on the physical stability of co-amorphous naproxen/indomethacin. *European Journal of Pharmaceutics and Biopharmaceutics*, *109*, 140–148. doi:10.1016/j.ejpb.2016.10.002 PMID:27746228

Beyer, A., Grohganz, H., Löbmann, K., Rades, T., & Leopold, C. S. (2017). Improvement Of The Physicochemical Properties Of Co-amorphous Naproxen-indomethacin By Naproxen-sodium. *International Journal of Pharmaceutics*, *526*(1-2), 88–94. doi:10.1016/j.ijpharm.2017.04.011 PMID:28392278

Beyer, A., Radi, L., Grohganz, H., Löbmann, K., Rades, T., & Leopold, C. S. (2016). Preparation and recrystallization behavior of spray-dried co-amorphous naproxen–indomethacin. *European Journal of Pharmaceutics and Biopharmaceutics*, *104*, 72–81. doi:10.1016/j.ejpb.2016.04.019 PMID:27130786

Bhatt, P. M., Azim, Y., Thakur, T. S., & Desiraju, G. R. (2008). Co-crystals of the anti-HIV drugs lamivudine and zidovudine. *Crystal Growth & Design*, *9*(2), 951–957. doi:10.1021/cg8007359

Bi, M., Hwang, S.-J., & Morris, K. R. (2003). Mechanism of eutectic formation upon compaction and its effects on tablet properties. *Thermochimica Acta*, *404*(1), 213–226. doi:10.1016/S0040-6031(03)00185-0

Braga, D., Grepioni, F., Maini, L., Capucci, D., Nanna, S., Wouters, J., ... Quéré, L. (2012). Combining piracetam and lithium salts: Ionic co-crystals and co-drugs? *Chemical Communications (Cambridge)*, *48*(66), 8219–8221. doi:10.1039/c2cc33855f PMID:22781963

Broberg, B. F., & Evers, H. C. (1985). *Local anesthetic mixture for topical application and method for obtaining local anesthesia*. Google Patents.

Burley, J. C., Alkhalil, A., Bloomfield, M., & Matousek, P. (2012). Transmission Raman spectroscopy for quality control in model cocrystal tablets. *Analyst (London)*, *137*(13), 3052–3057. doi:10.1039/c2an35216h PMID:22617192

Caira, M. R. (1992). Molecular complexes of sulfonamides. 2.1: 1 complexes between drug molecules: sulfadimidine-acetylsalicylic acid and sulfadimidine-4-aminosalicylic acid. *Journal of Chemical Crystallography*, *22*(2), 193–200.

Chandel, N., Gupta, V., Pandey, A., & Saxena, S. (2011). Co-crystallization of aceclofenac and paracetamol and their characterization. *Int. J. of Pharm. & Life Sci.*, *2*(8), 1020–1028.

Chavan, R. B., Thipparaboina, R., Kumar, D., & Shastri, N. R. (2016). Co amorphous systems: A product development perspective. *International Journal of Pharmaceutics*, *515*(1), 403–415. doi:10.1016/j.ijpharm.2016.10.043 PMID:27771485

Cheney, M. L., Weyna, D. R., Shan, N., Hanna, M., Wojtas, L., & Zaworotko, M. J. (2011). Coformer selection in pharmaceutical cocrystal development: A case study of a meloxicam aspirin cocrystal that exhibits enhanced solubility and pharmacokinetics. *Journal of Pharmaceutical Sciences*, *100*(6), 2172–2181. doi:10.1002/jps.22434 PMID:21491441

Cherukuvada, S., & Nangia, A. (2012). Fast dissolving eutectic compositions of two anti-tubercular drugs. *CrystEngComm*, *14*(7), 2579–2588. doi:10.1039/c2ce06391c

Cherukuvada, S., & Nangia, A. (2014). Eutectics as improved pharmaceutical materials: Design, properties and characterization. *Chemical Communications (Cambridge)*, *50*(8), 906–923. doi:10.1039/C3CC47521B PMID:24322207

Chieng, N., Aaltonen, J., Saville, D., & Rades, T. (2009). Physical characterization and stability of amorphous indomethacin and ranitidine hydrochloride binary systems prepared by mechanical activation. *European Journal of Pharmaceutics and Biopharmaceutics*, *71*(1), 47 54. doi:10.1016/j.ejpb.2008.06.022 PMID:18644443

Childs, S. L., Stahly, G. P., & Park, A. (2007). The salt– cocrystal continuum: The influence of crystal structure on ionization state. *Molecular Pharmaceutics*, *4*(3), 323–338. doi:10.1021/mp0601345 PMID:17461597

Conway, D., & Cohen, J. A. (2010). Combination therapy in multiple sclerosis. *Lancet Neurology*, *9*(3), 299–308. doi:10.1016/S1474-4422(10)70007-7 PMID:20170843

Cruz-Cabeza, A. J. (2012). Acid–base crystalline complexes and the p K a rule. *CrystEngComm*, *14*(20), 6362–6365. doi:10.1039/c2ce26055g

Delori, A., Galek, P. T., Pidcock, E., Patni, M., & Jones, W. (2013). Knowledge-based hydrogen bond prediction and the synthesis of salts and cocrystals of the anti-malarial drug pyrimethamine with various drug and GRAS molecules. *CrystEngComm*, *15*(15), 2916–2928. doi:10.1039/c3ce26765b

Dengale, S. J., Grohganz, H., Rades, T., & Löbmann, K. (2016). Recent advances in co-amorphous drug formulations. *Advanced Drug Delivery Reviews*, *100*, 116–125. doi:10.1016/j.addr.2015.12.009 PMID:26805787

Dengale, S. J., Hussen, S. S., Krishna, B., Musmade, P. B., Shenoy, G. G., & Bhat, K. (2015). Fabrication, solid state characterization and bioavailability assessment of stable binary amorphous phases of Ritonavir with Quercetin. *European Journal of Pharmaceutics and Biopharmaceutics*, *89*, 329–338. doi:10.1016/j.ejpb.2014.12.025 PMID:25542681

Dengale, S. J., Ranjan, O. P., Hussen, S. S., Krishna, B., Musmade, P. B., Shenoy, G. G., & Bhat, K. (2014). Preparation and characterization of co-amorphous Ritonavir–Indomethacin systems by solvent evaporation technique: Improved dissolution behavior and physical stability without evidence of intermolecular interactions. *European Journal of Pharmaceutical Sciences*, *62*, 57–64. doi:10.1016/j.ejps.2014.05.015 PMID:24878386

Desiraju, G. R. (1995). Supramolecular synthons in crystal engineering—a new organic synthesis. *Angewandte Chemie International Edition in English*, *34*(21), 2311–2327. doi:10.1002/anie.199523111

Drozd, K. V., Manin, A. N., Churakov, A. V., & Perlovich, G. L. (2017). Drug-drug cocrystals of antituberculous 4-aminosalicylic acid: Screening, crystal structures, thermochemical and solubility studies. *European Journal of Pharmaceutical Sciences*, *99*, 228–239. doi:10.1016/j.ejps.2016.12.016 PMID:28011126

Duggirala, N. K., Perry, M. L., Almarsson, Ö., & Zaworotko, M. J. (2016). Pharmaceutical cocrystals: Along the path to improved medicines. *Chemical Communications (Cambridge)*, *52*(4), 640–655. doi:10.1039/C5CC08216A PMID:26565650

Etter, M. C., MacDonald, J. C., & Bernstein, J. (1990). Graph-set analysis of hydrogen-bond patterns in organic crystals. *Acta Crystallographica. Section B, Structural Science*, *46*(2), 256–262. doi:10.1107/S0108768189012929 PMID:2344397

Évora, A. O., Castro, R. A., Maria, T. M., Rosado, M. T., Ramos Silva, M., Matos Beja, A., ... Eusébio, M. E. S. (2011). Pyrazinamide-diflunisal: A new dual-drug co-crystal. *Crystal Growth & Design*, *11*(11), 4780–4788. doi:10.1021/cg200288b

Figueirêdo, C. B. M., Nadvorny, D., de Medeiros Vieira, A. C. Q., Sobrinho, J. L. S., Neto, P. J. R., Lee, P. I., & Soares, M. F. L. R. (2017). Enhancement of dissolution rate through eutectic mixture and solid solution of posaconazole and benznidazole. *International Journal of Pharmaceutics*, *525*(1), 32–42. doi:10.1016/j.ijpharm.2017.04.021 PMID:28412452

Ganduri, R., Cherukuvada, S., & Guru Row, T. N. (2015). Multicomponent Adducts of Pyridoxine: An Evaluation of the Formation of Eutectics and Molecular Salts. *Crystal Growth & Design*, *15*(7), 3474–3480. doi:10.1021/acs.cgd.5b00546

Goldberg, A. H., Gibaldi, M., & Kanig, J. L. (1966). Increasing dissolution rates and gastrointestinal absorption of drugs via solid solutions and eutectic mixtures II: experimental evaluation of a eutectic mixture: urea-acetaminophen system. *Journal of Pharmaceutical Sciences*, *55*(5), 482–487. doi:10.1002/jps.2600550507

Gopi, S. P., Ganguly, S., & Desiraju, G. R. (2016). A Drug–Drug Salt Hydrate of Norfloxacin and Sulfathiazole: Enhancement of in Vitro Biological Properties via Improved Physicochemical Properties. *Molecular Pharmaceutics*, *13*(10), 3590–3594. doi:10.1021/acs.molpharmaceut.6b00320 PMID:27580175

Górniak, A., Karolewicz, B., Żurawska-Płaksej, E., & Pluta, J. (2013). Thermal, spectroscopic, and dissolution studies of the simvastatin–acetylsalicylic acid mixtures. *Journal of Thermal Analysis and Calorimetry*, *111*(3), 2125–2132. doi:10.100710973-012-2641-7

Górniak, A., Wojakowska, A., Karolewicz, B., & Pluta, J. (2011). Phase diagram and dissolution studies of the fenofibrate–acetylsalicylic acid system. *Journal of Thermal Analysis and Calorimetry*, *104*(3), 1195–1200. doi:10.100710973-010-1148-3

Goud, N. R., Suresh, K., Sanphui, P., & Nangia, A. (2012). Fast dissolving eutectic compositions of curcumin. *International Journal of Pharmaceutics*, *439*(1), 63–72. doi:10.1016/j.ijpharm.2012.09.045 PMID:23041131

Grobelny, P., Mukherjee, A., & Desiraju, G. R. (2011). Drug-drug co-crystals: Temperature-dependent proton mobility in the molecular complex of isoniazid with 4-aminosalicylic acid. *CrystEngComm*, *13*(13), 4358–4364. doi:10.1039/c0ce00842g

Haneef, J., & Chadha, R. (2017). Drug-Drug Multicomponent Solid Forms: Cocrystal, Coamorphous and Eutectic of Three Poorly Soluble Antihypertensive Drugs Using Mechanochemical Approach. *AAPS PharmSciTech*, 1–12. PMID:28101724

Issa, N., Karamertzanis, P. G., Welch, G. W., & Price, S. L. (2008). Can the formation of pharmaceutical cocrystals be computationally predicted? I. Comparison of lattice energies. *Crystal Growth & Design*, *9*(1), 442–453. doi:10.1021/cg800685z

Jain, H., Khomane, K. S., & Bansal, A. K. (2014). Implication of microstructure on the mechanical behaviour of an aspirin–paracetamol eutectic mixture. *CrystEngComm*, *16*(36), 8471–8478. doi:10.1039/C4CE00878B

Jensen, K. T., Blaabjerg, L. I., Lenz, E., Bohr, A., Grohganz, H., Kleinebudde, P., ... Lobmann, K. (2016). Preparation and characterization of spray-dried co-amorphous drug–amino acid salts. *The Journal of Pharmacy and Pharmacology*, *68*(5), 615–624. doi:10.1111/jphp.12458 PMID:26245703

Jiang, L., Huang, Y., Zhang, Q., He, H., Xu, Y., & Mei, X. (2014). Preparation and solid-state characterization of dapsone drug–drug co-crystals. *Crystal Growth & Design*, *14*(9), 4562–4573. doi:10.1021/cg500668a

Knapik, J., Wojnarowska, Z., Grzybowska, K., Jurkiewicz, K., Tajber, L., & Paluch, M. (2015). Molecular dynamics and physical stability of co-amorphous ezetimib and indapamide mixtures. *Molecular Pharmaceutics*, *12*(10), 3610–3619. doi:10.1021/acs.molpharmaceut.5b00334 PMID:26301858

Kojima, T., Tsutsumi, S., Yamamoto, K., Ikeda, Y., & Moriwaki, T. (2010). High-throughput cocrystal slurry screening by use of in situ Raman microscopy and multi-well plate. *International Journal of Pharmaceutics*, *399*(1), 52–59. doi:10.1016/j.ijpharm.2010.07.055 PMID:20696223

Lemmerer, A. (2012). Covalent assistance to supramolecular synthesis: Modifying the drug functionality of the antituberculosis API isoniazid in situ during co-crystallization with GRAS and API compounds. *CrystEngComm*, *14*(7), 2465–2478. doi:10.1039/C1CE06310C

Lenz, E., Jensen, K. T., Blaabjerg, L. I., Knop, K., Grohganz, H., Lobmann, K., ... Kleinebudde, P. (2015). Solid-state properties and dissolution behaviour of tablets containing co-amorphous indomethacin–arginine. *European Journal of Pharmaceutics and Biopharmaceutics*, *96*, 44–52. doi:10.1016/j.ejpb.2015.07.011 PMID:26197392

Leung, D. H., Lohani, S., Ball, R. G., Canfield, N., Wang, Y., Rhodes, T., & Bak, A. (2012). Two novel pharmaceutical cocrystals of a development compound–screening, scale-up, and characterization. *Crystal Growth & Design*, *12*(3), 1254–1262. doi:10.1021/cg201270s

Lim, A. W., Löbmann, K., Grohganz, H., Rades, T., & Chieng, N. (2016). Investigation of physical properties and stability of indomethacin–cimetidine and naproxen–cimetidine co-amorphous systems prepared by quench cooling, coprecipitation and ball milling. *The Journal of Pharmacy and Pharmacology*, *68*(1), 36–45. doi:10.1111/jphp.12494 PMID:26663364

Lobmann, K., Laitinen, R., Grohganz, H., Gordon, K. C., Strachan, C., & Rades, T. (2011). Coamorphous drug systems: Enhanced physical stability and dissolution rate of indomethacin and naproxen. *Molecular Pharmaceutics*, *8*(5), 1919–1928. doi:10.1021/mp2002973 PMID:21815614

Löbmann, K., Laitinen, R., Grohganz, H., Gordon, K. C., Strachan, C., & Rades, T. (2011). Coamorphous drug systems: Enhanced physical stability and dissolution rate of indomethacin and naproxen. *Molecular Pharmaceutics*, *8*(5), 1919–1928. doi:10.1021/mp2002973 PMID:21815614

Löbmann, K., Laitinen, R., Grohganz, H., Strachan, C., Rades, T., & Gordon, K. C. (2013). A theoretical and spectroscopic study of co-amorphous naproxen and indomethacin. *International Journal of Pharmaceutics*, *453*(1), 80–87. doi:10.1016/j.ijpharm.2012.05.016 PMID:22613066

Löbmann, K., Strachan, C., Grohganz, H., Rades, T., Korhonen, O., & Laitinen, R. (2012). Co-amorphous simvastatin and glipizide combinations show improved physical stability without evidence of intermolecular interactions. *European Journal of Pharmaceutics and Biopharmaceutics*, *81*(1), 159–169. doi:10.1016/j.ejpb.2012.02.004 PMID:22353489

Lu, E., Rodríguez-Hornedo, N., & Suryanarayanan, R. (2008). A rapid thermal method for cocrystal screening. *CrystEngComm*, *10*(6), 665–668. doi:10.1039/b801713c

Lu, J., & Rohani, S. (2010). Synthesis and preliminary characterization of sulfamethazine-theophylline co-crystal. *Journal of Pharmaceutical Sciences*, *99*(9), 4042–4047. doi:10.1002/jps.22142 PMID:20665847

Mohammad, M. A., Alhalaweh, A., & Velaga, S. P. (2011). Hansen solubility parameter as a tool to predict cocrystal formation. *International Journal of Pharmaceutics*, *407*(1), 63–71. doi:10.1016/j.ijpharm.2011.01.030 PMID:21256944

Mukherjee, A., Tothadi, S., Chakraborty, S., Ganguly, S., & Desiraju, G. R. (2013). Synthon identification in co-crystals and polymorphs with IR spectroscopy. Primary amides as a case study. *CrystEngComm*, *15*(23), 4640–4654. doi:10.1039/c3ce40286j

Nagapudi, K., Umanzor, E. Y., & Masui, C. (2017). High-throughput screening and scale-up of cocrystals using resonant acoustic mixing. *International Journal of Pharmaceutics*, *521*(1), 337–345. doi:10.1016/j.ijpharm.2017.02.027 PMID:28229947

Nakao, S., Fujii, S., Sakaki, T., & Tomita, K. I. (1977). The crystal and molecular structure of the 2: 1 molecular complex of theophylline with phenobarbital. *Acta Crystallographica. Section B, Structural Science*, *33*(5), 1373–1378. doi:10.1107/S0567740877006116

Nangia, A. (2010). Supramolecular chemistry and crystal engineering. *Journal of Chemical Sciences*, *122*(3), 295–310. doi:10.100712039-010-0035-6

Nechipadappu, S. K., Tekuri, V., & Trivedi, D. R. (2017). Pharmaceutical Co-Crystal of Flufenamic Acid: Synthesis and Characterization of Two Novel Drug-Drug Co-Crystal. *Journal of Pharmaceutical Sciences*, *106*(5), 1384–1390. doi:10.1016/j.xphs.2017.01.033 PMID:28185907

Pajula, K., Wittoek, L., Lehto, V.-P., Ketolainen, J., & Korhonen, O. (2014). Phase Separation in Coamorphous Systems: In Silico Prediction and the Experimental Challenge of Detection. *Molecular Pharmaceutics*, *11*(7), 2271–2279. doi:10.1021/mp400712m PMID:24824610

Pathak, C., Savjani, K., Gajjar, A. K., & Savjani, J. K. (2013). cocrystal formation of paracetamol with indomethacin and mefenamic acid: An efficient approach to enhance solubility. *International Journal of Pharmacy and Pharmaceutical Sciences*, *5*(4), 414–419.

Paudel, A., Worku, Z. A., Meeus, J., Guns, S., & Van den Mooter, G. (2013). Manufacturing of solid dispersions of poorly water soluble drugs by spray drying: Formulation and process considerations. *International Journal of Pharmaceutics*, *453*(1), 253–284. doi:10.1016/j.ijpharm.2012.07.015 PMID:22820134

Pinto Vitorino, G., Sperandeo, N. R., Caira, M. R., & Mazzieri, M. R. (2013). A supramolecular assembly formed by heteroassociation of ciprofloxacin and norfloxacin in the solid state: Co-crystal synthesis and characterization. *Crystal Growth & Design*, *13*(3), 1050–1058. doi:10.1021/cg301299e

Putra, O. D., Furuishi, T., Yonemochi, E., Terada, K., & Uekusa, H. (2016). Drug–Drug Multicomponent Crystals as an Effective Technique to Overcome Weaknesses in Parent Drugs. *Crystal Growth & Design*, *16*(7), 3577–3581. doi:10.1021/acs.cgd.6b00639

Qi, S., McAuley, W. J., Yang, Z., & Tipduangta, P. (2014). Physical stabilization of low-molecular-weight amorphous drugs in the solid state: A material science approach. *Therapeutic Delivery*, *5*(7), 817–841. doi:10.4155/tde.14.39 PMID:25287388

Rahman, Z., Siddiqui, A., Gupta, A., & Khan, M. (2014). Regulatory considerations in development of amorphous solid dispersions. In *Amorphous Solid Dispersions* (pp. 545–563). Springer. doi:10.1007/978-1-4939-1598-9_17

Ravikumar, N., Gaddamanugu, G., & Solomon, K. A. (2013). Structural, spectroscopic (FT-IR, FT-Raman) and theoretical studies of the 1: 1 cocrystal of isoniazid with p-coumaric acid. *Journal of Molecular Structure*, *1033*, 272–279. doi:10.1016/j.molstruc.2012.10.029

Renuka, Singh, S. K., Gulati, M., & Narang, R. (2015). Stable amorphous binary systems of glipizide and atorvastatin powders with enhanced dissolution profiles: Formulation and characterization. *Pharmaceutical Development and Technology*, 1–13. PMID:26708555

Renuka, S., Singh, S. K., Gulati, M., & Narang, R. (2017). Stable amorphous binary systems of glipizide and atorvastatin powders with enhanced dissolution profiles: Formulation and characterization. *Pharmaceutical Development and Technology*, *22*(1), 13–25. doi:10.3109/10837450.2015.1125921 PMID:26708555

Russo, M. G., Sancho, M. I., Silva, L. M., Baldoni, H. A., Venancio, T., Ellena, J., & Narda, G. E. (2016). Looking for the interactions between omeprazole and amoxicillin in a disordered phase. An experimental and theoretical study. *Spectrochimica Acta. Part A: Molecular and Biomolecular Spectroscopy*, *156*, 70–77. doi:10.1016/j.saa.2015.11.021 PMID:26654963

Sanphui, P., Goud, N. R., Khandavilli, U. R., & Nangia, A. (2011). Fast dissolving curcumin cocrystals. *Crystal Growth & Design*, *11*(9), 4135–4145. doi:10.1021/cg200704s

Sardone, N., Bettinetti, G., & Sorrenti, M. (1997). Trimethoprim–Sulfadimidine 1: 2 Molecular Complex Monohydrate. *Acta Crystallographica. Section C, Structural Chemistry*, *53*(9), 1295–1299. doi:10.1107/S0108270197000425

Schultheiss, N., Roe, M., & Boerrigter, S. X. (2011). Cocrystals of nutraceutical p-coumaric acid with caffeine and theophylline: Polymorphism and solid-state stability explored in detail using their crystal graphs. *CrystEngComm*, *13*(2), 611–619. doi:10.1039/C0CE00214C

Sekiguchi, K., & Obi, N. (1961). Studies on Absorption of Eutectic Mixture. I. A Comparison of the Behavior of Eutectic Mixture of Sulfathiazole and that of Ordinary Sulfathiazole in Man. *Chemical & Pharmaceutical Bulletin*, *9*(11), 866–872. doi:10.1248/cpb.9.866

Sekiguchi, K., Obi, N., & Ueda, Y. (1964). Studies on Absorption of Eutectic Mixture. II. Absorption of fused Conglomerates of Chloramphenicol and Urea in Rabbits. *Chemical & Pharmaceutical Bulletin*, *12*(2), 134–144. doi:10.1248/cpb.12.134 PMID:14126741

Shayanfar, A., & Jouyban, A. (2013). Drug–Drug Coamorphous Systems: Characterization and Physicochemical Properties of Coamorphous Atorvastatin with Carvedilol and Glibenclamide. *Journal of Pharmaceutical Innovation*, *8*(4), 218–228. doi:10.100712247-013-9162-1

Shin, H.-C., Alani, A. W., Rao, D. A., Rockich, N. C., & Kwon, G. S. (2009). Multi-drug loaded polymeric micelles for simultaneous delivery of poorly soluble anticancer drugs. *Journal of Controlled Release*, *140*(3), 294–300. doi:10.1016/j.jconrel.2009.04.024 PMID:19409432

Sinha, A. S., Khandavilli, U. R., O'Connor, E. L., Deadman, B. J., Maguire, A. R., & Lawrence, S. E. (2015). Novel co-crystals of the nutraceutical sinapic acid. *CrystEngComm*, *17*(26), 4832–4841. doi:10.1039/C5CE00777A

Sokal, A., Pindelska, E., Szeleszczuk, L., & Kolodziejski, W. (2017). Pharmaceutical properties of two ethenzamide-gentisic acid cocrystal polymorphs: Drug release profiles, spectroscopic studies and theoretical calculations. *International Journal of Pharmaceutics*, *522*(1), 80–89. doi:10.1016/j.ijpharm.2017.03.004 PMID:28274662

Stepanovs, D., & Mishnev, A. (2012). Multicomponent pharmaceutical cocrystals: Furosemide and pentoxifylline. *Acta Crystallographica. Section C, Structural Chemistry*, *68*(12), o488–o491. doi:10.1107/S0108270112045866 PMID:23221253

Suresh, K., Mannava, M. C., & Nangia, A. (2014). A novel curcumin–artemisinin coamorphous solid: Physical properties and pharmacokinetic profile. *RSC Advances*, *4*(102), 58357–58361. doi:10.1039/C4RA11935E

Surov, A. O., Voronin, A. P., Manin, A. N., Manin, N. G., Kuzmina, L. G., Churakov, A. V., & Perlovich, G. L. (2014). Pharmaceutical cocrystals of diflunisal and diclofenac with theophylline. *Molecular Pharmaceutics*, *11*(10), 3707–3715. doi:10.1021/mp5004652 PMID:25184906

Teja, A., Musmade, P. B., Khade, A. B., & Dengale, S. J. (2015). Simultaneous improvement of solubility and permeability by fabricating binary glassy materials of Talinolol with Naringin: Solid state characterization, in-vivo in-situ evaluation. *European Journal of Pharmaceutical Sciences*, *78*, 234–244. doi:10.1016/j.ejps.2015.08.002 PMID:26253355

Thipparaboina, R., Chavan, R. B., Kumar, D., Modugula, S., & Shastri, N. R. (2015). Micellar carriers for the delivery of multiple therapeutic agents. *Colloids and Surfaces. B, Biointerfaces*, *135*, 291–308. doi:10.1016/j.colsurfb.2015.07.046 PMID:26263217

Thipparaboina, R., Kumar, D., Chavan, R. B., & Shastri, N. R. (2016). Multidrug co-crystals: Towards the development of effective therapeutic hybrids. *Drug Discovery Today*, *21*(3), 481–490. doi:10.1016/j.drudis.2016.02.001 PMID:26869329

Thipparaboina, R., Thumuri, D., Chavan, R., Naidu, V., & Shastri, N. R. (2017). Fast dissolving drug-drug eutectics with improved compressibility and synergistic effects. *European Journal of Pharmaceutical Sciences*, *104*, 82–89. doi:10.1016/j.ejps.2017.03.042 PMID:28366649

Ueda, H., Kadota, K., Imono, M., Ito, T., Kunita, A., & Tozuka, Y. (2017). Co-amorphous formation induced by combination of tranilast and diphenhydramine hydrochloride. *Journal of Pharmaceutical Sciences*, *106*(1), 123–128. doi:10.1016/j.xphs.2016.07.009 PMID:27539557

Ueda, H., Muranushi, N., Sakuma, S., Ida, Y., Endoh, T., Kadota, K., & Tozuka, Y. (2016). A strategy for co-former selection to design stable co-amorphous formations based on physicochemical properties of non-steroidal inflammatory drugs. *Pharmaceutical Research*, *33*(4), 1018–1029. doi:10.100711095-015-1848-2 PMID:26700604

Vasconcelos, T., Marques, S., das Neves, J., & Sarmento, B. (2016). Amorphous solid dispersions: Rational selection of a manufacturing process. *Advanced Drug Delivery Reviews*, *100*, 85–101. doi:10.1016/j.addr.2016.01.012 PMID:26826438

Vishweshwar, P., McMahon, J. A., Peterson, M. L., Hickey, M. B., Shattock, T. R., & Zaworotko, M. J. (2005). Crystal engineering of pharmaceutical co-crystals from polymorphic active pharmaceutical ingredients. *Chemical Communications*, (36): 4601–4603. doi:10.1039/b501304f PMID:16158128

Vo, C. L.-N., Park, C., & Lee, B.-J. (2013). Current trends and future perspectives of solid dispersions containing poorly water-soluble drugs. *European Journal of Pharmaceutics and Biopharmaceutics*, *85*(3), 799–813. doi:10.1016/j.ejpb.2013.09.007 PMID:24056053

Vogt, F. G., Clawson, J. S., Strohmeier, M., Edwards, A. J., Pham, T. N., & Watson, S. A. (2008). Solid-state NMR analysis of organic cocrystals and complexes. *Crystal Growth & Design*, *9*(2), 921–937. doi:10.1021/cg8007014

Wairkar, S., & Gaud, R. (2015). Co-Amorphous Combination of Nateglinide-Metformin Hydrochloride for Dissolution Enhancement. *AAPS PharmSciTech*, 1–9. PMID:26314243

Wang, J.-R., Yu, Q., Dai, W., & Mei, X. (2016). Drug–drug co-crystallization presents a new opportunity for the development of stable vitamins. *Chemical Communications (Cambridge)*, *52*(17), 3572–3575. doi:10.1039/C5CC10297A PMID:26845759

Yamamura, S., Gotoh, H., Sakamoto, Y., & Momose, Y. (2000). Physicochemical properties of amorphous precipitates of cimetidine–indomethacin binary system. *European Journal of Pharmaceutics and Biopharmaceutics*, *49*(3), 259–265. doi:10.1016/S0939-6411(00)00060-6 PMID:10799818

Yamamura, S., Gotoh, H., Sakamoto, Y., & Momose, Y. (2002). Physicochemical properties of amorphous salt of cimetidine and diflunisal system. *International Journal of Pharmaceutics*, *241*(2), 213–221. doi:10.1016/S0378-5173(02)00195-3 PMID:12100849

Zaitu, S., Miwa, Y., & Taga, T. (1995). A 2: 1 molecular complex of theophylline and 5-fluorouracil as the monohydrate. *Acta Crystallographica. Section C, Structural Chemistry*, *51*(9), 1857–1859. doi:10.1107/S0108270195003295

Žegarac, M., Lekšić, E., Šket, P., Plavec, J., Bogdanović, M. D., Bučar, D.-K., ... Meštrović, E. (2014). A sildenafil cocrystal based on acetylsalicylic acid exhibits an enhanced intrinsic dissolution rate. *CrystEngComm*, *16*(1), 32–35. doi:10.1039/C3CE42013B

Chapter 11
Multifunctional Nanocarrier Systems for Effective Delivery of Drugs in Cancer Treatment

Brahmeshwar Mishra
IIT (BHU), India

Sathish Thokala
IIT (BHU), India

ABSTRACT

The drug delivery to the cancer sites, with maintained effective drug concentration for longer duration, using low dose of drug, with minimum side effects is the prime concern of formulation scientist today. In the recent times, the nanocarrier systems are not only being utilized for achieving targeted, sustained and controlled release of drug to the disease site, but also are used in imaging of diseases. An attempt has been made through this chapter to give a brief outline about the cancer and elaborate details on the various multifunctional nanocarriers researched till date for effective delivery of drugs in cancer treatment. Further, functionalization and surface modification of nanocarrier with various ligands like folate, transferrin, TPGS (d-α- Tocopheryl Polyethylene Glycol 1000 Succinate), trastuzumab and hyaluronic acid etc., that have specific receptor in the proximity of disease site have been explained along with pros and cons of such carrier systems.

INTRODUCTION

The delivery of drugs to specified cancer sites, in early phase of disease, in safe and effective mode, with drug concentration in therapeutic range, over a period of time is needed to mitigate the disease consequence and this could be possible with carrier system and that can target the cancer site (Cerqueira, Lasham, Shelling, & Al-Kassas, 2017; Kushwaha, Ghoshal, Rai, & Singh, 2013; Singh, Sharma, Singh, Kumar, Pandey, Koch, & Muthu, 2016). However, the existing drug delivery approaches do not fully meet the criteria; therefore development of an effective drug carrier system to effectively deliver drugs and treat cancer or other diseases is inevitable.

DOI: 10.4018/978-1-5225-4781-5.ch011

Copyright © 2018, IGI Global. Copying or distributing in print or electronic forms without written permission of IGI Global is prohibited.

Cancer

Cancer is stated as uncontrolled proliferation of cells and better known disease to almost all populations of the world. The development of cancer cells is different from normal healthy cells (Dhas, Ige, & Kudarha, 2015). Despite of availability of treatment approaches like chemotherapy, an effective method is not yet found to eradicate the cancer and the failure of chemotherapy may be due to non-specificity as well as inability of the anticancer agent(s) to target the cancer cells. Cancer can affect different organs of the body and leads to cancer of liver, lung, breast, prostate, gall-bladder, ovary, pancreas and colon etc (Sheikhpour, Golbabaie, & Kasaeian, 2017). About 7.6 million deaths (approximately 13% of all deaths) occurred in 2008 because of cancer, as per the recent fact sheet of World Health Organization (WHO) wherein approximately 70% deaths happened in low and middle income countries. By 2030, cancer deaths are expected to rise over 13.1 million, worldwide (Mehra & Jain, 2015). Cancer treatment is a challenging task because; chemotherapeutic agents are cytotoxic in nature and could rarely differentiates healthy cells from cancer cells. Thus, leads to damage of vital normal organ cells in addition to killing cancer cells even at therapeutic drug concentration range, if their distribution in the body is not properly maintained and targeted towards the cancer cells or tissues (Modi, Patel, Desai, & Murthy, 2011). Therefore, targeted drug delivery to target cancer sites is essential need of the hour.

Drug Delivery

Almost all the present, chemotherapeutic agents are having low molecular weight with good pharmacokinetic volume of distribution, both of them bestow to their cytotoxicity and make them easily excreted, Their low therapeutic index does not offer favourably to this issue, as the required concentration for the better efficacy should be maintained, therefore higher drug concentration is needed and consequently toxicity is inevitable but unfortunately the therapeutic levels often exceeds. Further, these drugs administered alone, possess lack of specificity and cause notable damage to healthy tissues (Bharali, Khalil, Gurbuz, Simone, & Mousa, 2009). The aim of today's researchers is to fabricate novel drug carrier systems to address the problems associated with existing non-functionalised nanoparticle therapy, such as high dose size, dosing frequency, lack of specificity and side effects etc. This objective driven the formulation scientists to fabricate a novel delivery approaches for effective delivery of drugs to cancer site and could be achieved by early detection/diagnosis/imaging of the cancer by ligand decorated multifunctional nanocarrier systems (Gindy & Prud'homme, 2009).

Nanocarrier System

The researchers have explored various micro and nanoparticulate carrier systems to overcome the problems associated with conventional chemotherapy in cancer. Different types of nanoparticulate system are available, such as polymeric nanoparticles, solid lipid nanoparticles, metal nanoparticles, liposomes, niosomes, nanofibers, nanocrystals, polymeric micelles, carbon nanotubes, nanostructured lipid carrier, quantum dots, dendrimers and lipoproteins etc (Torchilin, 2007). These carriers have become one of the most prominent systems for the diagnosis, treatment and prevention of cancer.

Loading of drugs in the nanocarrier system would protect them from the body's natural defences and improves their availability at disease site. In addition, nanoparticles offer high drug payload and can also be surface modified with various types of ligands that could act as targeting moieties to reach the desired disease site. These functionalised nanoparticulate drug formulations not only enhance the therapeutic efficacy but also offer internalization into cell via receptor associated endocytosis and minimizes the problems like lack of targeting ability, inadequate bioavailability and poor drug loading etc (Crucho & Barros, 2015).

CLASSIFICATION OF NANOCARRIER SYSTEMS

Nanocarrier systems are essentially consists of nanoparticles, nanofibers, nanotubes, nanocrystals, liposomes and dendrimers etc. These systems are classified (as given below) based on the material opted for fabrication and methods employed for their preparation i.e., polymeric nanoparticles (nanospheres and nanocapsules), solid lipid nanoparticles (SLN), metal nanoparticles, drug nanocrystals and carbon nanotubes (CNTs) etc. (Ding & Li, 2017). And different types of nanocarrier systems have shown in Figure 1.

- Nanoparticles
    - Polymeric Nanoparticles
    - Solid Lipid Nanoparticles
    - Gold Nanoparticles
- Carbon Nanotubes
- Liposomes
- Drug Nanocrystals
- Nanofibers
- Nanosuspension
- Nanoemulsion
- Dendrimers

Figure 1. Nanocarrier systems for drug delivery in cancer

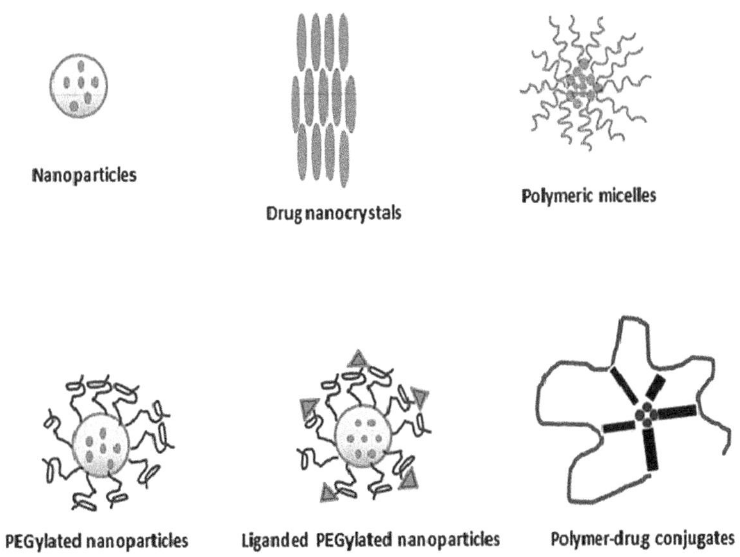

Nanoparticles

The nanoparticles further classified into different types as explained in detailed below.

Polymeric Nanoparticles

Polymeric nanoparticles have been widely explored for biomedical applications particularly in drug delivery and tissue engineering. Out of these applications, drug delivery by polymeric nanoparticles with specific internalization into a target cell has been taken into consideration (Esfandiarpour-Boroujeni, Bagheri-Khoulenjani, Mirzadeh, & Amanpour, 2017). It is well established that active targeting of polymeric nanoparticles by ligand conjugation enhances the specificity of nanoparticles to cancer cells. Ligands such as folic acid, antibiotics, sugars, aptamers and peptides etc. are being presently employed include polymeric nanoparticle functionalization with the aim of active targeting. Polymeric nanoparticles (PNPs) are favourable carriers for controlled drug delivery. Polymers employed in fabrication of PNP are natural polymers and synthetic polymers. Natural polymers include sodium alginate, albumin, chitosan and gelatine. And synthetic polymers include polylactides (PLA), poly (lactide coglycolides) (PLGA), polyglycolides (PGA), polyanhydrides, polycyanoacrylates, polycaprolactone (PCL), poly (malic acid) (PMLA), polyglutamic acid (PGA), poly (methyl methacrylate) (PMMA), poly (N-vinyl pyrrolidone) (PVP), poly (vinyl alcohol) (PVA), polyacrylamide (PAM), polyethylene glycol (PEG), polyacrylic acid (PAA) and poly (methacrylic acid) (PMAA) (Khalid & El-Sawy, 2017). Poly lactic-co-glycolic acid (PLGA) is the most regularly used biodegradable and biocompatible polymer in the fabrication of nanoparticles (Crucho & Barros, 2015).

Polymeric nanoparticles (PNPs) can be fabricated by different methods (mentioned below) based on their applications and the physicochemical characteristics of the drug. The methods include, emulsification-solvent evaporation, solvent diffusion, salting-out technique, nanoprecipitation method, dialysis and supercritical fluid process etc. out of the above methods emulsification-solvent evaporation is most widely used method. In brief, firstly the polymer(s) is solubilised in a volatile organic solvent. The resulting organic solution is emulsified with aqueous system contains surfactant(s) and homogenised with high-speed homogenizer or ultrasonicator, produces a dispersion of nanodroplets. From the above, suspension of nanoparticles is obtained by organic solvent evaporation; either by constant magnetic stirring at room temperature or under reduced pressure. After the complete removal of solvent, the solidified nanoparticles can be washed and collected by centrifuging, followed by lyophillization (Crucho & Barros, 2017).

Solid Lipid Nanoparticles

Solid lipid nanoparticles (SLN) were introduced in the early 1990s as an effective and non-toxic drug carrier system composed of natural lipids that are solids at body temperature. The lipophilic character of the SLN is well suited for loading of lipophilic drugs. On the other hand, hydrophilic drugs are poorly encapsulated in the core as they have a strong affinity to partition into the outer aqueous system during the preparation process, However, under optimized conditions, both hydrophilic and lipophilic drugs can be encapsulated into SLN (Peres, Peres, de Araújo, & Sayer, 2016). SLNs are better alternative drug carrier systems to conventional systems like solutions, suspensions and ointments etc. Physiological lipids and biocompatible surfactants are commonly employed to fabricate SLNs, which makes them well compatible with living systems and therefore, no acute toxicity is anticipated. Usually the mean diameter of SLN falls approximately in the size range of 50 and 1000 nm (Baig, Ahad, Aslam, Imam, Aqil, & Ali , 2016).

The preparation methods include the hot and cold homogenization techniques. In both methods the drug is solubilised or dispersed in the lipid phase being melted at approximately 5-10°C above its melting point. In hot homogenization procedure the drug dissolved melt is poured in a hot aqueous surfactant solution of identical temperature under stirring. Then the obtained pre-emulsion is homogenized, to produce hot O/W nanoemulsion and cooled at room temperature and further recrystallization of the lipid leads to formation of solid lipid nanoparticles. In cold homogenization method the drug dispersed lipid melt is cooled, the solidified lipid micronized to lipid microparticles (approximately 50-100 µm) and these lipid microparticles are poured in a cold surfactant solution to produce a pre suspension. Then this pre suspension is homogenized at or below room temperature, to obtained the solid lipid nanoparticles from lipid microparticles. This procedure avoids, or minimizes, melting of the lipids at higher temperature and therefore diminishes loss of hydrophilic drugs to the aqueous phase (MuÈller, MaÈder, & Gohla, 2000).

Gold Nanoparticles

Gold nanoparticles (AuNPs) are explored as a novel drug carrier system that could be utilized for both, imaging and treatment of cancer, referred to as theranostic application. AuNPs possess several physicochemical properties like (a) chemically inert, (b) easy surface functionalization, (c) electronic structure amenable for plasmon resonance and (d) optical properties that differentiate them from other nanocarrier systems and also make them as imaging agents. In addition, availability of AuNPs in different shapes and size makes them suitable for drug delivery applications. Different types of AuNPs have been reported based on methods of preparation and experimental conditions, i.e., gold nanospheres (AuNSs), nanoshells (AuNShs), nanorods (AuNRs), nanocages (AuNCgs), nanoboxes (AuNbs), nanostars (AuNSts), nanocubes (AuNCus), nanoclusters (AuNCls), nanocrystal (AuNCrs) and triangular bipyramaids (AuBps) (Muddineti, Ghosh, & Biswas, 2015).

AuNPs explored as radiosensitizers for X-radiation treatment of cancer due to their ability to convert low linear energy transfer (LET) X-rays into high LET and more radio biologically damaging photoelectrons. AuNPs may passively localize in tumours, following intravenous (i.v.) injection via enhanced permeation and retention (EPR) effect due to leaky tumour vascular endothelium and poor lymphatic drainage. AuNP can also be functionalised with monoclonal antibodies (mAbs), peptide and other ligands for active tumour targeting via associated antigens or receptors (Cai, Chattopadhya, Yang, Kwon, Yook, Pignol, & Reilly, 2016). Therefore, AuNPs extended researcher's interest owing to their remarkable applications in imaging, molecular diagnostics and drug delivery etc. Mainly, which NPs have been proved to be better effective against a wide range of human cancers such as breast, lung, prostate, colon and cervical etc. (Ramachandran, Krishnaraj, Sivakumar, Prasannakumar, Kumar, Shim, . . . Yun, 2017).

Carbon Nanotubes (Cnts)

CNTs were explored in 1991 by Sumio Iijima a Japanese scientist. Carbon nanotubes (CNTs) established as one of the most effective nanocarrier system for delivery of various drugs and bioactive owing to its large surface area with high aspect ratio, easy surface alteration, and higher loading capacity. The CNTs skeleton is made up of carbon atoms in hexagonal arrangement forming graphite sheet rolled up to seamless tubular cylinder. CNTs are classified into single-walled CNT (SWCNT), double-walled CNT (DWCNT) and multi-walled CNT (MWCNT) (Pruthi, Mehra, & Jain, 2012).

The non-functionalised MWCNTs often show some limitations because of traces of amorphous carbon obtained from catalysts in the synthesis process. This problem can be minimized or avoided by the purification and functionalization of MWCNTs by using hot nitric acid. MWCNTs, which are oxidised with nitric acid, the oxidised moieties can easily be modified with various organic and inorganic compounds. However, it is also reported that oxidation with nitric acid leads to increasing solubility and shortening of MWCNTs length, which expands their application, especially in drug delivery (Milosavljevic, Krejcova, Guran, Buchtelova, Wawrzak, Richtera, . . . Adam , 2017).

The MWCNT can be further decorated with various biologically active moieties such as drug, surfactant, imaging agents, antibody and targeting agents, which can target receptors that are over expressed on the cancer cells. The MWCNT can reside for longer period in the blood, evade host defences, and releases drug in the diseased cells and facilitate better *in-vitro* and *in-vivo* therapy. The *in-vivo* toxicity (both cellular and molecular levels) of pristine MWCNT, because of their hydrophobic nature can be reduced by surface activation strategies, i.e., oxidation, nitration and acylation techniques etc. (Singh, Sharma, Singh, Patne, Pandey, Koch, & Muthu , 2016)

Liposomes

Liposomes are concentric lipid bilayered vesicles that encompasses the aqueous phase and spherical in shape. Liposomes possess several significant properties compared to other drug delivery systems including bio-compatibility, non-immunogenicity, enhancement of the solubility, self-assembling ability, high drug payloads, protection of the drugs from degradation, minimize the toxicity of the drugs, site-specific delivery and improving penetration into tissues. Liposomes have the ability to deliver many pharmacologically active moieties and other macromolecules (e.g. DNA, peptides, proteins and imaging agents), both in their lipid bilayer (i.e., lipophilic molecules) and aqueous core (i.e., hydrophilic molecules). The basic preparation methods include, thin film hydration, sonication, high pressure homoginization, microfuidization, extrusioin method, reverse phase evaporation, ether injection and ethanol injection etc. In brief about ethanol injection, a predetermined volume of ethanol containing phospholipids is injected into an aqueous system under constant agitation via a syringe fixed with a needle (Sala, Miladi, Agusti, Elaissari, & Fessi, 2017).

The liposome size can range from very small (25 nm) to large (2.5 μm) vesicles. Based on their size and number of bilayer presence, liposomes are classified into two groups: (1) unilamellar vesicles and; (2) multilamellar vesicles (MLV). Unilamellar vesicles can be divided into two subgroups: (1) small unilamellar vesicles (SUV) and; (2) large unilamellar vesicles (LUV). Unilamellar vesicle consists of a single phospholipid bilayer surrounded by the aqueous environment. Generally, several unilamellar vesicles inside the larger vesicle, forming a multilamellar concentric phospholipid spheres separated by aqueous phase (Vahed, Salehi, Davaran, & Sharifi, 2016).

The targeted drug delivery via liposomes can diminish the side effects associated with drugs, which have a narrow therapeutic range, by circumventing drug distribution to the non-specific organs. PEGylated liposomes considerably minimize the cardiotoxicity of the incorporated anticancer agent (Tagami, Ando, & Ozeki, 2017).

Nanocrystals

Drug nanocrystals (NCs) are the nanoparticles of drug, which provide an additional benefit of 100% drug loading since they are carrier free nanoparticles. A NC formulation consists of drug and one/more stabilizers dispersed in aqueous or non-aqueous media. Stabilizers could be one or more generally regarded as safe (GRAS) excipients (surfactants or buffers, salts or sugars) (Srivalli & Mishra, 2016). Drug nanocrystals are the one of the most discussed approach for drug delivery in the last twenty years. As compared to other nanoparticulate systems, drug nanocrystals contains mainly pure API. They are often fabricated in aqueous system which contains one or more stabilizers for the dispersed state; therefore these systems sometimes can also be referred as nanosuspensions. Frequently, drug nanocrystals are also called as drug nanoparticles (Möschwitzer, 2013).

The basic strategies involved in fabrication of nanocrystals are the top-down technologies, nanosizing (drug powder size reduction, e.g. by mechanical attrition), the bottom–up technologies (regulated precipitation/ crystallization) and other production technologies including, supercritical fluid and solvent evaporation (Shegokar & Müller, 2010). The potential advantages of drug nanocrystals (NCs) include enhancing the solubility, dissolution and oral bioavailability of poorly soluble drugs. NC product regarded as "new drug" because of its superior and specific pharmacokinetic profile and not bioequivalent or resemble to any other solubilised dosage form of the same drug, not even to the micronized form of the drug (Srivalli & Mishra, 2015).

Nanofibers

In the recent times nanofibers (NFs) of polymers, metal oxides and composite metals with multifunctional properties have drawn greater attention of researches. Nanofibers are always being of interest due to their specific properties like high tensile strength, large surface area and porosity. In the last two decades, many researchers have shifted their attention from nanoparticles to nanofibers because of the prospective application. Electro spinning is the commonly used method in which strong electric fields are applied to produce large scale production of NFs, the mechanism involved in this method is electrostatic interaction. In brief, the peristaltic pump pushes the polymer solution via needle which connected by high voltage power supply. The NFs will be obtained at a counter electrode called collector as droplet ejected at the tip of needle and its advantages include, easy handling, minimum consumption of solution, controllable fiber diameter, easy surface alteration, stretchability, convenient to process, cost effective, simple and reproducible in processing the fibers (Thenmozhi, Dharmaraj, Kadirvelu, & Kim, 2017).

Polymeric nanofibers can also be prepared by the conventional technique i.e. extrusion of solutions or melts through spinnerets and produce fiber dimensions that are similar to natural fibers. However, the surface morphology and diameter (micro or nanostructures) of these fibers must be efficiently controlled to enhance their potential applications in drug delivery (Guimarães, Oliveira, Gomes, Gontijo, Cortés, Campos, . . . Sinisterra, 2015). The use of nanofibrous polymeric implantable device is a novel alternative method for local delivery. The higher surface area and fine pores of nanofibers prepared by electrospinning process leads to high drug payload compared to other drug formulations. The reduction of fiber diameter can also increase the possibility of higher drug loading in nanofibrous scaffolds (Irani, Sadeghi, & Haririan, 2017).

Nanosuspension

Nanosuspension is a relatively new concept in pharmaceutical technology for water insoluble drugs in which size reduction of drug particles happens to a nanorange. Nanosized particles can lead to an increase in the dissolution rate and bioavailability of a drug, especially one with stability and solubility problems. Additionally, particle size reduction can increase penetration through biological barriers and cell membranes, which can lead to an improved drug residence time in a specific tissue or organ. Other advantages include dose and toxicity reduction, increased drug concentration in affected tissues or organs, and better adhesion of nanoparticles to mucosal surfaces (Yin, Cai, Liu, Cui, Wang, Yin, . . . Huo, 2016). Nanosuspensions can be used to formulate the drugs that are poorly soluble in both water and oil. Therefore, nanosuspensions differ remarkably from other drug carriers such as colloidal polymeric nanoparticles etc. (Du, Li, Zhao, Zhou, Wang, Tian, & Wang, 2015).

The methods employed for preparation are top-down processes and bottom-up process, top-down process involves drug particle size reduction using various techniques, including media milling, micro fluidization and high-pressure homogenization. The wet milling and high-pressure homogenization methods are widely explored because they efficiently produce small particles and do not require organic solvents, making them more feasible for industry production. However, these techniques involve a high energy input, which generate heat, making it difficult to process thermo labile materials. (Dos Santos, Carvalho, Teixeira, Azevedo, de Barros, & Gremião , 2017).

The bottom up process, also known as the precipitation process, in which the particles are formed from a molecular state, based on the precipitation of particles from a supersaturated drug solution. The drug can be precipitated using methods such as solvent evaporation, supercritical fluid, antisolvent precipitation and chemical precipitation. The bottom-up method requires a low energy input, making it useful for thermo labile materials, and is also simple and inexpensive (Gao, Liu, Kang, Niu, Wang, Wang, . . . Wang, 2013).

Nanoemulsion

Nanoemulsions are oil-in-water (O/W) or water-in-oil (W/O) dispersion of two immiscible liquids stabilized by a surfactant or emulsifier. The mean droplet diameter attained is usually <500 nm. Small droplet size gives them a clear or hazy appearance which differs from milky white colour associated with coarse emulsion. The word nanoemulsion is sometimes used interchangeably with submicron emulsion or mini emulsion; however it should not be confused with microemulsion. Nanoemulsions despite of having the same droplet size range as microemulsions, differs tremendously in structural aspects and long term thermodynamic stability (Singh, Meher, Raval, Khan, Chaurasia, Jain, & Chourasia, 2017).

Nanoemulsions are composed of oils, surfactants and other functional materials, which can offer a promising stable vehicle for improving the aqueous solubility and oral bioavailability of lipophillic drugs, for diagnosis and targeted drug delivery and mentioned for overcoming multidrug resistance in cancer chemotherapy (Bu, He, Zhang, Yin, Yu, & Li, 2014). The preparation methods include either high energy dispersion technique or by spontaneous emulsification method such as a self nanoemulsifying drug delivery system (SNEDDS). The improved *in-vitro* dissolution and *in-vivo* bioavailability of poorly soluble drugs has been observed via nanoemulsion formulation (Fofaria, Qhattal, Liu, & Srivastava, 2016).

Dendrimers

Dendrimers are globular macro molecules characterised by high branching points, three-dimensional structure, nanometric size range (1–100 nm), monodispersity and are composed of three distinct domains i.e. core, branches, and other terminal functional groups at surface. They have been explored for their potential applications in the area of drug delivery, where by drugs could either be encapsulated into the dendrimer core or covalently attached to the surface. Dendrimer based drug delivery offers targeted delivery of drugs to disease sites such as tumour tissue or cells by the effect of enhanced permeation and retention, and thereby improves the pharmacological activities and reduces the unwanted side effects (Yuanjie Liu, Ng, Toh, & Chiu, 2015).

Different types of dendrimers have been explored for drug delivery i.e. polyamidoamine (PAMAM), poly-L-lysine (PLL), poly (glycerol-co-succinic acid), polypropyleneimine (PPI), melamine, triazine, poly (glycerol), poly [2, 2-bis (hydroxymethyl) propionic acid] and poly (ethylene glycol) (PEG) etc. Dendrimers have been explored among the researchers, in different pharmaceutical fields like drug delivery, gene delivery, solubility enhancement, diagnosis and tissue engineering etc (Patel, Gajbhiye, Kesharwani, & Jain, 2016).

Among various types of dendrimers, poly amidoamine (PAMAM) dendrimer have been extensively investigated and received greater interest of researchers for drug and gene delivery. However, the application of unmodified PAMAM dendrimer to achieve targeted delivery of anticancer drugs is limited by their intrinsic surface cationic charge, which leads to high cytotoxicity due to nonspecific interactions of PAMAM with both tumour and normal cells. A number of strategies including, PEGylation, conjugation with other polymers and ligand decoration, could be used to overcome the stated limitations. Out of these strategies, functionalization with ligands has been considered to be one of the most effective approach and benefits in improving the solubility, high drug payload, targeted, sustained and controlled drug delivery, enhancing stability as well as desired biodistribution and pharmacokinetic properties (Kesharwani, Xie, Banerjee, Mao, Padhye, Sarkar, & Iyer, 2015).

CONSTRAINTS OF NON-FUNCTIONALISED NANOCARRIERS

Traditional drug delivery approaches include oral and i.v. routes which have several constraints; for example, oral administration of tablets or capsules could results in unpredicted pharmacokinetics due to the exposure of drugs to the various metabolic pathways of the body. Cancer chemotherapy with non-functionalised carriers has few setbacks, i.e. poor target ability towards target site and rapid metabolism of drugs etc. Therefore, larger than required doses being administered, which can further results in serious toxicity. The specificity of non-functionalised carriers system is low, results in harmful effects to healthy normal tissues (Sinha, Kim, Nie, & Shin, 2006). The functionalization of nanocarrier system with ligands that have specific receptors at target site could resolve the said issue. The diagnosis/detection/imaging and drug delivery could simultaneously happen via multifunctional nanocarrier systems. (Kim, Lee, Lee, Yu, Lee, Park, & Hyeon , 2008)

The non-functionalised nanocarrier systems suffer from following issues:

- Poor drug target ability (Specificity)
- Failing to detect/diagnosis of cancer

- High drug toxic effects
- Poor drug payload
- Scale-up issues

Further, there is a probability that cancer nanotechnology could also pick up opportunities for personalized cancer diagnosis and treatment strategies by means of multifunctional nanoparticles in four main area: imaging of cancer disease-specific biomarkers, detection of tumours and their metastases, the functional delivery of drugs to target cells, and real-time monitoring of treatment in progression (Parvanian, Mostafavi, & Aghashiri, 2017).

FUNCTIONALIZED NANOCARRIER SYSTEMS

Nanoparticle system based drug delivery, using biodegradable polymers, metals, lipids etc. provides a more effective, less harmful; remedy to overcome the problems associated with cancer treatment. For example, the solubility of an insoluble drug can be enhanced by introducing solubilising agents into the polymer matrix, thereby improving its bioavailability, biodegradability and the possibility of modifying the surface properties of polymer increases their multifunctionality (Cabeza, Ortiz, Prados, Delgado, Martín-Villena, Clares, . . . Arias , 2017). Functionlalization of nanoparticle illustrsted in Figure 2.

The functionalization of nanocarrier system could be needed in order to tether the ligands i.e. proteins, peptides, carbohydrates, monoclonal antibodies etc. which possess specific receptors at cancer site, this would offer early detection/diagnosis of the cancer and provide targeted, sustained/prolonged and controlled delivery of therapeutic moieties, there by provide effective treatment, in addition to minimizing the drug wastage and drug related side effects (Gindy & Prud'homme, 2009).

Multifunctional nanostructured drug delivery systems, prepared by combining two or more components, have been widely studied with the purpose of improving the therapeutic activity and reducing

Figure 2. Multifunctionalised nanoparticle for drug delivery

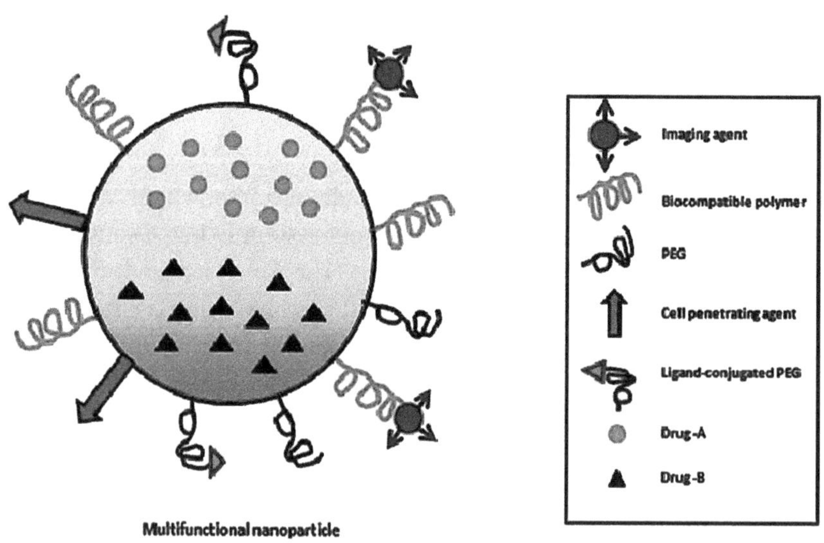

undesirable effects of highly toxic drugs by adding multiple functions to the nanoparticles. Nanoparticle system based diagnostics and therapeutics hold great promises because they are potential platforms for simultaneous therapy, biomedical imaging and diagnosis usually referred as nanotheranostics. The functionalised nanocarrier system based drug delivery would enhance the drug amount at the cancer affected site. The system also improves drug target ability by virtue of nanosize and ligand decoration. Cancer treatment could be achieved more prominently with targeted drug delivery via a functionalised nanocarrier (De Oliveira Freitas, de Melo Corgosinho, Faria, dos Santos, Resende, Leal, . . . de Sousa, 2017).

The functionalised nanocarrier systems could be employed in cancer diagnosis and imaging by means of attaching the detector molecules on surface of nanocarrier. The early detection of cancer would offer better treatment in concern of dose size; dosing frequency and dose related side effects. The brain cancer imaging and treatment has been carried by theranostic liosomes decorated with RGD TPGS (Singh, Sharma, Kumari, Koch, Singh, Bharti, . . . Muthu, 2016).

Aims and Characteristics of Multifunctional Nanocarrier System

- Increase drug concentration in the tumour via
    - Passive targeting
    - Active targeting
- Decrease drug concentration in normal healthy tissue or cells
- Increase the solubility of drug to allow i.v. administration
- Enhance pharmacokinetics and pharmacodynamics profiles
- Minimize the drug release during transit
- Enhance the drug release at the targeted site
- Reduce drug degradation to improve the stability
- Improve intracellular drug delivery
- To make the carrier biocompatible and biodegradable

Passive Targeting

The permeability virtue of tumour tissues offers the passive targeting of drugs. Hyper vasculature to serve rapid growing cancerous cells leads to formation of leaky and defective blood vessels. This in turn, can promote permeability of chemotherapeutic agents. The drug molecule physicochemical properties include molecular weight, charge, polarity, solubility and size, and surface properties of targeted cell mainly influence the passive targeting. Therefore, selective manipulation of drug molecules could offer effective targeting. Passive targeting offers the delivery of drugs to the tumour bed through several invasive modalities (Danhier, Feron, & Préat, 2010).

Active Targeting

The active targeting is generally achieved by tethering of targeting moieties/ligands on the surface of nanocarrier, thereby offers selective deposition of the drug in the specified cancer tissue, within individual cancer cells or intracellular organelles. The targeting moiety is chosen to bind to a receptor over expressed by cancer cells or tumour and not observed in normal cells. Active and passive targeting approaches are shown in Figure 3 and 4.

Figure 3. Mechanisms of nanoparticle drug delivery in cancer

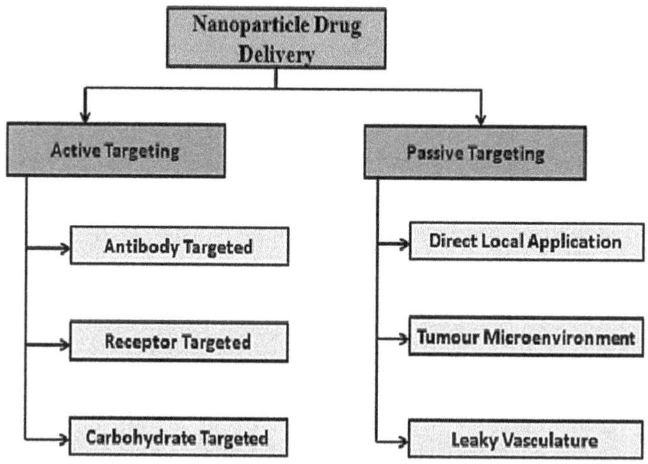

Figure 4. A. Passive targeting: Drugs (small molecules) and nanocarriers reach the tumours via leaky vasculature; drugs alone freely diffuse in and out of the tumour blood vessels because of their small size. Whereas, drug-loaded nanocarriers cannot diffuse back into the blood stream because of their large size. B. Active targeting: Ligand attached nanocarriers bind to receptors (over) expressed by tumour cells.

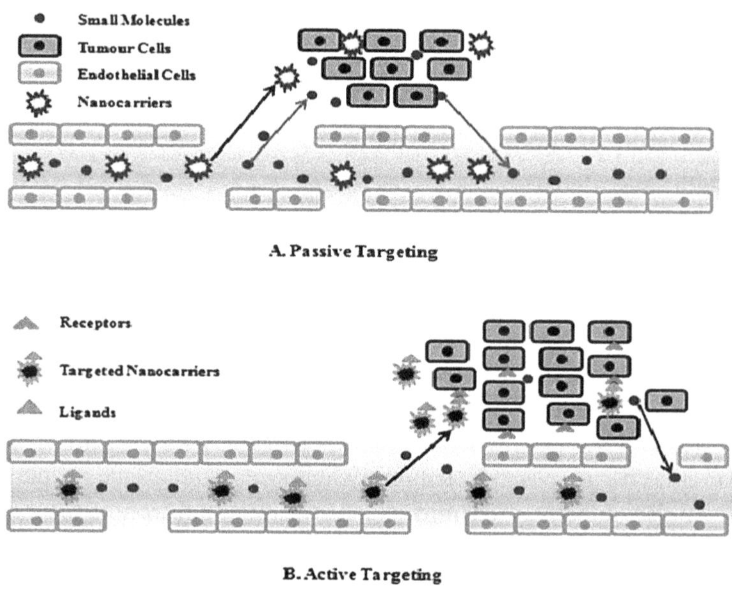

Surface Engineered/Functionalised Carbon Nanotubes (CNTS)

Carbon nanotubes (CNTs) have been employed as popular tool in cancer treatment, exhibiting considerable potentials in receptor oriented targeting owing to their unique properties such as high surface area and drug payload, membrane penetration, biocompatibility, easy surface alteration and non-immunogenicity etc. The hydrophilicity, is a major limitation associated with the first generation of CNTs i.e. pristine

CNTs, could be resolved by functionalization techniques (Mehra, Mishra, & Jain, 2014). Functionalization of (less toxicity) nanotubes makes them better and safer drug delivery system, surface functionalised CNTs are being explored for targeted, sustained and controlled drug delivery and have been reported to be non-toxic to normal human cells (Pan, Cui, Xu, Ozkan, Feng, Ozkan, He , 2009).

The multiwalled carbon nanotubes (MWCNTS) were utilized as drug carrier in the cancer treatment, the effective drug delivery has been achieved by functionalised/surface altered carbon nanotubes with specific targeting moieties (Jain, Dubey, Mehra, Lodhi, Nahar, Mishra, & Jain, 2009). Some of them are listed in Table 1.

Table 1. Functionalised carbon nanotubes (CNTS)

Drug	Ligands	Remarks	Reference
Docetaxel	Folate, PEG (for bridging)	Docetaxel loaded MWCNTS tethered with folate, anchored by poly ethylene glycol (PEG) for better cancer targeting.	(Mehra & Jain, 2015)
Doxorubicin	Vitamin E TPGS (d-α-Tocopheryl Polyethylene Glycol 1000 Succinate)	Doxorubicin loaded MWCNTS were conjugated with vitamin E TPGS for effective delivery in cancer.	(Mehra, Verma, Mishra, & Jain, 2014)
Methotrexate	DSPE-mPEG 2000	Methotrexate loaded multiwalled carbon nanotubes decorated with DSPE-mPEG 2000.	Modi et al., (2011)
Gemcitabine	Folate	Gemcitabine loaded smart nanotubes (folate attached) fabricated for breast cancer treatment.	(R. Singh, Mehra, Jain, & Jain, 2013)
Doxorubicin	Dexamethasone	Dexamethasone ligated, doxorubicin loaded MWCNTS were prepared for controlled delivery and to minimize drug toxicity.	(Lodhi, Mehra, & Jain, 2013)
Docetaxel	Chitosan-Folate	Chitosan-Folate conjugated multiwalled carbon nanotubes loaded with docetaxel for the lung cancer treatment.	R. P. Singh et al., (2017)
Docetaxel	Vitamin E TPGS (d-α-Tocopheryl polyethylene glycol 1000 succinate)	Multiwalled carbon nanotubes (MWCNT) tethered with d-α-Tocopheryl Polyethylene Glycol 1000 Succinate (TPGS) and loaded with docetaxel.	R. P. Singh, Sharma, Singh, Kumar, et al., (2016)
Docetaxel	Transferrin	Docetaxel loaded multiwalled carbon nanotubes (MWCNT) surface modified with transferrin	R. P. Singh, Sharma, Singh, Patne, et al., (2016)
Doxorubicin	Hyaluronic acid	Multifunctionality of MWCNTS achieved by polyethyleneimine (PEI) altered MWCNTs were attached with fluorescein isothiocyanate (FI) and hyaluronic acid (HA) and loaded with doxorubicin for targeted cancer therapy.	(Cao, Tao, Wen, Hou, & Shi, 2015)
Epirubicin	Distearoyl phosphatidyl ethanolamine-hyaluronic acid (DSPE-HA)	Distearoylphosphatidylethanolamine-hyaluronic acid (DSPE-HA) attached single walled carbon nanotubes (SWCNTs) to improve the biocompatibility and target CD44 receptors in MDR cancer cells for enhancement of intracellular drug uptake.	Yao et al., (2016)
--	Polyamidoamine (PAMAM)	Polyamidoamine (PAMAM) dendrimers tethered with multi-walled carbon nanotubes (MWCNTs) and cytotoxicity to human osteosarcoma MG-63 cells, and protein and DNA immobilization in cancer treatment.	Zhang et al., (2010)
--	Fluorescein isothiocyanate (FI), folic acid (FA) modified amine terminated generation 5 (G5) PAMAM dendrimers (G5 ·NH2-FI-FA)	Fluorescein isothiocyanate (FI) and folic acid (FA) modified amine terminated generation 5 (G5) PAMAM dendrimers (G5 ·NH2-FI-FA) attached to acid treated multiwalled carbon nanotubes (MWCNTs) for cancer targeting.	Shi et al., (2009)

Functionalised Polymeric Nanoparticles

Functionalised polymeric nanoparticles can be employed to deliver drugs, peptides, proteins, and nucleic acids. In comparison to conventional delivery approaches, they can enhance the solubility of poorly soluble drugs and improves drug half-life and selectivity towards the target sites. Further, most nanoparticles predominantly deposit within tumours via EPR effect because of virtue of their size and surface modification. Thus, a polymeric nanoparticle improves the intracellular drug accumulation in cancer cells and avoids toxicity to normal cells, resulting in potent therapeutic effects. (Park, Lee, Kang, Kim, Choi, & Kwon, 2009). Folic acid is a commonly used ligand for breast cancer targeting with polymeric nanoparticles because growing breast cancer cells over express folate receptors to maintain their folic acid requirement. Trastuzumab (Herceptin®), a monoclonal antibody, conjugated polymeric nanoparticles have been observed to specifically target HER2 receptors over expressed in breast cancer cells (Kumar, Lale, Alex, Choudhary, & Koul, 2017).

Table 2. Functionalised polymeric nanoparticles

Drug	Ligands	Remarks	Reference
Docetaxel	TPGS and Transferrin	Docetaxel loaded D-α Tocopherol Polyethylene Glycol 1000 Succinate tethered chitosan (TPGS chitosan) nanoparticles decorated with transferrin for cancer cells.	Agrawal et al., (2017)
Paclitaxel	Hyaluronic acid	Poly (lactic-co-glycolic acid) (PLGA) nanoparticles embedded with paclitaxel and coated with hyaluronic acid (HA-PTX PLGA)	Cerqueira et al., (2017)
Paclitaxel	Transferrin and PEG	Polyethylene glycol (PEG) attached chitosan nanoparticles (NPs) activated by transferrin (Tf) for prolonged and targeted drug delivery to tumour cells via transferrin receptor-mediated endocytosis.	(Nag, Gajbhiye, Kesharwani, & Jain, 2016)
Methotrexate	Trastuzumab	Methotrexate–human serum albumin conjugated nanoparticles (MTX–HSA NPs) surface modified with trastuzumab (TMAB) for caner targeting.	(Taheri, Dinarvand, Atyabi, Ghahremani, & Ostad, 2012)
Doxorubicin	N-acetyl-D-Glucosamine	Poly (styrene-alt-maleic anhydride $_{58}$-b-polystyrene$_{130}$ (P (St-alt-MA)$_{58}$-b-PSt$_{130}$) as a copolymer backbone, N-acetyl glucosamine (NAG) as a targeting moiety was designed and fabricated with doxorubicin.	Tian et al., (2015)
Bicalutamide (BCL)	Foli acid and Chitosan	(FA) attached chitosan (CS)-activated poly (D,L-lactide-co-glycolide) (PLGA) nanoparticles of bicalutamide (BCL) for cancer treatment.	Dhas et al., (2015)
Curcumin	Folic acid	Folate modified chitosan nanoparticles (NPs) were loaded with curcumin and fabricated via self assembling process.	Esfandiarpour-Boroujeni et al., (2017)
Lapatinib	Dextran-Chitosan	Dextran sulfate-chitosan (DS-CS) nanoparticles, possess properties such as nontoxicity, biocompatibility and biodegradability and employed as drug carrier in cancer therapy.	(Mobasseri, Karimi, Tian, Naderi-Manesh, & Ramakrishna, 2017)
5-Flurouracil	Chitosan	Chitosan (C) coated polylactic-co-glycolic acid (PLGA) and polycaprolactone [PCL] nanoparticles [NPs] were loaded with 5-Fluorouracil i.e. (C-5-FU PLGA NPs), (C-5-FU PCL NPs) and were fabricated as the carrier system for cancer treatment.	(Badran, Mady, Ghannam, & Shakeel, 2017)
Paclitaxel	Folate	Folate conjugated poly-lactide-co-glycolide & polyethylene glycol nanoparticles for effective delivery of paclitaxel (PTX) to endometrial carcinoma.	C. Liang et al., (2011)
Doxorubicin	Hyaluronic acid	Polyethylenimine (PEI) conjugated with methoxy poly (ethylene glycol) aldehyde (mPEG-CHO), poly (caprolactone) aldehyde (PCL-CHO) and pyrene-1-carboxaldehyde (Py-CHO) the conjugates self-assembled into nanoparticles to load with doxorubicin and coated with hyaluronic acid for tumour targeting.	Yan et al., (2017)

Functionalised Solid Lipid Nanoparticles

Solid lipid nanoparticles (SLNs) offer encapsulation of both lipophillic as well as hydrophilic drugs and provide sustained and controlled release pattern, targeting aspects and good encapsulation efficiency. Furthermore, SLNs have ability to protect the drug from chemical, photochemical or oxidative decomposition and has the ability to immobilize drug in the lipid matrix and therefore this delivery system has attracted much attention in recent times.

Many anticancer agents with wide variety of physiochemical properties have been incorporated in lipid nanoparticles with successful enhancement in stability, less toxicity, improved pharmacokinetics and improved efficacy (Soni, Soni, Pandey, Maheshwari, Kesharwani, & Tekade, 2016).

However, drug loading efficiency of hydrophilic drugs into SLN is low and the formation of an ion pairing with a lipophilic counter-ion has been proposed as an alternative to enhance the encapsulation. Fabricating with a lipophilic ion that also exhibits anticancer activity represents an interesting approach for the design of SLN (Oliveira, Mussi, Gomes, Yoshida, Frezard, Carregal, & Ferreira, 2016).

Functionalised Liposome Nanocarriers

Liposomes as an effective nanocarrier system has gained interest of researchers because of their non-toxicity and structural resemblance with biological components and well explored drug carrier system for cancer treatment. Liposomes are being reported in which the diagnostic and therapeutic agents are coated on surface, conjugated or encapsulated for diagnosis and treatment simultaneously at cellular and molecular levels and referred as theranostic liposomes.

The conjugation of liposomes with targeting ligands, can bind to over expressed receptors on the membrane of cancer cells for better drug delivery. The liposomes may circulate for longer periods of

Table 3. Functionalised solid lipid nanoparticles

Drug	Ligands	Remarks	Reference
Doxorubicin	Folate (FA)	Folate (FA) functionalized low density lipoproteins (LDL)/sodium carboxymethyl cellulose (CMC) nanoparticles (NP) loaded with doxorubicin were formulated, utilized in tumour targeting and pH-triggered drug release.	(H. Liang, He, Zhou, Li, & Li, 2017)
Gemcitabine	Mannose	Gemicitabine loaded mannosylated solid lipid nanoparticles (GmcH-SLNs) for enhancing drug internalization to the lung cancer cells.	Soni et al., (2016)
Doxorubicin	α- Tocopheryl Succinate (TS)	Tocopheryl Succinate (TS), coated solid lipid nanoparticles (SLN) loaded with doxorubicin for better anticancer activity and evaluating the effect of TS on drug loading efficiency.	Oliveira et al., (2016)
Curcumin	N-carboxymethyl chitosan (NCC)	N-carboxymethyl chitosan (NCC) coated curcumin-loaded SLN (NCC-SLN) to inhibit the immediate release of curcumin in acidic pH and to enhance the bioavailability.	(Baek & Cho, 2017)
Paclitaxel	Hyaluronic acid	Development of hyaluronic acid (HA) conjugated pluronic 85 (P85) coated solid lipid nanoparticles (SLN) encapsulated with paclitaxel.	(Fang Wang, Li, Liu, Chen, & Li, 2017)
DNA and siRNA	DEN-K (GALA)-TAT-K(STR)-CTP a peptide	A delivery system, consist of the fusogenic lipid 1,2-dioleoyl-sn-glycero-3-phosphoethanolamine (DOPE) with a synthetic multifunctional peptide, produced and optimized, with the aim to develop an effective gene delivery approach for breast cancer cells	(Wan, Dai, Nevagi, Toth, & Moyle, 2017)

time in the blood, evading host defences, and release drug and diagnostic agent together in the desired site and simultaneously facilitate *in-vivo* imaging and therapy. Incorporation of quantum dots within the lipophillic core or attached covalently on the surface of the liposomes with the therapeutic agents and ligands, recognised as effective approach for cellular and *in-vivo* tumour imaging with targeting and therapeutic modalities (Singh, Sharma, Kumari, Koch, Singh, Bharti, . . . Muthu, 2016).

Functionalised Metal Nanoparticles

The functionalised metal nanoparticles generally include gold, silver and iron nanoparticles etc. Gold nanoparticles can easily cross the blood vessels, tissue barriers and get into tumour vicinity and also possess several specific properties with multiple functions in therapeutics, imaging/dignosis, and surface modification. The surface alteration by specific ligands and coupled with various forms of therapeutics is a wide range of research and nanoparticle based drug delivery approach under development for cancer. The gold nanoparticle conjugates offer unique properties such as improved binding affinity and specific targeting to selective tissue or cells, leads to reduction in drug dose size for treatments and lessen toxicity to normal tissues coupled with lower side effects (Ajnai, Chiu, Kan, Cheng, Tsai, & Chang, 2014). Apart from gold nanoparticles other metal nanoparticles also mentioned in Table 5.

Miscellaneous Functionalised Nanocarriers

The functionalised nanoemulsion and mesoporous spheres have been explained in Table 6.

Table 4. Functionalised liposome nanocarriers

Drug	Ligands	Remarks	Reference
Doxorubicin	Hyaluronic acid	Hyaluronic acid tethered liposomes to study the uptake pathway in key cells in the brain including primary astrocytes, microglia and human GBM cells.	(Hayward, Wilson, & Kidambi, 2016)
Docetaxel	RGD-TPGS	RGD-TPGS conjugated theranostic liposomes contain both docetaxel (DTX) and quantum dots (QDs) for brain cancer diagnosis and treatment.	R. P. Singh, Sharma, Kumari, et al., (2016)
Paclitaxel	R8-RGD.	Cyclic RGD peptide was linked to a cell penetrating peptide R8 to develop a multifunctional peptide R8-RGD.	Yayuan Liu et al., (2014)
Doxorubicin	PEG, RNA-aptamer	Doxorubicin loaded PEGylated liposomes were conjugated with anti-breast cancer RNA aptamer for better treatment of breast cancer.	(Moosavian, Abnous, Badiee, & Jaafari, 2016)
--	RGD peptide	Liposomal delivery system conjugated with cyclic RGD peptide for $\alpha v\beta 3$ integrin, fabricated to enhance therapeutic efficacy in a mice model of bone metastasis from prostate cancer. Tumour cells are rich with $\alpha v\beta 3$ integrin.	(Fangfang Wang, Chen, Zhang, Chen, & Zhu, 2014)

Table 5. Functionalised metal nanoparticles

Drug	Ligands	Remarks	Reference
---	Trastuzumab	Polyethylene glycol (PEG) conjugated gold nanoparticles attached to trastuzumab to target HER2- receptors in breast cancer (BC) cells	Cai et al., (2016)
Doxorubicin Hydrochloride	Hyaluronan (HA)	Hyaluronan (HA) attached C60 fullerene silica nanoparticles loaded with doxorubicin hydrochloride (DOX) and indocyanine green (ICG) to target the CD44 receptors over expressed on breast cancer	H. Wang et al., (2016)
---	Anti-EGFR D-11	Functionalised gold nanoparticles consist of a monoclonal antibody against epidermal growth factor receptor (EGFR) (anti-EGFR D-11) for active tumour targeting.	Fernandes et al., (2017)
---	Heparin	Functionalised cerium oxide nanoparticles with either 130 or 880 molecules of un fractionated heparin using the organosilane linker, 3-aminopropyltriethoxysilane for cancer.	Lord et al., (2013)
Gemcitabine	Human epidermal growth factor receptor 2, (HER-2) antibody.	Fluorescent iron oxide (FIO) nanoparticles and gemcitabine (G) loaded poly (lactide-co-glycolide) (PLGA) nanospheres (PGFIO) were attached with human epidermal growth factor receptor 2, (HER-2) antibody for diagnosis and mitigation of pancreatic cancer.	Jaidev et al., (2017)
Doxorubicin	Biotin	Co-delivery of quercetin and doxorubicin via pH-sensitive Fe_3O_4@SiO_2 (FITC) multifunctional nanoparticles conjugated with biotin to potentiate the efficacy against chemoresistance.	(Daglioglu, 2017)
Paclitaxel	Chitosan Oligosaccharide (COS)	Chitosan oligosaccharide attached gold nanoparticles loaded with Paclitaxel and shown cytotoxic activity against MDA-MB-231 cells	(Manivasagan, Bharathiraja, Bui, Lim, & Oh, 2016)
Doxorubicin	PEG and PAMAM	Gold nanoparticles conjugated with thiolated polyethylene glycol (PEG) and covalently linked with a polyamidoamine (PAMAM) G4 dendrimer and doxorubicin was attached via amide bond	(Khutale & Casey, 2017)

Table 6. Miscellaneous functionalised nanoarriers

Drug	Ligand	Remarks	Reference
Docetaxel	Transferrin	Transferrin coupled docetaxel lipid nanoemulsion for improving tumour targeted delivery.	(Afzal, Shareef, & Kishan, 2016)
Doxorubicin	Hyaluronan (HA)	Calcium carbonate/hyaluronate/glutamate mesoporous hollow spheres are prepared and depicted that the mesoporous hollow spheres can efficiently load the anticancer drug doxorubicin.	Guo et al., (2017)
Doxorubicin	Folate	Functionalized, self-assembled metal organic nanotubes, SWMONTs loaded with doxorubicin via the modification of SWMONTs, DOX/SWMONTs-SiO2, DOX/SWMONTs-SiO2-NH2, DOX/SWMONTs-SiO2-NH2-FA for cancer treatment.	Yang et al., (2017)

LIMITATIONS

Though the multifunctional nanocarrier system has tremendous applications in cancer treatment but it also suffers with some bottlenecks. The functionalization/surface modification of nanocarrier system with ligands is a tedious process and limitations include stability, drug loading efficiency (in post conjugation), and scale-up process. The characterization and evaluation of multifunctional nanoparticulate system also a cumbersome process. The fabrication of functionalised nanocarrier systems into commercial scale is an expensive and time taking process. As the carrier system tethered with exogenous substances (ligands) the chances of occurrence of immune related issues such as hypersensitivity and auto immune disorders is quite likely. Thorough knowledge is needed to know compatibility of ligands with human models.

It has also been reported that, active targeting (ligand attachment) always doesn't improve the drug accumulation into tumour cells because of bulkier groups, and high density of cells and interstitial fluid pressure. Another challenge is retention of drug in the carrier system for longer period of time for sustained release (drug leakage may happens) (van Elk, Murphy, Eufrásio-da-Silva, O'Reilly, Vermonden, Hennink, . . . Ruiz-Hernández, 2016).

FUTURE PERSPECTIVES

The multifunctional nanocarrier systems explored much as an effective carrier system in both diagnosis and mitigation of cancer as discussed in this chapter. The decoration of specific liagands/proteins/peptides on the carrier surface would offer early detection/diagnosis and targets the cancer site efficiently. Therefore, the multifunctional carrier system would mitigate the dose size and dosing frequency, improves the patient compliance and diminish the dose related side effects. The said system can also explore as a drug carrier system for other typical diseases such as diabetes, tuberculosis, leishmaniasis and asthma etc. for efficient treatment.

Research has been carried on development of rifampicin loaded mannose-tethered chitosan nanoparticles for the visceral leishmaniasis treatment (Chaubey & Mishra, 2014). The exploration of novel nanocarriers and ligands in fabrication of multifunctional nanocarrier system with enhanced patient compliance and improved benefit to cost ratio is needed.

CONCLUSION

The drug delivery to the targeted cancer site, without accumulation in other parts of the body (non-cancerous tissue) is a primary prerequisite of current treatment approaches in order to minimize the formulation and patient related issues. And it's very much important in the case of potent anticancer drugs with narrow therapeutic range, since they produce serious toxic effects. The above, can be achieved via functionalised nanocarrier system as discussed in this chapter, which brings about early detection/diagnosis/imaging, targeted, sustained and controlled delivery of therapeutic moieties to the specific cancer site; therefore it circumvents the problems associated with the drug causing toxicity to healthy (normal) cells. In the present times, multifunctional nanocarrier system played a significant role in the cancer treatment, because of its specific advantages over conventional systems. In the near future, multifunctional nanocarrier systems may also take a major role in detection and mitigation of other diseases like diabetes, tuberculosis and leishmaniasis etc. via ligand-receptor based approaches.

REFERENCES

Afzal, S. M., Shareef, M. Z., & Kishan, V. (2016). Transferrin tagged lipid nanoemulsion of docetaxel for enhanced tumor targeting. *Journal of Drug Delivery Science and Technology*, *36*, 175–182. doi:10.1016/j.jddst.2016.10.008

Agrawal, P., Singh, R. P., Kumari, L., Sharma, G., Koch, B., Rajesh, C. V., ... Muthu, M. S. (2017). TPGS-chitosan cross-linked targeted nanoparticles for effective brain cancer therapy. *Materials Science and Engineering C*, *74*, 167–176. doi:10.1016/j.msec.2017.02.008 PMID:28254282

Ajnai, G., Chiu, A., Kan, T., Cheng, C.-C., Tsai, T.-H., & Chang, J. (2014). Trends of gold nanoparticle-based drug delivery system in cancer therapy. *Journal of Experimental and Clinical Medicine*, *6*(6), 172–178. doi:10.1016/j.jecm.2014.10.015

Badran, M. M., Mady, M. M., Ghannam, M. M., & Shakeel, F. (2017). Preparation and characterization of polymeric nanoparticles surface modified with chitosan for target treatment of colorectal cancer. *International Journal of Biological Macromolecules*, *95*, 643–649. doi:10.1016/j.ijbiomac.2016.11.098 PMID:27908720

Baek, J.-S., & Cho, C.-W. (2017). Surface modification of solid lipid nanoparticles for oral delivery of curcumin: Improvement of bioavailability through enhanced cellular uptake, and lymphatic uptake. *European Journal of Pharmaceutics and Biopharmaceutics*, *117*, 132–140. doi:10.1016/j.ejpb.2017.04.013 PMID:28412471

Baig, M. S., Ahad, A., Aslam, M., Imam, S. S., Aqil, M., & Ali, A. (2016). Application of Box–Behnken design for preparation of levofloxacin-loaded stearic acid solid lipid nanoparticles for ocular delivery: Optimization, in vitro release, ocular tolerance, and antibacterial activity. *International Journal of Biological Macromolecules*, *85*, 258–270. doi:10.1016/j.ijbiomac.2015.12.077 PMID:26740466

Bharali, D. J., Khalil, M., Gurbuz, M., Simone, T. M., & Mousa, S. A. (2009). Nanoparticles and cancer therapy: A concise review with emphasis on dendrimers. *International Journal of Nanomedicine*, *4*(1), 1–7. PMID:19421366

Bu, H., He, X., Zhang, Z., Yin, Q., Yu, H., & Li, Y. (2014). A TPGS-incorporating nanoemulsion of paclitaxel circumvents drug resistance in breast cancer. *International Journal of Pharmaceutics*, *471*(1), 206–213. doi:10.1016/j.ijpharm.2014.05.039 PMID:24866272

Cabeza, L., Ortiz, R., Prados, J., Delgado, Á. V., Martín-Villena, M. J., Clares, B., ... Arias, J. L. (2017). Improved antitumor activity and reduced toxicity of doxorubicin encapsulated in poly (ε-caprolactone) nanoparticles in lung and breast cancer treatment: An in vitro and in vivo study. *European Journal of Pharmaceutical Sciences*, *102*, 24–34. doi:10.1016/j.ejps.2017.02.026 PMID:28219748

Cai, Z., Chattopadhyay, N., Yang, K., Kwon, Y. L., Yook, S., Pignol, J.-P., & Reilly, R. M. (2016). 111 In-labeled trastuzumab-modified gold nanoparticles are cytotoxic in vitro to HER2-positive breast cancer cells and arrest tumor growth in vivo in athymic mice after intratumoral injection. *Nuclear Medicine and Biology*, *43*(12), 818–826. doi:10.1016/j.nucmedbio.2016.08.009 PMID:27788375

Cao, X., Tao, L., Wen, S., Hou, W., & Shi, X. (2015). Hyaluronic acid-modified multiwalled carbon nanotubes for targeted delivery of doxorubicin into cancer cells. *Carbohydrate Research*, *405*, 70–77. doi:10.1016/j.carres.2014.06.030 PMID:25500334

Cerqueira, B. B. S., Lasham, A., Shelling, A. N., & Al-Kassas, R. (2017). Development of biodegradable PLGA nanoparticles surface engineered with hyaluronic acid for targeted delivery of paclitaxel to triple negative breast cancer cells. *Materials Science and Engineering C*, *76*, 593–600. doi:10.1016/j.msec.2017.03.121 PMID:28482569

Chaubey, P., & Mishra, B. (2014). Mannose-conjugated chitosan nanoparticles loaded with rifampicin for the treatment of visceral leishmaniasis. *Carbohydrate Polymers*, *101*, 1101–1108. doi:10.1016/j.carbpol.2013.10.044 PMID:24299880

Crucho, C. I., & Barros, M. T. (2015). Formulation of functionalized PLGA polymeric nanoparticles for targeted drug delivery. *Polymer*, *68*, 41–46. doi:10.1016/j.polymer.2015.04.083

Crucho, C. I., & Barros, M. T. (2017). Polymeric nanoparticles: A study on the preparation variables and characterization methods. *Materials Science and Engineering C*. PMID:28866227

Daglioglu, C. (2017). Enhancing Tumor Cell Response to Multidrug Resistance with pH-Sensitive Quercetin and Doxorubicin Conjugated Multifunctional Nanoparticles. *Colloids and Surfaces. B, Biointerfaces*, *156*, 175–185. doi:10.1016/j.colsurfb.2017.05.012 PMID:28528134

Danhier, F., Feron, O., & Préat, V. (2010). To exploit the tumor microenvironment: Passive and active tumor targeting of nanocarriers for anti-cancer drug delivery. *Journal of Controlled Release*, *148*(2), 135–146. doi:10.1016/j.jconrel.2010.08.027 PMID:20797419

de Oliveira Freitas, L. B., de Melo Corgosinho, L., Faria, J. A. Q. A., dos Santos, V. M., Resende, J. M., Leal, A. S., ... de Sousa, E. M. B. (2017). Multifunctional mesoporous silica nanoparticles for cancer-targeted, controlled drug delivery and imaging. *Microporous and Mesoporous Materials*, *242*, 271–283. doi:10.1016/j.micromeso.2017.01.036

Dhas, N. L., Ige, P. P., & Kudarha, R. R. (2015). Design, optimization and in-vitro study of folic acid conjugated-chitosan functionalized PLGA nanoparticle for delivery of bicalutamide in prostate cancer. *Powder Technology*, *283*, 234–245. doi:10.1016/j.powtec.2015.04.053

Ding, C., & Li, Z. (2017). A review of drug release mechanisms from nanocarrier systems. *Materials Science and Engineering C*, *76*, 1440–1453. doi:10.1016/j.msec.2017.03.130 PMID:28482511

Dos Santos, A. M., Carvalho, F. C., Teixeira, D. A., Azevedo, D. L., de Barros, W. M., & Gremião, M. P. D. (2017). Computational and experimental approaches for development of methotrexate nanosuspensions by bottom-up nanoprecipitation. *International Journal of Pharmaceutics*, *524*(1), 330–338. doi:10.1016/j.ijpharm.2017.03.068 PMID:28359822

Du, J., Li, X., Zhao, H., Zhou, Y., Wang, L., Tian, S., & Wang, Y. (2015). Nanosuspensions of poorly water-soluble drugs prepared by bottom-up technologies. *International Journal of Pharmaceutics*, *495*(2), 738–749. doi:10.1016/j.ijpharm.2015.09.021 PMID:26383838

Esfandiarpour-Boroujeni, S., Bagheri-Khoulenjani, S., Mirzadeh, H., & Amanpour, S. (2017). Fabrication and study of curcumin loaded nanoparticles based on folate-chitosan for breast cancer therapy application. *Carbohydrate Polymers*, *168*, 14–21. doi:10.1016/j.carbpol.2017.03.031 PMID:28457434

Fernandes, A. R., Jesus, J., Martins, P., Figueiredo, S., Rosa, D., Martins, L. M., ... Baptista, P. V. (2017). Multifunctional gold-nanoparticles: A nanovectorization tool for the targeted delivery of novel chemotherapeutic agents. *Journal of Controlled Release*, *245*, 52–61. doi:10.1016/j.jconrel.2016.11.021 PMID:27871990

Fofaria, N. M., Qhattal, H. S. S., Liu, X., & Srivastava, S. K. (2016). Nanoemulsion formulations for anti-cancer agent piplartine—Characterization, toxicological, pharmacokinetics and efficacy studies. *International Journal of Pharmaceutics*, *498*(1), 12–22. doi:10.1016/j.ijpharm.2015.11.045 PMID:26642946

Gao, L., Liu, G., Kang, J., Niu, M., Wang, Z., Wang, H., ... Wang, X. (2013). Paclitaxel nanosuspensions coated with P-gp inhibitory surfactants: I. Acute toxicity and pharmacokinetics studies. *Colloids and Surfaces. B, Biointerfaces*, *111*, 277–281. doi:10.1016/j.colsurfb.2013.06.004 PMID:23838193

Gindy, M. E., & Prud'homme, R. K. (2009). Multifunctional nanoparticles for imaging, delivery and targeting in cancer therapy. *Expert Opinion on Drug Delivery*, *6*(8), 865–878. doi:10.1517/17425240902932908 PMID:19637974

Guimarães, P. P., Oliveira, M. F., Gomes, A. D., Gontijo, S. M., Cortés, M. E., Campos, P. P., ... Sinisterra, R. D. (2015). PLGA nanofibers improves the antitumoral effect of daunorubicin. *Colloids and Surfaces. B, Biointerfaces*, *136*, 248–255. doi:10.1016/j.colsurfb.2015.09.005 PMID:26402423

Guo, Y., Li, H., Shi, W., Zhang, J., Feng, J., Yang, X., ... Yang, L. (2017). Targeted Delivery and pH-Responsive Release of Doxorubicin to Cancer Cells Using Calcium Carbonate/Hyaluronate/Glutamate Mesoporous Hollow Spheres. *Journal of Colloid and Interface Science*, *502*, 59–66. doi:10.1016/j.jcis.2017.04.085 PMID:28477470

Hayward, S. L., Wilson, C. L., & Kidambi, S. (2016). Hyaluronic acid-conjugated liposome nanoparticles for targeted delivery to CD44 overexpressing glioblastoma cells. *Oncotarget*, *7*(23), 34158. doi:10.18632/oncotarget.8926 PMID:27120809

Irani, M., Sadeghi, G. M. M., & Haririan, I. (2017). The sustained delivery of temozolomide from electrospun PCL-Diol-b-PU/gold nanocompsite nanofibers to treat glioblastoma tumors. *Materials Science and Engineering C*, *75*, 165–174. doi:10.1016/j.msec.2017.02.029 PMID:28415451

Jaidev, L., Chellappan, D. R., Bhavsar, D. V., Ranganathan, R., Sivanantham, B., Subramanian, A., ... Sethuraman, S. (2017). Multi-functional nanoparticles as theranostic agents for the treatment & imaging of pancreatic cancer. *Acta Biomaterialia*, *49*, 422–433. doi:10.1016/j.actbio.2016.11.053 PMID:27890622

Jain, A. K., Dubey, V., Mehra, N. K., Lodhi, N., Nahar, M., Mishra, D. K., & Jain, N. K. (2009). Carbohydrate-conjugated multiwalled carbon nanotubes: Development and characterization. *Nanomedicine; Nanotechnology, Biology, and Medicine*, *5*(4), 432–442. doi:10.1016/j.nano.2009.03.001 PMID:19341818

Kesharwani, P., Xie, L., Banerjee, S., Mao, G., Padhye, S., Sarkar, F. H., & Iyer, A. K. (2015). Hyaluronic acid-conjugated polyamidoamine dendrimers for targeted delivery of 3, 4-difluorobenzylidene curcumin to CD44 overexpressing pancreatic cancer cells. *Colloids and Surfaces. B, Biointerfaces*, *136*, 413–423. doi:10.1016/j.colsurfb.2015.09.043 PMID:26440757

Khalid, M., & El-Sawy, H. S. (2017). Polymeric nanoparticles: Promising platform for drug delivery. *International Journal of Pharmaceutics*, *528*(1-2), 675–691. doi:10.1016/j.ijpharm.2017.06.052 PMID:28629982

Khutale, G. V., & Casey, A. (2017). Synthesis and characterization of a multifunctional gold-doxorubicin nanoparticle system for pH triggered intracellular drug release. *European Journal of Pharmaceutics and Biopharmaceutics*, *119*, 372–380. doi:10.1016/j.ejpb.2017.07.009 PMID:28736333

Kim, J., Lee, J. E., Lee, S. H., Yu, J. H., Lee, J. H., Park, T. G., & Hyeon, T. (2008). Designed fabrication of a multifunctional polymer nanomedical platform for simultaneous cancer-targeted imaging and magnetically guided drug delivery. *Advanced Materials*, *20*(3), 478–483. doi:10.1002/adma.200701726

Kumar, A., Lale, S. V., Alex, M. A., Choudhary, V., & Koul, V. (2017). Folic acid and trastuzumab conjugated redox responsive random multiblock copolymeric nanocarriers for breast cancer therapy: In-vitro and in-vivo studies. *Colloids and Surfaces. B, Biointerfaces*, *149*, 369–378. doi:10.1016/j.colsurfb.2016.10.044 PMID:27846450

Kushwaha, S. K. S., Ghoshal, S., Rai, A. K., & Singh, S. (2013). Carbon nanotubes as a novel drug delivery system for anticancer therapy: A review. *Brazilian Journal of Pharmaceutical Sciences*, *49*(4), 629–643. doi:10.1590/S1984-82502013000400002

Liang, C., Yang, Y., Ling, Y., Huang, Y., Li, T., & Li, X. (2011). Improved therapeutic effect of folate-decorated PLGA–PEG nanoparticles for endometrial carcinoma. *Bioorganic & Medicinal Chemistry*, *19*(13), 4057–4066. doi:10.1016/j.bmc.2011.05.016 PMID:21641806

Liang, H., He, L., Zhou, B., Li, B., & Li, J. (2017). Folate-functionalized assembly of low density lipoprotein/sodium carboxymethyl cellulose nanoparticles for targeted delivery. *Colloids and Surfaces. B, Biointerfaces*, *156*, 19–28. doi:10.1016/j.colsurfb.2017.05.004 PMID:28499201

Liu, Y., Ng, Y., Toh, M. R., & Chiu, G. N. (2015). Lipid-dendrimer hybrid nanosystem as a novel delivery system for paclitaxel to treat ovarian cancer. *Journal of Controlled Release*, *220*, 438–446. doi:10.1016/j.jconrel.2015.11.004 PMID:26551345

Liu, Y., Ran, R., Chen, J., Kuang, Q., Tang, J., Mei, L., ... He, Q. (2014). Paclitaxel loaded liposomes decorated with a multifunctional tandem peptide for glioma targeting. *Biomaterials*, *35*(17), 4835–4847. doi:10.1016/j.biomaterials.2014.02.031 PMID:24651033

Lodhi, N., Mehra, N. K., & Jain, N. K. (2013). Development and characterization of dexamethasone mesylate anchored on multi walled carbon nanotubes. *Journal of Drug Targeting*, *21*(1), 67–76. doi:10.3109/1061186X.2012.729213 PMID:23039174

Lord, M. S., Tsoi, B., Gunawan, C., Teoh, W. Y., Amal, R., & Whitelock, J. M. (2013). Anti-angiogenic activity of heparin functionalised cerium oxide nanoparticles. *Biomaterials*, *34*(34), 8808–8818. doi:10.1016/j.biomaterials.2013.07.083 PMID:23942211

Manivasagan, P., Bharathiraja, S., Bui, N. Q., Lim, I. G., & Oh, J. (2016). Paclitaxel-loaded chitosan oligosaccharide-stabilized gold nanoparticles as novel agents for drug delivery and photoacoustic imaging of cancer cells. *International Journal of Pharmaceutics*, *511*(1), 367–379. doi:10.1016/j.ijpharm.2016.07.025 PMID:27424169

Mehra, N. K., & Jain, N. (2015). Cancer targeting propensity of folate conjugated surface engineered multi-walled carbon nanotubes. *Colloids and Surfaces. B, Biointerfaces*, *132*, 17–26. doi:10.1016/j.colsurfb.2015.04.056 PMID:26001798

Mehra, N. K., Mishra, V., & Jain, N. (2014). A review of ligand tethered surface engineered carbon nanotubes. *Biomaterials*, *35*(4), 1267–1283. doi:10.1016/j.biomaterials.2013.10.032 PMID:24210872

Mehra, N. K., Verma, A. K., Mishra, P., & Jain, N. (2014). The cancer targeting potential of D-α-tocopheryl polyethylene glycol 1000 succinate tethered multi walled carbon nanotubes. *Biomaterials*, *35*(15), 4573–4588. doi:10.1016/j.biomaterials.2014.02.022 PMID:24612818

Milosavljevic, V., Krejcova, L., Guran, R., Buchtelova, H., Wawrzak, D., Richtera, L., ... Adam, V. (2017). Exceptional release kinetics and cytotoxic selectivity of oxidised MWCNTs double-functionalised with doxorubicin and prostate-homing peptide. *Colloids and Surfaces. B, Biointerfaces*, *156*, 123–132. doi:10.1016/j.colsurfb.2017.05.008 PMID:28527356

Mobasseri, R., Karimi, M., Tian, L., Naderi-Manesh, H., & Ramakrishna, S. (2017). Hydrophobic lapatinib encapsulated dextran-chitosan nanoparticles using a toxic solvent free method: Fabrication, release property & in vitro anti-cancer activity. *Materials Science and Engineering C*, *74*, 413–421. doi:10.1016/j.msec.2016.12.027 PMID:28254312

Modi, C. D., Patel, S. J., Desai, A. B., & Murthy, R. (2011). Functionalization and evaluation of PEGylated carbon nanotubes as novel drug delivery for methotrexate. *Journal of Applied Pharmaceutical Science*, *1*(5), 13.

Moosavian, S. A., Abnous, K., Badiee, A., & Jaafari, M. R. (2016). Improvement in the drug delivery and anti-tumor efficacy of PEGylated liposomal doxorubicin by targeting RNA aptamers in mice bearing breast tumor model. *Colloids and Surfaces. B, Biointerfaces*, *139*, 228–236. doi:10.1016/j.colsurfb.2015.12.009 PMID:26722819

Möschwitzer, J. P. (2013). Drug nanocrystals in the commercial pharmaceutical development process. *International Journal of Pharmaceutics*, *453*(1), 142–156. doi:10.1016/j.ijpharm.2012.09.034 PMID:23000841

Muddineti, O. S., Ghosh, B., & Biswas, S. (2015). Current trends in using polymer coated gold nanoparticles for cancer therapy. *International Journal of Pharmaceutics*, *484*(1), 252–267. doi:10.1016/j.ijpharm.2015.02.038 PMID:25701627

Muèller, R. H., MaÈder, K., & Gohla, S. (2000). Solid lipid nanoparticles (SLN) for controlled drug delivery–a review of the state of the art. *European Journal of Pharmaceutics and Biopharmaceutics*, *50*(1), 161–177. doi:10.1016/S0939-6411(00)00087-4 PMID:10840199

Nag, M., Gajbhiye, V., Kesharwani, P., & Jain, N. K. (2016). Transferrin functionalized chitosan-PEG nanoparticles for targeted delivery of paclitaxel to cancer cells. *Colloids and Surfaces. B, Biointerfaces*, *148*, 363–370. doi:10.1016/j.colsurfb.2016.08.059 PMID:27632697

Oliveira, M. S., Mussi, S. V., Gomes, D. A., Yoshida, M. I., Frezard, F., Carregal, V. M., & Ferreira, L. A. (2016). α-Tocopherol succinate improves encapsulation and anticancer activity of doxorubicin loaded in solid lipid nanoparticles. *Colloids and Surfaces. B, Biointerfaces*, *140*, 246–253. doi:10.1016/j.colsurfb.2015.12.019 PMID:26764108

Pan, B., Cui, D., Xu, P., Ozkan, C., Feng, G., Ozkan, M., & He, R. (2009). Synthesis and characterization of polyamidoamine dendrimer-coated multi-walled carbon nanotubes and their application in gene delivery systems. *Nanotechnology*, *20*(12), 125101. doi:10.1088/0957-4484/20/12/125101 PMID:19420458

Park, K., Lee, S., Kang, E., Kim, K., Choi, K., & Kwon, I. C. (2009). New generation of multifunctional nanoparticles for cancer imaging and therapy. *Advanced Functional Materials*, *19*(10), 1553–1566. doi:10.1002/adfm.200801655

Parvanian, S., Mostafavi, S. M., & Aghashiri, M. (2017). Multifunctional nanoparticle developments in cancer diagnosis and treatment. *Sensing and Bio-Sensing Research*, *13*, 81–87. doi:10.1016/j.sbsr.2016.08.002

Patel, H. K., Gajbhiye, V., Kesharwani, P., & Jain, N. K. (2016). Ligand anchored poly (propyleneimine) dendrimers for brain targeting: Comparative in vitro and in vivo assessment. *Journal of Colloid and Interface Science*, *482*, 142–150. doi:10.1016/j.jcis.2016.07.047 PMID:27501037

Peres, L. B., Peres, L. B., de Araújo, P. H. H., & Sayer, C. (2016). Solid lipid nanoparticles for encapsulation of hydrophilic drugs by an organic solvent free double emulsion technique. *Colloids and Surfaces. B, Biointerfaces*, *140*, 317–323. doi:10.1016/j.colsurfb.2015.12.033 PMID:26764112

Pruthi, J., Mehra, N. K., & Jain, N. K. (2012). Macrophages targeting of amphotericin B through mannosylated multiwalled carbon nanotubes. *Journal of Drug Targeting*, *20*(7), 593–604. doi:10.3109/1061186X.2012.697168 PMID:22690657

Ramachandran, R., Krishnaraj, C., Sivakumar, A. S., Prasannakumar, P., Kumar, V. A., Shim, K. S., ... Yun, S.-I. (2017). Anticancer activity of biologically synthesized silver and gold nanoparticles on mouse myoblast cancer cells and their toxicity against embryonic zebrafish. *Materials Science and Engineering C*, *73*, 674–683. doi:10.1016/j.msec.2016.12.110 PMID:28183660

Sala, M., Miladi, K., Agusti, G., Elaissari, A., & Fessi, H. (2017). Preparation of liposomes: A comparative study between the double solvent displacement and the conventional ethanol injection—From laboratory scale to large scale. *Colloids and Surfaces. A, Physicochemical and Engineering Aspects*, *524*, 71–78. doi:10.1016/j.colsurfa.2017.02.084

Shegokar, R., & Müller, R. H. (2010). Nanocrystals: Industrially feasible multifunctional formulation technology for poorly soluble actives. *International Journal of Pharmaceutics*, *399*(1), 129–139. doi:10.1016/j.ijpharm.2010.07.044 PMID:20674732

Sheikhpour, M., Golbabaie, A., & Kasaeian, A. (2017). Carbon nanotubes: A review of novel strategies for cancer diagnosis and treatment. *Materials Science and Engineering C*, *76*, 1289–1304. doi:10.1016/j.msec.2017.02.132 PMID:28482496

Shi, X., Wang, S. H., Shen, M., Antwerp, M. E., Chen, X., Li, C., ... Baker, J. R. Jr. (2009). Multifunctional dendrimer-modified multiwalled carbon nanotubes: Synthesis, characterization, and in vitro cancer cell targeting and imaging. *Biomacromolecules*, *10*(7), 1744–1750. doi:10.1021/bm9001624 PMID:19459647

Singh, R., Mehra, N. K., Jain, V., & Jain, N. K. (2013). Gemcitabine-loaded smart carbon nanotubes for effective targeting to cancer cells. *Journal of Drug Targeting*, *21*(6), 581–592. doi:10.3109/1061186X.2013.778264 PMID:23484494

Singh, R. P., Sharma, G., Kumari, L., Koch, B., Singh, S., Bharti, S., ... Muthu, M. S. (2016). RGD-TPGS decorated theranostic liposomes for brain targeted delivery. *Colloids and Surfaces. B, Biointerfaces*, *147*, 129–141. doi:10.1016/j.colsurfb.2016.07.058 PMID:27497076

Singh, R. P., Sharma, G., Singh, S., Bharti, S., Pandey, B. L., Koch, B., & Muthu, M. S. (2017). Chitosan-folate decorated carbon nanotubes for site specific lung cancer delivery. *Materials Science and Engineering C*, *77*, 446–458. doi:10.1016/j.msec.2017.03.225 PMID:28532051

Singh, R. P., Sharma, G., Singh, S., Kumar, M., Pandey, B. L., Koch, B., & Muthu, M. S. (2016). Vitamin E TPGS conjugated carbon nanotubes improved efficacy of docetaxel with safety for lung cancer treatment. *Colloids and Surfaces. B, Biointerfaces*, *141*, 429–442. doi:10.1016/j.colsurfb.2016.02.011 PMID:26895505

Singh, R. P., Sharma, G., Singh, S., Patne, S. C., Pandey, B. L., Koch, B., & Muthu, M. S. (2016). Effects of transferrin conjugated multi-walled carbon nanotubes in lung cancer delivery. *Materials Science and Engineering C*, *67*, 313–325. doi:10.1016/j.msec.2016.05.013 PMID:27287127

Singh, Y., Meher, J. G., Raval, K., Khan, F. A., Chaurasia, M., Jain, N. K., & Chourasia, M. K. (2017). Nanoemulsion: Concepts, development and applications in drug delivery. *Journal of Controlled Release*, *252*, 28–49. doi:10.1016/j.jconrel.2017.03.008 PMID:28279798

Sinha, R., Kim, G. J., Nie, S., & Shin, D. M. (2006). Nanotechnology in cancer therapeutics: Bioconjugated nanoparticles for drug delivery. *Molecular Cancer Therapeutics*, *5*(8), 1909–1917. doi:10.1158/1535-7163.MCT-06-0141 PMID:16928810

Soni, N., Soni, N., Pandey, H., Maheshwari, R., Kesharwani, P., & Tekade, R. K. (2016). Augmented delivery of gemcitabine in lung cancer cells exploring mannose anchored solid lipid nanoparticles. *Journal of Colloid and Interface Science*, *481*, 107–116. doi:10.1016/j.jcis.2016.07.020 PMID:27459173

Srivalli, K. M. R., & Mishra, B. (2015). Preparation and pharmacodynamic assessment of ezetimibe nanocrystals: Effect of P-gp inhibitory stabilizer on particle size and oral absorption. *Colloids and Surfaces. B, Biointerfaces*, *135*, 756–764. doi:10.1016/j.colsurfb.2015.08.042 PMID:26342321

Srivalli, K. M. R., & Mishra, B. (2016). Drug nanocrystals: A way toward scale-up. *Saudi Pharmaceutical Journal*, *24*(4), 386–404. doi:10.1016/j.jsps.2014.04.007 PMID:27330370

Tagami, T., Ando, Y., & Ozeki, T. (2017). Fabrication of liposomal doxorubicin exhibiting ultrasensitivity against phospholipase A 2 for efficient pulmonary drug delivery to lung cancers. *International Journal of Pharmaceutics*, *517*(1), 35–41. doi:10.1016/j.ijpharm.2016.11.039 PMID:27865984

Taheri, A., Dinarvand, R., Atyabi, F., Ghahremani, M. H., & Ostad, S. N. (2012). Trastuzumab decorated methotrexate–human serum albumin conjugated nanoparticles for targeted delivery to HER2 positive tumor cells. *European Journal of Pharmaceutical Sciences*, *47*(2), 331–340. doi:10.1016/j.ejps.2012.06.016 PMID:22771547

Thenmozhi, S., Dharmaraj, N., Kadirvelu, K., & Kim, H. Y. (2017). Electrospun nanofibers: New generation materials for advanced applications. *Materials Science and Engineering B*, *217*, 36–48. doi:10.1016/j.mseb.2017.01.001

Tian, B., Ding, Y., Han, J., Zhang, J., Han, Y., & Han, J. (2015). N-Acetyl-D-glucosamine decorated polymeric nanoparticles for targeted delivery of doxorubicin: Synthesis, characterization and in vitro evaluation. *Colloids and Surfaces. B, Biointerfaces*, *130*, 246–254. doi:10.1016/j.colsurfb.2015.04.019 PMID:25921641

Torchilin, V. P. (2007). Targeted pharmaceutical nanocarriers for cancer therapy and imaging. *The AAPS Journal*, *9*(2), E128–E147. doi:10.1208/aapsj0902015 PMID:17614355

Vahed, S. Z., Salehi, R., Davaran, S., & Sharifi, S. (2016). Liposome-based drug co-delivery systems in cancer cells. *Materials Science and Engineering C*, *71*, 1327–1341. doi:10.1016/j.msec.2016.11.073 PMID:27987688

van Elk, M., Murphy, B. P., Eufrásio-da-Silva, T., O'Reilly, D. P., Vermonden, T., Hennink, W. E., ... Ruiz-Hernández, E. (2016). Nanomedicines for advanced cancer treatments: Transitioning towards responsive systems. *International Journal of Pharmaceutics*, *515*(1), 132–164. doi:10.1016/j.ijpharm.2016.10.013 PMID:27725268

Wan, Y., Dai, W., Nevagi, R. J., Toth, I., & Moyle, P. M. (2017). Multifunctional peptide-lipid nanocomplexes for efficient targeted delivery of DNA and siRNA into breast cancer cells. *Acta Biomaterialia*, *59*, 257–268. doi:10.1016/j.actbio.2017.06.032 PMID:28655658

Wang, F., Chen, L., Zhang, R., Chen, Z., & Zhu, L. (2014). RGD peptide conjugated liposomal drug delivery system for enhance therapeutic efficacy in treating bone metastasis from prostate cancer. *Journal of Controlled Release*, *196*, 222–233. doi:10.1016/j.jconrel.2014.10.012 PMID:25456829

Wang, F., Li, L., Liu, B., Chen, Z., & Li, C. (2017). Hyaluronic acid decorated pluronic P85 solid lipid nanoparticles as a potential carrier to overcome multidrug resistance in cervical and breast cancer. *Biomedicine and Pharmacotherapy*, *86*, 595–604. doi:10.1016/j.biopha.2016.12.041 PMID:28027535

Wang, H., Agarwal, P., Zhao, S., Yu, J., Lu, X., & He, X. (2016). Combined cancer therapy with hyaluronan-decorated fullerene-silica multifunctional nanoparticles to target cancer stem-like cells. *Biomaterials*, *97*, 62–73. doi:10.1016/j.biomaterials.2016.04.030 PMID:27162075

Yan, J., Su, T., Cheng, F., Cao, J., Zhang, H., & He, B. (2017). Multifunctional nanoparticles self-assembled from polyethylenimine-based graft polymers as efficient anticancer drug delivery. *Colloids and Surfaces. B, Biointerfaces*, *155*, 118–127. doi:10.1016/j.colsurfb.2017.02.030 PMID:28415029

Yang, L., Liu, M., Huang, K., Ai, X., Li, C., Ma, J., ... Liu, X. (2017). Folate-targeted single-wall metal-organic nanotubes used as multifunctional drug carriers. *Applied Surface Science*, *392*, 189–195. doi:10.1016/j.apsusc.2016.09.030

Yao, H. J., Sun, L., Liu, Y., Jiang, S., Pu, Y., Li, J., & Zhang, Y. (2016). Monodistearoylphosphatidylethanolamine-hyaluronic acid functionalization of single-walled carbon nanotubes for targeting intracellular drug delivery to overcome multidrug resistance of cancer cells. *Carbon*, *96*, 362–376. doi:10.1016/j.carbon.2015.09.037

Yin, T., Cai, H., Liu, J., Cui, B., Wang, L., Yin, L., ... Huo, M. (2016). Biological evaluation of PEG modified nanosuspensions based on human serum albumin for tumor targeted delivery of paclitaxel. *European Journal of Pharmaceutical Sciences*, *83*, 79–87. doi:10.1016/j.ejps.2015.12.019 PMID:26699227

Zhang, B., Chen, Q., Tang, H., Xie, Q., Ma, M., Tan, L., ... Yao, S. (2010). Characterization of and biomolecule immobilization on the biocompatible multi-walled carbon nanotubes generated by functionalization with polyamidoamine dendrimers. *Colloids and Surfaces. B, Biointerfaces*, *80*(1), 18–25. doi:10.1016/j.colsurfb.2010.05.023 PMID:20542415

Chapter 12
Multifunctional Nanocomposites for Biotherapeutic Applications

Eliana B. Souto
University of Coimbra, Portugal

A. R. Fernandes
University of Coimbra, Portugal

J. Dias Ferreira
University of Coimbra, Portugal

C. F. da Silva
Federal University of Sao Paulo, Brazil

Patrícia Severino
Tiradentes University, Brazil

Carlos Martins-Gomes
University of Tras-os-Montes and Alto Douro, Portugal

Amélia M. Silva
University of Tras-os-Montes and Alto Douro, Portugal

ABSTRACT

The rationale for administering a drug is usually related to the increase of the drug bioavailability with the aim to achieve a therapeutic effect at a predetermined time. A drug delivery system consists of a formulation or even a device that introduces a drug into the organism being capable of assuring the efficacy and safety by controlling the rate, time, and place of release. With the field of multifunctional nanocomposites, crucial factors such as the improvement on the medicine's efficacy, reduced economic implications, extended life of product patent, better safety and efficacy profile, and increased compliance are the aim. Nowadays, nanocomposites and nanostructured materials are important for several biotherapeutic applications, including their use in drug delivery, in orthopaedics, and in dentistry.

DOI: 10.4018/978-1-5225-4781-5.ch012

Copyright © 2018, IGI Global. Copying or distributing in print or electronic forms without written permission of IGI Global is prohibited.

INTRODUCTION

In the dentistry, the dental materials that are used nowadays are greatly challenged by the secondary disease, e.g., caries. After an initial dental treatment, this disease is one of the main reasons for failures in dental materials previously applied (Mjör, Moorhead, & J.E. Dahl, 2000; Sarrett, 2005; Bernardo, 2007). Thus, there is an increasing interest in the bioactivity of dental materials as materials that need to go beyond the mechanical and physical aspects aiming the tissue repair. The new composite materials are essential in direct tooth restoration, however, is fundamental that things like wear resistance, fracture toughness and compression, surface hardness, tensile and flexural strengths are known due demands of mastication in the oral environment (Loguercio, 2006; Sadeghi, Lynch, & Shahamat, 2010). While improvements in these areas are being accomplished there are several limitations that still found for modern materials (Sadeghi, Lynch, & Shahamat, 2010). The principal difficulties include the adapting the material to the internal surfaces of a prepared cavity, the creation of an effective marginal seal in the cavity tooth interface, material discolouration over time, secondary decay caused by material microleakage and post-operative sensitivity (Korkmaz, 2010; Sadeghi, & Lynch, 2009).

Nanoscience or molecular engineering is also known as nanotechnology is characterised as the creation of materials and functional structures with characteristic dimensions in the nano range (0.1-100 nm). In case of inorganic phases in an organic/inorganic composite in nanosized, they are called nanocomposites (Chen, 2010). Nanocomposites, nowadays, are one of the biggest contribution to restorative and aesthetic dentistry for the restoration of tooth structure. Nanocomposites are characterised by filler-particle sizes ≤ 100 nm and present advantages faced to the current microfilled and hybrid resin-based composites, due to their aesthetic and strength advantages, as well as, have better polish-ability properties which produce a smoother surface with better shade characteristics and their microhardness (Ogle, & Byles, 2014).

Biomaterials are successfully integrated into surrounding tissue and should match tissue's topography and their mechanical properties. Nowadays there are some evidence that the cellular response to a biomaterial may be enhanced in the synthetic polymer formulations by mimicking the surface roughness associated with the nano-structured extra-cellular matrix components of natural tissue (Li, & Webster, 2007; Liu, Slamovich, & Webster, 2007). Although the some of the benefits from nanotechnology are known, relatively few advantages have been described for biological applications, such as bone regeneration. Despite the bone itself is a nano-structured material composed of biological entities like proteins (such as, collagen type I) and hydroxyapatite crystals that have nanometer dimensions (Taton, 2001). Then, cells are naturally accustomed to interacting with nano-structured surface roughness in the body. Conventional materials (rough at the micron scale but are usually smooth at the nanoscale) provide nonbiologically inspired surface roughness values to cells. Thus, the use of nano-structured materials in bone tissue engineering (and all of the tissue engineering) represents a challenge and a paradigm shift (Balasundaram, & Webster, 2007).

Nanocomposites are assemblies composed either by organic or inorganic materials being capable of a wide delivery of a set of molecules ranging different types and sizes. About the size, it is normally less than 1,000 nm (Soppimath, 2001). Such detail allows drug entrapment, adsorption and other techniques that would not be possible on bigger formulations (Shen, 2007). The inward structure of such particles is the verdict for their classification on vesicular or matrix system. The first one is also termed of nanocapsules being a heterogeneous system. In these conditions, the so-called drugs are kept in an aqueous or oily environment fenced by an organic or inorganic sheath (Manias, 2001). The second labels a homogeneous system in which the active agents are dissolved or dispersed. There are certain requirements to warrant to functionality of this formulation such as materials with precise and specific characteristics like having lack of natural immunogenicity; a good cellular adhesion; being capable to let cell perform endocytosis; biocompatible with human metabolic processes; easily and well-defined surface depending on the desired target; structural control regarding size and also drug shape; reduced protein binding and controlled triggering (Zare, Rhee, & Hui, 2017).

1. NANOCOMPOSITES IN DENTISTRY

Nanotechnology has the potential to bring improvements in various areas of study, included the physical properties of dental materials, however, the bioactivity aspect of the materials should not be overlooked in any step of the investigation. This might include nanomaterials coated, e.g., cytokines, compliment activation, to promote a beneficial immune response in the diseased tissue, as well as, subsequently growth factors to promote angiogenesis and wound faster repair (Cox, 2000). The choice of antibacterial nanomaterials mainly depends on the type of dentistry application. Nanoparticles composed of Ag, Zn and TiO2 are commonly incorporated in resin-based composites and/or used in the implants as an antimicrobial coating. Other components, such as bioactive glass nano-powders are mostly used as root canal disinfectants, e.g., composites that release chlorhexidine, used in the mouthwashes (Hook, 2014). Another study, in contrast, impregnation of bactericidal nanoparticles into resin-based composites has demonstrated a long-lasting effect against cariogenic bacteria without affecting the physical and mechanical properties of the teeth (Ahn, 2009). Composites used in dentistry generally consists of three main components which are chemically different from each other: the organic matrix, the inorganic matrix and a coupling agent. The organic matrix is usually a synthetic monomer or resin, the inorganic matrix is the filler and the coupling agent is normally the silane and is essential to bond the filler to the organic matrix. The resultant combination of these components determines the physical, chemical, mechanical and optimal properties of composites (as well as their clinical behaviour) and each of these phases can be modified. In the last few years have been introduced new materials, such as phosphine oxide initiators and monomethacrylate diluents. These compounds have led to dental composites with improved properties (Cramer, Stansbury, & Bowman, 2011). On the other side, the introduction of nano-fillers showed significant new advances in the composites that were developed. The characteristics of particles used in dental composites, such as the chemistry, the morphology and the size of filler vary significantly even within the nanoscale (Canche-Escamilla, Duarte-Aranda, & Toledano, 2014). The incorporation of fillers to the resin, regardless the type of filler, aiming to optimising the performance and properties of the final restorative material. Chen has described the advantages of addition of fillers as: 1) possibility to enhance the mechanical properties of dental composites; 2) modify the thermal expansion coefficient of the composite to match that of the tooth; 3) reduce the polymerisation shrinkage; 4) provide radio-opacity; 5) improve handling; 6) provide the composites with wear resistance and translucency (Chen, 2010). The dental composites present a system that reinforces fillers to the polymer matrix, once are composed of synthetic polymers, inorganic fillers, initiators, and activators that promote light-activated polymerization of the organic matrix to form cross-linked polymer networks and silane coupling agents (Chen, 2010). In terms of matrix, the most commercial dental composites use ethoxylated bisphenol-A-dimethacrylate (Bis-EMA) monomer as their organic matrix. This monomer has a very high viscosity due to the hydrogen bonding interactions that occur between the hydroxyl groups and the monomer molecules. The only way to provide the proper viscosity for use in dental composites must be dilute the monomer with more fluid monomers (Ferracane, 1995). Another base monomers that constitute the matrix that are used in current commercial composites are triethyleneglycol dimethacrylate (TEGDMA), urethane dimethacrylate (UDMA), decanediol dimethacrylate (D3MA), bis(methacryloyloxymethyl) tricyclodecane, and urethane tetramethacrylate (UTMA) (Chen, 2010).

To obtain good mechanical properties in dental composites is essential that exists the formation of a strong covalent bond between inorganic fillers and the organic matrix. Bonding of inorganic fillers and the organic matrix is achieved by coating the fillers with a silane coupling agent that has functional groups to link the two phases chemically. The typical coupling agent is 3-methacryloxypropyltrimethoxysilane (MPTS), once have one end of the molecule can be bonded to the hydroxyl groups of silica particles, and the other end is capable of copolymerizing into the polymer matrix (Karabela, & Sideridou).

The range of fillers that constitute the conventional composites includes colloidal silica, quartz, radiopaque silicate particles containing oxides of barium, strontium, zinc, aluminium and zirconium. These fillers have characteristics which permit that increase strength, modulus of elasticity, reduce polymerization shrinkage, the coefficient of thermal expansion, and water absorption. Lutz and Phillips has proposed a widely accepted classification based on filler particle size, where composites can be characterised as macro-filler composites (0.1-100 μm), microfiller composites (0.04-0.1 μm) and hybrid composites (fillers of different sizes) (Lutz, & Phillips, 1983). Resin-based composites can be classified according to their composition or the filler particle size (Lang, Jaarda, & Wang, 1992). The most conventional composites present a filler particle size in the range of 0.04-0.7 μm. The principal worry in the practical is that particles of these sizes cannot interact perfectly with the nanoscopic (1-10 nm) structural elements of enamel and dentin, e.g., dentinal tubules and collagen fibres, among others (Terry, 2004). As a consequence, the adhesion between the restorative material and the tissue can be greatly compromised. Then, the production of new advanced composites with unique properties became a possibility with the introduction of nano-fillers (1-100nm). The smaller particle size have some advantages, such as 1) reduces viscosity; 2) offers better handling, while the mechanical properties remain sufficiently competent; 3) allows a higher filler load (Terry, 2004). The filler size in nanocomposites is about 40nm. Filtek Supreme (3M ESPE, St. Paul, MN, USA) was the first dental nanocomposite in the market in 2002. Currently, there are other examples of commercially available nanocomposites such as Premise (Kerr/Sybron, Orange, CA, USA), GrandiO (Voco, Cuxhaven, Germany), Ceram-X (Dentsply DeTrey, Konstanz, Germany), and Palfique (Tokuyama Dental Corp., Tokyo, Japan) (Besinis, 2015).

Nanofillers can be produced by various techniques, such as flame pyrolysis, flame spray pyrolysis, and sol-gel processes. Once there are small filler particles that have dimensions below the wavelength of visible light (0.4-0.8 μm), they are unable to scatter or absorb visible light. Nanofillers due to their characteristics are usually invisible and offer the advantage of optical property improvement (Mitra, Wu, & Holmes). With the use of nanofillers, filler levels could be as high as 90-95% by weight. The increase of nanofillers also increases the surface area of the filler particles, which limits the total amount of filler particles because of the wettability of the fillers. As a consequence, the increase in filler level results in a lower amount of resin in nanocomposites and will also significantly reduce polymerization shrinkage and dramatically improve the physical properties of nanocomposites. Kasraei has shown that resin composite has antibacterial activity to inhibit the growth of oral cavity microorganisms. In this treatment, the antibacterial activity was tested against S. mutans and Lactobacillus after 12 hours of incubation. The results showed that the measurement of the active colonies formed on the surface of blood agar plates a significant antibacterial activity for the resin composites compared to the control group (Kasraei, 2014).

Figure 1. Main components of composites applied in dentistry

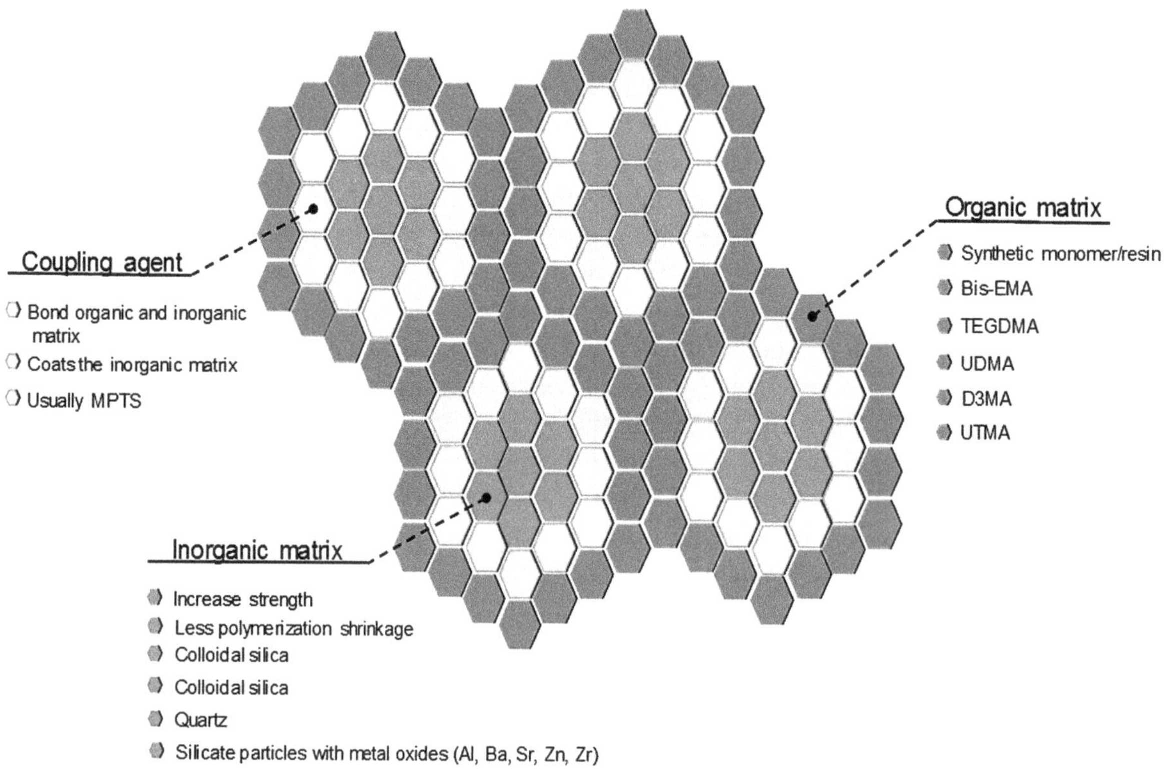

1.1 Restoration

Nanotechnology, nowadays, offers refinements to resin-based composite systems that already are clinically proven, what presents a huge impact on restorative dentistry. There are generally two types of composite restorative materials, such as nanohybrid and nanofilled resin-based composites. These particles are characterised by filler-particle sizes of ≤100nm (Chandki, 2012). Due to these characteristics, these materials can offer esthetic and strength advantages over conventional microfilled and hybrid resin-based composite systems. Primarily, nanohybrid and nanofilled composites are better in terms of smoothness, polishability, the precision of shade characterization and plus flexural strength and microhardness (Beun, 2007). So, in terms of restoration, the nanocomposites present advantages, such as 1) superior hardness; 2) superior Flexural strength, modulus of elasticity and translucency; 3) reduced filling shrinkage; 4) excellent handling properties.

Choosing a suitable resin-based composite for a restoration requires some functional properties, including enhanced longevity of the restoratives by excellent mechanical properties such as high strength, fracture toughness, surface hardness, optimized modulus of elasticity, low wear, water sorption, solubility, low polymerization shrinkage, low fatigue degradation, high radiopacity and a better detection of the material during removal of a composite restoration (Ilie, & Hickel, 2011). However, the biological properties are also essential, the materials need to have a good biocompatibility (both systemic and local), no postoperative pain or hypersensitivity, its necessary to preserve tooth integrity (not causing fractures or cracks), as well as caries-inhibiting abilities are required. In case of aesthetic considerations, the good colour matching and colour stability (translucency, shades), optimum polish ability, long-term surface gloss, the absence of marginal or surface staining and a good long-term anatomical form should also be taken into consideration (Frese, Staehle, & Wolff).

The resin-based composites showed several clinical negative effects, like marginal discrepancies (Irie, Suzuki, & Watts, 2002) marginal staining, white lines around the restoration, cusp fractures, debonding (Ferracane, 2008), microleakage, secondary caries, postoperative sensitivity or pain are still observed in restorations made using the modern resin-based composites. These effects are frequently associated with the polymerization shrinkage stress (Ferracane, & Mitchem, 2003).

The introduction of flowable resin-based composite material has the objective to be used as a liner in occlusal and posterior restorations. An example of this is the inclusion of a monomer having incorporated a photoactive group in urethane-based methacrylate resin, showing a 60–70% reduction when compared to conventional methacrylate-based resins, in shrinkage stress in the unfilled resin (Luan, 2009). When the resin was activated a relatively slow radical polymerization rate was demonstrated, suggesting that the photoinitiator incorporated into the resin is affecting the radical polymerization process. The filled compositions also showed a retained curing stress in cases of low filler loading (Luan, 2009).

Fillers are important once, allows the reduction in the monomer content and consequently the polymerization shrinkage, optimising wear, translucence, opalescence, radiopacity, intrinsic surface roughness and then polish ability, enhancing aesthetics and improving handling properties as well as, determines directly the mechanical properties of composite materials. Smaller particles are better in terms of polish and gloss. However, reduction of filler size and subsequent increase in surface area to volume ratio limited the achievable filler loading, what promote the decrease of handling and mechanical properties (Kwon, 2015). The microfill composites have, so far, better aesthetic qualities due to their excellent polish ability, as well as the capacity to retain surface smoothness over time.

1.2 Nanocomposites in Caries Inhibition

There are some fillers specially developed to control/inhibit dental caries. Calcium and phosphate ion-releasing fillers have been developed to increase mineral content and consequently control dental caries. Some examples are nanoparticles of dicalcium phosphate anhydrous (DCPA) (Xu, 2006; Xu, 2007) and tetracalcium phosphate [TTCP: Ca4(PO4)2O]-whiskers (Xu, Weir, & Sun, 2009).

DCPA-whiskers are another particles useful in the control of caries. Xu et al. (2006;2007) studied DCPA nanoparticles, two types of fillers were used: DCPA particles and nano-silica fused whisker. The results showed that decreasing the DCPA and consequently the particle size decreased the composite's strength, while whisker reinforcement more than doubled the composite's strength and significantly increased the elastic modulus. Also in this study was found that silanization of the DCPA particles increased the composite's strength, but decreased the calcium and phosphate ion release. The use of unsilanized nano DCPA with whisker reinforcement appeared to be the best method to produce a composite with high strength and ions release. There are some studies showed that when these ions were released from the composite restoration, they re-precipitated to form hydroxyapatite outside the composite and inside the tooth lesion which promotes significantly increasing the mineral content of the lesion (Skrtic, 2000; Dickens, Flaim, & Takagi, 2003). Nanocomposites with DCPA exhibited the highest release, due to their increased particle surface area. Improved DCPA particle surface increased significantly the calcium and phosphate ions (Xu, Weir, & Sun, 2007).

Another composites that release calcium and phosphate ion are constituted with fine TTCP particles and nanosilica-fused whiskers were developed (Xu, Weir, & Sun, 20009). The whiskers provided the needed load bearing ability while TTCP was enabled to promote the release of calcium and phosphate ions by the composites. The TTCP-whisker composite has shown strengths about two-fold those of the TTCP composite without whiskers. However, the TTCP-whisker composite increased ions release by about six-fold when the pH was reduced from neutral to four. Xu suggested that nanocomposites with fine TTCP may have the potential to provide the necessary combination of load-bearing and simultaneously have caries-inhibiting capability (Xu, Wier, & Sun, 2009).

The restorative material release calcium fluoride which is described in some studies as an inhibitor of tooth demineralization and have a fundamental role in caries development and also to strengthen the neighbouring enamel or dentin (Burke, Ray, & McConnell, 2006; Wang, 2007).

The addition of calcium fluoride nanoparticles and reinforce of whisker fillers in nanocomposites lead to the fluoride release. The fluoride release from this nanoparticles was better than that of traditional and resin-modified glass ionomer materials (Xu, 2008). Thus, nanocomposites containing calcium fluoride and DCPA, which can release fluoride, calcium, and phosphate ions for precipitation of fluoroapatite and inhibition of caries (Xu, 2008). The development strategy to this nanocomposite is to redirect the two major challenges, such as secondary caries and restoration fracture. Actually, the ion-releasing and caries-inhibiting restoratives have inadequate stress-bearing capabilities, especially in large posterior restorations. Then is essential the application of new mechanically strong nanocomposites with the release of these ions in posterior restorations where amalgam and hybrid composites are currently used (Xu, 2010).

Wang et al. described different types of fluoride-releasing polymer-kaolinite nanocomposites, including C(K-diamine), C(K-acrylamide), and C(K-acetate) (Wang, 2007). Due of its structural characteristics and its high surface area for adsorption of fluoride, kaolinite is an excellent carrier compared with the conventional filler used in composite resins. Polymer-kaolinite nanocomposites have a huge potential to provide sustained release of fluoride because present strong adsorption of kaolinite to fluoride during the fabrication process. According to some studies, C(K-acrylamide) might be a useful dental restorative material with caries-preventive properties (Wang, 2007).

1.3 Implants

In the denture teeth, wear resistance is the most important physical properties. On the one hand, porcelain denture teeth are most wear resistant, however, these teeth are brittle, lack bonding to the denture base, and difficult to polish. Another possibility is the acrylic resin denture teeth that are easier to recontour but undergo excessive wear (Freitas, 2005). The nanocomposite denture teeth comprise of polymethylmethacrylate and nanosized filler particles (uniformly dispersed). Nanocomposite denture teeth are the most advantageous solution once presents highly polishable, stain and impact resistant material, lively surface structure, superior surface hardness and wear resistance (Patil, Mehta, & Guuva, 2008). The principal preoccupation in any implant (whether metallic, ceramic or polymeric) are to prevent inflammatory responses, as well as the osteolysis, and to promote osseointegration and biological fixation. The aim of nanocoatings and nanocomposite coatings of implants are to achieve improvements in bioactivity, resistance to corrosion in oral medium, protection against metal ion release, biocompatibility, and an improved environment and structure for new bone growth. The advantages of nanocoatings and nanocomposite coatings are described as the opportunity that has in changing the surface properties of surgical-grade materials to attain improvements in clinical reliability, longevity and, most importantly, performance (Choi, 2013). Another advantages of nanocoatings include their purity due to the choice of raw materials and the ability to be mixed with other nanoparticles or compounds to produce nanocomposite coatings and if required, bulk nanocomposite materials (Choi, & Ben-Nissan, 2007).

The processing route, as well as the chemistry and the production methods, are essential to managing the microstructure and properties of nanostructured materials. Thus, is essential that the most appropriate technique is selected when synthesising nanomaterials with the desired properties and property combinations. Some techniques have been utilised to produce coatings at both micro and nanoscale, such as chemical, physical, electrochemical vapour depositions, metal-organic chemical vapour deposition, thermal or diffusion conversion, plasma, fusion coating and sol-gel processing. Modification and improvements in surfaces aiming increasing bioactivity with alterations in the chemical and morphological constitution of implants have been the main focus of the investigations in the biomedical field (Ben-Nissan, Choi, & Bendavid, 2013). Both nanocomposites and their coating are usually described as a combination of two or more materials, which includes a matrix material (can be a biocompatible polymer, metal or ceramic) and nanoscale secondary particles. The modification of composite allows manipulating the mechanical properties, such as strength and Young's modulus of the composites closer to those of natural bone, with the incorporation of secondary nanoparticles. This is an important hypothesis that is currently being explored in the development of a new generation of nanocomposite coatings containing nanomaterials such as bioglass and carbon nanotubes aiming to promote osseointegration. Some researchers are centred on improving the bioactivity of metallic dental implants with the application of nanocomposite coatings composed of hydroxyapatite nanoparticles and bioactive glass. This method was used, *in vitro* and *in vivo* studies that were carried out to investigate their suitability as a coating material in dental applications (Soundrapandian, 2011; Xie, 2012). However, there is evidence proved that the incorporation of bioactive glass into hydroxyapatite sputter coatings did not enhance the performance of a dental implant in implantations sites (van Oirshot, Narhi, Anil, Al Farraj Aldosari, van den Beucken, & Jansen, 2014).

The hypothesis of carbon nanotube composite coatings reinforced hydroxyapatite has been studied in order to research their biological characteristics (Facca, & Lahiri, 2012). The cell culture studies showed that did not have restricted growth of human osteoblasts close to carbon Nanotube regions and revealed the nontoxic nature of the carbon nanotube -hydroxyapatite coating. Facca has shown that did not observe any adverse effects or cytotoxicity *in vivo* caused by the addition of carbon nanotube to bone tissues when titanium implants coated with carbon nanotube -hydroxyapatite was implemented in rodent bone (Facca, & Lahiri, 2012).

The composite that has attracted much attention is the titanium dioxide composite as a bioactive coating, researchers believed that using titanium as reinforcement within the coating was one method for improving the mechanical reliability of hydroxyapatite. Aiming the use of Titanium Dioxide hydroxyapatite nanocomposite coating in an effort is to improve the strength and adhesion of the coating and increase the biological responses as well as reducing loosening of implants because of failure at the metal-coating interface (Kim, 2005; Kuwabara, 2012).

2. NANOCOMPOSITES IN ORTHOPAEDICS

Biodegradable polymeric materials are essential in orthopaedic tissue engineering, once, can be either natural (i.e., proteins) or synthetic. Nevertheless, synthetic polymers can offer better advantages than natural materials, once can be tailored to give a wider range of properties, are more predictable lot-to-lot uniformity and represent a more reliable source of raw materials, one often free from concerns of immunogenicity compared to materials from natural sources (Gunatillake, 2003). Based on these facts, the ideal polymer for an orthopaedic application need to have some characteristics such as, (1) does not present an inflammatory/toxic response, disproportionate to its beneficial effect; (2) is metabolized in the body after fulfilling its purpose leaving no trace components; (3) is easily processed into the final product form; (4) has acceptable shelf life; (5) is easily sterilized (Gunatillake, 2003). Another important factor is the mechanical properties, which must match the specific implant application so that sufficient strength remains until the surrounding tissue has healed.

The development of novel polymers that meet a number of demanding requirements aims to find tissue-engineered solutions to treat orthopaedic injuries/diseases. The principal characteristics required are the ability of polymer scaffolds to provide mechanical support during tissue growth, gradually degrade into natural biocompatible products to more demanding requirements (for example, the ability to incorporate cells, growth factors, etc.) and provide osteoconductive and osteoinductive environments. In the future is thought that form of an injectable liquid/paste in tissue engineering applications is a better way of tissue healing, once the development of in situ polymerisable compositions are becoming increasingly attractive due to their capability to functionalize as cell delivery systems (Portnov, Shulizmon, & Zilberman, 2016). The majority of the currently available degradable polymers do not fulfil all of these requirements and chemical changes to their structure may be required if they are to be formulated for such applications.

Most of the biodegradable polymers studied belong to the polyester family, which includes polyglycolides and polylactides (Gunatillake, 2003). However, these polymers present disadvantages in tissue engineering applications, such as their poor biocompatibility, the release of acidic degradation products, poor processability, and loss of mechanical properties very early during degradation.

In order to improve the properties of polymeric biomaterials, composites made from synthetic/natural polymers and ceramics have been investigated exhaustively for orthopaedic repair. Composites have advantages described as the ability to generate desired pore structures, matching size, shape, and mechanical properties to fit a variety of applications. As disadvantages stand out difficulty to shaping these scaffolds to fit cavities/defects with complicated geometries, bonding to the surrounding healthy bone tissues, and incorporating cells and growth factors (Balasundaram, & Webster, 2007).

Nanotechnology is important to tailor orthopaedic implant surfaces from the nanoscale structure of the extracellular matrix. The organic and inorganic components of a bone extracellular matrix form an environment replete with information for the cell types in bone tissue due to their three-dimensional architecture. The inorganic component of the bone extracellular matrix is composed with nanoscale calcium phosphate crystallites similar to hydroxyapatite (Hing, 2004). There are some techniques available for the deposition of calcium phosphate -coatings on metals, including plasma spraying, biomimetic deposition, laser deposition, ion beam deposition, radiofrequent magnetron sputter deposition, and electrostatic spray deposition. To the deposition of calcium phosphate -coatings on orthopaedic and dental implants, the plasma spraying is the most frequently used technique. However present some limitations including the lack of controlling coating structure, the relatively low cohesion within the thick coatings and the limited bond strength with the metallic implant substrate. The biomimetic deposition of calcium phosphate-coating is based on the deposition of calcium phosphate crystals with nanoscale dimensions (Barrere, 2003). The biomimetic process of calcium phosphate is important, once can be combined with the deposition of biologically active compounds (Liu, 2004). The resulting calcium phosphate coatings, produced by this co-precipitation process, do not only introduce bioactivity but can also actively influence cellular processes and reduce bacterial infections.

Nanocomposite bone grafts made of hydroxyapatite-collagen has shown some features of natural bone in composition and structure. Hydroxyapatite facilitates greater osteoconduction and related functions than conventional materials, however, its biodegradability is relatively slow and is not osteoinductive what are disadvantages (Kikuchi, 2001). In order to circumvent these disadvantages can be employed to make a composite in conjunction with osteogenic potential cells and osteoinductive growth factors, such as collagen. This tissue-engineered hydroxyapatite-collagen nanocomposite system can be very promising in engineering bone tissues (Liao, Cui, & Zhu, 2004). This nanocomposite construct was observed to support cellular adhesion, proliferation, and migration. *In vivo* tests showed that the system has great potential for the clinical repair of large bone defects according to the principles of bone tissue engineering.

2.1 Nanocomposites and Their Application

Nanomaterials, nanoparticles, nanofibers, nanosurfaces, nanocoatings, nanoscaffolds and nanocomposites are considered essential for various applications in orthopaedics and traumatology. Some studies support that nanomaterials in various physical forms are capable of enhancing the cell response selectively for biological tissue integration or improve the strength and wear resistance of current orthopaedic materials. Nowadays, orthopaedics are worried in prevention and correction of deformities, injuries and other disorders of the musculoskeletal system (Streicher, Schmidt, & Fiorito, 2007).

Nanoparticles have some characteristics essentials to be used in these treatments, i.e., a high specific surface area, for example, the reduction of particle size from micrometer to nanometer for a given quantity of material, the total surface increases a thousand times. Free nanoparticles are used as carriers because are small enough to move easily within cells, however, to achieve a specific task, they are coated and the coating is then functionalized. The bone loss, osteoporosis or osteolysis, are an important issue for which nanoparticles might offer a solution in orthopaedics. The use of crystalline hydroxyapatite and amorphous calcium phosphate nanoparticles and their functionalization by aminosilane chemistry with arginine-glycine-aspartate peptide facilitated attachment to cells, specifically to those of osteoporotic bone, according to some authors (Balasundaram, Sato, & Webster, 2006). When compared to the conventional hydroxyapatite, the amorphous nanoparticles was ten times higher degradation rates, suggesting their use for tailored drug release.

The term particle is associated with artificial joint wear, a major factor in aseptic loosening of orthopaedic implants (Gong, 2016). Nanosized abrasion particles have a bad reputation, once, as disadvantages, they tend to be highly inflammatory, leading to osteolysis, and are also able to migrate everywhere in the body with potentially adverse effects. Then, the nanoparticles in orthopaedics need to be differentiated from engineered nanoparticles and supported by extensive *in vivo* studies.

Many studies have being carried out looking at developing bone substitute composites for use in repairing bone defects (Wang, 2007; Wang, 2014). Nanocomposite bioactive materials are suitable for both bone and tissue applications, A novel biomedical composite, porous nano-hydroxyapatite/polyamide 66 (n-HA/PA66), has been developed, has good similarity to human bone, once n-HA has a similar composition and crystal structure to the mineral of natural bone as well as biocompatibility and bone regeneration, can prompt injured bone to reproduce (Wang, 2014). PA66 composite has good mechanical performance and can serve as a load-bearing bone substitute. The dense composite has been extensively used in repairing vertebral plates and has proven to have a good effect on bone reconstruction (Yang, 2012).

A scar is a deposition of connective tissue forms that allows that injured tissue return to normal function. The regeneration uninjured tissues within epithelia allow repairing tissue to function as normal without scar formation (Brown, 1992). Hench proposed a two-classification system for bioactive materials, where class A are osteoproductive, these materials possess a bioactive surface, which can be colonised by osteogenic stem cells due to the material inducing both intracellular and extracellular responses and the Class B which are osteoconductive, allowing a biocompatible surface for bone migration. For example, the hydroxyapatite (Class B), induces only extracellular responses from the target tissue (Hench, 1994). Nanocomposites are characterised into three categories depending on the matrix or continuous phase: ceramic-, metallic-, and polymer-based nanocomposites as we explained in Section 2 of this chapter.

Webster reported the advantages of nanocomposites in cell adhesion stated that osteoblast, fibroblast, and endothelial cell adhesion on nanophase materials (such as titania, alumina, hydroxyapatite) was significantly greater than that seen on conventional formulations of the same ceramic materials (Webster, 2000). In these study, the authors have shown that an increased adsorption of vitronectin on the nanophase material, which may facilitate the enhancement of the adhesion of osteoblast cells. Another interesting conclusion was that the analysis of a nanophase calcium phosphate-doped poly(lactic-co-glycolic acid) scaffold showed improved bioactivity, degradation rate and mechanical properties compared to that of the pure polymer (Webster, 2000).

The use of nanoparticles in biocomposites has numerous advantages, however, a poor dispersion of nanoparticles in the polymer solution or melt leading to agglomeration will negatively affect the final distribution of the nanoparticles in the matrix which promote materials with low mechanical properties (Boccaccini, & Ma, 2014). Thus, a cluster/aggregation of nanoparticles may prevent a proper interface with the polymeric matrix increasing the brittleness of the nanocomposite (Gloria, 2013).

2.2 Bone Tissue Engineering

The advantages of nanocomposites make them essential and with great potential for use in the treatment of critical size bone defects that occur due to trauma or disease. This treatment without nanocomposites would be based on tissue engineering approaches involving the use of engineered porous structures known as scaffolds. These scaffolds for bone tissue engineering are made of suitable bioceramics, polymers or combinations of them thus forming composites (Rezwan, 2006). Studies demonstrated that the interactions of the following four proteins, such as fibronectin, vitronectin, laminin and collagen, in bone regeneration enhance osteoblast function. Nanomaterials have greater integration of all these proteins which conduce to of cell growth and adhesion, as opposed to regular sized materials (Webster, 2000). When nanocomposites come into contact with physiological fluids strong bonds are formed with the bone via biological interactions because of their high surface reactivity (Hench, & Polak, 2002). Lysine, hydroxylysine, histidine, and arginine are all positively charged amino acids, which can participate in the formation of electrostatic chemical bonds that can occur between a positively charged amine group and a negatively charged oxygen surface of a ceramic. Hydrogen bonding from hydroxyl to carbonyl groups, or negatively charged surfaces, are considered the secondary types of chemical bonding and have the potential to attract organic components (Hench, 1971). The regeneration of bone requires: 1) osteoinduction; 2) the presence of cells that respond to osteogenesis signals; 3) a scaffold material to support the growth of cells, osteogenesis and subsequent matrix formation; 4) vascularisation of the treatment area (Burg, Porter, & Kellam, 2000).

The bioactive glass and glass ceramics are characterised due to their ability to chemically bond with living bone tissue and aiming this bond formation, a layer of biologically active hydroxycarbonate apatite (HCA) forms on the surface in response to exposure to physiological fluids (Ohtsuki, Kokubo, & Yamamuro, 1992). The HCA crystals are reinforced with collagen fibres, which form bonds between the bioactive material and the tissue (Hench, 1971). As the natural bone is composed of 70% inorganic component (apatite) and 30% organic component collagen, it seems logic that bioglasses have become the accepted treatment for bone repair (Park, & Lakes, 2007).

Nowadays there are more bioactive glasses/glass ceramics as well as sintered hydroxyapatite (Ca10(PO4)6(OH)2) [85]. Depending on their composition of bioactive glasses are silicate-based amorphous materials the properties change. When in contact with physiological fluids, bioactive glasses become coated with a layer of apatite which promote the formation of new bone. The apatite formation, however, depends on several factors, such as surface area and porosity (Balas, 2001). The use of silica-based bioactive glasses and ceramics promote a partial dissolution of the network at the surface followed by a polycondensation reaction. This last reaction induces the formation of a layer of silica on the surface, and consequently, a layer of calcium phosphate is formed (Hench, 1991). One of the most important biomaterials in the bone tissue engineering field, is the synthetic version of bone apatite, hydroxyapatite. The combination of hydroxyapatite with chitosan are essential for these two compounds once make them important for this application (Wang, 2003). Chitosan is a natural polymer, is biodegradable, does not induce an immune response during use or degradation and has advantageous mechanical properties, making it a widely used biomaterial for several applications. The addition of hydroxyapatite to chitosan is needed to provide sites for calcification consequently increase the osteoconductive behaviour of the material (Ogawa, 1984). Depan produced a chitosan-based hybrid nanocomposite, where the polymer was grafted onto propylene oxide forming a modified chitosan which was then bonded to ethylene glycol-functionalised hydroxyapatite, resulting in a highly porous structure. These structures supported adhesion, proliferation and viability of osteoblast cells. The osteoblast cells infiltrated and re-colonised the pores of the scaffold (Dapan, 2011). The utilisation of biodegradable polymers in biodegradable nanocomposites has huge potential as tissue repair and/or regeneration in orthopaedics. The filler content of the composite is usually low aiming provide and maintain suitable mechanical properties for specific target applications, once, a higher content may result in reduced biomimetic mechanical behaviour. However, a low volume fraction of hydroxyapatite within biodegradable composites may not support sufficient successful bone growth, then several factors to consider when developing nanocomposites for bone regeneration (Jayabalan, 2010). Wei et al. showed that nano-hydroxyapatite scaffolds, for bone tissue engineering, prepared using thermally-induced phase separation improved both the protein adsorption and mechanical properties of the scaffold (Wei, & Ma, 2004).

Bioglasses have also been used with biodegradable polymers, however, properties and biocompatibility of bioglass materials when prepared via a sol-gel method specifically reporting on the effect of aspect ratio of polycaprolactone/bioglass. These particles showed significant improvement biocompatibility and elastic modulus with only a small reduction in tensile strength, and osteoblast activity was also improved when compared to the microcomposite material (Jo, 2009).

Figure 2. Potential applications of nanocomposites in dentistry and orthopaedics

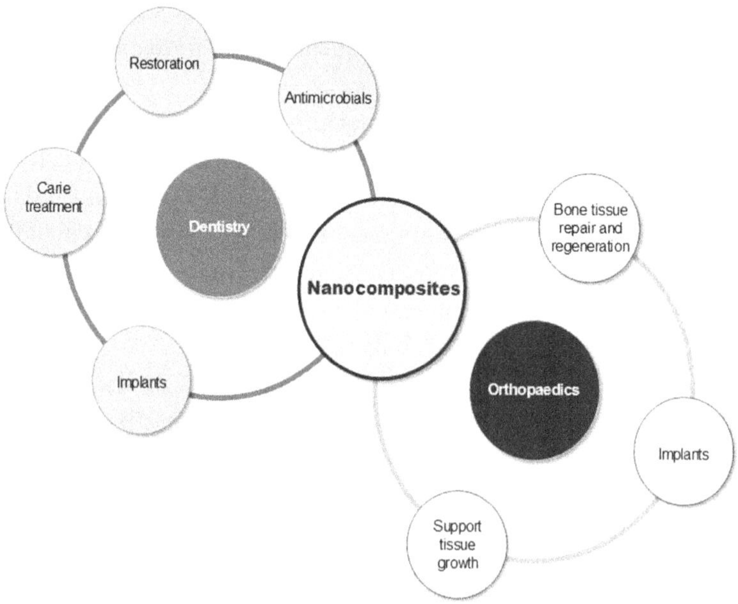

3. NANOCOMPOSITES IN DRUG DELIVERY SYSTEMS

3.1 Gene Delivery Systems

Gene therapy consists of the introduction of genomic material with specific purpose on the intracellular milieu of targeted cells being capable of remain innocuous to the non-targeted cells. This remarkable strategy can be used to treat a lot of diseases concerning cancer, neurodegenerative and autoimmune. Gene therapy can be divided into two main categories: germ cells therapy and somatic cell therapy (Nayerossadat, Maedeh, & Ali, 2012). Due to ethical implications, germ cells therapy cannot be performed and is forbidden by international Nonetheless, the progress made in the last two decades is not significant due to delays observed on the clinical protocols developments because such systems are required to be extremely safe and efficient. The perfect idealised vector would deliver the genetic material to the specific cell lineage, have the ability to lodge another kind of genes with enough size to achieve a positive introduction, be capable of inducing a transient expression of the interest genes and not be harmful/immunogenic to the host (Ibraheem, Elaissari, & Fessi, 2014). Two kinds of vectors exist in order to perform the referred task: viral and non-viral. The first one uses viruses' capacity to only infect a precise lineage of cells, replicating inside them and propagating virus genetic material obtaining the desired changes at a cellular level. When the gene of interest is introduced via this way the process is called transduction. Virus vectors used currently are adenovirus - types 2 and 5, adeno-associated virus, herpes virus, pox virus, retrovirus, human foamy virus (HFV), and lentivirus (Mali, 2013). The latter kind is the non-viral systems. In this assembly are covered physical and chemical systems excluding the prior referred viral systems. Physical systems are referent to techniques as electroporation, gene gun, particle bombardment, ultrasounds and magnetofection whilst chemical systems include cationic liposomes and polymers. This class of systems hold less efficacy than the viral when referring to expression capacity whereas another pattern contributed to create around them a reputation of more effectiveness with the capacity of genomic material delivery, as having a much lower potential to induce immune system, an optimal cost-effectiveness, availability, and presenting almost any limitations related to the size of transgenic DNA in comparison with viral system. The introduction of the interest genomic material via this way is termed transfection. Apropos of chemical systems they are most used than the referred physical. They include formulations like nanometric particles, liposomes, micelles and cationic polymers. When a system is engineered to transport, deliver and protect a nucleic acid from degradation, within a nanometric complex constituted by cationic polymers, it is designated by lipoplex (Ibraheem, Elaissari, & Fessi, 2014; Mali, 2013; Ramamoorth, & Narvekar, 2015).

3.2 Chitosan Composites

Drug delivery systems development requires the constant discovery of new materials with new properties ready to be tested and applied to new medicines research. Amongst these materials, natural polymers rise as unique objects with prodigious capacities (El-Nahrawy, 2016). Alginate, chitosan, hyaluronic acid are strong examples of what have been done on this field of research (Giannakas, 2016). Chitosan is a cationic substance with well-known mucoadhesive biological characteristics (Pradham, Dash, & Swain, 2015). A mixture-composite of chitosan and alginate demonstrated attractive results on insulin delivery by oral and nasal routes of administration with an additional application of antibiotics via ocular route (Sarmento, 2007; Goycoolea, 2009; Motwani, 2008). To stabilise the encapsulated drug, increase loading proficiency and even retard the remaining time at the desired action local of the drug a second natural polymer is often added to the formulation. Studies also demonstrated that during transfection of the desired gene, encapsulated on a composite mixture of chitosan and hyaluronic acid and then applied on human corneal epithelial and on a normal human conjunctival cell line, were notorious prominent level of transfection – ranging values up to 15% - without affecting cell viability (Krauland, & Alonso, 2008). Another composite mixture of chitosan and cyclodextrin was also taken for screening on basis of the possibility of this mixture increase the stability of protein (de la Fuente, Seijo, & Alonso, 2008).

3.3 Micellar Composites

Micellar formulations use usually amphiphilic copolymers which present unique properties as the high efficiency in loading with strategical molecules, appreciable stability, reliable production process and the low critical micelle concentration needed to form such structures (Wei, 2009; Kim, 2008). Consequently, micelles are one of most widely considered drug systems. Two sorts of polymers are held on these preparations – hydrophilic and lipophilic. Polyethylene glycol (PEG) is classically used as the hydrophilic segment of the copolymer, constituting the outmost layer of the structure. The inner core is surrounded by a lipophilic environment due to the hydrophobic segments resulting from the use of materials such polylactide. Amphiphilic copolymers have indeed the capacity of self-assembly with assured stability and a long half-time due to the presence of PEG, which delays the recognition of these particles by inner immune cells like macrophages. Recent researchers discovered new possibilities for these structures like pH-sensitive mixed micelles derive from combinations of poly(histidine)-b-polyethylene glycol and a copolymer such as PLA-PEG. Thermosensitive composite micelles are also reported in the literature with a constitution of pluronic F-127 and Tween 80 (Yang, 2009; Yin, & Bae, 2009; Oh, 2008).

3.4 Liposomal Composites

Liposomes are versatile structures, vesicular shaped, constituted by one or more bilayer membranes lipid-formed which border isolated hydrophilic partitions. Their spread for drug delivery systems is due to distinguished properties as biodegradability, biocompatibility and, additionally, the capacity for transport both kind of drugs on their inside – hydrophilic or lipophilic – being notorious such versatility (Huang, 2008). The prior referred capacity is a consequence of the amphipathic behaviour of these formulations – for lipophilic drugs the space between the bilayer is the preferential placement whilst hydrophilic drugs require the presence on the aqueous inner milieu. Submicron liposomes – ranging dimension from 1 nm to 1000 nm – are indeed considered a nanoparticle composite once to keep membrane fluidity – which is related to drug loading and drug release profile - cholesterol is required into the lipid bilayer to keep membrane stability and a mixture of several lipids is largely used to create the bilayer membrane (Sercombe, 2015; Allen, & Cullis, 2013). Exemplifying, antitumoral drug paclitaxel encapsulation efficiency raised from 60% to 95% when the liposomes until then structured with egg-yolk derived phosphatidylcholine were subjected to an addition of 10% with phosphatidylglycerol. Another policy is delaying the circulatory time of these medicines through their functionalization on the bilayer membrane with N-(carbonyl– methoxypolyethylene glycol 2000)-1,2-distearoyl-sn-glycero3-phosphoethanolamine sodium salt (MPEG - DSPE2000) (Crosasso, 2000).

3.5 Dendrimeric Composites

Dendrimer structures contain in their composition a sort of polymers possessing particular features which make them similar to biomolecules consenting their use as a widespread stand for antigen presenting cell directing also with regards to DNA vaccination (Boas, & Heegaard, 2004). Several studies revealed a magnificent capacity to induce immunogenicity with an in vitro and *in vivo* compatibility, stability and also a good permeability. Polypropylene imine – PPI – and polyamidoamine - PAMAM – are some examples of used polymers (Daftarian, 2011). Although very alike, dendrimers inside are made of covalent bonds and, consequently, a structure more rigid, less compact but with an increased number of a functional group on the surface available for posterior modifications. These kinds of formulations are also available as a source for the presentation of several epitopes (Caminade, 2014; Kesharwani, Jain, & Jain, 2014).

3.6 Solid Lipid Nanoparticle (SLN) Composites

Solid lipid nanoparticle (SLN) is formed by a lipid matrix solid at both room and body temperature made only with a solid lipid. The latter addition of surfactants has the main objective of stabilizing the formulation. Their firm nucleus of lipids warrants that SLN are much more stable than liposomes (Souto, & Doktorovova, 2009). The advantages in using such assemblies are vast: first of all, the versatility of being able to construct three different core compositions: 1) drug-enriched core; 2) drug-enriched shell; or even 3) a homogenous matrix (Faraji, & Wipf, 2009); then they can also be targeted to a specific place; they are easily biodegraded without toxicity associated (better than ceramic or polymeric nanoparticles); the possibility to control the pharmacokinetic parameters and at last the possible protection of drugs from enzymatic and/or chemical degradation (Hu, Tang, & Cui, 2004). Nevertheless, they have a restricted loading capacity once the lipids used to lead to perfect crystal matrix formation. The desire drugs are,

Figure 3. Examples of drug delivery systems based on nanocomposites

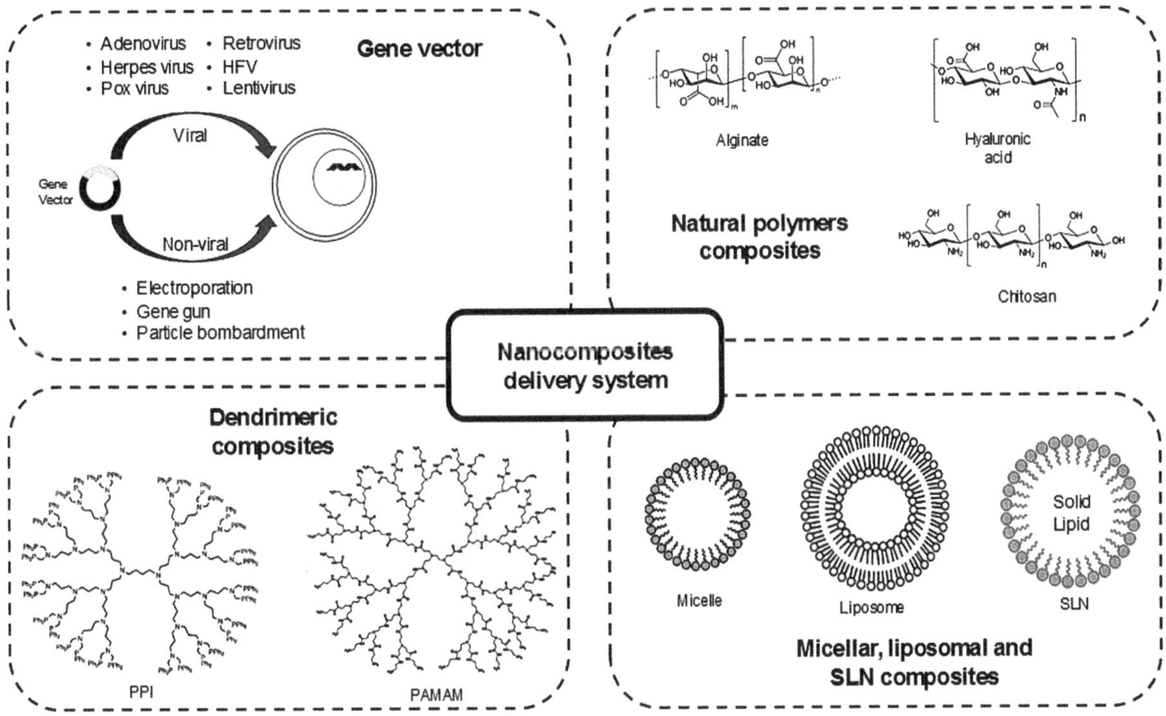

as referred on the construction possibilities above, incorporated among the lipids of the shell, in the core amorphous clusters or even between fatty acid chains. As an example, research work of Arias et al. could demonstrate that HIV-glycoprotein 140 formulated as adsorbed in carnauba wax was capable of inducing more solid in vitro T-cell proliferation than the self-antigen and exhibited their potential use as effective mucosal adjuvants for HIV vaccine (Arias, 2011).

3.7 Stimuli-Responsive Composites

Nanocomposites stimuli-responsive with a background of mesoporous materials possess ideal characteristics as drug delivery systems: have a high-load capacity, present the possibility of a controlled release and targeting to the desired places (Molina, 2015). A polymeric structure interposed and dispersed on mesoporous materials is used the get a full interface with the carrying drugs (Kuksenok, & Balazs, 2016; Meng, & Li, 2013). These nanocomposites are responsive to stimulus as pH, inner metabolites, solutes, temperature, ultrasounds or even electrical current. The mechanism of drugs releasing lies on the interaction forces stablished between polymer chains leading to a solubility dysregulation, distension performance of materials and a crystalline/amorphous transition. Many efforts have been made to achieve better results in this matter (Ding, 2016; Yao, Feng, & Chen, 2016). A research group published their studies on the effect of a system on which drug release is balanced by pH environment. To accomplish that purpose, a PBLG-g-PEG [poly(c-benzyl-L-glutamate)-poly(ethylene glycol)] copolymer was at first incorporated into an MBG and, after, gentamicin (hydrophilic antibiotic) and naproxen (lipophilic non-steroid anti-inflammatory) were used as model drugs to study this composite system (Xia, 2008).

3.8 Magnetic Composites

Magnetic particles with a mesoporous silica matrix constitute the so-called magnetic composites with wide applications among drug delivery systems, magnetic resonance imaging, hyperthermic treatment of tumors (Ruiz-Hernandez, 2007; Vestal, & Zhang, 2003). Although their high potential to aggregate when exposed to a biological environment, and so the less circulating periods, as drug delivery agents they are able to allow a selective targeting in the body via application of external orienting magnetic fields (Wei, 2012). The combination of a mesoporous silica matrix and magnetic particles as the ultimate goal of extend the circulating time by holding down the aggregation process. As referred previously such kind of therapy can also be applied to cancer cells chemotherapy on hyperthermic treatments once these cells cannot survive on a higher than 43 °C temperature generated by external application of a magnetic field (Ma, 2008).

3.9 Nanofiber Composites

Nanofiber composites are easy to produce, to control their size and shape, and have demonstrated valuable properties for sustained release. To produce such composites techniques as drawing, template synthesis, phase separation, self-assembly, and electrospinning were scrutinized (Hadjiargyrou, & Chiu,

Figure 4. Schematic representation of the use of magnetic composites for the treatment of tumors. Magnetic composites are guided through the bloodstream, by a magnetic field, to the lesion site
Modified after (Molina, 2015).

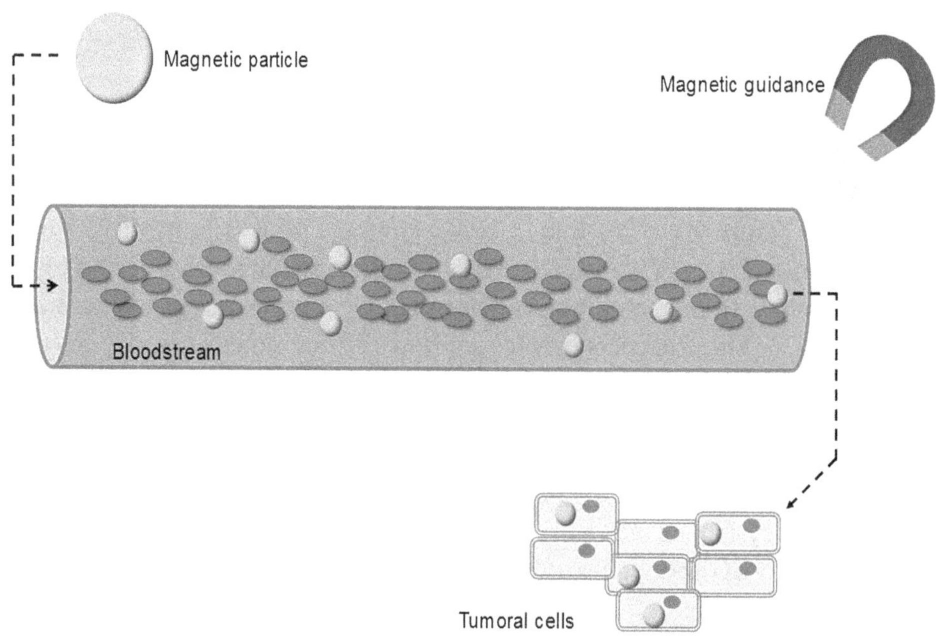

2008). Electrospinning at room temperature was the preferred method to generate this structure as the soft conditions used during the process allow the obtaining of an intact drug. Electrospun nanofiber mats used for drug delivery purposes offer a variety of advantages as a wide area of the surface with manageable properties of adsorption and release of drugs from the inner matrix which is controlled by diffusion and scaffold degradation (Jung, 2015; Sridhar, 2013).

3.10 Luminescent Mesoporous Composites

Nanoparticulate systems can also provide a good capacity for theranostic effects. Nanocomposites made of mesoporous silica with a mixture of fluorescent particles may be used as a tracker of disease on the human organism and also as a marker for drug release and bioavailability (Yang, 2009; Yang, 2011). Therefore, the development of these strategies has been under intense study in the last years.

4. CONCLUSION

In the future, there will be an increasing interest in the applications of dental materials and devices containing nanocoatings and nanocomposite coatings. The dental materials with potential will be used majority in bone grafts, biologically active membranes, implantable materials, slow drug delivery systems, stem cell- and biogenic material-containing multifunctional coatings and scaffolds. Nanocomposites that release fluorides has been studied. These nanocomposites contain calcium fluoride nanoparticles in a whisker-reinforced resin matrix that have the ability to sustain fluoride release. It is thought that decrease the incidence of caries. The use of nanotechnology to biomaterial science is a new frontier in orthopedic research, once, allows the development of new systems that mimic the complex, hierarchical structure of the native tissue to great effect. Bioglass was one of the earliest bioactive nanocomposite materials developed and still remains one of the most common used nanocomposite materials, particularly in bone tissue engineering uses. Greater physical and chemical control of structure will enable the interactions with body sites to be assessed in more detail and thus provide further advances in tissue engineering uses. Nanocomposites and bioactive materials have great potential, however, have the concern in the synthesis and subsequent therapeutic use in other biological environments that need to be investigated in the future in more studies. Pharmaceutical Industry focuses its devotion on the evolution (and revolution) of health products on a continuous manner. The development of new active pharmaceutical ingredients, so-called drugs, is a vital process from which society cannot hold itself nowadays. Although, the progression sightseeing in such a way requires tremendous amounts of investment by the order of billions, starting with new molecular entities discovery (drugs), through pre-clinical and final clinical trials, being lost with this slow process precious time for needed people, for market opportunities and on the product patent time. According to the prior, pharmaceuticals have been reacting and developing efforts to improve safety and efficacy parameters of some almost forgotten drugs and many others that are used on other purposes. To achieve such, the formulation process is the key point on the development of these new pharmaceutical systems. Different methods are employed to accomplish so, as sustain delivery, delayed delivery, rate controlled coating, nanoparticles production and the most recent targeted delivery of drugs. These approaches aim to overcome various difficulties related with the route of medicines administration and are so interesting that the number of published scientific papers all over the world regarding such subjects exponentially grown in the last decade. Following this pharmaceutical industry also finds striking prospects due to the possibility of having patents with extended lifetime and new products being born leading to tremendous amounts of receipts with a fraction of the total investment compared to the new entities discovery process. Significant advancements to realize the potential of nanobiomaterials are still needed to reach their full clinical use.

REFERENCES

Ahn, S.-J., Lee, S.-J., Kook, J.-K., & Lim, B.-S. (2009). Experimental antimicrobial orthodontic adhesives using nanofillers and silver nanoparticles. *Dental Materials*, *25*(2), 206–213. doi:10.1016/j.dental.2008.06.002 PMID:18632145

Allen, T. M., & Cullis, P. R. (2013). Liposomal drug delivery systems: From concept to clinical applications. *Advanced Drug Delivery Reviews*, *65*(1), 36–48. doi:10.1016/j.addr.2012.09.037 PMID:23036225

Arias, M. A., Loxley, A., Eatmon, C., Van Roey, G., Fairhurst, D., Mitchnick, M., ... Shattock, R. (2011). Carnauba wax nanoparticles enhance strong systemic and mucosal cellular and humoral immune responses to HIV-gp140 antigen. *Vaccine*, *29*(6), 1258–1269. doi:10.1016/j.vaccine.2010.11.084 PMID:21145913

Balas, F., Arcos, D., Pérez-Pariente, J., & Vallet-Regí, M. (2001). Textural properties of SiO 2· CaO· P 2 O 5 glasses prepared by the sol-gel method. *Journal of Materials Research*, *16*(05), 1345–1348. doi:10.1557/JMR.2001.0187

Balasundaram, G., Sato, M., & Webster, T. J. (2006). Using hydroxyapatite nanoparticles and decreased crystallinity to promote osteoblast adhesion similar to functionalizing with RGD. *Biomaterials*, *27*(14), 2798–2805. doi:10.1016/j.biomaterials.2005.12.008 PMID:16430957

Balasundaram, G., & Webster, T. J. (2007). An Overview of Nano-Polymers for Orthopedic Applications. *Macromolecular Bioscience*, *7*(5), 635–642. doi:10.1002/mabi.200600270 PMID:17477446

Barrère, F., van der Valk, C. M., Dalmeijer, R. A. J., van Blitterswijk, C. A., de Groot, K., & Layrolle, P. (2003). In vitro and in vivo degradation of biomimetic octacalcium phosphate and carbonate apatite coatings on titanium implants. *Journal of Biomedical Materials Research. Part A*, *64A*(2), 378–387. doi:10.1002/jbm.a.10291 PMID:12522826

Ben-Nissan, B., Choi, A. H., & Bendavid, A. (2013). Mechanical properties of inorganic biomedical thin films and their corresponding testing methods. *Surface and Coatings Technology*, *233*, 39–48. doi:10.1016/j.surfcoat.2012.11.020

Bernardo, M., Luis, H., Martin, M. D., Leroux, B. G., Rue, T., Leitão, J., & DeRouen, T. A. (2007). Survival and reasons for failure of amalgam versus composite posterior restorations placed in a randomized clinical trial. *The Journal of the American Dental Association*, *138*(6), 775–783. doi:10.14219/jada.archive.2007.0265 PMID:17545266

Besinis, A., De Peralta, T., Tredwin, C. J., & Handy, R. D. (2015). Review of Nanomaterials in Dentistry: Interactions with the Oral Microenvironment, Clinical Applications, Hazards, and Benefits. *ACS Nano*, *9*(3), 2255–2289. doi:10.1021/nn505015e PMID:25625290

Beun, S., Glorieux, T., Devaux, J., Vreven, J., & Leloup, G. (2007). Characterization of nanofilled compared to universal and microfilled composites. *Dental Materials*, *23*(1), 51–59. doi:10.1016/j.dental.2005.12.003 PMID:16423384

Boas, U., & Heegaard, P. M. (2004). Dendrimers in drug research. *Chemical Society Reviews*, *33*(1), 43–63. doi:10.1039/b309043b PMID:14737508

Boccaccini, A. R., & Ma, P. X. (2014). *Tissue engineering using ceramics and polymers*. Elsevier.

Bramhill, J., Ross, S., & Ross, G. (2017). Bioactive Nanocomposites for Tissue Repair and Regeneration: A Review. *International Journal of Environmental Research and Public Health*, *14*(1), 66. doi:10.3390/ijerph14010066 PMID:28085054

Brown, L. F., & … . (1992). Expression of vascular permeability factor (vascular endothelial growth factor) by epidermal keratinocytes during wound healing. *The Journal of Experimental Medicine*, *176*(5), 1375–1379. doi:10.1084/jem.176.5.1375 PMID:1402682

Burg, K. J., Porter, S., & Kellam, J. F. (2000). Biomaterial developments for bone tissue engineering. *Biomaterials*, *21*(23), 2347–2359. doi:10.1016/S0142-9612(00)00102-2 PMID:11055282

Burke, F., Ray, N., & McConnell, R. (2006). Fluoride-containing restorative materials. *International Dental Journal*, *56*(1), 33–43. doi:10.1111/j.1875-595X.2006.tb00072.x PMID:16515011

Caminade, A.-M., & Turrin, C.-O. (2014). Dendrimers for drug delivery. *Journal of Materials Chemistry. B, Materials for Biology and Medicine*, *2*(26), 4055–4066. doi:10.1039/C4TB00171K

Canché-Escamilla, G., Duarte-Aranda, S., & Toledano, M. (2014). Synthesis and characterization of hybrid silica/PMMA nanoparticles and their use as filler in dental composites. *Materials Science and Engineering C*, *42*, 161–167. doi:10.1016/j.msec.2014.05.016 PMID:25063106

Chandki, R., Kala, M., N, K. K., Brigit, B., Banthia, P., & Banthia, R. (2012). 'Nanodentistry': Exploring the beauty of miniature. *Journal of Clinical and Experimental Dentistry*, *4*(2), e119–e124. doi:10.4317/jced.50720 PMID:24558536

Chen, M.-H. (2010). Update on Dental Nanocomposites. *Journal of Dental Research*, *89*(6), 549–560. doi:10.1177/0022034510363765 PMID:20299523

Choi, A. H., & Ben-Nissan, B. (2007). Sol-gel production of bioactive nanocoatings for medical applications. Part II: Current research and development. *Nanomedicine (London)*, *2*(1), 51–61. doi:10.2217/17435889.2.1.51 PMID:17716190

Choi, A. H., Ben-Nissan, B., Matinlinna, J. P., & Conway, R. C. (2013). Current perspectives: Calcium phosphate nanocoatings and nanocomposite coatings in dentistry. *Journal of Dental Research*, *92*(10), 853–859. doi:10.1177/0022034513497754 PMID:23857642

Cox, M., & … . (2000). dental history: Eighteenth and nineteenth century dental restoration, treatment and consequences in a British nobleman. *British Dental Journal*, *189*(11), 593–596. PMID:11132689

Cramer, N. B., Stansbury, J. W., & Bowman, C. N. (2011). Recent Advances and Developments in Composite Dental Restorative Materials. *Journal of Dental Research*, *90*(4), 402–416. doi:10.1177/0022034510381263 PMID:20924063

Crosasso, P., Ceruti, M., Brusa, P., Arpicco, S., Dosio, F., & Cattel, L. (2000). Preparation, characterization and properties of sterically stabilized paclitaxel-containing liposomes. *Journal of Controlled Release*, *63*(1), 19–30. doi:10.1016/S0168-3659(99)00166-2 PMID:10640577

Daftarian, P., Kaifer, A. E., Li, W., Blomberg, B. B., Frasca, D., Roth, F., ... Serafini, P. (2011). Peptide-conjugated PAMAM dendrimer as a universal DNA vaccine platform to target antigen-presenting cells. *Cancer Research*, *71*(24), 7452–7462. doi:10.1158/0008-5472.CAN-11-1766 PMID:21987727

de la Fuente, M., Seijo, B., & Alonso, M. J. (2008). Novel hyaluronic acid-chitosan nanoparticles for ocular gene therapy. *Investigative Ophthalmology & Visual Science*, *49*(5), 2016–2024. doi:10.1167/iovs.07-1077 PMID:18436835

Depan, D., Venkata Surya, P. K. C., Girase, B., & Misra, R. D. K. (2011). Organic/inorganic hybrid network structure nanocomposite scaffolds based on grafted chitosan for tissue engineering. *Acta Biomaterialia*, *7*(5), 2163–2175. doi:10.1016/j.actbio.2011.01.029 PMID:21284959

Dickens, S. H., Flaim, G. M., & Takagi, S. (2003). Mechanical properties and biochemical activity of remineralizing resin-based Ca–PO 4 cements. *Dental Materials*, *19*(6), 558–566. doi:10.1016/S0109-5641(02)00105-7 PMID:12837405

Ding, C., Tong, L., Feng, J., & Fu, J. (2016). Recent Advances in Stimuli-Responsive Release Function Drug Delivery Systems for Tumor Treatment. *Molecules (Basel, Switzerland)*, *21*(12), 1715. doi:10.3390/molecules21121715 PMID:27999414

El-Nahrawy, A. M., Ali, A. I., Abou Hammad, A. B., & Youssef, A. M. (2016). Influences of Ag-NPs doping chitosan/calcium silicate nanocomposites for optical and antibacterial activity. *International Journal of Biological Macromolecules*, *93*, 267–275. doi:10.1016/j.ijbiomac.2016.08.045 PMID:27543348

Facca & Lahiri. (2012). Nanoreinforcement of hydroxyapatite coatings on titanium for osseointegration of orthopaedic implants. *Computer Methods in Biomechanics and Biomedical Engineering, 15*(sup1), 10-11.

Faraji, A. H., & Wipf, P. (2009). Nanoparticles in cellular drug delivery. *Bioorganic & Medicinal Chemistry*, *17*(8), 2950–2962. doi:10.1016/j.bmc.2009.02.043 PMID:19299149

Ferracane, J. L. (1995). Current Trends in Dental Composites. *Critical Reviews in Oral Biology and Medicine*, *6*(4), 302–318. doi:10.1177/10454411950060040301 PMID:8664421

Ferracane, J. L. (2008). Placing Dental Composites—A Stressful Experience. *Operative Dentistry*, *33*(3), 247–257. doi:10.2341/07-BL2 PMID:18505214

Ferracane, J. L., & Mitchem, J. C. (2003). Relationship between composite contraction stress and leakage in Class V cavities. *American Journal of Dentistry*, *16*(4), 239–243. PMID:14579877

Freitas, R. A. Jr. (2005). Nanotechnology, nanomedicine and nanosurgery. *International Journal of Surgery, 3*(4), 243–246. doi:10.1016/j.ijsu.2005.10.007 PMID:17462292

Frese, C., Staehle, H. J., & Wolff, D. (2012, May). The assessment of dentofacial esthetics in restorative dentistry. *The Journal of the American Dental Association, 143*(5), 461–466. doi:10.14219/jada.archive.2012.0205 PMID:22547716

Giannakas, A., Vlacha, M., Salmas, C., Leontiou, A., Katapodis, P., Stamatis, H., ... Ladavos, A. (2016). Preparation, characterization, mechanical, barrier and antimicrobial properties of chitosan/PVOH/clay nanocomposites. *Carbohydrate Polymers, 140*, 408–415. doi:10.1016/j.carbpol.2015.12.072 PMID:26876868

Gloria, A., Russo, T., D'Amora, U., Zeppetelli, S., D'Alessandro, T., Sandri, M., ... De Santis, R. (2013). Magnetic poly (ε-caprolactone)/iron-doped hydroxyapatite nanocomposite substrates for advanced bone tissue engineering. *Journal of the Royal Society, Interface, 10*(80), 20120833. doi:10.1098/rsif.2012.0833 PMID:23303218

Gong, K., Qu, S., Liu, Y., Wang, J., Zhang, Y., Jiang, C., & Shen, R. (2016). The mechanical and tribological properties of UHMWPE loaded ALN after mechanical activation for joint replacements. *Journal of the Mechanical Behavior of Biomedical Materials, 61*, 334–344. doi:10.1016/j.jmbbm.2016.03.023 PMID:27104932

Goycoolea, F. M., Lollo, G., Remuñán-López, C., Quaglia, F., & Alonso, M. J. (2009). Chitosan-alginate blended nanoparticles as carriers for the transmucosal delivery of macromolecules. *Biomacromolecules, 10*(7), 1736–1743. doi:10.1021/bm9001377 PMID:19545119

Gunatillake, P. A., & Adhikari, R. (2003). Biodegradable synthetic polymers for tissue engineering. *European Cells & Materials, 5*, 1–16. doi:10.22203/eCM.v005a01 PMID:14562275

Hadjiargyrou, M., & Chiu, J. B. (2008). Enhanced composite electrospun nanofiber scaffolds for use in drug delivery. *Expert Opinion on Drug Delivery, 5*(10), 1093–1106. doi:10.1517/17425247.5.10.1093 PMID:18817515

Hench, L. (1994). Bioactive ceramics: Theory and clinical applications. *Bioceramics, 7*, 3–14. doi:10.1016/B978-0-08-042144-5.50005-4

Hench, L. L. (1991). Bioceramics: From concept to clinic. *Journal of the American Ceramic Society, 74*(7), 1487–1510. doi:10.1111/j.1151-2916.1991.tb07132.x

Hench, L. L., & Polak, J. M. (2002). Third-generation biomedical materials. *Science, 295*(5557), 1014–1017. doi:10.1126cience.1067404 PMID:11834817

Hench, L. L., Splinter, R. J., Allen, W. C., & Greenlee, T. K. (1971). Bonding mechanisms at the interface of ceramic prosthetic materials. *Journal of Biomedical Materials Research, 5*(6), 117–141. doi:10.1002/jbm.820050611

Hing, K. A. (1825). *Bone repair in the twenty-first century: Biology, chemistry or engineering?* Philos Trans A Math Phys. *Engineering and Science, 2004*(362), 2821–2850.

Hook, E. R., Owen, O. J., Bellis, C. A., Holder, J. A., O'Sullivan, D. J., & Barbour, M. E. (2014). Development of a novel antimicrobial-releasing glass ionomer cement functionalized with chlorhexidine hexametaphosphate nanoparticles. *Journal of Nanobiotechnology*, *12*(1), 3. doi:10.1186/1477-3155-12-3 PMID:24456793

Hu, L., Tang, X., & Cui, F. (2004). Solid lipid nanoparticles (SLNs) to improve oral bioavailability of poorly soluble drugs. *The Journal of Pharmacy and Pharmacology*, *56*(12), 1527–1535. doi:10.1211/0022357044959 PMID:15563759

Huang, S.-L. (2008). Liposomes in ultrasonic drug and gene delivery. *Advanced Drug Delivery Reviews*, *60*(10), 1167–1176. doi:10.1016/j.addr.2008.03.003 PMID:18479776

Ibraheem, D., Elaissari, A., & Fessi, H. (2014). Gene therapy and DNA delivery systems. *International Journal of Pharmaceutics*, *459*(1), 70–83. doi:10.1016/j.ijpharm.2013.11.041 PMID:24286924

Ilie, N., & Hickel, R. (2011). Resin composite restorative materials. *Australian Dental Journal*, *56*, 59–66. doi:10.1111/j.1834-7819.2010.01296.x PMID:21564116

Irie, M., Suzuki, K., & Watts, D. C. (2002). Marginal gap formation of light-activated restorative materials: Effects of immediate setting shrinkage and bond strength. *Dental Materials*, *18*(3), 203–210. doi:10.1016/S0109-5641(01)00083-5 PMID:11823011

Jayabalan, M., Shalumon, K. T., Mitha, M. K., Ganesan, K., & Epple, M. (2010). Effect of hydroxyapatite on the biodegradation and biomechanical stability of polyester nanocomposites for orthopaedic applications. *Acta Biomaterialia*, *6*(3), 763–775. doi:10.1016/j.actbio.2009.09.015 PMID:19788944

Jo, J. H., Lee, E.-J., Shin, D.-S., Kim, H.-E., Kim, H.-W., Koh, Y.-H., & Jang, J.-H. (2009). In vitro/in vivo biocompatibility and mechanical properties of bioactive glass nanofiber and poly (ε-caprolactone) composite materials. *Journal of Biomedical Materials Research. Part B, Applied Biomaterials*, *91*(1), 213–220. doi:10.1002/jbm.b.31392 PMID:19422050

Jung, S.-M., Yoon, G. H., Lee, H. C., & Shin, H. S. (2015). Chitosan nanoparticle/PCL nanofiber composite for wound dressing and drug delivery. *Journal of Biomaterials Science. Polymer Edition*, *26*(4), 252–263. doi:10.1080/09205063.2014.996699 PMID:25573454

Karabela, M. M., & Sideridou, I. D. (2008, December). Effect of the structure of silane coupling agent on sorption characteristics of solvents by dental resin-nanocomposites. *Dental Materials*, *24*(12), 1631–1639. doi:10.1016/j.dental.2008.02.021 PMID:18462785

Kasraei, S., Sami, L., Hendi, S., AliKhani, M.-Y., Rezaei-Soufi, L., & Khamverdi, Z. (2014). Antibacterial properties of composite resins incorporating silver and zinc oxide nanoparticles on Streptococcus mutans and Lactobacillus. *Restorative Dentistry & Endodontics*, *39*(2), 109–114. doi:10.5395/rde.2014.39.2.109 PMID:24790923

Kesharwani, P., Jain, K., & Jain, N. K. (2014). Dendrimer as nanocarrier for drug delivery. *Progress in Polymer Science*, *39*(2), 268–307. doi:10.1016/j.progpolymsci.2013.07.005

Kikuchi, M., Itoh, S., Ichinose, S., Shinomiya, K., & Tanaka, J. (2001). Self-organization mechanism in a bone-like hydroxyapatite/collagen nanocomposite synthesized in vitro and its biological reaction in vivo. *Biomaterials*, *22*(13), 1705–1711. doi:10.1016/S0142-9612(00)00305-7 PMID:11396873

Kim, D., Lee, E. S., Oh, K. T., Gao, Z. G., & Bae, Y. H. (2008). Doxorubicin-loaded polymeric micelle overcomes multidrug resistance of cancer by double-targeting folate receptor and early endosomal pH. *Small*, *4*(11), 2043–2050. doi:10.1002mll.200701275 PMID:18949788

Kim, H.-W., Kim, H.-E., Salih, V., & Knowles, J. C. (2005). Hydroxyapatite and titania sol–gel composite coatings on titanium for hard tissue implants; Mechanical and in vitro biological performance. *Journal of Biomedical Materials Research. Part B, Applied Biomaterials*, *72B*(1), 1–8. doi:10.1002/jbm.b.30073 PMID:15481086

Korkmaz, Y., Ozel, E., Attar, N., Bicer, C. O., & Firatli, E. (2010). Microleakage and scanning electron microscopy evaluation of all-in-one self-etch adhesives and their respective nanocomposites prepared by erbium:yttrium–aluminum–garnet laser and bur. *Lasers in Medical Science*, *25*(4), 493–502. doi:10.100710103-009-0672-5 PMID:19396579

Krauland, A. H., & Alonso, M. J. (2007). Chitosan/cyclodextrin nanoparticles as macromolecular drug delivery system. *International Journal of Pharmaceutics*, *340*(1), 134–142. doi:10.1016/j.ijpharm.2007.03.005 PMID:17459620

Kuksenok, O., & Balazs, A. C. (2016). Stimuli-responsive behavior of composites integrating thermo-responsive gels with photo-responsive fibers. *Materials Horizons*, *3*(1), 53–62. doi:10.1039/C5MH00212E

Kuwabara, A., Hori, N., Sawada, T., Hoshi, N., Watazu, A., & Kimoto, K. (2012). Enhanced biological responses of a hydroxyapatite/TiO₂ hybrid structure when surface electric charge is controlled using radiofrequency sputtering. *Dental Materials Journal*, *31*(3), 368–376. doi:10.4012/dmj.2011-220 PMID:22673466

Kwon, H.-J., Oh, Y.-J., Jang, J.-H., Park, J.-E., Hwang, K.-S., & Park, Y.-D. (2015). The effect of polymerization conditions on the amounts of unreacted monomer and bisphenol A in dental composite resins. *Dental Materials Journal*, *34*(3), 327–335. doi:10.4012/dmj.2014-230 PMID:25904171

Lang, B. R., Jaarda, M., & Wang, R. F. (1992). Filler particle size and composite resin classification systems. *Journal of Oral Rehabilitation*, *19*(6), 569–584. doi:10.1111/j.1365-2842.1992.tb01487.x PMID:1469493

Liao, S. S., Cui, F. Z., & Zhu, Y. (2004). Osteoblasts Adherence and Migration through Three-dimensional Porous Mineralized Collagen Based Composite: nHAC/PLA. *Journal of Bioactive and Compatible Polymers*, *19*(2), 117–130. doi:10.1177/0883911504042643

Liu, H., Slamovich, E. B., & Webster, T. J. (2006). Increased osteoblast functions among nanophase titania/poly(lactide-co-glycolide) composites of the highest nanometer surface roughness. *Journal of Biomedical Materials Research. Part A*, *78*(4), 798–807. doi:10.1002/jbm.a.30734 PMID:16741979

Liu, H., & Webster, T. J. (2007). Nanomedicine for implants: A review of studies and necessary experimental tools. *Biomaterials*, *28*(2), 354–369. doi:10.1016/j.biomaterials.2006.08.049 PMID:21898921

Liu, Y., Hunziker, E. B., Layrolle, P., De Bruijn, J. D., & De Groot, K. (2004). Bone morphogenetic protein 2 incorporated into biomimetic coatings retains its biological activity. *Tissue Engineering*, *10*(1-2), 101–108. doi:10.1089/107632704322791745 PMID:15009935

Loguercio, A. D., Reis, A., Hernandez, P. A. G., Macedo, R. P., & Busato, A. L. S. (2006). 3-Year clinical evaluation of posterior packable composite resin restorations. *Journal of Oral Rehabilitation*, *33*(2), 144–151. doi:10.1111/j.1365-2842.2006.01539.x PMID:16457675

Luan, X., Dangaria, S., Ito, Y., Walker, C. G., Jin, T., Schmidt, M. K., ... Druzinsky, R. (2009). Neural crest lineage segregation: A blueprint for periodontal regeneration. *Journal of Dental Research*, *88*(9), 781–791. doi:10.1177/0022034509340641 PMID:19767574

Lutz, F., & Phillips, R. W. (1983). A classification and evaluation of composite resin systems. *The Journal of Prosthetic Dentistry*, *50*(4), 480–488. doi:10.1016/0022-3913(83)90566-8 PMID:6579287

Ma, H. (2008). Fabrication of magnetic porous hollow silica drug carriers using Ca CO 3/ Fe 3 O 4 composite nanoparticles and cationic surfactant double templates. *Journal of Applied Physics, 103*(7).

Mali, S. (2013). Delivery systems for gene therapy. *Indian Journal of Human Genetics*, *19*(1), 3. doi:10.4103/0971-6866.112870 PMID:23901186

Manias, E., Touny, A., Wu, L., Strawhecker, K., Lu, B., & Chung, T. C. (2001). Polypropylene/montmorillonite nanocomposites. Review of the synthetic routes and materials properties. *Chemistry of Materials*, *13*(10), 3516–3523. doi:10.1021/cm0110627

Meng, H., & Li, G. (2013). A review of stimuli-responsive shape memory polymer composites. *Polymer*, *54*(9), 2199–2221. doi:10.1016/j.polymer.2013.02.023

Mitra, S. B., Wu, D., & Holmes, B. N. (2003, October). An application of nanotechnology in advanced dental materials. *The Journal of the American Dental Association*, *134*(10), 1382–1390. doi:10.14219/jada.archive.2003.0054 PMID:14620019

Mjör, I. A., Moorhead, J. E., & Dahl, J. E. (2000). Reasons for replacement of restorations in permanent teeth in general dental practice. *International Dental Journal*, *50*(6), 361–366. doi:10.1111/j.1875-595X.2000.tb00569.x PMID:11197194

Molina, M., Asadian-Birjand, M., Balach, J., Bergueiro, J., Miceli, E., & Calderón, M. (2015). Stimuli-responsive nanogel composites and their application in nanomedicine. *Chemical Society Reviews*, *44*(17), 6161–6186. doi:10.1039/C5CS00199D PMID:26505057

Motwani, S. K., & .... (2008). Chitosan–sodium alginate nanoparticles as submicroscopic reservoirs for ocular delivery: Formulation, optimisation and in vitro characterisation. *European Journal of Pharmaceutics and Biopharmaceutics*, *68*(3), 513–525. PMID:17983737

Nayerossadat, N., Maedeh, T., & Ali, P. A. (2012). Viral and nonviral delivery systems for gene delivery. *Advanced Biomedical Research*, *1*(1), 27. doi:10.4103/2277-9175.98152 PMID:23210086

Ogawa, K., Hirano, S., Miyanishi, T., Yui, T., & Watanabe, T. (1984). A new polymorph of chitosan. *Macromolecules*, *17*(4), 973–975. doi:10.1021/ma00134a076

Ogle, O. E., & Byles, N. (2014). Nanotechnology in Dentistry Today. *The West Indian Medical Journal*, *63*(4), 344–348. PMID:25429479

Oh, K. T., Lee, E. S., Kim, D., & Bae, Y. H. (2008). L-histidine-based pH-sensitive anticancer drug carrier micelle: Reconstitution and brief evaluation of its systemic toxicity. *International Journal of Pharmaceutics*, *358*(1), 177–183. doi:10.1016/j.ijpharm.2008.03.003 PMID:18407443

Ohtsuki, C., Kokubo, T., & Yamamuro, T. (1992). Mechanism of apatite formation on CaOSiO2P2O5 glasses in a simulated body fluid. *Journal of Non-Crystalline Solids*, *143*, 84–92. doi:10.1016/S0022-3093(05)80556-3

Park, J., & Lakes, R. S. (2007). *Biomaterials: An introduction*. Springer Science & Business Media.

Patil, M., Mehta, D., & Guvva, S. (2008). Future impact of nanotechnology on medicine and dentistry. *Journal of Indian Society of Periodontology*, *12*(2), 34–40. doi:10.4103/0972-124X.44088 PMID:20142942

Portnov, T., Shulimzon, T., & Zilberman, M. (2016). Injectable hydrogel-based scaffolds for tissue engineering applications. *Reviews in Chemical Engineering*, *33*(1), 91–107. doi:10.1515/revce-2015-0074

Pradhan, G. C., Dash, S., & Swain, S. K. (2015). Barrier properties of nano silicon carbide designed chitosan nanocomposites. *Carbohydrate Polymers*, *134*, 60–65. doi:10.1016/j.carbpol.2015.06.081 PMID:26428100

Ramamoorth, M., & Narvekar, A. (2015). Non viral vectors in gene therapy-an overview. *Journal of Clinical and Diagnostic Research: JCDR*, *9*(1), GE01. PMID:25738007

Rezwan, K., Chen, Q. Z., Blaker, J. J., & Boccaccini, A. R. (2006). Biodegradable and bioactive porous polymer/inorganic composite scaffolds for bone tissue engineering. *Biomaterials*, *27*(18), 3413–3431. doi:10.1016/j.biomaterials.2006.01.039 PMID:16504284

Ruiz-Hernández, E., López-Noriega, A., Arcos, D., Izquierdo-Barba, I., Terasaki, O., & Vallet-Regí, M. (2007). Aerosol-assisted synthesis of magnetic mesoporous silica spheres for drug targeting. *Chemistry of Materials*, *19*(14), 3455–3463. doi:10.1021/cm0705789

Sadeghi, M., & Lynch, C. D. (2009). The Effect of Flowable Materials on the Microleakage of Class II Composite Restorations That Extend Apical to the Cemento-enamel Junction. *Operative Dentistry*, *34*(3), 306–311. doi:10.2341/08-91 PMID:19544820

Sadeghi, M., Lynch, C. D., & Shahamat, N. (2010). Eighteen-month clinical evaluation of microhybrid, packable and nanofilled resin composites in Class I restorations. *Journal of Oral Rehabilitation*, *37*(7), 532–537. doi:10.1111/j.1365-2842.2010.02073.x PMID:20202097

Sarmento, B., Ribeiro, A., Veiga, F., Sampaio, P., Neufeld, R., & Ferreira, D. (2007). Alginate/chitosan nanoparticles are effective for oral insulin delivery. *Pharmaceutical Research*, *24*(12), 2198–2206. doi:10.100711095-007-9367-4 PMID:17577641

Sarrett, D. C. (2005). Clinical challenges and the relevance of materials testing for posterior composite restorations. *Dental Materials*, *21*(1), 9–20. doi:10.1016/j.dental.2004.10.001 PMID:15680997

Sercombe, L., Veerati, T., Moheimani, F., Wu, S. Y., Sood, A. K., & Hua, S. (2015). Advances and challenges of liposome assisted drug delivery. *Frontiers in Pharmacology*, *6*, 286. doi:10.3389/fphar.2015.00286 PMID:26648870

Shen, S., & … . (2007). *Nanocomposites for drug delivery*. Nanotechnologies for the Life Sciences.

Skrtic, D., Antonucci, J. M., Eanes, E. D., Eichmiller, F. C., & Schumacher, G. E. (2000). Physicochemical evaluation of bioactive polymeric composites based on hybrid amorphous calcium phosphates. *Journal of Biomedical Materials Research*, *53*(4), 381–391. doi: PMID:10898879

Soppimath, K. S., Aminabhavi, T. M., Kulkarni, A. R., & Rudzinski, W. E. (2001). Biodegradable polymeric nanoparticles as drug delivery devices. *Journal of Controlled Release*, *70*(1), 1–20. doi:10.1016/S0168-3659(00)00339-4 PMID:11166403

Soundrapandian, C., Bharati, S., Basu, D., & Datta, S. (2011). Studies on novel bioactive glasses and bioactive glass–nano-HAp composites suitable for coating on metallic implants. *Ceramics International*, *37*(3), 759–769. doi:10.1016/j.ceramint.2010.10.025

Souto, E. B., & Doktorovová, S. (2009). Chapter Six-Solid Lipid Nanoparticle Formulations: Pharmacokinetic and Biopharmaceutical Aspects in Drug Delivery. *Methods in Enzymology*, *464*, 105–129. doi:10.1016/S0076-6879(09)64006-4 PMID:19903552

Sridhar, R., Sundarrajan, S., Venugopal, J. R., Ravichandran, R., & Ramakrishna, S. (2013). Electrospun inorganic and polymer composite nanofibers for biomedical applications. *Journal of Biomaterials Science. Polymer Edition*, *24*(4), 365–385. doi:10.1080/09205063.2012.690711 PMID:23565681

Streicher, R. M., Schmidt, M., & Fiorito, S. (2007). Nanosurfaces and nanostructures for artificial orthopedic implants. *Nanomedicine (London)*, *2*(6), 861–874. doi:10.2217/17435889.2.6.861 PMID:18095851

Taton, T. A. (2001). Nanotechnology: Boning up on biology. *Nature*, *412*(6846), 491–492. doi:10.1038/35087687 PMID:11484032

Terry, D. A. (2004). Applications of nanotechnology. *Pract Proced Aesthet Dent*, *16*(3), 220–222. PMID:15199697

van Oirschot, B. A. (2014). A.H., Närhi TO, Anil S, Al Farraj Aldosari A, van den Beucken JJ, Jansen JA, *In vivo evaluation of bioactive glassbased coatings on dental implants in a dog implantation model. Clinical Oral Implants Research*. doi:10.1111/clr.12060

Vestal, C. R., & Zhang, Z. J. (2003). Synthesis and magnetic characterization of Mn and Co spinel ferrite-silica nanoparticles with tunable magnetic core. *Nano Letters*, *3*(12), 1739–1743. doi:10.1021/nl034816k

Wang, H., Li, Y., Zuo, Y., Li, J., Ma, S., & Cheng, L. (2007). Biocompatibility and osteogenesis of biomimetic nano-hydroxyapatite/polyamide composite scaffolds for bone tissue engineering. *Biomaterials*, *28*(22), 3338–3348. doi:10.1016/j.biomaterials.2007.04.014 PMID:17481726

Wang, M. (2003). Developing bioactive composite materials for tissue replacement. *Biomaterials*, *24*(13), 2133–2151. doi:10.1016/S0142-9612(03)00037-1 PMID:12699650

Wang, W., Liao, S., Liu, M., Zhao, Q., & Zhu, Y. (2014). Polymer Composites Reinforced by Nanotubes as Scaffolds for Tissue Engineering. *International Journal of Polymer Science*, *2014*, 14. doi:10.1155/2014/805634

Wang, Y.-L., Lee, B.-S., Chang, K.-C., Chiu, H.-C., Lin, F.-H., & Lin, C.-P. (2007). Characterization, fluoride release and recharge properties of polymer–kaolinite nanocomposite resins. *Composites Science and Technology*, *67*(15), 3409–3416. doi:10.1016/j.compscitech.2007.03.018

Webster, T. J., Ergun, C., Doremus, R. H., Siegel, R. W., & Bizios, R. (2000). Specific proteins mediate enhanced osteoblast adhesion on nanophase ceramics. *Journal of Biomedical Materials Research. Part A*, *51*(3), 475–483. doi: PMID:10880091

Wei, G., & Ma, P. X. (2004). Structure and properties of nano-hydroxyapatite/polymer composite scaffolds for bone tissue engineering. *Biomaterials*, *25*(19), 4749–4757. doi:10.1016/j.biomaterials.2003.12.005 PMID:15120521

Wei, L., Cai, C., Lin, J., & Chen, T. (2009). Dual-drug delivery system based on hydrogel/micelle composites. *Biomaterials*, *30*(13), 2606–2613. doi:10.1016/j.biomaterials.2009.01.006 PMID:19162320

Wei, L., Shi, D., Zhou, Z., Ye, P., Wang, J., Zhao, J., ... Zhang, Y. (2012). Functionalized self-assembled monolayers on mesoporous silica nanoparticles with high surface coverage. *Nanoscale Research Letters*, *7*(1), 334. doi:10.1186/1556-276X-7-334 PMID:22720819

Xia, W., Chang, J., Lin, J., & Zhu, J. (2008). The pH-controlled dual-drug release from mesoporous bioactive glass/polypeptide graft copolymer nanomicelle composites. *European Journal of Pharmaceutics and Biopharmaceutics*, *69*(2), 546–552. doi:10.1016/j.ejpb.2007.11.018 PMID:18248801

Xie, X.-H., Wang, X.-L., He, Y.-X., Liu, Z., Sheng, H., Zhang, G., & Qin, L. (2012). Promotion of bone repair by implantation of cryopreserved bone marrow–derived mononuclear cells in a rabbit model of steroid-associated osteonecrosis. *Arthritis and Rheumatism*, *64*(5), 1562–1571. doi:10.1002/art.34525 PMID:22544527

Xu, H., Sun, L., Weir, M. D., Antonucci, J. M., Takagi, S., Chow, L. C., & Peltz, M. (2006). Nano DCPA-whisker composites with high strength and Ca and PO4 release. *Journal of Dental Research*, *85*(8), 722–727. doi:10.1177/154405910608500807 PMID:16861289

Xu, H., Weir, M. D., Sun, L., Takagi, S., & Chow, L. C. (2007). Effects of calcium phosphate nanoparticles on Ca-PO4 composite. *Journal of Dental Research*, *86*(4), 378–383. doi:10.1177/154405910708600415 PMID:17384036

Xu, H. H., Moreau, J. L., Sun, L., & Chow, L. C. (2008). Strength and fluoride release characteristics of a calcium fluoride based dental nanocomposite. *Biomaterials*, *29*(32), 4261–4267. doi:10.1016/j.biomaterials.2008.07.037 PMID:18708252

Xu, H. H., Weir, M. D., & Sun, L. (2007). Nanocomposites with Ca and PO 4 release: Effects of reinforcement, dicalcium phosphate particle size and silanization. *Dental Materials*, *23*(12), 1482–1491. doi:10.1016/j.dental.2007.01.002 PMID:17339048

Xu, H. H., Weir, M. D., & Sun, L. (2009). Calcium and phosphate ion releasing composite: Effect of pH on release and mechanical properties. *Dental Materials*, *25*(4), 535–542. doi:10.1016/j.dental.2008.10.009 PMID:19101026

Xu, H. H., Weir, M. D., Sun, L., Moreau, J. L., Takagi, S., Chow, L. C., & Antonucci, J. M. (2010). Strong nanocomposites with Ca, PO(4), and F release for caries inhibition. *Journal of Dental Research*, *89*(1), 19–28. doi:10.1177/0022034509351969 PMID:19948941

Yang, P., Quan, Z., Hou, Z., Li, C., Kang, X., Cheng, Z., & Lin, J. (2009). A magnetic, luminescent and mesoporous core–shell structured composite material as drug carrier. *Biomaterials*, *30*(27), 4786–4795. doi:10.1016/j.biomaterials.2009.05.038 PMID:19520428

Yang, P., Yang, P., Teng, X., Lin, J., & Huang, L. (2011). A novel luminescent mesoporous silica/apatite composite for controlled drug release. *Journal of Materials Chemistry*, *21*(14), 5505–5510. doi:10.1039/c0jm03878d

Yang, X., & ... . (2012). Anterior reconstruction with nano-hydroxyapatite/polyamide-66 cage after thoracic and lumbar corpectomy. *Orthopedics*, *35*(1), 01477447–20111122. PMID:22229617

Yang, Y., Wang, J. C., Zhang, X., Lu, W. L., & Zhang, Q. (2009). A novel mixed micelle gel with thermo-sensitive property for the local delivery of docetaxel. *Journal of Controlled Release*, *135*(2), 175–182. doi:10.1016/j.jconrel.2009.01.007 PMID:19331864

Yao, Feng, & Chen. (2016). External-stimuli responsive systems for cancer theranostic. *Asian Journal of Pharmaceutical Sciences, 11*(5), 585-595.

Yin, H., & Bae, Y. H. (2009). Physicochemical aspects of doxorubicin-loaded pH-sensitive polymeric micelle formulations from a mixture of poly (L-histidine)-b-poly (L-lactide)-b-poly (ethylene glycol). *European Journal of Pharmaceutics and Biopharmaceutics*, *71*(2), 223–230. doi:10.1016/j.ejpb.2008.08.013 PMID:18782616

Zare, Y., Rhee, K. Y., & Hui, D. (2017). Influences of nanoparticles aggregation/agglomeration on the interfacial/interphase and tensile properties of nanocomposites. *Composites. Part B, Engineering*, *122*, 41–46. doi:10.1016/j.compositesb.2017.04.008

Chapter 13
Nanocarriers as Non-Viral Vectors in Gene Delivery Application

Upendra Bulbake
NIPER Hyderabad, India

Anjali Jain
NIPER Hyderabad, India

Wahid Khan
NIPER Hyderabad, India

ABSTRACT

Gene therapy is the emerging trend in biomedical science for treatment of life-threatening diseases. This involves delivery of a therapeutic gene to the nucleus of an affected cell by a suitable vector. Gene delivery using non-viral vectors such as cationic polymer and lipid is gaining attention due to their favourable properties, including lack of immunogenicity, low toxicity, and potential for tissue specificity when compared with viral vectors. A variety of non-viral vectors have been proposed, most of which facilitate gene delivery by electrostatic interactions, encapsulation, and in some cases, condensing nucleic acids into nano-sized particles which can then be taken up by cells. Successful gene delivery within a cell is the nanocarrier's ability to protect its contents from degradation in the extracellular environment. A well-designed nanocarrier will promote cellular uptake and intracellular release of the nucleic acid. This chapter highlights different polymers, lipids, and their nanocarriers employed for gene delivery along with clinical trials.

1. INTRODUCTION

Gene therapy has gained significant attention over the past two decades as a potential method for treating life-threatening diseases (Swami, 2013). The idea of gene medicine is based on the utilization of nucleic acids as drugs for gene therapy with the hope of repairing or shutting down of a specific cellular function associated with the target gene (Cavazzana-Calvo, Thrasher, & Mavilio, 2004). It is now possible to treat diseases of genetic origin by administering healthy copies of mutated genes or promote a protective

DOI: 10.4018/978-1-5225-4781-5.ch013

Copyright © 2018, IGI Global. Copying or distributing in print or electronic forms without written permission of IGI Global is prohibited.

immune response by administering genes encoding for specific antigens. Currently, the research focused on designing effective carrier vectors that compact and protect oligonucleotides for gene therapy as free oligonucleotides are rapidly degraded by serum nucleases in the blood when injected intravenously (Anderson, 1985). Gene expression results when nucleic acid is transported inside the cell nucleus of the target cell and there is still a need for carriers, which perform this work safely and efficiently. An ideal carrier should be specific to the target cells and easy to enter the cell body. It should be able to express abundantly and continuously. Furthermore, it has to be safe, without showing any side effects, and be capable of large-scale production. Initial research concentrated on using viral carriers, including both retroviruses and adenoviruses, as these vectors exhibited high efficiency at delivering nucleic acids to numerous cell lines (Anderson, 1985). However, fundamental problems associated with viral vector systems, including toxicity, immunogenicity, and limitations with respect to scale-up procedures, encouraged the investigation of other potential carriers for the delivery of nucleic acids into targeted tissue (Verma, & Somia, 1997).

Non-viral gene delivery involves formulation of liposomes complexed with nucleic acid (lipoplexes) (Song, 1997), cationic polymers complexed with nucleic acid (polyplexes) (Ogris, 1999), polymeric vesicles complexed with nucleic acid (Brown, 2000) or a combination of both cationic lipids and cationic polymers complexed with nucleic acid (lipopolyplexes) (Kircheis, 1999). Figure 1 gives an overview of formation mechanism of gene-nonviral vector complex and release of gene followed by expression. After administration, these complexes were taken up by cells through endocytosis (Luo, & Saltzman, 2000). Cellular entry of these complexes is followed by endosomal escape and dissociation, which release nucleic acid into the nucleus from nonviral vectors complex for gene expression (Smyth, 2002). The lipids/polymers used are generally less toxic and immunogenic than the viral counterparts. Other advantages of nonviral approaches include ease of production and the potential for repeat administration. Nonviral gene delivery methods are generally viewed as less efficacious than the viral methods in terms of gene expression however, these methods are considered safer than methods involving viral vectors. The purpose of this chapter is to provide a concise overview of different polymers, lipids and their nanocarriers employed for gene delivery.

2. IDEAL PROPERTIES OF NON-VIRAL VECTORS FOR GENE DELIVERY

The key properties of non-viral gene delivery carrier are mentioned below (Ramamoorth, & Narvekar, 2015):

- The carrier should be biodegradable and biocompatible.
- The carrier should have appropriate circulating time and bio distribution in the body.
- The carrier should maintain the stability of gene in serum components.
- The carrier should be efficient for targeting and penetration through cell membrane.
- The carrier should possess the intracellular trafficking capacity (endosomal release and escape from degradation by cellular nucleases).

Apart from the above-mentioned properties, delivery systems should have capacity to be engineered for specific targeting, ability to permeate through blood vessels and different tissues, ability to evade

Figure 1. Various nonviral gene delivery vectors and sequential step in gene delivery. (A) siRNA complex formation by surface adsorption mechanism, (B) siRNA complex formation by entrapment mechanism (C) entry of gene-vector complex into cell, (D) endosomal escape, (E) entry of gene into cell nucleus and (F) gene expression.

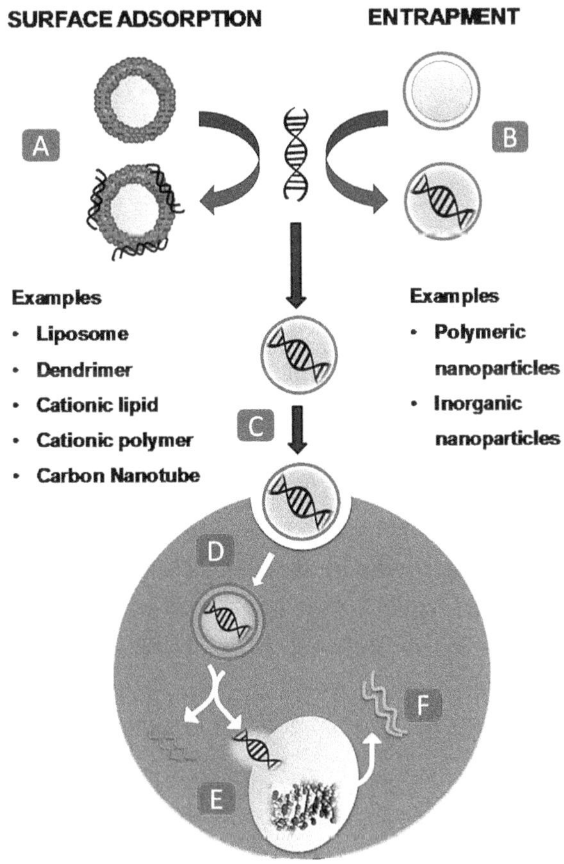

the immune system and nonspecific interactions with serum proteins and prevention of renal clearance (Pandi, 2017).

3. POLYMER AND LIPID USED FOR NON-VIRAL GENE DELIVERY VECTORS

Nanocarriers based on biodegradable and biocompatible polymeric systems have largely influenced the gene delivery concept. Polymers have been offered a great deal of promise for efficient transfection and release of nucleic acids (Gary, Puri, & Won, 2007). In 1987, Felgner and colleagues proposed lipids as an effective carrier for gene delivery for the first time as it was able to bind to the DNA and deliver the same to the cultured cells (Felgner, 1987). This has since resulted in the commercial production of *in vitro* gene delivery kits, e.g. lipofectin (*N*-[1-(2,3 - di - olyloxy)propyl -*N*,*N*,*N*- trimethylammonium-chloride, 1,2-dioleoylphosphatidylethanolamine-DOPE, 1:1) and the use of liposomal gene delivery in clinical trials (Porteous, 1997).

3.1 Polymers Used in Gene Delivery

Polymers have been explored in gene delivery, due to their molecular diversity, ease of structural modification, non-toxicity, biodegradability and excellent compatibility. They form smaller size complexes, which is crucial for gene transfer as small particle size may be favorable for improving transfection efficiency. Polymers most widely used for this purpose are Poly(L-Lysine) (PLL), Polyethylenimine (PEI), Chitosan, Cyclodextrins (CDs), Atelocollagen and Alginates (Khan, 2013; Jain, 2015). The structures of polymers used in gene therapy are given in Figure 2.

3.1.1. Poly(L-Lysine)

PLL is one of the most widely studied polypeptide with effective gene transfection activity. PLL is a synthetic repeat of the amino acid lysine, with the most commonly used PLLs ranging from a degree of polymerization (dp) of 90 to 450 (Wadhwa, 1997). The biodegradable nature of PLL makes it suitable for *in vivo* use. PLL possesses a high charge density essential for effective gene complexation and condensation (Kadlecova, 2012). Despite its effective complexation ability, PLL exhibits relatively low transfection efficiency. At physiological conditions (pH 7.4), some of the primary amine groups of PLL are protonated, with a low buffering capacity (pH 5.7–7.7); thus, PLL cannot efficiently escape the endosome without endosomolytic agents, the reason behind its low transfection ability (Martin, & Rice, 2007). Endosomal release can be improved with the addition of chloroquine or a fusogenic peptide to allow for release into the cytoplasm (Wolfert, & Seymour, 1998).

Figure 2. Chemical structures of polymers for the delivery of genes

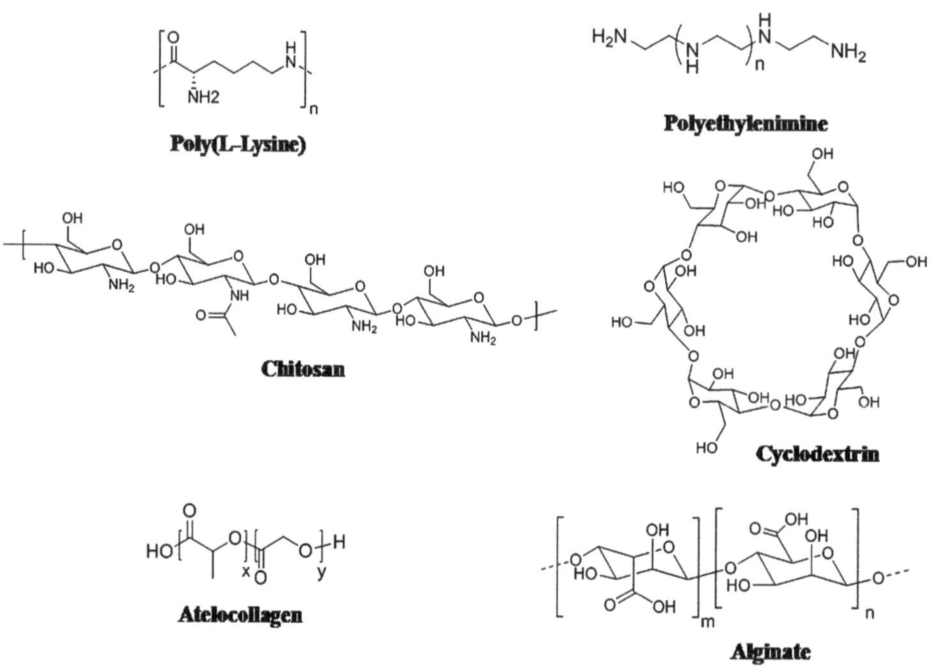

3.1.2. Polyethylenimine

PEI was introduced by Behr *et. al.* (1995) who considered it as a prototype for polymer-based gene carriers because of its relatively high transfection efficacy of its polyplexes of PLL with nucleic acid (Kichler, 2001). The success of PEI for gene transfection is primarily attributed to its composition of primary, secondary, and tertiary amines and high charge density (Gernett, 1999). PEI is available as linear and branched polymers. Several linear PEI transfection agents are commercially available, including ExGen500 and jetPEI, both of which are derivatives of linear polymer, with a *M*W of 22 KDa (Mn). The branched structure of PEI contains nitrogen at every third atom, resulting in high charge density. Primary amines are protonated at physiological pH 7.4 and enable PEI to bind negatively charged genes effectively into nano-sized complexes via electrostatic interactions. The secondary and tertiary amines are able to sequester protons in the endosomes, this phenomenon is termed as the proton-sponge effect.

3.1.3. Chitosan

Chitosan is a naturally occurring cationic polysaccharide. It has become one of the most prominent non-viral vectors for gene transfer due to its biodegradability and biocompatibility (Borchard, 2001; Khan, 2012). Chitosan consisting of repeating *D*-glucosamine and *N*-acetyl-*D*-glucosamine units that are linked via (1–4) glycosidic bonds (Onishi, & Machida, 1999). The protonated amine groups present in it allow transport of conjugated nucleic acids across cellular membranes and subsequent endocytosis into cells. Moreover, the positively charged amines (under slightly acidic conditions) allow electrostatic interaction with phosphate bearing nucleic acids to form polyelectrolyte complexes (Tong, 2009; Jain, 2014). The Mw and degree of deacetylation (DDA) of chitosan is an important factor that affects the gene transfer efficiency. Higher Mw and DDA are desirable characteristics for the formation of chitosan nanoparticles, higher Mw chitosan molecules are long and flexible while higher DDA enhances its electrostatic interaction with nucleic acids, thus synergically reducing the size of complexes and increasing their stability (Liu, 2007). A high charge ratio also enhances the stability of complexes because the loosely bound excess chitosan on the outer surface of nanoparticles can promote binding and uptake across anionic cell surfaces and also provide subsequent protection against nucleic acids degradation within endosome compartments (Liu, 2007). Oppositely, complexes formed with chitosans with low Mw are not sufficiently stable and cannot provide effective protection for nucleic acids due to early dissociation and therefore, exhibit little or no transgene expression (MacLaughlin, 1998). To obtain a high transfection efficiency, an intermediate degree of stability must be achieved with chitosan with an appropriate Mw between extracellular nucleic acids protection versus efficient intracellular nucleic acids release (Huang, 2005; Koping-Hoggard, 2004).

3.1.4. Cyclodextrins (CDs)

Cyclodextrins are cone-shaped natural cyclic oligomers of glucose where moieties of 6, 7, and 8 glucose units are termed alpha (α)-, beta (β)-, and gamma (γ)-CDs, respectively, joined by a-1,4 linkages (Davis, & Brewster, 2004). Of importance, CDs are known to lack immunogenicity [36]. The emergence of CDs in gene therapy has been considered since 1999 (Davis, 2004). Amongst a class of novel linear, cationic, β-CDs-containing polymers (β-CDPs) with 4, 5, 6, 7, 8, and 10 methylene units, the β-CDPs based on 6 methylene units (β-6CDP) has been found effective for nucleic acids delivery (Gonzalez, Hwang, &

Davis, 1999). However, CDPs do not contain any pH-buffering properties and are therefore unable to escape the endosomal pathway by themselves (Gonzalez, Hwang, & Davis, 1999; Kulkarni, 2005). To deal with endosomal and lysosomal entrapment and subsequent degradation, β-6CDPs have been modified with imidazole groups for improved intracellular delivery (Davis, 2004). The imidazole-containing form has been shown to buffer the pH inside endosomal vesicles, resulting in increased intracellular delivery compared with unmodified β-6CDPs (Koping-Hoggard, 2004).

3.1.5. Atelocollagen

Atelocollagen is very large protein (300 kDa) derived from pepsin treatment of type I collagen of calf dermis (Ochiya, 1999). Collagen is a fibrous protein in the connective tissue that plays an important role in the maintenance of the morphology of tissues and organs. A collagen molecule has an amino acid sequence called as telopeptide at both N- and C-terminals, which confers most of the collagen's antigenicity. Atelocollagen obtained by pepsin treatment is low in immunogenicity because it is free from telopeptides (Stenzel, Miyata, & Rubin, 1974). Upon mixing of atelocollagen with negatively charged nucleic acid molecules, different sizes of complex can be formed depending on the ratio between both components. It can be effectively used as a carrier for *in vivo* delivery of nucleic acid. Atelocollagen complexed with DNA molecules was efficiently transduced into mammalian cells (Honma, 2001) which resulted in long-term efficient gene expression (Ochiya, 1999). Since Atelocollagen allows increased cellular uptake, nuclease resistance and prolonged release of genes and oligonucleotides (Ochiya, 2001), an Atelocollagen complex is applicable for an efficient delivery of siRNA *in vitro*. Furthermore, Atelocollagen displays low-toxicity and low-immunogenicity when it is transplanted *in vivo* (Sano, 2003).

3.1.6. Alginates

Alginate is a water-soluble linear polysaccharide consisting of β-(1–4)-D-manuronic acid and α-(1–4)-L-guluronic acid units, which is derived from marine brown algae (laminariales) and some bacteria (Azotobacter vinelandii and Pseudomonas aeruginosa, among others) (Vold, Kristiansen, & Christensen, 2006). Alginate has shown low toxicity and good biocompatibility in drug delivery. Alginate has been employed to coat DNA/PEI complexes through ionic interaction in order to partially shield the positive charge of the complexes. It has been documented that such coating/shielding renders the DNA/PEI/alginate gene-delivery systems higher stability and higher transfection efficiency in serum conditions. Alginate was blended with high molecular weight PEI (25 kDa) (Patnaik, 2010) and PEI 750 kDa (Patnaik, 2006) through positive–negative electrostatic interaction. One of the drawbacks in such systems is that high molecular weight PEI is still needed as the DNA shrinkage. Thus, the severe cytotoxicity cannot be avoided after physical dissociation of alginate. Alternatively, it can be anticipated that using low-MW PEI rather than high-MW PEI might reduce the cytotoxicity of the alginate-PEI system.

3.1.7. Miscellaneous Polymers

Controlled release polymer vesicles comprised of block copolymers such as Poly Lactic-co-Glycolic Acid (PLGA), PEG-Polycaprolactone, PEG-Polylactic acid, inert PEG-polybutadiene etc., have been developed to deliver functional nucleic acid into cancer cells *in vitro* (Kim, 2009). These degradable carriers are taken up passively by cultured cells after which the vesicles transform into micelles that allow endolysosomal escape and delivery of nucleic acid into cytosol for gene knockdown.

3.2 Lipids Used in Gene Delivery

A large number of cationic lipids have been synthesized and studied for gene delivery (Felgner, 1994; Remy, 1994; Balasubramaniam, 1996). They share a common structure of positively charged hydrophilic head and hydrophobic tail that are connected via a linker structure. The hydrophobic moieties ensure that the cationic lipids assemble into bilayer vesicles on dispersion in aqueous media, effectively shielding the hydrophobic portion of the molecule and exposing the amine head groups to the aqueous medium. The amine group is an absolute necessity for transfection competence as this is the nucleic acid binding moiety interacting electrostatically with nucleic acid and condensing the large anionic molecule into small transportable units—lipoplexes. Table 1 summarizes some cationic lipids used in gene transfer.

Table 1. Lipids commonly used for gene delivery applications

S No.	Lipid	Abbreviation	Feature
1.	1,2-Dioleoyloxy-3-trimethylammonium-propane	DOTAP	Cationic
2.	N-[1-(2,3-Dioleyloxy)propyl]N,N,N-trimethylammonium chloride	DOTMA	Cationic
3.	1,2-Dioleyl-3-trimethylammonium-propane	DOPA	Cationic
4.	3β-[N-(N,N-Dimethylaminoethane)-carbamoyl]cholesterol	DC-Chol	Cationic
5.	Dioctadecylamidoglycylspermine	DOGS	Cationic
6.	Cetyltrimethylammonium bromide	CTAB	Cationic
7.	1,2-Dioleoyl-sn-glycero-3-phosphatidylcholine	DOPC	Helper
8.	1,2-Dioleoyl-sn-glycero-3-phosphatidylethanolamine	DOPE	Helper
9.	Cholesterol		Helper
10.	N-(3-Aminopropyl)-N,N-dimethyl-2,3-bis(dodecyloxy)-1-propanaminium bromide	GAP-DLRIE	Cationic
11.	2,3-Dioleyloxy-N-[2(sperminecarboxamido)-ethyl]-N,N-dimethyl-1-propanaminium trifluoroacetate	DOSPA	Cationic
12.	N-(2-Hydroxyethyl)-N,N-dimethyl-2,3-bis(tetradecyloxy)-1-propanaminium bromide	DMRIE	Cationic
13.	rac-[2(2,3-Dihexadecyloxypropyl-oxymethyloxy)ethyl]trimethylammonium bromide	CLIP-6	Cationic
14.	Dimyristooxypropyl dimethyl hydroxyethyl ammonium bromide	DMRI	Cationic
15.	Octadecenolyoxy[ethyl-2-heptadecenyl-3 hydroxyethyl] imidazolinium chloride	DOTIM	Cationic
16.	2-(3-[Bis-(3-amino-propyl)-amino]propylamino)-N-ditetradecylcarbamoylme-ethyl-acetamide	RPR209120	Cationic
17.	rac-[(2,3-Dioctadecyloxypropyl)(2-hydroxyethyl)]-dimethylammonium chloride	CLIP-1	Cationic
18.	1,3-Dioleoxy-2-(6-carboxy-spermyl)-propylamide	DOSPER	Cationic
19.	1,2-Dimyristoyl-trimethylammoniumpropane	DMTAP	Cationic

4. VARIOUS DELIVERY SYSTEMS USED FOR GENE DELIVERY

Selection of siRNA is based on target gene for different diseases. Multiple targets for a particular disease could be present based upon the mechanism and pathways involved in the pathophysiology of diseases. siRNAs are designed to bind and inhibit the target gene. Figure 3 illustrates commonly used genes with their reported nonviral nanocarriers.

4.1. Polymer Based Delivery Systems

Polymer based nanocarriers generally form two types of delivery systems i.e. polymeric nanoparticles and polyplexes. Some research findings based on polymeric nanocarrier for gene delivery are described in Table 2.

4.1.1. Polymeric Nanoparticles

Polymeric nanoparticles encapsulate the contents using hydrophobic interactions. For example, PLGA can encapsulate various nucleic acids by using a double emulsion-deposition technique (Khan, 2004). This formulation is attractive not only for its biodegradable properties, but also because it permits controlled release of the nucleic acid at the site of action via sustained diffusion through the polymer matrix due to degradation of the matrix.

4.1.2. Polyplexes

Polymer–nucleic acids complexes, termed polyplexes, are basically formed through the spontaneous electrostatic interaction between the positively charged polymer with the negatively charged phosphate backbone of the nucleic acid (Elouahabi, & Ruysscheart, 2005). The resulting polyplex can prevent nucleic acid molecules from degradation by metabolic enzymes, such as DNase or RNase, and overcome the electrostatic repulsion of the cell membrane, resulting in enhanced uptake by the cell. The molar ratio of cationic polymer to nucleic acid determines the proportion of electrostatic neutralization, which reflects the entire surface charge and the size of resulting polyplexes (De Smedt, Demeester, & Hennick, 2000). Polyplex formation is affected by experimental variables such as nucleic acid/cationic polymer concentration, time and medium for the complexation, the number and/or order of addition steps, and the presence of serum during polyplex formation (Luo, & Saltzman, 2000). Hence, these parameters should be optimized to obtain better transfection efficiency.

4.2. Lipid Based Delivery Systems

Cationic lipid-based nanocarriers represent one of the most intensively studied non-viral vectors. Lipid-based nanocarriers also forms two types of delivery systems i.e. lipoplex and lipopolyplexes. Few researches which include these two delivery systems are mentioned below in the Table 3.

Figure 3. Different target genes with their respective non-viral nanocarriers

Polymeric nanoparticle	Liposome	Lipid-polymer nanoparticle	Mesoporous-silica nanoparticle	Gold nanoparticle	Carbon nanotube	Dendrimer

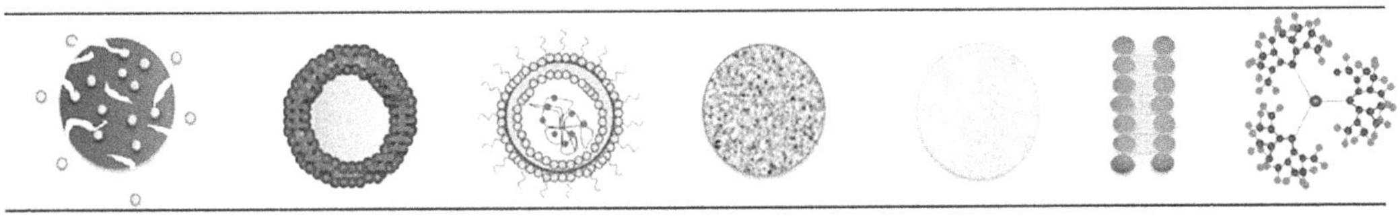

siRNA/shRNA

Polymeric nanoparticle	Liposome	Lipid-polymer nanoparticle	Mesoporous-silica nanoparticle	Gold nanoparticle	Carbon nanotube	Dendrimer
Bcl-2 [54, 55] Bcl-xL [56] Choline kinase [57] EGFR [58] MDR-1 [59, 60] MVP [61] Plk 1 [62] Survivnin [63] TNF-α [64]	Bcl-2 [65] MRP1/MDR1 [66] Cytosine deaminase [67] JIP1 [68] Mcl1 [69, 70] MDR-1 [71] Notch3 [72] Survivnin [73] STAT3 [74] TNF-α [12, 64]	c-Myc [75] VGRF [76] EGFR [77] IL-12 [78]	Bcl-2 [79] MDR-1 [80]	ASCL1[81] MDR-1[59]	Kinase [82]	Bcl-2 [83] Bcl-xL [83] Mcl-1 [83]

Table 2. Polymer based nano-carriers for gene delivery

S No.	Polymer	Gene Used	Delivery System/ Complex	Gene Delivery Application	
1.	PLL	siRNA	Nanoparticles	Targeted delivery system	[85]
		Plasmid DNA	Polyplex	Targeted delivery system	[86]
2.	PEI	Plasmid DNA	Polyplex	Human adipose tissue-derived stem cells	[87]
		Plasmid DNA	Micelle-like nanoparticle	Systemic gene therapy	[88]
3.	Chitosan	siRNA	Nanoparticle	Lung cancer	[31]
		Plasmid DNA	Polyplex	Targeted delivery system	[89]
4.	CDs	siRNA	Nanoparticle	Targeted delivery system	[90]
		siRNA	Nanoparticle	Targeted delivery system	[91]
5.	Atelocollagen	siRNA	Polyplex	Germ cell tumor	[92]
		siRNA	Polyplex	Human prostate cancer	[56]
6.	Alginate	Plasmid DNA	Nanocomposite	Gene transfection agent	[47]
7.	PLGA	siRNA	Nanoparticle	Gene transfection agent	[93]
	PLGA-PEI	siRNA	Nanoparticle	Gene transfection agent	[94]
8.	PEG-polybutadiene	siRNA	Nanoparticle	Germ cell tumor	[48]
9.	PEG polycaprolactone	siRNA	Nanoparticle	Germ cell tumor	[48]

Table 3. Lipid-based nano-carriers for gene delivery

S No.	Lipid	Gene Used	Delivery System/Complex	Gene Delivery Application	
1.	DOTMA	A1-Antitrypsin	Lipoplex	AAT deficiency	[103]
2.	DOTAP	CFTR	Lipoplex	Cystic fibrosis	[15]
3.	DC-chol	CFTR	Liposomes	Cystic fibrosis	[104]
4.	DMRIE	HLA-B7	Lipid nanoparticles	Cancer	[105]
5.	DC-chol	H-2K	Lipoplex	Cancer	[106]
6.	DC-chol	Adenovirus 5 E1A	Lipoplex	Cancer	[107]
7.	DMRIE	CFTR	Liposomes	Cancer	[108]
8.	DC-chol	Ad5 E1A	Lipoplex	Cancer	[109]
9.	DC-chol	HLA-B7	Liposomes	Cancer	[110]
10.	DMRIE	HLA-B7 + b2-microglobulin	Lipoplex	Cancer	[111]
11.	PLL/DOPE	Plasmid DNA	Lipopolyplex	Solid tumors	[82]

4.2.1. Lipoplexes

The nucleic acids such as siRNA when mixed with cationic liposomes, due to electrostatic interactions, they get condensed into small quasi-stable particles called lipoplexes (Montier, 2008) which protect them from nuclease degradation. In addition, the lipoplexes offer enhanced cellular uptake and facilitate release of nucleic acid from the intracellular vesicles before reaching destructive lysosomal compartments (Gao, Kim, & Liu, 2007). Various commercial transfection agents, such as Lipofectamine 2000 and Transit-TKO has been used as lipoplexes forming agents (de Fougerolles, 2007). Lipofectamine 2000 is a cationic liposome based reagent having high transfection efficiency and widely exploited for efficient transfection of synthetic siRNA into mammalian cells (Dalby, 2004), but its toxicity limits its application (Spagnou, 2004).

4.2.2. Lipopolyplexes

Lipopolyplex is a core-shell structure which have been prepared by condensing nucleic acid with a polycationic polymers such as poly-L-lysine (Guo, & Lee, 2000;Lee, & Huang, 1996) or polyethylenimine (Guo, & Lee, 2000), and entrapping this polyplex within anionic (Guo, & Lee, 2000) or neutral (Ibanez, 1996) liposomes. As a non-viral gene delivery vector, lipopolyplex combining the advantages of polyplex and lipoplex has shown superior colloidal stability, reduced cytotoxicity, extremely high gene transfection efficiency (Chen, 2016).

4.3. Miscelleneous Nanocarriers in Gene Delivery

4.3.1. Dendrimers

Dendrimers are a unique class of synthetic polymers utilized as a nanocarrier system (Khandare, 2012; Szymanski, Markowicz, & Mikiciuk-Olasik, 2011). A dendrimer is a macromolecule, which is characterized by its highly branched 3D structure with high degree of surface functionality and versatility.

A range of polyamidoamine (PAMAM) (Kukowska-Latallo, 1996; Du, Zhou, & Zhou, 1998) and phosphorous containing (Loup, 1999) dendrimers have been studied as gene delivery systems. Terminal amino groups bind with nucleic acid by electrostatic interaction (Bielinska, 1999) and the so formed positively charged complexes is known as dendriplex (Shah, 2000). Increased terminal amino groups with increased generation of dendrimer appears to enhance gene transfection efficiency (Toth, 1999). Dendriplexes are presumably internalized by endocytosis and there are also advantages associated with the dendritic shape of the polymer as nucleic acid appears to interact with the surface primary amines only, leaving the internal tertiary amines available for the neutralization of the acid pH within the endosomal/lysosomal compartment (Lee, Wang, & Low, 1996). Following internalization, the release of dendriplexes by the endosome has been attributed to the protonation of the internal tertiary nitrogens by endosomal protons which then results in a swelling of the endosome and the release of the nucleic acid to the cytoplasm (Tang, Redemann, & Szoka, 1996). Bielinska *et al.* (1996)have shown that PAMAM dendrimers can be complexed to antisense oligonucleotides or plasmid expression vectors coding antisense mRNA, to inhibit specific reporter luciferase gene expression by 30 to 60% (Bielinska, 1996). These results were obtained in several stable cell clones that demonstrate long-term luciferase expression of cDNA from mouse melanoma and rat embryonal fibroblast cells.

4.3.2. Inorganic Nanoparticles

Another widely employed non-viral approach for nucleic acid delivery is the use inorganic materials (Chowdhury, & Akaike, 2005). Most commonly used inorganic nanoparticles are gold, silica dioxide, iron oxide, calcium phosphate, biodegradable functional apatite particles fullerenes and quantum dots (e.g. carbon lattices, nanotubes). Due to their unique properties, applications of nanomaterials in gene delivery are increasing rapidly.

4.3.2.1. Gold Nanoparticles

Gold nanoparticles have also exhibited unique chemical and physical properties. They are essentially inert, non-toxic and in the size range of 1 to 150 nm. Moreover, they can be functionalized and modified to improve the versatility of gold nanoparticles. Significant efforts have been devoted over the past years to the fabrication of gold nanoparticles for the delivery of siRNA. Polyvalent RNA-gold nanoparticle conjugates has been designed to function in the RNAi pathway. The resultant conjugates have six times higher half-life than that of free dsRNA, and demonstrated high gene knockdown capability in a cell model (Giljohann, 2009). Several research groups have fabricated delivery systems based on gold nanoparticles bearing functional moieties. Polyethylene glycol modified gold nanoparticles has been developed for the delivery of siRNA. It was conjugated to the nanoparticles *via* biodegradable disulfide linkages, with approximately 30 strands of siRNA per nanoparticle. Developed functionalized nanoparticles facilitated better siRNA *in vitro* uptake as compared with lipofectamine 2000 (Lee, 2009).

4.3.2.2. Carbon Nanotubes

Carbon nanotubes (CNTs) have been utilized for various applications, including the delivery of nucleic acids in gene therapy. CNTs consist exclusively of carbon atoms arranged in condensed atomic rings which in turn are organized in one (single walled carbon nanotubes; SWNTs) or more (multi-walled carbon nanotubes; MWNTs) concentric sheets rolled up into cylinders. To avail various applications, it is necessary to chemically tailor the outer surfaces of the CNTs in order to maximize their unique properties (Bates, & Kostarelos, 2013). Functionalized SWNTs with hexamethylenediamine and polydiallyldimethylammonium chloride has been electrostatically complexed with extracellular signal-regulated kinase siRNA. These SWNTs demonstrated low cytotoxicity and better efficacy on isolated rat heart cells (Krajck, 2008).

4.3.2.3. Calcium Phosphate Nanoparticles

Calcium phosphate has excellent biocompatibility and bioresorbability due to its chemical similarity to human hard tissue (bone and teeth). In nanoparticulate dispersed form, it can be used as a carrier to transfer nucleic acids. Layered double hydroxide (LDH) nanoparticles have been developed to deliver siRNA to mammalian cells. Studies exhibited that siRNA-loaded LDH nanoparticles was tightly bind, protect, and release siRNA molecules and delivered siRNA via endosomal escape into the cytoplasm (Ladewig, 2010). Single-shell and multi-shell calcium phosphate nanoparticles has been prepared and functionalized with DNA and siRNA. Developed multi-shell nanoparticles were in nanometric size range (below 100nm) which protected genetic materials from the intracellular degradation by endonucleases and demonstrated better transfection efficiency of the nanoparticles in cell culture (Kovtun, Heumann, & Epple, 2009).

4.3.2.4. Other Inorganic Nanoparticles

Supermagnetic iron oxide nanoparticles have demonstrated potential for the delivery of biomolecules like siRNA. It can be utilized for concurrent diagnostic and therapeutic applications (Lee, 2009). Multifunctional magnetic nanocarriers have been designed for image-tagged siRNA delivery to intact pancreatic islets. Studies demonstrated that a magnetic nanoparticle carrying siRNA was efficiently taken up by murine pancreatic islets and visualized by magnetic resonance imaging and near-infrared fluorescence optical imaging. Thus, magnetic nanoparticles can overcome the challenges associated with genetic modification of intact pancreatic islets in a clinically acceptable manner (Medarova, 2008). Due to their unique properties, applications of iron oxide nanomaterials in the delivery, diagnosis and therapeutic applications of genetic material are increasing rapidly. Moreover, surface functionalized mesoporous silica nanoparticles (MSNP) can be used as an efficient and safe carrier for nucleic acids. Noncovalent attachment of polyethyleneimine polymers to the silica nanoparticles surface not only increases MSNP cellular uptake but also generates a cationic surface to which DNA and siRNA constructs has been attached.

5. CLINICAL TRIALS

Advances in non-viral vectors based nanocarriers have been rapidly translated into clinical practice. Today, there are good number of non-viral vectors based nanocarriers present in various clinical trials (Table 4).

6. CONCLUSION

Gene therapy demonstrates a variety of advantages over conventional therapeutic modalities, such as its specificity or selectivity toward objects, minimal side effects, correction of genetic causes, and per-

Table 4. Current non-viral vectors based nanocarriers mediated gene therapy clinical trials

S No.	Nanocarrier	Gene	Indication	Clinical Phase
1.	Liposome/Lipid NPs	Tumor suppressor gene FUS1	Non-small-cell lung cancer	Phase II
2.	Liposome/Lipid NPs	Nucleocapsid N gene siRNA	Respiratory syncytial virus infections	Phase II
3.	Liposome/Lipid NPs	CFTR gene	Cystic fibrosis	Phase II
4.	Transferrin Targeted Cyclodextrin Nanoparticle	CALAA-01	Solid tumors	Phase I
5.	Transferrin Targeted Liposome with p53 Gene	SGT53-01	Solid tumors	Phase I
6.	Liposome/Lipid NPs	siRNA targeting gene proprotein convertase subtilisn/kexin type 9	Hypercholesterolemia	Phase I
7.	Liposome/Lipid NPs	EGFR antisense DNA	Advanced head and neck cancer	Phase I
8.	Liposome/Lipid NPs	pGT-1 gene	Cystic fibrosis	Phase I
9.	Liposome/Lipid NPs	Bik gene	Pancreatic cancer	Phase I
10.	Stabilized Nanoparticles	M2 subunit of ribonucleotide reductase (R2) siRNA	Solid tumor cancers	Phase I
11.	Lipid Nanoparticles	VEGF and KSP siRNA	Advanced solid tumors with liver involvement	Phase I
12.	Liposome/Lipid NPs	PKN3 siRNA	Advanced solid cancer	Phase I
13.	Lipid Nanoparticles	Ttransthyretin gene siRNA	Transthyretin mediated amyloidosis	Phase I
14.	Liposome/Lipid NPs	siRNA targeting ApoB	Hypercholesterolemia	Phase I
15.	Liposome/Lipid NPs	siRNA directed against PLK1	Solid tumor cancers	Phase I

sistent therapeutic effects after single application. Numerous nonviral gene delivery systems have been developed in the last 20 to 25 years. This chapter has discussed polymer and lipid based nanocarriers as nonviral vectors. These naocarriers are vulnerable in the plasma, on arrival at the cell must be endocytosed, escape from the endosome and eventually deliver nucleic acid to the nucleus. Improvements in all these aspects of gene transport are required if efficient systems are to emerge from the current effort. The cell toxicity associated with the efficient polymeric and lipid systems hamper their widespread use but principally the main issues surrounding these systems concern their efficiency.

REFERENCES

Ahn, H. H., Lee, J. H., Kim, K. S., Lee, J. Y., Kim, M. S., Khang, G., ... Lee, H. B. (2008). Polyethylenei-mine-mediated gene delivery into human adipose derived stem cells. *Biomaterials*, *29*(15), 2415–2422. doi:10.1016/j.biomaterials.2008.02.006 PMID:18295879

Anderson, W. F. (1985). Human gene therapy: Scientific and ethical considerations. *The Journal of Medicine and Philosophy*, *10*(3), 275–292. doi:10.1093/jmp/10.3.275 PMID:3900264

Balasubramaniam, R., & ... . (1996). Structural and functional analysis of cationic transfection lipids: The hydrophobic domain. *Gene Therapy*, *3*(2), 163–172. PMID:8867864

Bartlett, D. W., & Davis, M. E. (2008). Impact of tumor-specific targeting and dosing schedule on tumor growth inhibition after intravenous administration of siRNA-containing nanoparticles. *Biotechnology and Bioengineering*, *99*(4), 975–985. doi:10.1002/bit.21668 PMID:17929316

Bates, K., & Kostarelos, K. (2013). Carbon nanotubes as vectors for gene therapy: Past achievements, present challenges and future goals. *Advanced Drug Delivery Reviews*, *65*(15), 2023–2033. doi:10.1016/j.addr.2013.10.003 PMID:24184373

Bielinska, A. (1996). Regulation of in vitro gene expression using antisense oligonucleotides or antisense expression plasmids transfected using starburst PAMAM dendrimers. *Nucleic Acids Research*, *24*(11), 2176–2182. doi:10.1093/nar/24.11.2176 PMID:8668551

Bielinska, A. U., Chen, C., Johnson, J., & Baker, J. R. (1999). DNA complexing with polyamidoamine dendrimers: Implications for transfection. *Bioconjugate Chemistry*, *10*(5), 843–850. doi:10.1021/bc990036k PMID:10502352

Borchard, G. (2001). Chitosans for gene delivery. *Advanced Drug Delivery Reviews*, *52*(2), 145–150. doi:10.1016/S0169-409X(01)00198-3 PMID:11718938

Boussif, O., Lezoualc'h, F., Zanta, M. A., Mergny, M. D., Scherman, D., Demeneix, B., & Behr, J. P. (1995). A versatile vector for gene and oligonucleotide transfer into cells in culture and in vivo: Polyethylenimine. *Proceedings of the National Academy of Sciences of the United States of America*, *92*(16), 7297–7301. doi:10.1073/pnas.92.16.7297 PMID:7638184

Brigham, K. L., Lane, K. B., Meyrick, B., Stecenko, A. A., Strack, S., Cannon, D. R., ... Canonico, A. E. (2000). Transfection of nasal mucosa with a normal alpha1-antitrypsin gene in alpha1-antitrypsin-deficient subjects: Comparison with protein therapy. *Human Gene Therapy*, *11*(7), 1023–1032. doi:10.1089/10430340050015338 PMID:10811231

Brown, M., Schätzlein, A., Brownlie, A., Jack, V., Wang, W., Tetley, L., ... Uchegbu, I. F. (2000). Preliminary characterization of novel amino acid based polymeric vesicles as gene and drug delivery agents. *Bioconjugate Chemistry*, *11*(6), 880–891. doi:10.1021/bc000052d PMID:11087338

Cao, N., Cheng, D., Zou, S., Ai, H., Gao, J., & Shuai, X. (2011). The synergistic effect of hierarchical assemblies of siRNA and chemotherapeutic drugs co-delivered into hepatic cancer cells. *Biomaterials*, *32*(8), 2222–2232. doi:10.1016/j.biomaterials.2010.11.061 PMID:21186059

Caplen, N. J., Alton, E. W. F. W., Mddleton, P. G., Dorin, J. R., Stevenson, B. J., Gao, X., ... Geddes, D. M. (1995). Liposome-mediated CFTR gene transfer to the nasal epithelium of patients with cystic fibrosis. *Nature Medicine*, *1*(1), 39–46. doi:10.1038/nm0195-39 PMID:7584951

Cavazzana-Calvo, M., Thrasher, A., & Mavilio, F. (2004). The future of gene therapy. *Nature*, *427*(6977), 779–781. doi:10.1038/427779a PMID:14985734

Chang, R. S., Suh, M. S., Kim, S., Shim, G., Lee, S., Han, S. S., ... Oh, Y.-K. (2011). Cationic drug-derived nanoparticles for multifunctional delivery of anticancer siRNA. *Biomaterials*, *32*(36), 9785–9795. doi:10.1016/j.biomaterials.2011.09.017 PMID:21937102

Chen, A. M., Zhang, M., Wei, D., Stueber, D., Taratula, O., Minko, T., & He, H. (2009). Co-delivery of doxorubicin and Bcl-2 siRNA by mesoporous silica nanoparticles enhances the efficacy of chemotherapy in multidrug-resistant cancer cells. *Small*, *5*(23), 2673–2677. doi:10.1002mll.200900621 PMID:19780069

Chen, W., Li, H., Liu, Z., & Yuan, W. (2016). Lipopolyplex for therapeutic gene delivery and its application for the treatment of Parkinson's disease. *Frontiers in Aging Neuroscience*, *8*, 68. doi:10.3389/fnagi.2016.00068 PMID:27092073

Chen, Y., Bathula, S. R., Li, J., & Huang, L. (2010). Multifunctional nanoparticles delivering small interfering RNA and doxorubicin overcome drug resistance in cancer. *The Journal of Biological Chemistry*, *285*(29), 22639–22650. doi:10.1074/jbc.M110.125906 PMID:20460382

Chen, Y., Sen, J., Bathula, S. R., Yang, Q., Fittipaldi, R., & Huang, L. (2009). Novel cationic lipid that delivers siRNA and enhances therapeutic effect in lung cancer cells. *Molecular Pharmaceutics*, *6*(3), 696–705. doi:10.1021/mp800136v PMID:19267451

Chen, Y., Wu, J. J., & Huang, L. (2010). Nanoparticles targeted with NGR motif deliver c-myc siRNA and doxorubicin for anticancer therapy. *Molecular Therapy*, *18*(4), 828–834. doi:10.1038/mt.2009.291 PMID:20068551

Chen, Z., Penet, M.-F., Nimmagadda, S., Li, C., Banerjee, S. R., Winnard, P. T. Jr, ... Bhujwalla, Z. M. (2012). PSMA-targeted theranostic nanoplex for prostate cancer therapy. *ACS Nano*, *6*(9), 7752–7762. doi:10.1021/nn301725w PMID:22866897

Chowdhury, E. H., & Akaike, T. (2005). Bio-functional inorganic materials: An attractive branch of gene-based nano-medicine delivery for 21st century. *Current Gene Therapy*, *5*(6), 669–676. doi:10.2174/156652305774964613 PMID:16457655

Cristiano, R. J., & Roth, J. A. (1995). Epidermal growth factor mediated DNA delivery into lung cancer cells via the epidermal growth factor receptor. *Cancer Gene Therapy*, *3*(1), 4–10. PMID:8785711

Dalby, B., & ... . (2004). Advanced transfection with Lipofectamine 2000 reagent: Primary neurons, siRNA, and high-throughput applications. *Methods (San Diego, Calif.)*, *33*(2), 95–103. doi:10.1016/j.ymeth.2003.11.023 PMID:15121163

Davis, M., Pun, S., Bellocq, N., Reineke, T., Popielarski, S., Mishra, S., & Heidel, J. (2004). Self-assembling nucleic acid delivery vehicles via linear, water-soluble, cyclodextrin-containing polymers. *Current Medicinal Chemistry*, *11*(2), 179–197. doi:10.2174/0929867043456179 PMID:14754416

Davis, M. E., & Brewster, M. E. (2004). Cyclodextrin-based pharmaceutics: Past, present and future. *Nature Reviews. Drug Discovery*, *3*(12), 1023–1035. doi:10.1038/nrd1576 PMID:15573101

De Boer, J. P., & ... . (2012). Targeting JNK-interacting protein 1 (JIP1) sensitises osteosarcoma to doxorubicin. *Oncotarget*, *3*(10), 1169. PMID:23045411

de Fougerolles, A., Vornlocher, H.-P., Maraganore, J., & Lieberman, J. (2007). Interfering with disease: A progress report on siRNA-based therapeutics. *Nature Reviews. Drug Discovery*, *6*(6), 443–453. doi:10.1038/nrd2310 PMID:17541417

De Smedt, S. C., Demeester, J., & Hennink, W. E. (2000). Cationic polymer based gene delivery systems. *Pharmaceutical Research*, *17*(2), 113–126. doi:10.1023/A:1007548826495 PMID:10751024

Du, B., Zhou, R., & Zhuo, R. (1998). Synthesis of cyclic core dendritic polymer and its usage as a vector for transferring foreign DNA into human cells. *Chinese Chemical Letters*, *9*(7), 635–638.

Elouahabi, A., & Ruysschaert, J.-M. (2005). Formation and intracellular trafficking of lipoplexes and polyplexes. *Molecular Therapy*, *11*(3), 336–347. doi:10.1016/j.ymthe.2004.12.006 PMID:15727930

Felgner, J. H., & ... . (1994). Enhanced gene delivery and mechanism studies with a novel series of cationic lipid formulations. *The Journal of Biological Chemistry*, *269*(4), 2550–2561. PMID:8300583

Felgner, P. L., Gadek, T. R., Holm, M., Roman, R., Chan, H. W., Wenz, M., ... Danielsen, M. (1987). Lipofection: A highly efficient, lipid-mediated DNA-transfection procedure. *Proceedings of the National Academy of Sciences of the United States of America*, *84*(21), 7413–7417. doi:10.1073/pnas.84.21.7413 PMID:2823261

Fetz, V., Bier, C., Habtemichael, N., Schuon, R., Schweitzer, A., Kunkel, M., ... Knauer, S. K. (2009). Inducible NO synthase confers chemoresistance in head and neck cancer by modulating survivin. *International Journal of Cancer*, *124*(9), 2033–2041. doi:10.1002/ijc.24182 PMID:19130609

Gao, X., Kim, K.-S., & Liu, D. (2007). Nonviral gene delivery: What we know and what is next. *The AAPS Journal*, *9*(1), E92–E104. doi:10.1208/aapsj0901009 PMID:17408239

Garnett, M.C. (1999). Gene-delivery systems using cationic polymers. *Critical Reviews™ in Therapeutic Drug Carrier Systems, 16*(2).

Gary, D. J., Puri, N., & Won, Y.-Y. (2007). Polymer-based siRNA delivery: Perspectives on the fundamental and phenomenological distinctions from polymer-based DNA delivery. *Journal of Controlled Release*, *121*(1), 64–73. doi:10.1016/j.jconrel.2007.05.021 PMID:17588702

Giljohann, D. A., Seferos, D. S., Prigodich, A. E., Patel, P. C., & Mirkin, C. A. (2009). Gene regulation with polyvalent siRNA-nanoparticle conjugates. *Journal of the American Chemical Society*, *131*(6), 2072–2073. doi:10.1021/ja808719p PMID:19170493

Gonzalez, H., Hwang, S. J., & Davis, M. (1999). New class of polymers for the delivery of macromolecular therapeutics. *Bioconjugate Chemistry*, *10*(6), 1068–1074. doi:10.1021/bc990072j PMID:10563777

Guo, W., & Lee, R. J. (2000). Efficient gene delivery using anionic liposome-complexed polyplexes (LPDII). *Bioscience Reports*, *20*(5), 419–432. doi:10.1023/A:1010338219401 PMID:11332603

Han, M., Lv, Q., Tang, X.-J., Hu, Y.-L., Xu, D.-H., Li, F.-Z., ... Gao, J.-Q. (2012). Overcoming drug resistance of MCF-7/ADR cells by altering intracellular distribution of doxorubicin via MVP knockdown with a novel siRNA polyamidoamine-hyaluronic acid complex. *Journal of Controlled Release*, *163*(2), 136–144. doi:10.1016/j.jconrel.2012.08.020 PMID:22940126

Honma, K., Ochiya, T., Nagahara, S., Sano, A., Yamamoto, H., Hirai, K., ... Terada, M. (2001). Atelocollagen-based gene transfer in cells allows high-throughput screening of gene functions. *Biochemical and Biophysical Research Communications*, *289*(5), 1075–1081. doi:10.1006/bbrc.2001.6133 PMID:11741301

Hortobagyi, G. N., Ueno, N. T., Xia, W., Zhang, S., Wolf, J. K., Putnam, J. B., ... Hung, M.-C. (2001). Cationic liposome-mediated E1A gene transfer to human breast and ovarian cancer cells and its biologic effects: A phase I clinical trial. *Journal of Clinical Oncology*, *19*(14), 3422–3433. doi:10.1200/JCO.2001.19.14.3422 PMID:11454891

Hu-Lieskovan, S., Heidel, J. D., Bartlett, D. W., Davis, M. E., & Triche, T. J. (2005). Sequence-specific knockdown of EWS-FLI1 by targeted, nonviral delivery of small interfering RNA inhibits tumor growth in a murine model of metastatic Ewing's sarcoma. *Cancer Research*, *65*(19), 8984–8992. doi:10.1158/0008-5472.CAN-05-0565 PMID:16204072

Huang, M., Fong, C.-W., Khor, E., & Lim, L.-Y. (2005). Transfection efficiency of chitosan vectors: Effect of polymer molecular weight and degree of deacetylation. *Journal of Controlled Release*, *106*(3), 391–406. doi:10.1016/j.jconrel.2005.05.004 PMID:15967533

Hui, K., Ang, P. T., Huang, L., & Tay, S. K. (1997). Phase I study of immunotherapy of cutaneous metastases of human carcinoma using allogeneic and xenogeneic MHC DNA-liposome complexes. *Gene Therapy*, *4*(8), 783–790. doi:10.1038j.gt.3300455 PMID:9338006

Hung, M.-C., Chang, J. Y., & Xing, X. (1998). Preclinical and clinical study of HER-2/neu-targeting cancer gene therapy. *Advanced Drug Delivery Reviews*, *30*(1), 219–227. doi:10.1016/S0169-409X(97)00118-X PMID:10837613

Ibanez, M., Santiago, R., Wong, C., Baeza, I., Gariglio, P., & Chávez, P. (1996). Spermidine-condensed DNA and cone-shaped lipids improve delivery and expression of exogenous DNA transfer by liposomes. *Biochemistry and Cell Biology*, *74*(5), 633–643. doi:10.1139/o96-068 PMID:9018370

Ionov, M., Lazniewska, J., Dzmitruk, V., Halets, I., Loznikova, S., Novopashina, D., ... Bryszewska, M. (2015). Anticancer siRNA cocktails as a novel tool to treat cancer cells. Part (A). Mechanisms of interaction. *International Journal of Pharmaceutics*, *485*(1), 261–269. doi:10.1016/j.ijpharm.2015.03.024 PMID:25791760

Jain, A. (2015). Cationic Polymers for the Delivery of Therapeutic Nucleotides. *Polysaccharides: Bioactivity and Biotechnology*, 1969-1990.

Jain, A. (2014). Cationic Polysaccharides in Gene Delivery. In Cationic Polymers in Regenerative Medicine. Royal Society of Chemistry.

Janát-Amsbury, M. M., Yockman, J. W., Lee, M., Kern, S., Furgeson, D. Y., Bikram, M., & Kim, S. W. (2004). Combination of local, nonviral IL12 gene therapy and systemic paclitaxel treatment in a metastatic breast cancer model. *Molecular Therapy*, *9*(6), 829–836. doi:10.1016/j.ymthe.2004.03.015 PMID:15194049

Jiang, H., Kwon, J.-T., Kim, Y.-K., Kim, E.-M., Arote, R., Jeong, H.-J., ... Cho, C.-S. (2007). Galactosylated chitosan-graft-polyethylenimine as a gene carrier for hepatocyte targeting. *Gene Therapy*, *14*(19), 1389–1398. doi:10.1038j.gt.3302997 PMID:17637795

Jiang, J., Yang, S., Wang, J., Yang, L., Xu, Z., Yang, T., ... Zhang, Q. (2010). Sequential treatment of drug-resistant tumors with RGD-modified liposomes containing siRNA or doxorubicin. *European Journal of Pharmaceutics and Biopharmaceutics*, *76*(2), 170–178. doi:10.1016/j.ejpb.2010.06.011 PMID:20600887

Kadlecova, Z., Rajendra, Y., Matasci, M., Hacker, D., Baldi, L., Wurm, F. M., & Klok, H.-A. (2012). Hyperbranched polylysine: A versatile, biodegradable transfection agent for the production of recombinant proteins by transient gene expression and the transfection of primary cells. *Macromolecular Bioscience*, *12*(6), 794–804. doi:10.1002/mabi.201100519 PMID:22496075

Khan, A., Benboubetra, M., Sayyed, P. Z., Wooi Ng, K., Fox, S., Beck, G., ... Akhtar, S. (2004). Sustained polymeric delivery of gene silencing antisense ODNs, siRNA, DNAzymes and ribozymes: In vitro and in vivo studies. *Journal of Drug Targeting*, *12*(6), 393–404. doi:10.1080/10611860400003858 PMID:15545089

Khan, W. (2013). Cationic polymers for the delivery of therapeutic nucleotides. *Nanotechnology for the Delivery of Therapeutic Nucleic Acids, 8*, 27-56.

Khan, W., Hosseinkhani, H., Ickowicz, D., Hong, P.-D., Yu, D.-S., & Domb, A. J. (2012). Polysaccharide gene transfection agents. *Acta Biomaterialia*, *8*(12), 4224–4232. doi:10.1016/j.actbio.2012.09.022 PMID:23022542

Khandare, J., Calderón, M., Dagia, N. M., & Haag, R. (2012). Multifunctional dendritic polymers in nanomedicine: Opportunities and challenges. *Chemical Society Reviews*, *41*(7), 2824–2848. doi:10.1039/C1CS15242D PMID:22158998

Kichler, A., Leborgne, C., Coeytaux, E., & Danos, O. (2001). Polyethylenimine-mediated gene delivery: A mechanistic study. *The Journal of Gene Medicine*, *3*(2), 135–144. doi:10.1002/jgm.173 PMID:11318112

Kim, C., Shah, B. P., Subramaniam, P., & Lee, K.-B. (2011). Synergistic induction of apoptosis in brain cancer cells by targeted codelivery of siRNA and anticancer drugs. *Molecular Pharmaceutics*, *8*(5), 1955–1961. doi:10.1021/mp100460h PMID:21793576

Kim, Y., Tewari, M., Pajerowski, J. D., Cai, S., Sen, S., Williams, J., ... Discher, D. E. (2009). Polymersome delivery of siRNA and antisense oligonucleotides. *Journal of Controlled Release*, *134*(2), 132–140. doi:10.1016/j.jconrel.2008.10.020 PMID:19084037

Kircheis, R., Schüller, S., Brunner, S., Ogris, M., Heider, K.-H., Zauner, W., & Wagner, E. (1999). Polycation-based DNA complexes for tumor-targeted gene delivery in vivo. *The Journal of Gene Medicine*, *1*(2), 111–120. doi: PMID:10738575

Ko, Y. T., Kale, A., Hartner, W. C., Papahadjopoulos-Sternberg, B., & Torchilin, V. P. (2009). Self-assembling micelle-like nanoparticles based on phospholipid–polyethyleneimine conjugates for systemic gene delivery. *Journal of Controlled Release*, *133*(2), 132–138. doi:10.1016/j.jconrel.2008.09.079 PMID:18929605

Köping-Höggård, M., Vårum, K. M., Issa, M., Danielsen, S., Christensen, B. E., Stokke, B. T., & Artursson, P. (2004). Improved chitosan-mediated gene delivery based on easily dissociated chitosan polyplexes of highly defined chitosan oligomers. *Gene Therapy*, *11*(19), 1441–1452. doi:10.1038j.gt.3302312 PMID:15269712

Kovtun, A., Heumann, R., & Epple, M. (2009). Calcium phosphate nanoparticles for the transfection of cells. *Bio-Medical Materials and Engineering*, *19*(2-3), 241–247. PMID:19581719

Krajcik, R., Jung, A., Hirsch, A., Neuhuber, W., & Zolk, O. (2008). Functionalization of carbon nanotubes enables non-covalent binding and intracellular delivery of small interfering RNA for efficient knock-down of genes. *Biochemical and Biophysical Research Communications*, *369*(2), 595–602. doi:10.1016/j.bbrc.2008.02.072 PMID:18298946

Kukowska-Latallo, J. F., Bielinska, A. U., Johnson, J., Spindler, R., Tomalia, D. A., & Baker, J. R. (1996). Efficient transfer of genetic material into mammalian cells using Starburst polyamidoamine dendrimers. *Proceedings of the National Academy of Sciences of the United States of America*, *93*(10), 4897–4902. doi:10.1073/pnas.93.10.4897 PMID:8643500

Kulkarni, R. P., Mishra, S., Fraser, S. E., & Davis, M. E. (2005). Single cell kinetics of intracellular, nonviral, nucleic acid delivery vehicle acidification and trafficking. *Bioconjugate Chemistry*, *16*(4), 986–994. doi:10.1021/bc050081u PMID:16029041

Ladewig, K., Niebert, M., Xu, Z. P., Gray, P. P., & Lu, G. Q. M. (2010). Efficient siRNA delivery to mammalian cells using layered double hydroxide nanoparticles. *Biomaterials*, *31*(7), 1821–1829. doi:10.1016/j.biomaterials.2009.10.058 PMID:19922997

Laitinen, M., Hartikainen, J., Hiltunen, M. O., Eranen, J., Kiviniemi, M., Narvanen, O., ... Yla-Herttuala, S. (2000). Catheter-mediated vascular endothelial growth factor gene transfer to human coronary arteries after angioplasty. *Human Gene Therapy*, *11*(2), 263–270. doi:10.1089/10430340050016003 PMID:10680840

Lee, E.-S., Ko, K.-K., Joe, Y. A., Kang, S.-G., & Hong, Y.-K. (2011). Inhibition of STAT3 reverses drug resistance acquired in temozolomide-resistant human glioma cells. *Oncology Letters*, *2*(1), 115–121. doi:10.3892/ol.2010.210 PMID:22870139

Lee, J. H., Lee, K., Moon, S. H., Lee, Y., Park, T. G., & Cheon, J. (2009). All-in-One Target-Cell-Specific Magnetic Nanoparticles for Simultaneous Molecular Imaging and siRNA Delivery. *Angewandte Chemie*, *121*(23), 4238–4243. doi:10.1002/ange.200805998 PMID:19408274

Lee, J.-S., Green, J. J., Love, K. T., Sunshine, J., Langer, R., & Anderson, D. G. (2009). Gold, poly (β-amino ester) nanoparticles for small interfering RNA delivery. *Nano Letters*, *9*(6), 2402–2406. doi:10.1021/nl9009793 PMID:19422265

Lee, R. J., & Huang, L. (1996). Folate-targeted, anionic liposome-entrapped polylysine-condensed DNA for tumor cell-specific gene transfer. *The Journal of Biological Chemistry*, *271*(14), 8481–8487. doi:10.1074/jbc.271.14.8481 PMID:8626549

Lee, R. J., Wang, S., & Low, P. S. (1996). Measurement of endosome pH following folate receptor-mediated endocytosis. *Biochimica et Biophysica Acta (BBA)- Molecular Cell Research*, *1312*(3), 237–242. PMID:8703993

Liu, X., Howard, K. A., Dong, M., Andersen, M. Ø., Rahbek, U. L., Johnsen, M. G., ... Kjems, J. (2007). The influence of polymeric properties on chitosan/siRNA nanoparticle formulation and gene silencing. *Biomaterials*, *28*(6), 1280–1288. doi:10.1016/j.biomaterials.2006.11.004 PMID:17126901

Loup, C., Zanta, M.-A., Caminade, A.-M., Majoral, J.-P., & Meunier, B. (1999). Preparation of Water-Soluble Cationic Phosphorus-Containing Dendrimers as DNA Transfecting Agents. *Chemistry (Weinheim an der Bergstrasse, Germany)*, *5*(12), 3644–3650. doi:

Luo, D., & Saltzman, W. M. (2000). Synthetic DNA delivery systems. *Nature Biotechnology*, *18*(1), 33–37. doi:10.1038/71889 PMID:10625387

MacLaughlin, F. C., Mumper, R. J., Wang, J., Tagliaferri, J. M., Gill, I., Hinchcliffe, M., & Rolland, A. P. (1998). Chitosan and depolymerized chitosan oligomers as condensing carriers for in vivo plasmid delivery. *Journal of Controlled Release*, *56*(1), 259–272. doi:10.1016/S0168-3659(98)00097-2 PMID:9801449

Martin, M. E., & Rice, K. G. (2007). Peptide-guided gene delivery. *The AAPS Journal*, *9*(1), E18–E29. doi:10.1208/aapsj0901003 PMID:17408236

McAuliffe, S. M., Morgan, S. L., Wyant, G. A., Tran, L. T., Muto, K. W., Chen, Y. S., ... Dinulescu, D. M. (2012). Targeting Notch, a key pathway for ovarian cancer stem cells, sensitizes tumors to platinum therapy. *Proceedings of the National Academy of Sciences of the United States of America*, *109*(43), E2939–E2948. doi:10.1073/pnas.1206400109 PMID:23019585

Medarova, Z., Kumar, M., Ng, S., Yang, J., Barteneva, N., Evgenov, N. V., ... Moore, A. (2008). Multifunctional magnetic nanocarriers for image-tagged SiRNA delivery to intact pancreatic islets. *Transplantation*, *86*(9), 1170–1177. doi:10.1097/TP.0b013e31818a81b2 PMID:19005396

Meng, H., Liong, M., Xia, T., Li, Z., Ji, Z., Zink, J. I., & Nel, A. E. (2010). Engineered design of mesoporous silica nanoparticles to deliver doxorubicin and P-glycoprotein siRNA to overcome drug resistance in a cancer cell line. *ACS Nano*, *4*(8), 4539–4550. doi:10.1021/nn100690m PMID:20731437

Minakuchi, Y., & ... . (2004). Atelocollagen-mediated synthetic small interfering RNA delivery for effective gene silencing in vitro and in vivo. *Nucleic Acids Research*, *32*(13), e109–e109. doi:10.1093/nar/gnh093 PMID:15272050

Montier, T., Benvegnu, T., Jaffres, P.-A., Yaouanc, J.-J., & Lehn, P. (2008). Progress in cationic lipid-mediated gene transfection: A series of bio-inspired lipids as an example. *Current Gene Therapy*, *8*(5), 296–312. doi:10.2174/156652308786070989 PMID:18855628

Mu, P., Nagahara, S., Makita, N., Tarumi, Y., Kadomatsu, K., & Takei, Y. (2009). Systemic delivery of siRNA specific to tumor mediated by atelocollagen: Combined therapy using siRNA targeting Bcl-xL and cisplatin against prostate cancer. *International Journal of Cancer*, *125*(12), 2978–2990. doi:10.1002/ijc.24382 PMID:19422046

Nabel, G. J., Gordon, D., Bishop, D. K., Nickoloff, B. J., Yang, Z., Aruga, A., ... Chang, A. E. (1996). Immune response in human melanoma after transfer of an allogeneic class I major histocompatibility complex gene with DNA–liposome complexes. *Proceedings of the National Academy of Sciences of the United States of America*, *93*(26), 15388–15393. doi:10.1073/pnas.93.26.15388 PMID:8986821

Nabel, G. J., Nabel, E. G., Yang, Z. Y., Fox, B. A., Plautz, G. E., Gao, X., ... Chang, A. E. (1993). Direct gene transfer with DNA-liposome complexes in melanoma: Expression, biologic activity, and lack of toxicity in humans. *Proceedings of the National Academy of Sciences of the United States of America*, *90*(23), 11307–11311. doi:10.1073/pnas.90.23.11307 PMID:8248244

Nakamura, K., Abu Lila, A. S., Matsunaga, M., Doi, Y., Ishida, T., & Kiwada, H. (2011). A double-modulation strategy in cancer treatment with a chemotherapeutic agent and siRNA. *Molecular Therapy*, *19*(11), 2040–2047. doi:10.1038/mt.2011.174 PMID:21878904

Nguyen, J., Steele, T. W. J., Merkel, O., Reul, R., & Kissel, T. (2008). Fast degrading polyesters as siRNA nano-carriers for pulmonary gene therapy. *Journal of Controlled Release*, *132*(3), 243–251. doi:10.1016/j.jconrel.2008.06.010 PMID:18619502

Ochiya, T., & .... (1999). New delivery system for plasmid DNA in vivo using atelocollagen as a carrier material: The Minipellet. *Nature Medicine*, *5*(6), 707–710. doi:10.1038/9560 PMID:10371512

Ochiya, T., Nagahara, S., Sano, A., Itoh, H., & Terada, M. (2001). Biomaterials for gene delivery atelocollagen-mediated controlled release of molecular medicines. *Current Gene Therapy*, *1*(1), 31–52. doi:10.2174/1566523013348887 PMID:12109137

Ogris, M., Brunner, S., Schüller, S., Kircheis, R., & Wagner, E. (1999). PEGylated DNA/transferrin-PEI complexes: Reduced interaction with blood components, extended circulation in blood and potential for systemic gene delivery. *Gene Therapy*, *6*(4), 595–605. doi:10.1038j.gt.3300900 PMID:10476219

Onishi, H., & Machida, Y. (1999). Biodegradation and distribution of water-soluble chitosan in mice. *Biomaterials*, *20*(2), 175–182. doi:10.1016/S0142-9612(98)00159-8 PMID:10022787

Pandi, P., Jain, A., Raju, S., & Khan, W. (2017). Therapeutic approaches for the delivery of TNF-α siRNA. *Therapeutic Delivery*, *8*(5), 343–355. doi:10.4155/tde-2017-0011 PMID:28361614

Patil, Y., & Panyam, J. (2009). Polymeric nanoparticles for siRNA delivery and gene silencing. *International Journal of Pharmaceutics*, *367*(1), 195–203. doi:10.1016/j.ijpharm.2008.09.039 PMID:18940242

Patil, Y. B., Swaminathan, S. K., Sadhukha, T., Ma, L., & Panyam, J. (2010). The use of nanoparticle-mediated targeted gene silencing and drug delivery to overcome tumor drug resistance. *Biomaterials*, *31*(2), 358–365. doi:10.1016/j.biomaterials.2009.09.048 PMID:19800114

Patnaik, S., Aggarwal, A., Nimesh, S., Goel, A., Ganguli, M., Saini, N., ... Gupta, K. C. (2006). PEI-alginate nanocomposites as efficient in vitro gene transfection agents. *Journal of Controlled Release*, *114*(3), 398–409. doi:10.1016/j.jconrel.2006.06.025 PMID:16891026

Patnaik, S., Arif, M., Pathak, A., Singh, N., & Gupta, K. C. (2010). PEI-alginate nanocomposites: Efficient non-viral vectors for nucleic acids. *International Journal of Pharmaceutics*, *385*(1), 194–202. doi:10.1016/j.ijpharm.2009.10.041 PMID:19874879

Porteous, D. J., Dorin, J. R., McLachlan, G., Davidson-Smith, H., Davidson, H., Stevenson, B. J., ... Innes, J. A. (1997). Evidence for safety and efficacy of DOTAP cationic liposome mediated CFTR gene transfer to the nasal epithelium of patients with cystic fibrosis. *Gene Therapy*, *4*(3), 210–218. doi:10.1038j.gt.3300390 PMID:9135734

Ramamoorth, M., & Narvekar, A. (2015). Non viral vectors in gene therapy-an overview. *Journal of Clinical and Diagnostic Research: JCDR*, *9*(1), GE01. PMID:25738007

Remy, J.-S., Sirlin, C., Vierling, P., & Behr, J.-P. (1994). Gene transfer with a series of lipophilic DNA-binding molecules. *Bioconjugate Chemistry*, *5*(6), 647–654. doi:10.1021/bc00030a021 PMID:7873668

Saad, M., Garbuzenko, O. B., & Minko, T. (2008). Co-delivery of siRNA and an anticancer drug for treatment of multidrug-resistant cancer. *Nanomedicine (London)*, *3*(6), 761–776. doi:10.2217/17435889.3.6.761 PMID:19025451

Sano, A. (2003). Atelocollagen for protein and gene delivery. *Advanced Drug Delivery Reviews*, *55*(12), 1651–1677. doi:10.1016/j.addr.2003.08.005 PMID:14623406

Shah, D. S., Sakthivel, T., Toth, I., Florence, A. T., & Wilderspin, A. F. (2000). DNA transfection and transfected cell viability using amphipathic asymmetric dendrimers. *International Journal of Pharmaceutics*, *208*(1), 41–48. doi:10.1016/S0378-5173(00)00534-2 PMID:11064210

Sher, Y.-P., Chang, C.-M., Juo, C.-G., Chen, C.-T., Hsu, J. L., Lin, C.-Y., ... Hung, M.-C. (2013). Targeted endostatin-cytosine deaminase fusion gene therapy plus 5-fluorocytosine suppresses ovarian tumor growth. *Oncogene*, *32*(9), 1082–1090. doi:10.1038/onc.2012.134 PMID:22562248

Singh, H. D., Wang, G., Uludağ, H., & Unsworth, L. D. (2010). Poly-L-lysine-coated albumin nanoparticles: Stability, mechanism for increasing in vitro enzymatic resilience, and siRNA release characteristics. *Acta Biomaterialia*, *6*(11), 4277–4284. doi:10.1016/j.actbio.2010.06.017 PMID:20601248

Smyth Templeton, N. (2002). Liposomal delivery of nucleic acids in vivo. *DNA and Cell Biology*, *21*(12), 857–867. doi:10.1089/104454902762053828 PMID:12573046

Song, Y. K., Liu, F., Chu, S., & Liu, D. (1997). Characterization of cationic liposome-mediated gene transfer in vivo by intravenous administration. *Human Gene Therapy*, *8*(13), 1585–1594. doi:10.1089/hum.1997.8.13-1585 PMID:9322091

Sorscher, E. J., Logan, J. J., Frizzell, R. A., Lyrene, R. K., Bebok, Z., Dong, J. Y., ... Wiatrak, B. J. (1994). Gene Therapy for Cystic Fibrosis Using Cationic Liposome Mediated Gene Transfer: A Phase I Trial of Safety and Efficacy in the Nasal Airway. University of Alabama at Birmingham, Birmingham, Alabama. *Human Gene Therapy*, *5*(10), 1259–1277. doi:10.1089/hum.1994.5.10-1259 PMID:7531503

Spagnou, S., Miller, A. D., & Keller, M. (2004). Lipidic carriers of siRNA: Differences in the formulation, cellular uptake, and delivery with plasmid DNA. *Biochemistry*, *43*(42), 13348–13356. doi:10.1021/bi048950a PMID:15491141

Stenzel, K. H., Miyata, T., & Rubin, A. L. (1974). Collagen as a biomaterial. *Annual Review of Biophysics and Bioengineering*, *3*(1), 231–253. doi:10.1146/annurev.bb.03.060174.001311 PMID:4607533

Stopeck, A. T. (2001). Phase II study of direct intralesional gene transfer of Allovectin-7, an HLA-B7/β2-microglobulin DNA-liposome complex, in patients with metastatic melanoma. *Clinical Cancer Research*, *7*(8), 2285–2291. PMID:11489803

Su, B., Cengizeroglu, A., Farkasova, K., Viola, J. R., Anton, M., Ellwart, J. W., ... Ogris, M. (2013). Systemic TNFα gene therapy synergizes with liposomal doxorubicine in the treatment of metastatic cancer. *Molecular Therapy*, *21*(2), 300–308. doi:10.1038/mt.2012.229 PMID:23299796

Sun, T.-M., Du, J.-Z., Yao, Y.-D., Mao, C.-Q., Dou, S., Huang, S.-Y., ... Wang, J. (2011). Simultaneous delivery of siRNA and paclitaxel via a "two-in-one" micelleplex promotes synergistic tumor suppression. *ACS Nano*, *5*(2), 1483–1494. doi:10.1021/nn103349h PMID:21204585

Swami, R., Singh, I., Khan, W., & Ramakrishna, S. (2013). Diseases originate and terminate by genes: Unraveling nonviral gene delivery. *Drug Delivery and Translational Research*, *3*(6), 593–610. doi:10.100713346-013-0159-6 PMID:25786377

Szejtli, J., & Osa, T. (1996). *Comprehensive Supramolecular Chemistry: Cyclodextrins* (Vol. 3). Oxford: Elsevier.

Szymański, P., Markowicz, M., & Mikiciuk-Olasik, E. (2011). Nanotechnology in pharmaceutical and biomedical applications: Dendrimers. *Nano*, *6*(06), 509–539. doi:10.1142/S1793292011002871

Tang, M. X., Redemann, C. T., & Szoka, F. C. (1996). In vitro gene delivery by degraded polyamidoamine dendrimers. *Bioconjugate Chemistry*, *7*(6), 703–714. doi:10.1021/bc9600630 PMID:8950489

Tong, H., Shi, Q., Fernandes, J., Liu, L., Dai, K., & Zhang, X. (2009). Progress and prospects of chitosan and its derivatives as non-viral gene vectors in gene therapy. *Current Gene Therapy*, *9*(6), 495–502. doi:10.2174/156652309790031111 PMID:19807649

Toth, I. (1999). Novel cationic lipidic peptide dendrimer vectors in vitro gene delivery. *STP Pharma Sciences, 9*(1), 93-99.

Verma, I. M., & Somia, N. (1997). Gene therapy-promises, problems and prospects. *Nature*, *389*(6648), 239–242. doi:10.1038/38410 PMID:9305836

Vold, I. M. N., Kristiansen, K. A., & Christensen, B. E. (2006). A study of the chain stiffness and extension of alginates, in vitro epimerized alginates, and periodate-oxidized alginates using size-exclusion chromatography combined with light scattering and viscosity detectors. *Biomacromolecules*, *7*(7), 2136–2146. doi:10.1021/bm060099n PMID:16827580

Wadhwa, M. S., Collard, W. T., Adami, R. C., McKenzie, D. L., & Rice, K. G. (1997). Peptide-mediated gene delivery: Influence of peptide structure on gene expression. *Bioconjugate Chemistry*, *8*(1), 81–88. doi:10.1021/bc960079q PMID:9026040

Wang, Y., Gao, S., Ye, W.-H., Yoon, H. S., & Yang, Y.-Y. (2006). Co-delivery of drugs and DNA from cationic core–shell nanoparticles self-assembled from a biodegradable copolymer. *Nature Materials*, *5*(10), 791–796. doi:10.1038/nmat1737 PMID:16998471

Wolfert, M., & Seymour, L. (1998). Chloroquine and amphipathic peptide helices show synergistic transfection in vitro. *Gene Therapy*, *5*(3), 409–414. doi:10.1038j.gt.3300606 PMID:9614562

Xiao, Y., Jaskula-Sztul, R., Javadi, A., Xu, W., Eide, J., Dammalapati, A., ... Gong, S. (2012). Co-delivery of doxorubicin and siRNA using octreotide-conjugated gold nanorods for targeted neuroendocrine cancer therapy. *Nanoscale*, *4*(22), 7185–7193. doi:10.1039/c2nr31853a PMID:23070403

Xiong, X.-B., & Lavasanifar, A. (2011). Traceable multifunctional micellar nanocarriers for cancer-targeted co-delivery of MDR-1 siRNA and doxorubicin. *ACS Nano*, *5*(6), 5202–5213. doi:10.1021/nn2013707 PMID:21627074

Yin, Q., Shen, J., Chen, L., Zhang, Z., Gu, W., & Li, Y. (2012). Overcoming multidrug resistance by co-delivery of Mdr-1 and survivin-targeting RNA with reduction-responsible cationic poly (β-amino esters). *Biomaterials*, *33*(27), 6495–6506. doi:10.1016/j.biomaterials.2012.05.039 PMID:22704597

Yu, Y. H., Kim, E., Park, D. E., Shim, G., Lee, S., Kim, Y. B., ... Oh, Y.-K. (2012). Cationic solid lipid nanoparticles for co-delivery of paclitaxel and siRNA. *European Journal of Pharmaceutics and Biopharmaceutics*, *80*(2), 268–273. doi:10.1016/j.ejpb.2011.11.002 PMID:22108492

Chapter 14
Nanocarriers for Vaccine and Gene Delivery Application

Behiye Şenel
Anadolu University, Turkey

Gülay Büyükköroğlu
Anadolu University, Turkey

ABSTRACT

Nanocarriers with various compositions and biological properties are frequently used systems for in-vitro/in-vivo vaccination and gene transfer. In recent years, developments in nanotechnology have focused on the design and synthesis of nanocarriers that have new properties and can be modified for gene and vaccine delivery. In the favorable results obtained from in-vivo studies performed, they increase interest in these developments and pave the way for their therapeutic use. Nanocarriers have become increasingly important because they can stabilize vaccine antigens and serve as adjuvants, with the advantage of easily transporting genetic material to the target site. In nanocarriers, the molecules involved are adsorbed to the surface or encapsulated in particulates. At the same time, surface modification of nanoparticles allows these systems to carry cargo molecules easily to target site. Among the most studied nanocarriers, lipidic and polymeric systems dendrimers, inorganic nanoparticles, cyclodextrins, cell penetration peptides, and ISCOMs are attracting attention.

INTRODUCTION

Gene therapy is a rapidly advancing field with great potential for treating genetic and acquired systemic diseases. This therapy involves the introduction of foreign genetic material into target cells to alter a genetic sequence. Viral and nonviral vectors are used for this purpose. Viral vectors are the most effective ones, but their applications are limited due to their immunogenicity, oncogenicity, and limited DNA size that they can carry. However, nonviral vectors are safer, less costly, and easier to produce. Moreover, the size of the genetic material that they carry is not limited. Despite improvements in the recent years, low transfection efficiency is still a disadvantage in nonviral systems (Dorraj, Carreras, Nunez, Abushammala, & Melero, 2017).

DOI: 10.4018/978-1-5225-4781-5.ch014

Copyright © 2018, IGI Global. Copying or distributing in print or electronic forms without written permission of IGI Global is prohibited.

Significant progress has been made in traditional vaccination strategies with the developments in biotechnology. In these strategies, the development of vaccine systems in combination with nanostructures, or the use of nanostructures as adjuvants, has facilitated an effective humoral, cellular, and mucosal immunity. These new approaches involve a variety of innovative methods producing effective host responses (Kalam, Khan, & Alshamsan, 2017).

Nanostructures can be designed in a complex manner to be used for treating various diseases. Especially having particles of nanosize in the designed nanocarrier systems affects the gene/vaccine-carrying capacity and the efficacy of these systems in the medical applications. The particle size in the transport systems is an important parameter for reaching the target area from the circulatory system and to be taken out of the cell. These carriers not only increase the effectiveness of the vaccine and genetic material, but also help to release them into the right place. Therefore, it is extremely important to know the physicochemical properties of the carrier system together with cellular and biological properties in nanostructure-mediated gene or vaccine transport, and to make a design by taking all these parameters into consideration.

The aim of this chapter is to provide information and examples of common nanocarriers currently used in gene and vaccine delivery. the general perspective of the article.

Gene Therapy: An Overview

The idea of using genes as medicines in treatments was first put forward in the United States in the 1970s. The emergence of this concept has led to the development of different technologies for determining human gene functions, the elucidation of effects of the mutant human genes with the updated information, and development of different technologies for DNA transmission to mammalian cells (Giacca, 2010).

Different gene manipulation methods can be applied in gene therapy to restore a specific gene function or to knock down a specific gene(s). This requires the transfer of an appropriate gene into a cell to replace a defective or a missing gene (Mellott, Forrest & Detamore, 2013).

Initially, gene therapy was used for treating inherited metabolic diseases such as autosomal or X-linked recessive single-gene disorders, cystic fibrosis), ADA-SCID, emphysema, retinitis pigmentosa, and sickle cell anemia. Later on, anemia, phenylketonuria, hemophilia, Duchenne muscular dystrophy, some autosomal dominant disorders, polygenic disorders, different cancer types, vascular disease, neurodegenerative disorders, inflammatory conditions, and other acquired diseases became targets of gene therapy (Nayerossadat, Maedeh & Ali, 2012; Dizaj, Jafari & Khosroushahi, 2014).

About 2335 studies on clinical gene therapy were performed between 1989 and 2015, and these studies continue worldwide (Hanna, Rémuzat, Auquier & Toumi, 2016).

Almost 38% of these clinical trials were performed with virus-mediated gene transfer. A vast majority of these trials (from phase II to phase III) also involved virus-mediated experiments. Only 24 of these clinical trials in the literature have been reported to reach phase III. The majority of gene therapy targets in the clinic are cancer diseases. The first gene therapy reported in the literature was approved for Glibera, which was given for an adeno-associated virus carrying a lipoprotein lipase gene. This drug was approved by the European Union in 2012 for treating a rare form of hereditary dyslipidemia. Moreover, ONYX-15 was a first-generation oncolytic adenovirus for the local treatment of head and neck cancers in China; however, its use has not been approved in other countries yet (Lukashev & Zamyatnin, 2016; Hanna, Rémuzat, Auquier & Toumi, 2016).

Gene therapy has two main categories: germline gene therapy and somatic gene therapy. The germline gene therapy has tremendous potential; however, these therapies could not be tested in humans due to many judicial, technical, and ethical difficulties predicted in the near future. Today, the human gene therapy is limited with the alterations in somatic cells (Misra, 2013).

Two major transfection strategies have been developed to transfer genetic material such as DNA or RNA to the cells. These are viral and nonviral vectors (Salimzadeh, Jaberipour, Hosseini & Avicenna, 2013).

Some successful viral vector systems used today include retroviruses, adenoviruses, adeno-associated viruses, herpes viruses, cough viruses, human foamy viruses (HFV), and lentiviruses (Nayerossadat, Maedeh & Ali, 2012).

In addition, some bacterial carriers such as *Listeria* and *Salmonella* can be used as a gene carrier system due to their ease of production and storage, capacity to carry a large amount of DNA, and ease of spread from one cell to another (Alpar, Cevher & Özsoy, 2014).

However, not all viruses are suitable for gene therapy. For example, murine leukemia virus and lentiviruses are retroviruses. Lentiviruses can infect nondividing cells; however, murine leukemia virus cannot infect cells. For this reason, these viruses cannot be used for treating neurological diseases (Pohl & Braz, 2001; Marshall, 2002).

Studies have shown that viral vectors are effective tools for transfection. However, their therapeutic use is limited due to serious safety concerns such as immunogenicity and viral insertional mutagenesis. For example, leukemia developed in 2 of 11 children who received a gene therapy using a retroviral vector. This was probably caused by the activation of oncogenes due to viral gene integration. This suggested that existing viral vectors should be used in humans with extreme caution and more vectors should be developed (Marshall, 2002, Pohl & Braz, 2001; Huang, Liu, Dong, Liu, He, & Liu, 2011).

Thus, although nonviral vectors capable of forming nanostructures for nucleic acid delivery are less effective, they are much more attractive due to their low or no immunogenicity, shortened transgenic expression time, cheaper and easier preparation, large-scale production, and vector modification (Elfinger, Uzgun & Rudolph, 2008; Lukashev & Zamyatnin, 2016). The advantages and disadvantages of viral and nonviral vectors are shown in Table 1.

Table 1. Advantages and disadvantages of the main viral and non-viral vectors

	Advantages	Disadvantages
Viral Vectors		
Adeno Virus	• High titers • Infects both dividing and non-dividing cells • Wide tissue tropism • Efficient gene transfer • Easily modify tissue tropism • Insertion of large DNA fragments	• Transient expression • Highly immunogenic • High titers of virus can be toxic • DNA size limitation • Short expression duration
Retrovirus	• Integration • Permanent expression • Pseudo-typed virus • Long term genetic alterations • Low immunogenicity • Insertion of large DNA fragments	• Only infecting dividing cells • Insertional mutagenesis (tumor formation) • Activate oncogenes • Inhibit tumor suppressor genes

continued on following page

Table 1. Continued

	Advantages	Disadvantages
AVV	• High titers • Integration and persistent expression • Low immunogenicity • No insertional mutagenesis • Infects both dividing and non-dividing cells • Safety	• DNA Size limitation ~4.9 kb • Low titer of virus • Low level of gene expression
Herpes Virus	• Prolonged gene expression • Safe for use in immunocompromised patients	• Common pathogen in humans • Difficult to produce in large amount
Pox Virus	• High stable insertion capacity	• Complex structure and biology • Low biosafety • Risk of cytopathic effects
	Non-Viral Vectors	
Lipidic Nanoparticles	• Safety • Carry large DNA molecules • No immune response • Stable complex • Targeting to specific cells • Simple and easy production • Structure and features well illuminated • Electrostatically bind to DNA • Biocompatibility and biodegradability	• Low transfection efficiency • Inhibited by serum nucleases • Limited stability for liposomes • Fast clearance
Polymeric Nanoparticles	• Stability • Simple and easy production • Natural polymer are safe for cytotoxicity • Structure and features well illuminated • Electrostatically bind to DNA • Make surface modification	• Destabilization of incorporated molecules during particle preparation • Rapid clearance • Synthetic polymers can be toxic
Dendrimers	• Very precise size and shape controllability • Water solubility • Biocompatibility • Low immune response • Easy electrostatic interaction with nucleic acid • Protection from nuclease activity	• Specific cytotoxicity • Limited release ability • Rapid clearance
Cyclodextrins (CD)	• Low toxicity • Acting as molecular containers that can help to increase the biological properties of the loaded molecules • Behavior of the immune stimulus at an unobservable level • *In vivo* stability	• High production costs • Security concerns • Limited dissolution properties
	Inorganic Materials	
CNTs	• Ultra-high functionalization and loading capacities • High penetration capacity for biological barriers • Encapsulation properties • Storage functions	• Difficulty in production • Cytotoxicity • Problems in biodegradability
Silica Nanoparticles	• Large surface area • Stability • Biocompatibility • Controllable porosity	• *In vivo* toxicity
Magnetic Nanoparticles	• Large surface area, • Long stay in circulation • Advanced tissue penetration • High magnetisation properties for remote controlled rapid transport, potential for multimodal applications (targeting, diagnosis and therapy etc.)	• Poor stability • Problems in biodegradability • High cost in large-scale of production • Limited biocompatibility

Liu, Chia & Tian, 2004; Ragusa, García, & Penadés, 2007; Elfinger, Uzgun & Rudolph, 2008; (Nayerossadat, Maedeh & Ali, 2012; Mellott, Forrest &Detamore, 2013; Dizaj, Jafari & Khosroushahi, 2014; Loh, Lee, Doua & Deene, 2016; Kalam, Khan, & Alshamsan, 2017.

What Are DNA Vaccines?

Vaccination plays a key role in public health in terms of being able to remove or control various infectious or epidemic diseases (Greenwood, 2014).

At the beginning of the 1990s, it was shown that plasmid DNA could be transfected directly into animal cells *in vivo*, and then plasmid DNA encoding antigenic proteins was directly injected into animals to induce immune responses. This method, called nucleic acid immunization, has been used in preclinical animal models to elicit various protective antibodies and cell-mediated immunological responses in viral, bacterial, and parasitic diseases (Donnelly, Ulmer, Shiver & Liu, 1997)

Conventional vaccines (or the first-generation vaccines) consist of live, attenuated, or dead microorganisms. The whole microorganism is needed to prepare the vaccine. Although the conventional vaccines are useful in preventing diseases, they have some limitations. For example, the attenuated forms of these pathogens may turn into a harmful form and cause disease. Unlike conventional vaccines, dead grafts do not show any characteristics of creating harmful forms. However, even if dead vaccines produce an antibody response, they do not produce a cellular response (T-killer response). Antibody production may or may not be sufficient for infection depending on the disease. Therefore, second-generation vaccines have been developed to reduce risk rates. These are subunit vaccines consisting of defined protein antigens or recombinant protein components (G. Kumar, S. Kumar, Varghese, Chamoli & Barthwal, 2013). Nucleic acid vaccines, referred to as third-generation vaccines, are among the simple but effective tools of stimulating broad-based immunity. Nucleic acid vaccines are a novel and important technology that uses DNA or RNA genetically engineered to produce an immunologic response. Unlike gene therapy, genetic integration is not aimed. They are designed to allow localized and short-term expression of the target antigen (Novicki, 2005; Hasson, Al-Busaidi & Sallam, 2015)

How Does It Work?

In classical vaccinations, antigens are used to produce immune responses in the body. No antigen is given in DNA- or RNA-based vaccines. Only genetic information–containing RNA or DNA is used to produce antigen. Thus, in this particular vaccination, instructions are given to the body to produce the antigen itself via the delivery of DNA and RNA. These vaccines may be injected in various ways. For example, intradermal, intravenous and intralymphatic injections can be given for their transfection. Transfected cells use the RNA sequence of the antigen to synthesize the protein. These cells then allow the excretion of the antigen exerting an immune response. Nucleic acid vaccines, such as live or attenuated virus vaccines, also affect the major histocompatibility complex (MHC)-I and MHC-II pathways that allow for the induction of CD8 + and CD4 + T cells. Antigenic molecules found in soluble form, such as the recombinant protein produced, often induce only antibody production in the immune system (Leitner, Ying & amp; Restifo, 1999).

One of the most important aspects of vaccination is the need for new adjuvants (immunostimulants) and delivery systems. Until recently, the adjuvants licensed for use in humans were aluminum, calcium hydroxide, and phosphate salts. However, the use of alum-type adjuvants for vaccination has some disadvantages. They are not effective for all antigens and induce local reactions and immunoglobulin E antibody responses. However, they do not induce cell-mediated immunity and specific cytotoxic T lymphocyte (CTL) responses. Therefore, more efficient and safe adjuvants and vaccine delivery systems need to be developed to achieve high and long-term immune responses (Brewer, 2006; Akagi, Baba & Akashi, 2012).

On the contrary, new strategies for developing protective and therapeutic vaccines have focused on targeting antigens to dendritic cells (DCs) and relocating these cells for an extended period of time. Nanostructures are used in these strategies. These carriers can stay with an antigen for a long time, without causing any deformation, to increase the possibility of antigen uptake and handling by DCs. DCs are the most effective antigen-presenting cells (APCs) implicating in initiating T-cell-mediated immunity. DCs shape T-cell-mediated immune responses by expressing both activating and inhibitory factors. For example, they can stimulate T-cell immune responses by means of the MHC Class I and II pathways (shown in Figure 1). They also establish the induction of activation-induced cell death through the Fas/Fas ligand (Fas/FasL) system and the inhibition of T-cell response (Termeer, Averbeck, Hara, Eibel, Herrlich, Sleeman, & Simon, 2003; Akagi, Baba & Akashi, 2012).

Recent developments have facilitated the understanding of antigen presentation by innate immune cells and their interaction with the adaptive immune system, thereby contributing to the design and development of vaccine delivery systems. The most important elements that an effective vaccine should have are as follows:

- Ability to have an antigen that elicits an adaptive immune response,
- Immunopotency to stimulate the innate immune system,
- The development of a delivery system to target APCs (Mohan, Verna & Nageswara, 2013).

From this point of view, nanoparticle-based vaccine delivery systems designed to meet these criteria have many advantages over conventional vaccines:

- They prevent deterioration of the antigen and increase its stability,
- They stimulate co-encapsulation of the antigen, and the immune-stimulating substance increases the immunogenicity and potency of the vaccines,

Figure 1. MHC I and MHC II pathways after transfection

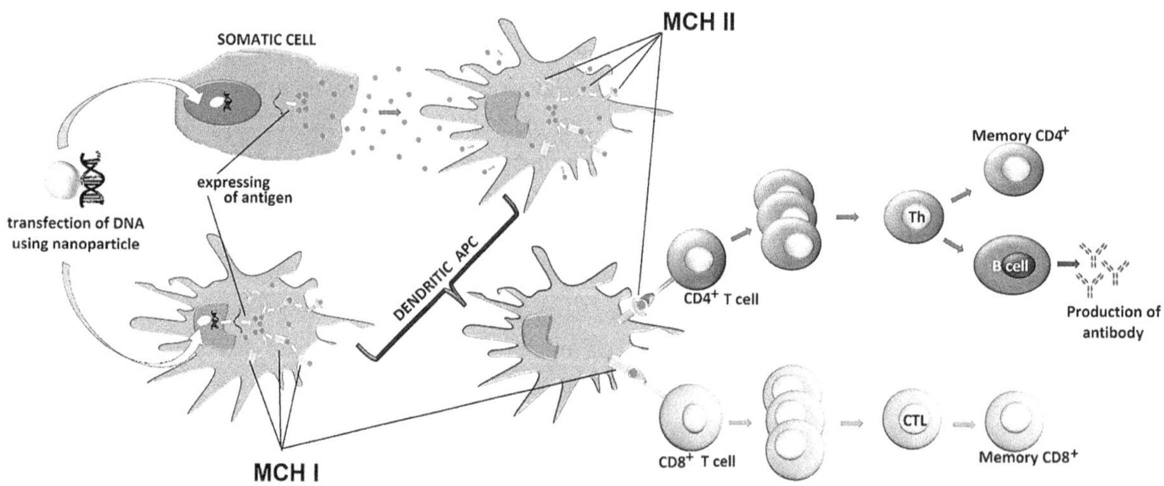

- APCs can phagocyte and process nanoparticles,
- They increase the MHC-I presentation of the antigens, thereby inducing CTL cell responses,
- Antigens on the surfaces of the particles allow an increase in humoral immunity,
- It facilitates targeting surface modifications in the particles (Mohan, Verna & Nageswara, 2013; Sahdev, Ochyl & Moon, 2014).

Cellular Uptake of Nanocarriers and Biological Barriers

The target of gene therapy is that the transferred gene works in the cell by reaching the cytoplasm or the nucleus. Although the targeted nanocarriers have many advantages, they have not been as effective as initially expected. The various barriers outside or inside the cell are important factors limiting the success of gene therapy.

When the genetic material is administered *in vivo*, it comes in contact with the intracellular environment, such as the bloodstream, stomach, intestines, and respiratory tract mucosa. Before reaching the target organ, the genetic material cannot stay in the bloodstream for a long time, especially due to enzymatic activities. The naked DNA applied via parenteral routes (i.v. or i.m.) has a half-life of 1.2–21 min (Alpar, Cevher & Özsoy, 2014).

Therefore, nanostructures have gained considerable interest in recent years, especially because they allow the therapeutic agents, such as proteins, peptides, and nucleic acids, to be stable against enzymatic degradation and enable (cellular/tissue) transportation and sustained release of these therapeutic agents to the target tissue (Dizaj, Jafari & Khosroushahi, 2014).

In addition, nanocarriers also enable passive targeting via enhanced permeability and retention (EPR) of tumoral tissues due to the small particle size (1–1000 nm), thus allowing the molecules they carry to reach the target region (Acharya & Sahoo, 2011; Nakamura & Maeda, 2011). The activities of these nanostructures are critically dependent on properties such as particle size, degradation, and clearance. For example, the nanocarrier should be within a size range of 10–100 nm to use the EPR effect efficiently. If the nanocarrier is less than 10 nm, it is rapidly cleared by the kidneys and larger carriers are cleared by the reticuloendothelial system. Additionally, the disintegration of particles also depends on particle size (Panyam, Dali, Sahoo, Ma, Chakravarthi, Amidon, & ...Labhasetvar, 2003). Besides particle size, particle shape of the nanostructures also has a strong effect on the carrier performance. For example, a study showed that long rod-shaped nanoparticles reduce cell viability compared with those with short rod and spherical shapes (Huang, Teng, Chen, Tang & He, 2010).

Nanostructures are introduced into the cell via a process called endocytosis. After carriers are successfully endocytosed depending on the intended target, they are directed to the relevant organelles of the cell. The endocytosis process is widely divided into two categories: (1) phagocytosis involving the uptake of large particles and; (2) pinocytosis involving the ingestion of liquids and solutes. Phagocytosis is mainly observed in special mammalian cells such as macrophages, whereas pinocytosis occurs in all cells. Pinocytosis is accomplished via four major mechanisms: macropinocytosis, clathrin-mediated endocytosis, caveolae-mediated endocytosis, and clathrin/caveolea-independent endocytosis (Palakurthi, Yellepeddi & Kumar, 2011). Particles of 2–3 µm size are taken up by macrophages via phagocytosis. Nanoparticles of almost 1 µm size are taken up via macropinocytosis. Particles of ~ 120 nm size are taken up via clathrin-mediated endocytosis, whereas nanoparticles less than ~90 nm are taken up via clathrin/caveolae-independent endocytosis, and particles of smaller nanosize range (~ 60 nm) are taken up via caveolin-mediated endocytosis (Petros & DeSimone, 2010). The most common endocytosis used by targeted nanocarriers is clathrin-mediated endocytosis through endocytic route receptor–ligand interaction (Palakurthi, Yellepeddi & Kumar, 2011). In Figure 2 shows a nanoparticle system, the pathways to the target tumor site and the uptake of nanoparticles from a cell after delivery to the body.

Figure 2. An example of a nanocarrier, condition in systemic circulation, different mechanisms of endocytosis

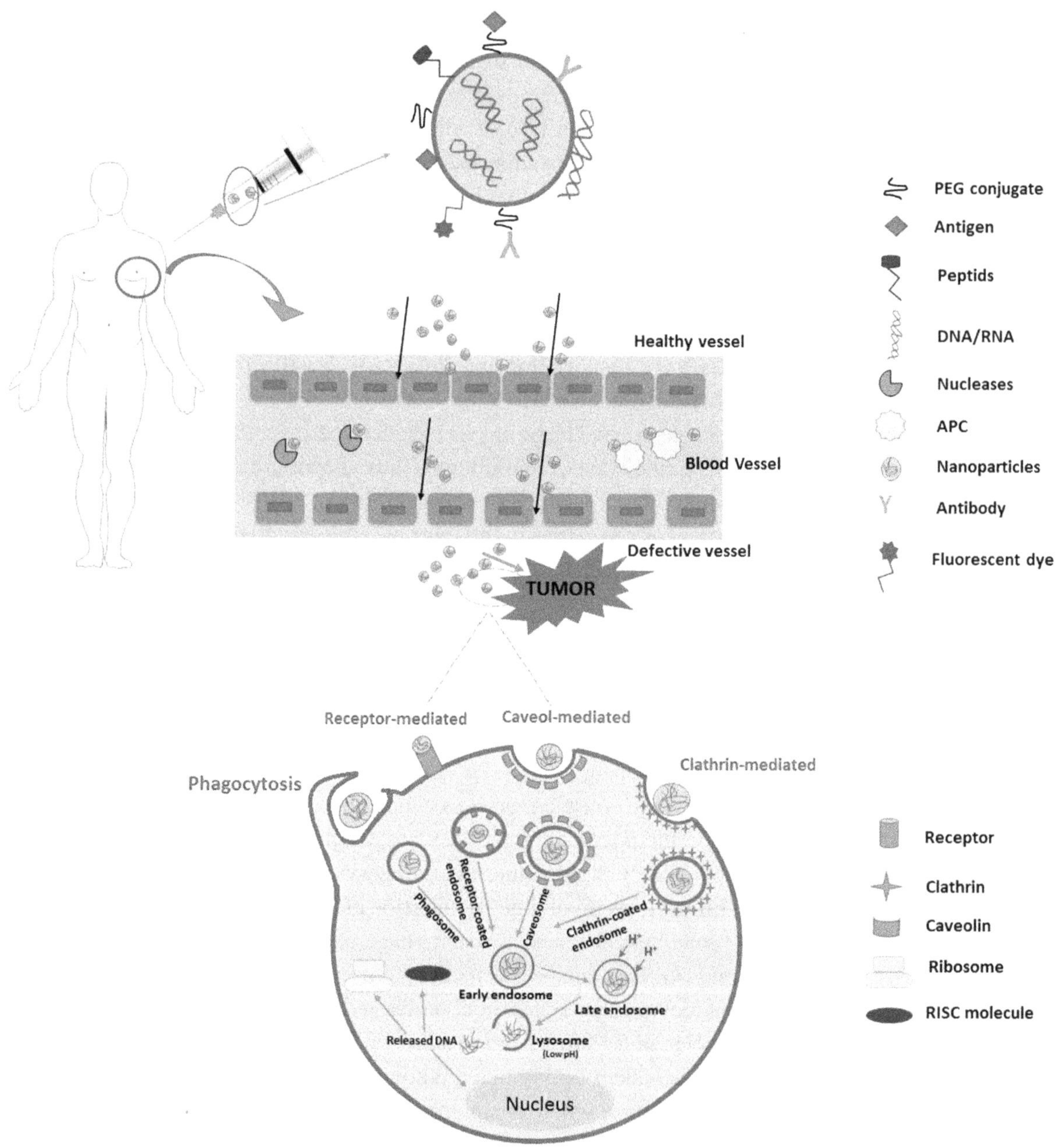

NANOCARRIERS USED FOR VACCINES AND NUCLEIC ACIDS

Various nanoparticles, nanocapsules, emulsions, micelle systems, metal ion nanoparticles, and nanoconjugates have been used for nucleic acids and vaccines so far (both carrier and adjuvant). It is important to use carrier systems to ensure that nucleic acids and vaccine antigens can stay in circulation and at the target site for a long period of time, preventing them from being cleaved by plasma nuclease or eliminated by immune system organelles (Storni, Kundig, Senti & Johansen, 2005).

This section described the nanocarriers used for vaccines and nucleic acids with examples.

Polymeric Nanocarriers

Systems comprise mostly spherical particles with a size range of 1–1000 nm carrying the relevant molecules. The materials to be transported can be encapsulated in polymeric matrices or adsorbed or conjugated on the surface of nanoparticles (Luten, van Nostrum, De Smed & Hennink, 2008). The most commonly used polymers include poly(lactic-co-glycolic acid) (PLGA), poly-L-lysine (PLL), PEI (Polyethylenimine), polyethylene glycol (PEG), dendrimers, and chitosan.

PLGA

PLGA-based nanoparticles appear to be a potential vector for gene delivery. Studies have shown that PLGA provides a better safety profile compared with high-molecular-weight PEIs and liposomes. Furthermore, it has been shown that these nanoparticles cannot interfere with the transfection efficiency of the serum (Dizaj, Jafari & Khosroushahi, 2014).

Nanoparticles such as PLGA coated with different lipid molecules to form hybrid nanostructures are available in recent years with the developments in surface engineering. It is stated that the target specificity of these hybrid carriers is high and the nanoparticle–cell relationship is also improved due to their physicochemical properties. Thus, these carriers have been reported to increase *in vivo* cellular permeability, formation of an immunological response, and also half-life in circulation (Bose, Lee & Park, 2016).

Biodegradable nanostructures produced from PLGA polymers exhibit a safety profile approved by the US, the Food and Drug Administration, and the European Medicine Agency. Besides good and controlled long-term release capabilities, these nano-sized carriers are frequently used as strong antigenic/adjuvant carriers. They also have biocompatible and degradable properties (Storni, Kundig, Senti & Johansen, 2005). Since the long-term release of antigens can provide more effective immune responses, long-term release aspect is an important parameter for grafting. Additionally, it also avoids the risk of tolerance and generally does not require boosting administrations to provide protective immunity. Some *in vitro* studies have also shown that long-term release is achieved from PLGA nanoparticles in which antigens are encapsulated (Danhier, Ansorena, Silva, Coco, Le Breton, & Preat, 2012).

Conjugations with two or more polymeric block copolymers such as PLGA-b-PEG and PLA-b-PEG have become remarkable in vaccine studies because the copolymers carry the combined advantages of individual polymers and maximize the uptake efficiency of the vaccine and cells (Cruz, Tacken, Fokkink & Figdor, 2011).

PEG

PEG is a good peptide and protein carrier. It maintains its own properties when covalently attached to another molecule. Coating the surface of the formed carrier system with PEG prevents the interference and binding of blood compounds to the surface of the nanoparticle sterically. This prevents the opsonization and recognition of the carriage system by the reticuloendothelial system elements. Thus, the PEG-conjugated carrier system can survive in the blood circulation for a long time. Accordingly, PEG is generally used for surface protection in carrier systems (Ramamoorth & Narvekar, 2015). The half-life of nanoparticles in circulation can vary according to the changes in the PEG chain length, PEG density, surface coverage, particle size, and surface load (Li & Huang, 2010).

The disadvantage of the PEGylated surface is that it reduces the efficiency of uptake by the target cells, thereby causing a decrease in biological activity. The PEG conjugation in nanoparticles reduces the cellular uptake capacity of nanoparticles and the ability to release charge from endosomes, inhibiting the formation of essential nonbilayer intermediates and fusion with the cell and/or endosomal membrane and eventually reducing transfection efficiency. Therefore, some neutral auxiliary lipids (such as cholesterol) are recommended to improve the ability of liposomes with PEG to be taken up by the target (Al-Dosari & Gao, 2009; Zhang, Satterlee & Huang, 2012; Ramamoorth & Narvekar, 2015).

Factors such as chain length, particle size, targeting, and surface properties of polymers in developing vaccine systems are crucial in cellular uptake and immunization of the antigen. For example, both PEG chain length and antibody conjugation for targeting these chains have been shown to be important parameters influencing vaccine delivery and immunological responses (Cruz, Tacken, Fokkink & Figdor, 2011).

PEI

PEI is a cationic polymer synthesized in various forms including linear or branched and high- or low-molecular-weight species. These polymers, which form nano-scale complexes (polyplexes) with nucleic acids and have high amine content, are widely used for gene transfer through electrostatic interactions (Wegmann, Gartlan, Harandi, Brinckmann, Coccia, Hillson, …Settantau, 2012).

These polyplexes can bind heparan sulfate proteoglycans present on the surface of cells, including APCs, and migrate into cells via endocytosis. During endosomal acidification (up to pH 3), the buffering effect of PEI (i.e., proton sponge effect, shown in Figure 3) causes osmotic tearing of endosomes and allows polyplexes to enter the cytosol and release their content. Thus, it is believed that PEI–DNA polyplexes increase plasmid DNA uptake and enhance immune responses in the cell (Grant, Thomas, Fortune, Klibanov & Letvin, 2012; Benjaminsen, Mattebjerg, Henriksen, Moghimi & Andresen, 2013).

High transfection efficiency and low cytotoxicity are two main targets in gene therapy research. However, the cytotoxicity and broad size distributions of polyplexes prepared using PEI alone are the limiting factors for the transport of genetic material. In particular, the high-molecular-weight PEI shows severe cytotoxicity and reduced blood compatibility due to its strong electrostatic interactions with cell membranes and extracellular matrix (Jäger, Schubert, Ochrimenko, Fischer, & Schubert, 2012; Wang, Niu, Hu & Li, 2015). In addition, endosomal swelling and rupture upon endocytotic PEI uptake cause some changes in intracellular stresses and mitochondria. As a result, high rates of apoptotic cell death are observed (Beyerle, Irmler, Beckers, Kissel, & Stoeger, 2010; Wang, Niu, Hu & Li, 2015).

Figure 3. Proton sponge effect

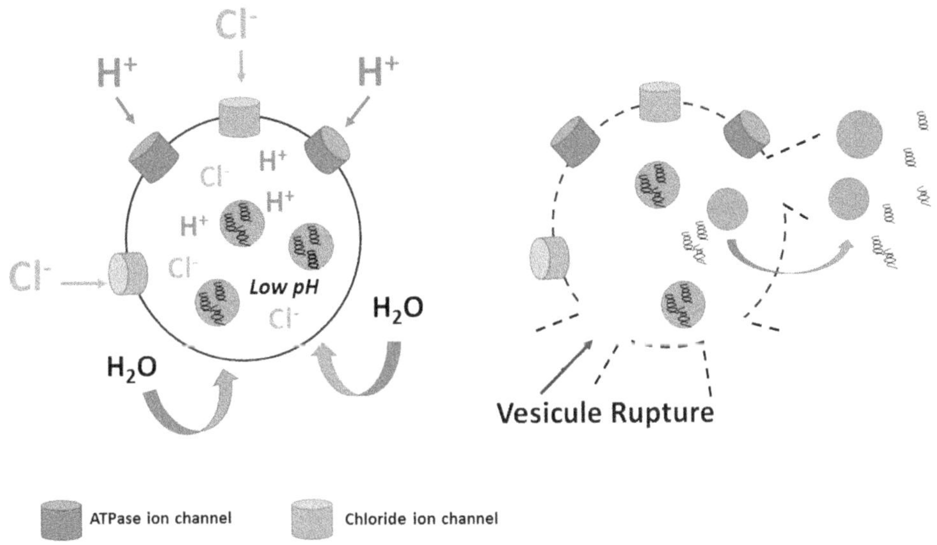

It has been determined that the three-dimensional structure and elasticity of PEI molecules affect the safety and efficacy of these molecules as well as many structural parameters such as molar mass, type, number, and charge density (Fischer, Li, Ahlemeyer, Krieglstein, & Kissel, 2003; Wang, Niu, Hu & Li, 2015). For example, branched polymers exhibit higher transfection efficiency because of the high cationic charge and are considered to be the "gold standard" for the delivery of genes with a molecular weight of 25 kDa (Patnaik & Gupta, 2013).

PEI is also implicated in the transport of PEI-based DNA vaccines. For example, a study reported that administration of intravenous PEI–DNA plasmid complexes increased gene expression levels 20- to 400-fold. It was also found that the DNA-induced epitope-specific CD8 T-cell responses also increased 10–25 times (Grant, Thomas, Fortune, Klibanov & Letvin, 2012).

However, recent studies have shown that PEI has a strong adjuvant effect. Conventional vaccines containing PEI as immunostimulant have been found to be more effective in treating infections or tumors (Shen, Li, Zhang, Li, Shen, Zhu, & Tao, 2017), thereby enhancing the production of antigen-specific antibodies, cytokines, and chemokines.

PLL

PLL is a biodegradable peptide synthesized by polymerization of lysine in N-carboxy-anhydride. It can form nanometer-sized complexes with nucleic acids due to the presence of protonatable amine groups on the lysine moiety. The most commonly used PLL has a degree of polymerization between 90 and 450. This property helps in the *in vivo* use of PLL, making this peptide structure suitable for biodegradation (Zhang, Xu,Wang, Qiao, Liu, & Li, 2004).

However, the low-molecular-weight PLL interacts with DNA at low rates and results in rapid excretion from Kupffer cells in the liver. The activity of PLL increases as the molecular weight increases, but it has been shown to increase cytotoxicity as well (Dizaj, Jafari & Khosroushahi 2014).

PLL has a low transfection rate when it is used alone. However, binding of PLL to plasma proteins and its rapid clearance from the systemic circulation limit the *in vivo* use of these polymers (Perera & Bernkop-Schnürch, 2012). It also requires the addition of an endosomolytic agent, such as chlorosine or a fusogenic peptide, to allow release into the cytoplasm. Forming a complex with PEG is preferred to prevent binding of plasma proteins and increase circulation half-life (Tiera, Winnik & Fernandes, 2006).

Chitosan

Chitosan is obtained by deacetylation of chitin. It is a biocompatible polysaccharide composed of repeating D-glucosamine and N-acetyl-glucosamine units linked to each other via glycosidic bonds (Mao, Sun & Kissel, 2010).

Chitosan has the ability to interact with negatively charged molecules such as DNA and RNA due to its highly cationic nature (Cheung, Ng, Wong, & Chan, 2015). The binding affinity, stability, and particle size of chitosan, and the activity and release of the complex in the cell depend on the parameters of the formulation prepared. These parameters are the molecular weight of chitosan, degree of deacetylation, stoichiometry of complex (N / P ratio), concentration of genetic material, serum concentration, pH of the transfection medium, and so forth (De Martimprey, Vauthier, Malvy & Couvreur, 2009).

Chitosan has been proposed as a safe alternative to other nonviral vectors for gene transfer. However, the poor water solubility of chitosan limits its biomedical applications. Various chemical modifications have been made to increase the solubility and variety of applications of chitosan since its discovery. The conversion of chitosan into chitooligosaccharide is the most remarkable one among these modifications(Alves & Mano, 2008). Chitooligosaccharides are partial hydrolysis products of chitosan. These products have antimicrobial, antioxidant, anti-inflammatory, and antitumor effects (Park & Kim, 2010).

Many studies have shown that chitosan nanoparticles loaded with genetic material can achieve high transfection levels in many cell lines. This is because they can open intracellular tight junctions (Illum, 1998).

Chitosan has various remarkable properties such as high availability, biodegradability and biocompatibility for vaccine delivery applications. In addition, it has some other features such as, the presence of high-density amino groups in chitosan, easy chemical modification, complexation with negatively charged antigens, and mucoadhesive properties (Islam, Firdous, Choi, Yun & Cho, 2012).

The antigen-loaded chitosan nanoparticles prepared by Koppolu et al. were compared with the soluble antigen. Eventually, chitosan particles were found to significantly increase the upregulation of co-stimulatory markers on APCs and the release of proinflammatory cytokines [e.g., interleukin (IL)-1β, IL-6, and tumor necrosis factor (TNF)-α]. Chitosan particles carrying ovalbumin (OVA) antigen promoted antigen delivery via MHC-I and MHC-II pathways in dendritic cells (DCs) compared with equivalent doses of soluble antigens and increased proliferation of antigen-specific CD4+ and CD8+ T cells. Interestingly, macrophages and DCs exhibited maximum antigen uptake by 1 μm chitosan particles, while 300 nm and 3 μm particles reduced the *in vitro* antigen uptake (Koppolu & Zaharoff, 2013).

Biopolymers such as chitosan can be used as stable carriers that trigger an immune response for diseases such as hepatitis B, tetanus, and leishmaniasis. For example, chitosan formulations prepared with ionic gelation have been tested for transport of TLR3 agonist poly (I:C) (pIC) and T-helper peptide (PADRE;Pan DR Epitope) to produce antibodies against the disease. Chitosan nanoparticles (CNPs) are important in achieving good immune responses in mice. The current state of the antigen in CNPs is an important factor influencing immune response. However, adsorption of the peptide on the CNP surface resulted in a higher antibody response to the entrapping counterpart (Correia-Pinto, Csaba, Schiller & Alonso, 2015).

Chitosan is a mucoadhesive adjuvant that has been shown to enhance the immunological response to various antigens in preclinical models and, more importantly, in human subjects. Also, alive virus studies have clearly demonstrated the effectiveness of chitosan-based vaccines in protective immunity. Depending on the vaccine antigen used, chitosan may function as an independent adjuvant or an auxiliary compound. The excellent safety profile of chitosan is of particular importance when considering the reactogenicity and/or toxicity of many of the alternative vaccine adjuvants (Smith, Perelman & Hinchcliffe, 2014; Kalam, Khan, & Alshamsan, 2017).

Dendrimers

Dendrimers are polymer-based molecules that have a functional terminal group as well as a symmetrical structure of definite size and shape. Dendrimers are composed of three parts. They are a central core consisting of a single atom or atom with two or more similar chemical functions, branching from the nucleus and repeating units, and terminal functional groups at the end (Nandy, Santosh & Maiti, 2012).

Dendrimers are synthetic and highly branched macromolecular compounds consisting of an inner core attached to a series of branches like a tree. Every monomer layer is called a generation. Polymer-based dendrimers may be hydrophilic or hydrophobic. Thus, genetic material/ns (polypeptide/polysaccharide) are incorporated into the nucleus or bound to the surface (Aulenta, Hayes & Rannard, 2003).

At physiological pH, positively charged peripheral groups of dendrimers and negatively charged phosphate groups of nucleic acids interact. Due to their nanometric dimensions, dendrimers can interact effectively with cell components such as organelles and proteins (Dutta, Jain, McMillan & Parekh, 2010).

Polyamidoamine (PAMAM) dendrimers are highly branched, spherical polymers having primary amino groups with high surface solubility and unique surface charge in aqueous solutions. They can be produced in large quantities and synthesized over a range of molecular weights. The structure starts with a core molecule and gradually grows during the polymerization process. The number of surface amine groups increases with each generation for the attachment of antibodies, contrast agents, and radiopharmaceuticals used in various applications. PAMAM dendrimers are of great interest because of their nano-spherical, hyperbranched and monodisperse molecules suitable for gene delivery (Jin, Zeng, Liu, Deng & He, 2014).

The toxicity profile of dendrimers is good, but it may vary depending on the number of terminal amino groups and the positive charge density. Furthermore, toxicity increases with an increase in concentration and generation because the number of surface groups doubles with increasing number of generations (Choi, Kang, Kim, Lim & Chung, 2010).

Several studies have reported the nanoparticle potentials of dendrimers to carry vaccines. Starburst dendrimers are patented systems as powerful adjuvants for influenza vaccination. Since the formulation is effective at small concentrations, no toxicity is reported. Moreover, the required dose of antigen has been reduced due to the strong adjuvant effect. Middle-generation dendrimers have been found to produce a stronger immune response. Belldegrum and colleagues were the first to investigate dendrimer-based anticancer vaccination against renal cell carcinoma using the G250 kidney cancer–specific antigen (Belldegrun & Tso, 2002; Jain, Khoane, Jain & Dani, 2011).

Lipidic Nanocarriers

Lipid-based systems have long been used in pharmaceutical preparations, such as drug/gene/vaccine delivery systems, because they are composed of well-conferred physiological lipids. Cationic liposomes, cationic lipids, cationic solid lipids, and cationic emulsions are lipid-based structures routinely used for antigen delivery to the cells by nucleic acids.

Cationic Lipids

Cationic lipids are amphiphilic molecules with a hydrophilic head and a hydrophobic tail. The hydrophobic chain is usually formed with fatty acyl, alkyl, or alcoxy chains and affects the physical properties of the lipid bilayer. The hydrophilic head group is composed of one or more amine groups comprising primary, secondary, and tertiary amines or quaternary ammonium salts. Also, a linker connects the hydrophobic tail to the hydrophilic head. This linker determines the biodegradability toxicity, and transfection efficiency of cationic lipids (Koynova & Tenchov, 2010; Thapa & Narain, 2016).

Quaternary ammonium detergents have been used for the transport of many solid lipid NPs such as cholesterol, cationic derivatives of diacylglycerol, and lipid derivatives of polyamines. Dioleylpropyl trimethylammonium chloride (DOTMA), DOTAP, and dioleoylphosphatidylethanolamine (DOPE) are three of the most popular cationic lipids (Liu & Zhang, 2011)

Cationic lipids have some disadvantages such as poor stability, rapid clearance, and low efficacy and anti-inflammatory response. Therefore, cationic lipids have failed in clinical trials. For example, Allovectin-7 Phase III, consisting of plasmid DNA/DOPE/DMRIE for treating metastatic melanoma, is a cationic lipid formulation that has reached the clinical stage but cannot overcome this stage (Yang, Leonand & Gan, 2017)

Lipid nanoparticles (LNPs) may have an adjuvant effect by themselves. Some lipids activate the immune system and can reduce inflammation. Activation of the immune system is a challenge in protein replacement therapy and gene therapy, but it is a desirable advantage for vaccination. In particular, LNPs containing cationic lipids, such as the DOTAP chloride salt, have been shown to activate Toll-like 4 (TLR 4) and produce a strong proinflammatory response with Th1-type cytokines such as IL-2, IFN-γ, and TNF-α (Kedmi, Arie & Peer, 2010; Reichmuth, Oberli, Jaklenec, Langer & Blankschtein, 2016).

TLRs are a class of receptors expressed in APCs. TLRs have become the target of adjuvant studies because inflammation-inducing cytokines are produced following the activation of TLRs. The use of TLR as an adjuvant to transport lipids further enhances the vaccine potential and provides an advantage in targeting the immune response in the desired direction (Akira, 2011).

Solid Lipid Nanoparticles

Solid lipid nanoparticles (SLNs) have been explored since the early 1990s and developed as an alternative to traditional carrier systems such as emulsion liposomes and polymeric systems (Chime & Onyishi, 2013).

A solid lipid nanoparticle is typically spherical and has a solid lipid core that can be dissolved in lipophilic molecules with a particle diameter ranging from about 10 to about 1000 nm.

SLNs are nano-sized particles prepared by using lipids that are solid at room and body temperatures and can be stabilized with surfactants. Triglycerides (tristearin, etc.), fatty acids (stearic acid, etc.), steroids (cholesterol, etc.), and waxes (cetyl palmitate, etc) are examples of the solid lipids used (Saupe & Rades, 2006).

SLNs can be prepared via high-pressure homogenization (hot or cold), microemulsion, solvent emulsification–evaporation, emulsification–diffusion and high-speed stirring, and ultrasonication methods (Chaturvedi & Kumar, 2012)

A variety of solid lipidic compounds have been used for preparing SLNs, including stearic acid, monostearin, Compritol 888 ATO, cetylpalmitate, Precirol ATO 5, glyceryl trioleate, cholesterol, soya lecithin, and glyceryl monostearate. The choice of the lipid is extremely important for the gene delivery properties of the SLN formulation. Moreover, the choice of the suitable method to prepare SLNs should be also considered. The issues such as size and stability of drugs during the production process may be affected by the composition (Şenel, Büyükköroğlu & Yazan, 2015; Büyükköroğlu, 2016)

SLNs are more advantageous compared with cationic lipids and cationic polymers due to their ease of manufacturing without the need for organic solvents, large-scale production possibilities with qualified production lines, and good stability under storage conditions with possibilities of steam sterilization and lyophilization (Pozo-Rodríguez, Solinís & Rodríguez-Gascón, 2016).

The uptake efficiency and immunogenicity of the antigen-loaded SLNs can be affected by size, lipid source, preparation method, and surface properties. For example, Bhargava et al. reported SLNs as tumor antigen carriers capable of inducing immune signals without any toxicity (Wen, Umeano, Francis, Sharma, Tundup, & Dhar, 2016)

Nanostructured lipid carriers (NLCs) have been developed as an alternative to SLNs due to their improved drug-loading capacity and release characteristics. The NLCs are different from SLNs in that in that they consist of solid and liquid lipid mixtures. Like other lipidic systems, NLCs can encapsulate a lipophilic drug in the nuclear region. They are also characterized by an ability to electrostatically bind nucleic acids (Pozo-Rodríguez, Solinís & Rodríguez-Gascón, 2016).

Studies are available on the encapsulation of low-molecular-weight proteins such as insulin and somatostatin using these lipid systems; however, studies on antigen proteins are limited. In one of these few studies, hepatitis B surface antigen was encapsulated in 90-nm SLNs. The release of antigens from lipid nanoparticles was not fully controlled in the study, leading to problems in dosing. They also noted that the methods to prepare formulations should be carefully assessed in terms of both protein degradation and damage to the epitope (Courant, Bayon, Reynaud-Dougier, Villiers, Menneteau, Marche, & Navarro, 2017).

Liposomes

A liposome is a spherical vesicle of the lamellar phase of the lipid bilayer. These lipid bilayer phospholipids, defined as the hydrophobic tail and the hydrophilic head, are amphiphilic molecules with hydrophilic (water-loving, polar) and lipophilic (lipid-loving) properties. Therefore, liposomes are artificial phospholipid bilayers. Consequently, liposomes have biocompatible properties. Moreover, liposomes have gained attention due to their remarkable features, such as no toxicity, low antigenicity, scalability and easy production, biodegradability, easy metabolism, and high membrane permeability (Wang, Rajala & Rajala, 2015).

Liposomes are commonly used for gene transfer. Many studies have shown that liposomes protect nucleic acids from enzymatic degradation and facilitate transfection by transporting nucleic acids to the target site. Lipofectamine 2000 and Lipofectin are some of the well-known liposomes. These systems have been successfully used for gene transfer in cultures, animals, and patients registered in phase I and II clinical trials and have been found to be more effective in naked gene transfer (Saffari, Moghimi & Dass, 2016). On the contrary, fast plasma clearance is one of the disadvantages of these systems (Thapa & Narain, 2016).

The acid dissociation constant (pKa) of the head group and the distance to the presented lipid bilayer interface were important parameters for *in vivo* gene delivery, eliminating biological barriers, and gene silencing with siRNA in particular. However, some studies indicate that a load on lipids can lead to toxic side effects and rapid clearance from circulation. Anionic lipids with a pKa value of 7 or less for both *in vitro* and *in vivo* activities are preferable, resulting in lower toxicity and effective encapsulation of nucleic acids (Zhao & Huang, 2014).

Cationic liposomes have been used in gene transfer to lung, skeletal muscles, spleen, kidney, liver, testis, heart, and skin cells. Liposome-based technology has progressed from first-generation classical vesicles to stealth liposomes, targeted liposomes, and, more recently, stimuli-sensitive liposomes. These new-generation liposomes have overcome many of the challenges faced by conventional liposomes, such as immune system avoidance, toxicity due to charged liposomes, and low half-life stability (Nayeros-sadat, Maedeh & Ali, 2012).

When administered *in vivo*, liposomes rapidly leak encapsulated macromolecules and cause premature vesicle rupture and antigen loss before reaching DCs in lymphoid organs. To address this limitation, Moon et al. (2011) formed cross-links between lipid head groups in multilamellar liposomes to stabilize lipid vesicles. Lipid nanoparticles termed interbilayer-crosslinked multilamellar vesicles, which are capable of encapsulating a large number of antigen proteins, have been shown to exhibit good serum stability for more than 30 days in the serum-containing medium with the zero-order antigen release. Furthermore, when the prepared liposomes were compared with conventional liposomal means, the activation of DCs in lymphoid tissues increased (Moon, Bershteyn, Stephan, Liu, Huang, …Irvine, 2011; Sahdev, Ochyl & Moon, 2014).

Liposomes are accepted as good antigen carriers owing to the aforementioned properties. It has been reported that these systems can carry antigens in a wide variety of channels. For example, these systems have been shown to work with a broad range of antigens, such as E7 peptide and heat shock protein 70 (HSP70), potentially vaccinable against many diseases such as cancer and human papillomavirus. The liposomal mucin 1 (MUC1) vaccine BLP25, which was prepared for a pilot study, was tried for about 1 year on about 20 patients, and no autoimmunity was observed with L-BLP25 in the study. L-BLP25 was then re-tested as an immunotherapeutic in a new international randomized and double-blind phase III clinical trial including 1513 patients with non-small cell third-stage lung cancer. Ultimately, the survival was found to be longer compared with placebo by a few months, requiring new clinical trials (Wen, Umeano, Francis, Sharma, Tundup, & Dhar, 2016).

Antigen persistence is important, but studies have shown that it is necessary to avoid antigen tolerance and adjuvant co-administration at high concentrations (Sahdev, Ochyl & Moon, 2014).

The PEG coating of liposomes may increase the time spent in blood circulation, and reduce complex activation. For this reason, the right amount of PEG coating is critical. In a literature review, the liposome surfaces were coated with various PEG fractions and the differences compared. As a result, 5% PEG liposome showed similar IgG2a and IgG2b primer response (after 7 days of vaccination). However, it increased antibody titers 1.5-fold after 3 weeks of inoculation compared with 1% PEG formulation. Both formulations indicated a twofold increase in IFN-γ production following antigen re-stimulation compared with non-PEG liposomes (Sahdev, Ochyl & Moon, 2014; Reichmuth, Oberli, Jaklenec, Langer & Blankschtein, 2016).

Emulsions

Emulsions are systems formed by dispersing two liquids insoluble in each other with the help of a surfactant. They are called macro-, micro-, and nanoemulsions depending on the size of droplets forming the emulsion. The addition of cationic lipids as surfactants to these dispersed systems makes them suitable for gene delivery (Martini, Fattal, de Oliveira & Teixeira, 2008; Pozo-Rodríguez, Solinís & Rodríguez-Gascón, 2016).

The presence of cationic surfactants such as DOTAP, DOTMA, or DC-Chol supports strong electrostatic interactions between the emulsion and the nucleic acid phosphate groups, leading to the formation of positively charged droplets. Co-lipid DOPE is frequently used to enhance the ability to transfect cells due to the fusogenic properties of cationic emulsions (Nam, Park, Kim, Kwon & Jeong, 2009; Verissimo, Lima, Egito, de Oliveira & do Egito, 2010)

The nanoemulsions most commonly used in gene delivery consist of oil, water, and surfactants and provide a drop size distribution of about 200 nm. These lipid-based delivery systems are seen as an ideal transport tool for the formation of physiological lipids such as cholesterol, cholesterol esters, phospholipids, and triglycerides (Verissimo, Lima, Egito, de Oliveira & do Egito, 2010; Verissimo, Lima, Egito, de Oliveira & do Egito, 2010; Pozo-Rodríguez, Solinís & Alicia Rodríguez-Gascón, 2016).

The emulsion-based dispensing system is attractive for a variety of reasons. For example, it can be used either orally or parenterally in a variety of gene delivery applications because it is a formulation in liquid form. The oil phase of the emulsion may also serve as a tool for the application of hydrophobic molecules, such as low-molecular-weight anti-inflammatory agents, for synergistic action. It also protects the lipid-phase encapsulated DNA from digestive enzymes (Verissimo, Lima, Egito, de Oliveira & do Egito, 2010; Attarwala & Amiji, 2012).

Some *in vitro* and *in vivo* studies have suggested that cationic nanoemulsions may be a more efficient carrier system than liposomes (Nam, Park, Kim, Kwon & Jeong, 2009) due to their physical properties and good stability in serum.

Nanoemulsion systems can also serve as a reservoir for sustained release of the antigen. The antigens may be incorporated into the internal aqueous phase of the w/o/w or w/o emulsion or may simply be mixed with the antigen. The emulsion-based Freund's vaccine adjuvant is still being used as the *gold standard* in developing new vaccine adjuvants (Jain, Khomane, Jain & Dani; 2011).

As an oil-in-water emulsion, MF59 is a commonly used emulsion of influenza vaccines licensed as a safe and potent vaccine adjuvant in more than 20 countries (O'Hagan, 2007). Moreover, Montanide is an oil-in-water and water-in-oil emulsion containing ISA 50 V, 51, 201, 206, and 720 in it. Montanide ISA 51 and 720 were used for malaria vaccines, and Montanide ISA 201 and 206 were used as hand-and foot-disease vaccines (Zhao, & Huang, 2014).

Niosomes

Niosomes have been used in the pharmaceutical field since the 1980s as a means of administering many drugs, such as chemotherapy drugs, peptides, antigens, hormones, and other bioactive agents. These systems are nonionic surfactant vesicles with a bilayer structure (Rajera, Nagpal, Singh & Mishra, 2011).

Compared with liposomes, niosomes were presented as an alternative to liposomes due to their low cost and superior chemical and storage stability. However, a few studies are available on gene transfer (Pardakhty & Moazeni, 2013).

For example, a niosome formulation was prepared and characterized by combining 2,3-di (tetradecyloxy) propane-1-amine–based cationic lipid with squalene and polysorbate 80 in one of the studies. This formulation transfected into the retina was effective depending on the route of administration. For example, it was detected that when the subretinal injections were essentially transfected into the retinal pigment epithelium (RPE) layer, the intravitreal injections were found to affect a large surface in the inner layers of the retina (Puras, Mashal, Zárate, Agirre, Ojeda, Grijalvo, …Pedraz, 2014).

Niosomes have also been used in vaccine applications other than DNA transport. For example, the first application on niosome antigen presentation was made against bovine serum albumin of BALB/c mice. Studies have shown that niosomes can potentially stimulate a subset of Th1 lymphocytes (Brewer & Alexander, 1992).

In another study, the herpes simplex 1 antigen was encapsulated in 1-monopalmitoyl glycerol (MP)/CHOL/DCP, resulting in better immunogenicity when it was administered to mice (Hassan, Brewer, Alexander & Jennings, 1996).

The niosomes prepared by Okrea et al. with a Span-20-based lipid film hydration technique were loaded with the vaccine against the Newcastle disease and assessed using adjuvanity and hemagglutination inhibition test. They found that the prepared niosomes exerted more immune response than the product in the market called L Sota and increased the immunogenicity of the Newcastle vaccine (Okore, Attama, Ofokansi, Esimone & Onuigbo, 2011).

In another study, Brij52-based nanoniosomes (Novasome) were prepared to protect guinea pigs from lethal tuberculosis. Single-dose subcutaneous administration of killed *Mycobacterium bovis* Bacille Calmette-Guerin (BCG) was explored. All formulations prepared at the end of the study were well tolerated, and high survival was observed in animals.

Other Nanocarriers

Inorganic Nanoparticles

Inorganic nanoparticle-based gene delivery vectors have attracted the attention of researchers in recent years due to their unique physical and chemical properties. Inorganic nanoparticles are nanoparticles of varying size, shape, and porosity that can be designed to avoid reticuloendothelial system or protect the trapped molecule from destruction or denaturation without degradation. They are also advantageous due to the ease of preparation and functionalization of their surfaces, showing good storage stability and not being exposed to microbial attacks (Guo & Huang, 2012).

Calcium phosphate, silica, gold-coated particles, semiconductor nanocrystals, hybrid nanoparticles, and several magnetic compounds are the most studied inorganic particles (Sokolova & Epple, 2007; Das, Han, Choi, Song, Cho, Park, … Kim, 2016).

A nonviral carrier system called NanoCeria (CeO_2) has been developed recently. DODAB cationic lipid was used to impart cationic properties to this system. Despite the high cytotoxicity characteristic of DODAB, NanoCeria, which mimics superoxide dismutase and has high antioxidant activity, has been shown to be highly effective in gene transfections of hybrid molecules due to its biocompatibility (Das, Han, Choi, Song, Cho, Park, … Kim, 2016).

Antigen transport agents also include many inorganic substances such as aluminum salt, silver, gold, carbon materials, silicon oxide, and iron oxide (Wen,Umeano, Francis, Sharma, Tundup, & Dhar, 2016).

Silica-Coated Nanoparticles are biocompatible structures used for a variety of biological applications, including gene therapy, due to their unique properties such as adjustable particle/pore size, biocompatibility, and low cost (Guo & Huang, 2012).

Generally, pure silica nanoparticles without surface modification do not appear to be effective in gene transfer due to the presence of hydroxy groups on their surface. Therefore, silica nanoparticles have to be modified to function by linking DNA via electrostatic interaction or surface group reactions (Liu, Lou, Yang, Shi & Miyoshi, 2011).

The first study on this topic reported that aminosilane-modified solid silica nanoparticles, which were 10–100 nm in diameter, could bind strongly to plasmid DNA (pDNA) and exhibit excellent in vitro gene transfection. Following this study, silica nanoparticles were used as gene delivery systems in many following studies (Yu, Niu, Zhang, Zhang, Yang, Taran, …Yu, 2016).

For example, a study showed that polycationic silica nanoparticles with larger particle diameters had a better gene transfection performance than their spherical counterparts (Lin, Zhao, Yan, Hu & Xu, 2015).

For example, a study showed that polycationic silica nanoparticles with larger particle diameters had a better gene transfection performance compared with their global counterparts (Lin, Zhao, Yan, Hu & Xu, 2015).

Recently, the synthesized mesoporous silica nanoparticles (MSNs) have attracted attention. In these nanoparticles, small molecules can be stored in the pores and dimensionally defined "caps" such as dendrimers, proteins, or semiconductor nanocrystals (quantum dots) can be used to close the openings of mesoporous channels covalently. Thus, they can physically prevent the infiltration of the drug (Vivero-Escoto, Slowing, Wu & Lin, 2007; Lu, Choi, Tamanoi & Zink, 2008; Vivero-Escoto, Slowing, 2009). From that perspective, the MSNs modified with azo-benzene derivatives can release their content following light irradiation (Trewyn, Giri, Slowing & Lin, 2007; Lu, Choi, Tamanoi & Zink, 2008; Vivero-Escoto, Slowing, Wu & Lin, 2009).

Silica particles have also been studied in vaccine transport and gene transfer. For example, Guo et al. (2012) reported effective immunization in porcine circovirus type II mice with mesoporous silica nanoparticles (Guo, & Huang, 2012).

Another study by Mody et al. has shown that albumin-loaded silica nanoparticles can induce humoral and cellular immunity (Mody, Popat, Mahony, Cavallaro, Yu, & Mitter, 2013). In another study, MSNs were used as carriers and adjuvants for the transport of active antigens derived from pig circovirus and human immunodeficiency virus in the range of 50–200 nm (Zhao, & Huang, 2014).

However, these MSNs have disadvantages when they are coated with cationic polymers, such as shrinking the pore volume, blocking the release of a gene due to highly cationic properties, increasing cytotoxicity, and rapid elimination from the kidneys. Recent studies showed that using ammonium salt–grafted MSNs instead of amino group–carrying types decreased cytotoxicity and induced gene transfection efficiency (Li, Hei, Xu, Qian & Zhu, 2016).

Another biologically compatible controlled-release system is the snap-top-covered silica nanocontainer, in which the snap ball depolarizes the molecules in the nanopores and the stopper cap is activated by an esterase, leading to release of contents by cleavage after activation (Patel, Angelos, Dichtel, Coskun, Yang, Zink, & Stoddart, 2008)

Magnetic Inorganic Nanoparticles (such as Fe_3O_4, MnO_2) have been used to carry cancer-targeted nucleic acids and perform simultaneous diagnosis with magnetic resonance imaging (Guo & Huang,

2012). Large surface areas allow for various modifications by making the transport of target molecules, drugs, and imaging agents possible (Peng, Qian, Mao, Wang, Chen, Nie, & Shin, 2008).

Nanoparticles are more reactive than bulk materials because they have a high surface/volume ratio. Hence, these magnetic core nanomaterials must be coated to protect against corrosion. This coating also prevents the penetration of potentially toxic components into the body during in vivo applications. Natural and synthetic polymers, silica, and gold can be used as coating materials. In addition, it requires an organic linker to bind to organic biomolecules. Among these linkers, the most commonly used are amine, carboxylic acid, thiol, and aldehydes (McBain, Yiu & Dobson, 2008).

In these transport systems, termed as magnetofection, the magnetic nanoparticles are combined with nucleic acid molecules to form a meniscal area to increase gene transfer. The method was first tried in cell culture plates by Christian Plank et al. and then carried out *in vivo*. Intravenously administered nanoparticles are retained in the target site by being held by an external magnet while traveling in the circulatory system, thus facilitating tissue uptake (Majidi, Sehrig, Samiei, Milani, Abbasi, Dadashzadeh & Akbarzadeh, 2016)

Gold Nanoparticles (AuNP) are a new type of material having many biological functions. These compounds can be metabolized by the urine and do not have a clear cytotoxicity. Studies have shown that unmodified gold nanoparticles are insufficient to transport DNA. However, an increase in gene transfection efficiency has been observed after surface modification. Gold nanoparticles have been reported to have properties such as good stability, high surface activity, strong ability to carry genes, and specific biological affinity. Therefore, they are currently used in several fields, such as DNA testing, rapid immunodiagnosis, biosensors, and drug delivery to targeted sites (Sun, Liu & Hu, 2013).

The activities of these systems have generally been shown by in vitro studies so far. However, some issues need to be solved before AuNP–nucleic acid conjugates can be transformed into clinical applications. First, it is essential to minimize the short- and long-term cytotoxicity of AuNPs. Although many studies have shown the biological compatibility of these therapeutic NPs using simple cytotoxicity assays, a detailed toxicological evaluation (cell membrane damage, oxidative stress, genotoxicity, etc.) has not been properly addressed. Second, these transport tools need to be targeted to specific organs and tissues to reduce side effects. Hence, several superficial modifications have to be made to coat the surfaces with antibodies or to avoid biological barriers (Ding, Jiang, Saha, Kim, Kim, Landis, & Rotello, 2014). For example, gold-cysteamine (AuCM)/plasmid DNA (pDNA)/polyTAT (pTAT)/hyaluronic acid (HA) nanocomplexes were developed for use in liver cancer in a recent study. Eventually, liver accumulation was achieved and gene transfer was completed successfully (Yu, Niu, Zhang, Zhang, Yang, Taran, … Yu, 2016).

AuNPs are also used in vaccine transport because they can be easily prepared in different shapes (spherical, rod, cubic, etc.) at a size range of 2–150 nm, and their surfaces can be modified with carbohydrates. Influenza has been used as an adjuvant for DNA vaccines for carriers or HIV for antigens from viruses that cause hand-and-foot disease (Zhao, & Huang, 2014).

Semiconductor Nanocrystals or Quantum Dots (QD), light-emitting nanoparticles successfully applied for in vitro and in vivo transfection. QDs are almost spherical semiconductor particles with a core-shell structure. The semiconductor structure of these nanocrystals and their fluorescence properties dependent on their size make them attractive for diagnosing diseases. Gene-related molecules can be loaded into a core of the QD or attached directly to the surface of these nanoparticles via conjugation or electrostatic interaction. QDs can protect genes from degradation by nuclease (Probst, Zrazhevskiy, Bagalkot & Gao, 2013; Biju, Mundayoor, Omkumar, Anas & Ishikawa, 2010).

QDs are widely used for carrying and imaging gene materials in vivo and in vitro depending on their excellent optical properties. They are ideal tools for discovering and validating in cells and small animals. However, since biologically conjugated QDs cannot be efficiently eliminated from the body, their potential use as drug delivery tools for human medicines is not clear yet (Zha & Zhu 2016).

Carbon Nanotubes (CNTs) are single-walled or multi-walled cylindrical structures formed by the rolling of carbon plates. Their diameters range from 2 to 100 nm, and the length varies between 2 and 500 nm (Değim, 2014).

The use of CNTs in in vitro applications is noteworthy. However, their potential to be used in in vivo applications is limited by their cytotoxicity and low bioavailability. Surface modification or functionalization can increase their solubility and bioaccumulation in aqueous solutions (Lee, Yoon & Cho, 2013)

CNTs are also used to prepare biomaterials such as conductive/polymer blends in drug and vaccine delivery systems. Various DNA and protein biosensors have been prepared using CNTs (Chang, 2014).

Villa et al. (2011) showed that single-walled carbon nanotubes caused an increase in mouse immune responses, without showing any toxicity or immunogenicity in vitro and in vivo (Villa, Dao, Ahearn, Fehrenbacher, Casey, Rey, ...Philips, 2011).

Another study reported that low surface load and size shortening facilitated cellular uptake and produced higher immune responses compared with positively charged long CNTs in multi-walled CNTs carrying OVA (Ovalbumin) (Hassan,, Smyth, Rubio, Ratnasothy, Wang, Bansal,...Al-Jamal, 2016).

Fullerenes, especially C60, are water-insoluble allotropic carbons. The dissolution of fullerenes in the water environment causes difficulties in cellular studies. Therefore, this characteristic can be improved by adding organic solvents such as dimethylformamide (DMF), which causes increased cytotoxicity and thus decreased cell viability (Katragaddai Choudhury & Murthy, 2010).

In this context, polyfunctionalized fullerenes carrying one or more positive charges in their structure, have been investigated as nucleic acid carriers. In one of the first studies, a "two-handed" fullerene derivative was synthesized. It was observed that that newly developed complex transfected plasmid DNA (pDNA) was as good as commercial reagents (Nakamura, Isobe, Tomita, Sawamura, Jinno, & Okayama, 2000)

In the first in vivo study conducted using fullerenes, a complex was formed with tetraaminofurans and the insulin-2 gene and this complex was compared with Lipofectamine. An acute toxicity was reported for the fullerenic complex compared with Lipofectamine administration. The in vivo administration of the insulin-2 gene resulted in increased plasma insulin levels and low blood glucose concentration. Finally, fullerenes have been reported to have a high potential to be used as gene carriers (Maeda-Mamiya, Noiri, Isobe, Nakanishi, Okamoto, Doi, ... Nakamura, 2010).

Calcium Phosphate gene transfer system was developed by Graham and Van Der Eb. Since then, this system has been extensively used as an easy-to-use, cost-effective, and highly reliable gene transfer system (Jin, Zeng, Liu, Deng & Nongyue, 2014).

These nanoparticles can be used alone or in combination with other vectors (viral or nonviral). They exhibit good gene transfer properties, especially when incorporated into colloidal particle systems. For example, divalent metal cations such as Ca^{2+}, Mg^{2+}, Mn^{2+}, and Ba^{2+} can form ionic complexes with DNA resulting in stabilized structures. These complexes can be further transported through the cell membrane via ion channel–mediated endocytosis (Maitra, 2005).

Calcium phosphate nanoparticles may be formed by mixing calcium chloride, dibasic sodium phosphate, and sodium citrate under certain conditions. They are not toxic and can be formed in sizes of 50–100 nm. These nanoparticles are useful adjuvants for DNA vaccines and mucosal immunity and exhibit excellent biocompatibility (Zhao, & Huang, 2014).

Cyclodextrins (CDs) are cyclic oligosaccharides obtained by enzymatic degradation of starch. The most frequently used CDs in the pharmaceutical field are α-CD, β-CD, and γ-CD with six, seven, and eight subunits, respectively (Jambhekar & Breen, 2016).

CDs are able to modulate the physiochemical properties of the molecules they carry, such as solubility and/or stability in the biological environment. Despite all these advantages, CDs have some limitations, too. For example, it is well known that β-CD has low water solubility, causing hemolysis in blood cells when administered via the parenteral route. The structures of natural CDs have been replaced with different chemical groups and their biocompatibility has been increased to overcome these difficulties (Varan, Benito, Mellet & Bilensoy, 2017). For example, CDs were administered to the mouse mesenchyme intravesically in a study conducted with DOTAP/DNA complex with methyl betacyclodextrin. Two days after the transfection, it was observed that the nanoparticles remained in the bladder and the gene expression could continue for up to 30 days (Nimesh, 2013).

Cell Penetrating Peptides

Cell-penetrating peptides (CPPs) are a class of nonviral transport vectors used extensively for the delivery of genetic molecules both *in vitro* and *in vivo* due to their remarkable translocation properties.

In 1988, the first CPP was sequenced from an HIV-1-encoded cell-penetrating transactivator of transcription (TAT) peptide and efficiently transferred through cell membranes. Since then, TAT has become a widely used application (Wang, A. Rajala & R. V. Rajala, 2015).

In particular, arginine-rich cell penetration peptides, such as TAT, can help in the successful transport of many biologically active macromolecules due to their ability to pass through plasma membranes easily (Schmidt, Mishra, Lai & Wong, 2010). These peptides are capable of directing a low-molecular-weight DNA and a synthetic RNA to the cytoplasm by direct delivery through energy-dependent macropinocytosis and lipid layer (Alpar, Cevher, Özsoy, 2014).

Some disadvantages associated with the use of peptides are lack of specificity, cytotoxicity, high cost, production of potent immunological responses *in vivo*, and proteolytic degradation in the bloodstream (Pujals & Giralt, 2008).

Immunostimulatory Complexes

Immunostimulatory complexes (ISCOMs) are clinically tested carriers with strong adjuvant effect. They are composed of Quil A, which is approximately 40 nm in size and a cage-like structure having antigens, cholesterol, phospholipids, and a saponin adjuvant. Antigens are bound to ISCOMs via hydrophobic or electrostatic interaction (Alpar, Cevher, Özsoy, 2014).

These spherical particles can capture the antigen via apolar interactions. ISCOMATRIX contains ISCOMs without antigen. It can be mixed with the antigen and provides a more flexible application by removing the restriction of hydrophobic antigens. Various antigens have been used to generate ISCOMs, including influenza, herpes simplex virus, HIV, and antigens derived from Newcastle disease (Zhao, & Huang, 2014).

CONCLUSION

Vectors are vehicles that carry genetic material or vaccine molecules to a variety of cells and tissues. To develop an optimal transport system, the targeted cell, the size of the genetic material to be transported, the duration of the expression, the physicochemical properties of the transport material are important. In particular, the size, surface charges and the materials in the composition affect access to target cell and uptake by cells. Existing vectors used for transport are divided into two as a viral vectors and non-viral vectors. Among them, the second group is generally preferred, due to the significant properties compared to the first. The most studied non-viral vectors are polymeric and lipidic carriers. But they are still not as effective as viral vectors. For this reason, non-viral vectors have been increased functionalitics with various surface modifications. Nanocarriers have been used in the clinical field to transport various drug molecules, so far. Likewise, the transport of genes and vaccine antigens via nanocarriers promises hope for the treatment of infectious and neurological diseases as well as cancer and genetic diseases. At the same time the fact that nano-carriers alone have adjuvant properties is considered an advantage in immunological studies. The positive results obtained in studies carried out worldwide in recent years demonstrate that this nanoscale transport system can be effective in clinical practice. Finally, combination approaches of the use of radiotherapy, immunotherapy and others with nanoparticle-based therapy containing different molecules (chemotherapeutic drugs, DNA, RNA, protein etc.) will have a very important spot in future clinical applications.

REFERENCES

Acharya, S., & Sahoo, S. K. (2011). PLGA nanoparticles containing various anticancer agents and tumour delivery by EPR effect. *Advanced Drug Delivery Reviews*, *63*(3), 170–183. doi:10.1016/j.addr.2010.10.008 PMID:20965219

Akagi, T., Baba, M., & Akashi, M. (2012). Biodegradable nanoparticles as vaccine adjuvants and delivery systems: Regulation of immune responses by nanoparticle-based vaccine. *Advances in Polymer Science*, *247*, 31–64. doi:10.1007/12_2011_150

Al-Dosari, M. S., & Gao, X. (2009). Non viral gene delivery: Principle, limitations and recent progress. *American Association of Pharmaceutical Scientists*, *11*(4), 671–681. PMID:19834816

Alpar, H. O., Cevher, E., & Özsoy, Y. (2014). Nanopartiküllerin gen tedavisinde kullanılması. In A. Zırh-Gülsoy (Ed), Nanofarmasötikler ve uygulamaları (pp. 261-276). İstanbul: Kontrollü Salım Derneği Yayını No: 3.

Alves, N. M., & Mano, J. F. (2008). Chitosan derivatives obtained by chemical modifications for biomedical and environmental applications. *International Journal of Biological Macromolecules*, *43*(5), 40–41. doi:10.1016/j.ijbiomac.2008.09.007 PMID:18838086

Attarwala, H., & Amiji, M. (2012). Multi-compartmental nanoparticles-in-emulsion formulation for macrophage-specific anti-inflammatory gene delivery. *Pharmaceutical Research*, *29*(6), 1637–1649. doi:10.100711095-012-0677-9 PMID:22281760

Aulenta, F., Hayes, W., & Rannard, S. (2003, September). Dendrimers: A new class of nanoscopic containers and delivery devices. *European Polymer Journal, 39*(9), 1741–1771. doi:10.1016/S0014-3057(03)00100-9

Belldegrun, A., & Tso, C. L. (2002). Kidney-specific tumor vaccine directed against kidney tumor antigen G-250. *U.S. Patent 2002/0058041-A1, May 16.*

Benjaminsen, R. V., Mattebjerg, M. A., Henriksen, J. R., Moghimi, S. M., & Andresen, T. L. (2013). The possible "Proton Sponge" effect of polyethylenimine (PEI) does not include change in lysosomal pH. *Molecular Therapy, 21*(1), 149–157. doi:10.1038/mt.2012.185 PMID:23032976

Beyerle, A., Irmler, M., Beckers, J., Kissel, T., & Stoeger, T. (2010). Toxicity pathway focused gene expression profiling of PEI-based polymers for pulmonary applications. *Molecular Pharmaceutics, 7*(3), 727–737. doi:10.1021/mp900278x PMID:20429563

Biju, V., Mundayoor, S., Omkumar, R. V., Anas, A., & Ishikawa, M. (2010). Bioconjugated quantum dots for cancer research: Present status, prospects and remaining issues. *Biotechnology Advances, 28*(2), 27.

Bose, R. J. C., Lee, S. H., & Park, H. (2016). Lipid-based surface engineering of PLGA nanoparticles for drug and gene delivery applications. *Biomaterials Research, 20*(34), 1–9. PMID:27807476

Brewer, J., & Alexander, J. (1992). The adjuvant activity of non-ionic surfactant vesicles (niosomes) on the BALB/c humoral response to bovine serum albumin. *Immunology, 75*, 570–575. PMID:1592432

Brewer, J. M. (2006). How do aluminium adjuvants work? *Immunology Letters, 102*(1), 10–15. doi:10.1016/j.imlet.2005.08.002 PMID:16188325

Büyükköroğlu, G. (2016). Development of solid lipid gene delivery system. *Turkish Journal of Pharmaceutical Sciences, 13*(2), 249–258.

Chaturvedi, S. P., & Kumar, V. (2012). Production techniques of lipid nanoparticles: A review. *Research Journal of Pharmaceutical, Biological and Chemical Sciences, 3*, 525–541.

Cheung, C. R. F., Ng, T. B., Wong, J. H., & Chan, W. Y. (2015). Chitosan: An Update on Potential Biomedical and Pharmaceutical Applications. *Marine Drugs, 13*(8), 5156–5186. doi:10.3390/md13085156 PMID:26287217

Chime, S. A., & Onyishi, V. I. (2013). Lipid-based drug delivery systems (LDDS): Recent advances and applications of lipids in drug delivery. *African Journal of Pharmacy and Pharmacology, 7*(48), 3034–3059. doi:10.5897/AJPPX2013.0004

Choi, Y. J., Kang, S. J., Kim, Y. J., Lim, Y. B., & Chung, H. W. (2010). Comparative studies on the genotoxicity and cytotoxicity of polymeric gene carriers polyethylenimine (PEI) and Polyamidoamine (PAMAM) dendrimer in jurkat T-cells. drug and chemical. *Toxicology, 33*(4), 357–366. PMID:20550436

Correia-Pinto, J. F., Csaba, N., Schiller, J. T., & Alonso, M. J. (2015). Chitosan-poly (I: C)-PADRE based nanoparticles as delivery vehicles for synthetic peptide vaccines. *Vaccines, 3*(3), 730–750. doi:10.3390/vaccines3030730 PMID:26378586

Courant, T., Bayon, E., Reynaud-Dougier, H. L., Villiers, C., Menneteau, M., Marche, P. N., & Navarro, F. P. (2017). Tailoring nanostructured lipid carriers for the delivery of protein antigens: Physicochemical properties versus immunogenicity studies. *Biomaterials*, *136*, 29–42. doi:10.1016/j.biomaterials.2017.05.001 PMID:28511142

Cruz, L. J., Tacken, P. J., Fokkink, R., & Figdor, C. G. (2011). The influence of PEG chain length and targeting moiety on antibody-mediated delivery of nanoparticle vaccines to human dendritic cells. *Biomaterials*, *32*(28), 6791–6803. doi:10.1016/j.biomaterials.2011.04.082 PMID:21724247

Danhier, F., Ansorena, E., Silva, J. M., Coco, R., Le Breton, A., & Préat, V. (2012). PLGA-based nanoparticles: An overview of biomedical applications. *Journal of Controlled Release*, *161*(2), 505–522. doi:10.1016/j.jconrel.2012.01.043 PMID:22353619

Das, J., Han, J. W., Choi, Y. J., Song, H., Cho, S. G., Park, C., ... Kim, J. H. (2016). Cationic lipid-nanoceria hybrids, a novel nonviral vector-mediated gene delivery into mammalian cells: Investigation of the cellular uptake mechanism. *Scientific Reports*, *6*(29197), 1–13. PMID:27380727

De Martimprey, H., Vauthier, C., Malvy, C., & Couvreur, P. (2009). Polymer nanocarriers for the delivery of small fragments of nucleic acids: Oligonucleotides and siRNA. *European Journal of Pharmaceutics and Biopharmaceutics*, *71*(3), 490–504. doi:10.1016/j.ejpb.2008.09.024 PMID:18977435

Değim, İ. T. (2014). Fulleren, karbon nanotüp, nanolif, nanokafesler. In A. Zırh-Gülsoy (Ed.), Nanofarmasötikler ve Uygulamaları (pp. 139-150). İstanbul: Kontrollü Salım Derneği Yayını No: 3.

Del Pozo-Rodríguez, A., Solinís, M. A., & Rodríguez-Gascón, A. (2016). Applications of lipid nanoparticles in gene therapy. *European Journal of Pharmaceutics and Biopharmaceutics*, *109*, 184–193. doi:10.1016/j.ejpb.2016.10.016 PMID:27789356

Ding, Y., Jiang, Z., Saha, K., Kim, C. S., Kim, S. T., Landis, R. F., & Rotello, V. M. (2014). Gold nanoparticles for nucleic acid delivery. *Molecular Therapy*, *22*(6), 1075–1083. doi:10.1038/mt.2014.30 PMID:24599278

Dizaj, S. M., Jafari, S., & Khosroushahi, A. Y. (2014). A sight on the current nanoparticle-based gene delivery vectors. *Nanoscale Research Letters*, *9*(252), 1–9. PMID:24936161

Donnelly, J. J., Ulmer, J. B., Shiver, J. W., & Liu, M. A. (1997). DNA vaccines. *Annual Review of Immunology*, *15*(1), 617–648. doi:10.1146/annurev.immunol.15.1.617 PMID:9143702

Dorraj, G., Carreras, J. J., Nunez, H., Abushammala, I., & Melero, A. (2017). Lipid nanoparticles as potential gene therapeutic delivery systems for oral administration. *Current Gene Therapy*, *17*(2), 89–104. doi:10.2174/1566523217666170510163038 PMID:28494737

Dutta, T., Jain, N. K., McMillan, N. A., & Parekh, H. S. (2010). Dendrimer nanocarriers as versatile vectors in gene delivery. *Nanomedicine (London)*, *6*(1), 25–34. doi:10.1016/j.nano.2009.05.005 PMID:19450708

Elfinger, M., Uzgun, S., & Rudolph, C. (2008). Nanocarriers for gene delivery - Polymer structure, targeting ligands and controlled-release devices. *Current Nanoscience*, *4*(4), 322–353. doi:10.2174/157341308786306062

Fang, J., Nakamura, H., & Maeda, H. (2011). The EPR effect unique features of tumor blood vessels for drug delivery, factors involved, and limitationsand augmentation of the effect. *Advanced Drug Delivery Reviews*, *63*(3), 136–151. doi:10.1016/j.addr.2010.04.009 PMID:20441782

Fischer, D., Li, Y. X., Ahlemeyer, B., Krieglstein, J., & Kissel, T. (2003). *In vitro* cytotoxicity testing of polycations: Influence of polymer structure on cell viability and hemolysis. *Biomaterials*, *24*(7), 1121–1131. doi:10.1016/S0142-9612(02)00445-3 PMID:12527253

Giacca, M. (2010). Introduction to gene therapy. In *Gene Therapy* (pp. 1–6). Springer Verlag. doi:10.1007/978-88-470-1643-9_1

Grant, E. V., Thomas, M., Fortune, J., Klibanov, A. M., & Letvin, N. L. (2012). Enhancement of plasmid DNA immunogenicity with linear polyethylenimine. *European Journal of Immunology*, *42*(11), 2937–2948. doi:10.1002/eji.201242410 PMID:22886924

Greenwood, B. (2014). The contribution of vaccination to global health: Past, present and future. *Philosophical Transactions of the Royal Society of London. Series B, Biological Sciences*, *369*(1645), 1–9. doi:10.1098/rstb.2013.0433 PMID:24821919

Guo, H. C., Feng, X. M., Sun, S. Q., Wei, Y. Q., Sun, D. H., Liu, X. T., ... Yin, H. (2012). Immunization of mice by hollow mesoporous silica nanoparticles as carriers of porcine circovirus type 2 ORF2 protein. *Virology Journal*, *9*(108), 1–10. PMID:22691538

Guo, X., & Huang, L. (2012). Recent advances in nonviral vectors for gene delivery. accounts of chemical research. *Accounts of Chemical Research*, *45*(7), 971–979. doi:10.1021/ar200151m PMID:21870813

Hanna, E., Rémuzat, C., Auquier, P., & Toumi, M. (2016). Gene therapies development: Slow progress and promising prospect. *Journal of Market Access & Health Policy*, *5*(1), 1–9. PMID:28265348

Hassan, H. A., Smyth, L., Rubio, N., Ratnasothy, K., Wang, J. T. W., Bansal, S. S., ... Al-Jamal, K. T. (2016). Carbon nanotubes' surface chemistry determines their potency as vaccine nanocarriers *in vitro* and *in vivo*. *Journal of Controlled Release*, *225*, 205–216. doi:10.1016/j.jconrel.2016.01.030 PMID:26802552

Hassan, Y., Brewer, J., Alexander, J., & Jennings, R. (1996). Immune responses in mice induced by HSV-1 glycoproteins presented with ISCOMs or NISV delivery systems. *Vaccine*, *14*(17), 1581–1589. doi:10.1016/S0264-410X(96)00155-7 PMID:9032885

Hasson, S. S. A. A., Al-Busaidi, J., & Sallam, T. A. (2015). The past, current and future trends in DNA vaccine immunisations. *Asian Pacific Journal of Tropical Biomedicine*, *5*(5), 344–353. doi:10.1016/S2221-1691(15)30366-X

Huang, X., Teng, X., Chen, D., Tang, F., & He, J. (2010). The effect of the shape of mesoporous silica nanoparticles on cellular uptake and cell function. *Biomaterials*, *31*(3), 438–448. doi:10.1016/j.biomaterials.2009.09.060 PMID:19800115

Huang, Y., Liu, X., Dong, L., Liu, Z., He, X., & Liu, W. (2011). Development of viral vectors for gene therapy for chronic pain. *Pain Research and Treatment*, *2011*, 1–8. doi:10.1155/2011/968218 PMID:22110937

Illum, L. (1998). Chitosan and its use as a pharmaceutical excipient. *Pharmaceutical Research, 15*(9), 1326–1331. doi:10.1023/A:1011929016601 PMID:9755881

Islam, M. A., Firdous, J., Choi, Y. J., Yun, C. H., & Cho, C. S. (2012). Design and application of chitosan microspheres as oral and nasal vaccine carriers: An updated review. *International Journal of Nanomedicine, 7*, 6077–6093. PMID:23271909

Jäger, M., Schubert, S., Ochrimenko, S., Fischer, D., & Schubert, U. S. (2012). Branched and linear poly(ethylene imine)-based conjugates: Synthetic modification, characterization, and application. *Chemical Society Reviews, 41*(13), 4755–4767. doi:10.1039/c2cs35146c PMID:22648524

Jain, S., Khomane, K., Jain, A. K., & Dani, P. (2011). Nanocarriers for transmucosal vaccine delivery. *Current Nanoscience, 7*, 160–177. doi:10.2174/157341311794653541

Jambhekar, S. S., & Breen, P. (2016). Cyclodextrins in pharmaceutical formulations I: Structure and physicochemical properties, formation of complexes, and types of complex. *Drug Discovery Today, 21*(2), 356–362. doi:10.1016/j.drudis.2015.11.017 PMID:26686054

Jin, L., Zeng, X., Liu, M., Deng, Y., & He, N. (2014). Current progress in gene delivery technology based on chemical methods and nano-carriers. *Theranostics, 4*(3), 240–255. doi:10.7150/thno.6914 PMID:24505233

Kalam, M. A., Khan, A. A., & Alshamsan, A. (2017). Non-invasive administration of biodegradable nano-carrier vaccines. *American Journal of Translational Research, 9*(1), 15–35. PMID:28123631

Katragadda, C. S., Choudhury, P. K., & Murthy, P. (2010). Nanoparticles as non-viral gene delivery vectors. *Indian Journal of Pharmaceutical Education and Research, 44*(2), 109–111.

Kawai, T., & Akira, S. (2011). Toll-like receptors and their crosstalk with other innate receptors in infection and immunity. *Immunity, 34*(5), 637–650. doi:10.1016/j.immuni.2011.05.006 PMID:21616434

Kedmi, R., Ben-Arie, N., & Peer, D. (2010, September). The systemic toxicity of positively charged lipid nanoparticles and the role of Toll-like receptor 4 in immune activation. *Biomaterials, 31*(26), 6867–6875. doi:10.1016/j.biomaterials.2010.05.027 PMID:20541799

Koppolu, B., & Zaharoff, D. A. (2013). The effect of antigen encapsulation in chitosan particles on uptake, activation and presentation by antigen presenting cells. *Biomaterials, 34*(9), 2359–2369. doi:10.1016/j.biomaterials.2012.11.066 PMID:23274070

Koynova, R., & Tenchov, B. (2010). Cationic lipids: Molecular structure/ transfection activity relationships and interactions with biomembranes. *Topics in Current Chemistry, 296*, 51–93. doi:10.1007/128_2010_67 PMID:21504100

Kumar, U., Kumar, S., Varghese, S., Chamoli, R., & Barthwal, P. (2013). DNA vaccine: A modern biotechnological approach towards human welfare and clinical trials. *International Journal of Research in Biomedicine and Biotechnology, 3*(1), 17–20.

Lee, J. M., Yoon, T. J., & Cho, Y. S. (2013). Recent developments in nanoparticle-based siRNA delivery for cancer therapy. *BioMed Research International, 2013*, 1–10. doi:10.1155/2013/310461 PMID:23844368

Leitner, W. W., Ying, H., & Restifo, N. P. (1999). DNA and RNA-based vaccines: Principles, progress and prospects. *Vaccine*, *18*(9-10), 765–777. doi:10.1016/S0264-410X(99)00271-6 PMID:10580187

Li, S. D., & Huang, L. (2010). Stealth nanoparticles: High density but sheddable PEG is a key for tumor targeting. *Journal of Controlled Release*, *145*(3), 178–181. doi:10.1016/j.jconrel.2010.03.016 PMID:20338200

Li, Y., Hei, M., Xu, Y., Qian, X., & Zhu, W. (2016). Ammonium salt modified mesoporous silica nanoparticles for dual intracellular-responsive gene delivery. *International Journal of Pharmaceutics*, *511*(2), 689–702. doi:10.1016/j.ijpharm.2016.07.029 PMID:27426108

Lin, X. Y., Zhao, N. N., Yan, P., Hu, H., & Xu, F. J. (2015). The shape and size effects of polycation functionalized silica nanoparticles on gene transfection. *Acta Biomaterialia*, *11*, 381–392. doi:10.1016/j.actbio.2014.09.004 PMID:25219349

Liu, C., & Zhang, N. (2011). Chapter 13-Nanoparticles in gene therapy: Principles, prospects, and challenges. *Progress in Molecular Biology and Translational Science*, *104*, 509–562. doi:10.1016/B978-0-12-416020-0.00013-9 PMID:22093228

Liu, D., Chia, E. F., & Tian, H. (2004). Chemical methods for DNA delivery, In W. C. Heiser (Ed.), Methods in Molecular Biology, Volume 1: Nonviral Gene Transfer Techniques (pp. 3-23). Totowa: Humana Press Inc.

Liu, Y., Lou, C., Yang, H., Shi, M., & Miyoshi, H. (2011). Silica nanoparticles as promising drug/gene delivery carriers and fluorescent nano-probes: Recent advances. *Current Cancer Drug Targets*, *11*(2), 156–163. doi:10.2174/156800911794328411 PMID:21158720

Loh, X. J., Lee, T. C., Doua, Q., & Deene, G. R. (2016). Utilising inorganic nanocarriers for gene delivery. *Biomaterials Science*, *4*(1), 70–86. doi:10.1039/C5BM00277J PMID:26484365

Lu, J., Choi, E., Tamanoi, F., & Zink, J. I. (2008). Light-activated nanoimpeller-controlled drug release in cancer cells. *Small*, *4*(4), 421–426. doi:10.1002mll.200700903 PMID:18383576

Lukashev, N., & Zamyatnin, A. A. (2016). Viral vectors for gene therapy: Current state and clinical perspectives. *Biochemistry (Moscow)*, *81*(7), 700–708. doi:10.1134/S0006297916070063 PMID:27449616

Luten, J., van Nostrum, C. F., De Smedt, S. C., & Hennink, W. E. (2008). Biodegradable polymers as non-viral carriers for plasmid DNA delivery. *Journal of Controlled Release*, *126*(2), 97–110. doi:10.1016/j.jconrel.2007.10.028 PMID:18201788

Maeda-Mamiya, R., Noiri, E., Isobe, H., Nakanishi, W., Okamoto, K., Doi, K., … Nakamura, E. (2010). *In vivo* gene delivery by cationic tetraamino fullerene. *Proceedings of the National Academy of Sciences of the United States of America*, *107*(12), 5339-5344. 10.1073/pnas.0909223107

Maitra, A. (2005). Calcium phosphate nanoparticles: Second-generation nonviral vectors in gene therapy. *Expert Review of Molecular Diagnostics*, *5*(6), 893–905. doi:10.1586/14737159.5.6.893 PMID:16255631

Majidi, S., Sehrig, F. Z., Samiei, M., Milani, M., Abbasi, E., Dadashzadeh, K., & Akbarzadeh, A. (2016). Magnetic nanoparticles: Applications in gene delivery and gene therapy. *Artificial Cells, Nanomedicine, and Biotechnology*, *4*(4), 1186–1193. PMID:25727710

Mao, S., Sun, W., & Kissel, T. (2010). Chitosan-based formulations for delivery of DNA and siRNA. *Advanced Drug Delivery Reviews*, *62*(1), 12–27. doi:10.1016/j.addr.2009.08.004 PMID:19796660

Marshall, E. (2002). Clinical research: Gene therapy a suspect in leukemia-like disease. *Science*, *298*(5591), 34–35. doi:10.1126cience.298.5591.34 PMID:12364755

McBain, S. C., Yiu, H. H. P., & Dobson, J. (2008). Magnetic nanoparticles for gene and drug delivery. *International Journal of Nanomedicine*, *3*(2), 169–180. PMID:18686777

Mellott, A. J., Forrest, M. L., & Detamore, M. S. (2013). Physical non-viral gene delivery methods for tissue engineering. *Annals of Biomedical Engineering*, *41*(3), 446–468. doi:10.100710439-012-0678-1 PMID:23099792

Misra, S. (2013). Human gene therapy: A brief overview of the genetic revolution. *The Journal of the Association of Physicians of India*, *61*(2), 127–133. PMID:24471251

Mody, K. T., Popat, A., Mahony, D., Cavallaro, A. S., Yu, C., & Mitter, N. (2013). Mesoporous silica nanoparticles as antigen carriers and adjuvants for vaccine delivery. *Nanoscale*, *5*(12), 5167–5179. doi:10.1039/c3nr00357d PMID:23657437

Mohan, T., Verma, P., & Rao, D. N. (2013). Novel adjuvants & delivery vehicles for vaccines development: A road ahead. *The Indian Journal of Medical Research*, *138*(5), 779–795. PMID:24434331

Moon, J. J., Suh, H., Bershteyn, A., Stephan, M. T., Liu, H., Huang, B., ... Irvine, D. C. (2011). Interbilayer-crosslinked multilamellar vesicles as synthetic vaccines for potent humoral and cellular immune responses. *Nature Materials*, *10*(3), 243–251. doi:10.1038/nmat2960 PMID:21336265

Nakamura, E., Isobe, H., Tomita, N., Sawamura, M., Jinno, S., & Okayama, H. (2000). Functionalized fullerene as a new artificial vector for transfection. *Angewandte Chemie International Edition in English*, *39*, 4254–4257.

Nam, H. Y., Park, J. H., Kim, K., Kwon, I. C., & Jeong, S. Y. (2009). Lipid-based emulsion system as non-viral gene carriers. *Archives of Pharmacal Research*, *32*(5), 639–646. doi:10.100712272-009-1500-y PMID:19471876

Nandy, B., Santosh, M., & Maiti, P. K. (2012). Interaction of nucleic acids with carbon nanotubes and dendrimers. *Journal of Biosciences*, *37*(3), 457–474. doi:10.100712038-012-9220-8 PMID:22750983

Nayerossadat, N., Maedeh, T., & Ali, P. A. (2012). Viral and nonviral delivery systems for gene delivery. *Advanced Biomedical Research*, (1): 1–27. PMID:23210086

Nımesh, S. (2013). Cyclodextrin and cyclodextrin containing polymers. In Gene theraphy: Potentail Application Of Nanotechnology (pp. 287-304). UK Woodhead Publishing Limited. doi:10.1533/9781908818645.287

Novicki, D. L. (2005). DNA vaccines. In H. V. Vohr (Ed.), *Encyclopedic reference of immunotoxicology* (pp. 212–215). Berlin: Springer. doi:10.1007/3-540-27806-0_396

O'Hagan, D. T. (2007). MF59 is a safe and potent vaccine adjuvant that enhances protection against influenza virus infection. *Expert Review of Vaccines*, *6*(5), 699–710. doi:10.1586/14760584.6.5.699 PMID:17931151

Ojeda, E., Puras, G., Agirre, M., Zárate, J., Grijalvo, S., Pons, R., ... Pedraz, J. L. (2015). Niosomes based on synthetic cationic lipids for gene delivery: The influence of polar head-groups on the transfection efficiency in HEK-293,ARPE-19 and MSC-D1 cells. *Organic & Biomolecular Chemistry*, *13*(4), 1068–1081. doi:10.1039/C4OB02087A PMID:25412820

Okore, V. C., Attama, A. A., Ofokansi, K. C., Esimone, C. O., & Onuigbo, E. B. (2011). Formulation and evaluation of niosomes. *Indian Journal of Pharmaceutical Sciences*, *73*(3), 323–328. PMID:22457561

Palakurthi, S., Yellepeddi, V. K., & Kumar, A. (2011). Nanocarriers for Cytosolic Drug and Gene Delivery in Cancer Therapy. In M. Anna & S. Olsztynska (Eds.), *Biomedical engineering, trends, research and technologies* (pp. 245–272). Croatia: InTech. doi:10.5772/12918

Panyam, J., Dali, M. M., Sahoo, S. K., Ma, W., Chakravarthi, S. S., Amidon, G. L., ... Labhasetvar, V. (2003). Polymer degradation and *in vitro* release of a model protein from poly(D,L-lactideco- glycolide) nano- and microparticles. *Journal of Controlled Release*, *92*(1-2), 173–187. doi:10.1016/S0168-3659(03)00328-6 PMID:14499195

Pardakhty, A., & Moazeni, E. (2013). Nano-niosomes in drug, vaccine and gene delivery: A rapid overview. *Nanomedicine Journal*, *1*(1), 1–12.

Park, B. K., & Kim, M. M. (2010). Applications of chitin and its derivatives in biological medicine. *International Journal of Molecular Sciences*, *11*(12), 5152–5164. doi:10.3390/ijms11125152 PMID:21614199

Patel, K., Angelos, S., Dichtel, W. R., Coskun, A., Yang, Y. W., Zink, J. I., & Stoddart, J. F. (2008). Enzyme-responsive snap-top covered silica nanocontainers. *Journal of the American Chemical Society*, *130*(8), 2382–2383. doi:10.1021/ja0772086 PMID:18232687

Patnaik, S., & Gupta, K. C. (2013). Novel polyethylenimine-derived nanoparticles for *in vivo* gene delivery. *Expert Opinion on Drug Delivery*, *10*(2), 215–228. doi:10.1517/17425247.2013.744964 PMID:23252504

Peng, X. H., Qian, X., Mao, H., Wang, A. Y., Chen, Z. G., Nie, S., & Shin, D. M. (2008). Targeted magnetic iron oxide nanoparticles for tumor imaging and therapy. *International Journal of Nanomedicine*, *3*(3), 311–321. PMID:18990940

Perera, G., & Bernkop-Schnürch, A. (2012). Pharmaceutical non-viral formulations for gene vaccines. In J. Thalhamer, R. Weiss, & S. Scheiblhofer (Eds.), *Gene Vaccine* (pp. 109–127). New York: Springer. doi:10.1007/978-3-7091-0439-2_5

Petros, R. A., & DeSimone, J. M. (2010). Strategies in the design of nanoparticles for therapeutic applications. *Nature Reviews. Drug Discovery*, *9*(8), 615–627. doi:10.1038/nrd2591 PMID:20616808

Pohl, M., & Braz, J. (2001). Gene therapy of pain: Emerging strategies and future directions. *European Journal of Pharmacology*, *429*(1–3), 39–48. doi:10.1016/S0014-2999(01)01304-8 PMID:11698025

Probst, C. E., Zrazhevskiy, P., Bagalkot, V., & Gao, X. (2013). Quantum dots as a platform for nanoparticle drug delivery vehicle design. *Advanced Drug Delivery Reviews*, *65*(5), 703–718. doi:10.1016/j.addr.2012.09.036 PMID:23000745

Pujals, S., & Giralt, E. (2008). Proline-rich, amphipathic cell-penetrating peptides. *Advanced Drug Delivery Reviews*, *60*(4-5), 473–484. doi:10.1016/j.addr.2007.09.012 PMID:18187229

Puras, G., Mashal, M., Zárate, J., Agirre, M., Ojeda, E., Grijalvo, S., ... Pedraz, J. L. (2014). A novel cationic niosome formulation for gene delivery to the retina. *Journal of Controlled Release*, *174*, 27–36. doi:10.1016/j.jconrel.2013.11.004 PMID:24231407

Ragusa, A., García, I., & Penadés, S. (2007). Nanoparticles as Nonviral Gene Delivery Vectors. *Transactions on Nanobioscience*, *6*(4), 319–330. doi:10.1109/TNB.2007.908996 PMID:18217625

Rajera, R., Nagpal, K., Singh, S. K., & Mishra, D. N. (2011). Niosomes: A controlled and novel drug delivery system. *Biological & Pharmaceutical Bulletin*, *34*(7), 945–953. doi:10.1248/bpb.34.945 PMID:21719996

Ramamoorth, M., & Narvekar, A. (2015). Non viral vectors in gene therapy- An overview. *Journal of Clinical and Diagnostic Research: JCDR*, *9*(1), 1–6. PMID:25738007

Reichmuth, A. M., Oberli, M. A., Jaklenec, A., Langer, R., & Blankschtein, D. (2016). mRNA vaccine delivery using lipid nanoparticles. *Therapeutic Delivery*, *7*(5), 319–334. doi:10.4155/tde-2016-0006 PMID:27075952

Saffari, M., Moghimi, H. R., & Dass, C. R. (2016). Barriers to liposomal gene delivery: From application site to the target. *Iranian Journal of Pharmaceutical Research*, *15*(Suppl), 3–17. PMID:28228799

Sahdev, P., Ochyl, L. J., & Moon, J. J. (2014). Biomaterials for nanoparticle vaccine delivery systems. *Pharmaceutical Research*, *31*(10), 2563–2582. doi:10.100711095-014-1419-y PMID:24848341

Salimzadeh, L., Jaberipour, M., Hosseini, A., & Avicenna, A. G. (2013). Non-viral transfection methods optimized for gene delivery to a lung cancer cell line. *Avicenna Journal of Medical Biotechnology*, *5*(2), 68–77. PMID:23799175

Sanna, V., Pala, N., & Sechi, M. (2014). Targeted therapy using nanotechnology: Focus on cancer. *International Journal of Nanomedicine*, *9*, 467–483. PMID:24531078

Saupe, A., & Rades, R. (2006). Solid lipid nanoparticles. In M. R. Mozafari (Ed.), *Nanocarrier technologies frontiers of nanotherapy* (pp. 41–43). Springer, Netherlands. doi:10.1007/978-1-4020-5041-1_3

Schmidt, N., Mishra, A., Lai, G. H., & Wong, G. C. L. (2010). Arginine-rich cell-penetrating peptides. *Federation of European Biochemical Societies*, *584*(9), 1806–1813. doi:10.1016/j.febslet.2009.11.046 PMID:19925791

Şenel, B., Büyükköroğlu, G., & Yazan, Y. (2015). Solid lipid and chitosan particulate systems for delivery of siRNA. *Die Pharmazie*, *70*, 698–705. PMID:26790185

Shen, C., Li, J., Zhang, Y., Li, Y., Shen, G., Zhu, J., & Tao, J. (2017). Polyethylenimine-based micro/nanoparticles as vaccine adjuvants. *International Journal of Nanomedicine*, *12*, 5443–5460. doi:10.2147/IJN.S137980 PMID:28814862

Smith, A., Perelman, M., & Hinchcliffe, M. (2014). Chitosan: A promising safe and immune-enhancing adjuvant for intranasal vaccines. *Human Vaccines & Immunotherapeutics*, *10*(3), 797–807. doi:10.4161/hv.27449 PMID:24346613

Sokolova, V., & Epple, M. (2007). Inorganic nanoparticles as carriers of nucleic acids into cells. *Angewandte Chemie International Edition in English*, *46*, 2–16.

Storni, T., Kündig, T. M., Senti, G., & Johansen, P. (2005). Immunity in response to particulate antigen-delivery systems. *Advanced Drug Delivery Reviews*, *57*(3), 333–355. doi:10.1016/j.addr.2004.09.008 PMID:15560945

Sun, N. F., Liu, Z. A., & Hu, S. Y. (2013). The application of nanoparticles for gene vector in tumor gene therapy. *Journal of Tumor*, *1*(5), 24–27.

Termeer, C., Averbeck, M., Hara, H., Eibel, H., Herrlich, P., Sleeman, J., & Simon, J. C. (2003). Targeting dendritic cells with CD44 monoclonal antibodies selectively inhibits the proliferation of naive $CD4^+$ T-helper cells by induction of FAS-independent T-cell apoptosis. *Immunology*, *109*(1), 32–40. doi:10.1046/j.1365-2567.2003.01617.x PMID:12709015

Thapa, B., & Narain, R. (2016). Mechanism, current challanges and new approaches for non viral gene delivery. In R. Narain (Ed.), *Polymer and Nanomaterials for gene therapy* (pp. 1–28). Elsevier. doi:10.1016/B978-0-08-100520-0.00001-1

Tiera, M. J., Winnik, F. O., & Fernandes, J. C. (2006). Synthetic and natural polycations for gene therapy: State of the art and new perspectives. *Current Gene Therapy*, *6*(1), 59–71. doi:10.2174/156652306775515510 PMID:16475946

Trewyn, B. G., Giri, S., Slowing, I. I., & Lin, V. S. (2007). Mesoporous silica nanoparticle based controlled release, drug delivery, and biosensor systems. *Chemical communications (Cambridge, England)*, *31*(31), 3236–3245. doi:10.1039/b701744h PMID:17668088

Verissimo, L. M., Lima, L. F. A., Egito, L. C. M., de Oliveira, A. G., & do Egito, E. S. T. (2010). Pharmaceutical emulsions: A new approach for gene therapy. *Journal of Drug Targeting*, *18*(5), 333–342. doi:10.3109/10611860903434019 PMID:19958051

Villa, C. H., Dao, T., Ahearn, I., Fehrenbacher, N., Casey, E., Rey, D. A., ... Philips, M. R. (2011). Single-walled carbon nanotubes deliver peptide antigen into dendritic cells and enhance IgG responses to tumor-associated antigens. *ACS Nano*, *5*(7), 5300–5311. doi:10.1021/nn200182x PMID:21682329

Vivero-Escoto, J. L., Slowing, I. I., Wu, C. W., & Lin, V. S. (2009). Photoinduced intracellular controlled release drug delivery in human cells by gold-capped mesoporous silica nanosphere. *Journal of the American Chemical Society*, *131*(10), 3462–3463. doi:10.1021/ja900025f PMID:19275256

Wang, X., Niu, D., Hu, C., & Li, P. (2015). Polyethyleneimine-based nanocarriers for gene delivery. *Current Pharmaceutical Design*, *21*(42), 6140–6156. doi:10.2174/1381612821666151027152907 PMID:26503146

Wang, Y., Rajala, A., & Rajala, R. V. S. (2015). Lipid nanoparticles for ocular gene delivery. *Journal of Functional Biomaterials*, *6*(2), 379–394. doi:10.3390/jfb6020379 PMID:26062170

Wegmann, F., Gartlan, K. H., Harandi, A. M., Brinckmann, S. A., Coccia, M., Hillson, W. R., ... Settantau, Q. J. (2012). Polyethyleneimine is a potentmucosal adjuvant for viral glycoprotein antigens. *Nature Biotechnology*, *30*(9), 883–888. doi:10.1038/nbt.2344 PMID:22922673

Wen, R., Umeano, A. C., Francis, L., Sharma, N., Tundup, S., & Dhar, S. (2016). Mitochondrion: A promising target for nanoparticle-based vaccine delivery systems. *Vaccines*, *4*(18), 1–25. PMID:27258316

Yang, Y., Leonand, M., & Gan, H. (n.d.). Viral and Non-Viral Cancer Gene Therapy. In D. Shi (Ed.), The World Scientific Encyclopedia of Nanomedicine and Bioengineering I: Nanotechnology for Translational Medicine: Tissue Engineering, Biological Sensing, Medical Imaging, and Therapeutics, Volume 3 Nanotechnology in Gene Delivery (pp. 1-33). Singapoure: World Scientific.

Yu, F., Huang, J., Yu, Y., Lu, Y., Chen, Y., Zhang, H., ... Zhong, Y. (2016). Glutathione-responsive multilayer coated gold nanoparticles for targeted gene delivery. *Journal of Biomedical Nanotechnology*, *12*(3), 503–515. doi:10.1166/jbn.2016.2177 PMID:27280248

Yu, M., Niu, Y., Zhang, J., Zhang, H., Yang, Y., Taran, E., ... Yu, C. (2016). Size-dependent gene delivery of amine-modified silica nanoparticles. *Nano Research*, *9*(2), 291–305. doi:10.100712274-015-0909-5

Zha, M. X., & Zhu, B. J. (2016). The research and applications of quantum dots as nano-carriers for targeted drug delivery and cancer therapy. *Nanoscale Research Letters*, *11*(207), 1–9. PMID:26729219

Zhang, S., Xu, Y., Wang, B., Qiao, W., Liu, D., & Li, Z. (2004). Cationic compounds used in lipoplexes and polyplexes for gene delivery. *Journal of Controlled Release*, *100*(2), 165–180. doi:10.1016/j.jconrel.2004.08.019 PMID:15544865

Zhang, Y., Satterlee, A., & Huang, L. (2012). *In vivo* gene delivery by nonviral vectors: Overcoming hurdles? *Molecular Therapy*, *20*(7), 1298–1304. doi:10.1038/mt.2012.79 PMID:22525514

Zhao, L., Seth, A., Wibowo, N., Zhao, C. X., Mitter, N., Yu, C., & Middelberg, A. P. J. (2014). Nanoparticle vaccines. *Vaccine*, *32*(3), 327–337. doi:10.1016/j.vaccine.2013.11.069 PMID:24295808

Zhao, Y., & Huang, L. (2014). Lipid nanoparticles for gene delivery. *Advances in Genetics*, *88*, 13–36. doi:10.1016/B978-0-12-800148-6.00002-X PMID:25409602

KEY TERMS AND DEFINITIONS

Adjuvant: Molecules that increase the power of immunity of vaccines.

Biodegradable: The ability of the active substance to fragment by the action of the organisms or their enzymes.

Cytotoxic: Substances causing damage or death in the structure and function of the cells.

EPR Effect: Enhanced permeability and retention of agent in the target site due to loose vascular occlusion in the tumor area.

Immunogen: Immune stimulating substance, antigen.

In-Vitro Study: Artificial environment study to investigate the effect of a chemical substance on tissue or cells.

In-Vivo Study: Work on living organisms to investigate the direct effects of an agent (chemical substance or microorganism) on a particular organism.

Transfection: Transfer of a genetic information or drug molecule into a cell with viral or non-viral substances.

Chapter 15
Nanocomposites in Drug Delivery and Imaging Applications

Dimple Sethi Chopra
Punjabi University, India

ABSTRACT

Nanocomposites are a class of materials in which one or more phases with nanoscale dimensions are embedded in a metal, ceramic, or polymer matrix. The properties of nanocomposites depend on matrix, loading, degree of dispersion, size, shape, and orientation of the nanoscale phase and interaction between the matrix and the nanoscale phase. Nanocomposites are generally prepared using direct melt intercalation. The formation of nanocomposite is ascertained by XRD pattern, FTIR spectra, electron microscopy, and thermal analysis like DSC and TGA. Nanocomposites have properties of nanoparticles, multifunctional capabilities, chemical functionalization, huge interphase zone. Novel nanomaterials offer a new chemotherapeutic route for cancer treatment by combining cell imaging and hyperthermia in a synergistic way. In spite of toxicity and safety concerns, multifunctional nanocomposite still interest the researchers because of emergence of versatile properties, better understanding of disease biomarkers, and quest for ways to improve biocompatibility.

1. INTRODUCTION

Targeted nano drug delivery envisage not only improved bioavailability but also safety of therapeutic agents. This may provide solution to problems associated with cancer treatment viz. dose-dependent cytotoxicity, drug resistance. Passive targeting is obtained by enhanced permeation and retention (EPR) effect while active targeting depends upon specific interaction between drug carrier and cellular target. Nanocarriers can be functionalized with ligands which bind specifically to receptors on cancer cells which enable them to undergo receptor mediated endocytosis. Tumor cells have been found to overexpress one of these receptors: lectin receptors, Fc receptors, complement receptors, interleukin receptors, lipoprotein receptors, transferrin receptors and dopamine receptors. It has been found that

DOI: 10.4018/978-1-5225-4781-5.ch015

Copyright © 2018, IGI Global. Copying or distributing in print or electronic forms without written permission of IGI Global is prohibited.

dopamine (DA) receptors are overex pressed in human colon adenocarcinoma cells and breast cancer cells. DA functionalized nanocarriers have been used to selectively deliver anticancer drugs curcumin, camptothecin and doxorubicin to human colon adenocarcinoma cells (Das, & Jana, 2015). Considerable efforts have been made towards translation of nanotechnology into medical practice specially for cancer management. The two main applications are diagnosis and therapy. The targets being same, the development of separate approaches can miss opportunity to improve efficacy. The physical properties of nanomaterials enable them to serve as the basis for superior imaging probes to simultaneously locate and deliver therapeutics to cancerous lesions. These technologies have resulted in development of nanotheranostics with both imaging and therapeutic functionalities. These multimodal platforms are valuable components for emerging trend towards personalized medicine (Xie, Liu, Eden, Ai, & Chen, 2011; Chen, Ai, Liu, & Lu, 2014).

Nanocomposites are a class of materials in which one or more phases with nanoscale dimensions are embedded in a metal, ceramic or polymer matrix. There are principally three types of nanocomposites metallic, ceramic, polymer matrix nanocomposites as shown in Figure 1. Polymer nanocomposites have been extensively used for biomedical applications. The possibility to form self-assembled and supramolecular morphologies makes organic polymers and inorganic nanoparticles desirable building blocks for the design of nanocomposite hydrogels. The properties of nanocomposite depend on matrix, loading, degree of dispersion, size, shape and orientation of the nanoscale phase and interaction between the matrix and the nanoscale phase (Kumar, & Krishhnamoorti, 2010). Nanocomposites are generally prepared using direct melt intercalation. Layered double hydroxides are used as nucleating agent which induces crystallization of biopolymers like poly (L-lactide), polycaprolactone. The formation of nanocomposite is ascertained by XRD pattern, FTIR spectra, electron microscopy and thermal analysis like DSC and TGA. Nanocomposites have properties of nanoparticles, multifunctional capabilities, chemical functionalization, huge interphase zone (Taneja, Pareeka, Vermaa, Jaina, Ratana, & Ashawatb, 2012). Many polymer nanocomposites have been used for improved drug delivery. Nanocomposite films of layered double hydroxide tethered with ibuprofen (IBU) blended into poly (l-lactide) polymer exhibited six times higher release rate than non-composite films. Mechanism of drug release changed to diffusion/ion exchange from diffusion controlled process. The prepared nanocomposite film had improved elastic

Figure 1. Schematic representation of a nanocomposite and its types. It is the matrix which determines the type of nanocomposite.

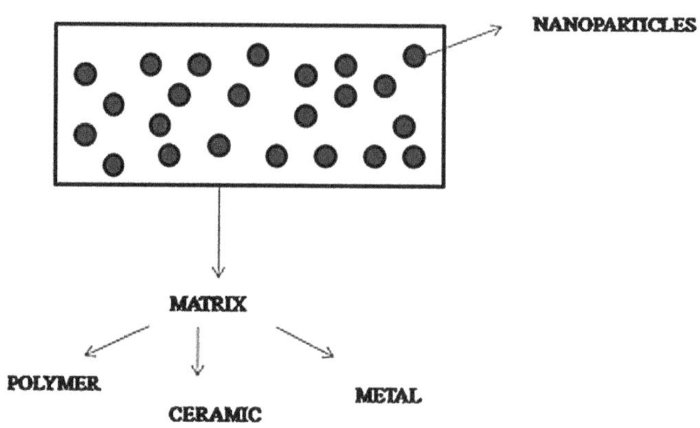

modulus. A new drug delivery system was developed by combining layered double hydroxides (LDH) with electrospinning. LDH-IBU nanoparticles were uniformly dispersed in the electrospun polycaprolactone (PCL) fibers even at a high loading level of 5%w/w. The initial burst release problem in IBU/PCL fibers was considerably reduced by using LDH-IBU. This new drug delivery system is anticipated for effective loading and sustained release of drugs. Recently sodium dodecyl sulfate (SDS) was used to obtain organically modified layered double hydroxide by anion-exchange reaction. The modified LDH provided a better nucleating effect than the unmodified LDH in poly (l-lactide) polymer matrix (Theiss, Avoko, & Frost, 2016).

Multifunctional magnetic nanocomposite can be prepared using a single step, microwave-assisted approach. This method results in higher degree of Fe_3O_4 nanoparticle crystallinity which leads to enhanced magnetic behavior and better relaxivity. Novel nanomaterials offer a new chemotherapeutic route for cancer treatment by combining cell imaging and hyperthermia in a synergistic way (Nalawade, Aware, Kadam, & Hirlekar, 2009). A multifunctional nanocarriers based on up-conversion luminescent nanoparticles of $NaYF_4$: Yb^{3+}/Er^{3+} (UCNPs) core and thermo/pH coupling sensitive polymer poly[(N-isopropylacrylamide)-co-(methacrylic acid)] [P(NIPAm-Co-MAA)] gated mesoporous silica shell represent a platform technology for simultaneous imaging and stimuli responsive controlled drug delivery. Specific functional groups are introduced into the stimuli responsive nanocomposites which can respond to external triggers such as pH, temperature, light, magnetic field, enzymes, reactive oxygen species (ROS). This regulates the movement of the drug payload, thus releasing the drug at a desired time in a desired spatial location. This plays a pivotal role in increasing anticancer drug efficacy. In case of enzyme responsive nanocomposites, drug or imaging agent is released due to specific peptide bond cleavage by enzymes such as cathepsin or matrix metalloproteinase. ROS generated from myeloperoxidase activates nanocomposites by oligomerization of monomers or releases fluorophores by chemical bond cleavage (Miao, Hong, Dan, Ruiyu, Tjiu, & Tianxi, 2012).

Up-conversion luminescent and porous $NaYF_4$: $Yb^{3+}/Er^{3+}@SiO_2$ nanocomposite fibers were prepared by electrospining process. These fibers were tested for biocompatibility on L929 fibroblast cells which revealed low cytotoxicity. Doxorubicin hydrochloride (DOX) a typical anticancer drug is introduced into nanocomposite fibers. The release of DOX exhibited sustained, pH sensitive release patterns. Confocal microscopy showed nanocomposites were successfully taken up by HeLa cells. Furthermore, the fibers show near-infrared UC luminescence and are successfully applied in bioimaging of HeLa cells. The results indicate the promise of using this nanocomposite fibre as multifunctional carriers for drug delivery and cell imaging. Lanthanide ion (Ln^{3+}) based up conversion nanomaterials emit high-energy visible light when excited by low energy near infrared (NIR) light. These nanomaterials have unique optical and chemical properties including minimum photodamage to living organisms, low auto fluorescence, high signal to noise ratio, high detection sensitivity and high penetration depth in biological samples. Many multifunctional (magnetic/up conversion luminescence and porous) composite materials based on Ln^{3+} have been designed for controlled drug delivery and multimodal bioimaging (Hou, Li, Ma, Cheng, Li, Zhang, Dai, Yang, Lian, & Lin, 2012).

Nanocomposites are thus hierarchical structures with tailored properties. Two dimensional materials like grapheme, clay and LDH possessing organized nanosheets act as building blocks for these nanostructures (Sirousazar, 2013). The goal of widespread biomedical application of multifunctional nanocomposite can be attained only after overcoming its potential toxicity. Metal oxides like Fe_3O_4, $MnFe_2O_4$, MnO for MRI purposes, dendrimers and biodegradable polymers for drug delivery and therapeutic biomolecules such as siRNA, antibodies do not exhibit any salient toxicity in short term studies. Hence they can be incorporated into nanocomposites without any potential future risk in human beings (Gaharwar, 2014). Porous silicon nanoparticles, silica nanospheres, carbon nanotubes, gold nanorods and nanoshells, lanthanide group metal oxides with less toxicity issues in short term studies, have yet to prove that they are safe for long-term and frequent administration (Shariatinia, & Zaharee, 2017). Nanocomposites for drug delivery have to be evaluated extensively as far as biocompatibility is concerned, whereas nanocomposites used as image contrast agents, in low doses and administered less frequently are accepted without much resistance (Bai, Muthoosamy, Shipton, Pandikumar, Rameshkumar, Huang, & Manickam, 2016). In spite of toxicity and safety concerns, multifunctional nanocomposite still charm the researchers because of emergence of new nanomaterials with versatile properties, better understanding of disease biomarkers and quest for ways to improve biocompatibility of nanocomposites (Gaharwar, Peppas, & Khademhosseini, 2014).

2. POLYMER MATRIX NANOCOMPOSITES

Recently, there has been significant increase in nanocomposites based on a hydrogel matrix and biopolymeric nanoparticles for controlled release of drugs. Biodegradable nanoparticles have been prepared using poly(α-hydroxy esters) like poly(lactic acid) (PLA) and poly(glycolic acid) (PGA), poly(lactic-co-glycolide) (PLGA) copolymers (Rescignano, Amelia, Credi, Kenny, & Armentano, 2012). They undergo hydrolytic degradation and are removed by natural pathways like tricarboxylic acid cycle. PLA, PGA, PLGA are approved for use in biomedical products and devices by the US Food and Drug Administration. The co-polymer PLGA is usually preferred as it offers a precise control on degradation rate by varying the ratio between its monomers lactic acid and glycolic acid (Ulery, Nair, & Laurencin, 2011). A nanocomposite hydrogel have been prepared by the incorporation of PLA nanoparticles into semi-interpenetrating polymer hydrogels of alginate and thermosensitive poly(N-isopropylacrylamide). The successful incorporation of PLLA nanoparticles into the semiIPN gels was confirmed by field emission scanning electron microscope (FESEM) and infrared spectroscopy (FT-IR). The introduction of PLLA nanoparticles does not affect the thermal stability of the gel and does not modify the lower critical solution temperature (LCST), while interferes with the contraction behavior of the gel, leading to a different thermal expansion coefficient observed for the nanocomposite. Furthermore, rheological results suggest a different degree of crosslinking for the nanocomposite gel, due to the presence of PLLA nanoparticles that probably hinders the reaction of crosslinking of PNIPAAm. The prepared NPs-AlgPNIPAAm-semi IPN gels with thermosensitive and biodegradable properties are very interesting from both applied and fundamental perspectives and make this system a good candidate for practical application in drug delivery and controlled drug release (Rescignano, Hernandez, Armentano, Puglia, Mijangos, & Kenny, 2014). The addition of polymer nanoparticles into hydrogels allows the local delivery of hydrophobic drugs loaded into nanoparticles. The advantages of such system over conventional hydrogels are superior control on the release of high molecular weight drugs. The drug first diffuse through the nanoparticles and then from the hydrogel network. Therefore, in case of nanocomposite hydrogel there are two barriers which control drug release (Laroui, Dalmasso, Nguyen, Yan, Sitaraman, & Merlin, 2010). A novel antibacterial polymeric nanocomposite was developed for co-delivery of anti cancer drugs doxorubicin (DOX) and methotrexate (MTX). The nanocarrier sustained the release of both drugs in a pH-triggered manner. Its antibacterial activity was assessed by minimum inhibitory concentration (MIC) values. Its anticancer performance to MCF7 cell lines was verified by qRT-PCR and MTT assay. The developed nanocomposite proved to be an efficient antibacterial and anticancer drug delivery system (Zakerzadeh, Alizadeh, Kafil, Hassanzadeh, Salehi, & Mahkam, 2016).

3. CHARACTERIZATION OF NANOCOMPOSITES

Nanoparticles are generally characterized by electron microscopy, dynamic light scattering, XRD, differential scanning calorimetry and thermogravimetry. The nanoporous structure of PLGA and PLA nanoparticles was ascertained by an innovative thermal method: thermoporosimetry, providing information about nanopore dimensions. In vitro degradation studies reveal gradual surface degradation of biodegradable nanoparticles. The prepared nanocomposite is characterized by FTIR, ^{1}H NMR, thermogravimetric analysis (TGA), and FESEM-EDX (Chen, Ai, Liu, & Lu, 2014; Kumar, & Krishnamoorti, 2010).

4. GELATIN BASED NANOCOMPOSITES

Gelatin is a natural polymer derived from collagen. It is commonly used for pharmaceutical and medical applications. It is biocompatible as well as biodegradable (Vandervoort, & Ludwig, 2004: Young, Wong, Tabata, & Mikos, 2005). During the fabrication process, the isoelectric point of gelatin can be modified to yield either a negatively charged acidic gelatin or a positively charged basic gelatin at physiological pH. This property forms the basis of electrostatic interactions between a charged biomolecule and gelatin, forming polyion complexes. Many types of gelatin matrices have been used for controlled release applications. The charged biomolecules like proteins and plasmid DNA were absorbed by gelatin matrix (Fukunaka, Iwanaga, Morimoto, Kakemi, & Tabata, 2002; Yamamoto, Takahashi, & Tabata, 2003). The complexed biomolecules are released by enzymatic degradation of the matrix which in turn depends upon crosslinking density of gelatin hydrogels (Yamamoto, Ikada, & Tabata, 2001).

Samba *et al.* prepared novel nanocomposites based on gelatin polymer networks containing poly(lactic-co-glycolide)(PLGA) nanoparticles (PLGA-NPs). Their morphological, chemical and rheological properties were investigated. The incorporation of PLGA nanoparticles into the gelatin gels was confirmed by field emission scanning electron microscope (FESEM) and infrared spectroscopy (FTIR). FESEM microscopy comparatively homogeneous pore structure of the nanocomposite with respect to the primary gel. The introduction of PLGA nanospheres at a 1% w/v with respect to gelatin weight does not influence the elastic modulus of the pristine gelatin but an increase in the amount of PLGA nanospheres had a negative effect on the elastic modulus. The prepared PLGA-NPs gelatin gels with biocompatible and biodegradable properties have potential for the control release of active molecules (Samba, Hernandez, Rescignano, Mijangos, & Kenny, 2015).

5. ALBUMIN BASED NANOCOMPOSITE

It has been found that inflammatory cells in rheumatoid arthritis (RA) patients metabolize more albumin than healthy cells. This was further confirmed by Wunder et al. They showed that fluorescence-labeled human serum albumin were concentrated in the arthritic regions of mouse compared to those without arthritis (Krukemeyer, Krenn, Jakobs, & Wagner, 2012). Cancer cells also require large amounts of nitrogen and energy for their fast replication and growth. Studies have suggested that cancer cells most likely utilize albumin as a source of nitrogen and energy. All these facts form the basis of inclusion of albumin within a drug delivery system to increase its retention in tumor and inflammatory tissues (Ryou, Park, Kim, Jeon, Yun, Han, Kim, Lee, Kim, Han, Bae, & Lee, 2011).

A variety of nanostructures have been designed to achieve magnetic resonance (MR) imaging, near-infrared fluorescence(NIRF), photoacoustics (PA), computed tomography (CT) for tumor detection (Misak, Zachariasb, Song, Hwangd, Mana, Asmatulua, & Yang, 2013; Wunder, Muller-Ladner, Stelzer, Funk, Neumann, Stehle, Pap, Sinn, Gay, & Fiehn, 2003; Misak, Asmatulu, Gopu, Man, Zacharias, Wooley, & Yang, 2014; Menon, Jadeja, Tambe, Vu, Yuan, & Nguyen, 2013). However, monomodal imaging of nanoparticles is difficult to satisfy spatial resolution and ultrasensitivity characteristics of an ideal imaging technique. MR imaging possesses high spatial resolution, but limited sensitivity; whereas fluorescent imaging has excellent sensitivity, but lacks spatial and anatomical resolution. PA imaging is a novel imaging modality that can visualize microscopic biological objects such as solid tumor and its inner vasculature through thermoelastic expansion and thereof photoacoustic waves, and thus is capable of providing anatomical localization and satisfactory spatial resolution at microscopic level (Misak, Asmatula, Gopu, Man, Zacharias, Wooley, & Yang, 2014). Recently, multifunctional nanoparticles have been explored for multimodal imaging (Wang, & Hu, 2012). Albumin scaffold of nanocomposites has the potential to biomineralize metal nanocrystals and simultaneously integrate various functional organic molecules for widespread theranostic applications. Bovine serum albumin (BSA) has been found to sequester inorganic ions such as Au ions through a simulative biomineralization process which triggers the formation of metal ion complexes and subsequent formation of protein coated nanoclusters. Albumin-based biomineralization have several advantages which includes reproducibility, stability. The amino acid residues on the surface are used to integrate cyanine dyes for designing effective theranostic nanocomposites (Menon, Jadeja, Tambe, Vu, Yuan, & Nguyen, 2013; Li, Anton, Zuber, Vandamme, 2014)

Wang et al. have successfully synthesized smart cyanine grafted gadolinium oxide nanocrystals (Cy-GdNCs) with largest hydrodynamic diameter of 20.3 nm using an optimized biomineralization process, in which albumin was complexed with Gd ions, resulting in formation of Gd_2O_3 nanocrystals within protein scaffold in basic environment, followed by conjugation of cyanine dye on protein scaffold. Cy-GdNCs exhibited ultrasensitivity, precise anatomical localization, and good spatial resolution, which resulted in successful attainment of multimodal (NIRF/PA/MR) imaging with precise tumor localization. Moreover, Cy-GdNCs show pH responsive photothermal effect, enhanced tumor accumulation, and increased cellular uptake, resulting in tumor ablation without regrowth (Li, Anton, Zuber, Vandamme, 2014).

6. MAGENTITE NANOCOMPOSITES

Magnetic nanoparticles, particularly superparamagnetic iron oxide nanoparticles (SPIONs), have been extensively studied as contrast agents for magnetic resonance imaging (MRI). Due to considerable progress in synthesis and surface modification of iron oxide nanoparticles, many opportunities exist for these biomaterials. These tiny magnetic crystals are potential platforms with large surface-to-volume ratios. The surface functionalization of SPION make them excellent scaffolds for the construction of theranostic agents. Researchers have developed many physicochemical methods to prepare magnetic nanoparticles that possess accurate sizes, shapes, compositions, magnetizations, relaxivities, and surface charges. These features can be used to reduce toxicity, improve stability of nanoparticles to further load functionalities, onto the nanoparticle surfaces (Xie, Liu, Eden, Ai, & Chen, 2011).

Magnetic drug targeting (MDT) is a new treatment principle for tumors. Passive MDT (pMDT) uses cytostatics coupled to ferromagnetic nanoparticles, whereas in active MDT (aMDT), extracorporeal magnets are placed over the tumor area. Krukemeyer *et al,* prepared mitoxantrone-magnetite-dextran composite particles to assess the distribution and effect of MDT in a rhabdomyosarcoma rat model. MDT exhibited higher levels of mitoxantrone in tumor tissue without increase in plasma drug concentration which subsequently resulted in reduced tumor volume (Krukemeyer, Krenn, Jakobs, & Wagner, 2012).

A magnetically targeted drug delivery system (DDS) with magnetic field strengths between 100 and 2500 Oersted is promising external force for drug localization due to higher magnetic targeting effectiveness, lower risk, and lower cost as compared to other targeted systems (Rescignano, Amelia, Credi, Kenny, & Armentano, 2012). 5-fluorouracil (5-Fu) loaded magnetic nanocomposite were prepared using an emulsion-solvent evaporation method, and tested on a mouse model of experimental squamous cell carcinoma (SCC) a type of skin cancer. The nanocomposite thus prepared was spherical in shape with a particle size of 750–1100 nm. It consisted of PLGA, HSA, 5-FU, magnetite nanoparticles (10 nm) and a fluorescent tracer (diphenylhexatriene). Diphenylhexatriene (DPH) helps in tracking the nanocomposite within the tumor tissue. The purpose of using albumin was to localize the nanocomposite in the tumor tissue once they it was globally guided by magnetic nanoparticles. It was found that magnetic targeted nanocomposite exhibited significantly superior therapeutic effects in treating the skin cancer in comparison to local subcutaneous injection of 5-FU. Moreover, it was found that magnetically targeted nanocomposite was able to treat the tumor for longer time with lower concentration of 5-FU. This further reduces the risk of drug toxicity (Misak, Zachariasb, Song, Hwangd, Mana, Asmatulua, & Yang, 2013).

7. METAL OXIDE-GRAPHENE OXIDE NANOCOMPOSITE

Graphene is one atom thick, two dimensional (2D) monolayer sheet of in-plane sp2 bonded carbons having unaffected p_z orbitals. Its derivative graphene oxide (GO), chemically converted graphene (CCG)/ reduced graphene oxide (rGO) are most commonly used. These derivatives are reported to form functional nanocomposites with polymers (e.g. polyaniline, polyvinylalcohol), metal/metal ions (e.g. Ag, Au, Pt/Eu ion) and metal oxides (e.g. ZnO, TiO2, Fe3O4, MnO2, SnO2, Co3O4) (Kundu, Layek, Kuila, Nandi, 2012; Son, Kwon, Park, Seo, Yi, Angadi, Lee, & Choi, 2012; Zhou, Wang, Li, Zhang, Li, Wu, Wen, Lu, & Cheng, 2010; Peng, Peng, Liu, Wu, Xie, Yu, 2013; Kim, Kim, Park, Gwon, Seo, Kim, Kang, 2010; Wu, Ren, Wen, Gao, Zhao, Chen, Zhou, Li, & Cheng, 2010). The nanocomposites thus formed have superior electrical, optical, electrochemical and mechanical properties resulting in widespread applications like cellular imaging, antibacterial property, drug delivery, enzyme sensing, photothermal therapy, photocatalytic activity, supercapacitors, photovoltaic devices (Wu, Xu, Yao, Liu, & Shi, 2010; Hu, Chen, Hung, Chen, & Chen, 2012; Huang, Qi, Boey, & Zhang, 2012). Graphene oxide (GO) and its derivatives are gaining importance to develop nanocarriers for drug delivery and biological imaging. They possess large specific surface area for entrapment of drugs. Surface functionalization of graphene sheets improves their selectivity, aqueous dispersibility, biocompatibility and reduces their aggregation (Bera, Ghosh, Pal, Das, Saha, Dutta, & Jana, 2014).

ZnO is a well-known functional semiconductor oxide having wide band gap (3.37 eV, at room temperature) and a large excitation binding energy (60 meV). Because of its characteristic UV emission,

ZnO could be an important material for optoelectronic application. Moreover, several visible emissions could be observed under a single light excitation due to the formation of surface defects in ZnO (Zhan, Zheng, Pan, Sun, & Li, 2012; Pal, Bera, Sarkar, & Jana, 2014). These emissions can be tuned through doping with Iron, europium or controlling parameters during material synthesis. Europium incorporated ZnO-chemically converted graphene (CCG) ternary nanocomposites (ZEG) were synthesized by varying europium nitrate to zinc acetate molar ratios with fixed amount of graphene oxide, using low temperature (95°C) solvothermal process. The change in crystallite/particle size of hexagonal ZnO was found to be dependent on the Eu incorporation level. There was evidence of chemical interaction/complexation between the oxygen functionalities of CCG and inorganic moieties (ZnO/Zn2+ and Eu ions). The nanocomposite formed was mesoporous with large specific surface area. the photoluminescence spectra of the nanocomposites exhibited UV emission, an orange emission at 595 nm and other visible emissions. Under a confocal laser scanning microscope, bright orange fluorescence images of human breast cancer cells (MCF7) with the ZEG nanocomposite indicated the internalization of nanomaterials within the cells. The nanocomposite also exhibited comparatively low in vitro cytotoxicity on the cells. Therefore ZEG nanocomposite are suitable for both cancer cell targeted optical imaging and drug delivery (Bera, Ghosh, Pal, Das, Saha, Dutta, & Jana, 2014).

Another method could be, through the formation of nanocomposite with graphene. The Zn^{2+} ions chemisorbed on the ZnO nanoparticles, react with the oxygen of carboxylic, hydroxyl and epoxide functional groups of GO, leading to the formation of Zn–O–C bonding. graphene shows better biocompatibility in comparison to ZnO as living cell can well adhere and proliferate on graphene sheets. The biocompatibility of ZnO nanoparticles is improved by surface modification with graphene. In the nanocomposites, GO get transformed into chemically converted graphene (CCG) also known as reduced graphene oxide, rGO with a lesser number of oxygen containing functional groups (Pal, Bera, Sarkar, & Jana, 2014). Zhao et al. studied carboxylated GO conjugated folate-terminated PEG (CG–PEG–FA) nanocarrier which exhibited good dispersibility in PBS media, high drug-loading efficiency, significant cytocompatibility, and precise targeting of folate receptors (Zhao, Li, & Lee, 2008). Masoudipour et al., conjugated dopamine onto nano graphene oxide (nGO) via amide bonding in order to design a targeted nanocarrier for anti-cancer drug, Methotrexate (MTX) for dopamine receptor positive cancer cells. The large number of carboxyl functional groups of nGO provide a suitable interface for conjugation with amino group of dopamine. The benzene ring and hydroxyl groups of dopamine provide another interface for hydrophobic interaction and hydrogen bonding with nGO respectively. MTX was loaded at pH equal to its pka (4.7) under acidic condition. The protonation of amino group present in MTX resulted in electrostatic interaction with negatively charged nGO. In vitro release study showed that the release profile of MTX from DA-nGO was diffusion controlled. In vitro cytotoxicity tests further supported the fact that the presence of DA on the surface of nanocarrier improved its uptake by DA receptor positive cancer cells (Masoudipour, Kashanian, & Maleki, 2017).

For biomedical applications like drug delivery, bioimaging, tissue engineering, bioimmobilization, biosensor metal oxide nanoparticles should possess adequate biocompatibility, particle size and surface for biofunctionalization. Biofunctionalization involves surface modification of nanoparticles for obtaining adequate biocompatibility. It is of utmost importance to study the interaction between metal oxide nanoparticles and protein as nanoparticles get surrounded by protein molecules in biological fluids. Recently Naskar *et al.* studied interaction between zinc oxide – reduced graphene oxide nanocomposite (ZG) with BSA by UV-visible and photoluminescence spectral studies. The interaction between the BSA protein increased with increasing ZG content. The ZnO nanoparticles were synthesized by polyvinylalcohol foam based precursor followed by coupling of the nanoparticles with in-situ formed reduced graphene oxide (rGO) from as-synthesized graphene oxide in presence of hydrazine. Field emission scanning and transmission electron microscopy revealed that ZnO/ZnO-rGO (ZG) nanoparticles are quasi-spherical. FTIR and Raman spectral analysis revealed existence of chemical interaction between the oxygen functional groups of rGO and the inorganic moiety (ZnO/Zn^{2+}) present in ZG nanocomposite (Naskar, Khan, Bera, & Jana, 2017). Quantum-dot-tagged reduced graphene oxide (QD-rGO) nanocomposites internalized into targeted tumor cells display bright fluorescence from the QDs by absorbing Near Infra Red (NIR) radiation incident on the rGO and convert it into heat. The cell death is revealed by simultaneous cell fluorescence reduction. Thus graphene nanocomposite is not only capable of tumor imaging, photothermal therapy but also in situ monitoring of treatment (Bera, Ghosh, Pal, Das, Saha, Dutta, & Jana, 2014).

8. MESOPOROUS NANOCOMPOSITE

Ordered mesoporous materials possess organized nanochannels, high pore volumes, narrow pore size distributions, and large surface area. This makes them suitable for controlled drug release.

The adsorption of drug molecules into the porous mesostructure is governed by textural features of the matrix such as mesopore diameter, type of mesostructure, surface area, and surface chemistry (Vallet-Regi, 2014). Development of inorganic-based drug delivery systems including mesoporous silica (Slowing, Trewyn, Giri, & Lin, 2007), hydroxyapatite (Itokazu, Yang, Aoki, Hara, & Kato, 1998), bioactive glass (Xia, & Chang, 2006), calcium phosphate cements (Del Real, Wolke, & Vallet-Regi, 2002), has led to considerable advances in the field of drug delivery (Arcos, Vallet-Regi, 2013). Magnesium-based biomaterials have received much attention due to their excellent bioactivity, biocompatibility, and mechanical properties as bone regeneration material and local drug delivery systems. These systems include magnesium-containing bioactive glasses, Mg-substituted calcium phosphate bone cements (Verron, Gauthier, Janvier, Pilet, Lesoeur, & Bujoli, 2010; Moscofian, Silva, & Airoldi, 2008), forsterite (Mg2SiO4)(Hassanzadeh-Tabrizi, Bigham, & Rafienia, 2016). Biomaterials that are ideally suitable for bone repair, should be both bioactive and have capacity for controllable drug delivery (Vallet-Regi, 2014). Moreover, magnesium is one of the important constituents of body fluids and bone tissue. It may improve bone mineral density and prevent bone fragility and plays a key role in the development of bony tissue by promoting the adhesion and growth of osteoblastic cells (Wu, Tang, Guo, Tang, Niu, Zhang, Zhang, Ma, Su, Liu, & Wei, 2014). Bigham *et al.* prepared ordered mesoporous magnesium silicate (OMMS) by sol-gel method and studied the effect of calcination temperature on release of ibuprofen (IBU).The prepared powders were calcined at 350, 550, 750°C and characterized by X-ray diffraction (XRD), Fourier transmissioninfrared spectroscopy (FTIR), N2 adsorption–desorption, and transmission electron microscopy (TEM). All samples demonstrated mesoporous characteristics with high specific surface area ranging from 386-504 m^2/g. It was found that the sample calcined at 350°C showed the slowest drug release among all samples, due to smaller pore size and the existence of larger amounts of intrawall microporosity. Cytotoxicity of MG63 osteoblast cell line was investigated by MTT assay, indicating no toxicity for IBU loaded sample calcined at 550 °C with a concentration less than 10 mg/ml. Thus, altering the calcination temperature changes the drug delivery behavior of OMMS by affecting textural properties and reveals OMMS as a promising local drug delivery system for bone tissue engineering applications (Bigham, Hassanzadeh-Tabrizi, Rafienia, & Salehi, 2016).

9. HYBRID NANOCOMPOSITE

A hybrid nanocomposite of silver nanoparticles (AgNPs) and clotrimazole was prepared to overcome clotrimazole resistance. An inclusion complex of clotrimazole with β-cyclodextrin was prepared to improve its water solubility. The drug loaded dextrin moiety was functionalized on the surface of bovine serum albumin (BSA)stabilized silver nanoparticles using 1-Ethyl-3-(3-dimethylaminopropyl) carbodiimide/N-hydroxysulfosuccinimide(EDC/NHS) chemistry. The use of BSA helped in preventing physical interaction of AgNPs with clotrimazole β-cyclodextrin complex. The idea is to totally disrupt the resistance development process by multi targeting approach. AgNPs because of its surface properties and sustained release of Ag^{+} induce direct disruption of fungal cell membrane,inhibition of DNA replication, ATP production and generation of reactive oxygen species. Clotrimazole released from this hybrid inhibit ergosterol biosynthesis, leading to leaky fungal plasma membrane (Chauhan, Gupta, Sehrawat, Karla, Rath, & Goyal, 2015). Such hybrid nanocomposites bear immense potential for antifungal therapy where chances of drug resistance are quite high. It has been found that silver based nanocomposites had shown significant inhibiton against microorganisms including 16 major species of bacteria (Perreault, Faria, Nejati, Elimelech, 2015). Moreover, AgNPs are known to be environmental friendly, non-toxic material for biomedical applications (Prabhu, & Poulose, 2012).

10. CONCLUSION AND FUTURE PROSPECTS

There is a great need for processing technologies that are able to create hierarchically organized nanostructured materials similar to those found in natural bio-nanocomposites like bone, teeth or antler. Such natural composites are typically made by 'bottom-up' self assembly processes rather than 'top-down' processes as often used in industrially relevant processes. 'Bottom-up' methods, many of which are related to chemical processes and self-assembly, have also been shown to be very attractive to create manmade organized nanostructured materials. Examples are layer-by-layer techniques to create brick-and-mortar structures similar to those found in abalone shells or sol-gel techniques to create nanostructured ceramic coatings. 'Top-down' processes that allow for microstructuration, remain however of great interest for the fabrication of nanostructured materials and devices as they are often more industrially relevant and allow for an almost perfect positioning and repeatability. It is clear that nanocomposite materials have a huge potential in future technologies but the creation of these materials with controlled structural organization in combination with engineered interfaces is still a great challenge. The future of nanocomposites research will therefore rely on our ability to create complex multifunctional structures with new capabilities such as self-sensing, self-healing, embedded power etc. Natural composites are here a great source of inspiration as they often exhibit high levels of hierarchy and structural organization at high filler loadings and the origin of toughness of many biological structures has been attributed to nanocomposite mechanism. Biopolymeric porous nano-systems of PLA, PLGA offer a great potential for substantial improvement in tissue engineering, diagnosis and targeted drug delivery systems. Successful targeting of various anticancer drugs have been achieved by incorporating albumin into magnetic nanocomposite. Thus, the future lies in successful design of theranostic nanocomposites, a novel approach for both multimodal imaging and cancer therapy.

REFERENCES

Anderson, J. M., & Shive, M. S. (2012). Biodegradation and biocompatibility of PLA and PLGA microspheres. *Advanced Drug Delivery Reviews*, *64*, 72–82. doi:10.1016/j.addr.2012.09.004

Arcos, D., & Vallet-Regi, M. (2013). Bioceramics for drug delivery. *Acta Materialia*, *61*(3), 890–911. doi:10.1016/j.actamat.2012.10.039

Bai, R. G., Muthoosamy, K., Shipton, F. N., Pandikumar, A., Rameshkumar, P., Huang, N. M., & Manickam, S. (2016). The biogenic synthesis of a reduced graphene oxide–silver (RGO–Ag) nanocomposite and its dual applications as an antibacterial agent and cancer biomarker. *RSC Advances*, *6*(43), 36576–36587. doi:10.1039/C6RA02928K

Bera, S., Ghosh, M., Pal, M., Das, N., Saha, S., Dutta, S. K., & Jana, S. (2014). Synthesis, characterization and cytotoxicity of europium incorporated ZnO–graphene nanocomposites on human MCF7 breast cancer cells. *RSC Advances*, *4*(71), 37479–37490. doi:10.1039/C4RA06243D

Bigham, A., Hassanzadeh-Tabrizi, S. A., Rafienia, M., & Salehi, H. (2016). Ordered Mesoporous Magnesium Silicate with Uniform Nanochannels as a Drug Delivery System:The Effect of Calcination Temperature on DrugDelivery Rate. *Ceramics International*, *42*(15), 17185–17191. doi:10.1016/j.ceramint.2016.08.009

Chauhan, G., Gupta, N., Sehrawat, D., Kalra, S., Rath, G. A., & Goyal, A. (2015). Albumin stabilized silver nanoparticles-clotrimazole β-cyclodextrin hybrid nanocomposite for enriched anti-fungal activity in normal and drug resistant Candida cells. *RSC Advances*, *5*(87), 71190–71202. doi:10.1039/C5RA08274A

Chen, Y., Ai, K., Liu, Y., & Lu, L. (2014). Tailor-made charge-conversional nanocomposite for pH-responsive drug delivery and cell imaging. *ACS Applied Materials & Interfaces*, *6*(1), 655–663. doi:10.1021/am404761h PMID:24308443

Das, P., & Jana, N. R. (2015). Dopamine functionalized polymeric nanoparticle for targeted drug delivery. *RSC Advances*, *5*(42), 33586–33594. doi:10.1039/C5RA03302K

Del Real, R. P., Wolke, J. G. C., Vallet-Regi, M., & Jansen, J. A. (2002). A new method to produce macropores in calcium–phosphate cements. *Biomaterials*, *17*(17), 3673–3680. doi:10.1016/S0142-9612(02)00101-1 PMID:12109693

Fukunaka, Y., Iwanaga, K., Morimoto, K., Kakemi, M., & Tabata, Y. (2002). Controlled release of plasmid DNA from cationized gelatin hydrogels based on hydrogel degradation *J. Controll. Rel.*, *2*(80), 333–343.

Gaharwar, A. K., Peppas, N. A., & Khademhosseini, A. (2014). Nanocomposite hydrogels for biomedical applications. *Biotechnology and Bioengineering*, *111*(3), 441–453. doi:10.1002/bit.25160 PMID:24264728

Hassanzadeh-Tabrizi, S. A., Bigham, A., & Rafienia, M. (2016). Surfactant-assisted sol–gel synthesis of forsterite nanoparticles as a novel drug delivery system. *Materials Science and Engineering C*, *58*, 737–741. doi:10.1016/j.msec.2015.09.020 PMID:26478366

Hou, Z., Li, C., Ma, P., Cheng, Z., Li, X., Zhang, X., ... Lin, J. (2012). Up-Conversion Luminescent and Porous NaYF 4:Yb 3 +, Er 3 + @SiO 2 Nanocomposite Fibers for Anti-Cancer Drug Delivery and Cell Imaging. *Advanced Functional Materials*, *22*(13), 2713–2722. doi:10.1002/adfm.201200082

Hu, S. H., Chen, Y. W., Hung, W. T., Chen, I. W., & Chen, S. Y. (2012). Quantum-dot-tagged reduced graphene oxide nanocomposites for bright fluorescence bioimaging and photothermal therapy monitored in situ. *Advanced Materials*, *24*(13), 1748–1754. doi:10.1002/adma.201104070 PMID:22422734

Huang, X., Qi, X., Boey, F., & Zhang, H. (2012). Graphene-based composites. *Chemical Society Reviews*, *41*(2), 666–686. doi:10.1039/C1CS15078B PMID:21796314

Itokazu, M., Yang, W., Aoki, T., Hara, A. O., & Kato, N. (1998). Synthesis of antibiotic-loaded interporous hydroxyapatite blocks by vacuum method and in vitro drug release testing. *Biomaterials*, *19*(7-9), 817–819. doi:10.1016/S0142-9612(97)00237-8 PMID:9663758

James, K. C., & Gaharwar, A. K. (2014). Bioinspired Polymeric Nanocomposites for Regenerative Medicine. *Macromolecular Chemistry and Physics*, *216*, 248–264.

Kim, H., Kim, S. W., Park, Y. U., Gwon, H., Seo, D. H., Kim, Y., & Kang, K. (2010). SnO_2/graphene composite with high lithium storage capability for lithium rechargeable batteries. *Nano Research*, *3*(11), 813–821. doi:10.100712274-010-0050-4

Krukemeyer, M. G., Krenn, V., Jakobs, M., & Wagner, W. (2012). Magnetic drug targeting in a rhabdomyosarcoma rat model using magnetite-dextran composite nanoparticle-bound mitoxantrone and 0.6 tesla extracorporeal magnets - sarcoma treatment in progress. *Journal of Drug Targeting*, *20*(2), 185–193. doi:10.3109/1061186X.2011.622399 PMID:22044194

Kumar, S. K., & Krishnamoorti, R. (2010). Nanocomposites: Structure, Phase Behavior, and Properties. *Annual Review of Chemical and Biomolecular Engineering*, *1*(1), 37–58. doi:10.1146/annurev-chembioeng-073009-100856 PMID:22432572

Kundu, A., Layek, R. K., Kuila, A., & Nandi, A. K. (2012). Highly Fluorescent Graphene Oxide-Poly(vinyl alcohol) Hybrid: An Effective Material for Specific Au3+ Ion Sensors. *ACS Applied Materials & Interfaces*, *4*(10), 5576–5582. doi:10.1021/am301467z PMID:23009213

Laroui, H., Dalmasso, G., Nguyen, H. T., Yan, Y., Sitaraman, S. V., & Merlin, D. (2010). Drug-loaded nanoparticles targeted to the colon with polysaccharide hydrogel reduce colitis in a mouse model. *Gastroenterology*, *138*(3), 843–853. doi:10.1053/j.gastro.2009.11.003 PMID:19909746

Li, X., Anton, N., Zuber, G., & Vandamme, T. (2014). Contrast agents for preclinical targeted X-ray imaging. *Advanced Drug Delivery Reviews*, *76*, 116–133. doi:10.1016/j.addr.2014.07.013 PMID:25086373

Luna, L. A. V., Moraes, A. C. M., Consonni, S. R., Pereira, C. D., Cadore, S., Giorgio, S., & Alves, O. L. (2016). Comparative in vitro toxicity of a graphene oxide-silver nanocomposite and the pristine counterparts toward macrophages. *Journal of Nanobiotechnology*, *14*, 1–17. PMID:26912341

Masoudipour, E., Kashanian, S., & Maleki, N. (2017). A targeted drug delivery system based on dopamine functionalized nano graphene oxide. *Chemical Physics Letters*, *668*, 56–63. doi:10.1016/j.cplett.2016.12.019

Menon, J. U., Jadeja, P., Tambe, P., Vu, K., Yuan, B., & Nguyen, K. T. (2013). Nanomaterials for photo-based diagnostic and therapeutic applications. *Theranostics*, *3*(3), 152–166. doi:10.7150/thno.5327 PMID:23471164

Miao, Y. E., Hong, Z., Dan, C., Ruiyu, W., Tjiu, W. W., & Tianxi, L. (2012). Electrospun fibers of layered double hydroxide/biopolymer nanocomposites as effective drug delivery systems. *Materials Chemistry and Physics*, *134*(2-3), 623–630. doi:10.1016/j.matchemphys.2012.03.041

Misak, H., Zachariasb, N., Song, Z., Hwangd, S., Mana, K. P., Asmatulua, R., & Yang, S. Y. (2013). Skin cancer treatment by albumin/5-Fu loaded magnetic nanocomposite spheres in a mouse model. *Journal of Biotechnology*, *164*(1), 130–136. doi:10.1016/j.jbiotec.2013.01.003 PMID:23395619

Misak, H. E., Asmatulu, R., Gopu, J. S., Man, K. P., Zacharias, N. M., Wooley, P. H., & Yang, S. Y. (2014). Albumin-based nanocomposite spheres for advanced drug delivery systems. *Biotechnology Journal*, *9*(1), 163–170. doi:10.1002/biot.201300150 PMID:24106002

Moscofian, A. S., Silva, C. R., & Airoldi, C. (2008). Stability of layered aluminum and magnesium organosilicates. *Microporous and Mesoporous Materials*, *107*(1-2), 113–120. doi:10.1016/j.micromeso.2007.05.047

Nalawade, P., Aware, B., Kadam, V. J., & Hirlekar, R. S. (2009). Layered double hydroxides: A review. *Journal of Scientific and Industrial Research*, *68*, 267–272.

Naskar, A., Khan, H., Bera, S., & Jana, S. (2017). Soft chemical synthesis, characterization and interaction of ZnO graphene nanocomposite with bovine serum albumin protein. *Journal of Molecular Liquids*, *237*, 113–119. doi:10.1016/j.molliq.2017.04.074

Pal, M., Bera, S., Sarkar, S., & Jana, S. (2014). Influence of Al doping on microstructural, optical and photocatalytic properties of sol–gel based nanostructured zinc oxide films on glass. *RSC Advances*, *4*(23), 11552–11563. doi:10.1039/C3RA44612C

Peng, L., Peng, X., Liu, B., Wu, C., Xie, Y., & Yu, G. (2013). Ultrathin Two-Dimensional MnO_2/Graphene Hybrid Nanostructures for High-Performance. *Flexible Planar Supercapacitors. Nano Lett.*, *13*, 2151–2157. PMID:23590256

Perreault, F., de Faria, A. F., Nejati, S., & Elimelech, M. (2015). Antimicrobial Properties of Graphene Oxide Nanosheets: Why Size Matters. *ACS Nano*, *9*(7), 7226–7236. doi:10.1021/acsnano.5b02067 PMID:26091689

Prabhu, S., & Poulose, E. K. (2012). Silver nanoparticles: Mechanism of antimicrobial action,synthesis, medical applications, and toxicity effects. *International Nano Letters*, *2*(1), 32–42. doi:10.1186/2228-5326-2-32

Rescignano, N., Amelia, M., Credi, A., Kenny, J. M., & Armentano, I. (2012). Morphological and thermal behavior of porous biopolymeric nanoparticle. *European Polymer Journal*, *48*(7), 1152–1159. doi:10.1016/j.eurpolymj.2012.05.005

Rescignano, N., Hernández, R., Armentano, I., Puglia, D., Mijangos, C., & Kenny, J. M. (2014). Inclusion of PLLA nanoparticles in thermosensitive semi-interpenetrating polymer. *Networks. Polymer Degradation & Stability*, *108*, 280–287. doi:10.1016/j.polymdegradstab.2014.03.007

Ryou, S. M., Park, M., Kim, J. M., Jeon, C. O., Yun, C. H., Han, S. H., ... Lee, K. (2011). Inhibition of xenograft tumor growthin mice by gold nanoparticle-assisted delivery of short hairpin RNAs against Mcl-1L. *Journal of Biotechnology*, *156*(2), 89–94. doi:10.1016/j.jbiotec.2011.07.037 PMID:21906638

Samba, I., Hernandez, R., Rescignano, N., Mijangos, C., & Kenny, J. M. (2015). Nanocomposite hydrogels based on embedded PLGA nanoparticles in gelatin. *Nanocomposites.*, *1*(1), 46–50. doi:10.1179/2055033214Y.0000000006

Shariatinia, Z., & Zahraee, Z. (2017). Controlled release of metformin from chitosan–based nanocomposite films containing mesoporous MCM-41 nanoparticles as novel drug delivery systems. *Journal of Colloid and Interface Science*, *501*, 60–76. doi:10.1016/j.jcis.2017.04.036 PMID:28433886

Sirousazar, M. (2013). Mechanism of gentamicin sulphate release in nanocomposite hydrogel drug delivery systems. *Journal of Drug Delivery Science and Technology*, *23*(6), 619–621. doi:10.1016/S1773-2247(13)50094-3

Slowing, I. I., Trewyn, B. G., Giri, S., & Lin, V. S. Y. (2007). Mesoporous silica nanoparticles for drug delivery and biosensing applications. *Advanced Functional Materials*, *17*(8), 1225–1236. doi:10.1002/adfm.200601191

Son, D. I., Kwon, B. W., Park, D. H., Seo, W. S., Yi, Y., Angadi, B., ... Choi, W. K. (2012). Emissive ZnO-graphene quantum dots for white-light-emitting diodes. *Nature Nanotechnology*, *7*(7), 465–471. doi:10.1038/nnano.2012.71 PMID:22635098

Taneja, K., Pareeka, A., Vermaa, P., Jaina, V., Yashumati Ratana, Y., & Ashawatb, M. S. (2012). Nanocomposite: An emerging tool for bone tissue transplantation and drug delivery. *Indian Journal of Transplantation.*, *6*(3), 88–96. doi:10.1016/j.ijt.2012.07.002

Theiss, F. L., Ayoko, G. A., & Frost, R. L. (2016). Synthesis of layered double hydroxides containing Mg^{2+}, Zn^{2+}, Ca^{2+} and Al^{3+} layer cations by co-precipitation methods—A review. *Applied Surface Science*, *383*, 200–213. doi:10.1016/j.apsusc.2016.04.150

Tkachenko, A. G., Xie, H., Coleman, D., Glomm, W., Ryan, J., Anderson, M. F., ... Feldheim, D. L. (2003). Multifunctional Gold Nanoparticle−Peptide Complexes for Nuclear Targeting. *Journal of the American Chemical Society*, *125*(16), 4700–4701. doi:10.1021/ja0296935 PMID:12696875

Ulery, B. D., Nair, L. S., & Laurencin, C. T. (2011). Biomedical applications of biodegradable polymers. *Journal of Polymer Science. Part B, Polymer Physics*, *49*(12), 832–864. doi:10.1002/polb.22259 PMID:21769165

Vallet-Regi, M. (2014). *Bio-ceramics with clinical applications*. John Wiley & Sons Ltd. doi:10.1002/9781118406748

Vandervoort, J., & Ludwig, A. (2004). Preparation and evaluation of drug-loaded gelatin nanoparticles for topical ophthalmic use. *European Journal of Pharmaceutics and Biopharmaceutics*, *57*(2), 251–261. doi:10.1016/S0939-6411(03)00187-5 PMID:15018982

Verron, E., Gauthier, O., Janvier, P., Pilet, P., Lesoeur, J., Bujoli, B., ... Bouler, J.-M. (2010). In vivo bone augmentation in an osteoporotic environment using bisphosphonate-loaded calcium deficient apatite. *Biomaterials*, *31*(30), 7776–7784. doi:10.1016/j.biomaterials.2010.06.047 PMID:20643480

Wang, L. V., & Hu, S. (2012). Photoacoustic Tomography: In Vivo Imaging from Organelles to Organs. *Science*, *335*(6075), 1458–1462. doi:10.1126cience.1216210 PMID:22442475

Wang, Y., Yang, T., Ke, H., Zhu, A., Wang, Y., Wang, J., ... Chen, H. (2015). Smart Albumin-Biomineralized Nanocomposites for Multimodal Imaging and Photothermal Tumor Ablation. *Advanced Materials*, *27*(26), 3874–3882. doi:10.1002/adma.201500229 PMID:25997571

Wu, Q., Xu, Y., Yao, Z., Liu, A., & Shi, G. (2010). Supercapacitors Based on Flexible Graphene/Polyaniline Nanofiber Composite Films. *ACS Nano*, *4*(4), 1963–1970. doi:10.1021/nn1000035 PMID:20355733

Wu, Z., Tang, T., Guo, H., Tang, S., Niu, Y., Zhang, J., ... Wei, J. (2014). In vitro degradability, bioactivity and cell responses to mesoporous magnesium silicate for the induction of bone regeneration. *Colloids and Surfaces. B, Biointerfaces*, *120*, 38–46. doi:10.1016/j.colsurfb.2014.04.010 PMID:24905677

Wu, Z. S., Ren, W., Wen, L., Gao, L., Zhao, J., Chen, Z., ... Cheng, H. M. (2010). Graphene Anchored with Co_3O_4 Nanoparticles as Anode of Lithium Ion Batteries with Enhanced Reversible Capacity and Cyclic Performance. *ACS Nano*, *4*(6), 3187–3194. doi:10.1021/nn100740x PMID:20455594

Wunder, A., Müller-Ladner, U., Stelzer, E. H., Funk, J., Neumann, E., Stehle, G., ... Fiehn, C. (2003). Albumin-based drug delivery as novel therapeutic approach for rheumatoid arthritis. *Journal of Immunology (Baltimore, Md.: 1950)*, *170*(9), 4793–4801. doi:10.4049/jimmunol.170.9.4793 PMID:12707361

Xia, W., & Chang, J. (2006). Well ordered mesoporous bioactive glasses (MBG): A promising bioactive drug delivery system. *Journal of Controlled Release*, *110*(3), 522–530. doi:10.1016/j.jconrel.2005.11.002 PMID:16375986

Xie, J., Liu, G., Eden, H. S., Ai, H., & Chen, X. (2011). Surface-engineered magnetic nanoparticle platforms for cancer imaging and therapy. *Accounts of Chemical Research*, *44*(10), 883–892. doi:10.1021/ar200044b PMID:21548618

Xie, J., Zheng, Y., & Ying, J. Y. (2009). Protein-directed synthesis of highly fluorescent gold nanoclusters. *Journal of the American Chemical Society*, *131*(3), 888–889. doi:10.1021/ja806804u PMID:19123810

Yamamoto, M., Ikada, Y., & Tabata, Y. (2001). Controlled release of growth factors based on biodegradation of gelatin hydrogel. Biomater. *Sci. Polym. Ed.*, *12*(1), 77–88. PMID:11334191

Yamamoto, M., Takahashi, Y., & Tabata, Y. (2003). Controlled release by biodegradable hydrogels enhances the ectopic bone formation of bone morphogenetic protein. *Biomaterials*, *24*(24), 4375–4383. doi:10.1016/S0142-9612(03)00337-5 PMID:12922150

Young, S., Wong, M., Tabata, Y., & Mikos, A. G. (2005). Gelatin as a delivery vehicle for the controlled release of bioactive molecules. *J. Controll. Rel.*, *109*(1-3), 256–274. doi:10.1016/j.jconrel.2005.09.023 PMID:16266768

Zakerzadeh, E., Alizadeh, E., Kafil, H. S., Hassanzadeh, A. M., Salehi, R., & Mahkam, M. (2016). Novel antibacterial polymeric nanocomposite for smart co-delivery of anticancer drugs. Artifical Cells [volume?]. *NanoBiotechnology*, *3*, 1–12. doi:10.1080/21691401.2016.1260576

Zhan, Z., Zheng, L., Pan, Y., Sun, G., & Li, L. (2012). Self-powered, visible-light photodetector based on thermally reduced graphene oxide–ZnO (rGO–ZnO) hybrid nanostructure. *Journal of Materials Chemistry*, *22*(6), 2589–2595. doi:10.1039/C1JM13920G

Zhao, X., Li, H., & Lee, R. J. (2008). Targeted drug delivery via folate receptors. *Expert Opinion on Drug Delivery*, *5*(3), 309–319. doi:10.1517/17425247.5.3.309 PMID:18318652

Zhou, G., Wang, D. W., Li, F., Zhang, L., Li, N., Wu, Z. S., ... Cheng, H. M. (2010). Graphene-Wrapped Fe_3O_4 Anode Material with Improved Reversible Capacity and Cyclic Stability for Lithium Ion Batteries Chem. *Mater.*, *22*, 5306–5313.

Chapter 16
Smart Mesoporous Nanomaterials With Improved Therapeutic Applications:
Therapeutic Application of MSN

Sandhya Sanand
ICAR-NRCPB, India

Anshika Tyagi
ICAR-NRCPB, India

Sandeep Kumar
National Institute of Virology, India

Gautam Kaul
National Dairy Research Institute, India

ABSTRACT

Nanomaterials have revolutionized the drug delivery and therapeutic industry due to their unique physical characteristics, which render them extremely manipulative at nano-scale. One such category of nanomaterials is mesoporous silica nanoparticles. Due to their small size and rigid honeycomb-like structure, they are highly conducive for packaging of drugs, dyes, antibodies, etc. In addition, they show excellent biocompatibility. These new generation nanomaterials can be further functionalized by incorporating surface modifications, thus increasing their acceptability as carriers for drugs and molecules. In this chapter, a brief and comprehensive review covering various aspects of the recent advancements in synthesis of mesoporous nanomaterials and post-synthesis strategies for functionalization has been presented. Further, it also sheds light on how efficiently these smart nano-carriers are involved in transport and site-specific delivery of highly toxic drugs, like chemotherapeutic agents for cancer treatment, and their biocompatibility evaluation from a biosafety point of view.

DOI: 10.4018/978-1-5225-4781-5.ch016

Copyright © 2018, IGI Global. Copying or distributing in print or electronic forms without written permission of IGI Global is prohibited.

BACKGROUND

Nanomaterials have revolutionized the drug delivery and therapeutic industry due to their unique physical characteristics which render them extremely manipulative at nano-scale. One such category of nanomaterials is mesoporous silica nanoparticles. Due to their small size and rigid honeycomb like structure, they are highly conducive for packaging of drugs, dyes, antibodies etc. Besides, they show excellent biocompatibility. These new generation nanomaterials can be further functionalized by incorporating surface modifications, thus increasing their acceptability as carriers for drugs and molecules. In this chapter, a brief and comprehensive review covering various aspects of the recent advancements in synthesis of mesoporous nanomaterials and post synthesis strategies for functionalization has been presented. Further, it also throws light on how efficiently these smart nano-carriers are involved in transport and site-specific delivery of highly toxic drugs, like chemotherapeutic agents for cancer treatment, and also, their cytocompatibility/ biocompatibility evaluation from biosafety point of view.

INTRODUCTION

In recent era, nanomaterials have got immense applications in healthcare, electronics, cosmetics and other areas (Xia, Yang, Sun, Wu, Mayers, Gates, Yin, Kim, & Yan, 2003; Sanchez, Belleville, Popall, & Nicole, 2011; Vallet-Regí & Arcos, 2015). They are widely used in nanomedicine which opens new range of solutions for different problems (Lanone, & Boczkowski, 2006; Shi, Votruba, Farokhzad, & Langer, 2010; Fernandez-Fernandez, Manchanda, & McGoron, 2011; Albanese, Tang, & Chan, 2012). Till date, more than 250 nanomedicine products have been developed that have been either accepted for use or are at different stages of clinical study (Etheridge, Campbell, Erdman, Haynes, Wolf, & McCullough, 2013). Besides, nanomaterials have also been employed in development of target-specific drug therapies and methods for early diagnosis of pathologies. Consequently, powerful new nano-devices for early diagnosis, prediction, prevention and personalized treatment of cancer tumors have been developed (Barreto, O'Malley, Kubeil, Graham, Stephan, & Spiccia, 2011; Xie, Liu, Eden, Ai, & Chen, 2011; Baeza, 2014). Use of nanoparticles (NPs) has allowed more effective and patient friendly treatment regimens by reducing drug concentration and dosing frequency, easy administrations and improved safety. Inorganic nanomaterials are highly advantageous as compared to the organic ones in terms of high thermal, chemical and mechanical stability under physiological conditions and biocompatibility. Among inorganic nanomaterials, mesoporous silica nanoparicles (MSNs) are one of the most promising drug carriers, and have attracted increasing attention in fields such as drug delivery, diagnostics, medical imaging and engineering due their unique properties (Figure 1) that include: large surface area (~1000 $m^2 \cdot g^{-1}$ for MCM-41 type particles) and large pore volumes (~1 $cm^3 \cdot g^{-1}$) providing high loading capacity, high degree of tunability, morphology and pore diameter, biocompatibility, bio distribution, biodegradation and excretion (Vallet-Regí, Balas, & Arcos, 2007; Manzano, Colilla, & Vallet-Regí, 2009; Gai, Yang, Li, Wang, Dai, Niu, & Lin, 2010; Yang, Gai, & Lin, 2012; Argyo, Weiss, Braeuchle, & Bein, 2014; Tang, Hu, Zhang, Song, Nie, Wang, Niu, Huang, Lu, & Chen, 2012; Li, Barnes, Bosoy, Stoddart, & Zink, 2012; Colilla, Baeza, & Vallet-Regí, 2015; Vallet-Regí, Manzano, & Colilla, 2012; Martínez, Fuentes-Paniagua, Baeza, Sánchez-Nieves, Cicuéndez, Gómez, de la Mata, González, & Vallet-Regí, 2015). Besides, the ease with which MSNs can be synthesized and that too with a range of

Figure 1. Unique properties of MSNs to be used as therapeutic agent

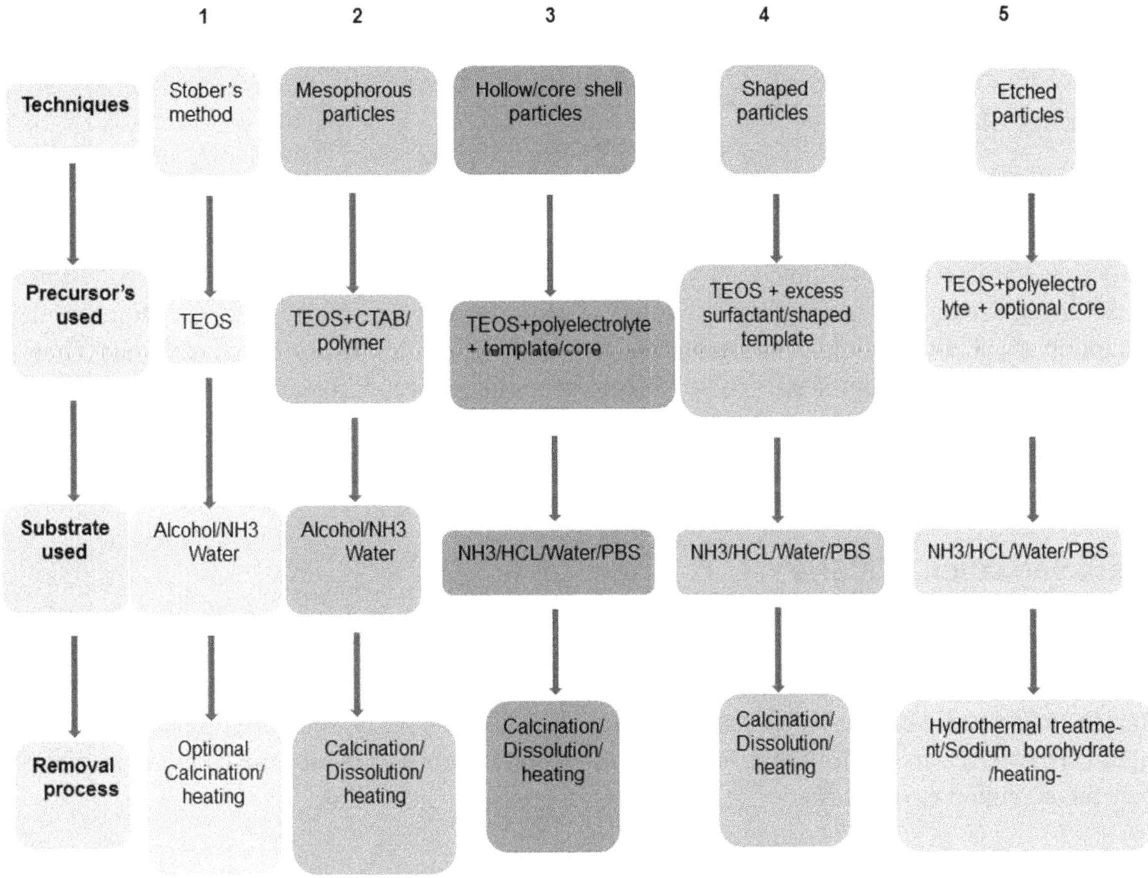

shapes and surface modifications adds to their advantages (Stöber, Fink, & Bohn, 1968; Muñoz, Rámila, Pérez-Pariente, Díaz, & Vallet-Regí, 2003; Trewyn, Slowing, Giri, Chen, & Lin, 2007; Vallet-Regí, & Ruiz-Hernandez, 2011). The following chapter throws light on these aspects as well as on the recent advancements in targeted delivery of therapeutics using MSNs.

Properties of MSNs

Although several carriers viz inorganic and organic NPs, lipid based nano-conjugates and polymeric NPs are used for targeting and delivery of molecules, but MSNs are considered as the most biocompatible and intelligent nano-carriers. Their unique characteristics make them more efficient and competent in drug delivery and imaging systems. The size of MSNs ranges from 5 to 300 nm and can be easily manipulated. Secondly, the uniform pore size of MSNs allows the loading of different kinds of small molecules, chemicals and drugs for targeted delivery. Moreover, the structure of pores in MSNs is very ordered which results imperfect capping and zero premature release of drug molecules. There is no chance of leakage of drug molecules unlike other carries e.g. Dendrimers. Thirdly, the high surface area by volume ratio permits loading of large amounts of drug molecules. The honey comb like structure of MSNs consists of cylindrical pores and external surface of particles can be used for effective functionalization using several functional groups which helps in selective targeting of drug loaded with MSNs. Overall these properties of MSNs make them more efficient carrier for targeted drug delivery.

Synthesis of MSNs

MSNs can be synthesized in two different ways: a) Modified Stöber method (Grun, lauer, & Unger, 1997): It involves cationic surfactants which cause condensation of silica under basic conditions, b) Aerosol-assisted synthesis: It utilizes cationic, anionic and non-ionic surfactants as well to obtain MSNs (Brinker, Lu, Sellinger, & Fan, 1999; Arcos, López-Noriega, & Ruiz-Hernández, 2009) These procedures result in generation of cylindrical mesopores arranged hexagonally, typical of MCM-41 type materials (Kresge, Leonowicz, Roth, & Vartuli, 1992). These MSNs can be subjected to further surface modifications.

There are several other methods also for MSNs synthesis including self-assembly by hard templating, self-assembly by soft templating, solution based synthesis, evaporation induced self-assembly etc. General outline of each method has given in Figure 2.

Characterization of MSNs

Following synthesis, characterization is the most important process which is essential for better understanding of nanomaterials and also to confirm the kind/ class/ size/ shape of nanomaterial we need. Though, many methods exist to characterize properties like nature of solubility, state (aggregation/ agglomeration), reactivity etc. Table1 shows the common methods used for characterization of physicochemical properties of MSNs.

Figure 2. Techniques used in the synthesis of mesoporous nanoparticles

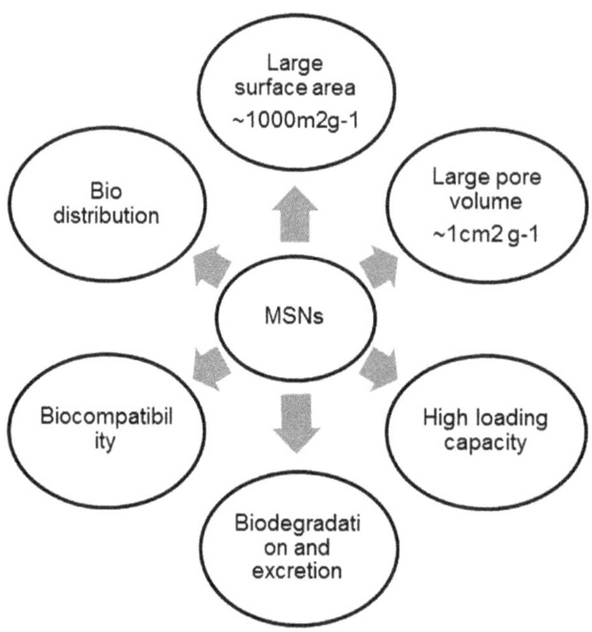

Table 1. Methods used for characterization of MSNs

Physicochemical Property	Methods
Size	DLS, TEM
Surface morphology	SEM, AFM, STM
Surface area and porosity	BET isotherm
Surface charge	Zeta Potential
Molecular structure	FTIR, EDS, SAXS
Surface chemistry	XPS

Functionalization of MSNs

Functionalization of MSNs can be achieved either during MSNs synthesis by co-condensation or post-synthesis using organo alkoxysilanes (Hoffmann, & Fröba, 2011). Specific functionalities can be incorporated for specific purposes like drug adsorption or conjugation of fluorophores for better imaging (Shahbazi, Herranz, & Santos, 2012). These features enhance the functional potential of MSNs. Besides, additional moieties such as targeting agents can also be incorporated into MSNs, thus providing them with multifunctional properties. Below mentioned methods can be used for functionalization.

Co-Condensation

It is widely used for the functionalization of several organoalkxysilane. This is called co- condensation because by introducing two organoalkxysilane, we can produce MSNs containing both acidic as well as basic groups (Huh, Chen, Wiench & J.W, 2005). In this process, functionalization of the silica surface happens simultan eously during the synthesis of the material. Functional groups such as organosilanes are added into the reaction solution together with TEOS or immediately after the addition of TEOS which helps in incorporation of organosilanes in the final material (Kennedy, Bickford, Lewinski, Coughlin, Hu, & Day, 2011).

Post Synthesis Strategies

Grafting Strategy

This strategy is employed where functionalizing molecules are not compatible with medium used for synthesis of mesoporous silicates. Grafting strategies uses commonly employed silane linkers.

Backfilling Strategy

This is also a post synthetic strategy of functionalization. In this approach, pores of mesostructured silica can be filled with functional molecules by incubating empty mesopores with solution or vapor of functional molecules (Rytkonen, Miettinen, Kaasalainen, Lehto, Salonen, & Narvanen, 2012).

Imprint Coating

It is based on the template method to prepare polymer containing organized structures. In this approach, mesoporous materials are coated with ligandspre-bound with metal ions. Recently, preparation of multibranched gold–silica–molecularly imprinted polymer (bAu@mSiO2@MIP) core–shell nanoparticles showed capability to identify the enrofloxacin (ENRO) (Sergio, Elena, Fernando, Judith, Marta, Luis, & María, 2016), thus highlighting the potential application as label-free nanosensors for the specific detection of antimicrobe.

Surface Functionalization as Step for Cell Targeting

One of the major challenges in cancer therapeutics is low concentration of drugs achieved in target tissues. To overcome this, nanomaterials can be functionalized which will improve the efficiency of target selection and delivery of drugs. Porous nanomaterials have the added advantage of being able to get modified with different surface modifications. It has been attempted in recent times using number of molecules viz. peptides, antibodies etc. and have been met with success (Yang, Quan, Lu, Huang, & Lin, 2008; Slowing, Vivero-Escoto, Wu, & Lin, 2008). For efficient tumor targeting, small molecules can be conjugated, preferably in aqueous solvent which has minimal effect on silica.

Selective Targeting

Targeted MSNs can effectively transport and guide the drugs to the site of tumor. Such strategies help to reduce the amount of cytotoxic drugs, thereby improving the therapeutic potential and at the same time reducing the adverse effects to minimal.

Passive Targeting

Tumors develop their own vasculature, but their lymphatic drainage is deficient. Because of this, nanoparticles less than 4 nm cannot diffuse into the tumor and instead accumulatein the tumor interstitium. This phenomenon is called *enhanced permeability and retention (EPR) effect.* Successful passive targeting depends on the circulation time of the nanoparticle and its ability to diffuse into the target tissues.

Active Targeting

Cancerous tissues are a mix of healthy and abnormal tissues. In this context, it is necessary on the part of nanocarriers to selectively target the diseased cells and spare the healthy ones. Active targeting implies modifying the periphery of the nanoparticle so that it preferentially selects the cancerous cells.

Different molecular targets for active targeting of cancer by MSNs are schematically displayed in Figure 3.

Stimuli-Responsive Mesoporous Silica Nanoparticles

In these systems, drug molecules are enclosed within the silica mesopores which are further modified in such a way that it prevents premature release of the drug. Drug release occurs under a given stimuli

Figure 3. Illustration of selective targeting and molecular targets for cancer by mesoporous silica nanoparticles

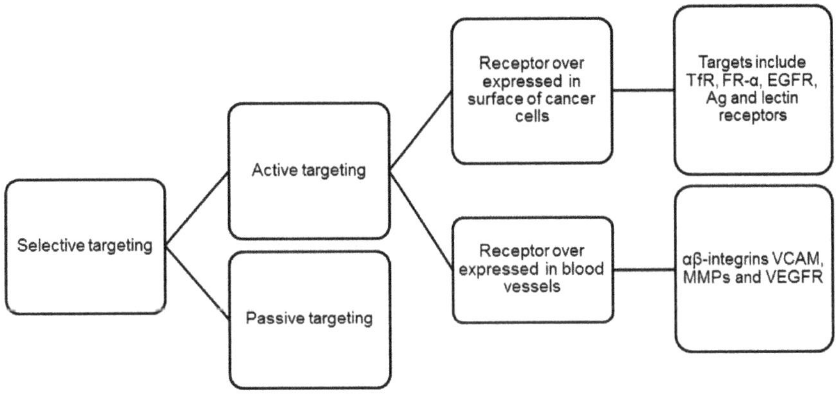

which leads to removal of protective covering and release of drug in the destined tissue. Commonly used linkers are Octadecyl (C18) chains, PNIPAm, DNA strands, Coiled-coil peptide motifs etc.

- **External Stimuli:** The main objective of using stimuli responsive drug delivery is to prevent the untargeted delivery. Stimuli responsive delivery enhances the targeted delivery to the specific site and at the same time minimizes the side effect of drugs. Drug-delivery systems that take advantage of externally applied stimuli, involve temperature changes, magnetic fields, ultrasounds, light

Figure 4. Stimuli-responsive strategies for smart drug delivery mesoporous silica nanoparticles

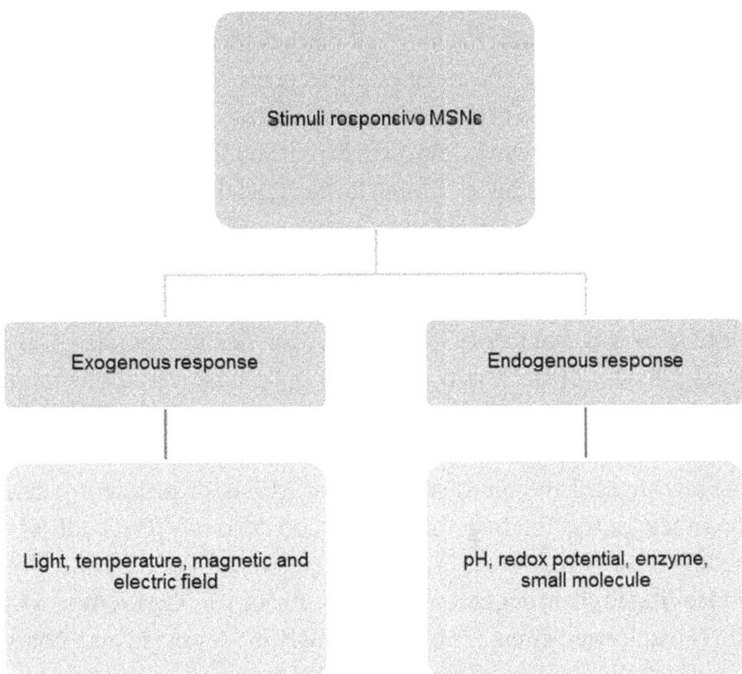

and electric fields. Use of linking and capping agents depends on the type of external stimuli and their compatibility with each other.

- **Internal Stimuli:** Internal stimuli are sensitive to chemical variations arising inside the organism. These stimuli don't rely on external sources for releasing drugs. Such stimuli include changes in pH, variations in the oxidation-reduction potential and presence of various biomolecules like hormone, enzymes etc.
- **Dual and Multi Responsive Stimuli:** Efficiency of drug delivery can be enhanced by increasing sensitivity to multiple stimuli e.g., sensitivity towards a combination of pH and temperature. Considering the complexity of the development of tumors, it is likely that a combination of different delivery approaches will increase the effectiveness of therapeutics multifold. MSNs that can respond to different stimuli like changes in pH, presence/ absence of glucose, temperature etc. have been developed and are significantly effective than their previous counterparts (Sun, Piao, Wang, Javed, Hong, & Pan, 2013, Zhao, Meng Wang, Donovan, Fu, You, Chen, Zhang, &Tan, 2013, Chen, Geng, Pu, Yang, Ren, & Qu, 2011, Zhang, Yang, Dai, Ma, Li Cheng, Hou, Kang, Li, & Lin, 2013). A dual stimuli MSNs involving azobenzene as light-activated nanoimpellers and pseudorotaxanes as pH-responsive nanovalves were developed by Angelos et al. (2009) where both the systems need to get activated for drug release. Another dual pH-responsive MSN-based drug release system has been developed.

Biocompatibility of MSNs

Biocompatibility and bio-distribution studies of nanomaterials need to be performed before using an organic compound in organisms. Silica based materials have been generally regarded as biocompatible and safe for use. Extensive usage of these nanomaterials and their applicability in living systems for drug delivery and other purposes has raised concerns from biosafety point of view. Physiochemical properties of materials like size shape and surface area are the major determinants of the toxic potential or biocompatibility of the nanomaterials. Various cell models have been used to study the mesoporous nanomaterials biosafety / cytotoxicity and most of the reports reflect excellent biocompatibility and smooth biodegradability characteristics of these materials. However, some contradictory reports are also available which show MSNs induced cytotoxicity in different cell lines in dose and time dependent effect. Pertinently, toxicity evaluation is imperative before allowing the development of clinical applications in the treatment and/or diagnosis of human diseases.

Differential conjugation of MSNs with different ligands can affect their distribution in different organ systems which in turn define their safety profile. Thus an extensive review of biocompatibility and biosafety assessment of MSNs is mandatory. (Fadeel, & García-Bennett, 2010). Biosafety assessment also becomes necessary because of the fact that there are immense variations in the characteristics of this class of materials. Such variations are a result of differences in the methods of production, size of the particle, its shape and surface modifications performed.

Meng et al.(2011) investigated the bio-distribution of MSNs of different particles sizes (80, 120, 200 and 360 nm) and their corresponding PEGylated counterparts (PEG-MSNs). As expected, the blood-circulation lifetime of PEG-MSNs was relatively longer. Both of them were more easily captured by the organs, which facilitated their degradation (Yang, Zhao, Li, Xu, Li, Wu, Miyoshi, & Li, 2013). Conjugated PEG-MSNs had longed circulation times, slowly biodegraded and, consequently, had lower excretion rates (Meng, Xue, Xia, Ji, Tarn, Zink, & Nel, 2011).

Table 2. Biocompatibility study of MSNs in various model systems

MSN/Polymer and Hybrid Materials	Loaded/Coated With	Cell Line	Parameter Assessed	Major Outcome	Applicable Field	Stimuli Response	References
Folic Acid- or N-Acetyl Glucosamine	Doxorubicin (DOX-FA-MSNPs or DOX-NAG-MSNPs)	Breast cancer cell lines.	Cellular uptake of FITC tagged FA-MSNPs and NAG-MSNPs	DOX-loaded NAG-MSNPs exerted significant higher cytotoxicity than DOX-FA-MSNPs	Drug delivery	-	Kumar et al., (2017)
Poly (Ethylene Glycol)-Poly (Ethylene Imine) (PEG-PEI)	Poly(ethylene glycol)-poly(ethylene imine) (PEG-PEI)	RBE4 rat brain endothelial cells and Madin-Darby canine kidney epithelial cells)	Cell viability, in vivo imaging. Cellular uptake	No cytotoxicity	Drug delivery	-	Baghir et al., (2016)
DOX@MSN-NH-N=C-PAD$_{10}$	Doxorubicin hydrochloride (Dox)	HeLa cells	Cytotoxicity test and cellular uptake	Excellent biocompatibility	Drug delivery	pH	Zhang et al., (2017)
MSN-Me-CPT and MSN-Et-CPT	Camptothecin	Cancer cell	MTT assays	functionalized nanoparticles more significantly involved controlled drug release.	Drug delivery	pH	Yan et al., (2017)
MSN-ss-GHA (DOX@MSN-ss-GHA)	Doxorubicin hydrochloride (DOX)	Murine breast cancer cell line (4T1 cells), (HeLa cells) and HUVEC cells	Cytotoxicity test and cellular uptake, hemolysis assay	Excellent biocompatibility	Drug delivery and MR imaging	Redox	Chen et al., (2016)
MSN-HA/Dox	Doxorubicin hydrochloride (Dox)	Cancer cells	Cellular uptake and apoptosis	MSN exhibited good biocompatibility in vitro and in vivo. MSN-HA/Dox nanoparticles induced apoptosis more efficiently than free doxorubicin and inhibited tumor growth with minimal systemic toxicity in vivo	Drug delivery	HAse	Zhan et al., (2016)
Composite of Poly(DL-Lactic-Co-Glycolic Acid) (PLGA)	and nHA) (PLGA-MSN/ nHA	Rabbit marrow-derived MSCs and New Zealand rabbits	Cell proliferation, Osteoinductive Ability Assay, histological observation	Good biocompatibility and osteoinductivity In vivo and in vitro	Bone regeneration		Shu et al., (2016)
C_{60}-TEG-COOH Modified MSN (MSN@C_{60})	doxorubicin hydrochloride (DOX)	HeLa cells	Cellular uptake/ cytotoxicity test CCK-8 assay	excellent biocompatibility and the DOX-loaded nanocarrier exhibited efficient anticancer ability.	Drug delivery and bioimaging system	pH	Tan. et al., (2016)
Mesoporous Silica-Coated Superparamagnetic Manganese Ferrite (MnFe2O4) Nanoparticles (M-MSN)	Doxorubicin	HeLa cells and in vivo mice model	In vitro cytotoxicity, fluorescence microscopy, and apoptosis studies.	Excellent biocompatibility	Drug delivery and MR imaging	CTAB	Saho et al., (2014)
Hybrid Mesoporous Silica Nanoparticles (MSNs) Modified with Polymer Polyethylene Glycol (PEG)	Rhodamine B (RhB)	Rabbit red blood cells (RBCs) and MCF-7 breast cancer cells	Hemolysis assay, serum protein adsorption and cell viability test	biocompatibility of silica carriers increased.	Drug delivery	Redox-responsive	Wang et al., (2015)

continued on following page

Table 2. Continued

MSN/Polymer and Hybrid Materials	Loaded/Coated With	Cell Line	Parameter Assessed	Major Outcome	Applicable Field	Stimuli Response	References
Hyaluronic Acid (HA)	doxorubicin (DOX)	HCT-116 cells	Confocal laser scanning microscopy (CLSM) and fluorescence-activated cell sorting (FACS)	The CMS-SS-oHA exhibited a higher cellular uptake via CD44 receptor-mediated endocytosis in HCT-116 cells than in NIH-3T3.	Drug release and targeted delivery.	Redox and enzyme Dual-stimuli responsive	Zhaoa et al., (2015)
Van-MSN-CaSO4 Composite	Vancomycin	MC3T3-E1cells and newzee land rabbit	In vitro cytotoxicity tests	MSN exhibited good biocompatibility	Bone grafting/ regeneration	-	Gu et al., (2016)
Oligo (Ethylene Glycol) Acrylate (OEGA) and Cross-Linker N,N'-CystaminebismEthacrylamide (CBMA)	Doxorubicin (DOX)		In vitro cytotoxicity assays, and endocytosis, cellular internalizatio	MSN exhibited good biocompatibility	Drug delivery	Redox Responsive	Sun et., (2013)
CuS@MSN-DOX	Doxorubicin (DOX	Mice model	Photothermal therapy and chemotherapy	MSN showed synergistic effect of chemo-photothermal therapy No cytotoxicity	Photothermal therapy and Chemotherapy	-	Peng et al., (2017)
Collagen/MSN/VEGF (CMV) Scaffold	Vascular endothelial growth factor (VEGF)	Mice model		EGF-releasing scaffold induced significantly increased number of blood vessel complexes when compared with VEGF-free scaffold	Angiogenesis and tissue repair		Kim et al., (2016)
MSN	Camptothecin	Mice model	Serological, hematological, histopathological examination and Bio distribution studies	MSNs are biocompatible and suppress tumor growth.	Drug delivery	-	Lu j., 2010
MSN-Dox@GO-Apt	Aptamer+ doxorubicin (Dox)	MCF-7 cells	MTT assay, Dox release and therapy efficacy	Synergism of chemotherapy and photothermal therapy of loaded MSN at a single platform led to much more effective cancer cell killing than monotherapies,	Drug deliver	Light/ photo	Tang et al., (2015)
Dendritic Mesoporous Silica Nanoparticles (DMSNs-CHO)	Protein/ drug	RAW 264.7 cells	In vitro cytotoxicity and cellular uptake	DMSNs-CHO nanoparticles had no cytotoxicity and could be efficiently taken up by cells	Drug/ Protein delivery	pH	Tian et al., (2016)
(Polyethylene Glycol-B-Polyaspartate-Modified Rose Bengal-Loaded Magnetic Mesoporous Silica [RB–MMSNs]	Rose bengal-loaded magnetic mesoporous silica [RB–MMSNs])	Mouse melanoma B16 cells and C57BL/6J male mice	Cellular uptake, Cytotoxicity and detection of cellular ROS	MMSNs effectively increased the therapeutical concentration of hydrophobic photosensitizer RB in the tumor site	Drug Delivery	Magnetic and pH dual-responsive	Jieqion et al., (2017)
Grafting Folic Acid (FA) onto the EuGd-MSN Surface (EuGd-FA-MSNs)	Camptothecin (CPT),	(Mus musculus fibroblast cell line) and HeLa (human epithelial carcinoma cell line) and Female BALB/c nude mice	In vitro cytotoxicity a		Disease diagnosis drug delivery		Chan & Lin 2015

Applications of MSNs

Several studies have demonstrated the successful use of MSNs in diagnostics and therapeutics (He & Shi, 2011; Slowing, Vivero-Escoto, Wu, & Lin, 2008) especially in drug delivery and biomedical imaging (Vallet-Regí, Manzano & Colilla, 2012; Taylor, 2008). Large pore size of MSNs allows them to accommodate large amounts of drug molecules. MSNs have been used to develop targeted drug delivery systems (He & Shi, 2011). They are also being used in medical imaging, usually in combination with magnetically active material such as gadolinium or manganese oxide (Taylor, 2008; Kim, 2011).

CONCLUSION

To summarize, this chapter describes the recent advances in synthesis of surface modified or functionalized MSNs and how these nanomaterials are being employed in targeted release of drugs and other therapeutic molecules in biological systems. Versatile approaches for the selective functionalization of MSNs have been developed that tends to make delivery of molecules to the targeted cell more efficient and at the same prevents undesirable side effects. Other important characteristics of silica nanoparticles are that they can be merged with other materials with different functionalities which add to their advantages. Since the development of MSNs as drug delivery systems almost 20 years ago, they have been subjected to extensive modifications which have been shown to be highly effective in diagnostics and therapeutics especially cancer.

REFERENCES

Albanese, A., Tang, P. S., & Chan, W. C. W. (2012). The Effect of Nanoparticle Size, Shape, and Surface Chemistry on Biological Systems. *Annual Review of Biomedical Engineering*, *14*(1), 1–16. doi:10.1146/annurev-bioeng-071811-150124 PMID:22524388

Angelos, S., Yang, Y.-W., Khashab, N. M., Stoddart, J. F., & Zink, J. I. (2009). Dual-controlled nanoparticles exhibiting AND logic. *Journal of the American Chemical Society*, *131*(32), 11344–11346. doi:10.1021/ja9042752 PMID:19624127

Arcos, D., López-Noriega, A., Ruiz-Hernández, E., Terasaki, O., & Vallet-Regí, M. (2009). Ordered mesoporous microspheres for bone grafting and drug delivery. *Chemistry of Materials*, *21*(6), 1000–1009. doi:10.1021/cm801649z

Argyo, C., Weiss, V., Braeuchle, C., & Bein, T. (2014). Multifunctional mesoporous silica nanoparticles as a universal platform for drug delivery. *Chemistry of Materials*, *26*(1), 435–451. doi:10.1021/cm402592t

Baeza, A. (2014). Ceramic Nanoparticles for Cancer Treatment. In *Bio-Ceramics with Clinical Application*. John Wiley & Sons, Ltd.

Baghirov, H., Karaman, D., Viitala, T., Duchanoy, A., Lou, Y. R., Mamaeva, V., ... Rosenholm, J. M. (2016). Feasibility Study of the Permeability and Uptake of Mesoporous Silica Nanoparticles across the Blood-Brain Barrier. *PLoS One*, *11*(8).

Barreto, J. A., O'Malley, W., Kubeil, M., Graham, B., Stephan, H., & Spiccia, L. (2011). Nanomaterials: Applications in cancer imaging and therapy. *Advanced Materials*, *23*(12), 18–40. doi:10.1002/adma.201100140 PMID:21433100

Brinker, C. J., Lu, Y. F., Sellinger, A., & Fan, H. Y. (1999). Evaporation-induced self-assembly: Nanostructures made easy. *Advanced Materials*, *11*(7), 579–585. doi:

Chan, M.H., & Lin, H.M. (2015). Preparation and identification of multifunctional mesoporous silica nanoparticles for in vitro and in vivo dual-mode imaging, theranostics, and targeted tracking. *Biomaterials, 46*, 149-158.

Chen, C., Geng, J., Pu, F., Yang, X., Ren, J., & Qu, X. (2011). Polyvalent nucleic acid/mesoporous silica nanoparticle conjugates: Dual stimuli-responsive vehicles for intracellular drug delivery. Angew. Chem. Int., 50, 882–886.

Chen, L., Zhou, X., Nie, W., Zhang, Q., Wang, W., Zhang, Y., & He, C. (2016). Multifunctional Redox-Responsive Mesoporous Silica Nanoparticles for Efficient Targeting Drug Delivery and Magnetic Resonance Imaging. *ACS Applied Materials & Interfaces*, *8*(49), 33829–33841. doi:10.1021/acsami.6b11802 PMID:27960384

Colilla, M., Baeza, A., & Vallet-Regí, M. (2015). Mesoporous Silica Nanoparticles for Drug Delivery and Controlled Release Applications. In The Sol-Gel Handbook. Wiley-VCH Verlag GmbH & Co. KGaA. doi:10.1002/9783527670819.ch42

Etheridge, M. L., Campbell, S. A., Erdman, A. G., Haynes, C. L., Wolf, S. M., & McCullough, J. (2013). The big picture on nanomedicine: The state of investigational and approved nanomedicine products. *Nanomedicine (London)*, *9*(1), 1–14. doi:10.1016/j.nano.2012.05.013 PMID:22684017

Fadeel, B., & García-Bennett, A. E. (2010). Better safe than sorry: Understanding the toxicological properties of inorganic nanoparticles manufactured for biomedical applications. *Advanced Drug Delivery Reviews*, *62*(3), 362–374. doi:10.1016/j.addr.2009.11.008 PMID:19900497

Fernandez-Fernandez, A., Manchanda, R., & McGoron, A. (2011). Theranostic applications of nanomaterials in cancer: Drug delivery, image-guided therapy, and multifunctional platforms. *Applied Biochemistry and Biotechnology*, *165*(7-8), 1628–1651. doi:10.100712010-011-9383-z PMID:21947761

Gai, S., Yang, P., Li, C., Wang, W., Dai, Y., Niu, N., & Lin, J. (2010). Synthesis of magnetic, up-conversion luminescent, and mesoporous core-shell-structured nanocomposites as drug carriers. *Advanced Functional Materials*, *20*(7), 1166–1172. doi:10.1002/adfm.200902274

Grun, M., Lauer, I., & Unger, K.K. (1997). The synthesis of miro meter and sub micrometer size sphere of ordered mesoporous oxide MCM -41. *Adv Matter*, *3*, 254-257.

Gu, J., Wang, T., Fan, G., Ma, J., Hu, W., & Cai, X. (2016). Biocompatibility of artificial bone based on vancomycin loaded mesoporous silica nanoparticles and calcium sulfate composites. *Journal of Materials Science. Materials in Medicine*, *27*(4), 64. doi:10.100710856-016-5671-z PMID:26883948

He, Q., & Shi, J. (2011). Mesoporous silica nanoparticle based nano drug delivery systems: Synthesis, controlled drug release and delivery, pharmacokinetics and biocompatibility. *Journal of Materials Chemistry*, *21*(16), 5845–5855. doi:10.1039/c0jm03851b

He Q & Shi J. (2014). MSN Anti-Cancer Nanomedicines: Chemotherapy Enhancement, Overcoming of Drug Resistance, and Metastasis Inhibition. *Advance Materials.*

He, S., Lin, K. F., Fan, J. J., Hu, G., Dong, X., Zhao, Y. N., ... Liu, J. (2016). Synergistic Effect of Mesoporous Silica and Hydroxyapatite in Loaded Poly(DL-lactic-co-glycolic acid) Microspheres on the Regeneration of Bone Defects. *BioMed Research International*. PMID:27652269

Hoffmann, F., & Fröba, M. (2011). Vitalising porous inorganic silica networks with organic functions-PMOs and related hybrid materials. *Chemical Society Reviews*, *40*(2), 608–620. doi:10.1039/C0CS00076K PMID:21180714

Huh, S., Chen, H. T., Wiench, J. W., Pruski, M., & Lin, V. S.-Y. (2005). Cooperative catalysis by general acid and base bifunctionalized mesoporous silica nanospheres. *Angewandte Chemie International Edition in English*, *44*(12), 1826–1830. doi:10.1002/anie.200462424 PMID:15712306

Kennedy, L. C., Bickford, L. R., Lewinski, N. A., Coughlin, A. J., Hu, Y., Day, E. S., ... Drezek, R. A. (2011). A new era for cancer treatment: Gold-nanoparticle mediated thermal therapies. *Small*, *7*(2), 169–183. doi:10.1002mll.201000134 PMID:21213377

Kim, J.H., Kim, T.H., Kang, M.S., & Kim, H.W. (2016). Angiogenic Effects of Collagen/Mesoporous Nanoparticle Composite Scaffold Delivering VEGF165. *Biomed Res Int.*

Kim, T., Momin, E., Choi, J., Yuan, K., Zaidi, H., Kim, J., ... Gilad, A. A. (2011). Mesoporous Silica-Coated Hollow Manganese Oxide Nanoparticles as Positive T1 Contrast Agents for Labeling and MRI Tracking of Adipose-Derived Mesenchymal Stem Cells. *Journal of the American Chemical Society*, *133*(9), 2955–2961. doi:10.1021/ja1084095 PMID:21314118

Kresge, C. T., Leonowicz, M. E., Roth, W. J., Vartuli, J. C., & Beck, J. S. (1992). Ordered mesoporous molecular sieves synthesized by a liquid-crystal template mechanism. *Nature*, *359*(6397), 710–712. doi:10.1038/359710a0

Kumar, P., Tambe, P., Paknikar, KM., & Gajbhiye V. (2017) Folate/N-acetyl glucosamine conjugated mesoporous silica nanoparticles for targeting breast cancer cells: A comparative study. *Colloids Surf B Biointerfaces*, *156*, 203-212.

Lanone, S., & Boczkowski, J. (2006). Biomedical applications and potential health risks of nanomaterials: Molecular mechanisms. *Current Molecular Medicine*, *6*(6), 651–663. doi:10.2174/156652406778195026 PMID:17022735

Li, Z., Barnes, J. C., Bosoy, A., Stoddart, J. F., & Zink, J. I. (2012). Mesoporous silica nanoparticles in biomedical applications. *Chemical Society Reviews*, *41*(7), 2590–2605. doi:10.1039/c1cs15246g PMID:22216418

Lu, J., Liong, M., Li, Z., Zink, J.I., & Tamanoi, F. (2010). Biocompatibility, biodistribution, and drug-delivery efficiency of mesoporous silica nanoparticles for cancer therapy in animals. *Small*, *6*(16), 1794-805.

Manzano, M., Colilla, M., & Vallet-Regí, M. (2009). Drug delivery from ordered mesoporous matrices. *Expert Opinion on Drug Delivery*, *6*(12), 1383–1400. doi:10.1517/17425240903304024 PMID:19941412

Martínez, Á., Fuentes-Paniagua, E., Baeza, A., Sánchez-Nieves, J., Cicuéndez, M., Gómez, R., ... Vallet-Regí, M. (2015). Mesoporous silica nanoparticles decorated with carbosilane dendrons as new non-viral oligonucleotide delivery carriers. *Chemistry*, *21*(44), 15651–15666. doi:10.1002/chem.201501966 PMID:26361378

Meng, H., Xue, M., Xia, T., Ji, Z., Tarn, D. Y., Zink, J. I., & Nel, A. E. (2011). Use of size and a copolymer design feature to improve the biodistribution and the enhanced permeability and retention effect of doxorubicin-loaded mesoporous silica nanoparticles in a murine xenograft tumor model. *ACS Nano*, *5*(5), 4131–4144. doi:10.1021/nn200809t PMID:21524062

Muñoz, B., Rámila, A., Pérez-Pariente, J., Díaz, I., & Vallet-Regí, M. (2003). MCM-41 Organic modification as drug delivery rate regulator. *Chemistry of Materials*, *15*(2), 500–503. doi:10.1021/cm021217q

Peng, S., He, Y., Er, M., Sheng, Y., & Chen, H. (2017). Biocompatible Cu S-based nanoplatforms for efficient photothermal therapy and chemotherapy *in vivo*. *Biomaterials Science*, *5*(3), 475–484. doi:10.1039/C6BM00626D PMID:28078340

Peng, S., He, Y., Er, M., Sheng, Y., Gu, Y. & Chen, H. (2017). Biocompatible CuS-based nanoplatforms for efficient photothermal therapy and chemotherapy in vivo. *Biomater Sci*, *5*(3), 475-484.

Royal Society of Chemistry. (2015). Nanoceramics in Clinical Use: From Materials to Applications (2nd ed.). Cambridge, UK: Author.

Rytkonen, J., Miettinen, R., Kaasalainen, M., Lehto, V., Salonen, J., & Narvanen, A. (2012). Functionalization of mesoporous silicon nanoparticles for targeting and bioimaging purposes. *Journal of Nanomaterials*, *2012*, 1–9. doi:10.1155/2012/896562

Sahoo, B., Devi, K. S., Dutta, S., Maiti, T. K., Pramanik, P., & Dhara, D. (2014). Biocompatible mesoporous silica-coated superparamagnetic manganese ferrite nanoparticles for targeted drug delivery and MR imaging applications. *Journal of Colloid and Interface Science*, *431*, 31–41. doi:10.1016/j.jcis.2014.06.003 PMID:24980623

Sanchez, C., Belleville, P., Popall, M., & Nicole, L. (2011). Applications of advanced hybrid organic-inorganic nanomaterials: From laboratory to market. *Chemical Society Reviews*, *40*(2), 696–753. doi:10.1039/c0cs00136h PMID:21229132

Sergio, C., Elena, B. P., Fernando, N. V., Judith, L., Marta, N., Luis, M. L. M., & María, C. M. B. (2016). Multibranched Gold–Mesoporous Silica Nanoparticles Coated with a Molecularly Imprinted Polymer for Label-Free Antibiotic Surface-Enhanced Raman Scattering Analysis. *Chemistry of Materials*, *28*(21), 7947–7954. doi:10.1021/acs.chemmater.6b03613

Shahbazi, M. A., Herranz, B., & Santos, H. A. (2012). Nanostructured porous Si-based nanoparticles for targeted drug delivery. *Biomatter*, *2*(4), 296–312. doi:10.4161/biom.22347 PMID:23507894

Shi, J., Votruba, A. R., Farokhzad, O. C., & Langer, R. (2010). Nanotechnology in drug delivery and tissue engineering: From discovery to applications. *Nano Letters*, *10*(9), 3223–3230. doi:10.1021/nl102184c PMID:20726522

Slowing, I. I., Vivero-Escoto, J. L., Wu, C.-W., & Lin, V. S. Y. (2008). Mesoporous silica nanoparticles as controlled release drug delivery and gene transfection carriers. *Advanced Drug Delivery Reviews*, *60*(11), 1278–1288. doi:10.1016/j.addr.2008.03.012 PMID:18514969

Stöber, W., Fink, A., & Bohn, E. (1968). Controlled growth of monodisperse silica spheres in the micron size range. *Journal of Colloid and Interface Science*, *26*(1), 62–69. doi:10.1016/0021-9797(68)90272-5

Sun, J. T., Piao, J. G., Wang, L. H., Javed, M., Hong, C. Y., & Pan, C. Y. (2013). One-pot synthesis of redox-responsive polymers-coated mesoporous silica nanoparticles and their controlled drug release. *Macromolecular Rapid Communications*, *34*(17), 1387–1394. doi:10.1002/marc.201300477 PMID:23881541

Sun, L., Zhang, X., Zheng, C., Wu, Z., & Li, C. (2013). A pH gated, glucose-sensitive nanoparticle based on worm-like mesoporous silica for controlled insulin release. *The Journal of Physical Chemistry B*, *117*(14), 3852–3860. doi:10.1021/jp400442x PMID:23517533

Tan, L., Wu, T., Tang, Z. W., Xiao, J. Y., Zhuo, R. X., Shi, B., & Liu, C. J. (2016). Water-soluble photoluminescent fullerene capped mesoporous silica for pH-responsive drug delivery and bioimaging. *Nanotechnology*, *27*(31), 315104. doi:10.1088/0957-4484/27/31/315104 PMID:27346782

Tang, F., Li, L., & Chen, D. (2012). Mesoporous silica nanoparticles: Synthesis, biocompatibility and drug delivery. *Advanced Materials*, *24*(12), 1504–1534. doi:10.1002/adma.201104763 PMID:22378538

Tang, Y., Hu, H., Zhang, M.G., Song, J., Nie, L., Wang, S., … Chen X. (2015). An aptamer-targeting photoresponsive drug delivery system using "off on" graphene oxide wrapped mesoporous silica nanoparticles. *Nanoscale*, *7*(14), 6304-10.

Tang, Y., Hu, H., Zhang, M. G., Song, J., Nie, L., Wang, S., ... Chen, X. (2015, April 14). An aptamer-targeting photoresponsive drug delivery system using "off-on" graphene oxide wrapped mesoporous silica nanoparticles. *Nanoscale*, *7*(14), 6304–6310. doi:10.1039/C4NR07493A PMID:25782595

Tang, Y., Hu, H., Zhang, M.H., Song, J., Nie, L., Wang, S., … Xiaoyuan, C. (2015). An aptamer-targeting photoresponsive drug delivery system using "off–on" graphene oxide wrapped mesoporous silica nanoparticles. *Nanoscale, 7*(14), 6304–6310.

Taylor, K. M. L., Kim, J. S., Rieter, W. J., An, H., Lin, W., & Lin, W. (2008). Mesoporous Silica Nanospheres as Highly Efficient MRI Contrast Agents. *Journal of the American Chemical Society*, *130*(7), 2154–2155. doi:10.1021/ja710193c PMID:18217764

Tian, Z. F., Yi, X. & Zhu, Y. (2017). Aldehyde-functionalized dendritic mesoporous silica nanoparticles as potential nanocarriers for pH-responsive protein drug delivery. *Materials Science & Engineering CInt J Nanomedicine*, *12*, 2733-2748.

Trewyn, B. G., Slowing, I. I., Giri, S., Chen, H.-T., & Lin, V. S. Y. (2007). Synthesis and functionalization of a mesoporous silica nanoparticle based on the sol-gel process and applications in controlled release. *Accounts of Chemical Research*, *40*(9), 846–853. doi:10.1021/ar600032u PMID:17645305

Vallet-Reg. (2012). *Mesoporous Silica Nanoparticles: Their Projection in Nanomedicine. Materials Science.*

Vallet-Regí, M., Balas, F., & Arcos, D. (2007). Mesoporous materials for drug delivery. *Angewandte Chemie International Edition*, *46*(40), 7548–7558. doi:10.1002/anie.200604488 PMID:17854012

Vallet-Regí, M., Manzano, M., & Colilla, M. (2012). Biomedical Applications of Mesoporous Ceramics: Drug Delivery, Smart Materials and Bone Tissue Engineering. CRC Press.

Vallet-Regí, M., & Ruiz-Hernandez, E. (2011). Bioceramics: From bone regeneration to cancer nanomedicine. *Advanced Materials*, *23*(44), 5177–5218. doi:10.1002/adma.201101586 PMID:22009627

Wang, Y., Han, N., Zhao, Q., Bai, L., Li, J., Jiang, T., & Wang, S. (2015). Redox-responsive mesoporous silica as carriers for controlled drug delivery: A comparative study based on silica and PEG gatekeepers. *European Journal of Pharmaceutical Sciences*, *25*(72), 12–20. doi:10.1016/j.ejps.2015.02.008 PMID:25701727

Xia, Y., Yang, P., Sun, Y., Wu, Y., Mayers, B., Gates, B., ... Yan, H. (2003). One-dimensional nanostructures: Synthesis, characterization, and applications. *Advanced Materials*, *15*(5), 353–389. doi:10.1002/adma.200390087

Xie, J., Liu, G., Eden, H. S., Ai, H., & Chen, X. (2011). Surface-engineered magnetic nanoparticle platforms for cancer imaging and therapy. *Accounts of Chemical Research*, *44*(10), 883–892. doi:10.1021/ar200044b PMID:21548618

Yan, Y., Fu, J., Wang, T., & Lu, X. (2017). Controlled release of silyl ether camptothecin from thiol-ene click chemistry-functionalized mesoporous silica nanoparticles. *Acta Biomaterialia*, *15*(51), 471–478. doi:10.1016/j.actbio.2017.01.062 PMID:28131940

Yang, H., Zhao, F., Li, Y., Xu, M., Li, L., Wu, C., ... Liu, Y. (2013). VCAM-1-targeted core/shell nanoparticles for selective adhesion and delivery to endothelial cells with lipopolysaccharide-induced inflammation under shear flow and cellular magnetic resonance imaging in vitro. *International Journal of Nanomedicine*, *8*, 1897–1906. PMID:23696701

Yang, P., Gai, S., & Lin, J. (2012). Functionalized mesoporous silica materials for controlled drug delivery. *Chemical Society Reviews*, *41*(9), 3679–3698. doi:10.1039/c2cs15308d PMID:22441299

Yang, P., Quan, Z., Lu, L., Huang, S., & Lin, J. (2008). Luminescence functionalization of mesoporous silica with different morphologies and applications as drug delivery systems. *Biomaterials*, *29*(6), 692–702. doi:10.1016/j.biomaterials.2007.10.019 PMID:17996294

Yao, X., Chen, X., He, C., Chen, L., & Chen, X. (2015). Dual pH-responsive mesoporous silica nanoparticles for efficient combination of chemotherapy and photodynamic therapy. *Journal of Materials Chemistry. B, Materials for Biology and Medicine*, *3*(23), 4707–4714. doi:10.1039/C5TB00256G

Zhan, J., Ma, Z., Wang, D., Li, X., Li, X., Le, L., ... Yang, F. (2017). Li, x., Le, li., Hu, P., She, L., & Yan· F.(2017) Magnetic and pH dual-responsive mesoporous silica nanocomposites for effective and low-toxic photodynamic therapy. *International Journal of Nanomedicine*, *12*, 2733–2748. doi:10.2147/IJN.S127528 PMID:28442903

Zhang, M., Liu, J., Kuang, Y., Li, Q., Zheng, D. W., Song, Q., ... Jiang, B. (2017). Ingenious pH-sensitive dextran/mesoporous silica nanoparticles based drug delivery systems for controlled intracellular drug release. *International Journal of Biological Macromolecules*, *98*, 691–700. doi:10.1016/j.ijbiomac.2017.01.136 PMID:28174081

Zhang, M., Xu, C., Wen, L., Han, M. K., Xiao, B., Zhou, J., ... Merlin, D. (2016). A Hyaluronidase-Responsive Nanoparticle-Based Drug Delivery System for Targeting Colon Cancer Cells. *Cancer Research*, *76*(24), 7208–7218. doi:10.1158/0008-5472.CAN-16-1681 PMID:27742685

Zhang, X., Yang, P., Dai, Y., Ma, P. A., Li, X., Cheng, Z., ... Lin, J. (2013). Multifunctional up-converting nanocomposites with smart polymer brushes gated mesopores for cell imaging and thermo/pH dual-responsive drug controlled release. *Advanced Functional Materials*, *23*(33), 4067–4078. doi:10.1002/adfm.201300136

Zhao, Q., Liu, J., Zhu, W., Sun, C., Di, D., Zhang, Y., ... Wang, S. (2015). Dual-stimuli responsive hyaluronic acid-conjugated mesoporous silica for targeted delivery to CD44-overexpressing cancer cells. *Acta Biomaterialia*, *23*, 147–156. doi:10.1016/j.actbio.2015.05.010 PMID:25985912

Zhao, Z., Meng, H., Wang, N., Donovan, M. J., Fu, T., You, M., . . . Tan, W. A. (2013). Controlled-release nanocarrier with extracellular pH value driven tumor targeting and translocation for drug delivery. Angew. Chem. Int., 52, 7487-7491.

Chapter 17
Emergence of Polymer-Lipid Hybrid Systems in Healthcare Scenario

Anamika Jain
Dr. H. S. Gour Vishwavidyalaya, India

Rajeev Sharma
Dr. H. S. Gour Vishwavidyalaya, India

Laxmikant Gautam
Dr. H. S. Gour Vishwavidyalaya, India

Nishi Mody
Dr. H. S. Gour Vishwavidyalaya, India

Nikhar Vishwakarma
Dr. H. S. Gour Vishwavidyalaya, India

Surbhi Dubey
Dr. H. S. Gour Vishwavidyalaya, India

Suresh P. Vyas
Dr. H. S. Gour Vishwavidyalaya, India

ABSTRACT

Nanotechnology has drawn the attention of many researchers for the delivery of therapeutics used in various medical applications. Liposomes and polymeric nanoparticles represent promising nanocarriers that efficiently encapsulate drugs, which prevents their degradation along with the control and sustained drug release. Despite the many advantages of these formulations, some of the drawbacks associated with them limit their application to a certain extent. Therefore, there is need for a novel nanocarrier that possesses all of their individual advantages and excludes their drawbacks. Currently, researchers are focused on developing a novel platform that is a hybrid of a polymeric and liposomal-based carrier that combines the peculiarity of both and excludes their shortcomings. Lipid hybrid polymer nanoparticles (LPNs) contain the hydrophobic biodegradable polymeric core surrounded by a lipid layer for intensification of biocompatibility. This chapter includes an introduction of LPNs along with their advantages, composition, and method of preparation.

DOI: 10.4018/978-1-5225-4781-5.ch017

Copyright © 2018, IGI Global. Copying or distributing in print or electronic forms without written permission of IGI Global is prohibited.

INTRODUCTION

Nanotechnology represents the most powerful tool in the field of drug delivery over the past decade (Dehaini, Fang, Luk, Pang, Hu, & Kroll, 2016). Nanotechnology deals with a nano-size range usually one billion of a meter. Nanotechnology has performed the miracle that the researcher could work at the atomic level which was not possible before (Liu, Miyoshi, & Nakamura, 2007). Newer generation nanocarriers have been structured, which proved to be a milestone in the field of nanotechnology. Recently a nanomedicine word has come into vogue, which is an engineered nano devices and nanostructured explored for treatment of various ailments (Ruggiero, & Pastorino, 2010). According to the National Institute of health, nanomedicine referred as the application of nanotechnology for the treatment, diagnosis, monitoring of disease and control of the biological system(Liu, Miyoshi, & Nakamura, 2007). Due to the poor bioavailability and pharmacokinetics of the available potential therapeutics, there is an urgent need of a delivery system which delivers the active molecule only to the target site, without side effects (Ruggiero, & Pastorino, 2010). Variety of drug delivery carriers has been introduced such as liposomes, dendrimers, quantum dots, carbon nanotubes and nanocapsules. During the last decade, various liposome and nanoparticles based formulations emerged into market and number of them are under clinical trials (Zhang, Chan, Gu, Rhee, Wang, & Radovic-Moreno, 2008). Liposomes and polymeric nanoparticles represent most promising carriers which deliver the active therapeutics. Liposomes and polymeric nanoparticles represent promising nanocarriers that efficiently encapsulate drug which prevents its degradation along with the control and sustained drug release. Despite the many advantages of these formulations, some of the drawbacks associated with them, which limit their application to a certain extent. Therefore there is need of a novel nanocarrier, which possesses all of their individual advantages and excluding their drawbacks. These novel nanocarriers based upon the traditional approaches with some of the modification in their preparation method, which enhances their therapeutic potential. Nowadays researchers focus to develop a novel platform that is hybrid of a polymeric and liposomal-based carrier which combined peculiarity of both the system and excluding their shortcomings (Zhang, & Zhang, 2010). Lipid hybrid polymer nanoparticles (PLNs) contain the hydrophobic biodegradable polymeric core surrounded by a lipid layer for intensification of biocompatibility. This book chapter includes the introduction of PLNs along with their advantages, composition, and method of preparation. Finally, we highlight application and future challenges associated with the PLNs.

POLYMERIC NANOCARRIERS

Polymeric nanocarriers are nanosized polymeric colloidal particles which encapsulate potential therapeutics within their polymeric matrix or conjugate or adsorbed onto their surface. Nanometer size range of these carriers offers distinct advantages for the delivery of therapeutics. Due to their nanosize, the nanoparticles can invade deep into the tissue and blood capillaries, thus enhance uptake by the cells (Panyam, & Labhasetwar, 2003). Particle size, surface modification, surface charge, and hydrophobicity are important characteristics of polymeric nanoparticles which directly affect targeting behavior of NPs. Interaction of the polymeric NPs with the cell membrane and its penetration is greatly affected by particle size and size distribution (Kumari, Yadav, & Yadav, 2010). Surface charge is important for cellular internalization, it is a deciding factor whether nanoparticle flows into the blood or would adhere to cell or interact with cell membrane. Cell membrane possesses negative charge due to which cationic surface charge is prerequisite for cellular internalization.

Numerous polymers are available for the preparation of NPs may be of natural or synthetic origin. Natural polymers include chitosan, dextrin, alginate, agar, among them chitosan is more popular. Synthetic polymers used for NPs preparation are poly(lactide-co-glycolide) (PLGA), poly (lactide-co-glycolide), polyethylenimine (PEI), Poly(lactide) (PLA), poly(glycolide) (PGA), poly(cyanoacrylates) (PCA), or polycaprolactone (PCL) etc (Plapied, Duhem, des Rieux, & Préat, 2011).

Prolong systemic circulation is required for targeted drug delivery. Conventional NPs are rapidly removed from the blood due to their hydrophobicity. They are rapidly opsonized by the macrophages and cleared from the blood. Surface functionalization of the conventional NPs is carried out to overcome these shortcomings. Coating of the NPs with hydrophilic polymer enhance the systemic circulation time.

Polymeric nanoparticles are superior to conventional dosage form due to the control and sustained drug release, targeted drug delivery, lesser side effects and enhance therapeutic effectiveness. Although it is not gaining much attention at scale up level due to the biocompatibility issue and thus further investigation in the area is needed to be done.

LIPID-BASED NANOCARRIERS

Lipid-based nanocarriers can be defined as colloidal carriers prepared with a view for providing the release of drug in a controlled manner, to enhance the bioavailability of certain drug substances and to minimize side effects for effective drug therapy as compared to that of conventional dosage forms already available in the market. Some of the examples of lipid-based nanocarriers are solid lipid nanoparticles, nano-liposomes, nano-emulsions, nano-suspensions, lipid nano-tubes, lipid nano-capsules. Lipid-based nanocarriers are preferred over normal carriers as they offer to enhance oral bioavailability and ease of characterization of lipoid excipients. Lipid-based nanocarriers are preferred more due to their good oral bioavailability, lesser fluctuation in plasma profile and better evaluation characteristics of lipoid adjuvants(Patidar, Thakur, Kumar, & Verma, 2010). Figure 1 is showing classification of lipid-based nanocarriers.

Solid Lipid Nanoparticles (SLN)

SLN are Nanoparticles consist of a core made up of solid lipid matrix which is surrounded by a phospholipid monolayer. Their size ranges from 10 to 1000 nanometers. Solid lipid nanoparticle offers several advantages over liposomes such as extended stability, enhanced bioavailability, ease of large-scale production, better release kinetics, etc. SLNs can be prepared by using methods such as hot homogenization technique, cold homogenization technique, ultrasonication or highspeed homogenization, solvent emulsification-diffusion technique, solvent emulsification-evaporation technique, double emulsion technique, membrane contractor technique, solvent injection technique, supercritical fluid technology, micro-emulsion based method, etc. SLNs are novel carriers which can be used for the targeted delivery of drugs to a tumour, in cosmeceuticals, in chemotherapy, for delivery of drugs through the oral route, topical route, ocular route and rectal route, etc. (H, JS, & Dhole, 2012).

Figure 1. Classification of lipid-based nanocarriers

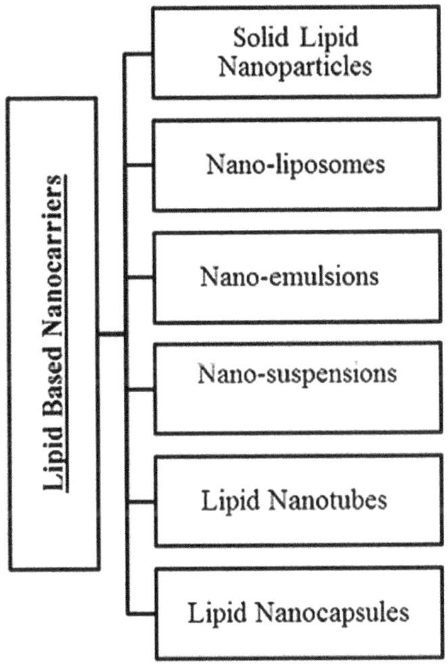

Nano-Liposomes

Nano-liposomes are nano-sized liposomes prepared in order to achieve delivery of various anticancer agents, proteins, amino acids and diagnostic agent. Nanoliposomes proved to be an efficient means for controlling the rate of release of medicament to a certain target.

Nano-Emulsions

Nano emulsions are biphasic colloidal dispersion of two immiscible liquids in which the dispersed phase or the internal phase is in the submicron size range of 20 to 600nm. Nanoemulsion can be of two types depending upon the internal phase i.e. either O/W when nano-sized oil droplets act as an internal phase or W/O when nano-sized water droplets act as an internal phase. Nanoemulsion can be prepared by ultrasonic emulsification, high-pressure homogenization, microfluidization, phase inversion temperature and spontaneous emulsification methods. Nanoemulsions can be used for targeted delivery of various pharmaceuticals (Jaiswal, & Dudhe, 2015).

Nano-Suspensions

Nano-suspensions are biphasic dispersion prepared by suspending poorly water-soluble drugs dispersed in the form of fine droplets in the continuous phase. Nanosuspensions can be prepared by the precipitation method, high-pressure homogenization, homogenization in aqueous media (Dissocubes), homogenization in non-aqueous media (Nanopure), microprecipitation (Nanoedge), nanojet technology and superficial critical fluid methods etc (Patel, & Agrawal, 2011).

Lipid Nanotubes

Lipid Nanotubes also known as tethers are open tubes of hollow cylindrical structures with their diameter in the size ranging from 10 to 100 nanometers. Lipid nanotubes are biocompatible molecules and are used for effective targeted delivery of drugs and encapsulated particles (Elia, Ubalek, Rown R, Erve, & Illigan, 1998).

Lipid Nanocapsules

Lipid Nanocapsules are nanosized capsule structures made in order to provide controlled release of medicaments, improved bioavailability, and diverse administration routes. Nanocapsules can be prepared by solvent-free phase inversion method, phase inversion temperature method. Figure 2 is showing different types of lipid-based nanocarriers.

BENEFITS OF MERGING THE POLYMERIC AND LIPID-BASED NANOCARRIERS

Many attractive features associated with the polymeric and lipid-based nanocarriers. Lipid-based carriers having excellent biocompatibility and ability to carry out hydrophilic drug into the core and hydrophobic drug into the surrounding lipid layer. Surface modification is easy to carry out with polyethylene glycol (PEG) and targeting ligands through which longer systemic circulation time and targeted drug delivery can be achieved. However many drawbacks associated with these formulations such as relatively complicated preparation steps, lesser loading efficiency for hydrophobic drugs, burst release and stability issues during storage. Lipid-based nanocarriers are only effective if they successfully cross the acidic gastric environment and drug maintain its structural integrity in the stomach. Enzymatic breakdown of the lipid occurs, which change structural integrity and leads to the burst drug release. These drawbacks limit their pharmaceutical application (Rao, & Prestidge, 2016).

Lipid-based nanocarriers have some drawbacks that have the advantages of polymeric nanoparticles. Polymeric nanocarriers have some excellent features such as high structural integrity, stability during storage, high loading efficiency of hydrophobic drugs and the capability to remain stable in the gastrointestinal tract (GIT). The rate of the drug release depends on polymer degradation, which can be controlled by choosing an appropriate polymer with required degradation rate and binding affinity towards the entrapped drug. Furthermore, it can be synthesized by self-assembly of the polymer by a simple

Figure 2. Different types of lipid-based nanocarriers

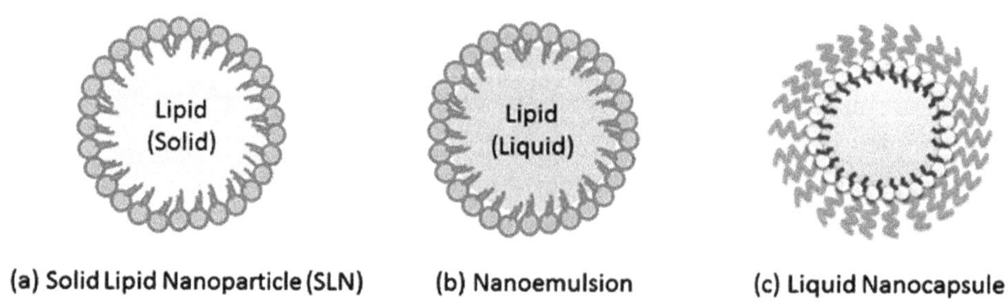

nano precipitation method, which is a cost-effective method. Despite all attractive features, polymeric nanoparticles do not get success as the liposome has received probably due to the biocompatibility issue and limited systemic circulation time (Chan, Zhang, Yuet, Liao, Rhee, & Langer, 2009).

PLN combining the positive attributes of both the polymeric NPs and lipid-based nanocarriers. On combining both the carriers, the hybrid system is formed which is superior to both of them in terms of biocompatibility and release profile. These PLN are characterize by their simple preparation method, favorable pharmacokinetic profile, biocompatibility, prolong shelf life and cost-effective. Active targeting can be achieved by conjugating molecular probes on the surface of nanoparticle, which shows an attractive approach for the targeted drug delivery in cancer through which the drug is released in control and sustained manner. (Hu, Kaushal, Cao, Aryal, Sartor, Esener, 2010). And the drug is released in control and sustained manner. So, by using PLN both the targeted and controlled drug delivery can be achieved. Effective cancer treatment can be achieved by combining antibodies through the PLN (Gao, Feng, & Guo, 2010). Figure 3 is showing the limitations of polymeric NPs and lipid-based nanocarriers.

EMERGENCE AND PROGRESS OF PLN DEVELOPMENT

In the early 1990's R.H. Muller introduced the Solid Lipid Nanoparticle (SLN), which consist of a matrix of solid lipid such as glycerides in which lipophilic drugs can be incorporated. SLN is suitable for the delivery of hydrophobic drugs but hydrophilic drugs cannot be loaded due to the hydrophobic matrix. Thus to overcome these limitations a new system was introduced in 2002, wherein a charged polymer (*i.e.* dextran sulphate) was incorporated into the SLN, which allows the high drug loading and sustained drug release of hydrophilic drugs (Wong, Bendayan, Rauth, & Wu, 1993-2008). Then after PLN is gain the attention of many researchers in order to deliver various hydrophilic, hydrophobic drugs, nucleic acid delivery, protein delivery, a diagnostic agent such as imaging probes (Rao, & Prestidge, 2016).

Various PLN formulations have been investigated for the delivery of the single drug, a combination of drugs, and drugs with P-glycoprotein inhibitor. PLN formulation is effective and reduces the side effects in the treatment of multidrug resistance (MDR) in cancer cells. It was observed that PLN facilitated drug uptake and localized at the P-gp overexpressing cells. Due to the P-gp inhibitor, intracellular

Figure 3. Limitations of polymeric NPs and lipid-based nanocarriers

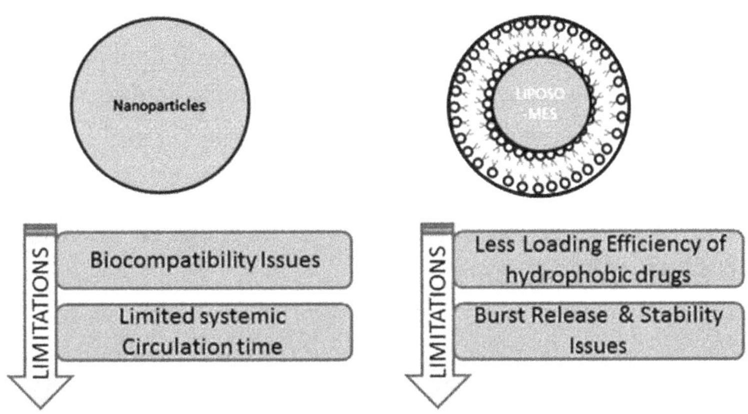

drug release can be achieved and drug transported to the nuclei where its target is located (DNA). This enables local bioavailability of the anticancer drugs to the tumors and malignant cells. PLN possess these unique features and better pharmacokinetic profile than the marketed approved drug Doxorubicin (Doxil®/Caelyx®), which has a long biological half-life of 118 hrs, synergistic anticancer drugs such as doxorubicin and mitomycin C encapsulated in the PLN formulation gives superior results as compare to marketed formulation in the MDR cancer cells and in preclinical models of tumor (Prasad, Shuhendler, Cai, Rauth, & Wu, 2013; Zhang, Cai, Zhang, Chen, Li, & Cheng, 2016).

HYBRID LIPID POLYMER NANOPARTICLE COMPOSITION

PLN mitigate the drawbacks of the two established nanocarriers liposome and nanoparticle. PLN composed of three functional domains:

1. Inner hydrophobic polymer core where poorly water-soluble drugs can be incorporated.
2. A highly biocompatible lipid layer that surrounds the polymeric core, it prevents the drug leaking, thus increase the drug retention time.
3. The outer most layer is the hydrophilic polymer stealth layer, that enhances the systemic circulation time and PLN stability (Fang, Aryal, Hu, & Zhang, 2010).

Depending on the preparation method, lipid layers in the PLN may be monolayer, bilayer or multilayer (Zhao, Li, Li, Wang, Ren, & Chen, 2015). Inner polymeric core and outer lipid layer are associated with different forces such as van der Wal force, electrostatic interaction, hydrophobic interactions and other non-covalent forces. Lipid layer and hydrophilic polymeric stealth layer often conjugated with covalent forces (Zhang, & Zhang, 2010).

Polymer and lipids used in the formulation of PLN should be GRAS substances and should be approved by the FDA for clinical use (Zhao, Li, Li, Wang, Ren, & Chen, 2015). Polymer used in the preparation of PLN should be biocompatible such as poly (lactic-co-glycolic acid) (PLGA), polyethylenimine (PEI), dextran sulphate, gelatin soybean oil etc. Lipids used in the PLN preparation are those already used in the marketed products, like phospholipids, lecithin, found in the body (endogenous fatty acids), 1,2-distearoyl-sn-glycero-3-phosphoethanolamine (DSPE) and polyethylene glycol (PEG)-lipid etc (Wu, 2016).

PLN formulation can be divided into two basic categories. Type A - monolithic matrix PLN, in which drug and polymer is uniformly distributed throughout the solid lipid matrix. Type B – core-shell PLN, where drug polymeric core is encapsulated within the within a lipid layer. The latter is sometimes referred as hybrid lipid polymer nanoparticles (PLN). Table 1 shows the different lipids and polymer used in the preparation of PLN.

MECHANISM OF FORMATION OF PLN

PLN is prepared by the mixing of the two components at the molecular level. These two components organized cooperatively into a new structure, form a hybrid which is superior to them. The hybrid is not only superior in terms of functionalities or properties of the respective constituents but also shows

Table 1. Different types of lipids and polymer used in the preparation of PLN

Component	Examples
Polymer	Poly(lactic-co-glycolic acid) (PLGA) (Zhao, Li, Li, Wang, Ren, & Chen, 2015; Shi, Xiao, Votruba, Vilos, Farokhzad, 2011). Polycaprolactone, Polyethylenimine (PEI), Polymer derived from soy bean oil, Dextran sulfate, Gelatin, poly(dimethyl siloxane) (PDMS)(Wu, 2016), poly(isobutylene) (PIB) (Olubummo, Schulz, Lechner, Scholtysek, Bacia, & Blume,2012) or poly(butadiene) (PBut) (Nam, Vanderlick, & Beales, 2012), poly(ethylene oxide) (PEO) or poly(2-methyloxazoline) (PMOXA)
Lipid	Phospholipids, Polyethylene glycol (PEG)–lipid, Lecithin (Zhao, Li, Li, Wang, Ren, & Chen, 2015; Shi, Xiao, Votruba, Vilos, & Farokhzad, 2011; Salvador-Morales, Zhang, Langer, & Farokhzad, 2009), Glyceryl tripalmitate (tripalmitin), 1,2-distearoyl-sn-glycero-3-phosphoethanolamine (DSPE) (Salvador-Morales, Zhang, Langer, & Farokhzad, 2009), Myristic acid (Prasad, Shuhendler, Cai, Rauth, Wu, 2013).

synergistic actions arising from their collective interaction or supramolecular assemblies at the higher levels (Lin, Chen, Hashimoto, & Chen, 2016). Core-shell nanoparticles formed in two different steps: (a) Cross-links likely to be occurring within the shell in the nucleation and particle growth step, both the steps occur simultaneously; (b) Cross-link structure seems to be occur during the slow particle growth.

A critical parameter that is necessary to the formation of stable hybrid vesicles chemical composition and size of hydrophobic segments between lipids and polymers. Apart from this thermodynamic incompatibility, due to the differences between entropy and enthalpy between the hydrophobic blocks, may lead to the phase separation. All the polymers used in the PLN formulations exhibit a low glass transition temperature (Tg), that allows the dynamic exchange of chains and leads to the equilibrium structure of the membrane when it forms. The solubility parameter of hydrocarbon moiety in phospholipids and hydrophobic polymer blocks should be relatively close. These relatively close values suggest chemical compatibility between polymer and lipids. This is the important criteria for the formation of PLN, although the lateral phase separation may occur for other reasons. (Le Meins, Schatz, Lecommandoux, & Sandre, 2013).

Apart from the gel or fluid state of the lipid, other factors also determine the formation of stable hybrid vesicles such as size mismatch between the lipid chain and polymer. Membrane thickness of the liposomes should be 3 5 nm and for polymerosomes (either graft copolymer, monolayer for triblock or bilayer for diblock) it should vary from 5 to 50 nm. Large size gap would lead to the high line tension at the polymer/lipid boundaries arising due to the thickness mismatch between domain and polymer membrane with a co-occurance exposure of hydrophobic polymer to the water. To avoid this exposure and energetic cost of the boundary edges, there are two possibilities; (a) Conformational adaptation through elastic deformation of the polymer chains at the boundary at an entropic cost for the polymer chains (but globally reducing the line tension). This scenario is analogous to the elastic deformation of the membrane. (b) Coalescence into domains of a larger area (Kuzmin, Akimov, Chizmadzhev, Zimmerberg, & Cohen, 2005).

Effect of the composition, polymer/lipid molar ratio on the formation of PLN is rarely investigated in a systemic manner. When polymers or nanoparticles interact with the lipid membrane final morphology is strongly determined by their charge, composition, and size of the interacting components.

TYPES OF LIPID POLYMER HYBRID NANOPARTICLES

Polymer Core-Lipid Shell Nanoparticles

This type of system usually consists of the polymeric core inside, surrounded by the single or multiple layers of lipid. Lipid layer prevents the penetration of the water into the polymeric core, modulate polymer degradation, restrict the drug leakage and allows the sustained drug release. Polymeric core aid in the structural integrity of the lipid layer in the PLNs (Pandita, Kumar, & Lather, 2015). The drug can be encapsulated in the core or both in the core and lipid layer. The space between the core and lipid layer is occupied with the aqueous phase or water. Cationic or zwitterionic phospholipids have been used to form the outer lipid layer. Electrostatic interactions are present in between lipid and opposite charge polymers. The ratio of drug to polymer is a very critical parameter in the preparation of PLNs. An improper ratio may lead to the formation of lumps and thus fails the formation of PLNs. This system is can easily encapsulate the hydrophobic drugs but it is not a suitable carrier for the hydrophilic drugs (Mandal, Bhattacharjee, Mittal, Sah, Balabathula, & Thoma, 2013).

Lipid Core Polymer Shell Systems

The lipid core polymer shell system is composed of 3 domains:

1. Inner hollow core made up of positive charge containing lipid layer.
2. Middle layer made up of the polymeric layer (*i.e.* PLGA), which is hydrophobic in nature.
3. The interface formed in between polymer and outer PEG layer by neutral lipids.

This type of system differs from the conventional PLNs because they contain properties of both the PEGylated lipoplexes and PLGA NPs. It can be prepared by the double emulsification solvent evaporation method (Zhang, Chan, Gu, Rhee, Wang, & Radovic-Moreno, 2008). PEGylation of this system is necessary in order to avoid recognition by the immune system and thus improve the stability during circulation (Davis, 2009). Sustained drug release can be obtained by the middle polymer layer. (Zhang, Chan, Gu, Rhee, Wang, & Radovic-Moreno, 2008). Moreover, inner hollow core made up of the cationic lipids, able to encapsulate anionic drugs more efficiently as compared to polymer alone. The advantage of this system includes more than one active moiety or combination of two active moieties can deliver efficiently. For example, it is helpful for the treatment of several diseases such as multidrug resistant cancer due to the incorporation of the combination of si-RNA and small drug molecule within the hydrophobic PLGA layer (Zhao, Li, Li, Wang, Ren, & Chen, 2015).

Polymer Caged Nanoparticles

These systems are composed of polymers anchored at the surface of the liposome to provide the stability and to get better results (Lee, Chen, Dettmer, O'Halloran, & Nguyen, 2007). Polymer caged nanoparticles are more stable and exhibit pH-sensitive behavior. Both the drug release and surface properties can be modified by this method. pH-responsive cross-linked polymer enhance the stability, prevent drug leakage and allows the release of drug at low pH, thus it is beneficial for tumor therapy (Casey, Grinstein, & Orlowski, 2010). Circulation lifetime of these nanocarriers can also modify by varying the degree of cross-linking in polymer cage. Nowadays researcher focus to enhance the drug release by using pH-sensitive lipid (Gerasimov, Boomer, Quall, & Thompson, 1999) such as phosphatidylethanolamine (Bergstrand, Arfvidsson, Kim, Thompson, & Edwards, 2003) and acid labile PEG, which is also called polymer-caged nanobin (PCN) (Lee, Chen, O'Halloran, & Nguyen, 2009). Steric stability provided by the polymer cage around the lipid shell.

For the preparation of polymer caged nanoparticles, first liposomes are prepared then cholesterol-functionalized poly(acrylic acid) joined to its exterior part, which gives surface active carboxylate groups through which linkers such as telechelic 2,2-(ethylenedioxy) bis(ethylamine) can be attached. This free carboxylate group are protonated in the acidic environments, which leads to the pocket of increased local hydrophobicity on the surface of polymer cage nanobin, leads to the collapse of vesicle and release their content (Tannock, & Rotin, 1989).

METHODS OF PREPARATION OF PLN

In general, there are two distinct approaches through which PLN can be prepared. In two step method both the lipid shell and polymeric nanoparticles are prepared separately and then merged together. In one step method, PLN can be prepared by nanoprecipitation and self-assembly method. For the biomedical application, the surface of the PLN can be modified by using appropriate targeting ligand for the targeted delivery of PLN. Figure 4 showing the preparation methods of PLN.

Two Step Method

Conventional Two Step Method

Two-step approaches are typically used to prepare PLN in the early stage of PLN development. In this method, preformed lipid shell is mixed with the preformed polymeric nanoparticle. Lipid shell is

Figure 4. Preparation methods of PLN

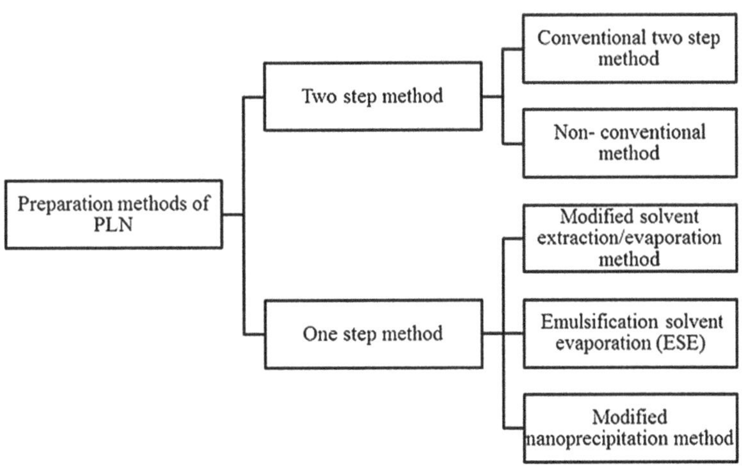

adsorbed on the polymeric nanoparticles through the electrostatic interaction. In this method, the liposome is formed by the sonication method or extrusion method. Polymeric nanoparticles are formed by the high pressure homogenization method (Fenart, Casanova, Dehouck, Duhem, Slupek, & Cecchelli, 1999) emulsification solvent evaporation (Mieszawska, Gianella, Cormode, Zhao, Meijerink, & Langer, 2012) and nanoprecipitation method (Thevenot, Troutier, David, Delair, & Ladavière, 2007). Previously formed nanoparticles can be merged with lipid shell in the following manner:

- A polymeric nanoparticle can be added to dried thin lipid film (Thevenot, Troutier, David, Delair, & Ladavière, 2007).
- Alternatively, a polymeric nanoparticle can be added to preformed lipid vesicles, which is prepared by hydration of lipid film.

In both the above process, PLNs are prepared by either ultrasonication or vortexing of the lipid-polymer suspension at a temperature higher than the gel-to-liquid transition temperature of the lipid. After that PLNs are separated by unadsorbed lipid by the centrifugation method. Monodisperse PLNs size can be obtained by subjected PLNs to homogenization or extrusion steps after their synthesis. In the extrusion step, PLNs suspension is passed through a porous membrane to prepare PLNs in the size range of membrane's pore size.

Nonconventional Two Step Method

In the non-conventional method, other methods apart from the conventional methods such as spray drying and soft lithography particle molding have been employed. Hitzman et al. (Nidhi, Indrajeet, Khushboo, Gauri, & Sen, 2011) prepared polymeric nanoparticles by spray drying method, then after dispersed in the dichloromethane solution containing the lipids (i.e., tripalmitin, tristearin, cetyl alcohol). This lipid-polymer suspension is then spray dried to prepare lipid coated polymeric nanoparticles (Li, Anton, Arpagaus, Belleteix, & Vandamme, 2010).

For the gene delivery researcher employed a new technique which is a soft lithography particle molding technique termed as particle replication in non-wetting templates (PRINT) (Hasan, Chu, Gullapalli, Dunn, Elizabeth, & Enlow, 2012). In this technique, a polymer is dissolved in organic solvent with the genetic material and cast onto a polyethylene terephthalate (PET) sheet. The PET sheet was then heated while in conformal contact with a PRINT mold containing 80-320 nm patterns, allowing the PLGA to flow into the mold and to solidify upon being returned to ambient temperature, thereby forming the PLGA nanoparticles. Next, the nanoparticles were harvested from the mold by having the mold in conformal contact with a poly(vinyl alcohol) (PVA)-coated PET sheet. The nanoparticles were then released from the PVA-coated PET sheet using an aqueous solution of the lipids (i.e., 1,2-dioleoyl-3-trimethylammonium-propane (DOTAP) and 1,2-dioleoyl-sn-glycero-3-phosphoethanolamine (DOPE)), which dissolved the PVA layer, hence removing the nanoparticles from the mold, and simultaneously forming lipid-coated PLGA nanoparticles. The PLNs produced after freeze-drying were needle-shaped with the length of 200 nm and zeta potential of (+) 5 mV. Importantly, the PRINT technique enables precise control over size and shape of the PLNs as these properties are governed by the size and shape of the mold cavity.

Figure 5. Schematic representation of formation of PLNs by the two-step method

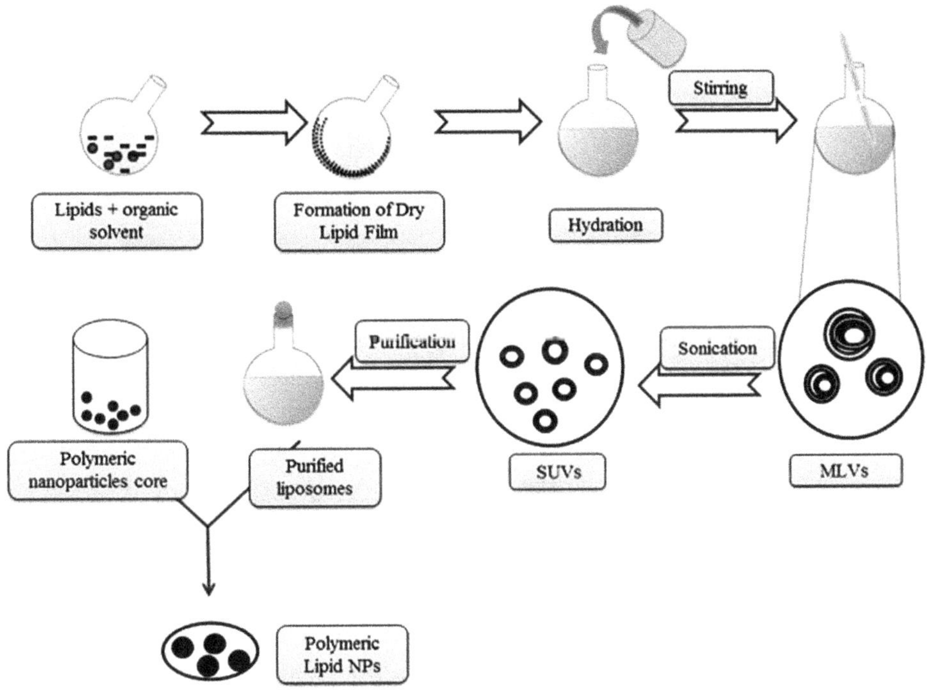

One Step Method

Despite the new techniques involve in the synthesis of PLNs in a two-step method, drawbacks remain the same. In this method, lipid shell and polymeric nanoparticles are prepared separately which is a time and energy consuming process. This method gives rise to a bilayer or multilayer containing PLNs. Thus to overcome the limitations of this method, relatively simple approach has been applied that merged these two steps into a single step. This method requires only mixing of lipid and polymer solution, after which they self-assembled to form the PLNs by either emulsification solvent evaporation or nanoprecipitation method. Figure 6 shows the schematic representation of the steps involved in the formation PLNs by the one-step method.

Nanoprecipitation

In this method polymer and drug or encapsulated substance are dissolved in the water-miscible organic solvent such as acetone, acetonitrile, while the lipid-PEG conjugate or lipid are dispersed in the water Zhang, Chan, Gu, Rhee, Wang, & Radovic-Moreno, 2008). In order to facilitate the solubilization of phospholipid into the aqueous dispersion, a small amount of water-miscible organic solvent can be added to the aqueous dispersion. To form a homogenous dispersion of lipid and lipid-PEG solution, it is heated up to 60-70°C. Polymer solution is then added dropwise to the aqueous solution under continuous stirring, organic solvent diffuses into the aqueous solution, leads to the precipitate the polymer into the nanoparticle. This mixture is then vortexed and subsequently homogenized or ultrasonicated in order to reduce the particle size in the nanometer range (Valencia, Basto, Zhang, Rhee, Langer, & Farokhzad,

Figure 6. Schematic representation of formation of PLNs by the one-step method

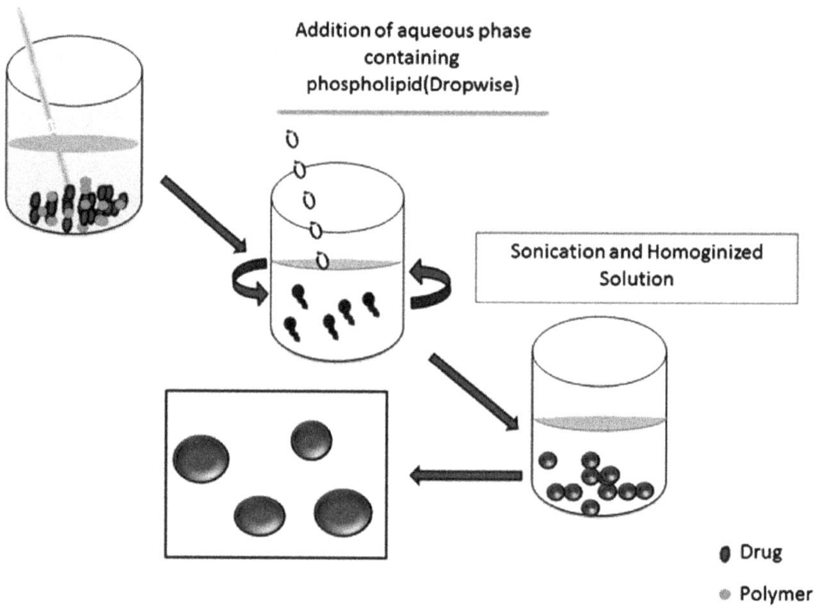

2010). Simultaneously lipids self-assemble around the polymeric core through the hydrophobic interaction in order to reduce the system's free energy. Hydrophobic tail of the lipids is joined with the polymeric nanoparticle and hydrophilic head faces towards the external aqueous surroundings, leads to the formation of PLNs that are further stabilized by the lipid. This one-step method is a cost-effective, time saving, scalable and predictable formulation strategies of PLNs (Zhang & Zhang, 2010).

Emulsification–Solvent–Evaporation (ESE)

ESE method is divided into two categories: single and double emulsification method. Single ESE method is used when drug substance is soluble in the hydrophobic solvent such as oil phase. In this method water, the immiscible solvent which contains the drug and polymer is added dropwise to the hydrophilic solvent containing the lipid which forms an o/w emulsion under constant stirring. When the hydrophobic phase is removed by evaporation, polymer core is formed and then lipid is self-assembled around the polymeric core to form PLNs (Irvine, 2009).

A double ESE method is used when the drug is insoluble in organic solvents, it cannot be dissolved in any solvent together with polymer. For such type of drugs, it is dissolved in hydrophilic solvent and then emulsified with oil phase which contains the lipid and polymer. This emulsion is then further emulsified in an aqueous phase containing lipid-PEG which forms the w/o/w emulsion, which gives PLNs after the evaporation of the oil phase (Cheow, & Hadinoto, 2011). In this method PLNs which are synthesized is somewhat different in terms of its composition as described here:

- Aqueous hollow core which is surrounded by the inner lipid layer,
- Polymer layer in the middle,
- The outer most layer which contains the lipid-PEG.

Modified Solvent Extraction/Evaporation Method

This method is a slight alteration of the ESE method introduced by the Gurny et al.(Gurny, Peppas, Harrington, & Banker, 1981). This method has been used to synthesize PLNs loaded with paclitaxel (Liu, Pan, & Feng, 2010) and docetaxel (Chan, Zhang, Yuet, Liao, Rhee, & Langer, 2009; Liu, Li, Pan, Liu, & Feng, 2010). In this method, polymer and drug are dissolved in water immiscible solvents such as ethyl acetate, chloroform, and dichloromethane. Then a fixed amount lipid is dispersed through the bath mechanical stirring, heat or sonication. After this oil, phase is mixed with the aqueous phase, and sonication is performed by using probe sonicator and ice bath. After the sonication organic dispersed phase is broken into mini nanodroplets, which congeal into a nanosphere surrounded by a lipid layer. The rotary evaporator is used to remove the organic solvent under reduced pressure or stirred overnight. The particle suspension is further purified by centrifugation followed by freeze-drying to obtain a dry powder.

APPLICATIONS

Researchers focus on the PLN for effective treatment of many diseases particularly cancer due to its unique features discussed in the previous section. Drug delivery applications of PLNs are dominated by the anticancer drugs due to the delivery of a combination of drugs within a single carrier, which is an effective therapy for the multidrug resistance cancer. Figure 7 shows the applications of PLN.

Delivery of Small Molecules for Cancer Therapy

Single Drug Delivery

Treatment of the cancer is largely occupied by the chemotherapy. However, number of biological barriers is present in the body which decreases the drug accumulation within tumor and cancer cell thus decline

Figure 7. Applications of PLNs

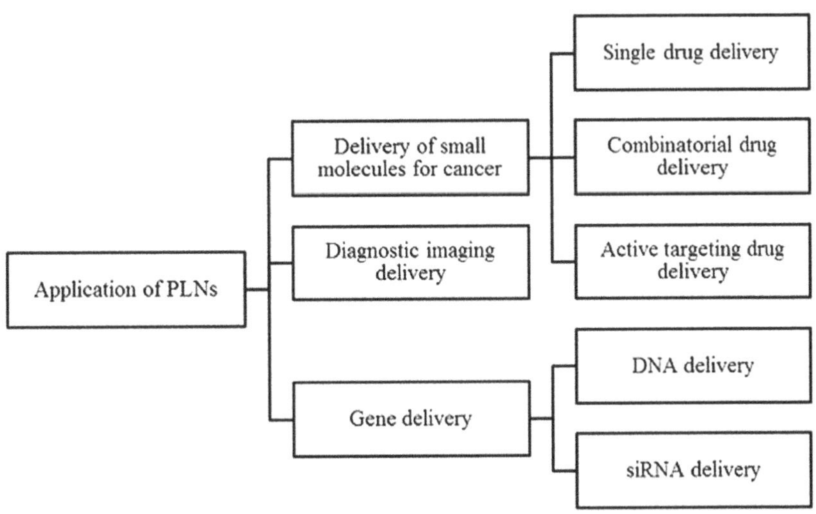

the efficacy of the chemotherapeutic agents (Zhang, Wong, Xue, Eoh, & Wu, 2016; Wong, Bendayan, Rauth, Li, & Wu, 2007). Researchers have carried out numerous studies to develop PLNs for the delivery of different drugs against the various cancers such as prostate, breast, pancreatic, lung and cervical cancer etc. Various PLN formulations have been used to conquer these limitations of chemotherapy.

Chan et al. prepared PLNs for single drug delivery, in which "nanoburr" system was devised for delivery of paclitaxel for the cure of injured vasculature. This system contains a core made up of paclitaxel-conjugated PLA and a shell of lecithin/DSPE-PEG, which is again modified with basement membrane targeting peptide. The resultant PLNs having a size of 100nm concentrated at injured vasculature in the rat model and release the drug content over two weeks (Chan, Zhang, Tong, Ghosh, Gao, & Liao, 2010).

Another example of single drug delivery of a doxorubicin was developed by the Wong et.al. against the MDR breast cancer. Cellular uptake of PLNs is significantly increased as compared to solution formulation. Two possible mechanisms of cytotoxicity are proposed:

- The free drug was released from PLNs and kill the cancer cells.
- PLNs itself entered into the cell and release the active moiety there, thus bypass the P-gp efflux pump.

The drug in the PLNs is entered into the cell via a combination of both the phagocytosis and diffusion. Due to the physical association of the drug and polymer, the drug is not effluxed due to the P-gp pump. Therefore chronic suppression of MDR cell proliferation occurs due to the continuous supply of a drug to the cancer cell. (Liu, Pan, & Feng, 2010).

Combinatorial Drug Delivery

For the effective treatment of cancer, the combination of the different drugs or chemotherapeutic drug with another therapeutic agent (gene, magnetic nanoparticle) or diagnostic agent (^{90}Y,^{131}I) is required. Thus there is a need for a nanocarrier system that can carry multiple therapeutic agents within one carrier at the precise molar ratio, which is also biocompatible and provide controlled release. PLNs provide a way to overcome these obstacles and show promising results. Multiple drugs can be incorporated into PLNs in different ways such as:

For One-Step Method

- Before the lipid/polymer mixing, one therapeutic agent is covalently linked to the polymer while other linked to the lipid precursors.
- In other method, different chemotherapeutic agents are separately covalently conjugated with polymer chain of the similar length before to the lipid/polymer mixing step.

For Two-Step Method

- Separately chemotherapeutic agents are encapsulated in preformed polymeric NPs and preformed lipid vesicles.

- For one step and two step methods, one of the drugs is entrapped into the PLNs, while the other drugs can be covalently linked or adsorbed electrostatically to the lipid layer after the PLNs preparation.

After reaching the target site (tumor cell), these drug conjugate linkers are hydrolyzed and release the individual drug.

Sengupta *et al.* designed a nanocell system for the tumor. It consists of a core made up of PLGA containing doxorubicin and multilayered lipid shell containing anti-angiogenic agent (combretastatin). This nanocell system is very effective in tumor reduction and enhances the survival rate of rats as compare to single drug treatment. The synergistic effect shown by the temporal release of anti-angiogenesis agent from the outer lipid shell, prevent the formation of new blood vessels; polymer core releasing the doxorubicin further destroy the cancer cells. (Sengupta, Eavarone, Capila, Zhao, Watson, & Kiziltepe, 2005).

Another PLNs system designed for the prostate cancer is a chemorad NPs. Chemorad composed of PLGA core and lecithin/DMPE-DTPA lipid shell, designed for the codelivery of chemotherapeutic agent (docetaxel) and therapeutic radionuclide yttrium 90 (^{90}Y). An oligonucleotide aptamer A10, which is having high affinity and selectivity to the PSMA-positive prostate cancer cells, attached to the outer surface of PLNs via a coupling reaction with DSPE-PEG to generate a targeted particles (Apt-Dtxl-^{90}Y-NPs). Chemorad NPs improve the chemoradiotherapy against the prostate cancer (Wang, Yuet, Zhang, Gu, Huynh-Le, & Radovic-Moreno, 2010).

Active Targeted Drug Delivery

In the anticancer therapy active targeted drug delivery is prerequisite for the effective treatment and to minimize the exposure of chemotherapeutic agents to healthy cells. Through the PLNs nanocarrier, it can be achieved by functionalizing the PLNs via targeting ligands, which have a special affinity for the tumor cell. Folic acid (FA) is an example of such a targeting moiety because folic acid receptors are highly expressed on the surface of cancer cells so active targeting can be achieved by this strategy. In this regard PEG end groups are particularly suitable for the conjugation of targeting ligand (Kanwar, 2012). This insertion may be achieved via pre-insertion technique (prior to PLNs preparation) or post-insertion technique (post PLNs preparation).

Apart from the FA, other active targeting ligands single chain variable fragment (Messerschmidt, Musyanovych, Altvater, Scheurich, Pfizenmaier, & Landfester, 2009), antibody (Hu, Kaushal, Cao, Aryal, Sartor, & Esener, 2010) aptamer, (Zhang, Chan, Gu, Rhee, & Wang, 2008), transferrin (Zheng, Yu, Weecharangsan, Piao, Darby, & Mao, 2010), and peptides (Chan, Rhee, Drum, Bronson, Golomb, & Langer, 2011) have been attached to the PLNs and active targeting is successfully achieved.

Gene Delivery

Delivery of the gene through the non viral vectors such as cationic lipids (DOTAB) (i.e., lipoplex) and cationic polymer (PEI) (i.e., polyplex) offers a many advantages such as low toxicity, low immunogenicity and feasibility for large-scale production etc (Parker, Newman, Briggs, Seymour, & Sheridan, 2003). Even though the lipoplex and polyplex show promising results in *in vivo* and *in vitro* studies, they are not clinically manifested due to the instability during systemic administration. Their cationic surface prone to non specific binding of the serum protein and rapidly cleared from the systemic circulation (Al-Dosari,

& Gao, 2009). However coating of the lipoplex with the polymer, protect the binding of serum protein to it (Papanicolaou, Briggs, & Alpar, 2004). Another approach to preventing rapid systemic clearance is by using lipid-PEG, where PEG reduces the surface charge of the lipoplex (Ambegia, Ansell, Cullis, Heyes, Palmer, & MacLachlan, 2005).

DNA Delivery

"One-bullet" dosage of PLNs has the combination of chemotherapeutic agent and gene, which provides synergistic cytotoxicity through the different mechanisms of drug action (Kang, Gao, Huang, Jin, & Wang, 2015). A "triple-punch" PLNs was developed for the loading of *survivin* siRNA, paclitaxel and indocyanine green (ICG) for an intereated gene, chemotherapy, and phototherapy within a single system. The release of the paclitaxel is thermally controlled by laser irradiated ICG. This "triple punch" PLNs carrier shows the sequential therapies by first inhibiting anti-apoptotic gene *surviving* and then releasing anticancer drug paclitaxel into tumor cells, showing the effective antitumor activity with minimum side effects in the breast tumor model (Antitumor, Su, Tian, Li, Ding, & Ji, 2015).

Another researcher reported a PLNs formulation with plasmid DNA encoded luciferase receptor gene composed of PLGA core and cationic lipids DOTAP/DC cholesterol. This PLNs formulation transfects the luciferase gene in prostate cancer cells 500-600 times more efficiently than the unbound DNA (Zhong, Chinta, Pamujula, Wang, Yao, & Mandal, 2010).

siRNA Delivery

siRNA shows the promising results in gene therapy by suppressing the expression of a specific gene via RNA interference. siRNA inhibits the protein expression that is involved in tumor initiation and progression (Li, & Rana, 2012). Through the lipoplex (Nourbakhsh, Jaafari, Lage, Abnous, Mosaffa, & Badiee, 2015), and polyplex (Gary, Puri, & Won, 2007), several formulations have been developed for the delivery of siRNA, although faces the same challenges as in the case of DNA delivery (poor stability in systemic circulation). Thus the better siRNA delivery can be achieved by a PLNs formulation.

A hybrid nanostructure developed by the Shi et.al. that is capable of protecting siRNA and lipoplexes from physiological environment. The system is referred as *Differentially charged hollow core/shell lipid-polymer-lipid hybrid nanoparticles*, which contain the four functional building blocks: an inner hollow core made up of cationic lipids, hydrophobic PLGA layer and an outer lipid layer containing the PEG chains. This hybrid system releases siRNA in a sustained manner and increased in vivo gene silencing and further inhibited luciferase gene expression in the murine xenograft tumors. This strategy shows the potential success in the gene delivery for the treatment of MDR cancer (Shi, Xiao, Votruba, Vilos, & Farokhzad, 2011).

Diagnostic Imaging Agent Delivery

Apart from the delivery of therapeutic agents, PLNs can also deliver imaging agents such as fluorescent dyes, iron oxide and quantum dots (QDs) by entrapping into the polymeric core. Application of the PLNs in bioimaging is a very attractive approach due to the high stability and biocompatibility of the PLNs (Zhang & Zhang, 2010).

CHALLENGES AND FUTURE DIRECTION

The concept of the drug delivery through the PLN system is relatively new as compared to established formulations like liposomes and nanoparticles. It is an alternative approach for the treatment of life-threatening diseases, particularly cancer. Because of the incorporation of multiple drugs within one system offers many advantages over other systems. Incorporation of different drugs within core and lipid layer provide exclusivity to this system and very effective in the treatment of MDR and life threatening diseases. Apart from this, delivery of the small molecular drugs, incorporation of genes, proteins and diagnostic agents like quantum dots often makes a promising carrier (Mandal, Bhattacharjee, Mittal, Sah, Balabathula, & Thoma, 2013). Still, there are many challenges associated with these formulations regarding stability profile, release kinetics, and drug loading efficiency. Apart from this combination of different surfactant, lipid and polymer could alter the stability of individual excipient. So excipients used in the formulation of the PLN, still should be GRAS substances (Zhang, Ahmed, Li, Li, Abbasi, & Wu, 2017). Although huge success made in formulation parameters of PLN, still there are many unmeet challenges associated with this formulation.

Although a number of researchers are attempting to investigate the mechanism of formation of PLN, but still researchers have not met the answers to many questions such as:

- At what concentration polymer and lipids need to be mixed and what is the impact of the change in size (molecular weight) and polymer structure?
- Whether these PLN formulations are stable for long-term storage?
- Is it possible to get control over membrane structure and composition, meaning a homogenous distribution of both components or the formation of heterogeneous domain?

REFERENCES

Al-Dosari, M. S., & Gao, X. (2009). Nonviral Gene Delivery: Principle, Limitations, and Recent Progress. *The AAPS Journal, 11*(4), 671–681. doi:10.120812248-009-9143-y PMID:19834816

Bergstrand, N., Arfvidsson, M. C., Kim, J. M., Thompson, D. H., & Edwards, K. (2003). Interactions between pH-sensitive liposomes and model membranes. *Biophysical Chemistry, 104*(1), 361–379. doi:10.1016/S0301-4622(03)00011-5 PMID:12834854

Casey, J. R., Grinstein, S., & Orlowski, J. (2010). Sensors and regulators of intracellular pH. *Nat Rev Mol Cell Biol, 11*(1), 50–61. Available from: http://www.nature.com/doifinder/10.1038/nrm2820

Chan, J. M., Rhee, J.-W., Drum, C. L., Bronson, R. T., Golomb, G., Langer, R., & Farokhzad, O. C. (2011). In vivo prevention of arterial restenosis with paclitaxel-encapsulated targeted lipid-polymeric nanoparticles. *Proceedings of the National Academy of Sciences of the United States of America, 108*(48), 19347–19352. doi:10.1073/pnas.1115945108 PMID:22087004

Chan, J. M., Zhang, L., Tong, R., Ghosh, D., Gao, W., Liao, G., ... Farokhzad, O. C. (2010). Spatiotemporal controlled delivery of nanoparticles to injured vasculature. *Proceedings of the National Academy of Sciences of the United States of America, 107*(5), 2213–2218. doi:10.1073/pnas.0914585107 PMID:20133865

Chemin, M., Brun, P.-M., Lecommandoux, S., Sandre, O., & Le Meins, J.-F. (2012). Hybrid polymer/lipid vesicles: Fine control of the lipid and polymer distribution in the binary membrane. *Soft Matter*, *8*(10), 2867. doi:10.1039/c2sm07188f

Cheow, W. S., & Hadinoto, K. (2011). Factors affecting drug encapsulation and stability of lipid-polymer hybrid nanoparticles. *Colloids Surfaces B Biointerfaces*, *85*(2), 214–220. doi:10.1016/j.colsurfb.2011.02.033 PMID:21439797

Davis, M. E. (2009). The first targeted delivery of siRNA in humans via a self-assembling, cyclodextrin polymer-based nanoparticle: From concept to clinic. *Molecular Pharmaceutics*, *6*(3), 659–668. doi:10.1021/mp900015y PMID:19267452

Dehaini, D., Fang, R. H., Luk, B. T., Pang, Z., Hu, C.-M. J., Kroll, A. V., ... Zhang, L. (2016). Ultra-small lipid–polymer hybrid nanoparticles for tumor-penetrating drug delivery. *Nanoscale*, *8*(30), 14411–14419. doi:10.1039/C6NR04091H PMID:27411852

Fang, R. H., Aryal, S., Hu, C. M. J., & Zhang, L. (2010). Quick synthesis of lipid-polymer hybrid nanoparticles with low polydispersity using a single-step sonication method. *Langmuir*, *26*(22), 16958–16962. doi:10.1021/la103576a PMID:20961057

Fenart, L., Casanova, A., Dehouck, B., Duhem, C., Slupek, S., & Cecchelli, R. (1999). Evaluation of effect of charge and lipid coating on ability of 60-nm nanoparticles to cross an in vitro model of the blood-brain barrier. *The Journal of Pharmacology and Experimental Therapeutics*, *291*(3), 1017–1022. PMID:10565819

Gao, J., Feng, S.-S., & Guo, Y. (2010). Antibody engineering promotes nanomedicine for cancer treatment. *Nanomedicine (London)*, *5*(8), 1141–1145. Available from http://www.futuremedicine.com/doi/10.2217/nnm.10.94. doi:10.2217/nnm.10.94 PMID:21039191

Gary, D. J., Puri, N., & Won, Y. Y. (2007). Polymer-based siRNA delivery: Perspectives on the fundamental and phenomenological distinctions from polymer-based DNA delivery. *Journal of Controlled Release*, *121*(1–2), 64–73. doi:10.1016/j.jconrel.2007.05.021 PMID:17588702

Gerasimov, O. V., Boomer, J. A., Qualls, M. M., & Thompson, D. H. (1999). Cytosolic drug delivery using pH- and light-sensitive liposomes. *Advanced Drug Delivery Reviews*, *38*(3), 317–338. doi:10.1016/S0169-409X(99)00035-6 PMID:10837763

Gurny, R., Peppas, N. A., Harrington, D., & Banker, G. S. (1981). Development of Biodegradable and Injectable Latices for Controlled Release of Potent Drugs. *Drug Development and Industrial Pharmacy*, *7*(1), 1–25. doi:10.3109/03639048109055684

H, R.K. (2012). Solid Lipid Nanoparticle: A Review. *IOSR J Pharm.*, *2*(6), 2250–3013.

Hasan, W., Chu, K., Gullapalli, A., Dunn, S. S., Elizabeth, M., & Enlow. (2012). Nanoparticles for Treatment of Prostate Cancer. *Nano Letters*, *12*(1), 287–292. doi:10.1021/nl2035354 PMID:22165988

Hu, C. J., Kaushal, S., Cao, H. S. T., Aryal, S., Sartor, M., Esener, S., ... Zhang, L. (2010). Half-Antibody Functionalized Lipid - Polymer Hybrid Nanoparticles for Targeted Drug Delivery to Carcinoembryonic Antigen Presenting Pancreatic Cancer Cells. *Molecular Pharmaceutics*, *7*(3), 914–920. doi:10.1021/mp900316a PMID:20394436

Kanwar, J. R. (2012). Cancer nanotechnology. *Journal of Cancer Science & Therapy*, *4*(1), 249–265. doi:10.4172/1948-5956.1000e104

Kumari, A., Yadav, S. K., & Yadav, S. C. (2010). Biodegradable polymeric nanoparticles based drug delivery systems. *Colloids and Surfaces. B, Biointerfaces*, *75*(1), 1–18. doi:10.1016/j.colsurfb.2009.09.001 PMID:19782542

Kuzmin, P. I., Akimov, S. A., Chizmadzhev, Y. A., Zimmerberg, J., & Cohen, F. S. (2005). Line Tension and Interaction Energies of Membrane Rafts Calculated from Lipid Splay and Tilt. *Biophys J, 88*(2), 1120–33. Available from: http://linkinghub.elsevier.com/retrieve/pii/S0006349505731817

Le Meins, J.F., Schatz, C., Lecommandoux, S., & Sandre, O. (2013). Hybrid polymer/lipid vesicles: State of the art and future perspectives. *Mater Today, 16*(10), 397–402. 10.1016/j.mattod.2013.09.002

Lee, S. M., Chen, H., Dettmer, C. M., O'Halloran, T. V., & Nguyen, S. T. (2007). Polymer-caged lipsomes: A pH-responsive delivery system with high stability. *Journal of the American Chemical Society*, *129*(49), 15096–15097. doi:10.1021/ja070748i PMID:17999499

Lee, S. M., Chen, H., O'Halloran, T. V., & Nguyen, S. B. T. (2009). "Clickable" polymer-caged nanobins as a modular drug delivery platform. *Journal of the American Chemical Society*, *131*(26), 9311–9320. doi:10.1021/ja9017336 PMID:19527027

Li, X., Anton, N., Arpagaus, C., Belleteix, F., & Vandamme, T. F. (2010). Nanoparticles by spray drying using innovative new technology: The Büchi Nano Spray Dryer B-90. *J Control Release*, *147*(2), 304–310. doi:10.1016/j.jconrel.2010.07.113 PMID:20659510

Li, Z., & Rana, T. M. (2012). Molecular mechanisms of RNA-triggered gene silencing machineries. *Accounts of Chemical Research*, *45*(7), 1122–1131. doi:10.1021/ar200253u PMID:22304792

Lin, Y. C., Chen, H. L., Hashimoto, T., & Chen, S. A. (2016). Mechanism of hierarchical structure formation of polymer/nanoparticle hybrids. *Macromolecules*, *49*(19), 7535–7550. doi:10.1021/acs.macromol.6b01531

Liu, Y., Miyoshi, H., & Nakamura, M. (2007). Nanomedicine for drug delivery and imaging: A promising avenue for cancer therapy and diagnosis using targeted functional nanoparticles. *International Journal of Cancer*, *120*(12), 2527–2537. doi:10.1002/ijc.22709 PMID:17390371

Liu, Y., Pan, J., & Feng, S. S. (2010). Nanoparticles of lipid monolayer shell and biodegradable polymer core for controlled release of paclitaxel: Effects of surfactants on particles size, characteristics and in vitro performance. *International Journal of Pharmaceutics*, *395*(1–2), 243–250. doi:10.1016/j.ijpharm.2010.05.008 PMID:20472049

Messerschmidt, S. K. E., Musyanovych, A., Altvater, M., Scheurich, P., Pfizenmaier, K., Landfester, K., & Kontermann, R. E. (2009). Targeted lipid-coated nanoparticles: Delivery of tumor necrosis factor-functionalized particles to tumor cells. *Journal of Controlled Release*, *137*(1), 69–77. doi:10.1016/j.jconrel.2009.03.010 PMID:19306900

Mieszawska, A. J., Gianella, A., Cormode, D. P., Zhao, Y., Meijerink, A., Langer, R., ... Mulder, W. J. M. (2012). Engineering of lipid-coated PLGA nanoparticles with a tunable payload of diagnostically active nanocrystals for medical imaging. *Chemical Communications (Cambridge)*, *48*(47), 5835. doi:10.1039/c2cc32149a PMID:22555311

Nam, J., Vanderlick, T. K., & Beales, P. A. (2012). Formation and dissolution of phospholipid domains with varying textures in hybrid lipo-polymersomes. *Soft Matter*, *8*(30), 7982. doi:10.1039/c2sm25646k

Nidhi, K., Indrajeet, S., Khushboo, M., Gauri, K., & Sen, D. J. (2011). Hydrotropy: A promising tool for solubility enhancement: A review. *Int J Drug Dev Res.*, *3*(2), 26–33.

Nourbakhsh, M., Jaafari, M. R., Lage, H., Abnous, K., Mosaffa, F., Badiee, A, & … . (2015). Nanolipoparticles-mediated MDR1 siRNA delivery reduces doxorubicin resistance in breast cancer cells and silences MDR1 expression in xenograft model of human breast cancer. *Iran J Basic Med Sci*, *18*(4), 385–392. doi:10.1038/nbt.1602 PMID:26019802

Olubummo, A., Schulz, M., Lechner, B., Scholtysek, P., Bacia, K., & Blume, A. (2012). Controlling the Localization of in Mixed Lipid / Polymer Membranes. *ACS Nano*, (10), 8713–8727. doi:10.1021/nn3023602 PMID:22950802

Panyam, J., & Labhasetwar, V. (2003). Biodegradable nanoparticles for drug and gene delivery to cells and tissue. *Advanced Drug Delivery Reviews*, *55*(3), 329–347. doi:10.1016/S0169-409X(02)00228-4 PMID:12628320

Papanicolaou, I., Briggs, S., & Alpar, H. O. (2004). Increased Resistance of DNA Lipoplexes to Protein Binding In Vitro by Surface-modification with a Multivalent Hydrophilic Polymer. *Journal of Drug Targeting*, *12*(8), 541–547. doi:10.1080/10611860400011950 PMID:15621679

Parker, A. L., Newman, C., Briggs, S., Seymour, L., & Sheridan, P. J. (2003). Nonviral gene delivery: Techniques and implications for molecular medicine. *Expert Reviews in Molecular Medicine*, *5*(22). doi:10.1017/S1462399403006562 PMID:14585173

Patidar, A., Thakur, D. S., Kumar, P., & Verma, J. (2010). A review on novel lipid based nanocarriers. *International Journal of Pharmacy and Pharmaceutical Sciences*, *2*(4), 30–35.

Plapied, L., Duhem, N., des Rieux, A., & Préat, V. (2011). Fate of polymeric nanocarriers for oral drug delivery. *Curr Opin Colloid Interface Sci.*, *16*(3), 228–37. Available from: 10.1016/j.cocis.2010.12.005

Prasad, P., Shuhendler, A., Cai, P., Rauth, A. M., & Wu, X. Y. (2013). Doxorubicin and mitomycin C co-loaded polymer-lipid hybrid nanoparticles inhibit growth of sensitive and multidrug resistant human mammary tumor xenografts. *Cancer Lett*, *334*(2), 263–273. doi:10.1016/j.canlet.2012.08.008 PMID:22902994

Rao, S., & Prestidge, C. A. (2016). Polymer-lipid hybrid systems: Merging the benefits of polymeric and lipid-based nanocarriers to improve oral drug delivery. *Expert Opinion on Drug Delivery*, *13*(5), 691–707. doi:10.1517/17425247.2016.1151872 PMID:26866382

Salvador-Morales, C., Zhang, L., Langer, R., & Farokhzad, O.C. (2009). Immunocompatibility properties of lipid-polymer hybrid nanoparticles with heterogeneous surface functional groups. *Biomaterials, 30*(12), 2231–40. 10.1016/j.biomaterials.2009.01.005

Sengupta, S., Eavarone, D., Capila, I., Zhao, G., Watson, N., Kiziltepe, T., & Sasisekharan, R. (2005). Temporal targeting of tumour cells and neovasculature with a nanoscale delivery system. *Nature*, *436*(7050), 568–572. doi:10.1038/nature03794 PMID:16049491

Shi, J., Xiao, Z., Votruba, A. R., Vilos, C., & Farokhzad, O. C. (2011). Differentially Charged Hollow Core / Shell Lipid – Polymer – Lipid Hybrid Nanoparticles for Small Interfering RNA Delivery. *Angewandte Chemie International Edition*, *50*(31), 7027–7031. doi:10.1002/anie.201101554 PMID:21698724

Tannock, I. F., & Rotin, D. (1989). Acid pH in tumors and its potential for therpeutic exploitation. [Internet]. *Cancer Research*, *49*(16), 4373–4384. Available from http://www.scopus.com/inward/record.url?eid=2-s2.0-0024379967&partnerID=40&md5=9790fdf29f52b21920045c832198f74c PMID:2545340

Thevenot, J., Troutier, A. L., David, L., Delair, T., & Ladavière, C. (2007). Steric stabilization of lipid/polymer particle assemblies by poly(ethylene glycol)-lipids. *Biomacromolecules*, *8*(11), 3651–3660. doi:10.1021/bm700753q PMID:17958441

Valencia, P. M., Basto, P. A., Zhang, L., Rhee, M., Langer, R., Farokhzad, O. C., & Karnik, R. (2010). Single-step assembly of homogenous lipid-polymeric and lipid-quantum dot nanoparticles enabled by microfluidic rapid mixing. *ACS Nano*, *4*(3), 1671–1679. doi:10.1021/nn901433u PMID:20166699

Wang, A. Z., Yuet, K., Zhang, L., Gu, F. X., Huynh-Le, M., Radovic-Moreno, A. F., ... Farokhzad, O. C. (2010). ChemoRad nanoparticles: A novel multifunctional nanoparticle platform for targeted delivery of concurrent chemoradiation. *Nanomedicine (London)*, *5*(3), 361–368. doi:10.2217/nnm.10.6 PMID:20394530

Wong, H. L., Bendayan, R., Rauth, A. M., Li, Y., & Wu, X. Y. (2007). Chemotherapy with anticancer drugs encapsulated in solid lipid nanoparticles. *Advanced Drug Delivery Reviews*, *59*(6), 491–504. doi:10.1016/j.addr.2007.04.008 PMID:17532091

Wong, H. L., Bendayan, R., Rauth, A. M., & Wu, X. Y. (2004). Development of solid lipid nanoparticles containing ionically complexed chemotherapeutic drugs and chemosensitizers. *Journal of Pharmaceutical Sciences*, *93*(8), 1993–2008. doi:10.1002/jps.20100 PMID:15236449

Wu, X. Y. (2016). Strategies for optimizing polymer-lipid hybrid nanoparticle-mediated drug delivery. [Internet]. *Expert Opinion on Drug Delivery*, *13*(5), 609–612. doi:10.1517/17425247.2016.1165662 PMID:26978527

Zhang, L., Chan, J.M., Gu, F.X., Rhee, J., Wang, A.Z., & Radovic-moreno, A.F. (2008). Self-Assembled Lipid Polymer Hybrid Nanoparticles: A Robust Drug Delivery Platform. *ACS Nano, 2*(8), 1696–702.

Zhang, L., & Zhang, L. (2010). Lipid–Polymer Hybrid Nanoparticles: Synthesis, Characterization and Applications. *Nano Life, 1*(1-2), 163–73. Available from: http://www.worldscientific.com/doi/abs/10.1142/S179398441000016X

Zhang, R. X., Ahmed, T., Li, L. Y., Li, J., Abbasi, A. Z., & Wu, X. Y. (2017). Design of nanocarriers for nanoscale drug delivery to enhance cancer treatment using hybrid polymer and lipid building blocks. *Nanoscale*, *9*(4), 1334–1355. doi:10.1039/C6NR08486A PMID:27973629

Zhang, R. X., Cai, P., Zhang, T., Chen, K., Li, J., & Cheng, J. (2016). Polymer-lipid hybrid nanoparticles synchronize pharmacokinetics of co-encapsulated doxorubicin-mitomycin C and enable their spatiotemporal co-delivery and local bioavailability in breast tumor. *Nanomedicine Nanotechnology, Biol Med*, *12*(5), 1279–1290. doi:10.1016/j.nano.2015.12.383

Zhang, R. X., Wong, H. L., Xue, H. Y., Eoh, J. Y., & Wu, X. Y. (2016). Nanomedicine of synergistic drug combinations for cancer therapy??? Strategies and perspectives. *J Control Release*, *240*, 489–503. doi:10.1016/j.jconrel.2016.06.012 PMID:27287891

Zheng, Y., Yu, B., Weecharangsan, W., Piao, L., Darby, M., Mao, Y., & … . (2010). Transferrin-conjugated lipid-coated PLGA nanoparticles for targeted delivery of aromatase inhibitor 7α-APTADD to breast cancer cells. *Int J Pharm*, *390*(2), 234–241. doi:10.1016/j.ijpharm.2010.02.008 PMID:20156537

Zhong, Q., Chinta, D., Pamujula, S., Wang, H., Yao, X., Mandal, T. K., & Luftig, R. B. (2010). Optimization of DNA delivery by three classes of hybrid nanoparticle/DNA complexes. *Journal of Nanobiotechnology*, *8*(1), 6. doi:10.1186/1477-3155-8-6 PMID:20181278

Compilation of References

Abbasi, E., Aval, S. F., Akbarzadeh, A., Milani, M., Nasrabadi, H. T., Joo, S. W., ... Pashaei-Asl, R. (2014). Dendrimers: Synthesis, applications, and properties. *Nanoscale Research Letters*, *9*(1), 247. doi:10.1186/1556-276X-9-247 PMID:24994950

Abd El-Fattah, A. I., Fathy, M. M., Ali, Z. Y., El-Garawany, A. E. A., & Mohamed, E. K. (2017). Enhanced therapeutic benefit of quercetin-loaded phytosome nanoparticles in ovariectomized rats. *Chemico-Biological Interactions*, *271*, 30–38. doi:10.1016/j.cbi.2017.04.026 PMID:28460884

Abdelkader, H., Longman, M. R., Alany, R. G., & Pierscionek, B. (2016). Phytosome-hyaluronic acid systems for ocular delivery of L-carnosine. *International Journal of Nanomedicine*, *11*, 2815–2827. doi:10.2147/IJN.S104774 PMID:27366062

Abdous, B., Sajjadi, S. M., & Mamani, L. (2017). β-Cyclodextrin modified mesoporous silica nanoparticles as a nano-carrier: Response surface methodology to investigate and optimize loading and release processes for curcumin delivery. *Journal of Applied Biomedicine*, *133*, 1–9.

Abothu, I. R. (2007). Processing, Properties and Electrical Reliability of Embedded Ultra - Thin Film Ceramic Capacitors in Organic Packages. *Electronic Components and Technology Conference*, 1014 – 1018.

Acharya, S., & Sahoo, S. K. (2011). PLGA nanoparticles containing various anticancer agents and tumour delivery by EPR effect. *Advanced Drug Delivery Reviews*, *63*(3), 170–183. doi:10.1016/j.addr.2010.10.008 PMID:20965219

Afzal, S. M., Shareef, M. Z., & Kishan, V. (2016). Transferrin tagged lipid nanoemulsion of docetaxel for enhanced tumor targeting. *Journal of Drug Delivery Science and Technology*, *36*, 175–182. doi:10.1016/j.jddst.2016.10.008

Agarwal, R., Jurney, P., Raythatha, M., Singh, V., Sreenivasan, S., Shi, L., & Roy, K. (2015). Effect of shape, size, and aspect ratio on nanoparticle penetration and distribution inside solid tissues using 3D spheroid models. *Advanced Healthcare Materials*, *4*(15), 2269–2280. doi:10.1002/adhm.201500441 PMID:26376024

Agarwal, R., Singh, V., Jurney, P., Shi, L., Sreenivasan, S. V., & Roy, K. (2013). Mammalian cells preferentially internalize hydrogel nanodiscs over nanorods and use shape-specific uptake mechanisms. *Proceedings of the National Academy of Sciences of the United States of America*, *110*(43), 17247–17252. doi:10.1073/pnas.1305000110 PMID:24101456

Agostinis, P., Berg, K., Cengel, K. A., Foster, T. H., Girotti, A. W., Gollnick, S. O., ... Korbelik, M. (2011). Photodynamic therapy of cancer: An update. *CA: a Cancer Journal for Clinicians*, *61*(4), 250–281. doi:10.3322/caac.20114 PMID:21617154

Agrawal, O. P., & Agrawal, S. (2012). An overview of new drug delivery system: Microemulsions. *Asian Journal of Pharmaceutical Science & Technology*, *2*(1), 5–12.

Agrawal, P., Singh, R. P., Kumari, L., Sharma, G., Koch, B., Rajesh, C. V., ... Muthu, M. S. (2017). TPGS-chitosan cross-linked targeted nanoparticles for effective brain cancer therapy. *Materials Science and Engineering C*, *74*, 167–176. doi:10.1016/j.msec.2017.02.008 PMID:28254282

Ahmad, N., Ahmad, R., Naqvi, A. A., Alam, M. A., Ashafaq, M., Abdur Rub, R., & Ahmad, F. J. (2017). Intranasal delivery of quercetin-loaded mucoadhesive nanoemulsion for treatment of cerebral ischaemia. *Artificial Cells, Nanomedicine, and Biotechnology*, *12*, 1–13. PMID:28604104

Ahmad, T., Bae, H., Rhee, I., Chang, Y., Jin, S. U., & Hong, S. (2012). Gold-coated iron oxide nanoparticles as a T 2 contrast agent in magnetic resonance imaging. *Journal of Nanoscience and Nanotechnology*, *12*(7), 5132–5137. doi:10.1166/jnn.2012.6368 PMID:22966533

Ahn, H. H., Lee, J. H., Kim, K. S., Lee, J. Y., Kim, M. S., Khang, G., ... Lee, H. B. (2008). Polyethyleneimine-mediated gene delivery into human adipose derived stem cells. *Biomaterials*, *29*(15), 2415–2422. doi:10.1016/j.biomaterials.2008.02.006 PMID:18295879

Ahn, S.-J., Lee, S.-J., Kook, J.-K., & Lim, B.-S. (2009). Experimental antimicrobial orthodontic adhesives using nanofillers and silver nanoparticles. *Dental Materials*, *25*(2), 206–213. doi:10.1016/j.dental.2008.06.002 PMID:18632145

Ainbinder, D., Godin, B., & Touitou, E. (2016). Ethosomes: Enhanced Delivery of Drugs to and Across the Skin. In Percutaneous Penetration Enhancers Chemical Methods in Penetration Enhancement (pp. 61–75). Berlin: Springer Berlin Heidelberg. doi:10.1007/978-3-662-47862-2_4

Aitipamula, S., Banerjee, R., Bansal, A. K., Biradha, K., Cheney, M. L., Choudhury, A. R., ... Duggirala, N. (2012). Polymorphs, salts, and cocrystals: What's in a name? *Crystal Growth & Design*, *12*(5), 2147–2152. doi:10.1021/cg3002948

Aitipamula, S., Chow, P. S., & Tan, R. B. (2009). Theophylline–gentisic acid (1/1). *Acta Crystallogr. E: Struct. Rep. Online*, *65*(9), o2126–o2127. doi:10.1107/S1600536809031031 PMID:21577539

Aizik, G., Waiskopf, N., Agbaria, M., Levi-Kalisman, Y., Banin, U., & Golomb, G. (2017). Delivery of Liposomal Quantum Dots via Monocytes for Imaging of Inflamed Tissue. *ACS Nano*, *11*(3), 3038–3051. doi:10.1021/acsnano.7b00016 PMID:28196324

Ajnai, G., Chiu, A., Kan, T., Cheng, C.-C., Tsai, T.-H., & Chang, J. (2014). Trends of gold nanoparticle-based drug delivery system in cancer therapy. *Journal of Experimental and Clinical Medicine*, *6*(6), 172–178. doi:10.1016/j.jecm.2014.10.015

Akagi, T., Baba, M., & Akashi, M. (2012). Biodegradable nanoparticles as vaccine adjuvants and delivery systems: Regulation of immune responses by nanoparticle-based vaccine. *Advances in Polymer Science*, *247*, 31–64. doi:10.1007/12_2011_150

Akbarzadeh, A., Rezaei-Sadabady, R., Davaran, S., Joo, S. W., Zarghami, N., Hanifehpour, Y., ... Nejati-Koshki, K. (2013). Liposome: Classification, preparation, and applications. *Nanoscale Research Letters*, *8*(1), 102. doi:10.1186/1556-276X-8-102 PMID:23432972

Akbarzadeh, A., Samiei, M., & Davaran, S. (2012). Magnetic nanoparticles: Preparation, physical properties, and applications in biomedicine. *Nanoscale Research Letters*, *7*(1), 144. doi:10.1186/1556-276X-7-144 PMID:22348683

Al Shuwaili, A. H., Rasool, B. K., & Abdulrasool, A. A. (2016). Optimization of elastic transfersomes formulations for transdermal delivery of pentoxifylline. *European Journal of Pharmaceutics and Biopharmaceutics*, *102*, 101–114. doi:10.1016/j.ejpb.2016.02.013 PMID:26925505

Alavi, S. E., Mansouri, H., Esfahani, M. K., Movahedi, F., Akbarzadeh, A., & Chiani, M. (2014). Archaeosome: As new drug carrier for delivery of Paclitaxel to breast cancer. *Indian Journal of Clinical Biochemistry*, *29*(2), 150–153. doi:10.100712291-013-0305-4 PMID:24757295

Albanese, A., Tang, P. S., & Chan, W. C. (2012). The effect of nanoparticle size, shape, and surface chemistry on biological systems. *Annual Review of Biomedical Engineering*, *14*(1), 1–16. doi:10.1146/annurev-bioeng-071811-150124 PMID:22524388

Al-Dosari, M. S., & Gao, X. (2009). Non viral gene delivery: Principle, limitations and recent progress. *American Association of Pharmaceutical Scientists*, *11*(4), 671–681. PMID:19834816

Al-Dosari, M. S., & Gao, X. (2009). Nonviral Gene Delivery: Principle, Limitations, and Recent Progress. *The AAPS Journal*, *11*(4), 671–681. doi:10.120812248-009-9143-y PMID:19834816

Alexander, P., Kucera, G., & Pardee, T. S. (2016). Improving nucleoside analogs via lipid conjugation: Is fatter any better? *Critical Reviews in Oncology/Hematology*, *100*, 46–56. doi:10.1016/j.critrevonc.2016.01.015 PMID:26829896

Ali, A., & Hira Zafar, M. Z. (2016). Synthesis, characterization, applications, and challenges of iron oxide nanoparticles. *Nanotechnology, Science and Applications*, *9*, 49–67. doi:10.2147/NSA.S99986 PMID:27578966

Alibolandi, M., Taghdisi, S. M., Ramezani, P., Hosseini Shamili, F., Farzad, S. A., Abnous, K., & Ramezani, M. (2017). Smart AS1411-aptamer conjugated pegylated PAMAM dendrimer for the superior delivery of camptothecin to colon adenocarcinoma in vitro and in vivo. *International Journal of Pharmaceutics*, *519*(1-2), 352–364. doi:10.1016/j.ijpharm.2017.01.044 PMID:28126548

Ali, M. F., Salem, H. F., Abdelmohsen, H. F., & Attia, S. K. (2015). Preparation and clinical evaluation of nano-transferosomes for treatment of erectile dysfunction. *Drug Design, Development and Therapy*, *9*, 2431–2447. doi:10.2147/DDDT.S81236 PMID:25995616

Allam, A. N., Komeil, I. A., & Abdallah, O. Y. (2015). Curcumin phytosomal softgel formulation: Development, optimization and physicochemical characterization. *Acta Pharmaceutica (Zagreb, Croatia)*, *65*(3), 285–297. doi:10.1515/acph-2015-0029 PMID:26431106

Allen, T. M., & Cullis, P. R. (2013). Liposomal drug delivery systems: From concept to clinical applications. *Advanced Drug Delivery Reviews*, *65*(1), 36–48. doi:10.1016/j.addr.2012.09.037 PMID:23036225

Alleso, M., Chieng, N., Rehder, S., Rantanen, J., Rades, T., & Aaltonen, J. (2009). Enhanced dissolution rate and synchronized release of drugs in binary systems through formulation: Amorphous naproxen–cimetidine mixtures prepared by mechanical activation. *Journal of Controlled Release*, *136*(1), 45–53. doi:10.1016/j.jconrel.2009.01.027 PMID:19331842

Allesø, M., Velaga, S., Alhalaweh, A., Cornett, C., Rasmussen, M. A., Berg, F., ... Rantanen, J. (2008). Near-infrared spectroscopy for cocrystal screening. A comparative study with Raman spectroscopy. *Analytical Chemistry*, *80*(20), 7755–7764. doi:10.1021/ac8011329 PMID:18798651

Alpar, H. O., Cevher, E., & Özsoy, Y. (2014). Nanopartiküllerin gen tedavisinde kullanılması. In A. Zırh-Gülsoy (Ed), Nanofarmasötikler ve uygulamaları (pp. 261-276). İstanbul: Kontrollü Salım Derneği Yayını No: 3.

Alves, N. M., & Mano, J. F. (2008). Chitosan derivatives obtained by chemical modifications for biomedical and environmental applications. *International Journal of Biological Macromolecules*, *43*(5), 40–41. doi:10.1016/j.ijbiomac.2008.09.007 PMID:18838086

Amidon, G. L., Lennernas, H., Shah, V. P., & Crison, J. R. (1995). A theoretical basis for a biopharmaceutic drug classification: The correlation in vitro drug product dissolution and in vivo bioavailability. *Pharmaceutical Research*, *12*(3), 413–420. doi:10.1023/A:1016212804288 PMID:7617530

Anderson, D. L., Cheng, C. H., & Nacht, S. (1994). Flow characteristics of loosely compacted macroporous microsponge polymeric systems. *Powder Technology*, *78*(1), 15–18. doi:10.1016/0032-5910(93)02764-2

Anderson, J. M., & Shive, M. S. (2012). Biodegradation and biocompatibility of PLA and PLGA microspheres. *Advanced Drug Delivery Reviews*, *64*, 72–82. doi:10.1016/j.addr.2012.09.004

Anderson, W. F. (1985). Human gene therapy: Scientific and ethical considerations. *The Journal of Medicine and Philosophy*, *10*(3), 275–292. doi:10.1093/jmp/10.3.275 PMID:3900264

Angelos, S., Yang, Y.-W., Khashab, N. M., Stoddart, J. F., & Zink, J. I. (2009). Dual-controlled nanoparticles exhibiting AND logic. *Journal of the American Chemical Society*, *131*(32), 11344–11346. doi:10.1021/ja9042752 PMID:19624127

Ansari, K. A., Vavia, P. R., Trotta, F., & Cavalli, R. (2011). Cyclodextrin-based nanosponges for delivery of resveratrol: In vitro characterization, stability, cytotoxicity and permeation study. *AAPS PharmSciTech*, *12*(1), 279–286. doi:10.120812249-011-9584-3 PMID:21240574

Anselmo, A. C., Zhang, M., Kumar, S., Vogus, D. R., Menegatti, S., Helgeson, M. E., & Mitragotri, S. (2015). Elasticity of nanoparticles influences their blood circulation, phagocytosis, endocytosis, and targeting. *ACS Nano*, *9*(3), 3169–3177. doi:10.1021/acsnano.5b00147 PMID:25715979

Anwekar, H., Patel, S., & Singhai, A. (2011). Liposome- as drug carriers. *International Journal of Pharmacy & Life Sciences*, *2*, 945–951.

Apolinario, A. C., de Lima Damasceno, B. P., de Macedo Beltrao, N. E., Pessoa, A., Converti, A., & da Silva, J. A. (2014). Inulin-type fructans: A review on different aspects of biochemical and pharmaceutical technology. *Carbohydrate Polymers*, *101*, 368–378. doi:10.1016/j.carbpol.2013.09.081 PMID:24299785

Arachchige, M. C. M., Reshetnyak, Y. K., & Andreev, O. A. (2015). Advanced Targeted Nanomedicine. *Journal of Biotechnology*, *202*, 88–97. doi:10.1016/j.jbiotec.2015.01.009 PMID:25615945

Araújo, R. S., Silveira, A. L. M., De Sales, E., Souza, É. L., Freire, R. H., De Souza, C. M., ... Cardoso, V. N. (2017). Intestinal toxicity evaluation of long-circulating and pH sensitive liposomes loaded with cisplatin. *European Journal of Pharmaceutical Sciences*, *106*, 142–151. doi:10.1016/j.ejps.2017.05.046 PMID:28546107

Arcos, D., López-Noriega, A., Ruiz-Hernández, E., Terasaki, O., & Vallet-Regí, M. (2009). Ordered mesoporous microspheres for bone grafting and drug delivery. *Chemistry of Materials*, *21*(6), 1000–1009. doi:10.1021/cm801649z

Arcos, D., & Vallet-Regi, M. (2013). Bioceramics for drug delivery. *Acta Materialia*, *61*(3), 890–911. doi:10.1016/j.actamat.2012.10.039

Argyo, C., Weiss, V., Braeuchle, C., & Bein, T. (2014). Multifunctional mesoporous silica nanoparticles as a universal platform for drug delivery. *Chemistry of Materials*, *26*(1), 435–451. doi:10.1021/cm402592t

Arias, M. A., Loxley, A., Eatmon, C., Van Roey, G., Fairhurst, D., Mitchnick, M., ... Shattock, R. (2011). Carnauba wax nanoparticles enhance strong systemic and mucosal cellular and humoral immune responses to HIV-gp140 antigen. *Vaccine*, *29*(6), 1258–1269. doi:10.1016/j.vaccine.2010.11.084 PMID:21145913

Aritomi, H., Yamasaki, Y., Yamada, K., Honda, H., & Koshi, M. (1996). Development of sustained release formulation of chlorpheniramine maleate using powder coated microsponges prepared by dry impact blending method. *Journal of Pharmaceutical Science and Technology*, *56*(1), 49–56.

Arvizo, R. R., Miranda, O. R., Thompson, M. A., Pabelick, C. M., Bhattacharya, R., Robertson, J. D., & Mukherjee, P. (2010). Effect of nanoparticle surface charge at the plasma membrane and beyond. *Nano Letters*, *10*(7), 2543–2548. doi:10.1021/nl101140t PMID:20533851

Arya, P., & Pathak, K. (n.d.). Assessing the viability of microsponges as gastro retentive drug delivery system of curcumin: Optimization and pharmacokinetics. *International Journal of Pharmaceutics*, *2*, 1–12. PMID:24184218

Asefa, T., & Tao, Z. (2012). Biocompatibility of Mesoporous Silica Nanoparticles. *Chemical Research in Toxicology*, *25*(11), 2265–2284. doi:10.1021/tx300166u PMID:22823891

Asghar, L. F. A., & Chandran, S. (2006). Multiparticulate formulation approach to colon specific drug delivery: Current perspectives. *Journal of Pharmacy & Pharmaceutical Sciences*, *9*(3), 327–338. PMID:17207416

Attama, A. A., Momoh, M. A., & Builders, P. F. (2012). *Lipid nanoparticulate drug delivery systems: a revolution in dosage form design and development in: recent advances in novel drug carrier systems* (A. D. Sezer, Ed.). InTech.

Attarwala, H., & Amiji, M. (2012). Multi-compartmental nanoparticles-in-emulsion formulation for macrophage-specific anti-inflammatory gene delivery. *Pharmaceutical Research*, *29*(6), 1637–1649. doi:10.100711095-012-0677-9 PMID:22281760

Aulenta, F., Hayes, W., & Rannard, S. (2003, September). Dendrimers: A new class of nanoscopic containers and delivery devices. *European Polymer Journal*, *39*(9), 1741–1771. doi:10.1016/S0014-3057(03)00100-9

Averous, L., & Pollet, E. (2012). Biodegradable polymers. In *Environmental silicate nano-biocomposites* (pp. 13–39). Springer. doi:10.1007/978-1-4471-4108-2_2

Awasthi, R., Kulkarni, G. T., & Pawar, V. K. (2011). Phytosomes: An approach to increase the bioavailability of plant extracts. *International Journal of Pharmacy and Pharmaceutical Sciences*, *3*(2), 1–3.

Babu, A., Templeton, A. K., Munshi, A., & Ramesh, R. (2013). Nanoparticle-based drug delivery for therapy of lung cancer: Progress and challenges. *Journal of Nanomaterials*, *2013*, 14. doi:10.1155/2013/863951

Bacri, J. C., Perzynski, R., Salin, D., Cabuil, V., & Massart, R. (1990). Ionic ferrofluids: A crossing of chemistry and physics. *Journal of Magnetism and Magnetic Materials*, *85*(1-3), 27–32. doi:10.1016/0304-8853(90)90010-N

Badran, M. M., Mady, M. M., Ghannam, M. M., & Shakeel, F. (2017). Preparation and characterization of polymeric nanoparticles surface modified with chitosan for target treatment of colorectal cancer. *International Journal of Biological Macromolecules*, *95*, 643–649. doi:10.1016/j.ijbiomac.2016.11.098 PMID:27908720

Baek, J. S., & Cho, C. W. (2017). Surface modification of solid lipid nanoparticles for oral delivery of curcumin: Improvement of bioavailability through enhanced cellular uptake, and lymphatic uptake. *European Journal of Pharmaceutics and Biopharmaceutics*, *117*, 132–140. doi:10.1016/j.ejpb.2017.04.013 PMID:28412471

Bae, S. E., Son, J. S., Park, K., & Han, D. K. (2009). Fabrication of covered porous PLGA microspheres using hydrogen peroxide for controlled drug delivery and regenerative medicine. *Journal of Controlled Release*, *133*(1), 37–43. doi:10.1016/j.jconrel.2008.09.006 PMID:18838089

Baeza, A. (2014). Ceramic Nanoparticles for Cancer Treatment. In *Bio-Ceramics with Clinical Application*. John Wiley & Sons, Ltd.

Baeza, A., Guisasola, E., Ruiz-Hernández, E., & Vallet-Regí, M. (2012). Magnetically Triggered Multidrug Release by Hybrid Mesoporous Silica Nanoparticles. *Chemistry of Materials*, *24*(3), 517–524. doi:10.1021/cm203000u

Baghirov, H., Karaman, D., Viitala, T., Duchanoy, A., Lou, Y. R., Mamaeva, V., ... Rosenholm, J. M. (2016). Feasibility Study of the Permeability and Uptake of Mesoporous Silica Nanoparticles across the Blood-Brain Barrier. *PLoS One*, *11*(8).

Bahadur, D., & Giri, J. (2003). Biomaterials and magnetism. *Sadhana*, *28*(3-4), 639–656. doi:10.1007/BF02706451

Baig, M. S., Ahad, A., Aslam, M., Imam, S. S., Aqil, M., & Ali, A. (2016). Application of Box–Behnken design for preparation of levofloxacin-loaded stearic acid solid lipid nanoparticles for ocular delivery: Optimization, in vitro release, ocular tolerance, and antibacterial activity. *International Journal of Biological Macromolecules*, *85*, 258–270. doi:10.1016/j.ijbiomac.2015.12.077 PMID:26740466

Bai, R. G., Muthoosamy, K., Shipton, F. N., Pandikumar, A., Rameshkumar, P., Huang, N. M., & Manickam, S. (2016). The biogenic synthesis of a reduced graphene oxide–silver (RGO–Ag) nanocomposite and its dual applications as an antibacterial agent and cancer biomarker. *RSC Advances*, *6*(43), 36576–36587. doi:10.1039/C6RA02928K

Balas, F., Arcos, D., Pérez-Pariente, J., & Vallet-Regí, M. (2001). Textural properties of SiO 2· CaO· P 2 O 5 glasses prepared by the sol-gel method. *Journal of Materials Research*, *16*(05), 1345–1348. doi:10.1557/JMR.2001.0187

Balasubramaniam, R., & … . (1996). Structural and functional analysis of cationic transfection lipids: The hydrophobic domain. *Gene Therapy*, *3*(2), 163–172. PMID:8867864

Balasundaram, G., Sato, M., & Webster, T. J. (2006). Using hydroxyapatite nanoparticles and decreased crystallinity to promote osteoblast adhesion similar to functionalizing with RGD. *Biomaterials*, *27*(14), 2798–2805. doi:10.1016/j.biomaterials.2005.12.008 PMID:16430957

Balasundaram, G., & Webster, T. J. (2007). An Overview of Nano-Polymers for Orthopedic Applications. *Macromolecular Bioscience*, *7*(5), 635–642. doi:10.1002/mabi.200600270 PMID:17477446

Ballesteros-Gómez, A., & Rubio, S. (2009). Hemimicelles of alkyl carboxylates chemisorbed onto magnetic nanoparticles: Study and application to the extraction of carcinogenic polycyclic aromatic hydrocarbons in environmental water samples. *Analytical Chemistry*, *81*(21), 9012–9020. doi:10.1021/ac9016264 PMID:19785448

Bamrungsap, S., Chen, T., Shukoor, M. I., Chen, Z., Sefah, K., Chen, Y., & Tan, W. (2012). Pattern recognition of cancer cells using aptamer-conjugated magnetic nanoparticles. *ACS Nano*, *6*(5), 3974–3981. doi:10.1021/nn3002328 PMID:22424140

Banerjee, R., Katsenovich, Y., Lagos, L., McIintosh, M., Zhang, X., & Li, C. Z. (2010). Nanomedicine: Magnetic nanoparticles and their biomedical applications. *Current Medicinal Chemistry*, *17*(27), 3120–3141. doi:10.2174/092986710791959765 PMID:20629620

Bangham, A. D., & Horne, R. W. (1964). Negative staining of phospholipids and their structural modification by surface-active agents as observed in the electron microscope. *Journal of Molecular Biology*, *8*(5), 660–IN10. doi:10.1016/S0022-2836(64)80115-7 PMID:14187392

Banquy, X., Suarez, F., Argaw, A., Rabanel, J. M., Grutter, P., Bouchard, J. F., ... Giasson, S. (2009). Effect of mechanical properties of hydrogel nanoparticles on macrophage cell uptake. *Soft Matter*, *5*(20), 3984–3991. doi:10.1039/b821583a

Baowan, D., & Thamwattana, N. (2014). Modelling encapsulation of gold and silver nanoparticles inside lipid nanotubes. *Physica A*, *396*, 149–154. doi:10.1016/j.physa.2013.11.003

Barakat, N. S. (2009). Magnetically modulated nanosystems: A unique drug-delivery platform. *Nanomedicine (London)*, *4*(7), 799–812. doi:10.2217/nnm.09.66 PMID:19839815

Baroli, B., Ennas, M. G., Loffredo, F., Isola, M., Pinna, R., & López-Quintela, M. A. (2007). Penetration of metallic nanoparticles in human full-thickness skin. *The Journal of Investigative Dermatology*, *127*(7), 1701–1712. doi:10.1038j.jid.5700733 PMID:17380118

Barrère, F., van der Valk, C. M., Dalmeijer, R. A. J., van Blitterswijk, C. A., de Groot, K., & Layrolle, P. (2003). In vitro and in vivo degradation of biomimetic octacalcium phosphate and carbonate apatite coatings on titanium implants. *Journal of Biomedical Materials Research. Part A*, *64A*(2), 378–387. doi:10.1002/jbm.a.10291 PMID:12522826

Barreto, J. A., O'Malley, W., Kubeil, M., Graham, B., Stephan, H., & Spiccia, L. (2011). Nanomaterials: Applications in cancer imaging and therapy. *Advanced Materials*, *23*(12), 18–40. doi:10.1002/adma.201100140 PMID:21433100

Bartlett, D. W., & Davis, M. E. (2008). Impact of tumor-specific targeting and dosing schedule on tumor growth inhibition after intravenous administration of siRNA-containing nanoparticles. *Biotechnology and Bioengineering*, *99*(4), 975–985. doi:10.1002/bit.21668 PMID:17929316

Bates, K., & Kostarelos, K. (2013). Carbon nanotubes as vectors for gene therapy: Past achievements, present challenges and future goals. *Advanced Drug Delivery Reviews*, *65*(15), 2023–2033. doi:10.1016/j.addr.2013.10.003 PMID:24184373

Batista-Duharte, A., Lastre, M., Romeu, B., Portuondo, D. L., Téllez-Martínez, D., & Manente, F. A. … Carlos, I. Z. (2016). Antifungal and immunomodulatory activity of a novel cochleate for amphotericin B delivery against Sporothrix schenckii. *International Immunopharmacology*. doi:10.1016/j.intimp.2016.09.008

Battaglia, L., & Gallarate, M. (2012). Lipid nanoparticles: State of the art, new preparation methods and challenges in drug delivery. *Expert Opinion on Drug Delivery*, *9*(5), 497–508. doi:10.1517/17425247.2012.673278 PMID:22439808

Baudry, J., Bertrand, E., Rouzeau, C., Greffier, O., Koenig, A., Dreyfus, R., ... Lequeux, N. (2004). Colloids for studying molecular recognition. [). Lavoisier.]. *Annales de chimie*, *29*(1), 97–106. doi:10.3166/acsm.29.97-106

Bawarski, W. E., Chidlowsky, E., Bharali, D. J., & Mousa, S. A. (2008). Emerging nanopharmaceuticals. *Nanomedicine; Nanotechnology, Biology, and Medicine*, *4*(4), 273–282. doi:10.1016/j.nano.2008.06.002 PMID:18640076

Belldegrun, A., & Tso, C. L. (2002). Kidney-specific tumor vaccine directed against kidney tumor antigen G-250. *U.S. Patent 2002/0058041-A1, May 16.*

Belletti, D., Riva, G., Luppi, M., Tosi, G., Forni, F., Vandelli, M. A., ... Pederzoli, F. (2017). Anticancer drug-loaded quantum dots engineered polymeric nanoparticles: Diagnosis/therapy combined approach. *European Journal of Pharmaceutical Sciences*, *107*, 230–239. doi:10.1016/j.ejps.2017.07.020 PMID:28728978

Beloqui, A., Solinis, M. A., Rodriguez-Gascon, A., Almeida, A. J., & Preat, V. (2016). Nanostructured lipid carriers: Promising drug delivery systems for future clinics. *Nanomedicine; Nanotechnology, Biology, and Medicine*, *12*(1), 143–161. doi:10.1016/j.nano.2015.09.004 PMID:26410277

Benjaminsen, R. V., Mattebjerg, M. A., Henriksen, J. R., Moghimi, S. M., & Andresen, T. L. (2013). The possible "Proton Sponge" effect of polyethylenimine (PEI) does not include change in lysosomal pH. *Molecular Therapy*, *21*(1), 149–157. doi:10.1038/mt.2012.185 PMID:23032976

Benmerah, A., & Lamaze, C. (2007). Clathrin-Coated Pits: Vive La Différence? *Traffic (Copenhagen, Denmark)*, *8*(8), 970–982. doi:10.1111/j.1600-0854.2007.00585.x PMID:17547704

Ben-Nissan, B., Choi, A. H., & Bendavid, A. (2013). Mechanical properties of inorganic biomedical thin films and their corresponding testing methods. *Surface and Coatings Technology*, *233*, 39–48. doi:10.1016/j.surfcoat.2012.11.020

Benson, H. A. (2006). Transfersomes for transdermal drug delivery. *Expert Opinion on Drug Delivery*, *3*(6), 727–737. doi:10.1517/17425247.3.6.727 PMID:17076595

Bera, S., Ghosh, M., Pal, M., Das, N., Saha, S., Dutta, S. K., & Jana, S. (2014). Synthesis, characterization and cytotoxicity of europium incorporated ZnO–graphene nanocomposites on human MCF7 breast cancer cells. *RSC Advances*, *4*(71), 37479–37490. doi:10.1039/C4RA06243D

Bergstrand, N., Arfvidsson, M. C., Kim, J. M., Thompson, D. H., & Edwards, K. (2003). Interactions between pH-sensitive liposomes and model membranes. *Biophysical Chemistry*, *104*(1), 361–379. doi:10.1016/S0301-4622(03)00011-5 PMID:12834854

Bernardo, M., Luis, H., Martin, M. D., Leroux, B. G., Rue, T., Leitão, J., & DeRouen, T. A. (2007). Survival and reasons for failure of amalgam versus composite posterior restorations placed in a randomized clinical trial. *The Journal of the American Dental Association*, *138*(6), 775–783. doi:10.14219/jada.archive.2007.0265 PMID:17545266

Bertacco, R. (2014). Electric control of magnetism at the Fe / BaTiO3 interface. *Nature Communications*, *5*(3404). PMID:24584546

Berutoa, D. T., Bottera, R., & Milena, M. (2002). The effect of water in inorganic microsponges of calcium phosphates on the porosity and permeability of composites made with polymethylmethacrylate. *Biomaterials*, *23*(12), 2509–2517. doi:10.1016/S0142-9612(01)00385-4 PMID:12033598

Besinis, A., De Peralta, T., Tredwin, C. J., & Handy, R. D. (2015). Review of Nanomaterials in Dentistry: Interactions with the Oral Microenvironment, Clinical Applications, Hazards, and Benefits. *ACS Nano*, *9*(3), 2255–2289. doi:10.1021/nn505015e PMID:25625290

Bettinetti, G., Caira, M. R., Callegari, A., Merli, M., Sorrenti, M., & Tadini, C. (2000). Structure and solid-state chemistry of anhydrous and hydrated crystal forms of the trimethoprim-sulfamethoxypyridazine 1: 1 molecular complex. *Journal of Pharmaceutical Sciences*, *89*(4), 478–489. doi: PMID:10737909

Beun, S., Glorieux, T., Devaux, J., Vreven, J., & Leloup, G. (2007). Characterization of nanofilled compared to universal and microfilled composites. *Dental Materials*, *23*(1), 51–59. doi:10.1016/j.dental.2005.12.003 PMID:16423384

Beyer, A., Grohganz, H., Löbmann, K., Rades, T., & Leopold, C. S. (2016). Influence of the cooling rate and the blend ratio on the physical stability of co-amorphous naproxen/indomethacin. *European Journal of Pharmaceutics and Biopharmaceutics*, *109*, 140–148. doi:10.1016/j.ejpb.2016.10.002 PMID:27746228

Beyer, A., Grohganz, H., Löbmann, K., Rades, T., & Leopold, C. S. (2017). Improvement Of The Physicochemical Properties Of Co-amorphous Naproxen-indomethacin By Naproxen-sodium. *International Journal of Pharmaceutics*, *526*(1-2), 88–94. doi:10.1016/j.ijpharm.2017.04.011 PMID:28392278

Beyer, A., Radi, L., Grohganz, H., Löbmann, K., Rades, T., & Leopold, C. S. (2016). Preparation and recrystallization behavior of spray-dried co-amorphous naproxen–indomethacin. *European Journal of Pharmaceutics and Biopharmaceutics*, *104*, 72–81. doi:10.1016/j.ejpb.2016.04.019 PMID:27130786

Beyerle, A., Irmler, M., Beckers, J., Kissel, T., & Stoeger, T. (2010). Toxicity pathway focused gene expression profiling of PEI-based polymers for pulmonary applications. *Molecular Pharmaceutics*, *7*(3), 727–737. doi:10.1021/mp900278x PMID:20429563

Bharali, D. J., Khalil, M., Gurbuz, M., Simone, T. M., & Mousa, S. A. (2009). Nanoparticles and cancer therapy: A concise review with emphasis on dendrimers. *International Journal of Nanomedicine*, *4*(1), 1–7. PMID:19421366

Bharaniraja, B., Jayaram Kumar, K., Prasad, C., & Sen, A. (2011). Modified katira gum for colon targeted drug delivery. *Journal of Applied Polymer Science*, *119*(5), 2644–2651. doi:10.1002/app.32829

Bhatia, S. (2016). Nanoparticles Types, Classification, Characterization, Fabrication Methods and Drug Delivery Applications. In *Natural Polymer Drug Delivery Systems* (pp. 33–93). Springer International Publishing. doi:10.1007/978-3-319-41129-3_2

Bhattacharya, S. (2007). Optimization of Epoxy - Barium Titanate Nanocomposite for High Performance Embedded Capacitor Components. *IEEE Transactions on Components and Packaging Technologies, 30*(2).

Bhattacharya, S. (2009). Phytosomes: The new technology for enhancement of bioavailability of botanicals and nutraceuticals. *International Journal of Health Research*, *2*(3), 225–232. doi:10.4314/ijhr.v2i3.47905

Bhatt, P. M., Azim, Y., Thakur, T. S., & Desiraju, G. R. (2008). Co-crystals of the anti-HIV drugs lamivudine and zidovudine. *Crystal Growth & Design*, *9*(2), 951–957. doi:10.1021/cg8007359

Bielinska, A. (1996). Regulation of in vitro gene expression using antisense oligonucleotides or antisense expression plasmids transfected using starburst PAMAM dendrimers. *Nucleic Acids Research*, *24*(11), 2176–2182. doi:10.1093/nar/24.11.2176 PMID:8668551

Bielinska, A. U., Chen, C., Johnson, J., & Baker, J. R. (1999). DNA complexing with polyamidoamine dendrimers: Implications for transfection. *Bioconjugate Chemistry*, *10*(5), 843–850. doi:10.1021/bc990036k PMID:10502352

Bigham, A., Hassanzadeh-Tabrizi, S. A., Rafienia, M., & Salehi, H. (2016). Ordered Mesoporous Magnesium Silicate with Uniform Nanochannels as a Drug Delivery System:The Effect of Calcination Temperature on DrugDelivery Rate. *Ceramics International*, *42*(15), 17185–17191. doi:10.1016/j.ceramint.2016.08.009

Biju, V., Mundayoor, S., Omkumar, R. V., Anas, A., & Ishikawa, M. (2010). Bioconjugated quantum dots for cancer research: Present status, prospects and remaining issues. *Biotechnology Advances, 28*(2), 27.

Bi, M., Hwang, S.-J., & Morris, K. R. (2003). Mechanism of eutectic formation upon compaction and its effects on tablet properties. *Thermochimica Acta*, *404*(1), 213–226. doi:10.1016/S0040-6031(03)00185-0

Blasiak, B., van Veggel, F. C., & Tomanek, B. (2013). Applications of nanoparticles for MRI cancer diagnosis and therapy. *Journal of Nanomaterials*, *2013*, 12. doi:10.1155/2013/148578

Boas, U., & Heegaard, P. M. (2004). Dendrimers in drug research. *Chemical Society Reviews*, *33*(1), 43–63. doi:10.1039/b309043b PMID:14737508

Bobic, J. D. (2008). History and Challenges of Barium Titanate: Part I I -. *Science of Sintering*, *40*(3), 235–244. doi:10.2298/SOS0803235V

Bobo, D., Robinson, K. J., Islam, J., Thurecht, K. J., & Corrie, S. R. (2016). Nanoparticle-Based Medicines: A Review of FDA-Approved Materials and Clinical Trials to Date. *Pharmaceutical Research*, *33*(10), 2373–2387. doi:10.100711095-016-1958-5 PMID:27299311

Boccaccini, A. R., & Ma, P. X. (2014). *Tissue engineering using ceramics and polymers*. Elsevier.

Boge, L., Umerska, A., Matougui, N., Bysell, H., Ringstad, L., Davoudi, M., ... Andersson, M. (2017). Cubosomes post-loaded with antimicrobial peptides: Characterization, bactericidal effect and proteolytic stability. *International Journal of Pharmaceutics*, *526*(1-2), 400–412. doi:10.1016/j.ijpharm.2017.04.082 PMID:28476579

Boissenot, T., Bordat, A., Fattal, E., & Tsapis, N. (2016). Ultrasound-triggered drug delivery for cancer treatment using drug delivery systems: From theoretical considerations to practical applications. *Journal of Controlled Release*, *241*, 144–163. doi:10.1016/j.jconrel.2016.09.026 PMID:27667179

Bollu, V. S., Barui, A. K., Mondal, S. K., Prashar, S., Fajardo, M., Briones, D., ... Gomez-Ruiz, S. (2016). Curcumin-loaded silica-based mesoporous materials: Synthesis, characterization and cytotoxic properties against cancer cells. *Materials Science and Engineering C*, *63*, 393–410. doi:10.1016/j.msec.2016.03.011 PMID:27040234

Bonnemain, B. (1998). Superparamagnetic agents in magnetic resonance imaging: Physicochemical characteristics and clinical applications a review. *Journal of Drug Targeting*, *6*(3), 167–174. doi:10.3109/10611869808997890 PMID:9888302

Borchard, G. (2001). Chitosans for gene delivery. *Advanced Drug Delivery Reviews*, *52*(2), 145–150. doi:10.1016/S0169-409X(01)00198-3 PMID:11718938

Bose, R. J. C., Lee, S. H., & Park, H. (2016). Lipid-based surface engineering of PLGA nanoparticles for drug and gene delivery applications. *Biomaterials Research*, *20*(34), 1–9. PMID:27807476

Boukany, P. E., Wu, Y., Zhao, X., Kwak, K. J., Glazer, P. J., Leong, K., & Lee, L. J. (2014). Nonendocytic delivery of lipoplex nanoparticles into living cells using nanochannel electroporation. *Advanced Healthcare Materials*, *3*(5), 682–689. doi:10.1002/adhm.201300213 PMID:23996973

Boussif, O., Lezoualc'h, F., Zanta, M. A., Mergny, M. D., Scherman, D., Demeneix, B., & Behr, J. P. (1995). A versatile vector for gene and oligonucleotide transfer into cells in culture and in vivo: Polyethylenimine. *Proceedings of the National Academy of Sciences of the United States of America*, *92*(16), 7297–7301. doi:10.1073/pnas.92.16.7297 PMID:7638184

Bouwstra, J. A., Honeywell-Nguyen, P. L., & Gooris, G. M. (2003). Structure of the skin barrier and its modulation by vesicular formulations. *Progress in Lipid Research*, *42*(1), 1–36. doi:10.1016/S0163-7827(02)00028-0 PMID:12467638

Bouwstra, J. A., & Ponec, M. (2006). The skin barrier in healthy and diseased state. *Biochimica et Biophysica Acta*, *1758*(12), 2080–2095. doi:10.1016/j.bbamem.2006.06.021 PMID:16945325

Braga, D., Grepioni, F., Maini, L., Capucci, D., Nanna, S., Wouters, J., ... Quéré, L. (2012). Combining piracetam and lithium salts: Ionic co-crystals and co-drugs? *Chemical Communications (Cambridge)*, *48*(66), 8219–8221. doi:10.1039/c2cc33855f PMID:22781963

Bramhill, J., Ross, S., & Ross, G. (2017). Bioactive Nanocomposites for Tissue Repair and Regeneration: A Review. *International Journal of Environmental Research and Public Health*, *14*(1), 66. doi:10.3390/ijerph14010066 PMID:28085054

Bremmell, K. E., Tan, A., Martin, A., & Prestidge, C. A. (2013). Tableting lipid-based formulations for oral drug delivery: A case study with silica nanoparticle-lipid-mannitol hybrid microparticles. *Journal of Pharmaceutical Sciences*, *102*(2), 684–693. doi:10.1002/jps.23406 PMID:23242712

Brewer, J. M. (2006). How do aluminium adjuvants work? *Immunology Letters*, *102*(1), 10–15. doi:10.1016/j.imlet.2005.08.002 PMID:16188325

Brewer, J., & Alexander, J. (1992). The adjuvant activity of non-ionic surfactant vesicles (niosomes) on the BALB/c humoral response to bovine serum albumin. *Immunology*, *75*, 570–575. PMID:1592432

Brigham, K. L., Lane, K. B., Meyrick, B., Stecenko, A. A., Strack, S., Cannon, D. R., ... Canonico, A. E. (2000). Transfection of nasal mucosa with a normal alpha1-antitrypsin gene in alpha1-antitrypsin-deficient subjects: Comparison with protein therapy. *Human Gene Therapy*, *11*(7), 1023–1032. doi:10.1089/10430340050015338 PMID:10811231

Brinker, C. J., Lu, Y. F., Sellinger, A., & Fan, H. Y. (1999). Evaporation-induced self-assembly: Nanostructures made easy. *Advanced Materials*, *11*(7), 579–585. doi:

Broberg, B. F., & Evers, H. C. (1985). *Local anesthetic mixture for topical application and method for obtaining local anesthesia*. Google Patents.

Brown, L. F., & ... . (1992). Expression of vascular permeability factor (vascular endothelial growth factor) by epidermal keratinocytes during wound healing. *The Journal of Experimental Medicine*, *176*(5), 1375–1379. doi:10.1084/jem.176.5.1375 PMID:1402682

Brown, M., Schätzlein, A., Brownlie, A., Jack, V., Wang, W., Tetley, L., ... Uchegbu, I. F. (2000). Preliminary characterization of novel amino acid based polymeric vesicles as gene and drug delivery agents. *Bioconjugate Chemistry*, *11*(6), 880–891. doi:10.1021/bc000052d PMID:11087338

Bruley, J. (2013). Switching of ferroelectric in without epitaxial conducting without bottom electrode a conducting BaTiO3 films on silicon bottom electrode. *Nature Nanotechnology*.

Brunella, V., Jadhav, S. A., Miletto, I., Berlier, G., Ugazio, E., Sapino, S., & Scalarone, D. (2016). Hybrid drug carriers with temperature-controlled on–off release: A simple and reliable synthesis of PNIPAM-functionalized mesoporous silica nanoparticles. *Reactive & Functional Polymers*, *98*, 31–37. doi:10.1016/j.reactfunctpolym.2015.11.006

Bu, H., He, X., Zhang, Z., Yin, Q., Yu, H., & Li, Y. (2014). A TPGS-incorporating nanoemulsion of paclitaxel circumvents drug resistance in breast cancer. *International Journal of Pharmaceutics*, *471*(1), 206–213. doi:10.1016/j.ijpharm.2014.05.039 PMID:24866272

Burg, K. J., Porter, S., & Kellam, J. F. (2000). Biomaterial developments for bone tissue engineering. *Biomaterials*, *21*(23), 2347–2359. doi:10.1016/S0142-9612(00)00102-2 PMID:11055282

Burke, F., Ray, N., & McConnell, R. (2006). Fluoride-containing restorative materials. *International Dental Journal*, *56*(1), 33–43. doi:10.1111/j.1875-595X.2006.tb00072.x PMID:16515011

Burleigh, M. C., Dai, S., Hagaman, E. W., Barnes, C. E., & Xue, Z. L. (2000). *Stepwise Assembly of Surface Imprint Sites on MCM-41 for Selective Metal Ion Separations. In Nuclear Site Remediation* (pp. 146–158). American Chemical Society.

Burley, J. C., Alkhalil, A., Bloomfield, M., & Matousek, P. (2012). Transmission Raman spectroscopy for quality control in model cocrystal tablets. *Analyst (London)*, *137*(13), 3052–3057. doi:10.1039/c2an35216h PMID:22617192

Businova, P., Chomoucka, J., Prasek, J., Hrdy, R., Drbohlavova, J., Sedlacek, P., & Hubalek, J. (2011). Polymer coated iron oxide magnetic nanoparticles: Preparation and characterization. *Nanocon*, *9*, 21–23.

Büyükköroğlu, G. (2016). Development of solid lipid gene delivery system. *Turkish Journal of Pharmaceutical Sciences*, *13*(2), 249–258.

Cabeza, L., Ortiz, R., Prados, J., Delgado, Á. V., Martín-Villena, M. J., Clares, B., ... Arias, J. L. (2017). Improved antitumor activity and reduced toxicity of doxorubicin encapsulated in poly (ε-caprolactone) nanoparticles in lung and breast cancer treatment: An in vitro and in vivo study. *European Journal of Pharmaceutical Sciences*, *102*, 24–34. doi:10.1016/j.ejps.2017.02.026 PMID:28219748

Cabral, H., & Kataoka, K. (2014). Progress of drug-loaded polymeric micelles into clinical studies. *Journal of Controlled Release*, *190*, 465–476. doi:10.1016/j.jconrel.2014.06.042 PMID:24993430

Caira, M. R. (1992). Molecular complexes of sulfonamides. 2.1: 1 complexes between drug molecules: sulfadimidine-acetylsalicylic acid and sulfadimidine-4-aminosalicylic acid. *Journal of Chemical Crystallography*, *22*(2), 193–200.

Cai, Z., Chattopadhyay, N., Yang, K., Kwon, Y. L., Yook, S., Pignol, J.-P., & Reilly, R. M. (2016). 111 In-labeled trastuzumab-modified gold nanoparticles are cytotoxic in vitro to HER2-positive breast cancer cells and arrest tumor growth in vivo in athymic mice after intratumoral injection. *Nuclear Medicine and Biology*, *43*(12), 818–826. doi:10.1016/j.nucmedbio.2016.08.009 PMID:27788375

Calvin, S., Miller, M. M., Goswami, R., Cheng, S. F., Mulvaney, S. P., Whitman, L. J., & Harris, V. G. (2003). Determination of crystallite size in a magnetic nanocomposite using extended x-ray absorption fine structure. *Journal of Applied Physics*, *94*(1), 778–783. doi:10.1063/1.1581344

Caminade, A.-M., & Turrin, C.-O. (2014). Dendrimers for drug delivery. *Journal of Materials Chemistry. B, Materials for Biology and Medicine*, *2*(26), 4055–4066. doi:10.1039/C4TB00171K

Canché-Escamilla, G., Duarte-Aranda, S., & Toledano, M. (2014). Synthesis and characterization of hybrid silica/PMMA nanoparticles and their use as filler in dental composites. *Materials Science and Engineering C*, *42*, 161–167. doi:10.1016/j.msec.2014.05.016 PMID:25063106

Canton, I., & Battaglia, G. (2012). Endocytosis at the nanoscale. *Chemical Society Reviews*, *41*(7), 2718–2739. doi:10.1039/c2cs15309b PMID:22389111

Cao, N., Cheng, D., Zou, S., Ai, H., Gao, J., & Shuai, X. (2011). The synergistic effect of hierarchical assemblies of siRNA and chemotherapeutic drugs co-delivered into hepatic cancer cells. *Biomaterials*, *32*(8), 2222–2232. doi:10.1016/j.biomaterials.2010.11.061 PMID:21186059

Cao, X., Tao, L., Wen, S., Hou, W., & Shi, X. (2015). Hyaluronic acid-modified multiwalled carbon nanotubes for targeted delivery of doxorubicin into cancer cells. *Carbohydrate Research*, *405*, 70–77. doi:10.1016/j.carres.2014.06.030 PMID:25500334

Cao, Y., Marra, M., & Anderson, B. D. (2004). Predictive relationships for the effects of triglyceride ester concentration and water uptake on solubility and partitioning of small molecules into lipid vehicles. *Journal of Pharmaceutical Sciences*, *93*(11), 2768–2779. doi:10.1002/jps.20126 PMID:15389678

Caplen, N. J., Alton, E. W. F. W., Mddleton, P. G., Dorin, J. R., Stevenson, B. J., Gao, X., ... Geddes, D. M. (1995). Liposome-mediated CFTR gene transfer to the nasal epithelium of patients with cystic fibrosis. *Nature Medicine*, *1*(1), 39–46. doi:10.1038/nm0195-39 PMID:7584951

Cartmell, S. H., & Dobson, J. (2009) The use of magnetic particles in tissue engineering. In Nanomaterials for Life Sciences: Magnetic Nanomaterials (pp. 293-308). Wiley-VCH.

Casadei, M. A., Pitarresi, G., Calabrese, R., Paolicelli, P., & Giammona, G. (2008). Biodegradable and pH-sensitive hydrogels for potential colon-specific drug delivery: Characterization and in vitro release studies. *Biomacromolecules*, *9*(1), 43–49. doi:10.1021/bm700716c PMID:18052027

Casey, J. R., Grinstein, S., & Orlowski, J. (2010). Sensors and regulators of intracellular pH. *Nat Rev Mol Cell Biol, 11*(1), 50–61. Available from: http://www.nature.com/doifinder/10.1038/nrm2820

Castilho-Fernandes, A., Lopes, T. G., Primo, F. L., Pinto, M. R., & Tedesco, A. C. (2017). Photodynamic process induced by chloro-aluminum phthalocyanine nanoemulsion in glioblastoma. *Photodiagnosis and Photodynamic Therapy,* S1572-1000(17)30195-3.

Cavalli Roberta, C. (1993). Solid lipospheres of doxorubicin and idarubicin. *International Journal of Pharmaceutics*, *89*(1), R9–R12. doi:10.1016/0378-5173(93)90313-5

Cavalli, R., Trotta, F., & Tumiatti, W. (2006). Cyclodextrin-based nanosponges for drug delivery. *Journal of Inclusion Phenomena and Macrocyclic Chemistry*, *56*(1-2), 209–213. doi:10.100710847-006-9085-2

Cavalli, R., Trotta, F., Tumiatti, W., Serpe, L., & Zara, G. P. (2006). 5-Fluorouracile loaded β-cyclodextrin nanosponges: invitro characterization and cytotoxicity. *International Cyclodextrin Symposium*, *13*, 207.

Cavazzana-Calvo, M., Thrasher, A., & Mavilio, F. (2004). The future of gene therapy. *Nature*, *427*(6977), 779–781. doi:10.1038/427779a PMID:14985734

Cerchiara, T., Abruzzo, A., Parolin, C., Vitali, B., Bigucci, F., Gallucci, M. C., ... Luppi, B. (2016). Microparticles based on chitosan/carboxymethylcellulose polyelectrolyte complexes for colon delivery of vancomycin. *Carbohydrate Polymers*, *143*, 124–130. doi:10.1016/j.carbpol.2016.02.020 PMID:27083351

Cerqueira, B. B. S., Lasham, A., Shelling, A. N., & Al-Kassas, R. (2017). Development of biodegradable PLGA nanoparticles surface engineered with hyaluronic acid for targeted delivery of paclitaxel to triple negative breast cancer cells. *Materials Science and Engineering C*, *76*, 593–600. doi:10.1016/j.msec.2017.03.121 PMID:28482569

Cevc, G., & Chopra, A. (2016). Deformable (Transfersome®) vesicles for improved drug delivery into and through the skin. In Percutaneous Penetration Enhancers Chemical Methods in Penetration Enhancement (pp. 39–59). Berlin: Springer Berlin Heidelberg. doi:10.1007/978-3-662-47862-2_3

Chadawar, V., & Shaji, J. (2007). Microsponge delivery system. *Current Drug Delivery*, *4*(2), 123–129. doi:10.2174/156720107780362320 PMID:17456031

Chambin, O., & Jannin, V. (2005). Interest of multifunctional lipid excipients: Case of Gelucire 44/14. *Drug Development and Industrial Pharmacy*, *31*(6), 527–534. doi:10.1080/03639040500215750 PMID:16109625

Champion, J. A., & Mitragotri, S. (2006). Role of target geometry in phagocytosis. *Proceedings of the National Academy of Sciences of the United States of America*, *103*(13), 4930–4934. doi:10.1073/pnas.0600997103 PMID:16549762

Chan, M.H., & Lin, H.M. (2015). Preparation and identification of multifunctional mesoporous silica nanoparticles for in vitro and in vivo dual-mode imaging, theranostics, and targeted tracking. *Biomaterials, 46*, 149-158.

Chandel, N., Gupta, V., Pandey, A., & Saxena, S. (2011). Co-crystallization of aceclofenac and paracetamol and their characterization. *Int. J. of Pharm. & Life Sci.*, *2*(8), 1020–1028.

Chandki, R., Kala, M., N, K. K., Brigit, B., Banthia, P., & Banthia, R. (2012). 'Nanodentistry': Exploring the beauty of miniature. *Journal of Clinical and Experimental Dentistry*, *4*(2), e119–e124. doi:10.4317/jced.50720 PMID:24558536

Chang, C. C., Liu, D. Z., Lin, S. Y., Liang, H. J., Hou, W. C., Huang, W. J., ... Liang, Y. C. (2008). Liposome encapsulation reduces cantharidin toxicity. *Food and Chemical Toxicology*, *46*(9), 3116–3121. doi:10.1016/j.fct.2008.06.084 PMID:18652872

Chang, R. S., Suh, M. S., Kim, S., Shim, G., Lee, S., Han, S. S., ... Oh, Y.-K. (2011). Cationic drug-derived nanoparticles for multifunctional delivery of anticancer siRNA. *Biomaterials*, *32*(36), 9785–9795. doi:10.1016/j.biomaterials.2011.09.017 PMID:21937102

Chang, Y. J., Liu, X. Z., Zhao, Q., Yang, X. H., Wang, K. M., Wang, Q., ... Yang, M. (2015). P(VPBA-DMAEA) as a pH-sensitive nanovalve for mesoporous silica nanoparticles based controlled release. *Chinese Chemical Letters*, *26*(10), 1203–1208. doi:10.1016/j.cclet.2015.08.005

Chan, J. M., Rhee, J.-W., Drum, C. L., Bronson, R. T., Golomb, G., Langer, R., & Farokhzad, O. C. (2011). In vivo prevention of arterial restenosis with paclitaxel-encapsulated targeted lipid-polymeric nanoparticles. *Proceedings of the National Academy of Sciences of the United States of America*, *108*(48), 19347–19352. doi:10.1073/pnas.1115945108 PMID:22087004

Chan, J. M., Zhang, L., Tong, R., Ghosh, D., Gao, W., Liao, G., ... Farokhzad, O. C. (2010). Spatiotemporal controlled delivery of nanoparticles to injured vasculature. *Proceedings of the National Academy of Sciences of the United States of America*, *107*(5), 2213–2218. doi:10.1073/pnas.0914585107 PMID:20133865

Chan, M. H., & Lin, H. M. (2015). Preparation and identification of multifunctional mesoporous silica nanoparticles for in vitro and in vivo dual-mode imaging, theranostics, and targeted tracking. *Biomaterials*, *46*, 149–158. doi:10.1016/j.biomaterials.2014.12.034 PMID:25678124

Cha, R., Li, J., Liu, Y., Zhang, Y., Xie, Q., & Zhang, M. (2017). Fe3O4 nanoparticles modified by CD-containing star polymer for MRI and drug delivery. *Colloids and Surfaces. B, Biointerfaces*, *158*, 213–221. doi:10.1016/j.colsurfb.2017.06.049 PMID:28697436

Charman, W. N., Porter, C. J., Mithani, S., & Dressman, J. B. (1997). Physiochemical and physiological mechanisms for the effects of food on drug absorption: The role of lipids and pH. *Journal of Pharmaceutical Sciences*, *86*(3), 269–282. doi:10.1021/js960085v PMID:9050793

Charron, D. M., Chen, J., & Zheng, G. (2015). Theranostic lipid nanoparticles for cancer medicine. *Cancer Treatment and Research*, *166*, 103–127. doi:10.1007/978-3-319-16555-4_5 PMID:25895866

Chaturvedi, S. P., & Kumar, V. (2012). Production techniques of lipid nanoparticles: A review. *Research Journal of Pharmaceutical, Biological and Chemical Sciences*, *3*, 525–541.

Chaubey, P., & Mishra, B. (2014). Mannose-conjugated chitosan nanoparticles loaded with rifampicin for the treatment of visceral leishmaniasis. *Carbohydrate Polymers*, *101*, 1101–1108. doi:10.1016/j.carbpol.2013.10.044 PMID:24299880

Chauhan, B., Shimpi, S., & Paradkar, A. (2005a). Preparation and evaluation of glibenclamidepolyglycolized glycerides solid dispersions with silicon dioxide by spray drying technique. *European Journal of Pharmaceutical Sciences*, *26*(2), 219–230. doi:10.1016/j.ejps.2005.06.005 PMID:16087324

Chauhan, B., Shimpi, S., & Paradkar, A. (2005b). Preparation and characterization of etoricoxib solid dispersions using lipid carriers by spray drying technique. *AAPS PharmSciTech*, *6*(3), E405–E409. doi:10.1208/pt060350 PMID:16353998

Chauhan, G., Gupta, N., Sehrawat, D., Kalra, S., Rath, G. A., & Goyal, A. (2015). Albumin stabilized silver nanoparticles-clotrimazole β-cyclodextrin hybrid nanocomposite for enriched anti-fungal activity in normal and drug resistant Candida cells. *RSC Advances*, *5*(87), 71190–71202. doi:10.1039/C5RA08274A

Chavan, R. B., Thipparaboina, R., Kumar, D., & Shastri, N. R. (2016). Co amorphous systems: A product development perspective. *International Journal of Pharmaceutics*, *515*(1), 403–415. doi:10.1016/j.ijpharm.2016.10.043 PMID:27771485

Che, E., Wan, L., Zhang, Y., Zhao, Q., Han, X., Li, J., ... Wang, S. (2014). Development of phosphonate-terminated magnetic mesoporous silica nanoparticles for pH-controlled release of doxorubicin and improved tumor accumulation. *Asian Journal of Pharmaceutical Sciences*, *9*(6), 317–323. doi:10.1016/j.ajps.2014.07.003

Chemin, M., Brun, P.-M., Lecommandoux, S., Sandre, O., & Le Meins, J.-F. (2012). Hybrid polymer/lipid vesicles: Fine control of the lipid and polymer distribution in the binary membrane. *Soft Matter*, *8*(10), 2867. doi:10.1039/c2sm07188f

Chen, C., Geng, J., Pu, F., Yang, X., Ren, J., & Qu, X. (2011). Polyvalent nucleic acid/mesoporous silica nanoparticle conjugates: Dual stimuli-responsive vehicles for intracellular drug delivery. Angew. Chem. Int., 50, 882–886.

Chen, Guizhi, Jin, & Xiaoyuan. (2017). Rethinking cancer nanotheranostics. *Nature Reviews Materials, 2.*

Chen, H., & Sun, D. (2017). U.*S. Patent No. 9,533,045.* Washington, DC: U.S. Patent and Trademark Office.

Chen, A. M., Zhang, M., Wei, D., Stueber, D., Taratula, O., Minko, T., & He, H. (2009). Co-delivery of doxorubicin and Bcl-2 siRNA by mesoporous silica nanoparticles enhances the efficacy of chemotherapy in multidrug-resistant cancer cells. *Small*, *5*(23), 2673–2677. doi:10.1002mll.200900621 PMID:19780069

Cheney, M. L., Weyna, D. R., Shan, N., Hanna, M., Wojtas, L., & Zaworotko, M. J. (2011). Coformer selection in pharmaceutical cocrystal development: A case study of a meloxicam aspirin cocrystal that exhibits enhanced solubility and pharmacokinetics. *Journal of Pharmaceutical Sciences*, *100*(6), 2172–2181. doi:10.1002/jps.22434 PMID:21491441

Chen, G., Sato, T., Ohgusi, H., Ushida, T., Tateishi, T., & Tanaka, J. (2005). Culturing of skin fibroblasts in a thin PLGA_collagen hybrid mesh. *Biomaterials*, *26*(15), 2559–2566. doi:10.1016/j.biomaterials.2004.07.034 PMID:15585258

Cheng, G., Ushida, T., & Tateishi, T. (2000, August). A Biodegradable Hybrid Sponge Nested with collagen microsponges. *Journal of Biomedical Materials Research*, *51*(2), 273–279. doi: PMID:10825227

Cheng, Y. J., Zeng, X., Cheng, D. B., Xu, X. D., Zhang, X. Z., Zhuo, R. X., & He, F. (2016). Functional mesoporous silica nanoparticles (MSNs) for highly controllable drug release and synergistic therapy. *Colloids and Surfaces. B, Biointerfaces*, *145*, 217–225. doi:10.1016/j.colsurfb.2016.04.051 PMID:27182657

Chen, H., Burnett, J., Zhang, F., Zhang, J., Paholak, H., & Sun, D. (2014). Highly crystallized iron oxide nanoparticles as effective and biodegradable mediators for photothermal cancer therapy. *Journal of Materials Chemistry. B, Materials for Biology and Medicine*, *2*(7), 757–765. doi:10.1039/C3TB21338B

Chen, H., Ebner, A. D., Bockenfeld, D., Ritter, J. A., Kaminski, M. D., Liu, X., ... Rosengart, A. J. (2007). A comprehensive in vitro investigation of a portable magnetic separator device for human blood detoxification. *Physics in Medicine and Biology*, *52*(19), 6053–6072. doi:10.1088/0031-9155/52/19/023 PMID:17881819

Chen, H., Qi, F., Zhou, H., Jia, S., Gao, Y., Koh, K., & Yin, Y. (2015). Fe 3 O 4@ Au nanoparticles as a means of signal enhancement in surface plasmon resonance spectroscopy for thrombin detection. *Sensors and Actuators. B, Chemical*, *212*, 505–511. doi:10.1016/j.snb.2015.02.062

Chen, H., Zheng, D., Liu, J., Kuang, Y., Li, Q., Zhang, M., ... Jiang, B. (2016). pH-Sensitive drug delivery system based on modified dextrin coated mesoporous silica nanoparticles. *International Journal of Biological Macromolecules*, *85*, 596–603. doi:10.1016/j.ijbiomac.2016.01.038 PMID:26776872

Chen, H., Zhen, Z., Tang, W., Todd, T., Chuang, Y. J., Wang, L., ... Xie, J. (2013). Label-free luminescent mesoporous silica nanoparticles for imaging and drug delivery. *Theranostics*, *3*(9), 650–657. doi:10.7150/thno.6668 PMID:24052805

Chen, J. P., Yang, P. C., Ma, Y. H., & Wu, T. (2011). Characterization of chitosan magnetic nanoparticles for in situ delivery of tissue plasminogen activator. *Carbohydrate Polymers*, *84*(1), 364–372. doi:10.1016/j.carbpol.2010.11.052

Chen, L., Zhang, Z., Yao, X., Chen, X., & Chen, X. (2015). Intracellular pH-operated mechanized mesoporous silica nanoparticles as potential drug carries. *Microporous and Mesoporous Materials*, *201*, 169–175. doi:10.1016/j.micromeso.2014.09.023

Chen, L., Zheng, Z., Wang, J., & Wang, X. (2014). Mesoporous SBA-15 end-capped by PEG via l-cystine based linker for redox responsive controlled release. *Microporous and Mesoporous Materials*, *185*, 7–15. doi:10.1016/j.micromeso.2013.10.025

Chen, L., Zhou, X., Nie, W., Zhang, Q., Wang, W., Zhang, Y., & He, C. (2016). Multifunctional Redox-Responsive Mesoporous Silica Nanoparticles for Efficient Targeting Drug Delivery and Magnetic Resonance Imaging. *ACS Applied Materials & Interfaces*, *8*(49), 33829–33841. doi:10.1021/acsami.6b11802 PMID:27960384

Chen, M. (2008). Lipid excipients and delivery systems for pharmaceutical development: A regulatory perspective. *Advanced Drug Delivery Reviews*, *60*(6), 768–777. doi:10.1016/j.addr.2007.09.010 PMID:18077051

Chen, M.-H. (2010). Update on Dental Nanocomposites. *Journal of Dental Research*, *89*(6), 549–560. doi:10.1177/0022034510363765 PMID:20299523

Chen, M., He, X., Wang, K., He, D., Yang, S., Qiu, P., & Chen, S. (2014). A pH-responsive polymer/mesoporous silica nano-container linked through an acid cleavable linker for intracellular controlled release and tumor therapy in vivo. *Journal of Materials Chemistry. B, Materials for Biology and Medicine*, *2*(4), 428–436. doi:10.1039/C3TB21268H

Chen, W. H., Luo, G. F., Qiu, W. X., Lei, Q., Liu, L. H., Wang, S. B., & Zhang, X. Z. (2017). Mesoporous silica-based versatile theranostic nanoplatform constructed by layer-by-layer assembly for excellent photodynamic/chemo therapy. *Biomaterials*, *117*, 54–65. doi:10.1016/j.biomaterials.2016.11.057 PMID:27936417

Chen, W., Li, H., Liu, Z., & Yuan, W. (2016). Lipopolyplex for therapeutic gene delivery and its application for the treatment of Parkinson's disease. *Frontiers in Aging Neuroscience*, *8*, 68. doi:10.3389/fnagi.2016.00068 PMID:27092073

Chen, W., Zhang, S., Yu, Y., Zhang, H., & He, Q. (2016). Structural-Engineering Rationales of Gold Nanoparticles for Cancer Theranostics. *Advanced Materials*, *28*(39), 8567–8585. doi:10.1002/adma.201602080 PMID:27461909

Chen, X., Sun, H., Hu, J., Han, X., Liu, H., & Hu, Y. (2017). Transferrin gated mesoporous silica nanoparticles for redox-responsive and targeted drug delivery. *Colloids and Surfaces. B, Biointerfaces*, *152*, 77–84. doi:10.1016/j.colsurfb.2017.01.010 PMID:28088015

Chen, X., Yao, X., Wang, C., Chen, L., & Chen, X. (2015). Mesoporous silica nanoparticles capped with fluorescence-conjugated cyclodextrin for pH-activated controlled drug delivery and imaging. *Microporous and Mesoporous Materials*, *217*, 46–53. doi:10.1016/j.micromeso.2015.06.012

Chen, Y., Ai, K., Liu, Y., & Lu, L. (2014). Tailor-made charge-conversional nanocomposite for pH-responsive drug delivery and cell imaging. *ACS Applied Materials & Interfaces*, *6*(1), 655–663. doi:10.1021/am404761h PMID:24308443

Chen, Y., Bathula, S. R., Li, J., & Huang, L. (2010). Multifunctional nanoparticles delivering small interfering RNA and doxorubicin overcome drug resistance in cancer. *The Journal of Biological Chemistry*, *285*(29), 22639–22650. doi:10.1074/jbc.M110.125906 PMID:20460382

Chen, Y., Chen, H., Guo, L., He, Q., Chen, F., Zhou, J., ... Shi, J. (2010). Hollow/Rattle-Type Mesoporous Nanostructures by a Structural Difference-Based Selective Etching Strategy. *ACS Nano*, *4*(1), 529–539. doi:10.1021/nn901398j PMID:20041633

Chen, Y., Ma, P., & Gui, S. (2014). *Cubic and hexagonal liquid crystals as drug delivery systems*. BioMed Research International.

Chen, Y., Sen, J., Bathula, S. R., Yang, Q., Fittipaldi, R., & Huang, L. (2009). Novel cationic lipid that delivers siRNA and enhances therapeutic effect in lung cancer cells. *Molecular Pharmaceutics*, *6*(3), 696–705. doi:10.1021/mp800136v PMID:19267451

Chen, Y., Wu, J. J., & Huang, L. (2010). Nanoparticles targeted with NGR motif deliver c-myc siRNA and doxorubicin for anticancer therapy. *Molecular Therapy*, *18*(4), 828–834. doi:10.1038/mt.2009.291 PMID:20068551

Chen, Y., Yin, Q., Ji, X., Zhang, S., Chen, H., Zheng, Y., ... Shi, J. (2012). Manganese oxide-based multifunctionalized mesoporous silica nanoparticles for pH-responsive MRI, ultrasonography and circumvention of MDR in cancer cells. *Biomaterials*, *33*(29), 7126–7137. doi:10.1016/j.biomaterials.2012.06.059 PMID:22789722

Chen, Z., Penet, M.-F., Nimmagadda, S., Li, C., Banerjee, S. R., Winnard, P. T. Jr, ... Bhujwalla, Z. M. (2012). PSMA-targeted theranostic nanoplex for prostate cancer therapy. *ACS Nano*, *6*(9), 7752–7762. doi:10.1021/nn301725w PMID:22866897

Cheow, W. S., & Hadinoto, K. (2011). Factors affecting drug encapsulation and stability of lipid-polymer hybrid nanoparticles. *Colloids Surfaces B Biointerfaces*, *85*(2), 214–220. doi:10.1016/j.colsurfb.2011.02.033 PMID:21439797

Cherukuri, P., Glazer, E. S., & Curley, S. A. (2010). Targeted hyperthermia using metal nanoparticles. *Advanced Drug Delivery Reviews*, *62*(3), 339–345. doi:10.1016/j.addr.2009.11.006 PMID:19909777

Cherukuvada, S., & Nangia, A. (2012). Fast dissolving eutectic compositions of two anti-tubercular drugs. *CrystEngComm*, *14*(7), 2579–2588. doi:10.1039/c2ce06391c

Cherukuvada, S., & Nangia, A. (2014). Eutectics as improved pharmaceutical materials: Design, properties and characterization. *Chemical Communications (Cambridge)*, *50*(8), 906–923. doi:10.1039/C3CC47521B PMID:24322207

Cheung, C. R. F., Ng, T. B., Wong, J. H., & Chan, W. Y. (2015). Chitosan: An Update on Potential Biomedical and Pharmaceutical Applications. *Marine Drugs*, *13*(8), 5156–5186. doi:10.3390/md13085156 PMID:26287217

Chicheł, A., Skowronek, J., Kubaszewska, M., & Kanikowski, M. (2007). Hyperthermia–description of a method and a review of clinical applications. *Reports of Practical Oncology and Radiotherapy: Journal of Greatpoland Cancer Center in Poznan and Polish Society of Radiation Oncology*, *12*(5), 267–275. doi:10.1016/S1507-1367(10)60065-X

Chidambaram, M., Manavalan, R., & Kathiresan, K. (2011). Nanotherapeutics to overcome conventional cancer chemotherapy limitations. *Journal of Pharmacy & Pharmaceutical Sciences*, *14*(1), 67–77. doi:10.18433/J30C7D PMID:21501554

Chieng, N., Aaltonen, J., Saville, D., & Rades, T. (2009). Physical characterization and stability of amorphous indomethacin and ranitidine hydrochloride binary systems prepared by mechanical activation. *European Journal of Pharmaceutics and Biopharmaceutics*, *71*(1), 47–54. doi:10.1016/j.ejpb.2008.06.022 PMID:18644443

Childs, S. L., Stahly, G. P., & Park, A. (2007). The salt– cocrystal continuum: The influence of crystal structure on ionization state. *Molecular Pharmaceutics*, *4*(3), 323–338. doi:10.1021/mp0601345 PMID:17461597

Chime, S. A., Onyishi, I. V., Obitte, N. C., Onunkwo, G. C., & Odo, G. I. (2013). Sustained release artemether-loaded solid lipid microparticles based on solidified reverse micellar solution (SRMS). *Innovare J Sci.*, *1*, 1–7.

Chime, S. A., & Onyishi, V. I. (2013). Lipid-based drug delivery systems (LDDS): Recent advances and applications of lipids in drug delivery. *African Journal of Pharmacy and Pharmacology*, *7*(48), 3034–3059. doi:10.5897/AJPPX2013.0004

Chinchamalatpure & Ramkrishna. (2010). Synthesis and Electrical Characterization of BaTiO3 Thin Films on Si (100). *Materials Sciences and Applications*, *1*, 187-190.

Chocat, N. (2012). *Multimaterial Acoustic Fibers* (PhD Thesis). Massachusetts Institute of Technology.

Choi, A. H., & Ben-Nissan, B. (2007). Sol-gel production of bioactive nanocoatings for medical applications. Part II: Current research and development. *Nanomedicine (London)*, *2*(1), 51–61. doi:10.2217/17435889.2.1.51 PMID:17716190

Choi, A. H., Ben-Nissan, B., Matinlinna, J. P., & Conway, R. C. (2013). Current perspectives: Calcium phosphate nanocoatings and nanocomposite coatings in dentistry. *Journal of Dental Research*, *92*(10), 853–859. doi:10.1177/0022034513497754 PMID:23857642

Choi, Y. J., Kang, S. J., Kim, Y. J., Lim, Y. B., & Chung, H. W. (2010). Comparative studies on the genotoxicity and cytotoxicity of polymeric gene carriers polyethylenimine (PEI) and Polyamidoamine (PAMAM) dendrimer in jurkat T-cells. drug and chemical. *Toxicology*, *33*(4), 357–366. PMID:20550436

Cho, K., Wang, X., Nie, S., Chen, Z. G., & Shin, D. M. (2008). Therapeutic nanoparticles for drug delivery in cancer. *Clinical Cancer Research*, *14*(5), 1310–1316. doi:10.1158/1078-0432.CCR-07-1441 PMID:18316549

Chono, S., Tanino, T., Seki, T., & Morimoto, K. (2007). Uptake characteristics of liposomes by rat alveolar macrophages: Influence of particle size and surface mannose modification. *The Journal of Pharmacy and Pharmacology*, *59*(1), 75–80. doi:10.1211/jpp.59.1.0010 PMID:17227623

Chorny, M., Polyak, B., Alferiev, I. S., Walsh, K., Friedman, G., & Levy, R. J. (2007). Magnetically driven plasmid DNA delivery with biodegradable polymeric nanoparticles. *The FASEB Journal*, *21*(10), 2510–2519. doi:10.1096/fj.06-8070com PMID:17403937

Cho, S. H., Kim, A., Shin, W., Heo, M. B., Noh, H. J., Hong, K. S., ... Lim, Y. T. (2017). Photothermal-modulated drug delivery and magnetic relaxation based on collagen/poly(gamma-glutamic acid) hydrogel. *International Journal of Nanomedicine*, *12*, 2607–2620. doi:10.2147/IJN.S133078 PMID:28408827

Choudhury, H., Gorain, B., Karmakar, S., Biswas, E., Dey, G., Barik, R., & Pal, T. K. (2014). Improvement of cellular uptake, in vitro antitumor activity and sustained release profile with increased bioavailability from a nanoemulsion platform. *International Journal of Pharmaceutics*, *460*(1), 131–143. doi:10.1016/j.ijpharm.2013.10.055 PMID:24239580

Chourasia, M. K., & Jain, S. K. (2003). Pharmaceutical approaches to colon targeted drug delivery systems. *Journal of Pharmacy & Pharmaceutical Sciences*, *6*(1), 33–66. PMID:12753729

Chourasia, M. K., Kang, L., & Chan, S. Y. (2011). Nanosized ethosomes bearing ketoprofen for improved transdermal delivery. *Results in Pharma Sciences*, *1*(1), 60–67. doi:10.1016/j.rinphs.2011.10.002 PMID:25755983

Chowdhury, E. H., & Akaike, T. (2005). Bio-functional inorganic materials: An attractive branch of gene-based nano-medicine delivery for 21st century. *Current Gene Therapy*, *5*(6), 669–676. doi:10.2174/156652305774964613 PMID:16457655

Christie, W.W., (1987). *High-performance liquid chromatography and lipids: a practical guide.* Oxford, UK: Pergamon Press.

Cisterna, B. A., Kamaly, N., Choi, W. I., Tavakkoli, A., Farokhzad, O. C., & Vilos, C. (2016). Targeted nanoparticles for colorectal cancer. *Nanomedicine (London)*, *11*(18), 2443–2456. doi:10.2217/nnm-2016-0194 PMID:27529192

Cole, E. T., Cade, D., & Benameur, H. (2008). Challenges and opportunities in the encapsulation of liquid and semi-solid formulations into capsules for oral administration. *Advanced Drug Delivery Reviews*, *60*(6), 747–756. doi:10.1016/j.addr.2007.09.009 PMID:18096270

Colilla, M., Baeza, A., & Vallet-Regí, M. (2015). Mesoporous Silica Nanoparticles for Drug Delivery and Controlled Release Applications. In The Sol-Gel Handbook. Wiley-VCH Verlag GmbH & Co. KGaA. doi:10.1002/9783527670819.ch42

Collins, D. E., & Slamovich, E. B. (1999). Preparation of a Homogeneously Dispersed BaTiO3 Polymer Nanocomposite Thin Film. *Chemistry of Materials*, *11*(9), 2319–2321. doi:10.1021/cm990349p

Comoglu, C. T., Gonul, N., & Baykara, T. Preparation and *in vitro* evaluation of modified release ketoprofen microsponges. *ILFarmaco, 58,* 101–106.

Comoglu, T., Gonul, N., & Baykara, T. (2002). The effects of pressure and direct compression on tabletting of microsponges. *International Journal of Pharmaceutics*, *242*(1-2), 191–195. doi:10.1016/S0378-5173(02)00155-2 PMID:12176245

Conway, D., & Cohen, J. A. (2010). Combination therapy in multiple sclerosis. *Lancet Neurology*, *9*(3), 299–308. doi:10.1016/S1474-4422(10)70007-7 PMID:20170843

Copland, M. J., Rades, T., Davies, N. M., & Baird, M. A. (2005). Lipid based particulate formulations for the delivery of antigen. *Immunology and Cell Biology*, *89*(2), 97–105. doi:10.1111/j.1440-1711.2005.01315.x PMID:15748206

Correia-Pinto, J. F., Csaba, N., Schiller, J. T., & Alonso, M. J. (2015). Chitosan-poly (I: C)-PADRE based nanoparticles as delivery vehicles for synthetic peptide vaccines. *Vaccines*, *3*(3), 730–750. doi:10.3390/vaccines3030730 PMID:26378586

Coupe, A. J., Davis, S. S., & Wilding, I. R. (1991). Variation in gastrointestinal transit of pharmaceutical dosage forms in healthy subjects. *Pharmaceutical Research*, *8*(3), 360–364. doi:10.1023/A:1015849700421 PMID:2052525

Courant, T., Bayon, E., Reynaud-Dougier, H. L., Villiers, C., Menneteau, M., Marche, P. N., & Navarro, F. P. (2017). Tailoring nanostructured lipid carriers for the delivery of protein antigens: Physicochemical properties versus immunogenicity studies. *Biomaterials*, *136*, 29–42. doi:10.1016/j.biomaterials.2017.05.001 PMID:28511142

Couvreur, P. (2013). Nanoparticles in drug delivery: Past, present and future. *Advanced Drug Delivery Reviews*, *65*(1), 21–23. doi:10.1016/j.addr.2012.04.010 PMID:22580334

Cox, M., & … . (2000). dental history: Eighteenth and nineteenth century dental restoration, treatment and consequences in a British nobleman. *British Dental Journal*, *189*(11), 593–596. PMID:11132689

Craig, D. Q. M., Agnes Chan, K. Y., & Khan, N. (1995). Article. *Pharmacy and Pharmacology Communications*, *1*, 559.

Cramer, N. B., Stansbury, J. W., & Bowman, C. N. (2011). Recent Advances and Developments in Composite Dental Restorative Materials. *Journal of Dental Research*, *90*(4), 402–416. doi:10.1177/0022034510381263 PMID:20924063

Cristiano, R. J., & Roth, J. A. (1995). Epidermal growth factor mediated DNA delivery into lung cancer cells via the epidermal growth factor receptor. *Cancer Gene Therapy*, *3*(1), 4–10. PMID:8785711

Croissant, J., Chaix, A., Mongin, O., Wang, M., Clément, S., Raehm, L., ... Zink, J. I. (2014). Two-Photon-Triggered Drug Delivery via Fluorescent Nanovalves. *Small*, *10*(9), 1752–1755. doi:10.1002mll.201400042 PMID:24678053

Crosasso, P., Ceruti, M., Brusa, P., Arpicco, S., Dosio, F., & Cattel, L. (2000). Preparation, characterization and properties of sterically stabilized paclitaxel-containing liposomes. *Journal of Controlled Release*, *63*(1), 19–30. doi:10.1016/S0168-3659(99)00166-2 PMID:10640577

Crowley, M. (2013). Solutions, Emulsions, Suspensions, and Extracts. In L. Felton (Ed.), Remington: Essentials of Pharmaceutics (Vol. 1st, pp. 435–468). Pharmaceutical Press.

Croy, S. R., & Kwon, G. S. (2006). Polymeric micelles for drug delivery. *Current Pharmaceutical Design*, *12*(36), 4669–4684. doi:10.2174/138161206779026245 PMID:17168771

Crucho, C. I., & Barros, M. T. (2015). Formulation of functionalized PLGA polymeric nanoparticles for targeted drug delivery. *Polymer*, *68*, 41–46. doi:10.1016/j.polymer.2015.04.083

Crucho, C. I., & Barros, M. T. (2017). Polymeric nanoparticles: A study on the preparation variables and characterization methods. *Materials Science and Engineering C*. PMID:28866227

Cruz-Cabeza, A. J. (2012). Acid–base crystalline complexes and the p K a rule. *CrystEngComm*, *14*(20), 6362–6365. doi:10.1039/c2ce26055g

Cruz, L. J., Tacken, P. J., Fokkink, R., & Figdor, C. G. (2011). The influence of PEG chain length and targeting moiety on antibody-mediated delivery of nanoparticle vaccines to human dendritic cells. *Biomaterials*, *32*(28), 6791–6803. doi:10.1016/j.biomaterials.2011.04.082 PMID:21724247

Cui, Y., Dong, H., Cai, X., Wang, D., & Li, Y. (2012). Mesoporous silica nanoparticles capped with disulfide-linked PEG gatekeepers for glutathione-mediated controlled release. *ACS Applied Materials & Interfaces*, *4*(6), 3177–3183. doi:10.1021/am3005225 PMID:22646097

Cvec, G. (1992). *Preparation for drug application in minute droplet form*. European Patent Office.

Daftarian, P., Kaifer, A. E., Li, W., Blomberg, B. B., Frasca, D., Roth, F., ... Serafini, P. (2011). Peptide-conjugated PAMAM dendrimer as a universal DNA vaccine platform to target antigen-presenting cells. *Cancer Research*, *71*(24), 7452–7462. doi:10.1158/0008-5472.CAN-11-1766 PMID:21987727

Daglioglu, C. (2017). Enhancing Tumor Cell Response to Multidrug Resistance with pH-Sensitive Quercetin and Doxorubicin Conjugated Multifunctional Nanoparticles. *Colloids and Surfaces. B, Biointerfaces*, *156*, 175–185. doi:10.1016/j.colsurfb.2017.05.012 PMID:28528134

Dahl, O., & Overgaard, J. (1995). A century with hyperthermic oncology in Scandinavia. *Acta Oncologica*, *34*(8), 1075–1083. doi:10.3109/02841869509127234 PMID:8608032

Dakwar, G. R., Hammad, I. A., Popov, M., Linder, C., Grinberg, S., Heldman, E., & Stepensky, D. (2012). Delivery of proteins to the brain by bolaamphiphilic nano-sized vesicles. *Journal of Controlled Release*, *160*(2), 315–321. doi:10.1016/j.jconrel.2011.12.042 PMID:22261280

Dal Magro, R., Ornaghi, F., Cambianica, I., Beretta, S., Re, F., Musicanti, C., ... Sancini, G. (2017). ApoE-modified solid lipid nanoparticles: A feasible strategy to cross the blood-brain barrier. *Journal of Controlled Release*, *249*, 103–110. doi:10.1016/j.jconrel.2017.01.039 PMID:28153761

Dalby, B., & ... . (2004). Advanced transfection with Lipofectamine 2000 reagent: Primary neurons, siRNA, and high-throughput applications. *Methods (San Diego, Calif.)*, *33*(2), 95–103. doi:10.1016/j.ymeth.2003.11.023 PMID:15121163

Dang, L., Liu, J., Li, F., Wang, L., Li, D., Guo, B., ... Badshah, S. A. (2016). Targeted delivery systems for molecular therapy in skeletal disorders. *International Journal of Molecular Sciences*, *17*(3), 428. doi:10.3390/ijms17030428 PMID:27011176

Danhier, F., Ansorena, E., Silva, J. M., Coco, R., Le Breton, A., & Préat, V. (2012). PLGA-based nanoparticles: An overview of biomedical applications. *Journal of Controlled Release*, *161*(2), 505–522. doi:10.1016/j.jconrel.2012.01.043 PMID:22353619

Danhier, F., Feron, O., & Préat, V. (2010). To exploit the tumor microenvironment: Passive and active tumor targeting of nanocarriers for anti-cancer drug delivery. *Journal of Controlled Release*, *148*(2), 135–146. doi:10.1016/j.jconrel.2010.08.027 PMID:20797419

Dan, N. (2002). Effect of liposome charge and PEG polymer layer thickness on cell? liposome electrostatic interactions. *Biochimica et Biophysica Acta (BBA) - Biomembranes*, *1564*(2), 343–348. doi:10.1016/S0005-2736(02)00468-6 PMID:12175916

Dar, M. J., Ali, H., Khan, A., & Khan, G. M. (2017). Polymer-based drug delivery: The quest for local targeting of inflamed intestinal mucosa. *Journal of Drug Targeting*, *25*(7), 582–596. doi:10.1080/1061186X.2017.1298601 PMID:28277824

Das, B., Sen, S. O., Maji, R., Nayak, A. K., & Sen, K. K. (2017). Transferosomal gel for transdermal delivery of risperidone: Formulation optimization and ex vivo permeation. *Journal of Drug Delivery Science and Technology*, *38*, 59–71. doi:10.1016/j.jddst.2017.01.006

Dasgupta, S., Auth, T., & Gompper, G. (2014). Shape and orientation matter for the cellular uptake of nonspherical particles. *Nano Letters*, *14*(2), 687–693. doi:10.1021/nl403949h PMID:24383757

Das, J., Han, J. W., Choi, Y. J., Song, H., Cho, S. G., Park, C., ... Kim, J. H. (2016). Cationic lipid-nanoceria hybrids, a novel nonviral vector-mediated gene delivery into mammalian cells: Investigation of the cellular uptake mechanism. *Scientific Reports*, *6*(29197), 1–13. PMID:27380727

Das, P., & Jana, N. R. (2015). Dopamine functionalized polymeric nanoparticle for targeted drug delivery. *RSC Advances*, *5*(42), 33586–33594. doi:10.1039/C5RA03302K

Das, R., & Pal, S. (2015). Modified hydroxypropyl methyl cellulose: Efficient matrix for controlled release of 5-amino salicylic acid. *International Journal of Biological Macromolecules*, *77*, 207–213. doi:10.1016/j.ijbiomac.2015.03.015 PMID:25796452

Davis, M. E. (2009). The first targeted delivery of siRNA in humans via a self-assembling, cyclodextrin polymer-based nanoparticle: From concept to clinic. *Molecular Pharmaceutics*, *6*(3), 659–668. doi:10.1021/mp900015y PMID:19267452

Davis, M. E., & Brewster, M. E. (2004). Cyclodextrin-based pharmaceutics: Past, present and future. *Nature Reviews. Drug Discovery*, *3*(12), 1023–1035. doi:10.1038/nrd1576 PMID:15573101

Davis, M., Pun, S., Bellocq, N., Reineke, T., Popielarski, S., Mishra, S., & Heidel, J. (2004). Self-assembling nucleic acid delivery vehicles via linear, water-soluble, cyclodextrin-containing polymers. *Current Medicinal Chemistry*, *11*(2), 179–197. doi:10.2174/0929867043456179 PMID:14754416

De Boer, J. P., & … . (2012). Targeting JNK-interacting protein 1 (JIP1) sensitises osteosarcoma to doxorubicin. *Oncotarget*, *3*(10), 1169. PMID:23045411

de Fougerolles, A., Vornlocher, H.-P., Maraganore, J., & Lieberman, J. (2007). Interfering with disease: A progress report on siRNA-based therapeutics. *Nature Reviews. Drug Discovery*, *6*(6), 443–453. doi:10.1038/nrd2310 PMID:17541417

de Ilarduya, C. T., Sun, Y., & Düzgüneş, N. (2010). Gene delivery by lipoplexes and polyplexes. *European Journal of Pharmaceutical Sciences*, *40*(3), 159–170. doi:10.1016/j.ejps.2010.03.019 PMID:20359532

de la Fuente, M., Seijo, B., & Alonso, M. J. (2008). Novel hyaluronic acid-chitosan nanoparticles for ocular gene therapy. *Investigative Ophthalmology & Visual Science*, *49*(5), 2016–2024. doi:10.1167/iovs.07-1077 PMID:18436835

De Martimprey, H., Vauthier, C., Malvy, C., & Couvreur, P. (2009). Polymer nanocarriers for the delivery of small fragments of nucleic acids: Oligonucleotides and siRNA. *European Journal of Pharmaceutics and Biopharmaceutics*, *71*(3), 490–504. doi:10.1016/j.ejpb.2008.09.024 PMID:18977435

de Oliveira Freitas, L. B., de Melo Corgosinho, L., Faria, J. A. Q. A., dos Santos, V. M., Resende, J. M., Leal, A. S., … de Sousa, E. M. B. (2017). Multifunctional mesoporous silica nanoparticles for cancer-targeted, controlled drug delivery and imaging. *Microporous and Mesoporous Materials*, *242*, 271–283. doi:10.1016/j.micromeso.2017.01.036

De Smedt, S. C., Demeester, J., & Hennink, W. E. (2000). Cationic polymer based gene delivery systems. *Pharmaceutical Research*, *17*(2), 113–126. doi:10.1023/A:1007548826495 PMID:10751024

De Volder, M. F., Tawfick, S. H., Baughman, R. H., & Hart, A. J. (2013). Carbon nanotubes: Present and future commercial applications. *Science*, *339*(6119), 535–539. doi:10.1126cience.1222453 PMID:23372006

Deatsch, A. E., & Evans, B. A. (2014). Heating efficiency in magnetic nanoparticle hyperthermia. *Journal of Magnetism and Magnetic Materials*, *354*, 163–172. doi:10.1016/j.jmmm.2013.11.006

Debbage, P., & Jaschke, W. (2008). Molecular imaging with nanoparticles: Giant roles for dwarf actors. *Histochemistry and Cell Biology*, *130*(5), 845–875. doi:10.100700418-008-0511-y PMID:18825403

Değim, İ. T. (2014). Fulleren, karbon nanotüp, nanolif, nanokafesler. In A. Zırh-Gülsoy (Ed.), Nanofarmasötikler ve Uygulamaları (pp. 139-150). İstanbul: Kontrollü Salım Derneği Yayını No: 3.

Dehaini, D., Fang, R. H., Luk, B. T., Pang, Z., Hu, C.-M. J., Kroll, A. V., ... Zhang, L. (2016). Ultra-small lipid–polymer hybrid nanoparticles for tumor-penetrating drug delivery. *Nanoscale*, *8*(30), 14411–14419. doi:10.1039/C6NR04091H PMID:27411852

Del Campo, J., Lindqvist, M., Cuello, M., Bäckström, M., Cabrerra, O., Persson, J., ... Harandi, A. M. (2010). Intranasal immunization with a proteoliposome-derived cochleate containing recombinant gD protein confers protective immunity against genital herpes in mice. *Vaccine*, *28*(5), 1193–1200. doi:10.1016/j.vaccine.2009.11.035 PMID:19945418

Del Pozo-Rodríguez, A., Solinís, M. A., & Rodríguez-Gascón, A. (2016). Applications of lipid nanoparticles in gene therapy. *European Journal of Pharmaceutics and Biopharmaceutics*, *109*, 184–193. doi:10.1016/j.ejpb.2016.10.016 PMID:27789356

Del Real, R. P., Wolke, J. G. C., Vallet-Regi, M., & Jansen, J. A. (2002). A new method to produce macropores in calcium–phosphate cements. *Biomaterials*, *17*(17), 3673–3680. doi:10.1016/S0142-9612(02)00101-1 PMID:12109693

Delori, A., Galek, P. T., Pidcock, E., Patni, M., & Jones, W. (2013). Knowledge-based hydrogen bond prediction and the synthesis of salts and cocrystals of the anti-malarial drug pyrimethamine with various drug and GRAS molecules. *CrystEngComm*, *15*(15), 2916–2928. doi:10.1039/c3ce26765b

Del, R. J. Q. (2009). Benzoyl peroxide formulations: What is the science supporting microsphere vehicle technology and clinical use. *The Journal of Clinical and Aesthetic Dermatology*, *2*(9), 46–54. PMID:20729960

Dengale, S. J., Grohganz, H., Rades, T., & Löbmann, K. (2016). Recent advances in co-amorphous drug formulations. *Advanced Drug Delivery Reviews*, *100*, 116–125. doi:10.1016/j.addr.2015.12.009 PMID:26805787

Dengale, S. J., Hussen, S. S., Krishna, B., Musmade, P. B., Shenoy, G. G., & Bhat, K. (2015). Fabrication, solid state characterization and bioavailability assessment of stable binary amorphous phases of Ritonavir with Quercetin. *European Journal of Pharmaceutics and Biopharmaceutics*, *89*, 329–338. doi:10.1016/j.ejpb.2014.12.025 PMID:25542681

Dengale, S. J., Ranjan, O. P., Hussen, S. S., Krishna, B., Musmade, P. B., Shenoy, G. G., & Bhat, K. (2014). Preparation and characterization of co-amorphous Ritonavir–Indomethacin systems by solvent evaporation technique: Improved dissolution behavior and physical stability without evidence of intermolecular interactions. *European Journal of Pharmaceutical Sciences*, *62*, 57–64. doi:10.1016/j.ejps.2014.05.015 PMID:24878386

Dening, T. J., Rao, S., Thomas, N., & Prestidge, A. (2016). Novel Nanostructured Solid Materials for Modulating Oral Drug Delivery from Solid-State Lipid-Based Drug Delivery Systems. *The AAPS Journal*, *18*(1), 23–40. doi:10.120812248-015-9824-7 PMID:26354801

Depan, D., Venkata Surya, P. K. C., Girase, B., & Misra, R. D. K. (2011). Organic/inorganic hybrid network structure nanocomposite scaffolds based on grafted chitosan for tissue engineering. *Acta Biomaterialia*, *7*(5), 2163–2175. doi:10.1016/j.actbio.2011.01.029 PMID:21284959

Derjaguin, B. V. (1941). Theory of the stability of strongly charged lyophobic sols and the adhesion of strongly charged particles in solutions of electrolytes. *Acta Physicochim. USSR*, *14*, 633–662.

des Rieux, A., Fievez, V., Garinot, M., Schneider, Y. J., & Preat, V. (2006). Nanoparticles as potential oral delivery systems of proteins and vaccines: A mechanistic approach. *Journal of Controlled Release*, *116*(1), 1–27. doi:10.1016/j.jconrel.2006.08.013 PMID:17050027

Desai, P., Patlolla, R. R., & Singh, M. (2010). Interaction of nanoparticles and cell-penetrating peptides with skin for transdermal drug delivery. *Molecular Membrane Biology*, *27*(7), 247–259. doi:10.3109/09687688.2010.522203 PMID:21028936

Deshmukh, A., Nakhat, P., & Yeole, P. (2010). Formulation and in-vitro evaluation of self microemulsifying drug delivery system (SMEDDS) of Furosemide. *Der Pharm Lett*, *2*(2), 94–106.

Deshpande, S., & Singh, N. (2017). Influence of cubosome surface architecture on its cellular uptake mechanism. *Langmuir*, *33*(14), 3509–3516. doi:10.1021/acs.langmuir.6b04423 PMID:28325047

Desiraju, G. R. (1995). Supramolecular synthons in crystal engineering—a new organic synthesis. *Angewandte Chemie International Edition in English*, *34*(21), 2311–2327. doi:10.1002/anie.199523111

Devrim, B., & Canefe, K. (2006). Preparation and evaluation of modified release ibuprofen microspheres with acrylic polymers (Eudragit) by quasi-emulsion solvent diffusion method: Effect of variables. *Acta Poloniae Pharmaceutica*, *63*(6), 521–534. PMID:17438870

Dhas, N. L., Ige, P. P., & Kudarha, R. R. (2015). Design, optimization and in-vitro study of folic acid conjugated-chitosan functionalized PLGA nanoparticle for delivery of bicalutamide in prostate cancer. *Powder Technology*, *283*, 234–245. doi:10.1016/j.powtec.2015.04.053

Dhawale, S. C., Bankar, A. S., & Patro, M. N. (2010). Formulation and evaluation porous microspheres of 5- Fluorouracil for colon targeting. *International Journal of Pharm Tech Research*, *2*(2), 1112–1118.

Di Marco, M., Guilbert, I., Port, M., Robic, C., Couvreur, P., & Dubernet, C. (2007). Colloidal stability of ultrasmall superparamagnetic iron oxide (USPIO) particles with different coatings. *International Journal of Pharmaceutics*, *331*(2), 197–203. doi:10.1016/j.ijpharm.2006.11.002 PMID:17141984

Dickens, S. H., Flaim, G. M., & Takagi, S. (2003). Mechanical properties and biochemical activity of remineralizing resin-based Ca–PO4 cements. *Dental Materials*, *19*(6), 558–566. doi:10.1016/S0109-5641(02)00105-7 PMID:12837405

Ding, B. S., Dziubla, T., Shuvaev, V. V., Muro, S., & Muzykantov, V. R. (2006). Advanced drug delivery systems that target the vascular endothelium. *Molecular Interventions*, *6*(2), 98–112. doi:10.1124/mi.6.2.7 PMID:16565472

Ding, C., & Li, Z. (2017). A review of drug release mechanisms from nanocarrier systems. *Materials Science and Engineering C*, *76*, 1440–1453. doi:10.1016/j.msec.2017.03.130 PMID:28482511

Ding, C., Tong, L., Feng, J., & Fu, J. (2016). Recent Advances in Stimuli-Responsive Release Function Drug Delivery Systems for Tumor Treatment. *Molecules (Basel, Switzerland)*, *21*(12), 1715. doi:10.3390/molecules21121715 PMID:27999414

Ding, Y., Jiang, Z., Saha, K., Kim, C. S., Kim, S. T., Landis, R. F., & Rotello, V. M. (2014). Gold nanoparticles for nucleic acid delivery. *Molecular Therapy*, *22*(6), 1075–1083. doi:10.1038/mt.2014.30 PMID:24599278

Dizaj, S. M., Jafari, S., & Khosroushahi, A. Y. (2014). A sight on the current nanoparticle-based gene delivery vectors. *Nanoscale Research Letters*, *9*(252), 1–9. PMID:24936161

DM, S. (1969). Surface and bulk interactions of lipids and water with a classification of biologically active lipids based on these interactions. *Federation Proceedings*, *29*(4), 1320–1326. PMID:5459881

Doadrio, A. L., Sánchez-Montero, J. M., Doadrio, J. C., Salinas, A. J., & Vallet-Regí, M. (2017). Mesoporous silica nanoparticles as a new carrier methodology in the controlled release of the active components in a polypill. *European Journal of Pharmaceutical Sciences*, *97*, 1–8. doi:10.1016/j.ejps.2016.11.002 PMID:27818251

Doherty, G. J., & McMahon, H. T. (2009). Mechanisms of endocytosis. *Annual Review of Biochemistry*, *78*(1), 857–902. doi:10.1146/annurev.biochem.78.081307.110540 PMID:19317650

Donnelly, J. J., Ulmer, J. B., Shiver, J. W., & Liu, M. A. (1997). DNA vaccines. *Annual Review of Immunology*, *15*(1), 617–648. doi:10.1146/annurev.immunol.15.1.617 PMID:9143702

Dorraj, G., Carreras, J. J., Nunez, H., Abushammala, I., & Melero, A. (2017). Lipid nanoparticles as potential gene therapeutic delivery systems for oral administration. *Current Gene Therapy*, *17*(2), 89–104. doi:10.2174/1566523217666170510163038 PMID:28494737

Dos Santos, A. M., Carvalho, F. C., Teixeira, D. A., Azevedo, D. L., de Barros, W. M., & Gremião, M. P. D. (2017). Computational and experimental approaches for development of methotrexate nanosuspensions by bottom-up nanoprecipitation. *International Journal of Pharmaceutics*, *524*(1), 330–338. doi:10.1016/j.ijpharm.2017.03.068 PMID:28359822

Dos Santos, R., Thies, J., Richard, T. C., Le Meurlay, D., Gajan, V., Vandevelde, V., & Benoit, J.-P. (2003). A supercritical fluid-based coating technology. 2: Solubility considerations. *Journal of Microencapsulation*, *20*(1), 97–109. doi:10.3109/02652040309178052 PMID:12519705

Dragicevic, N., Verma, D. D., & Fahr, A. (2016). Invasomes: Vesicles for enhanced skin delivery of drugs. In Percutaneous Penetration Enhancers Chemical Methods in Penetration Enhancement (pp. 77–92). Berlin: Springer Berlin Heidelberg. doi:10.1007/978-3-662-47862-2_5

Dragicevic-Curic, N., Gräfe, S., Gitter, B., & Fahr, A. (2010). Efficacy of temoporfin-loaded invasomes in the photodynamic therapy in human epidermoid and colorectal tumour cell lines. *Journal of Photochemistry and Photobiology. B, Biology*, *101*(3), 238–250. doi:10.1016/j.jphotobiol.2010.07.009 PMID:20797872

Dragicevic-Curic, N., Scheglmann, D., Albrecht, V., & Fahr, A. (2008). Temoporfin-loaded invasomes: Development, characterization and in vitro skin penetration studies. *Journal of Controlled Release*, *127*(1), 59–69. doi:10.1016/j.jconrel.2007.12.013 PMID:18281119

Drechsler, M., Garbacz, G., Thomann, R., & Schubert, R. (2014). Development and evaluation of chitosan and chitosan/Kollicoat® Smartseal 30 D film-coated tablets for colon targeting. *European Journal of Pharmaceutics and Biopharmaceutics*, *88*(3), 807–815. doi:10.1016/j.ejpb.2014.09.006 PMID:25301294

Drozd, K. V., Manin, A. N., Churakov, A. V., & Perlovich, G. L. (2017). Drug-drug cocrystals of antituberculous 4-aminosalicylic acid: Screening, crystal structures, thermochemical and solubility studies. *European Journal of Pharmaceutical Sciences*, *99*, 228–239. doi:10.1016/j.ejps.2016.12.016 PMID:28011126

Dua, J. S., Rana, A. C., & Bhandari, A. K. (2012). Liposome: Methods of preparation and applications. *International Journal of Pharmaceutical Studies and Research*, *3*(2), 14–20.

Duangjit, S., Nimcharoenwan, T., Chomya, N., Locharoenrat, N., & Ngawhirunpat, T. (2016). Design and development of optimal invasomes for transdermal drug delivery using computer program. *Asian Journal of Pharmaceutical Sciences*, *11*(1), 52–53. doi:10.1016/j.ajps.2015.10.039

Du, B., Zhou, R., & Zhuo, R. (1998). Synthesis of cyclic core dendritic polymer and its usage as a vector for transferring foreign DNA into human cells. *Chinese Chemical Letters*, *9*(7), 635–638.

Duggirala, N. K., Perry, M. L., Almarsson, Ö., & Zaworotko, M. J. (2016). Pharmaceutical cocrystals: Along the path to improved medicines. *Chemical Communications (Cambridge)*, *52*(4), 640–655. doi:10.1039/C5CC08216A PMID:26565650

Du, J., Li, X., Zhao, H., Zhou, Y., Wang, L., Tian, S., & Wang, Y. (2015). Nanosuspensions of poorly water-soluble drugs prepared by bottom-up technologies. *International Journal of Pharmaceutics*, *495*(2), 738–749. doi:10.1016/j.ijpharm.2015.09.021 PMID:26383838

Dumoga, S., Rai, Y., Bhatt, A. N., Tiwari, A. K., Singh, S., Mishra, A. K., & Kakkar, D. (2017). Block Copolymer Based Nanoparticles for Theranostic Intervention of Cervical Cancer: Synthesis, Pharmacokinetics, and in Vitro/in Vivo Evaluation in HeLa Xenograft Models. *ACS Applied Materials & Interfaces*, *9*(27), 22195–22211. doi:10.1021/acsami.7b04982 PMID:28608677

Duncan, R., & Richardson, S. C. (2012). Endocytosis and intracellular trafficking as gateways for nanomedicine delivery: Opportunities and challenges. *Molecular Pharmaceutics*, *9*(9), 2380–2402. doi:10.1021/mp300293n PMID:22844998

Du, P., Zhao, X., Zeng, J., Guo, J., & Liu, P. (2015). Layer-by-layer engineering fluorescent polyelectrolyte coated mesoporous silica nanoparticles as pH-sensitive nanocarriers for controlled release. *Applied Surface Science*, *345*, 90–98. doi:10.1016/j.apsusc.2015.03.151

Dutta, T., Jain, N. K., McMillan, N. A., & Parekh, H. S. (2010). Dendrimer nanocarriers as versatile vectors in gene delivery. *Nanomedicine (London)*, *6*(1), 25–34. doi:10.1016/j.nano.2009.05.005 PMID:19450708

Dwivedi, M., Sharma, V., & Pathak, K. (2017). Pilosebaceous targeting by isotretenoin-loaded invasomal gel for the treatment of eosinophilic pustular folliculitis: Optimization, efficacy and cellular analysis. *Drug Development and Industrial Pharmacy*, *43*(2), 293–304. doi:10.1080/03639045.2016.1239628 PMID:27649797

Edwards, G. A., Porter, C. J. H., Caliph, S. M., Khoo, S., & Charman, W. N. (2001). Animal models for the study of intestinal lymphatic drug transport. *Advanced Drug Delivery Reviews*, *50*(1-2), 45–60. doi:10.1016/S0169-409X(01)00148-X PMID:11489333

Eisenmenger, W. (1998). Internal Charge Generation in Polyvinylidene Fluoride Films during Poling Observed By Raman Spectroscopy. *Proceedings of International Symposium on Electrical Insulating Materials*, 399 – 401. 10.1109/ISEIM.1998.741767

El Laithy, H. M., & El-Shaboury, K. M. (2002). The development of cutinalipogels and gel micromeulsion for topical administration of fluconazole. *AAPS PharmSciTech*, *3*, E35. PMID:12916929

El-Aassar, M. R., & Mo, X. (2016). Development of porous alginate microbeads containing silver nanoparticles and their antibacterial efficacy. *Advances in Polymer Technology*, *35*(3), 298–306. doi:10.1002/adv.21555

Elfinger, M., Uzgun, S., & Rudolph, C. (2008). Nanocarriers for gene delivery - Polymer structure, targeting ligands and controlled-release devices. *Current Nanoscience*, *4*(4), 322–353. doi:10.2174/157341308786306062

El-Hammadi, M. M., Delgado, A. V., Melguizo, C., Prados, J. C., & Arias, J. L. (2017). Folic acid-decorated and PEGylated PLGA nanoparticles for improving the antitumour activity of 5-fluorouracil. *International Journal of Pharmaceutics*, *516*(1-2), 61–70. doi:10.1016/j.ijpharm.2016.11.012 PMID:27825867

Elitez, Y., Ekinci, M., Ilem-Ozdemir, D., Gundogdu, E., & Asikoglu, M. (2017). Tc-99m Radiolabeled Alendronate Sodium Microemulsion: Characterization and Permeability Studies across Caco-2 Cells. *Current Drug Delivery*. doi:10.2174/1567201814666170613082752 PMID:28606033

El-Komy, M., Shalaby, S., Hegazy, R., Abdel Hay, R., Sherif, S., & Bendas, E. (2016). Assessment of cubosomal alpha lipoic acid gel efficacy for the aging face: A single-blinded, placebo-controlled, right-left comparative clinical study. *Journal of Cosmetic Dermatology*. doi:10.1111/jocd.12298 PMID:27873449

ElMaghraby, G. M., Barry, B. W., & Williams, A. C. (2008). Liposomes and skin: From drug delivery to model membranes. *European Journal of Pharmaceutical Sciences*, *34*(4-5), 203–222. doi:10.1016/j.ejps.2008.05.002 PMID:18572392

El-Nahrawy, A. M., Ali, A. I., Abou Hammad, A. B., & Youssef, A. M. (2016). Influences of Ag-NPs doping chitosan/calcium silicate nanocomposites for optical and antibacterial activity. *International Journal of Biological Macromolecules, 93*, 267–275. doi:10.1016/j.ijbiomac.2016.08.045 PMID:27543348

Elouahabi, A., & Ruysschaert, J.-M. (2005). Formation and intracellular trafficking of lipoplexes and polyplexes. *Molecular Therapy, 11*(3), 336–347. doi:10.1016/j.ymthe.2004.12.006 PMID:15727930

El-Sayed, A., & Harashima, H. (2013). Endocytosis of gene delivery vectors: From clathrin-dependent to lipid raft-mediated endocytosis. *Molecular Therapy, 21*(6), 1118–1130. doi:10.1038/mt.2013.54 PMID:23587924

Eltohamy, M., Seo, J. W., Hwang, J. Y., Jang, W. C., Kim, H. W., & Shin, U. S. (2016). Ionic and thermo-switchable polymer-masked mesoporous silica drug-nanocarrier: High drug loading capacity at 10 degrees C and fast drug release completion at 40 degrees C. *Colloids and Surfaces. B, Biointerfaces, 144*, 229–237. doi:10.1016/j.colsurfb.2016.04.023 PMID:27092438

Elzoghby, A. O., Samy, W. M., & Elgindy, N. A. (2012). Albumin-based nanoparticles as potential controlled release drug delivery systems. *Journal of Controlled Release, 157*(2), 168–182. doi:10.1016/j.jconrel.2011.07.031 PMID:21839127

Embil, V. P. (2000). OTC external analgesic cream/topical analgesic anti-inflammatory, counter irritant utilizing the microsponge delivery system for controlled release of actives. *UK Patent 01010586.*

Embil, K., & Nacht, S. (1996). The microsponge delivery system (MDS) a Topical Delivery System with reduced irritancy incorporating multiple triggering Mechanisms for the release of actives. *Journal of Microencapsulation, 13*(5), 575–588. doi:10.3109/02652049609026042 PMID:8864994

Erb, R. M. Y. B. (2009). Magnetic Manipulation of Colloidal Particles. Nanoscale Magnetic Materials and Applications, 19, 563-590.

Erlanson-Albertsson, C. (1992). Pancreatic colipase. Structural and physiological aspects. *Biochimica et Biophysica Acta, 1125*(1), 1–7. doi:10.1016/0005-2760(92)90147-N PMID:1567900

Esfandiarpour-Boroujeni, S., Bagheri-Khoulenjani, S., Mirzadeh, H., & Amanpour, S. (2017). Fabrication and study of curcumin loaded nanoparticles based on folate-chitosan for breast cancer therapy application. *Carbohydrate Polymers, 168*, 14–21. doi:10.1016/j.carbpol.2017.03.031 PMID:28457434

Etheridge, M. L., Campbell, S. A., Erdman, A. G., Haynes, C. L., Wolf, S. M., & McCullough, J. (2013). The big picture on nanomedicine: The state of investigational and approved nanomedicine products. *Nanomedicine (London), 9*(1), 1–14. doi:10.1016/j.nano.2012.05.013 PMID:22684017

Etter, M. C., MacDonald, J. C., & Bernstein, J. (1990). Graph-set analysis of hydrogen-bond patterns in organic crystals. *Acta Crystallographica. Section B, Structural Science, 46*(2), 256–262. doi:10.1107/S0108768189012929 PMID:2344397

Évora, A. O., Castro, R. A., Maria, T. M., Rosado, M. T., Ramos Silva, M., Matos Beja, A., ... Eusébio, M. E. S. (2011). Pyrazinamide-diflunisal: A new dual-drug co-crystal. *Crystal Growth & Design, 11*(11), 4780–4788. doi:10.1021/cg200288b

Evrard, B., Amighi, K., Beten, D., Delattre, L., & Moës, A. J. (1999). Influence of melting and rheological properties of fatty binders on the melt granulation process in a high-shear mixer. *Drug Development and Industrial Pharmacy, 25*(11), 1177–1184. doi:10.1081/DDC-100102285 PMID:10596355

Facca & Lahiri. (2012). Nanoreinforcement of hydroxyapatite coatings on titanium for osseointegration of orthopaedic implants. *Computer Methods in Biomechanics and Biomedical Engineering, 15*(sup1), 10-11.

Fadeel, B., & García-Bennett, A. E. (2010). Better safe than sorry: Understanding the toxicological properties of inorganic nanoparticles manufactured for biomedical applications. *Advanced Drug Delivery Reviews*, *62*(3), 362–374. doi:10.1016/j.addr.2009.11.008 PMID:19900497

Fang, J., Nakamura, H., & Maeda, H. (2011). The EPR effect unique features of tumor blood vessels for drug delivery, factors involved, and limitationsand augmentation of the effect. *Advanced Drug Delivery Reviews*, *63*(3), 136–151. doi:10.1016/j.addr.2010.04.009 PMID:20441782

Fang, R. H., Aryal, S., Hu, C. M. J., & Zhang, L. (2010). Quick synthesis of lipid-polymer hybrid nanoparticles with low polydispersity using a single-step sonication method. *Langmuir*, *26*(22), 16958–16962. doi:10.1021/la103576a PMID:20961057

Fanun, M. (2012). Microemulsions as delivery systems. *Current Opinion in Colloid & Interface Science*, *17*(5), 306–313. doi:10.1016/j.cocis.2012.06.001

Faraji, A. H., & Wipf, P. (2009). Nanoparticles in cellular drug delivery. *Bioorganic & Medicinal Chemistry*, *17*(8), 2950–2962. doi:10.1016/j.bmc.2009.02.043 PMID:19299149

Faraji, M., Yamini, Y., & Rezaee, M. (2010). Magnetic nanoparticles: Synthesis, stabilization, functionalization, characterization, and applications. *Journal of the Indian Chemical Society*, *7*(1), 1–37.

Fariya, M., Jain, A., Dhawan, V., Shah, S., & Nagarsenker, M. S. (2014). Bolaamphiphiles: A Pharmaceutical Review. *Advanced Pharmaceutical Bulletin*, *4*(Suppl 2), 483–491. PMID:25671179

Farooq, A., Tosheva, L., Azzawi, M., & Whitehead, D. (2016). Real-time observation of aortic vessel dilation through delivery of sodium nitroprusside via slow release mesoporous nanoparticles. *Journal of Colloid and Interface Science*, *478*, 127–135. doi:10.1016/j.jcis.2016.06.004 PMID:27288578

Felgner, J. H., & … . (1994). Enhanced gene delivery and mechanism studies with a novel series of cationic lipid formulations. *The Journal of Biological Chemistry*, *269*(4), 2550–2561. PMID:8300583

Felgner, P. L., Gadek, T. R., Holm, M., Roman, R., Chan, H. W., Wenz, M., ... Danielsen, M. (1987). Lipofection: A highly efficient, lipid-mediated DNA-transfection procedure. *Proceedings of the National Academy of Sciences of the United States of America*, *84*(21), 7413–7417. doi:10.1073/pnas.84.21.7413 PMID:2823261

Fenart, L., Casanova, A., Dehouck, B., Duhem, C., Slupek, S., & Cecchelli, R. (1999). Evaluation of effect of charge and lipid coating on ability of 60-nm nanoparticles to cross an in vitro model of the blood-brain barrier. *The Journal of Pharmacology and Experimental Therapeutics*, *291*(3), 1017–1022. PMID:10565819

Feng, Y., Panwar, N., Tng, D. J. H., Tjin, S. C., Wang, K., & Yong, K. T. (2016). The application of mesoporous silica nanoparticle family in cancer theranostics. *Coordination Chemistry Reviews*, *319*, 86–109. doi:10.1016/j.ccr.2016.04.019

Fernandes, A. R., Jesus, J., Martins, P., Figueiredo, S., Rosa, D., Martins, L. M., ... Baptista, P. V. (2017). Multifunctional gold-nanoparticles: A nanovectorization tool for the targeted delivery of novel chemotherapeutic agents. *Journal of Controlled Release*, *245*, 52–61. doi:10.1016/j.jconrel.2016.11.021 PMID:27871990

Fernandes, C. B., Mandawgade, S., & Patravale, V. B. (2013). Solid lipid nanoparticles of etoposide using solvent emulsification diffusion technique for parenteral administration. *International Journal of Pharma Bioscience and Technology*, *1*(1), 27–33.

Fernandes, C. B., Prabhu, P. S., Guggulothu, D., & Patravale, V. B. (2011). Lipid Nanocarriers for Topical Anti-cancer Therapy: An Update. In E. B. Souto & E. B. Souto (Eds.), *Lipid Nanocarriers in Cancer Diagnosis and Therapy* (pp. 461–491). New York: Smithers Rapra Technology.

Fernandes, C., Soni, U., & Patravale, V. (2010). Nano-interventions for neurodegenerative disorders. *Pharmacological Research*, *62*(2), 166–178. doi:10.1016/j.phrs.2010.02.004 PMID:20153429

Fernandez-Fernandez, A., Manchanda, R., & McGoron, A. (2011). Theranostic applications of nanomaterials in cancer: Drug delivery, image-guided therapy, and multifunctional platforms. *Applied Biochemistry and Biotechnology*, *165*(7-8), 1628–1651. doi:10.100712010-011-9383-z PMID:21947761

Ferracane, J. L. (1995). Current Trends in Dental Composites. *Critical Reviews in Oral Biology and Medicine*, *6*(4), 302–318. doi:10.1177/10454411950060040301 PMID:8664421

Ferracane, J. L. (2008). Placing Dental Composites—A Stressful Experience. *Operative Dentistry*, *33*(3), 247–257. doi:10.2341/07-BL2 PMID:18505214

Ferracane, J. L., & Mitchem, J. C. (2003). Relationship between composite contraction stress and leakage in Class V cavities. *American Journal of Dentistry*, *16*(4), 239–243. PMID:14579877

Ferrari, M. (2005). Cancer nanotechnology: Opportunities and challenges. *Nature Reviews. Cancer*, *5*(3), 161–171. doi:10.1038/nrc1566 PMID:15738981

Fetz, V., Bier, C., Habtemichael, N., Schuon, R., Schweitzer, A., Kunkel, M., ... Knauer, S. K. (2009). Inducible NO synthase confers chemoresistance in head and neck cancer by modulating survivin. *International Journal of Cancer*, *124*(9), 2033–2041. doi:10.1002/ijc.24182 PMID:19130609

Figueirêdo, C. B. M., Nadvorny, D., de Medeiros Vieira, A. C. Q., Sobrinho, J. L. S., Neto, P. J. R., Lee, P. I., & Soares, M. F. L. R. (2017). Enhancement of dissolution rate through eutectic mixture and solid solution of posaconazole and benznidazole. *International Journal of Pharmaceutics*, *525*(1), 32–42. doi:10.1016/j.ijpharm.2017.04.021 PMID:28412452

Fischer, D., Li, Y. X., Ahlemeyer, B., Krieglstein, J., & Kissel, T. (2003). *In vitro* cytotoxicity testing of polycations: Influence of polymer structure on cell viability and hemolysis. *Biomaterials*, *24*(7), 1121–1131. doi:10.1016/S0142-9612(02)00445-3 PMID:12527253

Fofaria, N. M., Qhattal, H. S. S., Liu, X., & Srivastava, S. K. (2016). Nanoemulsion formulations for anti-cancer agent piplartine—Characterization, toxicological, pharmacokinetics and efficacy studies. *International Journal of Pharmaceutics*, *498*(1), 12–22. doi:10.1016/j.ijpharm.2015.11.045 PMID:26642946

Fortin, M. (n.d.). *Magnetic nanoparticles for MRI applications in medicine*. Retrieved from http://www.cqmfscience.com/wpcontent/uploads/2013/05/Fortin_Chapter.pdf

Frangioni, J. V. (2008). New technologies for human cancer imaging. *Journal of Clinical Oncology*, *26*(24), 4012–4021. doi:10.1200/JCO.2007.14.3065 PMID:18711192

Freitas, J. C. D., Branco, R. M., Lisboa, I. G. O., Costa, T. P. D., Campos, M. G. N., Jafelicci Júnior, M., & Marques, R. F. C. (2015). Magnetic Nanoparticles Obtained by Homogeneous Coprecipitation Sonochemically Assisted. *Materials Research*, *18*(suppl 2), 220–224. doi:10.1590/1516-1439.366114

Freitas, R. A. Jr. (2005). Nanotechnology, nanomedicine and nanosurgery. *International Journal of Surgery*, *3*(4), 243–246. doi:10.1016/j.ijsu.2005.10.007 PMID:17462292

Frese, C., Staehle, H. J., & Wolff, D. (2012, May). The assessment of dentofacial esthetics in restorative dentistry. *The Journal of the American Dental Association*, *143*(5), 461–466. doi:10.14219/jada.archive.2012.0205 PMID:22547716

Fricker, J., & Writer, F. (2001). Drugs with a magnetic attraction to tumours. *Drug Discovery Today*, *6*(8), 387–389. doi:10.1016/S1359-6446(01)01771-8 PMID:11301276

Fritz, G., Schädler, V., Willenbacher, N., & Wagner, N. J. (2002). Electrosteric stabilization of colloidal dispersions. *Langmuir*, *18*(16), 6381–6390. doi:10.1021/la015734j

Fuhrhop, J. H., & Wang, T. (2004). Bolaamphiphiles. *Chemical Reviews*, *104*(6), 2901–2938. doi:10.1021/cr030602b PMID:15186184

Fukunaka, Y., Iwanaga, K., Morimoto, K., Kakemi, M., & Tabata, Y. (2002). Controlled release of plasmid DNA from cationized gelatin hydrogels based on hydrogel degradation *J. Controll. Rel.*, *2*(80), 333–343.

Fu, X., Wang, X., Zhou, S., & Zhang, Y. (2017). IONP-doped nanoparticles for highly effective NIR-controlled drug release and combination tumor therapy. *International Journal of Nanomedicine*, *12*, 3751–3766. doi:10.2147/IJN.S113963 PMID:28553112

Gaharwar, A. K., Peppas, N. A., & Khademhosseini, A. (2014). Nanocomposite hydrogels for biomedical applications. *Biotechnology and Bioengineering*, *111*(3), 441–453. doi:10.1002/bit.25160 PMID:24264728

Gai, S., Yang, P., Li, C., Wang, W., Dai, Y., Niu, N., & Lin, J. (2010). Synthesis of magnetic, up-conversion luminescent, and mesoporous core-shell-structured nanocomposites as drug carriers. *Advanced Functional Materials*, *20*(7), 1166–1172. doi:10.1002/adfm.200902274

Galbiati, A., Tabolacci, C., Morozzo Della Rocca, B., Mattioli, P., Beninati, S., Paradossi, G., & Desideri, A. (2011). Targeting tumor cells through chitosan-folate modified microcapsules loaded with camptothecin. *Bioconjugate Chemistry*, *22*(6), 1066–1072. doi:10.1021/bc100546s PMID:21545180

Ganduri, R., Cherukuvada, S., & Guru Row, T. N. (2015). Multicomponent Adducts of Pyridoxine: An Evaluation of the Formation of Eutectics and Molecular Salts. *Crystal Growth & Design*, *15*(7), 3474–3480. doi:10.1021/acs.cgd.5b00546

Gans, E. H. (1999). Polymer developments of cosmetic interest. *Cosmetics & Toiletries*, *114*, 53–60.

Gao, J., Feng, S.-S., & Guo, Y. (2010). Antibody engineering promotes nanomedicine for cancer treatment. *Nanomedicine (London)*, *5*(8), 1141–1145. Available from http://www.futuremedicine.com/doi/10.2217/nnm.10.94. doi:10.2217/nnm.10.94 PMID:21039191

Gao, L., Liu, G., Kang, J., Niu, M., Wang, Z., Wang, H., ... Wang, X. (2013). Paclitaxel nanosuspensions coated with P-gp inhibitory surfactants: I. Acute toxicity and pharmacokinetics studies. *Colloids and Surfaces. B, Biointerfaces*, *111*, 277–281. doi:10.1016/j.colsurfb.2013.06.004 PMID:23838193

Gao, N., Bozeman, E. N., Qian, W., Wang, L., Chen, H., Lipowska, M., ... Yang, L. (2017). Tumor Penetrating Theranostic Nanoparticles for Enhancement of Targeted and Image-guided Drug Delivery into Peritoneal Tumors following Intraperitoneal Delivery. *Theranostics*, *7*(6), 1689–1704. doi:10.7150/thno.18125 PMID:28529645

Gao, Q., Xu, Y., Wu, D., Sun, Y., & Li, X. (2009). pH-Responsive Drug Release from Polymer-Coated Mesoporous Silica Spheres. *The Journal of Physical Chemistry C*, *113*(29), 12753–12758. doi:10.1021/jp9043978

Gao, X., Kim, K.-S., & Liu, D. (2007). Nonviral gene delivery: What we know and what is next. *The AAPS Journal*, *9*(1), E92–E104. doi:10.1208/aapsj0901009 PMID:17408239

Gao, Y., Yang, R., Zhang, Z., Chen, L., Sun, Z., & Li, Y. (2011). Solid lipid nanoparticles reduce systemic toxicity of docetaxel: Performance and mechanism in animal. *Nanotoxicology*, *5*(4), 636–649. doi:10.3109/17435390.2010.551427 PMID:21306192

Garg, G., Saraf, S., & Saraf, S. (2007). Cubosomes: An Overview. *Biological & Pharmaceutical Bulletin*, *30*(2), 350–353. doi:10.1248/bpb.30.350 PMID:17268078

Garg, N. K., Singh, B., Jain, A., Nirbhavane, P., Sharma, R., Tyagi, R. K., ... Katare, O. P. (2016). Fucose decorated solid-lipid nanocarriers mediate efficient delivery of methotrexate in breast cancer therapeutics. *Colloids and Surfaces. B, Biointerfaces*, *146*, 114–126. doi:10.1016/j.colsurfb.2016.05.051 PMID:27268228

Garnett, M.C. (1999). Gene-delivery systems using cationic polymers. *Critical Reviews™ in Therapeutic Drug Carrier Systems, 16*(2).

Gary-Bobo, M., Hocine, O., Brevet, D., Maynadier, M., Raehm, L., Richeter, S., ... Durand, J. O. (2012a). Cancer therapy improvement with mesoporous silica nanoparticles combining targeting, drug delivery and PDT. *International Journal of Pharmaceutics*, *423*(2), 509–515. doi:10.1016/j.ijpharm.2011.11.045 PMID:22178618

Gary-Bobo, M., Mir, Y., Rouxel, C., Brevet, D., Hocine, O., Maynadier, M., ... Durand, J. O. (2012b). Multifunctionalized mesoporous silica nanoparticles for the in vitro treatment of retinoblastoma: Drug delivery, one and two-photon photodynamic therapy. *International Journal of Pharmaceutics*, *432*(1-2), 99–104. doi:10.1016/j.ijpharm.2012.04.056 PMID:22569231

Gary, D. J., Puri, N., & Won, Y.-Y. (2007). Polymer-based siRNA delivery: Perspectives on the fundamental and phenomenological distinctions from polymer-based DNA delivery. *Journal of Controlled Release*, *121*(1), 64–73. doi:10.1016/j.jconrel.2007.05.021 PMID:17588702

Gaucher, G., Dufresne, M. H., Sant, V. P., Kang, N., Maysinger, D., & Leroux, J. C. (2005). Block copolymer micelles: Preparation, characterization and application in drug delivery. *Journal of Controlled Release*, *109*(1-3), 169–188. doi:10.1016/j.jconrel.2005.09.034 PMID:16289422

Gaur, U., Sahoo, S. K., De Tapas, K., Ghosh, P. C., Maitra, A., & Ghosh, P. K. (2000). Biodistribution of fluoresceinated dextran using novel nanoparticles evading reticuloendothelial system. *International Journal of Pharmaceutics*, *202*(1), 1–10. doi:10.1016/S0378-5173(99)00447-0 PMID:10915921

Ge, K., Zhang, C., Jia, G., Ren, H., Wang, J., Tan, A., ... Zhang, J. (2015). Defect-Related Luminescent Mesoporous Silica Nanoparticles Employed for Novel Detectable Nanocarrier. *ACS Applied Materials & Interfaces*, *7*(20), 10905–10914. doi:10.1021/acsami.5b02146 PMID:25943277

Gerasimov, O. V., Boomer, J. A., Qualls, M. M., & Thompson, D. H. (1999). Cytosolic drug delivery using pH- and light-sensitive liposomes. *Advanced Drug Delivery Reviews*, *38*(3), 317–338. doi:10.1016/S0169-409X(99)00035-6 PMID:10837763

Gershkovich, P., Wasan, K. M., & Barta, C. A. (2008). A review of the application of lipid-based systems in systemic, dermal/ transdermal, and ocular drug delivery. *Critical Reviews in Therapeutic Drug Carrier Systems*, *25*(6), 545–584. doi:10.1615/CritRevTherDrugCarrierSyst.v25.i6.20 PMID:19166393

Geusens, B., Strobbe, T., Bracke, S., Dynoodt, P., Sanders, N., ... VanGele, M. (2011). Lipid-mediated gene delivery to the skin. *European Journal of Pharmaceutical Sciences*, *43*(4), 199–211. doi:10.1016/j.ejps.2011.04.003 PMID:21515366

Ghanbarzadeh, S., & Arami, A. (2013). Formulation and evaluation of piroxicam transferosomal gel: An approach for penetration enhancement. *Journal of Drug Delivery Science and Technology*, *23*(6), 587–590. doi:10.1016/S1773-2247(13)50089-X

Ghanbarzadeh, S., Hariri, R., Kouhsoltani, M., Shokri, J., Javadzadeh, Y., & Hamishehkar, H. (2015). Enhanced stability and dermal delivery of hydroquinone using solid lipid nanoparticles. *Colloids and Surfaces. B, Biointerfaces*, *136*, 1004–1010. doi:10.1016/j.colsurfb.2015.10.041 PMID:26579567

Ghorbani, M., Hamishehkar, H., Arsalani, N., & Entezami, A. A. (2015). Preparation of thermo and pH-responsive polymer@ Au/Fe3O4 core/shell nanoparticles as a carrier for delivery of anticancer agent. *Journal of Nanoparticle Research*, *17*(7), 305. doi:10.100711051-015-3097-z

Giacca, M. (2010). Introduction to gene therapy. In *Gene Therapy* (pp. 1–6). Springer Verlag. doi:10.1007/978-88-470-1643-9_1

Giannakas, A., Vlacha, M., Salmas, C., Leontiou, A., Katapodis, P., Stamatis, H., ... Ladavos, A. (2016). Preparation, characterization, mechanical, barrier and antimicrobial properties of chitosan/PVOH/clay nanocomposites. *Carbohydrate Polymers*, *140*, 408–415. doi:10.1016/j.carbpol.2015.12.072 PMID:26876868

Gibson, L. (2007). Lipid-based excipients for oral drug delivery. In D. J. Hauss (Ed.), *Oral lipid-based formulations: enhancing the bioavailability of poorly water soluble drugs* (pp. 33–61). InformaHealthcare.

Gilchrist, R. K., Medal, R., Shorey, W. D., Hanselman, R. C., Parrott, J. C., & Taylor, C. B. (1957). Selective inductive heating of lymph nodes. *Annals of Surgery*, *146*(4), 596–606. doi:10.1097/00000658-195710000-00007 PMID:13470751

Giljohann, D. A., Seferos, D. S., Prigodich, A. E., Patel, P. C., & Mirkin, C. A. (2009). Gene regulation with polyvalent siRNA-nanoparticle conjugates. *Journal of the American Chemical Society*, *131*(6), 2072–2073. doi:10.1021/ja808719p PMID:19170493

Gill, K. K., Kaddoumi, A., & Nazzal, S. (2015). PEG–lipid micelles as drug carriers: Physiochemical attributes, formulation principles and biological implication. *Journal of Drug Targeting*, *23*(3), 222–231. doi:10.3109/1061186X.2014.997735 PMID:25547369

Gindy, M. E., & Prud'homme, R. K. (2009). Multifunctional nanoparticles for imaging, delivery and targeting in cancer therapy. *Expert Opinion on Drug Delivery*, *6*(8), 865–878. doi:10.1517/17425240902932908 PMID:19637974

Gionchetti, P., Rizzello, F., Annese, V., Armuzzi, A., Biancone, L., Castiglione, F., ... Daperno, M. (2017). Use of corticosteroids and immunosuppressive drugs in inflammatory bowel disease: Clinical practice guidelines of the Italian Group for the Study of Inflammatory Bowel Disease. *Digestive and Liver Disease*, *49*(6), 604–617. doi:10.1016/j.dld.2017.01.161 PMID:28254463

Giovagnoli, S., Blasi, P., Schoubben, A., Rossi, C., & Ricci, M. (2007). Preparation of large porous biodegradable microspheres by using a simple double-emulsion method for capreomycin sulfate pulmonary delivery. *International Journal of Pharmaceutics*, *333*(1-2), 103–111. doi:10.1016/j.ijpharm.2006.10.005 PMID:17079101

Girgis, M. D., Federman, N., Rochefort, M. M., McCabe, K. E., Wu, A. M., Nagy, J. O., ... Tomlinson, J. S. (2013). An engineered anti-CA19-9 cys-diabody for positron emission tomography imaging of pancreatic cancer and targeting of polymerized liposomal nanoparticles. *The Journal of Surgical Research*, *185*(1), 45–55. doi:10.1016/j.jss.2013.05.095 PMID:23827791

Gizurarson, S. (2004). A bioadhesive agent. *European Patent 1480673A1*.

Glenn, G. M., & Kenney, R. T. (2006). Mass vaccination: Solutions in the skin. *Current Topics in Microbiology and Immunology*, *304*, 247–268. doi:10.1007/3-540-36583-4_14 PMID:16989274

Gloria, A., Russo, T., D'Amora, U., Zeppetelli, S., D'Alessandro, T., Sandri, M., ... De Santis, R. (2013). Magnetic poly (ε-caprolactone)/iron-doped hydroxyapatite nanocomposite substrates for advanced bone tissue engineering. *Journal of the Royal Society, Interface*, *10*(80), 20120833. doi:10.1098/rsif.2012.0833 PMID:23303218

Gnanavel, V., Palanichamy, V., & Roopan, S. M. (2017). Biosynthesis and characterization of copper oxide nanoparticles and its anticancer activity on human colon cancer cell lines (HCT-116). *Journal of Photochemistry and Photobiology. B, Biology*, *171*, 133–138. doi:10.1016/j.jphotobiol.2017.05.001 PMID:28501691

Goldberg, A. H., Gibaldi, M., & Kanig, J. L. (1966). Increasing dissolution rates and gastrointestinal absorption of drugs via solid solutions and eutectic mixtures II: experimental evaluation of a eutectic mixture: urea-acetaminophen system. *Journal of Pharmaceutical Sciences*, *55*(5), 482–487. doi:10.1002/jps.2600550507

Gollnick, H. P. M., & Krautheim, A. (2003). Topical Treatment in Acne: Current Status and Future Aspects. *Dermatology (Basel, Switzerland)*, *206*(1), 29–36. doi:10.1159/000067820 PMID:12566803

Gomes, M. J., Martins, S., Ferreira, D., Segundo, M. A., & Reis, S. (2014). Lipid nanoparticles for topical and transdermal application for alopecia treatment: Development, physicochemical characterization, and in vitro release and penetration studies. *International Journal of Nanomedicine*, *9*, 1231–1242. PMID:24634584

Gong, K., Qu, S., Liu, Y., Wang, J., Zhang, Y., Jiang, C., & Shen, R. (2016). The mechanical and tribological properties of UHMWPE loaded ALN after mechanical activation for joint replacements. *Journal of the Mechanical Behavior of Biomedical Materials*, *61*, 334–344. doi:10.1016/j.jmbbm.2016.03.023 PMID:27104932

Gonzalez, H., Hwang, S. J., & Davis, M. (1999). New class of polymers for the delivery of macromolecular therapeutics. *Bioconjugate Chemistry*, *10*(6), 1068–1074. doi:10.1021/bc990072j PMID:10563777

Gopi, S. P., Ganguly, S., & Desiraju, G. R. (2016). A Drug–Drug Salt Hydrate of Norfloxacin and Sulfathiazole: Enhancement of in Vitro Biological Properties via Improved Physicochemical Properties. *Molecular Pharmaceutics*, *13*(10), 3590–3594. doi:10.1021/acs.molpharmaceut.6b00320 PMID:27580175

Górniak, A., Karolewicz, B., Żurawska-Płaksej, E., & Pluta, J. (2013). Thermal, spectroscopic, and dissolution studies of the simvastatin–acetylsalicylic acid mixtures. *Journal of Thermal Analysis and Calorimetry*, *111*(3), 2125–2132. doi:10.100710973-012-2641-7

Górniak, A., Wojakowska, A., Karolewicz, B., & Pluta, J. (2011). Phase diagram and dissolution studies of the fenofibrate–acetylsalicylic acid system. *Journal of Thermal Analysis and Calorimetry*, *104*(3), 1195–1200. doi:10.100710973-010-1148-3

Goscianska, J., Olejnik, A., Nowak, I., Marciniak, M., & Pietrzak, R. (2015). Ordered mesoporous silica modified with lanthanum for ibuprofen loading and release behaviour. *European Journal of Pharmaceutics and Biopharmaceutics*, *94*, 550–558. doi:10.1016/j.ejpb.2015.07.003 PMID:26170160

Goud, N. R., Suresh, K., Sanphui, P., & Nangia, A. (2012). Fast dissolving eutectic compositions of curcumin. *International Journal of Pharmaceutics*, *439*(1), 63–72. doi:10.1016/j.ijpharm.2012.09.045 PMID:23041131

Goycoolea, F. M., Lollo, G., Remuñán-López, C., Quaglia, F., & Alonso, M. J. (2009). Chitosan-alginate blended nanoparticles as carriers for the transmucosal delivery of macromolecules. *Biomacromolecules*, *10*(7), 1736–1743. doi:10.1021/bm9001377 PMID:19545119

Goyel, M., Prajapati, R., Purohit, K. K., & Mehta, S. C. (2010). Floating drug delivery system. *Journal of Current Pharma Research*, *5*, 7–18.

Grabow, W. W., & Jaeger, L. (2012). siRNA delivery: Loaded-up microsponges. *Nature Materials*, *11*(4), 268–269. doi:10.1038/nmat3286 PMID:22437781

Grange, C., Geninatti-Crich, S., Esposito, G., Alberti, D., Tei, L., Bussolati, B., ... Camussi, G. (2010). Combined delivery and magnetic resonance imaging of neural cell adhesion molecule-targeted doxorubicin-containing liposomes in experimentally induced Kaposi's sarcoma. *Cancer Research*, *70*(6), 2180–2190. doi:10.1158/0008-5472.CAN-09-2821 PMID:20215497

Grant, E. V., Thomas, M., Fortune, J., Klibanov, A. M., & Letvin, N. L. (2012). Enhancement of plasmid DNA immunogenicity with linear polyethylenimine. *European Journal of Immunology*, *42*(11), 2937–2948. doi:10.1002/eji.201242410 PMID:22886924

Greenwood, B. (2014). The contribution of vaccination to global health: Past, present and future. *Philosophical Transactions of the Royal Society of London. Series B, Biological Sciences*, *369*(1645), 1–9. doi:10.1098/rstb.2013.0433 PMID:24821919

Gref, R., Minamitake, Y., Peracchia, M. T., Trubetskoy, V., Torchilin, V., & Langer, R. (1994). Biodegradable long-circulating polymeric nanospheres. *Science*, *263*(5153), 1600–1603. doi:10.1126cience.8128245 PMID:8128245

Grimes, P. E. (2004). A microsponge formulation of hydroquinone 4% and retinol 0.15% in the treatment of melasma and post inflammatory hyperpigmentation. *Cutis*, *74*(6), 362–368. PMID:15663072

Grobelny, P., Mukherjee, A., & Desiraju, G. R. (2011). Drug-drug co-crystals: Temperature-dependent proton mobility in the molecular complex of isoniazid with 4-aminosalicylic acid. *CrystEngComm*, *13*(13), 4358–4364. doi:10.1039/c0ce00842g

Grun, M., Lauer, I., & Unger, K.K. (1997). The synthesis of miro meter and sub micrometer size sphere of ordered mesoporous oxide MCM -41. *Adv Matte*r, *3*, 254-257.

Guimarães, P. P., Oliveira, M. F., Gomes, A. D., Gontijo, S. M., Cortés, M. E., Campos, P. P., ... Sinisterra, R. D. (2015). PLGA nanofibers improves the antitumoral effect of daunorubicin. *Colloids and Surfaces. B, Biointerfaces*, *136*, 248–255. doi:10.1016/j.colsurfb.2015.09.005 PMID:26402423

Guin, D., & Manorama, S. V. (2008). Room temperature synthesis of monodispersed iron oxide nanoparticles. *Materials Letters*, *62*(17), 3139–3142. doi:10.1016/j.matlet.2008.02.005

Guin, S., Ma, Q., Padhye, S., Zhou, Y. Q., Yao, H. P., & Wang, M. H. (2011). Targeting acute hypoxic cancer cells by doxorubicin-immunoliposomes directed by monoclonal antibodies specific to RON receptor tyrosine kinase. *Cancer Chemotherapy and Pharmacology*, *67*(5), 1073–1083. doi:10.100700280-010-1408-8 PMID:20658288

Guin, S., Yao, H. P., & Wang, M. H. (2010). RON receptor tyrosine kinase as a target for delivery of chemodrugs by antibody directed pathway for cancer cell cytotoxicity. *Molecular Pharmaceutics*, *7*(2), 386–397. doi:10.1021/mp900168v PMID:20039696

Gu, J., Wang, T., Fan, G., Ma, J., Hu, W., & Cai, X. (2016). Biocompatibility of artificial bone based on vancomycin loaded mesoporous silica nanoparticles and calcium sulfate composites. *Journal of Materials Science. Materials in Medicine*, *27*(4), 64. doi:10.100710856-016-5671-z PMID:26883948

Gunatillake, P. A., & Adhikari, R. (2003). Biodegradable synthetic polymers for tissue engineering. *European Cells & Materials*, *5*, 1–16. doi:10.22203/eCM.v005a01 PMID:14562275

Gunn, J., Wallen, H., Veiseh, O., Sun, C., Fang, C., Cao, J., ... Zhang, M. (2008). A multimodal targeting nanoparticle for selectively labeling T cells. *Small*, *4*(6), 712–715. doi:10.1002mll.200701103 PMID:18528851

Guo, H. C., Feng, X. M., Sun, S. Q., Wei, Y. Q., Sun, D. H., Liu, X. T., ... Yin, H. (2012). Immunization of mice by hollow mesoporous silica nanoparticles as carriers of porcine circovirus type 2 ORF2 protein. *Virology Journal*, *9*(108), 1–10. PMID:22691538

Guo, W., & Lee, R. J. (2000). Efficient gene delivery using anionic liposome-complexed polyplexes (LPDII). *Bioscience Reports*, *20*(5), 419–432. doi:10.1023/A:1010338219401 PMID:11332603

Guo, W., Yang, C., Cui, L., Lin, H., & Qu, F. (2014). An Enzyme-Responsive Controlled Release System of Mesoporous Silica Coated with Konjac Oligosaccharide. *Langmuir*, *30*(1), 243–249. doi:10.1021/la403494q PMID:24380643

Guo, X., & Huang, L. (2012). Recent advances in nonviral vectors for gene delivery. accounts of chemical research. *Accounts of Chemical Research*, *45*(7), 971–979. doi:10.1021/ar200151m PMID:21870813

Guo, Y., Li, H., Shi, W., Zhang, J., Feng, J., Yang, X., ... Yang, L. (2017). Targeted Delivery and pH-Responsive Release of Doxorubicin to Cancer Cells Using Calcium Carbonate/Hyaluronate/Glutamate Mesoporous Hollow Spheres. *Journal of Colloid and Interface Science*, *502*, 59–66. doi:10.1016/j.jcis.2017.04.085 PMID:28477470

Gupta, A. S., Kshirsagar, S. J., Bhalekar, M. R., & Saldanha, T. (2013). Design and development of liposomes for colon targeted drug delivery. *Journal of Drug Targeting*, *21*(2), 146–160. doi:10.3109/1061186X.2012.734311 PMID:23373543

Gupta, A., Eral, H. B., Hatton, T. A., & Doyle, P. S. (2016). Nanoemulsions: Formation, properties and applications. *Soft Matter*, *12*(11), 2826–2841. doi:10.1039/C5SM02958A PMID:26924445

Gupta, G., Arora, S., Singh, S., & Singh, N. (2014). Advances in magnetofection magnetically guided nucleic acid delivery: A review. *Journal of Pharmaceutical Technology. Research Management*, *1*, 19–29.

Gurka, M. K., Pender, D., Chuong, P., Fouts, B. L., Sobelov, A., McNally, M. W., ... McNally, L. R. (2016). Identification of pancreatic tumors in vivo with ligand-targeted, pH responsive mesoporous silica nanoparticles by multispectral optoacoustic tomography. *Journal of Controlled Release*, *231*, 60–67. doi:10.1016/j.jconrel.2015.12.055 PMID:26763377

Gurny, R., Peppas, N. A., Harrington, D., & Banker, G. S. (1981). Development of Biodegradable and Injectable Latices for Controlled Release of Potent Drugs. *Drug Development and Industrial Pharmacy*, *7*(1), 1–25. doi:10.3109/03639048109055684

Gutiérrez, L., Mejías, R., Barber, D. F., Veintemillas-Verdaguer, S., Serna, C. J., Lázaro, F. J., & Morales, M. P. (2012, February). Fighting cancer with magnetic nanoparticles and immunotherapy. In *SPIE BiOS* (pp. 82320X–82320X). International Society for Optics and Photonics. doi:10.1117/12.905890

Guven, B., Basaran-Akgul, N., Temur, E., Tamer, U., & Boyacı, İ. H. (2011). SERS-based sandwich immunoassay using antibody coated magnetic nanoparticles for Escherichia coli enumeration. *Analyst (London)*, *136*(4), 740–748. doi:10.1039/C0AN00473A PMID:21125089

Gu, W. X., Li, Q. L., Lu, H., Fang, L., Chen, Q., Yang, Y. W., & Gao, H. (2015). Construction of stable polymeric vesicles based on azobenzene and beta-cyclodextrin grafted poly(glycerol methacrylate)s for potential applications in colon-specific drug delivery. *Chemical Communications (Cambridge)*, *51*(22), 4715–4718. doi:10.1039/C5CC00628G PMID:25692460

Gu, Y., Guo, Y., Wang, C., Xu, J., Wu, J., Kirk, T. B., ... Xue, W. (2017). A polyamidoamne dendrimer functionalized graphene oxide for DOX and MMP-9 shRNA plasmid co-delivery. *Materials Science and Engineering C*, *70*(Pt 1), 572–585. doi:10.1016/j.msec.2016.09.035 PMID:27770930

Guy, R. H., & Hadgraft, J. (2003). *New York: Marcel Dekker, 2003. Transdermal Drug Delivery, Williams, A.* London: Pharmaceutical Press.

H, R.K. (2012). Solid Lipid Nanoparticle: A Review. *IOSR J Pharm.*, *2*(6), 2250–3013.

Hadjiargyrou, M., & Chiu, J. B. (2008). Enhanced composite electrospun nanofiber scaffolds for use in drug delivery. *Expert Opinion on Drug Delivery*, *5*(10), 1093–1106. doi:10.1517/17425247.5.10.1093 PMID:18817515

Hammond, P. T. (2016). Shooting for the moon: Nanoscale approaches to cancer. *ACS Nano*, *10*(2), 1711–1713. doi:10.1021/acsnano.6b01095 PMID:26902596

Haneef, J., & Chadha, R. (2017). Drug-Drug Multicomponent Solid Forms: Cocrystal, Coamorphous and Eutectic of Three Poorly Soluble Antihypertensive Drugs Using Mechanochemical Approach. *AAPS PharmSciTech*, 1–12. PMID:28101724

Han, M., Lv, Q., Tang, X.-J., Hu, Y.-L., Xu, D.-H., Li, F.-Z., ... Gao, J.-Q. (2012). Overcoming drug resistance of MCF-7/ADR cells by altering intracellular distribution of doxorubicin via MVP knockdown with a novel siRNA polyamidoamine-hyaluronic acid complex. *Journal of Controlled Release*, *163*(2), 136–144. doi:10.1016/j.jconrel.2012.08.020 PMID:22940126

Han, N., Wang, Y., Bai, J., Liu, J., Wang, Y., Gao, Y., ... Wang, S. (2016). Facile synthesis of the lipid bilayer coated mesoporous silica nanocomposites and their application in drug delivery. *Microporous and Mesoporous Materials*, *219*, 209–218. doi:10.1016/j.micromeso.2015.08.006

Hanna, E., Rémuzat, C., Auquier, P., & Toumi, M. (2016). Gene therapies development: Slow progress and promising prospect. *Journal of Market Access & Health Policy*, *5*(1), 1–9. PMID:28265348

Hansen, J., Neilsen, L. S., & Norling, T. (1999). Use of fatty acid esters as bioadhesive substances. *U.S. Patent 5955502A*.

Hansen, C. G., & Nichols, B. J. (2009). Molecular mechanisms of clathrin-independent endocytosis. *Journal of Cell Science*, *122*(11), 1713–1721. doi:10.1242/jcs.033951 PMID:19461071

Han, Y., Zhang, P., Chen, Y., Sun, J., & Kong, F. (2014). Co-delivery of plasmid DNA and doxorubicin by solid lipid nanoparticles for lung cancer therapy. *International Journal of Molecular Medicine*, *34*(1), 191–196. doi:10.3892/ijmm.2014.1770 PMID:24804644

Hao, N., Sun, C., Wu, Z., Xu, L., Gao, W., Cao, J., ... He, B. (2017). Fabrication of Polymeric Micelles with Aggregation-Induced Emission and Forster Resonance Energy Transfer for Anticancer Drug Delivery. *Bioconjugate Chemistry*, *28*(7), 1944–1954. doi:10.1021/acs.bioconjchem.7b00274 PMID:28570043

Hao, W., Shen, Y., Liu, D., Shang, Y., Zhang, J., Xu, S., & Liu, H. (2017). Dual-pH-sensitivity and tumour targeting core-shell particles for intracellular drug delivery. *RSC Advances*, *7*(2), 851–860. doi:10.1039/C6RA25224A

Hao, Y., & Teja, A. S. (2003). Continuous hydrothermal crystallization of α–Fe_2O_3 and Co_3O_4 nanoparticles. *Journal of Materials Research*, *18*(02), 415–422. doi:10.1557/JMR.2003.0053

Hardy, J. G., Wilson, C. G., & Wood, E. (1985). Drug delivery to the proximal colon. *The Journal of Pharmacy and Pharmacology*, *37*(12), 874–877. doi:10.1111/j.2042-7158.1985.tb04992.x PMID:2868094

Harisinghani, M. G., Barentsz, J., Hahn, P. F., Deserno, W. M., Tabatabaei, S., van de Kaa, C. H., ... Weissleder, R. (2003). Noninvasive detection of clinically occult lymph-node metastases in prostate cancer. *The New England Journal of Medicine*, *348*(25), 2491–2499. doi:10.1056/NEJMoa022749 PMID:12815134

Harms, M., & Müller-Goymann, C. C. (2011). Solid lipid nanoparticles for drug delivery. *Journal of Drug Delivery Science and Technology*, *21*(1), 89–99. doi:10.1016/S1773-2247(11)50008-5

Hartono, S. B., Hadisoewignyo, L., Yang, Y., Meka, A. K., Antaresti, & Yu, C. (2016). Amine functionalized cubic mesoporous silica nanoparticles as an oral delivery system for curcumin bioavailability enhancement. *Nanotechnology*, *27*(50), 505–605. doi:10.1088/0957-4484/27/50/505605 PMID:27875331

Harush-Frenkel, O., Debotton, N., Benita, S., & Altschuler, Y. (2007). Targeting of nanoparticles to the clathrin-mediated endocytic pathway. *Biochemical and Biophysical Research Communications*, *353*(1), 26–32. doi:10.1016/j.bbrc.2006.11.135 PMID:17184736

Hasan, W., Chu, K., Gullapalli, A., Dunn, S. S., Elizabeth, M., & Enlow. (2012). Nanoparticles for Treatment of Prostate Cancer. *Nano Letters*, *12*(1), 287–292. doi:10.1021/nl2035354 PMID:22165988

Hasany, S. F., Ahmed, I., Rajan, J., & Rehman, A. (2012). Systematic review of the preparation techniques of iron oxide magnetic nanoparticles. *Nanoscience and Nanotechnology*, *2*(6), 148–158. doi:10.5923/j.nn.20120206.01

Hassan, H. A., Smyth, L., Rubio, N., Ratnasothy, K., Wang, J. T. W., Bansal, S. S., ... Al-Jamal, K. T. (2016). Carbon nanotubes' surface chemistry determines their potency as vaccine nanocarriers *in vitro* and *in vivo*. *Journal of Controlled Release*, *225*, 205–216. doi:10.1016/j.jconrel.2016.01.030 PMID:26802552

Hassan, Y., Brewer, J., Alexander, J., & Jennings, R. (1996). Immune responses in mice induced by HSV-1 glycoproteins presented with ISCOMs or NISV delivery systems. *Vaccine*, *14*(17), 1581–1589. doi:10.1016/S0264-410X(96)00155-7 PMID:9032885

Hassanzadeh-Tabrizi, S. A., Bigham, A., & Rafienia, M. (2016). Surfactant-assisted sol–gel synthesis of forsterite nanoparticles as a novel drug delivery system. *Materials Science and Engineering C*, *58*, 737–741. doi:10.1016/j.msec.2015.09.020 PMID:26478366

Hasson, S. S. A. A., Al-Busaidi, J., & Sallam, T. A. (2015). The past, current and future trends in DNA vaccine immunisations. *Asian Pacific Journal of Tropical Biomedicine*, *5*(5), 344–353. doi:10.1016/S2221-1691(15)30366-X

Hauss, D. J. (2007). *Oral lipid-based formulations: enhancing the bioavailability of poorly water soluble drugs*. New York, NY: Informa Healthcare.

Hayward, S. L., Wilson, C. L., & Kidambi, S. (2016). Hyaluronic acid-conjugated liposome nanoparticles for targeted delivery to CD44 overexpressing glioblastoma cells. *Oncotarget*, *7*(23), 34158. doi:10.18632/oncotarget.8926 PMID:27120809

He Q & Shi J. (2014). MSN Anti-Cancer Nanomedicines: Chemotherapy Enhancement, Overcoming of Drug Resistance, and Metastasis Inhibition. *Advance Materials*.

He, B., Hu, H. Y., Tan, T., Wang, H., Sun, K. X., Li, Y. P. (2017). IR-780-loaded polymeric micelles enhance the efficacy of photothermal therapy in treating breast cancer lymphatic metastasis in mice. *Acta Pharmacol Sin*.

Head, K. A., & Jurenka, J. S. (2003). Inflammatory bowel disease Part 1: Ulcerative colitis--pathophysiology and conventional and alternative treatment options. *Alternative Medicine Review*, *8*(3), 247–283. PMID:12946238

Hegde, S. (2014). Effect of BaTiO3 Nanoparticle on Electro - Optical Properties of Polymer Dispersed Liquid Crystal Displays. *Journal of Crystallization Process and Technology, 4*, 60 - 63.

Hein, C. D., Liu, X. M., & Wang, D. (2008). Click chemistry, a powerful tool for pharmaceutical sciences. *Pharmaceutical Research*, *25*(10), 2216–2230. doi:10.100711095-008-9616-1 PMID:18509602

Hench, L. (1994). Bioactive ceramics: Theory and clinical applications. *Bioceramics*, *7*, 3–14. doi:10.1016/B978-0-08-042144-5.50005-4

Hench, L. L. (1991). Bioceramics: From concept to clinic. *Journal of the American Ceramic Society*, *74*(7), 1487–1510. doi:10.1111/j.1151-2916.1991.tb07132.x

Hench, L. L., & Polak, J. M. (2002). Third-generation biomedical materials. *Science*, *295*(5557), 1014–1017. doi:10.1126cience.1067404 PMID:11834817

Hench, L. L., Splinter, R. J., Allen, W. C., & Greenlee, T. K. (1971). Bonding mechanisms at the interface of ceramic prosthetic materials. *Journal of Biomedical Materials Research*, *5*(6), 117–141. doi:10.1002/jbm.820050611

He, Q., Ma, M., Wei, C., & Shi, J. (2012). Mesoporous carbon@silicon-silica nanotheranostics for synchronous delivery of insoluble drugs and luminescence imaging. *Biomaterials*, *33*(17), 4392–4402. doi:10.1016/j.biomaterials.2012.02.056 PMID:22425026

He, Q., & Shi, J. (2011). Mesoporous silica nanoparticle based nano drug delivery systems: Synthesis, controlled drug release and delivery, pharmacokinetics and biocompatibility. *Journal of Materials Chemistry*, *21*(16), 5845–5855. doi:10.1039/c0jm03851b

He, Q., Shi, J., Cui, X., Wei, C., Zhang, L., Wu, W., ... Wu, H. (2011). Synthesis of oxygen-deficient luminescent mesoporous silica nanoparticles for synchronous drug delivery and imaging. *Chemical Communications*, *47*(28), 7947–7949. doi:10.1039/c1cc11479d PMID:21499640

He, Q., Zhang, J., Chen, F., Guo, L., Zhu, Z., & Shi, J. (2010). An anti-ROS/hepatic fibrosis drug delivery system based on salvianolic acid B loaded mesoporous silica nanoparticles. *Biomaterials*, *31*(30), 7785–7796. doi:10.1016/j.biomaterials.2010.07.008 PMID:20674009

He, R., Cui, D., & Gao, F. (2009). Preparation of fluorescence ethosomes based on quantum dots and their skin scar penetration properties. *Materials Letters*, *63*(20), 1662–1664. doi:10.1016/j.matlet.2009.05.003

Hernandes, M. R. G., Moraes, L. C. A., Ribeiro, E. B., Fagundes, D. L. G., Honorio-França, A. C., & França, E. L. (2017). In vitro immunomodulatory effects of microemulsions with levamisole delivery systems on blood phagocytes interacting with Giardia lamblia. *Parasitology International*, *66*(3), 299–304. doi:10.1016/j.parint.2017.02.005 PMID:28257952

He, S., Lin, K. F., Fan, J. J., Hu, G., Dong, X., Zhao, Y. N., ... Liu, J. (2016). Synergistic Effect of Mesoporous Silica and Hydroxyapatite in Loaded Poly(DL-lactic-co-glycolic acid) Microspheres on the Regeneration of Bone Defects. *BioMed Research International*. PMID:27652269

Heurtault, B., Saulnier, P., Pech, B., Proust, J. E., & Benoit, J. P. (2002). A novel phase inversion-based process for the preparation of lipid nanocarriers. *Pharmaceutical Research*, *19*(6), 875–880. doi:10.1023/A:1016121319668 PMID:12134960

Hillaireau, H., & Couvreur, P. (2009). Nanocarriers' entry into the cell: Relevance to drug delivery. *Cellular and Molecular Life Sciences*, *66*(17), 2873–2896. doi:10.100700018-009-0053-z PMID:19499185

Hing, K. A. (1825). *Bone repair in the twenty-first century: Biology, chemistry or engineering?* Philos Trans A Math Phys. *Engineering and Science*, *2004*(362), 2821–2850.

Hinton, T. M., Grusche, F., Acharya, D., Shukla, R., Bansal, V., Waddington, L. J., ... Muir, B. W. (2014). Bicontinuous cubic phase nanoparticle lipid chemistry affects toxicity in cultured cells. *Toxicology Research*, *3*(1), 11–22. doi:10.1039/C3TX50075F

Hirota, K., & Terada, H. (2012). Endocytosis of particle formulations by macrophages and its application to clinical treatment. INTECH Open Access Publisher, 414-428.

Hirsjärvi, S., Belloche, C., Hindré, F., Garcion, E., & Benoit, J. P. (2014). Tumour targeting of lipid nanocapsules grafted with cRGD peptides. *European Journal of Pharmaceutics and Biopharmaceutics*, *87*(1), 152–159. doi:10.1016/j.ejpb.2013.12.006 PMID:24361535

Hirunpanich, V., & Sato, H. (2009). Improvement of cyclosporine A bioavailability by incorporating ethyl docosahexaenoate in the microemulsion as an oil excipient. *European Journal of Pharmaceutics and Biopharmaceutics*, *73*(2), 247–252. doi:10.1016/j.ejpb.2009.06.011 PMID:19560537

Hoffmann, F., Cornelius, M., Morell, J., & Fröba, M. (2006). Silica-Based Mesoporous Organic–Inorganic Hybrid Materials. *Angewandte Chemie International Edition*, *45*(20), 3216–3251. doi:10.1002/anie.200503075 PMID:16676373

Hoffmann, F., & Fröba, M. (2011). Vitalising porous inorganic silica networks with organic functions-PMOs and related hybrid materials. *Chemical Society Reviews*, *40*(2), 608–620. doi:10.1039/C0CS00076K PMID:21180714

Hong, C. Y., Li, X., & Pan, C. Y. (2009). Fabrication of smart nanocontainers with a mesoporous core and a pH-responsive shell for controlled uptake and release. *Journal of Materials Chemistry*, *19*(29), 5155–5160. doi:10.1039/b820534e

Hong, S., Leroueil, P. R., Majoros, I. J., Orr, B. G., Baker, J. R., & Holl, M. M. B. (2007). The binding avidity of a nanoparticle-based multivalent targeted drug delivery platform. *Chemistry & Biology*, *14*(1), 107–115. doi:10.1016/j.chembiol.2006.11.015 PMID:17254956

Honma, K., Ochiya, T., Nagahara, S., Sano, A., Yamamoto, H., Hirai, K., ... Terada, M. (2001). Atelocollagen-based gene transfer in cells allows high-throughput screening of gene functions. *Biochemical and Biophysical Research Communications*, *289*(5), 1075–1081. doi:10.1006/bbrc.2001.6133 PMID:11741301

Hook, E. R., Owen, O. J., Bellis, C. A., Holder, J. A., O'Sullivan, D. J., & Barbour, M. E. (2014). Development of a novel antimicrobial-releasing glass ionomer cement functionalized with chlorhexidine hexametaphosphate nanoparticles. *Journal of Nanobiotechnology*, *12*(1), 3. doi:10.1186/1477-3155-12-3 PMID:24456793

Horcajada, P., Rámila, A., Pérez-Pariente, J., & Vallet, M. (2004). Influence of pore size of MCM-41 matrices on drug delivery rate. *Microporous and Mesoporous Materials*, *68*(1-3), 105–109. doi:10.1016/j.micromeso.2003.12.012

Hortobagyi, G. N., Ueno, N. T., Xia, W., Zhang, S., Wolf, J. K., Putnam, J. B., ... Hung, M.-C. (2001). Cationic liposome-mediated E1A gene transfer to human breast and ovarian cancer cells and its biologic effects: A phase I clinical trial. *Journal of Clinical Oncology*, *19*(14), 3422–3433. doi:10.1200/JCO.2001.19.14.3422 PMID:11454891

Hosseini, M., Memari, Z., Ganjali, M. R., Khoobi, M., Faridbod, F., Shafiee, A., ... Hajinezhad, A. (2014). A novel mercury-sensitive fluorescent nano-chemosensor using new functionalized magnetic core-shell Fe3O4@ SiO2 nanoparticles. *International Journal of Environmental of Research*, *8*(4), 861–870.

Hou, Z., Li, C., Ma, P., Cheng, Z., Li, X., Zhang, X., ... Lin, J. (2012). Up-Conversion Luminescent and Porous NaYF 4:Yb 3 +, Er 3 + @SiO 2 Nanocomposite Fibers for Anti-Cancer Drug Delivery and Cell Imaging. *Advanced Functional Materials*, *22*(13), 2713–2722. doi:10.1002/adfm.201200082

Hsiao, S. M., Peng, B. Y., Tseng, Y. S., Liu, H. T., Chen, C. H., & Lin, H. M. (2017). Preparation and characterization of multifunctional mesoporous silica nanoparticles for dual magnetic resonance and fluorescence imaging in targeted cancer therapy. *Microporous and Mesoporous Materials*, *250*, 210–220. doi:10.1016/j.micromeso.2017.04.050

Huang, J., Peng, T., Li, Y., Zhan, Z., Zeng, Y., & Huang, Y., … Wu, C. (2017). Ocular cubosome drug delivery system for timolol maleate: Preparation, characterization, cytotoxicity, ex vivo, and in vivo evaluation. *AAPS PharmSciTech*. doi:10.120812249-017-0763-8

Huang, M., Fong, C.-W., Khor, E., & Lim, L.-Y. (2005). Transfection efficiency of chitosan vectors: Effect of polymer molecular weight and degree of deacetylation. *Journal of Controlled Release*, *106*(3), 391–406. doi:10.1016/j.jconrel.2005.05.004 PMID:15967533

Huang, P., Li, Z., Lin, J., Yang, D., Gao, G., Xu, C., ... Hu, H. (2011). Photosensitizer-conjugated magnetic nanoparticles for in vivo simultaneous magnetofluorescent imaging and targeting therapy. *Biomaterials*, *32*(13), 3447–3458. doi:10.1016/j.biomaterials.2011.01.032 PMID:21303717

Huang, Q., Bao, C., Lin, Y., Chen, J., Liu, Z., & Zhu, L. (2013). Disulfide-phenylazide: A reductively cleavable photoreactive linker for facile modification of nanoparticle surfaces. *Journal of Materials Chemistry. B, Materials for Biology and Medicine*, *1*(8), 1125–1132. doi:10.1039/c2tb00420h

Huang, S.-L. (2008). Liposomes in ultrasonic drug and gene delivery. *Advanced Drug Delivery Reviews*, *60*(10), 1167–1176. doi:10.1016/j.addr.2008.03.003 PMID:18479776

Huang, X., Li, L., Liu, T., Hao, N., Liu, H., Chen, D., & Tang, F. (2011). The Shape Effect of Mesoporous Silica Nanoparticles on Biodistribution, Clearance, and Biocompatibility in Vivo. *ACS Nano*, *5*(7), 5390–5399. doi:10.1021/nn200365a PMID:21634407

Huang, X., Qi, X., Boey, F., & Zhang, H. (2012). Graphene-based composites. *Chemical Society Reviews*, *41*(2), 666–686. doi:10.1039/C1CS15078B PMID:21796314

Huang, X., Teng, X., Chen, D., Tang, F., & He, J. (2010). The effect of the shape of mesoporous silica nanoparticles on cellular uptake and cell function. *Biomaterials*, *31*(3), 438–448. doi:10.1016/j.biomaterials.2009.09.060 PMID:19800115

Huang, Y., Liu, X., Dong, L., Liu, Z., He, X., & Liu, W. (2011). Development of viral vectors for gene therapy for chronic pain. *Pain Research and Treatment*, *2011*, 1–8. doi:10.1155/2011/968218 PMID:22110937

Hua, S., & Wu, S. Y. (2013). The use of lipid-based nanocarriers for targeted pain therapies. *Frontiers in Pharmacology*, *4*, 143. doi:10.3389/fphar.2013.00143 PMID:24319430

Hu, C. J., Kaushal, S., Cao, H. S. T., Aryal, S., Sartor, M., Esener, S., ... Zhang, L. (2010). Half-Antibody Functionalized Lipid - Polymer Hybrid Nanoparticles for Targeted Drug Delivery to Carcinoembryonic Antigen Presenting Pancreatic Cancer Cells. *Molecular Pharmaceutics*, *7*(3), 914–920. doi:10.1021/mp900316a PMID:20394436

Hudson, S. P., Padera, R. F., Langer, R., & Kohane, D. S. (2008). The biocompatibility of mesoporous silicates. *Biomaterials*, *29*(30), 4045–4055. doi:10.1016/j.biomaterials.2008.07.007 PMID:18675454

Hughes, S., El Haj, A. J., & Dobson, J. (2005). Magnetic micro-and nanoparticle mediated activation of mechanosensitive ion channels. *Medical Engineering & Physics*, *27*(9), 754–762. doi:10.1016/j.medengphy.2005.04.006 PMID:15985383

Huh, S., Chen, H. T., Wiench, J. W., Pruski, M., & Lin, V. S.-Y. (2005). Cooperative catalysis by general acid and base bifunctionalized mesoporous silica nanospheres. *Angewandte Chemie International Edition in English*, *44*(12), 1826–1830. doi:10.1002/anie.200462424 PMID:15712306

Huh, S., Wiench, J. W., Trewyn, B. G., Song, S., Pruski, M., & Lin, V. S. Y. (2003a). Tuning of particle morphology and pore properties in mesoporous silicas with multiple organic functional groups. *Chemical Communications*, (18), 2364–2365. doi:10.1039/b306255d PMID:14518916

Huh, S., Wiench, J. W., Yoo, J. C., Pruski, M., & Lin, V. S. Y. (2003b). Organic Functionalization and Morphology Control of Mesoporous Silicas via a Co-Condensation Synthesis Method. *Chemistry of Materials*, *15*(22), 4247–4256. doi:10.1021/cm0210041

Hui, K., Ang, P. T., Huang, L., & Tay, S. K. (1997). Phase I study of immunotherapy of cutaneous metastases of human carcinoma using allogeneic and xenogeneic MHC DNA-liposome complexes. *Gene Therapy*, *4*(8), 783–790. doi:10.1038j.gt.3300455 PMID:9338006

Hu, J. J., Liu, L. H., Li, Z. Y., Zhuo, R. X., & Zhang, X. Z. (2016). MMP-responsive theranostic nanoplatform based on mesoporous silica nanoparticles for tumor imaging and targeted drug delivery. *Journal of Materials Chemistry. B, Materials for Biology and Medicine*, *4*(11), 1932–1940. doi:10.1039/C5TB02490K

Hu, L., Tang, X., & Cui, F. (2004). Solid lipid nanoparticles (SLNs) to improve oral bioavailability of poorly soluble drugs. *The Journal of Pharmacy and Pharmacology*, *56*(12), 1527–1535. doi:10.1211/0022357044959 PMID:15563759

Hu-Lieskovan, S., Heidel, J. D., Bartlett, D. W., Davis, M. E., & Triche, T. J. (2005). Sequence-specific knockdown of EWS-FLI1 by targeted, nonviral delivery of small interfering RNA inhibits tumor growth in a murine model of metastatic Ewing's sarcoma. *Cancer Research*, *65*(19), 8984–8992. doi:10.1158/0008-5472.CAN-05-0565 PMID:16204072

Humberstone, A. J., & Charman, W. N. (1997). Lipid-based vehicles for the oral delivery of poorly water soluble drugs. *Advanced Drug Delivery Reviews*, *25*(1), 103–128. doi:10.1016/S0169-409X(96)00494-2

Hung, M.-C., Chang, J. Y., & Xing, X. (1998). Preclinical and clinical study of HER-2/neu-targeting cancer gene therapy. *Advanced Drug Delivery Reviews*, *30*(1), 219–227. doi:10.1016/S0169-409X(97)00118-X PMID:10837613

Hunt, J. N., & Knox, M. T. (1968). A relation between the chain length of fatty acids and the slowing of gastric emptying. *The Journal of Physiology*, *194*(2), 327–336. doi:10.1113/jphysiol.1968.sp008411 PMID:5639357

Hu, S. H., Chen, Y. W., Hung, W. T., Chen, I. W., & Chen, S. Y. (2012). Quantum-dot-tagged reduced graphene oxide nanocomposites for bright fluorescence bioimaging and photothermal therapy monitored in situ. *Advanced Materials*, *24*(13), 1748–1754. doi:10.1002/adma.201104070 PMID:22422734

Hu, S. H., Liu, T. Y., Liu, D. M., & Chen, S. Y. (2007). Nanoferrosponges for controlled drug release. *Journal of Controlled Release*, *121*(3), 181–189. doi:10.1016/j.jconrel.2007.06.002 PMID:17644206

Hussain, S. M., & Krestin, G. P. (2001). Superparamagnetic iron oxide contrast agents: Physicochemical characteristics and application in MR imaging. *European Journal of Radiology*, *11*(11), 2319–2331. doi:10.1007003300100908

Huwyler, J., Drewe, J., & Krähenbühl, S. (2008). Tumor targeting using liposomal antineoplastic drugs. *International Journal of Nanomedicine*, *3*(1), 21–29. doi:10.2147/IJN.S1253 PMID:18488413

Hu, Y., Meng, L., Niu, L., & Lu, Q. (2013). Facile synthesis of superparamagnetic Fe3O4@ polyphosphazene@ Au shells for magnetic resonance imaging and photothermal therapy. *ACS Applied Materials & Interfaces*, *5*(11), 4586–4591. doi:10.1021/am400843d PMID:23659588

Huynh, N. T., Passirani, C., Saulnier, P., & Benoît, J. P. (2009). Lipid nanocapsules: A new platform for nanomedicine. *International Journal of Pharmaceutics*, *379*(2), 201–209. doi:10.1016/j.ijpharm.2009.04.026 PMID:19409468

Hyeon, T. (2003). Chemical synthesis of magnetic nanoparticles. *Chemical Communications*, (8): 927–934. doi:10.1039/b207789b PMID:12744306

Ibanez, M., Santiago, R., Wong, C., Baeza, I., Gariglio, P., & Chávez, P. (1996). Spermidine-condensed DNA and cone-shaped lipids improve delivery and expression of exogenous DNA transfer by liposomes. *Biochemistry and Cell Biology*, *74*(5), 633–643. doi:10.1139/o96-068 PMID:9018370

Ibraheem, D., Elaissari, A., & Fessi, H. (2014). Gene therapy and DNA delivery systems. *International Journal of Pharmaceutics*, *459*(1), 70–83. doi:10.1016/j.ijpharm.2013.11.041 PMID:24286924

Ilbasmis-Tamer, S., Unsal, H., Tugcu-Demiroz, F., Kalaycioglu, G. D., Degim, I. T., & Aydogan, N. (2016). Stimuli-responsive lipid nanotubes in gel formulations for the delivery of doxorubicin. *Colloids and Surfaces. B, Biointerfaces*, *143*, 406–414. doi:10.1016/j.colsurfb.2016.03.070 PMID:27037777

Ilie, N., & Hickel, R. (2011). Resin composite restorative materials. *Australian Dental Journal*, *56*, 59–66. doi:10.1111/j.1834-7819.2010.01296.x PMID:21564116

Illum, L. (1998). Chitosan and its use as a pharmaceutical excipient. *Pharmaceutical Research*, *15*(9), 1326–1331. doi:10.1023/A:1011929016601 PMID:9755881

Indena. (2017). *Phytosome*. Retrieved June 26, 2017, from https://www.phytosome.info/

Ionov, M., Lazniewska, J., Dzmitruk, V., Halets, I., Loznikova, S., Novopashina, D., ... Bryszewska, M. (2015). Anticancer siRNA cocktails as a novel tool to treat cancer cells. Part (A). Mechanisms of interaction. *International Journal of Pharmaceutics*, *485*(1), 261–269. doi:10.1016/j.ijpharm.2015.03.024 PMID:25791760

Iqbal, J., & Hussain, M. M. (2009). Intestinal lipid absorption. *American Journal of Physiology. Endocrinology and Metabolism*, *296*(6), E1183–E1194. doi:10.1152/ajpendo.90899.2008 PMID:19158321

Irani, M., Sadeghi, G. M. M., & Haririan, I. (2017). The sustained delivery of temozolomide from electrospun PCL-Diol-b-PU/gold nanocompsite nanofibers to treat glioblastoma tumors. *Materials Science and Engineering C*, *75*, 165–174. doi:10.1016/j.msec.2017.02.029 PMID:28415451

Irby, D., Du, C., & Li, F. (2017). Lipid-drug conjugate for enhancing drug delivery. *Molecular Pharmaceutics*, *14*(5), 1325–1338. doi:10.1021/acs.molpharmaceut.6b01027 PMID:28080053

Irie, M., Suzuki, K., & Watts, D. C. (2002). Marginal gap formation of light-activated restorative materials: Effects of immediate setting shrinkage and bond strength. *Dental Materials*, *18*(3), 203–210. doi:10.1016/S0109-5641(01)00083-5 PMID:11823011

Islam, M. A., Firdous, J., Choi, Y. J., Yun, C. H., & Cho, C. S. (2012). Design and application of chitosan microspheres as oral and nasal vaccine carriers: An updated review. *International Journal of Nanomedicine*, *7*, 6077–6093. PMID:23271909

Issa, B., Obaidat, I. M., Albiss, B. A., & Haik, Y. (2013). Magnetic nanoparticles: Surface effects and properties related to biomedicine applications. *International Journal of Molecular Sciences*, *14*(11), 21266–21305. doi:10.3390/ijms141121266 PMID:24232575

Issa, N., Karamertzanis, P. G., Welch, G. W., & Price, S. L. (2008). Can the formation of pharmaceutical cocrystals be computationally predicted? I. Comparison of lattice energies. *Crystal Growth & Design*, *9*(1), 442–453. doi:10.1021/cg800685z

Ito, A., & Honda, H. (2006). Magnetic nanoparticles for tissue engineering. In *Nanotechnologies for the Life Sciences*. Wiley-VCH Verlag GmbH & Co. KGaA.

Itoh, K., Hirayama, T., Takahashi, A., Kubo, W., Miyazaki, S., Dairaku, M., ... Attwood, D. (2007). In situ gelling pectin formulations for oral drug delivery at high gastric pH. *International Journal of Pharmaceutics*, *335*(1), 90–96. doi:10.1016/j.ijpharm.2006.10.042 PMID:17141988

Itokazu, M., Yang, W., Aoki, T., Hara, A. O., & Kato, N. (1998). Synthesis of antibiotic-loaded interporous hydroxyapatite blocks by vacuum method and in vitro drug release testing. *Biomaterials*, *19*(7-9), 817–819. doi:10.1016/S0142-9612(97)00237-8 PMID:9663758

Ito, Y., Kusawake, T., Ishida, M., Tawa, R., Shibata, N., & Takada, K. (2005). Oral solid gentamicin preparation using emulsifier and adsorbent. *Journal of Controlled Release*, *105*(1-2), 23–31. doi:10.1016/j.jconrel.2005.03.017 PMID:15908031

Iversen, T. G., Skotland, T., & Sandvig, K. (2011). Endocytosis and intracellular transport of nanoparticles: Present knowledge and need for future studies. *Nano Today*, *6*(2), 176–185. doi:10.1016/j.nantod.2011.02.003

Iwai, S., Sawa, Y., Ichikawa, H., Taketani, S., Uchimura, E., Chen, G., ... Matsuda, H. (2004). Biodegradable polymer with collagen microsponge serves as a new bioengineered cardiovascular prosthesis. *The Journal of Thoracic and Cardiovascular Surgery*, *128*(3), 472–479. doi:10.1016/j.jtcvs.2004.04.013 PMID:15354111

Iyer, A. K., Khaled, G., Fang, J., & Maeda, H. (2006). Exploiting the enhanced permeability and retention effect for tumor targeting. *Drug Discovery Today*, *11*(17-18), 812–818. doi:10.1016/j.drudis.2006.07.005 PMID:16935749

Izadi, Z., Divsalar, A., Saboury, A. A., & Sawyer, L. (2016). beta-lactoglobulin-pectin Nanoparticle-based Oral Drug Delivery System for Potential Treatment of Colon Cancer. *Chemical Biology & Drug Design*, *88*(2), 209–216. doi:10.1111/cbdd.12748 PMID:26896377

Jadhav, S. A., Brunella, D. S. V., Ugazio, E., Sapino, S., & Berlier, G. (2017a). Thermoresponsive copolymer-grafted SBA-15 porous silica particles for temperature-triggered topical delivery systems. *Express Polymer Letters*, *11*(2), 96–105. doi:10.3144/expresspolymlett.2017.11

Jadhav, S. A., Brunella, V., Scalarone, D., & Berlier, G. (2017b). Poly(NIPAM-co-MPS)-grafted multimodal porous silica nanoparticles as reverse thermoresponsive drug delivery system. *Asian Journal of Pharmaceutical Sciences*, *12*(3), 279–284. doi:10.1016/j.ajps.2017.02.002

Jäger, M., Schubert, S., Ochrimenko, S., Fischer, D., & Schubert, U. S. (2012). Branched and linear poly(ethylene imine)-based conjugates: Synthetic modification, characterization, and application. *Chemical Society Reviews*, *41*(13), 4755–4767. doi:10.1039/c2cs35146c PMID:22648524

Jaidev, L., Chellappan, D. R., Bhavsar, D. V., Ranganathan, R., Sivanantham, B., Subramanian, A., ... Sethuraman, S. (2017). Multi-functional nanoparticles as theranostic agents for the treatment & imaging of pancreatic cancer. *Acta Biomaterialia*, *49*, 422–433. doi:10.1016/j.actbio.2016.11.053 PMID:27890622

Jain, A. (2014). Cationic Polysaccharides in Gene Delivery. In Cationic Polymers in Regenerative Medicine. Royal Society of Chemistry.

Jain, A. (2015). Cationic Polymers for the Delivery of Therapeutic Nucleotides. *Polysaccharides: Bioactivity and Biotechnology*, 1969-1990.

Jain, A. K., Dubey, V., Mehra, N. K., Lodhi, N., Nahar, M., Mishra, D. K., & Jain, N. K. (2009). Carbohydrate-conjugated multiwalled carbon nanotubes: Development and characterization. *Nanomedicine; Nanotechnology, Biology, and Medicine*, *5*(4), 432–442. doi:10.1016/j.nano.2009.03.001 PMID:19341818

Jain, A., Gulbake, A., Jain, A., Shilpi, S., Hurkat, P., & Jain, S. K. (2013). Dual drug delivery using "smart" liposomes for triggered release of anticancer agents. *Journal of Nanoparticle Research*, *15*(7), 1–12. doi:10.100711051-013-1772-5

Jain, A., Gupta, Y., & Jain, S. K. (2007). Perspectives of biodegradable natural polysaccharides for site-specific drug delivery to the colon. *Journal of Pharmacy & Pharmaceutical Sciences*, *10*(1), 86–128. PMID:17498397

Jain, A., & Jain, S. K. (2015). Colon Targeted Liposomal Systems (CTLS): Theranostic Potential. *Current Molecular Medicine*, *15*(7), 621–633. doi:10.2174/1566524015666150831131320 PMID:26321756

Jain, A., & Jain, S. K. (2016a). Liposomes in Cancer Therapy. In *Nanocarrier Systems for Drug Delivery* (pp. 1–42). Nova Science Publishers. Retrieved from https://www.novapublishers.com/catalog/product_info.php?products_id=59761&osCsid=e7d370318f328e75748328a1e44e48aa

Jain, A., & Jain, S. K. (2016b). Multipronged, strategic delivery of paclitaxel-topotecan using engineered liposomes to ovarian cancer. *Drug Development and Industrial Pharmacy*, *42*(1), 136–149. doi:10.3109/03639045.2015.1036066 PMID:26006330

Jain, A., Jain, S. K., Ganesh, N., Barve, J., & Beg, A. M. (2010). Design and development of ligand-appended polysaccharidic nanoparticles for the delivery of oxaliplatin in colorectal cancer. *Nanomedicine (London)*, *6*(1), 179–190. doi:10.1016/j.nano.2009.03.002 PMID:19447205

Jain, H., Khomane, K. S., & Bansal, A. K. (2014). Implication of microstructure on the mechanical behaviour of an aspirin–paracetamol eutectic mixture. *CrystEngComm*, *16*(36), 8471–8478. doi:10.1039/C4CE00878B

Jain, J., Fernandes, C., & Patravale, V. (2010). Formulation development of parenteral phospholipid-based microemulsion of etoposide. *AAPS PharmSciTech*, *11*(2), 826–831. doi:10.120812249-010-9440-x PMID:20464537

Jain, R. K., & Stylianopoulos, T. (2010). Delivering nanomedicine to solid tumors. *Nature Reviews. Clinical Oncology*, *7*(11), 653–664. doi:10.1038/nrclinonc.2010.139 PMID:20838415

Jain, S. A., Basu, H., Prabhu, P. S., Soni, U., Joshi, M. D., Mathur, D., ... Sharma, S. (2014). Parasite impairment by targeting Plasmodium-infected RBCs using glyceryl-dilaurate nanostructured lipid carriers. *Biomaterials*, *35*(24), 6636–6645. doi:10.1016/j.biomaterials.2014.04.058 PMID:24818881

Jain, S., Garg, T., Kushwah, V., Thanki, K., Agrawal, A. K., & Dora, C. P. (2017). 1.α-Tocopherol as functional excipient for resveratrol and coenzyme Q10-loaded SNEDDS for improved bioavailability and prophylaxis of breast cancer. *Journal of Drug Targeting*, *25*(6), 554–565. doi:10.1080/1061186X.2017.1298603 PMID:28274130

Jain, S., Khomane, K., Jain, A. K., & Dani, P. (2011). Nanocarriers for transmucosal vaccine delivery. *Current Nanoscience*, *7*, 160–177. doi:10.2174/157341311794653541

Jain, V., Jain, D., & Singh, R. (2010). Factors affecting the morphology of Eudragit RS100 based microsponges bearing dicyclomine for colonic delivery. *Journal of Pharmaceutical Sciences*, *100*(4), 1–8. PMID:20960455

Jain, V., & Singh, R. (2010). Development and characterization of Eudragit RS 100 loaded microsponges and its colonic delivery using natural polysaccharides. *Acta Poloniae Pharma-Drug Research*, *67*, 407–415. PMID:20635537

Jain, V., & Singh, R. (2010). Dicyclomine loaded Eudragit based microsponge with potential for colonic delivery: Preparation and characterization. *Tropical Journal of Pharmaceutical Research*, *9*(1), 67–72. doi:10.4314/tjpr.v9i1.52039

Jambhekar, S. S., & Breen, P. (2016). Cyclodextrins in pharmaceutical formulations I: Structure and physicochemical properties, formation of complexes, and types of complex. *Drug Discovery Today*, *21*(2), 356–362. doi:10.1016/j.drudis.2015.11.017 PMID:26686054

Jambhrunkar, S., Qu, Z., Popat, A., Karmakar, S., Xu, C., & Yu, C. (2014). Modulating in vitro release and solubility of griseofulvin using functionalized mesoporous silica nanoparticles. *Journal of Colloid and Interface Science*, *434*, 218–225. doi:10.1016/j.jcis.2014.08.019 PMID:25203914

James, K. C., & Gaharwar, A. K. (2014). Bioinspired Polymeric Nanocomposites for Regenerative Medicine. *Macromolecular Chemistry and Physics*, *216*, 248–264.

Janát-Amsbury, M. M., Yockman, J. W., Lee, M., Kern, S., Furgeson, D. Y., Bikram, M., & Kim, S. W. (2004). Combination of local, nonviral IL12 gene therapy and systemic paclitaxel treatment in a metastatic breast cancer model. *Molecular Therapy*, *9*(6), 829–836. doi:10.1016/j.ymthe.2004.03.015 PMID:15194049

Janib, S. M., Moses, A. S., & MacKay, J. A. (2010). Imaging and drug delivery using theranostic nanoparticles. *Advanced Drug Delivery Reviews*, *62*(11), 1052–1063. doi:10.1016/j.addr.2010.08.004 PMID:20709124

Jannin, V., Musakhanian, J., & Marchaud, D. (2008). Approaches for the development of solid and semi-solid lipid-based formulations. *Advanced Drug Delivery Reviews*, *60*(6), 734–746. doi:10.1016/j.addr.2007.09.006 PMID:18045728

Jaque, D., Maestro, L. M., Del Rosal, B., Haro-Gonzalez, P., Benayas, A., Plaza, J. L., ... Sole, J. G. (2014). Nanoparticles for photothermal therapies. *Nanoscale*, *6*(16), 9494–9530. doi:10.1039/C4NR00708E PMID:25030381

Jaspart, S., Bertholet, P., Piel, G., Dogné, J. M., Delattre, L., & Evrard, B. (2007). Solid lipid microparticles as a sustained release system for pulmonary drug delivery. *European Journal of Pharmaceutics and Biopharmaceutics*, *65*(1), 47–56. doi:10.1016/j.ejpb.2006.07.006 PMID:16962749

Javadi, M., Pitt, W. G., Belnap, D. M., Tsosie, N. H., & Hartley, J. M. (2012). Encapsulating nanoemulsions inside eLiposomes for ultrasonic drug delivery. *Langmuir*, *28*(41), 14720–14729. doi:10.1021/la303464v PMID:22989347

Jayabalan, M., Shalumon, K. T., Mitha, M. K., Ganesan, K., & Epple, M. (2010). Effect of hydroxyapatite on the biodegradation and biomechanical stability of polyester nanocomposites for orthopaedic applications. *Acta Biomaterialia*, *6*(3), 763–775. doi:10.1016/j.actbio.2009.09.015 PMID:19788944

Jayakody, L., & Hoover, R. (2008). Effect of annealing on the molecular structure and physicochemical properties of starches from different botanical origins–A review. *Carbohydrate Polymers*, *74*(3), 691–703. doi:10.1016/j.carbpol.2008.04.032

Jeevanandam, J., Chan, Y. S., & Danquah, M. K. (2016). Nano-formulations of drugs: Recent developments, impact and challenges. *Biochimie*, *128-129*, 99–112. doi:10.1016/j.biochi.2016.07.008 PMID:27436182

Jelvehgari, M., Siahi-Shadbad, M. R., Azarmi, S., Martin, G. P., & Nokhodchi, A. (2006). The microsponge delivery system of benzoyl peroxide: Preparation, characterization and release studies. *International Journal of Pharmaceutics*, *308*(1-2), 124–132. doi:10.1016/j.ijpharm.2005.11.001 PMID:16359833

Jensen, K. T., Blaabjerg, L. I., Lenz, E., Bohr, A., Grohganz, H., Kleinebudde, P., ... Lobmann, K. (2016). Preparation and characterization of spray-dried co-amorphous drug–amino acid salts. *The Journal of Pharmacy and Pharmacology*, *68*(5), 615–624. doi:10.1111/jphp.12458 PMID:26245703

Jeong, E. H., Jung, G., Hong, C. A., & Lee, H. (2014). Gold nanoparticle (AuNP)-based drug delivery and molecular imaging for biomedical applications. *Archives of Pharmacal Research*, *37*(1), 53–59. doi:10.100712272-013-0273-5 PMID:24214174

Jhaveri, A., & Torchilin, V. (2016). Intracellular delivery of nanocarriers and targeting to subcellular organelles. *Expert Opinion on Drug Delivery*, *13*(1), 49–70. doi:10.1517/17425247.2015.1086745 PMID:26358656

Jia, L., Li, Z., Shen, J., Zheng, D., Tian, X., Guo, H., & Chang, P. (2015). Multifunctional mesoporous silica nanoparticles mediated co-delivery of paclitaxel and tetrandrine for overcoming multidrug resistance. *International Journal of Pharmaceutics*, *489*(1-2), 318–330. doi:10.1016/j.ijpharm.2015.05.010 PMID:25956050

Jia, L., Shen, J., Li, Z., Zhang, D., Zhang, Q., Duan, C., ... Tian, X. (2012). Successfully tailoring the pore size of mesoporous silica nanoparticles: Exploitation of delivery systems for poorly water-soluble drugs. *International Journal of Pharmaceutics*, *439*(1-2), 81–91. doi:10.1016/j.ijpharm.2012.10.011 PMID:23078857

Jia, L., Shen, J., Li, Z., Zhang, D., Zhang, Q., Liu, G., ... Tian, X. (2013). In vitro and in vivo evaluation of paclitaxel-loaded mesoporous silica nanoparticles with three pore sizes. *International Journal of Pharmaceutics*, *445*(1-2), 12–19. doi:10.1016/j.ijpharm.2013.01.058 PMID:23384728

Jiang, H., Kwon, J.-T., Kim, Y.-K., Kim, E.-M., Arote, R., Jeong, H.-J., ... Cho, C.-S. (2007). Galactosylated chitosan-graft-polyethylenimine as a gene carrier for hepatocyte targeting. *Gene Therapy*, *14*(19), 1389–1398. doi:10.1038j.gt.3302997 PMID:17637795

Jiang, J., Yang, S., Wang, J., Yang, L., Xu, Z., Yang, T., ... Zhang, Q. (2010). Sequential treatment of drug-resistant tumors with RGD-modified liposomes containing siRNA or doxorubicin. *European Journal of Pharmaceutics and Biopharmaceutics*, *76*(2), 170–178. doi:10.1016/j.ejpb.2010.06.011 PMID:20600887

Jiang, L., Huang, Y., Zhang, Q., He, H., Xu, Y., & Mei, X. (2014). Preparation and solid-state characterization of dapsone drug–drug co-crystals. *Crystal Growth & Design*, *14*(9), 4562–4573. doi:10.1021/cg500668a

Jiang, W., Kim, B. Y., Rutka, J. T., & Chan, W. C. (2008). Nanoparticle-mediated cellular response is size-dependent. *Nature Nanotechnology*, *3*(3), 145–150. doi:10.1038/nnano.2008.30 PMID:18654486

Jiao, J., Liu, C., Li, X., Liu, J., Di, D., Zhang, Y., ... Wang, S. (2016b). Fluorescent carbon dot modified mesoporous silica nanocarriers for redox-responsive controlled drug delivery and bioimaging. *Journal of Colloid and Interface Science*, *483*, 343–352. doi:10.1016/j.jcis.2016.08.033 PMID:27569517

Jiao, J., Li, X., Zhang, S., Liu, J., Di, D., Zhang, Y., ... Wang, S. (2016a). Redox and pH dual-responsive PEG and chitosan-conjugated hollow mesoporous silica for controlled drug release. *Materials Science and Engineering C*, *67*, 26–33. doi:10.1016/j.msec.2016.04.091 PMID:27287095

Jin, H., Zhao, G., Hu, J., Ren, Q., Yang, K., Wan, C., ... Zou, Z. (2017). Melittin-Containing Hybrid Peptide Hydrogels for Enhanced Photothermal Therapy of Glioblastoma. *ACS Applied Materials & Interfaces*, *9*(31), 25755–25766. doi:10.1021/acsami.7b06431 PMID:28714303

Jin, L., Zeng, X., Liu, M., Deng, Y., & He, N. (2014). Current progress in gene delivery technology based on chemical methods and nano-carriers. *Theranostics*, *4*(3), 240–255. doi:10.7150/thno.6914 PMID:24505233

Jin, Y., Zhang, N., Li, C., Pu, K., Ding, C., & Zhu, Y. (2017). Nanosystem composed with MSNs, gadolinium, liposome and cytotoxic peptides for tumor theranostics. *Colloids and Surfaces. B, Biointerfaces*, *151*, 240–248. doi:10.1016/j.colsurfb.2016.12.024 PMID:28024200

Jo, J. H., Lee, E.-J., Shin, D.-S., Kim, H.-E., Kim, H.-W., Koh, Y.-H., & Jang, J.-H. (2009). In vitro/in vivo biocompatibility and mechanical properties of bioactive glass nanofiber and poly (ε-caprolactone) composite materials. *Journal of Biomedical Materials Research. Part B, Applied Biomaterials*, *91*(1), 213–220. doi:10.1002/jbm.b.31392 PMID:19422050

Joseyphus, R. J., Kodama, D., Matsumoto, T., Sato, Y., Jeyadevan, B., & Tohji, K. (2007). Role of polyol in the synthesis of Fe particles. *Journal of Magnetism and Magnetic Materials*, *310*(2), 2393–2395. doi:10.1016/j.jmmm.2006.10.1132

Joshi, R. P., Negi, G., Kumar, A., Pawar, Y. B., Munjal, B., Bansal, A. K., & Sharma, S. S. (2013). SNEDDS curcumin formulation leads to enhanced protection from pain and functional deficits associated with diabetic neuropathy: An insight into its mechanism for neuroprotection. *Nanomedicine (London)*, *9*(6), 776–785. doi:10.1016/j.nano.2013.01.001 PMID:23347896

Jung, S.-M., Yoon, G. H., Lee, H. C., & Shin, H. S. (2015). Chitosan nanoparticle/PCL nanofiber composite for wound dressing and drug delivery. *Journal of Biomaterials Science. Polymer Edition*, *26*(4), 252–263. doi:10.1080/09205063.2014.996699 PMID:25573454

Juškaitė, V., Ramanauskienė, K., & Briedis, V. (2017). Testing of resveratrol microemulsion photostability and protective effect against UV induced oxidative stress. *Acta Pharmaceutica (Zagreb, Croatia)*, *67*(2), 247–256. doi:10.1515/acph-2017-0018 PMID:28590913

Jyoti, W., Anroop, N., & Rachna, K. (2012). Emulsion forming drug delivery system for lipophilic drugs. *Acta Pol. Pharm. Drug Res.*, *69*(2), 179–191. PMID:22568032

Kadlecova, Z., Rajendra, Y., Matasci, M., Hacker, D., Baldi, L., Wurm, F. M., & Klok, H.-A. (2012). Hyperbranched polylysine: A versatile, biodegradable transfection agent for the production of recombinant proteins by transient gene expression and the transfection of primary cells. *Macromolecular Bioscience*, *12*(6), 794–804. doi:10.1002/mabi.201100519 PMID:22496075

Kagadis, G. C., Ford, N. L., Karnabatidis, D. N., & Loudos, G. K. (Eds.). (2016). *Handbook of Small Animal Imaging: Preclinical Imaging, Therapy, and Applications*. CRC Press. doi:10.1201/b19052

Kaity, S., Maiti, S., Ghosh, A. K., Pal, D., Ghosh, A., & Banerjee, S. (2010). Microsponges: A novel strategy for drug delivery system. *Journal of Advanced Pharmaceutical Technology & Research*, *1*(3), 283–290. doi:10.4103/0110-5558.72416 PMID:22247859

Kalam, M. A., Khan, A. A., & Alshamsan, A. (2017). Non-invasive administration of biodegradable nano-carrier vaccines. *American Journal of Translational Research*, *9*(1), 15–35. PMID:28123631

Kalepu, S., Manthina, M., & Padavala, V. (2013). Oral lipid-based drug delivery systems – an overview. *Acta Pharmaceutica Sinica. B*, *3*(6), 361–372. doi:10.1016/j.apsb.2013.10.001

Kamarudin, N. H. N., Jalil, A. A., Triwahyono, S., Salleh, N. F. M., Karim, A. H., Mukti, R. R., ... Ahmad, A. (2013). Role of 3-aminopropyltriethoxysilane in the preparation of mesoporous silica nanoparticles for ibuprofen delivery: Effect on physicochemical properties. *Microporous and Mesoporous Materials*, *180*, 235–241. doi:10.1016/j.micromeso.2013.06.041

Kam, N. W. S., Liu, Z., & Dai, H. (2005). Functionalization of Carbon Nanotubes via Cleavable Disulfide Bonds for Efficient Intracellular Delivery of siRNA and Potent Gene Silencing. *Journal of the American Chemical Society*, *127*(36), 12492–12493. doi:10.1021/ja053962k PMID:16144388

Kam, N. W., O'Connell, M., Wisdom, J. A., & Dai, H. (2005). Carbon nanotubes as multifunctional biological transporters and near-infrared agents for selective cancer cell destruction. *Proceedings of the National Academy of Sciences of the United States of America*, *102*(33), 11600–11605. doi:10.1073/pnas.0502680102 PMID:16087878

Kamps, J. A., Koning, G. A., Velinova, M. J., Morselt, H. W., Wilkens, M., Gorter, A., ... Scherphof, G. L. (2000). Uptake of long-circulating immunoliposomes, directed against colon adenocarcinoma cells, by liver metastases of colon cancer. *Journal of Drug Targeting*, *8*(4), 235–245. doi:10.3109/10611860008997902 PMID:11144234

Kanematsu, A., Marui, A., Yamamoto, S., Ozeki, K., Hirano, Y., Yamamoto, M., ... Tabata, Y. (2004, September). Type 1 collagen can function as a reservoir of basic fibroblast growth factor. *Journal of Controlled Release*, *99*(2), 281–292. doi:10.1016/j.jconrel.2004.07.008 PMID:15380637

Kang, M. S., Singh, R. K., Kim, T. H., Kim, J. H., Patel, K. D., & Kim, H. W. (2017). Optical imaging and anticancer chemotherapy through carbon dot created hollow mesoporous silica nanoparticles. *Acta Biomaterialia*, *55*, 466–480. doi:10.1016/j.actbio.2017.03.054 PMID:28373086

Kanwar, J. R. (2012). Cancer nanotechnology. *Journal of Cancer Science & Therapy*, *4*(1), 249–265. doi:10.4172/1948-5956.1000e104

Karabela, M. M., & Sideridou, I. D. (2008, December). Effect of the structure of silane coupling agent on sorption characteristics of solvents by dental resin-nanocomposites. *Dental Materials*, *24*(12), 1631–1639. doi:10.1016/j.dental.2008.02.021 PMID:18462785

Karaki, S., Benizri, S., Mejías, R., Baylot, V., Branger, N., Nguyen, T., ... Rocchi, P. (2017). Lipid-oligonucleotide conjugates improve cellular uptake and efficiency of TCTP-antisense in castration-resistant prostate cancer. *Journal of Controlled Release*, *258*, 1–9. doi:10.1016/j.jconrel.2017.04.042 PMID:28472637

Karaman, D. S., Desai, D., Senthilkumar, R., Johansson, E. M., Ratts, N., Oden, M., ... Rosenholm, J. M. (2012). Shape engineering vs organic modification of inorganic nanoparticles as a tool for enhancing cellular internalization. *Nanoscale Research Letters*, *7*(1), 358. doi:10.1186/1556-276X-7-358 PMID:22747910

Karami, Z., & Hamidi, M. (2016). Cubosomes: Remarkable drug delivery potential. *Drug Discovery Today*, *21*(5), 789–801. doi:10.1016/j.drudis.2016.01.004 PMID:26780385

Kasraei, S., Sami, L., Hendi, S., AliKhani, M.-Y., Rezaei-Soufi, L., & Khamverdi, Z. (2014). Antibacterial properties of composite resins incorporating silver and zinc oxide nanoparticles on Streptococcus mutans and Lactobacillus. *Restorative Dentistry & Endodontics*, *39*(2), 109–114. doi:10.5395/rde.2014.39.2.109 PMID:24790923

Katragadda, C. S., Choudhury, P. K., & Murthy, P. (2010). Nanoparticles as non-viral gene delivery vectors. *Indian Journal of Pharmaceutical Education and Research*, *44*(2), 109–111.

Katz, M. A., Cheng, C. H., & Nacht, S. (1999). Methods and composition for topical delivery of benzoyl peroxide. US5879716.

Kaukonen, A. M., Boyd, B. J., Porter, C. J., & Charman, W. N. (2004). Drug solubilization behavior during *in vitro* digestion of simple triglyceride lipid solution formulations. *Pharmaceutical Research*, *21*(2), 245–253. doi:10.1023/B:PHAM.0000016282.77887.1f PMID:15032305

Kaur, R., & Kaur, S. (2014). Role of polymers in drug delivery. *Journal of Drug Delivery and Therapeutics*, *4*(3), 32–36.

Kawai, T., & Akira, S. (2011). Toll-like receptors and their crosstalk with other innate receptors in infection and immunity. *Immunity*, *34*(5), 637–650. doi:10.1016/j.immuni.2011.05.006 PMID:21616434

Kawashima, Y., Niwa, T., Handa, T., Takeuchi, H., Iwamoto, T., & Itoh, K. (n.d.). Preparation of controlled-release microspheres of ibuprofen with acrylic polymers by a novel quasi-emulsion solvent diffusion method. Journal of Pharmaceutical Sciences, 78, 68–72.

Kawashima, Y., Niwa, T., Takeuchi, H., Hino, T., & Itoh, Y. (1992). Control of prolonged drug release and compression properties of ibuprofen microsponges with acrylic polymer, Eudragit RS, by changing their intraparticle density. *Chemical & Pharmaceutical Bulletin*, *40*(1), 196–201. doi:10.1248/cpb.40.196 PMID:1576674

Kedmi, R., Ben-Arie, N., & Peer, D. (2010, September). The systemic toxicity of positively charged lipid nanoparticles and the role of Toll like receptor 4 in immune activation. *Biomaterials*, *31*(26), 6867–6875. doi:10.1016/j.biomaterials.2010.05.027 PMID:20541799

Kenmotsu, H., Yasunaga, M., Goto, K., Nagano, T., Kuroda, J., Koga, Y., ... Matsumura, Y. (2010). The antitumor activity of NK012, an SN-38-incorporating micelle, in combination with bevacizumab against lung cancer xenografts. *Cancer*, *116*(19), 4597–4604. doi:10.1002/cncr.25233 PMID:20572031

Kennedy, L. C., Bickford, L. R., Lewinski, N. A., Coughlin, A. J., Hu, Y., Day, E. S., ... Drezek, R. A. (2011). A new era for cancer treatment: Gold-nanoparticle mediated thermal therapies. *Small*, *7*(2), 169–183. doi:10.1002mll.201000134 PMID:21213377

Kesharwani, P., Jain, K., & Jain, N. K. (2014). Dendrimer as nanocarrier for drug delivery. *Progress in Polymer Science*, *39*(2), 268–307. doi:10.1016/j.progpolymsci.2013.07.005

Kesharwani, P., Xie, L., Banerjee, S., Mao, G., Padhye, S., Sarkar, F. H., & Iyer, A. K. (2015). Hyaluronic acid-conjugated polyamidoamine dendrimers for targeted delivery of 3,4-difluorobenzylidene curcumin to CD44 overexpressing pancreatic cancer cells. *Colloids and Surfaces. B, Biointerfaces*, *136*, 413–423. doi:10.1016/j.colsurfb.2015.09.043 PMID:26440757

Khalid, M., & El-Sawy, H. S. (2017). Polymeric nanoparticles: Promising platform for drug delivery. *International Journal of Pharmaceutics*, *528*(1-2), 675–691. doi:10.1016/j.ijpharm.2017.06.052 PMID:28629982

Khan, W. (2013). Cationic polymers for the delivery of therapeutic nucleotides. *Nanotechnology for the Delivery of Therapeutic Nucleic Acids, 8*, 27-56.

Khan, A., Benboubetra, M., Sayyed, P. Z., Wooi Ng, K., Fox, S., Beck, G., ... Akhtar, S. (2004). Sustained polymeric delivery of gene silencing antisense ODNs, siRNA, DNAzymes and ribozymes: In vitro and in vivo studies. *Journal of Drug Targeting*, *12*(6), 393–404. doi:10.1080/10611860400003858 PMID:15545089

Khandare, J., Calderón, M., Dagia, N. M., & Haag, R. (2012). Multifunctional dendritic polymers in nanomedicine: Opportunities and challenges. *Chemical Society Reviews*, *41*(7), 2824–2848. doi:10.1039/C1CS15242D PMID:22158998

Khandelia, R., Bhandari, S., Pan, U. N., Ghosh, S. S., & Chattopadhyay, A. (2015). Gold Nanocluster Embedded Albumin Nanoparticles for Two-Photon Imaging of Cancer Cells Accompanying Drug Delivery. *Small*, *11*(33), 4075–4081. doi:10.1002mll.201500216 PMID:25939342

Khan, W., Hosseinkhani, H., Ickowicz, D., Hong, P.-D., Yu, D.-S., & Domb, A. J. (2012). Polysaccharide gene transfection agents. *Acta Biomaterialia*, *8*(12), 4224–4232. doi:10.1016/j.actbio.2012.09.022 PMID:23022542

Khopade, A. J., Jain, S., & Jain, N. K. (1996). The microsponge. *Eastern Pharmacist*, *39*, 49–53.

Khosravian, P., Shafiee Ardestani, M., Khoobi, M., Ostad, S. N., Dorkoosh, F. A., Akbari Javar, H., & Amanlou, M. (2016). Mesoporous silica nanoparticles functionalized with folic acid/methionine for active targeted delivery of docetaxel. *OncoTargets and Therapy*, *9*, 7315–7330. doi:10.2147/OTT.S113815 PMID:27980423

Khutale, G. V., & Casey, A. (2017). Synthesis and characterization of a multifunctional gold-doxorubicin nanoparticle system for pH triggered intracellular drug release. *European Journal of Pharmaceutics and Biopharmaceutics*, *119*, 372–380. doi:10.1016/j.ejpb.2017.07.009 PMID:28736333

Kichler, A., Leborgne, C., Coeytaux, E., & Danos, O. (2001). Polyethylenimine-mediated gene delivery: A mechanistic study. *The Journal of Gene Medicine*, *3*(2), 135–144. doi:10.1002/jgm.173 PMID:11318112

Kikuchi, M., Itoh, S., Ichinose, S., Shinomiya, K., & Tanaka, J. (2001). Self-organization mechanism in a bone-like hydroxyapatite/collagen nanocomposite synthesized in vitro and its biological reaction in vivo. *Biomaterials*, *22*(13), 1705–1711. doi:10.1016/S0142-9612(00)00305-7 PMID:11396873

Kilina, S. V., Tamukong, P. K., & Kilin, D. S. (2016). Surface Chemistry of Semiconducting Quantum Dots: Theoretical Perspectives. *Accounts of Chemical Research*, *49*(10), 2127–2135. doi:10.1021/acs.accounts.6b00196 PMID:27669357

Kim, J.H., Kim, T.H., Kang, M.S., & Kim, H.W. (2016). Angiogenic Effects of Collagen/Mesoporous Nanoparticle Composite Scaffold Delivering VEGF165. *Biomed Res Int.*

Kim, C., Shah, B. P., Subramaniam, P., & Lee, K.-B. (2011). Synergistic induction of apoptosis in brain cancer cells by targeted codelivery of siRNA and anticancer drugs. *Molecular Pharmaceutics*, *8*(5), 1955–1961. doi:10.1021/mp100460h PMID:21793576

Kim, D., Lee, E. S., Oh, K. T., Gao, Z. G., & Bae, Y. H. (2008). Doxorubicin-loaded polymeric micelle overcomes multidrug resistance of cancer by double-targeting folate receptor and early endosomal pH. *Small*, *4*(11), 2043–2050. doi:10.1002mll.200701275 PMID:18949788

Kim, H., Chung, K., Lee, S., Kim, D. H., & Lee, H. (2016). Near-infrared light-responsive nanomaterials for cancer theranostics. *Wiley Interdisciplinary Reviews. Nanomedicine and Nanobiotechnology*, *8*(1), 23–45. doi:10.1002/wnan.1347 PMID:25903643

Kim, H., Kim, S. W., Park, Y. U., Gwon, H., Seo, D. H., Kim, Y., & Kang, K. (2010). SnO_2/graphene composite with high lithium storage capability for lithium rechargeable batteries. *Nano Research*, *3*(11), 813–821. doi:10.100712274-010-0050-4

Kim, H.-W., Kim, H.-E., Salih, V., & Knowles, J. C. (2005). Hydroxyapatite and titania sol–gel composite coatings on titanium for hard tissue implants; Mechanical and in vitro biological performance. *Journal of Biomedical Materials Research. Part B, Applied Biomaterials*, *72B*(1), 1–8. doi:10.1002/jbm.b.30073 PMID:15481086

Kim, J. H., Eguchi, H., & Ishikawa, Y. (2017). Anticancer luminescent gold quantum clusters for in situ cancer-selective marking-imaging-targeting. *Nanoscale*, *9*(26), 9071–9082. doi:10.1039/C7NR02229H PMID:28639680

Kim, J., Kim, H. S., Lee, N., Kim, T., Kim, H., Yu, T., ... Hyeon, T. (2008). Multifunctional uniform nanoparticles composed of a magnetite nanocrystal core and a mesoporous silica shell for magnetic resonance and fluorescence imaging and for drug delivery. *Angewandte Chemie International Edition in English*, *47*(44), 8438–8441. doi:10.1002/anie.200802469 PMID:18726979

Kim, J., Lee, J. E., Lee, S. H., Yu, J. H., Lee, J. H., Park, T. G., & Hyeon, T. (2008). Designed fabrication of a multifunctional polymer nanomedical platform for simultaneous cancer-targeted imaging and magnetically guided drug delivery. *Advanced Materials*, *20*(3), 478–483. doi:10.1002/adma.200701726

Kim, T. H., Lee, S., & Chen, X. (2013). Nanotheranostics for personalized medicine. *Expert Review of Molecular Diagnostics*, *13*(3), 257–269. doi:10.1586/erm.13.15 PMID:23570404

Kim, T., & Hyeon, T. (2014). Applications of inorganic nanoparticles as therapeutic agents. *Nanotechnology*, *25*(1), 012001. doi:10.1088/0957-4484/25/1/012001 PMID:24334327

Kim, T., Momin, E., Choi, J., Yuan, K., Zaidi, H., Kim, J., ... Gilad, A. A. (2011). Mesoporous Silica-Coated Hollow Manganese Oxide Nanoparticles as Positive T1 Contrast Agents for Labeling and MRI Tracking of Adipose-Derived Mesenchymal Stem Cells. *Journal of the American Chemical Society*, *133*(9), 2955–2961. doi:10.1021/ja1084095 PMID:21314118

Kim, Y., Tewari, M., Pajerowski, J. D., Cai, S., Sen, S., Williams, J., ... Discher, D. E. (2009). Polymersome delivery of siRNA and antisense oligonucleotides. *Journal of Controlled Release*, *134*(2), 132–140. doi:10.1016/j.jconrel.2008.10.020 PMID:19084037

Kircheis, R., Schüller, S., Brunner, S., Ogris, M., Heider, K.-H., Zauner, W., & Wagner, E. (1999). Polycation-based DNA complexes for tumor-targeted gene delivery in vivo. *The Journal of Gene Medicine*, *1*(2), 111–120. doi: PMID:10738575

Knapik, J., Wojnarowska, Z., Grzybowska, K., Jurkiewicz, K., Tajber, L., & Paluch, M. (2015). Molecular dynamics and physical stability of co-amorphous ezetimib and indapamide mixtures. *Molecular Pharmaceutics*, *12*(10), 3610–3619. doi:10.1021/acs.molpharmaceut.5b00334 PMID:26301858

Kogan, G., Soltes, L., Stern, R., & Gemeiner, P. (2007). Hyaluronic acid: A natural biopolymer with a broad range of biomedical and industrial applications. *Biotechnology Letters*, *29*(1), 17–25. doi:10.100710529-006-9219-z PMID:17091377

Kohler, N., Sun, C., Wang, J., & Zhang, M. (2005). Methotrexate-modified superparamagnetic nanoparticles and their intracellular uptake into human cancer cells. *Langmuir*, *21*(19), 8858–8864. doi:10.1021/la0503451 PMID:16142971

Kohli, K., Chopra, S., Dhar, D., Arora, S., & Khar, R. K. (2010). Self-emulsifying drug delivery systems: An approach to enhance oral bioavailability. *Drug Discovery Today*, *15*(21–22), 958–965. doi:10.1016/j.drudis.2010.08.007 PMID:20727418

Kojima, T., Tsutsumi, S., Yamamoto, K., Ikeda, Y., & Moriwaki, T. (2010). High-throughput cocrystal slurry screening by use of in situ Raman microscopy and multi-well plate. *International Journal of Pharmaceutics*, *399*(1), 52–59. doi:10.1016/j.ijpharm.2010.07.055 PMID:20696223

Kolb, H. C., Finn, M. G., & Sharpless, K. B. (2001). Click chemistry: Diverse chemical function from a few good reactions. *Angewandte Chemie International Edition*, *40*(11), 2004–2021. doi: PMID:11433435

Kolhatkar, A. G., Jamison, A. C., Litvinov, D., Willson, R. C., & Lee, T. R. (2013). Tuning the magnetic properties of nanoparticles. *International Journal of Molecular Sciences*, *14*(8), 15977–16009. doi:10.3390/ijms140815977 PMID:23912237

Komarneni, S. (1996). Nanophase and Nanocomposite Materials II. *Materials Research Society Symposium Proceedings, 457.*

Koneru, B., Shi, Y., Wang, Y. C., Chavala, S. H., Miller, M. L., Holbert, B., ... Di Pasqua, A. J. (2015). Tetracycline-Containing MCM-41 Mesoporous Silica Nanoparticles for the Treatment of Escherichia coli. *Molecules (Basel, Switzerland)*, *20*(11), 19690–19698. doi:10.3390/molecules201119650 PMID:26528964

Koning, G. A., Kamps, J. A., & Scherphof, G. L. (2002). Efficient intracellular delivery of 5-fluorodeoxyuridine into colon cancer cells by targeted immunoliposomes. *Cancer Detection and Prevention*, *26*(4), 299–307. doi:10.1016/S0361-090X(02)00087-9 PMID:12430634

Koning, G. A., & Storm, G. (2003). Targeted drug delivery systems for the intracellular delivery of macromolecular drugs. *Drug Discovery Today*, *8*(11), 482–483. doi:10.1016/S1359-6446(03)02699-0 PMID:12818515

Kopecek, J. (2007). Hydrogel biomaterials: A smart future? *Biomaterials*, *28*(34), 5185–5192. doi:10.1016/j.biomaterials.2007.07.044 PMID:17697712

Kopecek, J., & Yang, J. (2007). Hydrogels as smart biomaterials. *Polymer International*, *56*(9), 1078–1098. doi:10.1002/pi.2253

Köping-Höggård, M., Vårum, K. M., Issa, M., Danielsen, S., Christensen, B. E., Stokke, B. T., & Artursson, P. (2004). Improved chitosan-mediated gene delivery based on easily dissociated chitosan polyplexes of highly defined chitosan oligomers. *Gene Therapy*, *11*(19), 1441–1452. doi:10.1038j.gt.3302312 PMID:15269712

Koppolu, B., & Zaharoff, D. A. (2013). The effect of antigen encapsulation in chitosan particles on uptake, activation and presentation by antigen presenting cells. *Biomaterials*, *34*(9), 2359–2369. doi:10.1016/j.biomaterials.2012.11.066 PMID:23274070

Korkmaz, Y., Ozel, E., Attar, N., Bicer, C. O., & Firatli, E. (2010). Microleakage and scanning electron microscopy evaluation of all-in-one self-etch adhesives and their respective nanocomposites prepared by erbium:yttrium–aluminum–garnet laser and bur. *Lasers in Medical Science*, *25*(4), 493–502. doi:10.100710103-009-0672-5 PMID:19396579

Kotov, N. A. (2008). *Nanoscale Design of Ultra strong Materials by L B L Assembly - Biomedical Circuits and Systems Conference*. Baltimore, MD: IEEE.

Kou, L., Sun, J., Zhai, Y., & He, Z. (2013). The endocytosis and intracellular fate of nanomedicines: Implication for rational design. *Asian Journal of Pharmaceutical Sciences*, *8*(1), 1–10. doi:10.1016/j.ajps.2013.07.001

Kovtun, A., Heumann, R., & Epple, M. (2009). Calcium phosphate nanoparticles for the transfection of cells. *Bio-Medical Materials and Engineering*, *19*(2-3), 241–247. PMID:19581719

Ko, Y. T., Kale, A., Hartner, W. C., Papahadjopoulos-Sternberg, B., & Torchilin, V. P. (2009). Self-assembling micelle-like nanoparticles based on phospholipid–polyethyleneimine conjugates for systemic gene delivery. *Journal of Controlled Release*, *133*(2), 132–138. doi:10.1016/j.jconrel.2008.09.079 PMID:18929605

Koynova, R., & Tenchov, B. (2010). Cationic lipids: Molecular structure/ transfection activity relationships and interactions with biomembranes. *Topics in Current Chemistry*, *296*, 51–93. doi:10.1007/128_2010_67 PMID:21504100

Koynova, R., & Tenchov, B. (2013). Recent patents on nonlamellar liquid crystalline lipid phases in drug delivery. *Recent Patents on Drug Delivery & Formulation*, *7*(3), 165–173. doi:10.2174/187221131130799900011 PMID:23829393

Krajcik, R., Jung, A., Hirsch, A., Neuhuber, W., & Zolk, O. (2008). Functionalization of carbon nanotubes enables non-covalent binding and intracellular delivery of small interfering RNA for efficient knock-down of genes. *Biochemical and Biophysical Research Communications*, *369*(2), 595–602. doi:10.1016/j.bbrc.2008.02.072 PMID:18298946

Krauland, A. H., & Alonso, M. J. (2007). Chitosan/cyclodextrin nanoparticles as macromolecular drug delivery system. *International Journal of Pharmaceutics*, *340*(1), 134–142. doi:10.1016/j.ijpharm.2007.03.005 PMID:17459620

Kresge, C. T., Leonowicz, M. E., Roth, W. J., Vartuli, J. C., & Beck, J. S. (1992). Ordered mesoporous molecular sieves synthesized by a liquid-crystal template mechanism. *Nature*, *359*(6397), 710–712. doi:10.1038/359710a0

Krishnan, L., & Sprott, G. D. (2008). Archaeosome adjuvants: Immunological capabilities and mechanism(s) of action. *Vaccine*, *26*(17), 2043–2055. doi:10.1016/j.vaccine.2008.02.026 PMID:18343538

Krukemeyer, M. G., Krenn, V., Jakobs, M., & Wagner, W. (2012). Magnetic drug targeting in a rhabdomyosarcoma rat model using magnetite-dextran composite nanoparticle-bound mitoxantrone and 0.6 tesla extracorporeal magnets - sarcoma treatment in progress. *Journal of Drug Targeting*, *20*(2), 185–193. doi:10.3109/1061186X.2011.622399 PMID:22044194

Kuang, Y., Zhang, K., Cao, Y., Chen, X., Wang, K., Liu, M., & Pei, R. (2017). Hydrophobic IR-780 Dye Encapsulated in cRGD-Conjugated Solid Lipid Nanoparticles for NIR Imaging-Guided Photothermal Therapy. *ACS Applied Materials & Interfaces*, *9*(14), 12217–12226. doi:10.1021/acsami.6b16705 PMID:28306236

Kukowska-Latallo, J. F., Bielinska, A. U., Johnson, J., Spindler, R., Tomalia, D. A., & Baker, J. R. (1996). Efficient transfer of genetic material into mammalian cells using Starburst polyamidoamine dendrimers. *Proceedings of the National Academy of Sciences of the United States of America*, *93*(10), 4897–4902. doi:10.1073/pnas.93.10.4897 PMID:8643500

Kukowska-Latallo, J. F., Candido, K. A., Cao, Z., Nigavekar, S. S., Majoros, I. J., Thomas, T. P., ... Baker, J. R. Jr. (2005). Nanoparticle targeting of anticancer drug improves therapeutic response in animal model of human epithelial cancer. *Cancer Research*, *65*(12), 5317–5324. doi:10.1158/0008-5472.CAN-04-3921 PMID:15958579

Kuksenok, O., & Balazs, A. C. (2016). Stimuli-responsive behavior of composites integrating thermo-responsive gels with photo-responsive fibers. *Materials Horizons*, *3*(1), 53–62. doi:10.1039/C5MH00212E

Kulkarni, R. P., Mishra, S., Fraser, S. E., & Davis, M. E. (2005). Single cell kinetics of intracellular, nonviral, nucleic acid delivery vehicle acidification and trafficking. *Bioconjugate Chemistry*, *16*(4), 986–994. doi:10.1021/bc050081u PMID:16029041

Kumar, N. (2010). Ferroelectric properties of KNO3 - polymer composite films. *J. Pure Appl. & Ind. Phys.*, *1*, 21 – 35.

Kumar, P., Tambe, P., Paknikar, KM., & Gajbhiye V. (2017) Folate/N-acetyl glucosamine conjugated mesoporous silica nanoparticles for targeting breast cancer cells: A comparative study. *Colloids Surf B Biointerfaces*, *156*, 203-212.

Kumar, A., Lale, S. V., Alex, M. A., Choudhary, V., & Koul, V. (2017). Folic acid and trastuzumab conjugated redox responsive random multiblock copolymeric nanocarriers for breast cancer therapy: In-vitro and in-vivo studies. *Colloids and Surfaces. B, Biointerfaces*, *149*, 369–378. doi:10.1016/j.colsurfb.2016.10.044 PMID:27846450

Kumar, B., Kulanthaivel, S., Mondal, A., Mishra, S., Banerjee, B., Bhaumik, A., ... Giri, S. (2017). Mesoporous silica nanoparticle based enzyme responsive system for colon specific drug delivery through guar gum capping. *Colloids and Surfaces. B, Biointerfaces*, *150*, 352–361. doi:10.1016/j.colsurfb.2016.10.049 PMID:27847225

Kumari, A., Jain, A., Hurkat, P., Verma, A., & Jain, S. K. (2016). Microsponges: A Pioneering Tool for Biomedical Applications. *Critical Reviews in Therapeutic Drug Carrier Systems*, *33*(1), 77–105. doi:10.1615/CritRevTherDrugCarrierSyst.v33.i1.40 PMID:27279339

Kumari, A., & Yadav, S. K. (2011). Cellular interactions of therapeutically delivered nanoparticles. *Expert Opinion on Drug Delivery*, *8*(2), 141–151. doi:10.1517/17425247.2011.547934 PMID:21219249

Kumari, A., Yadav, S. K., & Yadav, S. C. (2010). Biodegradable polymeric nanoparticles based drug delivery systems. *Colloids and Surfaces. B, Biointerfaces*, *75*(1), 1–18. doi:10.1016/j.colsurfb.2009.09.001 PMID:19782542

Kumari, B., & Kesavan, K. (2017). Effect of chitosan coating on microemulsion for effective dermal clotrimazole delivery. *Pharmaceutical Development and Technology*, *22*(4), 617–626. doi:10.1080/10837450.2016.1230629 PMID:27574791

Kumar, N., Rai, A., Reddy, N. D., Raj, P. V., Jain, P., Deshpande, P., ... Rao, C. M. (2014). Silymarin liposomes improves oral bioavailability of silybin besides targeting hepatocytes, and immune cells. *Pharmacological Reports*, *66*(5), 788–798. doi:10.1016/j.pharep.2014.04.007 PMID:25149982

Kumar, P., Tambe, P., Paknikar, K. M., & Gajbhiye, V. (2017). Folate/N-acetyl glucosamine conjugated mesoporous silica nanoparticles for targeting breast cancer cells: A comparative study. *Colloids and Surfaces. B, Biointerfaces*, *156*, 203–212. doi:10.1016/j.colsurfb.2017.05.032 PMID:28531877

Kumar, S. K., & Krishnamoorti, R. (2010). Nanocomposites: Structure, Phase Behavior, and Properties. *Annual Review of Chemical and Biomolecular Engineering*, *1*(1), 37–58. doi:10.1146/annurev-chembioeng-073009-100856 PMID:22432572

Kumar, U., Kumar, S., Varghese, S., Chamoli, R., & Barthwal, P. (2013). DNA vaccine: A modern biotechnological approach towards human welfare and clinical trials. *International Journal of Research in Biomedicine and Biotechnology*, *3*(1), 17–20.

Kundu, A., Layek, R. K., Kuila, A., & Nandi, A. K. (2012). Highly Fluorescent Graphene Oxide-Poly(vinyl alcohol) Hybrid: An Effective Material for Specific Au3+ Ion Sensors. *ACS Applied Materials & Interfaces*, *4*(10), 5576–5582. doi:10.1021/am301467z PMID:23009213

Kushwaha, S. K. S., Ghoshal, S., Rai, A. K., & Singh, S. (2013). Carbon nanotubes as a novel drug delivery system for anticancer therapy: A review. *Brazilian Journal of Pharmaceutical Sciences*, *49*(4), 629–643. doi:10.1590/S1984-82502013000400002

Kuthati, Y., Kankala, R. K., Busa, P., Lin, S. X., Deng, J. P., Mou, C. Y., & Lee, C. H. (2017). Phototherapeutic spectrum expansion through synergistic effect of mesoporous silica trio-nanohybrids against antibiotic-resistant gram-negative bacterium. *Journal of Photochemistry and Photobiology. B, Biology*, *169*, 124–133. doi:10.1016/j.jphotobiol.2017.03.003 PMID:28319867

Kuwabara, A., Hori, N., Sawada, T., Hoshi, N., Watazu, A., & Kimoto, K. (2012). Enhanced biological responses of a hydroxyapatite/TiO₂ hybrid structure when surface electric charge is controlled using radiofrequency sputtering. *Dental Materials Journal*, *31*(3), 368–376. doi:10.4012/dmj.2011-220 PMID:22673466

Kuzmin, P. I., Akimov, S. A., Chizmadzhev, Y. A., Zimmerberg, J., & Cohen, F. S. (2005). Line Tension and Interaction Energies of Membrane Rafts Calculated from Lipid Splay and Tilt. *Biophys J*, *88*(2), 1120–33. Available from: http://linkinghub.elsevier.com/retrieve/pii/S0006349505731817

Kwon, H.-J., Oh, Y.-J., Jang, J.-H., Park, J.-E., Hwang, K.-S., & Park, Y.-D. (2015). The effect of polymerization conditions on the amounts of unreacted monomer and bisphenol A in dental composite resins. *Dental Materials Journal*, *34*(3), 327–335. doi:10.4012/dmj.2014-230 PMID:25904171

Kwon, S., Singh, R. K., Perez, R. A., Abou Neel, E. A., Kim, H. W., & Chrzanowski, W. (2013). Silica-based mesoporous nanoparticles for controlled drug delivery. *Journal of Tissue Engineering*, *4*, 204–211. doi:10.1177/2041731413503357 PMID:24020012

Ladewig, K., Niebert, M., Xu, Z. P., Gray, P. P., & Lu, G. Q. M. (2010). Efficient siRNA delivery to mammalian cells using layered double hydroxide nanoparticles. *Biomaterials*, *31*(7), 1821–1829. doi:10.1016/j.biomaterials.2009.10.058 PMID:19922997

Laga, R., Janoušková, O., Ulbrich, K., Pola, R., Blažková, J., Filippov, S. K., ... Pechar, M. (2015). Thermoresponsive Polymer Micelles as Potential Nanosized Cancerostatics. *Biomacromolecules*, *16*(8), 2493–2505. doi:10.1021/acs.biomac.5b00764 PMID:26153904

Laitinen, M., Hartikainen, J., Hiltunen, M. O., Eranen, J., Kiviniemi, M., Narvanen, O., ... Yla-Herttuala, S. (2000). Catheter-mediated vascular endothelial growth factor gene transfer to human coronary arteries after angioplasty. *Human Gene Therapy*, *11*(2), 263–270. doi:10.1089/10430340050016003 PMID:10680840

Lakshmi, P., Kalpana, B., & Prasanthi, D. (2013). Invasomes-novel vesicular carriers for enhanced skin permeation. *Systematic Reviews in Pharmacy*, *4*(1), 26. doi:10.4103/0975-8453.135837

Lamprecht, A., Ubrich, N., Yamamoto, H., Schafer, U., Takeuchi, H., Maincent, P., ... Lehr, C. M. (2001). Biodegradable nanoparticles for targeted drug delivery in treatment of inflammatory bowel disease. *The Journal of Pharmacology and Experimental Therapeutics*, *299*(2), 775–781. PMID:11602694

Lang, B. R., Jaarda, M., & Wang, R. F. (1992). Filler particle size and composite resin classification systems. *Journal of Oral Rehabilitation*, *19*(6), 569–584. doi:10.1111/j.1365-2842.1992.tb01487.x PMID:1469493

Langer, R., & Vancanti, J. P. (1993). Tissue engineering. *Science*, *260*(5110), 920–926. doi:10.1126cience.8493529 PMID:8493529

Lanone, S., & Boczkowski, J. (2006). Biomedical applications and potential health risks of nanomaterials: Molecular mechanisms. *Current Molecular Medicine*, *6*(6), 651–663. doi:10.2174/156652406778195026 PMID:17022735

Laouini, A., Sfar, S., Charcosset, C., Fessi, H., Jaafar-Maalej, C., & Limayem-Blouza, I. (2012). Preparation, characterization and applications of liposomes. *Journal of Colloid Science and Biotechnology*, *1*(2), 147–168. doi:10.1166/jcsb.2012.1020

Laroui, H., Dalmasso, G., Nguyen, H. T., Yan, Y., Sitaraman, S. V., & Merlin, D. (2010). Drug-loaded nanoparticles targeted to the colon with polysaccharide hydrogel reduce colitis in a mouse model. *Gastroenterology*, *138*(3), 843–853. doi:10.1053/j.gastro.2009.11.003 PMID:19909746

Larsen, D. B., Joergensen, S., Olsen, N. V., Hansen, S. H., & Larsen, C. (2002). *In vivo* release of bupivacaine from subcutaneously administered oily solution: Comparison with *in vitro* release. *Journal of Controlled Release*, *81*(1-2), 145–154. doi:10.1016/S0168-3659(02)00055-X PMID:11992687

Laurent, S., Forge, D., Port, M., Roch, A., Robic, C., Vander Elst, L., & Muller, R. N. (2008). Magnetic iron oxide nanoparticles: Synthesis, stabilization, vectorization, physicochemical characterizations, and biological applications. *Chemical Reviews*, *108*(6), 2064–2110. doi:10.1021/cr068445e PMID:18543879

Lawrence, M. J., & Rees, G. D. (2000). Microemulsion-based media as novel drug delivery systems. *Advanced Drug Delivery Reviews*, *45*(1), 89–121. doi:10.1016/S0169-409X(00)00103-4 PMID:11104900

Le Meins, J.F., Schatz, C., Lecommandoux, S., & Sandre, O. (2013). Hybrid polymer/lipid vesicles: State of the art and future perspectives. *Mater Today, 16*(10), 397–402. 10.1016/j.mattod.2013.09.002

Le, D. H., Lee, K. L., Shukla, S., Commandeur, U., & Steinmetz, N. F. (2017). Potato virus X, a filamentous plant viral nanoparticle for doxorubicin delivery in cancer therapy. *Nanoscale*, *9*(6), 2348–2357. doi:10.1039/C6NR09099K PMID:28144662

Lee, E.-S., Ko, K.-K., Joe, Y. A., Kang, S.-G., & Hong, Y.-K. (2011). Inhibition of STAT3 reverses drug resistance acquired in temozolomide-resistant human glioma cells. *Oncology Letters*, *2*(1), 115–121. doi:10.3892/ol.2010.210 PMID:22870139

Lee, J. B., Hong, J., Bonner, D. K., Poon, Z., & Hammond, P. T. (2012). Self-assembled RNA interference microsponges for efficient siRNA delivery. *Nature Materials*, *11*(4), 316–322. doi:10.1038/nmat3253 PMID:22367004

Lee, J. H., Lee, K., Moon, S. H., Lee, Y., Park, T. G., & Cheon, J. (2009). All-in-One Target-Cell-Specific Magnetic Nanoparticles for Simultaneous Molecular Imaging and siRNA Delivery. *Angewandte Chemie*, *121*(23), 4238–4243. doi:10.1002/ange.200805998 PMID:19408274

Lee, J. M., Yoon, T. J., & Cho, Y. S. (2013). Recent developments in nanoparticle-based siRNA delivery for cancer therapy. *BioMed Research International*, *2013*, 1–10. doi:10.1155/2013/310461 PMID:23844368

Lee, J. Y., Termsarasab, U., Lee, M. Y., Kim, D. H., Lee, S. Y., Kim, J. S., ... Kim, D.-D. (2017). Chemosensitizing indomethacin-conjugated chitosan oligosaccharide nanoparticles for tumor-targeted drug delivery. *Acta Biomaterialia*, *57*, 262–273. doi:10.1016/j.actbio.2017.05.012 PMID:28483700

Lee, J.-S., Green, J. J., Love, K. T., Sunshine, J., Langer, R., & Anderson, D. G. (2009). Gold, poly (β-amino ester) nanoparticles for small interfering RNA delivery. *Nano Letters*, *9*(6), 2402–2406. doi:10.1021/nl9009793 PMID:19422265

Lee, K.-Y., Chiang, Y.-T., Hsu, N.-Y., Yang, C.-Y., Lo, C.-L., & Ku, C.-A. (2015). Vitamin E containing polymer micelles for reducing normal cell cytotoxicity and enhancing chemotherapy efficacy. *Acta Biomaterialia*, *24*, 286–296. doi:10.1016/j.actbio.2015.06.014 PMID:26087112

Lee, R. J., & Huang, L. (1996). Folate-targeted, anionic liposome-entrapped polylysine-condensed DNA for tumor cell-specific gene transfer. *The Journal of Biological Chemistry*, *271*(14), 8481–8487. doi:10.1074/jbc.271.14.8481 PMID:8626549

Lee, R. J., Wang, S., & Low, P. S. (1996). Measurement of endosome pH following folate receptor-mediated endocytosis. *Biochimica et Biophysica Acta (BBA)- Molecular Cell Research*, *1312*(3), 237–242. PMID:8703993

Lee, S. M., Chen, H., Dettmer, C. M., O'Halloran, T. V., & Nguyen, S. T. (2007). Polymer-caged lipsomes: A pH-responsive delivery system with high stability. *Journal of the American Chemical Society*, *129*(49), 15096–15097. doi:10.1021/ja070748i PMID:17999499

Lee, S. M., Chen, H., O'Halloran, T. V., & Nguyen, S. B. T. (2009). "Clickable" polymer-caged nanobins as a modular drug delivery platform. *Journal of the American Chemical Society*, *131*(26), 9311–9320. doi:10.1021/ja9017336 PMID:19527027

Leitner, W. W., Ying, H., & Restifo, N. P. (1999). DNA and RNA-based vaccines: Principles, progress and prospects. *Vaccine*, *18*(9-10), 765–777. doi:10.1016/S0264-410X(99)00271-6 PMID:10580187

Lemmerer, A. (2012). Covalent assistance to supramolecular synthesis: Modifying the drug functionality of the anti-tuberculosis API isoniazid in situ during co-crystallization with GRAS and API compounds. *CrystEngComm*, *14*(7), 2465–2478. doi:10.1039/C1CE06310C

Lenz, E., Jensen, K. T., Blaabjerg, L. I., Knop, K., Grohganz, H., Lobmann, K., ... Kleinebudde, P. (2015). Solid-state properties and dissolution behaviour of tablets containing co-amorphous indomethacin–arginine. *European Journal of Pharmaceutics and Biopharmaceutics*, *96*, 44–52. doi:10.1016/j.ejpb.2015.07.011 PMID:26197392

Lesniak, A., Salvati, A., Santos-Martinez, M. J., Radomski, M. W., Dawson, K. A., & Åberg, C. (2013). Nanoparticle adhesion to the cell membrane and its effect on nanoparticle uptake efficiency. *Journal of the American Chemical Society*, *135*(4), 1438–1444. doi:10.1021/ja309812z PMID:23301582

Leung, D. H., Lohani, S., Ball, R. G., Canfield, N., Wang, Y., Rhodes, T., & Bak, A. (2012). Two novel pharmaceutical cocrystals of a development compound–screening, scale-up, and characterization. *Crystal Growth & Design*, *12*(3), 1254–1262. doi:10.1021/cg201270s

Leyden, J. J., Tanghetti, E. A., Miller, B., Ung, M., Berson, D., & Lee, J. (2002). Once-daily tazarotene 0.1% gel versus once-daily tretinoin 0.1% microsponge gel for the treatment of facial acne vulgaris: A double-blind randomized trial. *Cutis*, *69*, 12–19. PMID:12095064

Li, N. J. (Ed.). (2013). Biosensors based on nanomaterials and nanodevices. CRC Press.

Liang, C., Song, X., Chen, Q., Liu, T., Song, G., Peng, R., & Liu, Z. (2015). Magnetic Field-Enhanced Photothermal Ablation of Tumor Sentinel Lymph Nodes to Inhibit Cancer Metastasis. *Small*, *11*(37), 4856–4863. doi:10.1002mll.201501197 PMID:26179806

Liang, C., Yang, Y., Ling, Y., Huang, Y., Li, T., & Li, X. (2011). Improved therapeutic effect of folate-decorated PLGA–PEG nanoparticles for endometrial carcinoma. *Bioorganic & Medicinal Chemistry*, *19*(13), 4057–4066. doi:10.1016/j.bmc.2011.05.016 PMID:21641806

Liang, H., He, L., Zhou, B., Li, B., & Li, J. (2017). Folate-functionalized assembly of low density lipoprotein/sodium carboxymethyl cellulose nanoparticles for targeted delivery. *Colloids and Surfaces. B, Biointerfaces*, *156*, 19–28. doi:10.1016/j.colsurfb.2017.05.004 PMID:28499201

Liang, T.-J., Zhou, Z.-M., Cao, Y.-Q., Ma, M.-Z., Wang, X.-J., & Jing, K. (2016). Gemcitabine-based polymer-drug conjugate for enhanced anticancer effect in colon cancer. *International Journal of Pharmaceutics*, *513*(1), 564–571. doi:10.1016/j.ijpharm.2016.09.018 PMID:27613255

Liang, X., Fan, J., Wang, Y., Zhao, Y., Jin, R., Sun, T., ... Wang, X. (2017). Synthesis of hollow and mesoporous structured NaYF4:Yb,Er upconversion luminescent nanoparticles for targeted drug delivery. *Journal of Rare Earths*, *35*(5), 419–429. doi:10.1016/S1002-0721(17)60929-3

Liang, X., Shang, W., Chi, C., Zeng, C., Wang, K., Fang, C., ... Tian, J. (2016). Dye-conjugated single-walled carbon nanotubes induce photothermal therapy under the guidance of near-infrared imaging. *Cancer Letters*, *383*(2), 243–249. doi:10.1016/j.canlet.2016.09.006 PMID:27693557

Liao, S. S., Cui, F. Z., & Zhu, Y. (2004). Osteoblasts Adherence and Migration through Three-dimensional Porous Mineralized Collagen Based Composite: nHAC/PLA. *Journal of Bioactive and Compatible Polymers*, *19*(2), 117–130. doi:10.1177/0883911504042643

Libster, D., Aserin, A., & Garti, N. (2015). Lipid Nano-Vehicles Based on Lyotropic Liquid crystals as drug delivery vehicles. *Lipids in Nanotechnology*, 191.

Li, F., Hu, R., Wang, B., Gui, Y., Cheng, G., Gao, S., ... Tang, J. (2017). Self-microemulsifying drug delivery system for improving the bioavailability of huperzine A by lymphatic uptake. *Acta Pharmaceutica Sinica. B*, *7*(3), 353–360. doi:10.1016/j.apsb.2017.02.002 PMID:28540173

Li, G., Fan, Y., Fan, C., Li, X., Wang, X., Li, M., & Liu, Y. (2012). Tacrolimus-loaded ethosomes: Physicochemical characterization and in vivo evaluation. *European Journal of Pharmaceutics and Biopharmaceutics*, *82*(1), 49–57. doi:10.1016/j.ejpb.2012.05.011 PMID:22705640

Li, H., Yu, H., Zhu, C., Hu, J., Du, M., Zhang, F., & Yang, D. (2016). Cisplatin and doxorubicin dual-loaded mesoporous silica nanoparticles for controlled drug delivery. *RSC Advances*, *6*(96), 94160–94169. doi:10.1039/C6RA17213J

Li, J., Xu, L., Wang, H., Yang, B., Liu, H., Pan, W., & Li, S. (2016). Comparison of bare and amino modified mesoporous silica@poly(ethyleneimine)s xerogel as indomethacin carrier: Superiority of amino modification. *Materials Science and Engineering C*, *59*, 710–716. doi:10.1016/j.msec.2015.10.072 PMID:26652425

Li, L., Liu, T., Fu, C., Tan, L., Meng, X., & Liu, H. (2015). Biodistribution, excretion, and toxicity of mesoporous silica nanoparticles after oral administration depend on their shape. *Nanomedicine; Nanotechnology, Biology, and Medicine*, *11*(8), 1915–1924. doi:10.1016/j.nano.2015.07.004 PMID:26238077

Lim, J. B. (2008). Dielectric Behavior in the BiSc03 - BaTi03 - (K1I2Bi1l2) Ti03 Ternary System. *IEEE Transactions.*

Li, M., Xu, G., Gong, Y., Wang, W., Liu, Y., & Guo, J. (2017). Green preparation of hollow mesoporous silica nanosphere inside-loaded gold nanoparticles and the catalytic activity. *Journal of Macromolecular Science, Part A.*, *54*(6), 376–381. doi:10.1080/10601325.2017.1313128

Lim, A. W., Löbmann, K., Grohganz, H., Rades, T., & Chieng, N. (2016). Investigation of physical properties and stability of indomethacin–cimetidine and naproxen–cimetidine co-amorphous systems prepared by quench cooling, coprecipitation and ball milling. *The Journal of Pharmacy and Pharmacology*, *68*(1), 36–45. doi:10.1111/jphp.12494 PMID:26663364

Linares, N., Silvestre-Albero, A. M., Serrano, E., Silvestre-Albero, J., & Garcia-Martinez, J. (2014). Mesoporous materials for clean energy technologies. *Chemical Society Reviews*, *43*(22), 7681–7717. doi:10.1039/C3CS60435G PMID:24699503

Lin, C. Y., Javadi, M., Belnap, D. M., Barrow, J. R., & Pitt, W. G. (2014). Ultrasound sensitive eLiposomes containing doxorubicin for drug targeting therapy. *Nanomedicine; Nanotechnology, Biology, and Medicine*, *10*(1), 67–76. doi:10.1016/j.nano.2013.06.011 PMID:23845926

Lin, C.-W., Lu, K.-Y., Wang, S.-Y., Sung, H.-W., & Mi, F.-L. (2016). CD44-specific nanoparticles for redox-triggered reactive oxygen species production and doxorubicin release. *Acta Biomaterialia*, *35*, 280–292. doi:10.1016/j.actbio.2016.02.005 PMID:26853764

Lindh, J., Ruan, C., Strømme, M., & Mihranyan, A. (2016). Preparation of porous cellulose beads via introduction of diamine spacers. *Langmuir*, *32*(22), 5600–5607. doi:10.1021/acs.langmuir.6b01288 PMID:27181427

Lindner, P. (2002). Scattering experiments: experimental aspects, initial data reduction and absolute calibration. *Neutrons, X-Rays and Light: Scattering methods applied to soft condensed matter*, 23-48.

Lin, J. T., Liu, Z. K., Zhu, Q. L., Rong, X. H., Liang, C. L., Wang, J., ... Wang, G. H. (2017). Redox-responsive nanocarriers for drug and gene co-delivery based on chitosan derivatives modified mesoporous silica nanoparticles. *Colloids and Surfaces. B, Biointerfaces*, *155*, 41–50. doi:10.1016/j.colsurfb.2017.04.002 PMID:28407530

Lin, J., Zhou, W., Kumbhar, A., Wiemann, J., Fang, J., Carpenter, E. E., & O'Connor, C. J. (2001). Gold-coated iron (Fe@ Au) nanoparticles: Synthesis, characterization, and magnetic field-induced self-assembly. *Journal of Solid State Chemistry*, *159*(1), 26–31. doi:10.1006/jssc.2001.9117

Lin, W., Hyeon, T., Lanza, G. M., Zhang, M., & Meade, T. J. (2009). Magnetic Nanoparticles for Early Detection of Cancer by Magnetic Resonance Imaging. *MRS Bulletin*, *34*(06), 441–448. doi:10.1557/mrs2009.120 PMID:26166945

Lin, W., Yao, N., Qian, L., Zhang, X., Chen, Q., Wang, J., & Zhang, L. (2017). pH-responsive unimolecular micelle-gold nanoparticles-drug nanohybrid system for cancer theranostics. *Acta Biomaterialia*, *58*, 455–465. doi:10.1016/j.actbio.2017.06.003 PMID:28583900

Lin, X. M., & Samia, A. C. (2006). Synthesis, assembly and physical properties of magnetic nanoparticles. *Journal of Magnetism and Magnetic Materials*, *305*(1), 100–109. doi:10.1016/j.jmmm.2005.11.042

Lin, X. Y., Zhao, N. N., Yan, P., Hu, H., & Xu, F. J. (2015). The shape and size effects of polycation functionalized silica nanoparticles on gene transfection. *Acta Biomaterialia*, *11*, 381–392. doi:10.1016/j.actbio.2014.09.004 PMID:25219349

Lin, Y. C., Chen, H. L., Hashimoto, T., & Chen, S. A. (2016). Mechanism of hierarchical structure formation of polymer/nanoparticle hybrids. *Macromolecules*, *49*(19), 7535–7550. doi:10.1021/acs.macromol.6b01531

Lin, Y. S., & Haynes, C. L. (2010). Impacts of Mesoporous Silica Nanoparticle Size, Pore Ordering, and Pore Integrity on Hemolytic Activity. *Journal of the American Chemical Society*, *132*(13), 4834–4842. doi:10.1021/ja910846q PMID:20230032

Li, S. D., & Huang, L. (2010). Stealth nanoparticles: High density but sheddable PEG is a key for tumor targeting. *Journal of Controlled Release*, *145*(3), 178–181. doi:10.1016/j.jconrel.2010.03.016 PMID:20338200

Li, S., Liu, H., & He, N. (2010). Covalent binding of streptavidin on gold magnetic nanoparticles for bead array fabrication. *Journal of Nanoscience and Nanotechnology*, *10*(8), 4875–4882. doi:10.1166/jnn.2010.2385 PMID:21125822

Li, T., Chen, X., Liu, Y., Fan, L., Lin, L., Xu, Y., ... Shao, J. (2017). pH-Sensitive mesoporous silica nanoparticles anticancer prodrugs for sustained release of ursolic acid and the enhanced anti-cancer efficacy for hepatocellular carcinoma cancer. *European Journal of Pharmaceutical Sciences*, *96*, 456–463. doi:10.1016/j.ejps.2016.10.019 PMID:27771513

Liu, D., Chia, E. F., & Tian, H. (2004). Chemical methods for DNA delivery, In W. C. Heiser (Ed.), Methods in Molecular Biology, Volume 1: Nonviral Gene Transfer Techniques (pp. 3-23). Totowa: Humana Press Inc.

Liu, C., & Zhang, N. (2011). Chapter 13-Nanoparticles in gene therapy: Principles, prospects, and challenges. *Progress in Molecular Biology and Translational Science*, *104*, 509–562. doi:10.1016/B978-0-12-416020-0.00013-9 PMID:22093228

Liu, C., Zou, B., Rondinone, A. J., & Zhang, Z. J. (2000). Reverse micelle synthesis and characterization of superparamagnetic MnFe2O4 spinel ferrite nanocrystallites. *The Journal of Physical Chemistry B*, *104*(6), 1141–1145. doi:10.1021/jp993552g

Liu, D., Lu, K., Poon, C., & Lin, W. (2014). Metal–Organic Frameworks as Sensory Materials and Imaging Agents. *Inorganic Chemistry*, *53*(4), 1916–1924. doi:10.1021/ic402194c PMID:24251853

Liu, G., Ma, J., Li, Y., Li, Q., Tan, C., Song, H., ... Zhu, X. (2017). Core-interlayer-shell Fe3O4@mSiO2@lipid-PEG-methotrexate nanoparticle for multimodal imaging and multistage targeted chemo-photodynamic therapy. *International Journal of Pharmaceutics*, *521*(1-2), 19–32. doi:10.1016/j.ijpharm.2017.01.068 PMID:28163230

Liu, H. L., Ko, S. P., Wu, J. H., Jung, M. H., Min, J. H., Lee, J. H., ... Kim, Y. K. (2007). One-pot polyol synthesis of monosize PVP-coated sub-5nm Fe 3 O 4 nanoparticles for biomedical applications. *Journal of Magnetism and Magnetic Materials*, *310*(2), e815–e817. doi:10.1016/j.jmmm.2006.10.776

Liu, H., Slamovich, E. B., & Webster, T. J. (2006). Increased osteoblast functions among nanophase titania/poly(lactide-co-glycolide) composites of the highest nanometer surface roughness. *Journal of Biomedical Materials Research. Part A*, *78*(4), 798–807. doi:10.1002/jbm.a.30734 PMID:16741979

Liu, H., & Webster, T. J. (2007). Nanomedicine for implants: A review of studies and necessary experimental tools. *Biomaterials*, *28*(2), 354–369. doi:10.1016/j.biomaterials.2006.08.049 PMID:21898921

Liu, L. S., Liu, S. Q., Ng, S. Y., Froix, M., Ohno, T., & Heller, J. (1997). Controlled release of interleukin-2 for tumour immunotherapy using alginate/chitosan porous microspheres. *Journal of Controlled Release*, *43*(1), 65–74. doi:10.1016/S0168-3659(96)01471-X

Liu, Q., Xu, Z., Finch, J. A., & Egerton, R. (1998). A novel two-step silica-coating process for engineering magnetic nanocomposites. *Chemistry of Materials*, *10*(12), 3936–3940. doi:10.1021/cm980370a

Liu, R., Zhao, X., Wu, T., & Feng, P. (2008). Tunable Redox-Responsive Hybrid Nanogated Ensembles. *Journal of the American Chemical Society*, *130*(44), 14418–14419. doi:10.1021/ja8060886 PMID:18841893

Liu, T. Y., Hu, S. H., Liu, K. H., Liu, D. M., & Chen, S. Y. (2006). Preparation and characterization of smart magnetic hydrogels and its use for drug release. *Journal of Magnetism and Magnetic Materials*, *304*(1), e397–e399. doi:10.1016/j.jmmm.2006.01.203

Liu, X., Howard, K. A., Dong, M., Andersen, M. Ø., Rahbek, U. L., Johnsen, M. G., ... Kjems, J. (2007). The influence of polymeric properties on chitosan/siRNA nanoparticle formulation and gene silencing. *Biomaterials*, *28*(6), 1280–1288. doi:10.1016/j.biomaterials.2006.11.004 PMID:17126901

Liu, Y. S., Wen, C. F., & Yang, Y. M. (2012). Development of ethosome-like catanionic vesicles for dermal drug delivery. *Journal of the Taiwan Institute of Chemical Engineers*, *43*(6), 830–838. doi:10.1016/j.jtice.2012.06.008

Liu, Y., Chen, Q., Xu, M., Guan, G., Hu, W., Liang, Y., ... Liu, H. (2015). Single peptide ligand-functionalized uniform hollow mesoporous silica nanoparticles achieving dual-targeting drug delivery to tumor cells and angiogenic blood vessel cells. *International Journal of Nanomedicine*, *10*, 1855–1867. doi:10.2147/IJN.S75098 PMID:25834425

Liu, Y., Hunziker, E. B., Layrolle, P., De Bruijn, J. D., & De Groot, K. (2004). Bone morphogenetic protein 2 incorporated into biomimetic coatings retains its biological activity. *Tissue Engineering*, *10*(1-2), 101–108. doi:10.1089/107632704322791745 PMID:15009935

Liu, Y., Hu, Y., & Huang, L. (2014). Influence of polyethylene glycol density and surface lipid on pharmacokinetics and biodistribution of lipid-calcium-phosphate nanoparticles. *Biomaterials*, *35*(9), 3027–3034. doi:10.1016/j.biomaterials.2013.12.022 PMID:24388798

Liu, Y., Lou, C., Yang, H., Shi, M., & Miyoshi, H. (2011). Silica nanoparticles as promising drug/gene delivery carriers and fluorescent nano-probes: Recent advances. *Current Cancer Drug Targets*, *11*(2), 156–163. doi:10.2174/156800911794328411 PMID:21158720

Liu, Y., Miyoshi, H., & Nakamura, M. (2007). Nanomedicine for drug delivery and imaging: A promising avenue for cancer therapy and diagnosis using targeted functional nanoparticles. *International Journal of Cancer*, *120*(12), 2527–2537. doi:10.1002/ijc.22709 PMID:17390371

Liu, Y., Ng, Y., Toh, M. R., & Chiu, G. N. (2015). Lipid-dendrimer hybrid nanosystem as a novel delivery system for paclitaxel to treat ovarian cancer. *Journal of Controlled Release*, *220*, 438–446. doi:10.1016/j.jconrel.2015.11.004 PMID:26551345

Liu, Y., Pan, J., & Feng, S. S. (2010). Nanoparticles of lipid monolayer shell and biodegradable polymer core for controlled release of paclitaxel: Effects of surfactants on particles size, characteristics and in vitro performance. *International Journal of Pharmaceutics*, *395*(1–2), 243–250. doi:10.1016/j.ijpharm.2010.05.008 PMID:20472049

Liu, Y., Ran, R., Chen, J., Kuang, Q., Tang, J., Mei, L., ... He, Q. (2014). Paclitaxel loaded liposomes decorated with a multifunctional tandem peptide for glioma targeting. *Biomaterials*, *35*(17), 4835–4847. doi:10.1016/j.biomaterials.2014.02.031 PMID:24651033

Li, X., Anton, N., Arpagaus, C., Belleteix, F., & Vandamme, T. F. (2010). Nanoparticles by spray drying using innovative new technology: The Büchi Nano Spray Dryer B-90. *J Control Release*, *147*(2), 304–310. doi:10.1016/j.jconrel.2010.07.113 PMID:20659510

Li, X., Anton, N., Zuber, G., & Vandamme, T. (2014). Contrast agents for preclinical targeted X-ray imaging. *Advanced Drug Delivery Reviews*, *76*, 116–133. doi:10.1016/j.addr.2014.07.013 PMID:25086373

Li, X., Wu, M., Pan, L., & Shi, J. (2016). Tumor vascular-targeted co-delivery of anti-angiogenesis and chemotherapeutic agents by mesoporous silica nanoparticle-based drug delivery system for synergetic therapy of tumor. *International Journal of Nanomedicine*, *11*, 93–105. PMID:26766908

Li, X., Xue, M., Raabe, O. G., Aaron, H. L., Eisen, E. A., Evans, J. E., ... Pinkerton, K. E. (2015). Aerosol droplet delivery of mesoporous silica nanoparticles: A strategy for respiratory-based therapeutics. *Nanomedicine (London)*, *11*(6), 1377–1385. doi:10.1016/j.nano.2015.03.007 PMID:25819886

Li, Y., Hei, M., Xu, Y., Qian, X., & Zhu, W. (2016). Ammonium salt modified mesoporous silica nanoparticles for dual intracellular-responsive gene delivery. *International Journal of Pharmaceutics*, *511*(2), 689–702. doi:10.1016/j.ijpharm.2016.07.029 PMID:27426108

Li, Y., Lai, Y., Xu, X., Zhang, X., Wu, Y., & Hu, C. (2016). Capsid-like supramolecular dendritic systems as pH-responsive nanocarriers for drug penetration and site-specific delivery. *Nanomedicine (London)*, *12*(2), 355–364. doi:10.1016/j.nano.2015.09.015 PMID:26711961

Li, Z. Y., Liu, Y., Hu, J. J., Xu, Q., Liu, L. H., Jia, H. Z., ... Zhang, X. Z. (2014). Stepwise-Acid-Active Multifunctional Mesoporous Silica Nanoparticles for Tumor-Specific Nucleus-Targeted Drug Delivery. *ACS Applied Materials & Interfaces*, *6*(16), 14568–14575. doi:10.1021/am503846p PMID:25103086

Li, Z., Barnes, J. C., Bosoy, A., Stoddart, J. F., & Zink, J. I. (2012). Mesoporous silica nanoparticles in biomedical applications. *Chemical Society Reviews*, *41*(7), 2590–2605. doi:10.1039/c1cs15246g PMID:22216418

Li, Z., & Rana, T. M. (2012). Molecular mechanisms of RNA-triggered gene silencing machineries. *Accounts of Chemical Research*, *45*(7), 1122–1131. doi:10.1021/ar200253u PMID:22304792

Li, Z.-Y., Liu, Y., Wang, X. Q., Liu, L. H., Hu, J. J., Luo, G. F., ... Zhang, X. Z. (2013). One-Pot Construction of Functional Mesoporous Silica Nanoparticles for the Tumor-Acidity-Activated Synergistic Chemotherapy of Glioblastoma. *ACS Applied Materials & Interfaces*, *5*(16), 7995–8001. doi:10.1021/am402082d PMID:23869943

Lobmann, K., Laitinen, R., Grohganz, H., Gordon, K. C., Strachan, C., & Rades, T. (2011). Coamorphous drug systems: Enhanced physical stability and dissolution rate of indomethacin and naproxen. *Molecular Pharmaceutics*, *8*(5), 1919–1928. doi:10.1021/mp2002973 PMID:21815614

Löbmann, K., Laitinen, R., Grohganz, H., Strachan, C., Rades, T., & Gordon, K. C. (2013). A theoretical and spectroscopic study of co-amorphous naproxen and indomethacin. *International Journal of Pharmaceutics*, *453*(1), 80–87. doi:10.1016/j.ijpharm.2012.05.016 PMID:22613066

Löbmann, K., Strachan, C., Grohganz, H., Rades, T., Korhonen, O., & Laitinen, R. (2012). Co-amorphous simvastatin and glipizide combinations show improved physical stability without evidence of intermolecular interactions. *European Journal of Pharmaceutics and Biopharmaceutics*, *81*(1), 159–169. doi:10.1016/j.ejpb.2012.02.004 PMID:22353489

Lobovkina, T., Jacobson, G. B., Gonzalez-Gonzalez, E., Hickerson, R. P., Leake, D., Kaspar, R. L., ... Zare, R. N. (2011). In vivo sustained release of sirna from solid lipid nanoparticles. *ACS Nano*, *5*(12), 9977–9983. doi:10.1021/nn203745n PMID:22077198

Lodhia, J., Mandarano, G., Ferris, N., Eu, P., & Cowell, S. (2010). Development and use of iron oxide nanoparticles (Part 1): Synthesis of iron oxide nanoparticles for MRI. *Biomed Imaging Interv J*, *6*(2), e12. doi:10.2349/biij.6.2.e12 PMID:21611034

Lodhi, N., Mehra, N. K., & Jain, N. K. (2013). Development and characterization of dexamethasone mesylate anchored on multi walled carbon nanotubes. *Journal of Drug Targeting*, *21*(1), 67–76. doi:10.3109/1061186X.2012.729213 PMID:23039174

Loguercio, A. D., Reis, A., Hernandez, P. A. G., Macedo, R. P., & Busato, A. L. S. (2006). 3-Year clinical evaluation of posterior packable composite resin restorations. *Journal of Oral Rehabilitation*, *33*(2), 144–151. doi:10.1111/j.1365-2842.2006.01539.x PMID:16457675

Loh, X. J., Lee, T. C., Doua, Q., & Deene, G. R. (2016). Utilising inorganic nanocarriers for gene delivery. *Biomaterials Science*, *4*(1), 70–86. doi:10.1039/C5BM00277J PMID:26484365

Longo, E. (2013). Fabrication and Characterization of PZT – Pani / PVDF Based Nano composite. *Joint UFFD, EFTF, and PFM Symposium.*

Lord, M. S., Tsoi, B., Gunawan, C., Teoh, W. Y., Amal, R., & Whitelock, J. M. (2013). Anti-angiogenic activity of heparin functionalised cerium oxide nanoparticles. *Biomaterials*, *34*(34), 8808–8818. doi:10.1016/j.biomaterials.2013.07.083 PMID:23942211

Loup, C., Zanta, M.-A., Caminade, A.-M., Majoral, J.-P., & Meunier, B. (1999). Preparation of Water-Soluble Cationic Phosphorus-Containing Dendrimers as DNA Transfecting Agents. *Chemistry (Weinheim an der Bergstrasse, Germany)*, *5*(12), 3644–3650. doi:

Lou, X. W., Archer, L. A., & Yang, Z. (2008). Hollow Micro-/Nanostructures: Synthesis and Applications. *Advanced Materials*, *20*(21), 3987–4019. doi:10.1002/adma.200800854

Lozano, N., Al-Ahmady, Z. S., Beziere, N. S., Ntziachristos, V., & Kostarelos, K. (2015). Monoclonal antibody-targeted PEGylated liposome-ICG encapsulating doxorubicin as a potential theranostic agent. *International Journal of Pharmaceutics*, *484*(1-2), 2–10. doi:10.1016/j.ijpharm.2014.10.045 PMID:25445515

Lu, J., Liong, M., Li, Z., Zink, J.I., & Tamanoi, F. (2010). Biocompatibility, biodistribution, and drug-delivery efficiency of mesoporous silica nanoparticles for cancer therapy in animals. *Small*, *6*(16), 1794-805.

Lu, A. H., Salabas, E. E., & Schüth, F. (2007). Magnetic nanoparticles: Synthesis, protection, functionalization, and application. *Angewandte Chemie International Edition*, *46*(8), 1222–1244. doi:10.1002/anie.200602866 PMID:17278160

Luan, X., Dangaria, S., Ito, Y., Walker, C. G., Jin, T., Schmidt, M. K., ... Druzinsky, R. (2009). Neural crest lineage segregation: A blueprint for periodontal regeneration. *Journal of Dental Research*, *88*(9), 781–791. doi:10.1177/0022034509340641 PMID:19767574

Lu, E., Rodríguez-Hornedo, N., & Suryanarayanan, R. (2008). A rapid thermal method for cocrystal screening. *CrystEngComm*, *10*(6), 665–668. doi:10.1039/b801713c

Lu, J., Choi, E., Tamanoi, F., & Zink, J. I. (2008). Light-activated nanoimpeller-controlled drug release in cancer cells. *Small*, *4*(4), 421–426. doi:10.1002mll.200700903 PMID:18383576

Lu, J., Liong, M., Zink, J. I., & Tamanoi, F. (2007). Mesoporous silica nanoparticles as a delivery system for hydrophobic anticancer drugs. *Small*, *3*(8), 1341–1346. doi:10.1002mll.200700005 PMID:17566138

Lu, J., Li, Z., Zink, J. I., & Tamanoi, F. (2012). In vivo tumor suppression efficacy of mesoporous silica nanoparticles-based drug-delivery system: Enhanced efficacy by folate modification. *Nanomedicine; Nanotechnology, Biology, and Medicine*, *8*(2), 212–220. doi:10.1016/j.nano.2011.06.002 PMID:21703996

Lu, J., & Rohani, S. (2010). Synthesis and preliminary characterization of sulfamethazine-theophylline co-crystal. *Journal of Pharmaceutical Sciences*, *99*(9), 4042–4047. doi:10.1002/jps.22142 PMID:20665847

Lukashev, N., & Zamyatnin, A. A. (2016). Viral vectors for gene therapy: Current state and clinical perspectives. *Biochemistry (Moscow)*, *81*(7), 700–708. doi:10.1134/S0006297916070063 PMID:27449616

Lu, L., Chen, G., Qiu, Y., Li, M., Liu, D., Hu, D., ... Xiao, Z. (2016). Nanoparticle-based oral delivery systems for colon targeting: Principles and design strategies. *Science Bulletin*, *61*(9), 670–681. doi:10.100711434-016-1056-4

Luna, L. A. V., Moraes, A. C. M., Consonni, S. R., Pereira, C. D., Cadore, S., Giorgio, S., & Alves, O. L. (2016). Comparative in vitro toxicity of a graphene oxide-silver nanocomposite and the pristine counterparts toward macrophages. *Journal of Nanobiotechnology*, *14*, 1–17. PMID:26912341

Lungare, S., Hallam, K., & Badhan, R. K. (2016). Phytochemical-loaded mesoporous silica nanoparticles for nose-to-brain olfactory drug delivery. *International Journal of Pharmaceutics*, *513*(1-2), 280–293. doi:10.1016/j.ijpharm.2016.09.042 PMID:27633279

Luo, D., & Saltzman, W. M. (2000). Synthetic DNA delivery systems. *Nature Biotechnology*, *18*(1), 33–37. doi:10.1038/71889 PMID:10625387

Luo, Q., Lin, T., Zhang, C. Y., Zhu, T., Wang, L., Ji, Z., ... Chen, W. (2015). A novel glyceryl monoolein-bearing cubosomes for gambogenic acid: Preparation, cytotoxicity and intracellular uptake. *International Journal of Pharmaceutics*, *493*(1), 30–39. doi:10.1016/j.ijpharm.2015.07.036 PMID:26209071

Lu, P. S., Inbaraj, B. S., & Chen, B. H. (2017). Determination of oral bioavailability of curcuminoid dispersions and nanoemulsions prepared from curcuma longa linnaeus. *Journal of the Science of Food and Agriculture*. doi:10.1002/jsfa.8437 PMID:28516478

Luten, J., van Nostrum, C. F., De Smedt, S. C., & Hennink, W. E. (2008). Biodegradable polymers as non-viral carriers for plasmid DNA delivery. *Journal of Controlled Release*, *126*(2), 97–110. doi:10.1016/j.jconrel.2007.10.028 PMID:18201788

Lutz, F., & Phillips, R. W. (1983). A classification and evaluation of composite resin systems. *The Journal of Prosthetic Dentistry*, *50*(4), 480–488. doi:10.1016/0022-3913(83)90566-8 PMID:6579287

Lu, Y., Fan, H., Stump, A., Ward, T. L., Rieker, T., & Brinker, C. J. (1999). Aerosol-assisted self-assembly of mesostructured spherical nanoparticles. *Nature*, *398*(6724), 223–226. doi:10.1038/18410

Lu, Y., Yin, Y., Mayers, B. T., & Xia, Y. (2002). Modifying the surface properties of superparamagnetic iron oxide nanoparticles through a sol– gel approach. *Nano Letters*, *2*(3), 183–186. doi:10.1021/nl015681q

Lyer, S., Singh, R., Tietze, R., & Alexiou, C. (2015). Magnetic nanoparticles for magnetic drug targeting. *Biomedical Engineering/Biomedizinische Technik*, *60*(5), 465-475.

Ma, H. (2008). Fabrication of magnetic porous hollow silica drug carriers using Ca CO 3/ Fe 3 O 4 composite nanoparticles and cationic surfactant double templates. *Journal of Applied Physics*, *103*(7).

MacGregor, K. J., Embleton, J. K., Lacy, J. E., Perry, E. A., Solomon, L. J., Seager, H., & Pouton, C. W. (1997). Influence of lipolysis on drug absorption from the gastro-intestinal tract. *Advanced Drug Delivery Reviews*, *25*(1), 33–46. doi:10.1016/S0169-409X(96)00489-9

Mackay, M., & Tomlinson, E. (1993). Colonic delivery of therapeutic peptides and proteins. *Drugs and the Pharmaceutical Sciences*, *60*, 159–176.

MacLaughlin, F. C., Mumper, R. J., Wang, J., Tagliaferri, J. M., Gill, I., Hinchcliffe, M., & Rolland, A. P. (1998). Chitosan and depolymerized chitosan oligomers as condensing carriers for in vivo plasmid delivery. *Journal of Controlled Release*, *56*(1), 259–272. doi:10.1016/S0168-3659(98)00097-2 PMID:9801449

Mäder, K., & Mehnert, W. (2001). Solid lipid nanoparticles: Production, characterization and applications. *Advanced Drug Delivery Reviews*, *47*(2–3), 165–196. doi:10.1016/S0169-409X(01)00105-3 PMID:11311991

Maeda-Mamiya, R., Noiri, E., Isobe, H., Nakanishi, W., Okamoto, K., Doi, K., … Nakamura, E. (2010). *In vivo* gene delivery by cationic tetraamino fullerene. *Proceedings of the National Academy of Sciences of the United States of America*, *107*(12), 5339-5344. 10.1073/pnas.0909223107

Maincent, P. (2007). The regulatory environment: The challenges for lipid-based formulations. *Bulletin Technique Gattefossé*, *100*, 47–49.

Maiti, S., Kaity, S., Ray, S., & Sa, B. (2011). Development and evaluation of xanthan gum-facilitated ethyl cellulose microsponges for controlled percutaneous delivery of diclofenac sodium. *Acta Pharmaceutica (Zagreb, Croatia)*, *61*(3), 257–270. doi:10.2478/v10007-011-0022-6 PMID:21945905

Maitra, A. (2005). Calcium phosphate nanoparticles: Second-generation nonviral vectors in gene therapy. *Expert Review of Molecular Diagnostics*, *5*(6), 893–905. doi:10.1586/14737159.5.6.893 PMID:16255631

Majidi, S., Sehrig, F. Z., Samiei, M., Milani, M., Abbasi, E., Dadashzadeh, K., & Akbarzadeh, A. (2016). Magnetic nanoparticles: Applications in gene delivery and gene therapy. *Artificial Cells, Nanomedicine, and Biotechnology*, *4*(4), 1186–1193. PMID:25727710

Malakar, J., Sen, S., Nayak, A. K., & Sen, K. K. (2012). Formulation, optimization and evaluation of transferosomal gel for transdermal insulin delivery. *Saudi Pharmaceutical Journal*, *20*(4), 355–363. doi:10.1016/j.jsps.2012.02.001 PMID:23960810

Malam, Y., Loizidou, M., & Seifalian, A. M. (2009). Liposomes and nanoparticles: Nanosized vehicles for drug delivery in cancer. *Trends in Pharmacological Sciences*, *30*(11), 592–599. doi:10.1016/j.tips.2009.08.004 PMID:19837467

Malik, N., Evagorou, E. G., & Duncan, R. (1999). Dendrimer-platinate: A novel approach to cancer chemotherapy. *Anti-Cancer Drugs*, *10*(8), 767–776. doi:10.1097/00001813-199909000-00010 PMID:10573209

Malinovsky, V. K. (1990). The Prospects of ferroelectrics applications. *IEEE 7th International Symposium on Applications of Ferroelectrics*, 11 – 13.

Mali, S. (2013). Delivery systems for gene therapy. *Indian Journal of Human Genetics*, *19*(1), 3. doi:10.4103/0971-6866.112870 PMID:23901186

Ma, N., Ma, C., Li, C., Wang, T., Tang, Y., Wang, H., ... He, N. (2013). Influence of nanoparticle shape, size, and surface functionalization on cellular uptake. *Journal of Nanoscience and Nanotechnology*, *13*(10), 6485–6498. doi:10.1166/jnn.2013.7525 PMID:24245105

Ma, N., Wang, W. J., Chen, S., Wang, X. S., Wang, X. Q., Wang, S. B., ... Zhang, X. Z. (2015). Cucurbit[8]uril-mediated supramolecular photoswitching for self-preservation of mesoporous silica nanoparticle delivery system. *Chemical Communications*, *51*(65), 12970–12973. doi:10.1039/C5CC04631A PMID:26176026

Mandal, S. M., Ghosh, A. K., & Mandal, M. (2008). Iron oxide nanoparticle assisted purification and mass spectrometry based proteolytic mapping of intact CD4+ T cells from human blood. *Preparative Biochemistry & Biotechnology*, *39*(1), 20–31. doi:10.1080/10826060802589510 PMID:19090418

Mandal, T. K., Bostanian, L. A., Graves, R. A., Chapman, S. R., & Idodo, T. U. (2001). Porous biodegradable microparticles for delivery of pentamidine. *European Journal of Pharmaceutics and Biopharmaceutics*, *52*(1), 91–96. doi:10.1016/S0939-6411(01)00150-3 PMID:11438428

Manias, E., Touny, A., Wu, L., Strawhecker, K., Lu, B., & Chung, T. C. (2001). Polypropylene/montmorillonite nanocomposites. Review of the synthetic routes and materials properties. *Chemistry of Materials*, *13*(10), 3516–3523. doi:10.1021/cm0110627

Manivasagan, P., Bharathiraja, S., Bui, N. Q., Jang, B., Oh, Y. O., Lim, I. G., & Oh, J. (2016). Doxorubicin-loaded fucoidan capped gold nanoparticles for drug delivery and photoacoustic imaging. *International Journal of Biological Macromolecules*, *91*, 578–588. doi:10.1016/j.ijbiomac.2016.06.007 PMID:27267570

Manivasagan, P., Bharathiraja, S., Bui, N. Q., Lim, I. G., & Oh, J. (2016). Paclitaxel-loaded chitosan oligosaccharide-stabilized gold nanoparticles as novel agents for drug delivery and photoacoustic imaging of cancer cells. *International Journal of Pharmaceutics*, *511*(1), 367–379. doi:10.1016/j.ijpharm.2016.07.025 PMID:27424169

Manjunath, K., Reddy, J., & Venkateswarlu, V. (2005). Solid lipid nanoparticles as drug delivery systems. *Methods and Findings in Experimental and Clinical Pharmacology*, *27*(2), 127–144. doi:10.1358/mf.2005.27.2.876286 PMID:15834465

Mannix, R. J., Kumar, S., Cassiola, F., Montoya-Zavala, M., Feinstein, E., Prentiss, M., & Ingber, D. E. (2008). Nanomagnetic actuation of receptor-mediated signal transduction. *Nature Nanotechnology*, *3*(1), 36–40. doi:10.1038/nnano.2007.418 PMID:18654448

Mano, J., Silva, G., Azevedo, H. S., Malafaya, P., Sousa, R., Silva, S., ... Marques, A. (2007). Natural origin biodegradable systems in tissue engineering and regenerative medicine: Present status and some moving trends. *Journal of the Royal Society, Interface*, *4*(17), 999–1030. doi:10.1098/rsif.2007.0220 PMID:17412675

Manzano, M., Colilla, M., & Vallet-Regí, M. (2009). Drug delivery from ordered mesoporous matrices. *Expert Opinion on Drug Delivery*, *6*(12), 1383–1400. doi:10.1517/17425240903304024 PMID:19941412

Mao, S., Sun, W., & Kissel, T. (2010). Chitosan-based formulations for delivery of DNA and siRNA. *Advanced Drug Delivery Reviews*, *62*(1), 12–27. doi:10.1016/j.addr.2009.08.004 PMID:19796660

Marino, N., Illingworth, S., Kodialbail, P., Patel, A., Calderon, H., Lear, R., ... Brown, A. C. N. (2017). Development of a versatile oncolytic virus platform for local intra-tumoural expression of therapeutic transgenes. *PLoS One*, *12*(5), e0177810. doi:10.1371/journal.pone.0177810 PMID:28542292

Markman, M. (2006). Pegylated liposomal doxorubicin in the treatment of cancers of the breast and ovary. *Expert Opinion on Pharmacotherapy*, *7*(11), 1469–1474. doi:10.1517/14656566.7.11.1469 PMID:16859430

Marshall, E. (2002). Clinical research: Gene therapy a suspect in leukemia-like disease. *Science*, *298*(5591), 34–35. doi:10.1126cience.298.5591.34 PMID:12364755

Martínez, Á., Fuentes-Paniagua, E., Baeza, A., Sánchez-Nieves, J., Cicuéndez, M., Gómez, R., ... Vallet-Regí, M. (2015). Mesoporous silica nanoparticles decorated with carbosilane dendrons as new non-viral oligonucleotide delivery carriers. *Chemistry*, *21*(44), 15651–15666. doi:10.1002/chem.201501966 PMID:26361378

Martin, M. E., & Rice, K. G. (2007). Peptide-guided gene delivery. *The AAPS Journal*, *9*(1), E18–E29. doi:10.1208/aapsj0901003 PMID:17408236

Martins, S., Costa-Lima, S., Carneiro, T., Cordeiro-da-Silva, A., Souto, E. B., & Ferreira, D. C. (2012). Solid lipid nanoparticles as intracellular drug transporters: An investigation of the uptake mechanism and pathway. *International Journal of Pharmaceutics*, *430*(1), 216–227. doi:10.1016/j.ijpharm.2012.03.032 PMID:22465548

Marto, J., Vitor, C., Guerreiro, A., Severino, C., Eleutério, C., Ascenso, A., & Simões, S. (2016). Ethosomes for enhanced skin delivery of griseofulvin. *Colloids and Surfaces. B, Biointerfaces*, *146*, 616–623. doi:10.1016/j.colsurfb.2016.07.021 PMID:27429295

Masoudipour, E., Kashanian, S., & Maleki, N. (2017). A targeted drug delivery system based on dopamine functionalized nano graphene oxide. *Chemical Physics Letters*, *668*, 56–63. doi:10.1016/j.cplett.2016.12.019

Matsumura, Y. (2011). Preclinical and clinical studies of NK012, an SN-38-incorporating polymeric micelles, which is designed based on EPR effect. *Advanced Drug Delivery Reviews*, *63*(3), 184–192. doi:10.1016/j.addr.2010.05.008 PMID:20561951

May, G. S. (2007). Optimization of Nanocomposite Integral Capacitor Fabrication Using Neural Networks and Genetic Algorithms. *27th Annual IEEE/SEMI International Electronics Manufacturing Technology Symposium*, 123 – 129.

Mayor, S., & Pagano, R. E. (2007). Pathways of clathrin-independent endocytosis. *Nature Reviews. Molecular Cell Biology*, *8*(8), 603–612. doi:10.1038/nrm2216 PMID:17609668

Ma, Z. G., Ma, R., Xiao, X. L., Zhang, Y. H., Zhang, X. Z., Hu, N., ... Sun, Z. J. (2016). Azo polymeric micelles designed for colon-targeted dimethyl fumarate delivery for colon cancer therapy. *Acta Biomaterialia*, *44*, 323–331. doi:10.1016/j.actbio.2016.08.021 PMID:27544813

Ma, Z., Bai, J., Wang, Y., & Jiang, X. (2014). Impact of Shape and Pore Size of Mesoporous Silica Nanoparticles on Serum Protein Adsorption and RBCs Hemolysis. *ACS Applied Materials & Interfaces*, *6*(4), 2431–2438. doi:10.1021/am404860q PMID:24460090

Mazumder, A., Dwivedi, A., Du Preez, J. L., & Du Plessis, J. (2016). In vitro wound healing and cytotoxic effects of sinigrin–phytosome complex. *International Journal of Pharmaceutics*, *498*(1-2), 283–293. doi:10.1016/j.ijpharm.2015.12.027 PMID:26706438

McAuliffe, S. M., Morgan, S. L., Wyant, G. A., Tran, L. T., Muto, K. W., Chen, Y. S., ... Dinulescu, D. M. (2012). Targeting Notch, a key pathway for ovarian cancer stem cells, sensitizes tumors to platinum therapy. *Proceedings of the National Academy of Sciences of the United States of America*, *109*(43), E2939–E2948. doi:10.1073/pnas.1206400109 PMID:23019585

McBain, S. C., Yiu, H. H. P., & Dobson, J. (2008). Magnetic nanoparticles for gene and drug delivery. *International Journal of Nanomedicine*, *3*(2), 169–180. PMID:18686777

McCarter, M. D., Clarke, J. H., & Harken, A. H. (2004). Lymphangiogenesis is pivotal to the trials of a successful cancer metastasis. *Surgery*, *135*(2), 121–124. doi:10.1016/S0039-6060(03)00342-8 PMID:14739845

McQuaid, R. G. P., McGilly, L. J., Sharma, P., Gruverman, A., & Gregg, J. M. (2011). Mesoscale flux - closure domain formation in single - crystal BaTiO3. *Nature Communications*, *2*, 404. doi:10.1038/ncomms1413 PMID:21792183

Medarova, Z., Kumar, M., Ng, S., Yang, J., Barteneva, N., Evgenov, N. V., ... Moore, A. (2008). Multifunctional magnetic nanocarriers for image-tagged SiRNA delivery to intact pancreatic islets. *Transplantation*, *86*(9), 1170–1177. doi:10.1097/TP.0b013e31818a81b2 PMID:19005396

Medina-Kauwe, L. K. (2007). "Alternative" endocytic mechanisms exploited by pathogens: New avenues for therapeutic delivery? *Advanced Drug Delivery Reviews*, *59*(8), 798–809. doi:10.1016/j.addr.2007.06.009 PMID:17707545

Mehra, N. K., & Jain, N. (2015). Cancer targeting propensity of folate conjugated surface engineered multi-walled carbon nanotubes. *Colloids and Surfaces. B, Biointerfaces*, *132*, 17–26. doi:10.1016/j.colsurfb.2015.04.056 PMID:26001798

Mehra, N. K., Mishra, V., & Jain, N. (2014). A review of ligand tethered surface engineered carbon nanotubes. *Biomaterials*, *35*(4), 1267–1283. doi:10.1016/j.biomaterials.2013.10.032 PMID:24210872

Mehra, N. K., Verma, A. K., Mishra, P., & Jain, N. (2014). The cancer targeting potential of D α tocopheryl polyethylene glycol 1000 succinate tethered multi walled carbon nanotubes. *Biomaterials*, *35*(15), 4573–4588. doi:10.1016/j.biomaterials.2014.02.022 PMID:24612818

Meister, A., & Blume, A. (2007). Self-assembly of bipolar amphiphiles. *Current Opinion in Colloid & Interface Science*, *12*(3), 138–147. doi:10.1016/j.cocis.2007.05.003

Mei, X., Chen, D., Li, N., Xu, Q., Ge, J., Li, H., & Lu, J. (2012). Hollow mesoporous silica nanoparticles conjugated with pH-sensitive amphiphilic diblock polymer for controlled drug release. *Microporous and Mesoporous Materials*, *152*, 16–24. doi:10.1016/j.micromeso.2011.12.015

Mellaerts, R., Mols, R., Jammaer, J. A., Aerts, C. A., Annaert, P., Van Humbeeck, J., ... Martens, J. A. (2008). Increasing the oral bioavailability of the poorly water soluble drug itraconazole with ordered mesoporous silica. *European Journal of Pharmaceutics and Biopharmaceutics*, *69*(1), 223–230. doi:10.1016/j.ejpb.2007.11.006 PMID:18164930

Mellott, A. J., Forrest, M. L., & Detamore, M. S. (2013). Physical non-viral gene delivery methods for tissue engineering. *Annals of Biomedical Engineering*, *41*(3), 446–468. doi:10.100710439-012-0678-1 PMID:23099792

Meng, F., Engbers, G. H., & Feijen, J. (2004). Polyethylene glycol–grafted polystyrene particles. *Journal of Biomedical Materials Research. Part A*, *70*(1), 49–58. doi:10.1002/jbm.a.30056 PMID:15174108

Meng, H., & Li, G. (2013). A review of stimuli-responsive shape memory polymer composites. *Polymer*, *54*(9), 2199–2221. doi:10.1016/j.polymer.2013.02.023

Meng, H., Liong, M., Xia, T., Li, Z., Ji, Z., Zink, J. I., & Nel, A. E. (2010). Engineered Design of Mesoporous Silica Nanoparticles to Deliver Doxorubicin and P-Glycoprotein siRNA to Overcome Drug Resistance in a Cancer Cell Line. *ACS Nano*, *4*(8), 4539–4550. doi:10.1021/nn100690m PMID:20731437

Meng, H., Mai, W. X., Zhang, H., Xue, M., Xia, T., Lin, S., ... Nel, A. E. (2013). Codelivery of an optimal drug/siRNA combination using mesoporous silica nanoparticles to overcome drug resistance in breast cancer in vitro and in vivo. *ACS Nano*, *7*(2), 994–1005. doi:10.1021/nn3044066 PMID:23289892

Meng, H., Xue, M., Xia, T., Ji, Z., Tarn, D. Y., Zink, J. I., & Nel, A. E. (2011). Use of size and a copolymer design feature to improve the biodistribution and the enhanced permeability and retention effect of doxorubicin-loaded mesoporous silica nanoparticles in a murine xenograft tumor model. *ACS Nano*, *5*(5), 4131–4144. doi:10.1021/nn200809t PMID:21524062

Menon, J. U., Jadeja, P., Tambe, P., Vu, K., Yuan, B., & Nguyen, K. T. (2013). Nanomaterials for photo-based diagnostic and therapeutic applications. *Theranostics*, *3*(3), 152–166. doi:10.7150/thno.5327 PMID:23471164

Mercer, J., & Helenius, A. (2009). Virus entry by macropinocytosis. *Nature Cell Biology*, *11*(5), 510–520. doi:10.1038/ncb0509-510 PMID:19404330

Messerschmidt, S. K. E., Musyanovych, A., Altvater, M., Scheurich, P., Pfizenmaier, K., Landfester, K., & Kontermann, R. E. (2009). Targeted lipid-coated nanoparticles: Delivery of tumor necrosis factor-functionalized particles to tumor cells. *Journal of Controlled Release*, *137*(1), 69–77. doi:10.1016/j.jconrel.2009.03.010 PMID:19306900

Miao, Y. E., Hong, Z., Dan, C., Ruiyu, W., Tjiu, W. W., & Tianxi, L. (2012). Electrospun fibers of layered double hydroxide/biopolymer nanocomposites as effective drug delivery systems. *Materials Chemistry and Physics*, *134*(2-3), 623–630. doi:10.1016/j.matchemphys.2012.03.041

Miclea, R. D., Varma, P. R., Peng, A., & Balu-Iyer, S. V. (2007). Development and characterization of lipidic cochleate containing recombinant factor VIII. *Biochimica et Biophysica Acta (BBA) -. Biomembranes*, *1768*(11), 2890–2898. doi:10.1016/j.bbamem.2007.08.001 PMID:17936245

Mieszawska, A. J., Gianella, A., Cormode, D. P., Zhao, Y., Meijerink, A., Langer, R., ... Mulder, W. J. M. (2012). Engineering of lipid-coated PLGA nanoparticles with a tunable payload of diagnostically active nanocrystals for medical imaging. *Chemical Communications (Cambridge)*, *48*(47), 5835. doi:10.1039/c2cc32149a PMID:22555311

Miller, C. R., Bondurant, B., McLean, S. D., McGovern, K. A., & O'Brien, D. F. (1998). Liposome-cell interactions in vitro: Effect of liposome surface charge on the binding and endocytosis of conventional and sterically stabilized liposomes. *Biochemistry*, *37*(37), 12875–12883. doi:10.1021/bi980096y PMID:9737866

Milosavljevic, V., Krejcova, L., Guran, R., Buchtelova, H., Wawrzak, D., Richtera, L., ... Adam, V. (2017). Exceptional release kinetics and cytotoxic selectivity of oxidised MWCNTs double-functionalised with doxorubicin and prostate-homing peptide. *Colloids and Surfaces. B, Biointerfaces*, *156*, 123–132. doi:10.1016/j.colsurfb.2017.05.008 PMID:28527356

Minakuchi, Y., & ... . (2004). Atelocollagen-mediated synthetic small interfering RNA delivery for effective gene silencing in vitro and in vivo. *Nucleic Acids Research*, *32*(13), e109–e109. doi:10.1093/nar/gnh093 PMID:15272050

Minati, L., Antonini, V., Dalla Serra, M., Speranza, G., Enrichi, F., & Riello, P. (2013). pH-activated doxorubicin release from polyelectrolyte complex layer coated mesoporous silica nanoparticles. *Microporous and Mesoporous Materials*, *180*, 86–91. doi:10.1016/j.micromeso.2013.06.016

Mirzaei, H., Shakeri, A., Rashidi, B., Jalili, A., Banikazemi, Z., & Sahebkar, A. (2017). Phytosomal curcumin: A review of pharmacokinetic, experimental and clinical studies. *Biomedicine and Pharmacotherapy*, *85*, 102–112. doi:10.1016/j.biopha.2016.11.098 PMID:27930973

Misak, H. E., Asmatulu, R., Gopu, J. S., Man, K. P., Zacharias, N. M., Wooley, P. H., & Yang, S. Y. (2014). Albumin-based nanocomposite spheres for advanced drug delivery systems. *Biotechnology Journal*, *9*(1), 163–170. doi:10.1002/biot.201300150 PMID:24106002

Misak, H., Zachariasb, N., Song, Z., Hwangd, S., Mana, K. P., Asmatulua, R., & Yang, S. Y. (2013). Skin cancer treatment by albumin/5-Fu loaded magnetic nanocomposite spheres in a mouse model. *Journal of Biotechnology*, *164*(1), 130–136. doi:10.1016/j.jbiotec.2013.01.003 PMID:23395619

Misra, R., Acharya, S., & Sahoo, S. K. (2010). Cancer nanotechnology: Application of nanotechnology in cancer therapy. *Drug Discovery Today*, *15*(19-20), 842–850. doi:10.1016/j.drudis.2010.08.006 PMID:20727417

Misra, S. (2013). Human gene therapy: A brief overview of the genetic revolution. *The Journal of the Association of Physicians of India*, *61*(2), 127–133. PMID:24471251

Mitchell, R. D., Vogl, A. W., & Adam, W. M. (2009). *Gray's Anatomy for Students E-Book*. Academic Press.

Miteva, D. O., Rutkowski, J. M., Dixon, J. B., Kilarski, W., Shields, J. D., & Swartz, M. A. (2010). Transmural flow modulates cell and fluid transport functions of lymphatic endothelium. *Circulation Research, 106*(5), 920–931. doi:10.1161/CIRCRESAHA.109.207274 PMID:20133901

Mitra, S. B., Wu, D., & Holmes, B. N. (2003, October). An application of nanotechnology in advanced dental materials. *The Journal of the American Dental Association, 134*(10), 1382–1390. doi:10.14219/jada.archive.2003.0054 PMID:14620019

Mjör, I. A., Moorhead, J. E., & Dahl, J. E. (2000). Reasons for replacement of restorations in permanent teeth in general dental practice. *International Dental Journal, 50*(6), 361–366. doi:10.1111/j.1875-595X.2000.tb00569.x PMID:11197194

Mobasseri, R., Karimi, M., Tian, L., Naderi-Manesh, H., & Ramakrishna, S. (2017). Hydrophobic lapatinib encapsulated dextran-chitosan nanoparticles using a toxic solvent free method: Fabrication, release property & in vitro anti-cancer activity. *Materials Science and Engineering C, 74*, 413–421. doi:10.1016/j.msec.2016.12.027 PMID:28254312

Modest, D., Kasper, S., Stintzing, S., Prasnikar, N., Müller, L., Caca, K., . . . Trarbach, T. (2016). Randomized phase II study of maintenance treatment with 5-FU/FA plus panitumumab vs 5-FU/FA alone after induction (mFOLFOX6 plus panitumumab) in patients with RAS WT metastatic colorectal cancer. *Annals of Oncology, 27*(suppl 6), 605TiP.

Modi, C. D., Patel, S. J., Desai, A. B., & Murthy, R. (2011). Functionalization and evaluation of PEGylated carbon nanotubes as novel drug delivery for methotrexate. *Journal of Applied Pharmaceutical Science, 1*(5), 13.

Mody, K. T., Popat, A., Mahony, D., Cavallaro, A. S., Yu, C., & Mitter, N. (2013). Mesoporous silica nanoparticles as antigen carriers and adjuvants for vaccine delivery. *Nanoscale, 5*(12), 5167–5179. doi:10.1039/c3nr00357d PMID:23657437

Mognetti, B., Barberis, A., Marino, S., Berta, G., Francia, D. S., Trotta, F., & Cavalli, R. J. (2012). *In vitro* enhancement of anticancer activity of paclitaxel by a Cremophor free cyclodextrin-based nanosponge formulation. *Journal of Inclusion Phenomena and Macrocyclic Chemistry, 74*(1-4), 201–210. doi:10.100710847-011-0101-9

Mohammad, M. A., Alhalaweh, A., & Velaga, S. P. (2011). Hansen solubility parameter as a tool to predict cocrystal formation. *International Journal of Pharmaceutics, 407*(1), 63–71. doi:10.1016/j.ijpharm.2011.01.030 PMID:21256944

Mohan, T., Verma, P., & Rao, D. N. (2013). Novel adjuvants & delivery vehicles for vaccines development: A road ahead. *The Indian Journal of Medical Research, 138*(5), 779–795. PMID:24434331

Mohanty, C., Das, M., & Sahoo, S. K. (2012). Emerging role of nanocarriers to increase the solubility and bioavailability of curcumin. *Expert Opinion on Drug Delivery, 9*(11), 1347–1364. doi:10.1517/17425247.2012.724676 PMID:22971222

Molina, M., Asadian-Birjand, M., Balach, J., Bergueiro, J., Miceli, E., & Calderón, M. (2015). Stimuli-responsive nanogel composites and their application in nanomedicine. *Chemical Society Reviews, 44*(17), 6161–6186. doi:10.1039/C5CS00199D PMID:26505057

Monteiro, N., Martins, A., Reis, R. L., & Neves, N. M. (2014). Liposomes in tissue engineering and regenerative medicine. *Journal of the Royal Society, Interface, 11*(101), 1–23. doi:10.1098/rsif.2014.0459 PMID:25401172

Montier, T., Benvegnu, T., Jaffres, P.-A., Yaouanc, J.-J., & Lehn, P. (2008). Progress in cationic lipid-mediated gene transfection: A series of bio-inspired lipids as an example. *Current Gene Therapy, 8*(5), 296–312. doi:10.2174/156652308786070989 PMID:18855628

Moon, J. J., Suh, H., Bershteyn, A., Stephan, M. T., Liu, H., Huang, B., ... Irvine, D. C. (2011). Interbilayer-crosslinked multilamellar vesicles as synthetic vaccines for potent humoral and cellular immune responses. *Nature Materials, 10*(3), 243–251. doi:10.1038/nmat2960 PMID:21336265

Moosavian, S. A., Abnous, K., Badiee, A., & Jaafari, M. R. (2016). Improvement in the drug delivery and anti-tumor efficacy of PEGylated liposomal doxorubicin by targeting RNA aptamers in mice bearing breast tumor model. *Colloids and Surfaces. B, Biointerfaces*, *139*, 228–236. doi:10.1016/j.colsurfb.2015.12.009 PMID:26722819

Mo, R., Sun, Q., Li, N., & Zhang, C. (2013). Intracellular delivery and antitumor effects of pH-sensitive liposomes based on zwitterionic oligopeptide lipids. *Biomaterials*, *34*(11), 2773–2786. doi:10.1016/j.biomaterials.2013.01.030 PMID:23352118

Moreno, L. C., Cavalcanti, I. M., Satyal, P., Santos-Magalhães, N. S., Rolim, H. M., & Freitas, R. M. (2015). Acute toxicity and anticonvulsant activity of liposomes containing nimodipine on pilocarpine-induced seizures in mice. *Neuroscience Letters*, *585*, 38–42. doi:10.1016/j.neulet.2014.11.025 PMID:25445375

Morgado, L. F., Trávolo, A. R. F., Muehlmann, L. A., Narcizo, P. S., Nunes, R. B., Pereira, P. A. G., & Longo, J. P. F. (2017). Photodynamic Therapy treatment of onychomycosis with Aluminium-Phthalocyanine Chloride nanoemulsions: A proof of concept clinical trial. *Journal of Photochemistry and Photobiology. B, Biology*, *173*, 266–270. doi:10.1016/j.jphotobiol.2017.06.010 PMID:28622558

Morgan, C. J., Renwick, A. G., & Friedmann, P. S. (2003). The role of stratum corneum and dermal microvascular perfusion in penetration and tissue levels of water-soluble drugs investigated by microdialysis. *British Journal of Dermatology*, *148*(3), 434–443. doi:10.1046/j.1365-2133.2003.05163.x PMID:12653734

Moros, E. (2012). *Physics of thermal therapy: fundamentals and clinical applications*. Taylor & Francis.

Morse, D. E. (2011). First Large - Scale Engineered Synthesis of BaTiO3 Nanoparticles Using Low Temperature Bio-inspired Principles. *Nature Protocols*, *6*(1), 97–104. doi:10.1038/nprot.2010.138 PMID:21212785

Möschwitzer, J. P. (2013). Drug nanocrystals in the commercial pharmaceutical development process. *International Journal of Pharmaceutics*, *453*(1), 142–156. doi:10.1016/j.ijpharm.2012.09.034 PMID:23000841

Moscofian, A. S., Silva, C. R., & Airoldi, C. (2008). Stability of layered aluminum and magnesium organosilicates. *Microporous and Mesoporous Materials*, *107*(1-2), 113–120. doi:10.1016/j.micromeso.2007.05.047

Motwani, S. K., & … . (2008). Chitosan–sodium alginate nanoparticles as submicroscopic reservoirs for ocular delivery: Formulation, optimisation and in vitro characterisation. *European Journal of Pharmaceutics and Biopharmaceutics*, *68*(3), 513–525. PMID:17983737

Moulik, P. S., & Kumar, R. A. (2008). Physicochemistry of W/O Microemulsions. In M. Fanun (Ed.), *Microemulsions: Properties and Applications* (pp. 17–40). Taylor and Francis Group, LLC; doi:10.1201/9781420089608.ch2

Mozafari, M. R., Pardakhty, A., Azarmi, S., Jazayeri, J. A., Nokhodchi, A., & Omri, A. (2009). Role of nanocarrier systems in cancer nanotherapy. *Journal of Liposome Research*, *19*(4), 310–321. doi:10.3109/08982100902913204 PMID:19863166

Muddineti, O. S., Ghosh, B., & Biswas, S. (2015). Current trends in using polymer coated gold nanoparticles for cancer therapy. *International Journal of Pharmaceutics*, *484*(1), 252–267. doi:10.1016/j.ijpharm.2015.02.038 PMID:25701627

Mueller-Goymann, C., & Hamann, H. J. (1991). Pharmacosomes - multilamellar vesicles consisting of pure drug. *European Journal of Pharmaceutics and Biopharmaceutics*, *37*(2), 113–117.

Mukherjee, A., Tothadi, S., Chakraborty, S., Ganguly, S., & Desiraju, G. R. (2013). Synthon identification in co-crystals and polymorphs with IR spectroscopy. Primary amides as a case study. *CrystEngComm*, *15*(23), 4640–4654. doi:10.1039/c3ce40286j

Mukherjee, S., Ray, S., & Thakur, R. S. (2009). Solid Lipid Nanoparticles: A Modern Formulation Approach in Drug Delivery System. *Indian Journal of Pharmaceutical Sciences*, *71*(4), 349–358. doi:10.4103/0250-474X.57282 PMID:20502539

Müller, R. H., Radtke, M., & Wissing, S. A. (2002). Solid lipid nanoparticles (SLN) and nanostructured lipid carriers (NLC) in cosmetic and dermatological preparations. *Advanced Drug Delivery Reviews*, *54*(Suppl 1), S131–S155. doi:10.1016/S0169-409X(02)00118-7 PMID:12460720

Müller, R., Mäder, K., & Gohla, S. (2000). Solid lipid nanoparticles (SLN) for controlled drug delivery: A review of the state of the art. *European Journal of Pharmaceutics and Biopharmaceutics*, *50*(1), 161–177. doi:10.1016/S0939-6411(00)00087-4 PMID:10840199

Muñoz, B., Rámila, A., Pérez-Pariente, J., Díaz, I., & Vallet-Regí, M. (2003). MCM-41 Organic modification as drug delivery rate regulator. *Chemistry of Materials*, *15*(2), 500–503. doi:10.1021/cm021217q

Mu, P., Nagahara, S., Makita, N., Tarumi, Y., Kadomatsu, K., & Takei, Y. (2009). Systemic delivery of siRNA specific to tumor mediated by atelocollagen: Combined therapy using siRNA targeting Bcl-xL and cisplatin against prostate cancer. *International Journal of Cancer*, *125*(12), 2978–2990. doi:10.1002/ijc.24382 PMID:19422046

Mura, S., Nicolas, J., & Couvreur, P. (2013). Stimuli-responsive nanocarriers for drug delivery. *Nature Materials*, *12*(11), 991–1003. doi:10.1038/nmat3776 PMID:24150417

Muro, S., Garnacho, C., Champion, J. A., Leferovich, J., Gajewski, C., Schuchman, E. H., ... Muzykantov, V. R. (2008). Control of endothelial targeting and intracellular delivery of therapeutic enzymes by modulating the size and shape of ICAM-1-targeted carriers. *Molecular Therapy*, *16*(8), 1450–1458. doi:10.1038/mt.2008.127 PMID:18560419

Murugan, K., Choonara, Y. E., Kumar, P., Bijukumar, D., du Toit, L. C., & Pillay, V. (2015). Parameters and characteristics governing cellular internalization and trans-barrier trafficking of nanostructures. *International Journal of Nanomedicine*, *10*, 2191. PMID:25834433

Mylon, S. E., Chen, K. L., & Elimelech, M. (2004). Influence of natural organic matter and ionic composition on the kinetics and structure of hematite colloid aggregation: Implications to iron depletion in estuaries. *Langmuir*, *20*(21), 9000–9006. doi:10.1021/la049153g PMID:15461479

Nabel, G. J., Gordon, D., Bishop, D. K., Nickoloff, B. J., Yang, Z., Aruga, A., ... Chang, A. E. (1996). Immune response in human melanoma after transfer of an allogeneic class I major histocompatibility complex gene with DNA–liposome complexes. *Proceedings of the National Academy of Sciences of the United States of America*, *93*(26), 15388–15393. doi:10.1073/pnas.93.26.15388 PMID:8986821

Nabel, G. J., Nabel, E. G., Yang, Z. Y., Fox, B. A., Plautz, G. E., Gao, X., ... Chang, A. E. (1993). Direct gene transfer with DNA-liposome complexes in melanoma: Expression, biologic activity, and lack of toxicity in humans. *Proceedings of the National Academy of Sciences of the United States of America*, *90*(23), 11307–11311. doi:10.1073/pnas.90.23.11307 PMID:8248244

Nacht, S., & Kantz, M. (1992). The microsponge: A novel topical programmable delivery system. *Topical Drug Delivery Systems*, *42*, 299–325.

Naessens, M., Cerdobbel, A., Soetaert, W., & Vandamme, E. J. (2005). Leuconostoc dextransucrase and dextran: Production, properties and applications. *Journal of Chemical Technology and Biotechnology (Oxford, Oxfordshire)*, *80*(8), 845–860. doi:10.1002/jctb.1322

Nagabandi, V., & Sambaraj, S. (2013). Silica-Lipid Hybrid Microparticles for Improved Bioavailability of Bcs Class IV Drugs. *Am J Adv Drug Deliv*, *1*(5), 663–681.

Nagapudi, K., Umanzor, E. Y., & Masui, C. (2017). High-throughput screening and scale-up of cocrystals using resonant acoustic mixing. *International Journal of Pharmaceutics*, *521*(1), 337–345. doi:10.1016/j.ijpharm.2017.02.027 PMID:28229947

Nagia, A., Iqbala, B., Kumara, S., Sharmaa, S., Alib, J., & Babootab, S. (2017). Quality by design based silymarin nanoemulsion for enhancement of oral bioavailability. *Journal of Drug Delivery Science and Technology*, *40*, 35–44. doi:10.1016/j.jddst.2017.05.019

Nag, M., Gajbhiye, V., Kesharwani, P., & Jain, N. K. (2016). Transferrin functionalized chitosan-PEG nanoparticles for targeted delivery of paclitaxel to cancer cells. *Colloids and Surfaces. B, Biointerfaces*, *148*, 363–370. doi:10.1016/j.colsurfb.2016.08.059 PMID:27632697

Nairi, V., Medda, L., Monduzzi, M., & Salis, A. (2017). Adsorption and release of ampicillin antibiotic from ordered mesoporous silica. *Journal of Colloid and Interface Science*, *497*, 217–225. doi:10.1016/j.jcis.2017.03.021 PMID:28285049

Nakamura, E., Isobe, H., Tomita, N., Sawamura, M., Jinno, S., & Okayama, H. (2000). Functionalized fullerene as a new artificial vector for transfection. *Angewandte Chemie International Edition in English*, *39*, 4254–4257.

Nakamura, K., Abu Lila, A. S., Matsunaga, M., Doi, Y., Ishida, T., & Kiwada, H. (2011). A double-modulation strategy in cancer treatment with a chemotherapeutic agent and siRNA. *Molecular Therapy*, *19*(11), 2040–2047. doi:10.1038/mt.2011.174 PMID:21878904

Nakao, S., Fujii, S., Sakaki, T., & Tomita, K. I. (1977). The crystal and molecular structure of the 2: 1 molecular complex of theophylline with phenobarbital. *Acta Crystallographica. Section B, Structural Science*, *33*(5), 1373–1378. doi:10.1107/S0567740877006116

Nalawade, P., Aware, B., Kadam, V. J., & Hirlekar, R. S. (2009). Layered double hydroxides: A review. *Journal of Scientific and Industrial Research*, *68*, 267–272.

Nam, H. Y., Park, J. H., Kim, K., Kwon, I. C., & Jeong, S. Y. (2009). Lipid-based emulsion system as non-viral gene carriers. *Archives of Pharmacal Research*, *32*(5), 639–646. doi:10.100712272-009-1500-y PMID:19471876

Nam, J., Vanderlick, T. K., & Beales, P. A. (2012). Formation and dissolution of phospholipid domains with varying textures in hybrid lipo-polymersomes. *Soft Matter*, *8*(30), 7982. doi:10.1039/c2sm25646k

Nandy, B., Santosh, M., & Maiti, P. K. (2012). Interaction of nucleic acids with carbon nanotubes and dendrimers. *Journal of Biosciences*, *37*(3), 457–474. doi:10.100712038-012-9220-8 PMID:22750983

Nangia, A. (2010). Supramolecular chemistry and crystal engineering. *Journal of Chemical Sciences*, *122*(3), 295–310. doi:10.100712039-010-0035-6

Nanjwade Basavaraj, K. (2009). Dendrimers: Emerging polymers for drug-delivery systems. *European Journal of Pharmaceutical Sciences*, *38*(3), 185–196. doi:10.1016/j.ejps.2009.07.008 PMID:19646528

Napper, D. H. (1970). Flocculation studies of sterically stabilized dispersions. *Journal of Colloid and Interface Science*, *32*(1), 106–114. doi:10.1016/0021-9797(70)90107-4

Naseri, N., Valizadeh, H., & Zakeri-Milani, P. (2015). Solid lipid nanoparticles and nanostructured lipid carriers: Structure preparation and application. *Advanced Pharmaceutical Bulletin*, *5*(3), 305–313. doi:10.15171/apb.2015.043 PMID:26504751

Naskar, A., Khan, H., Bera, S., & Jana, S. (2017). Soft chemical synthesis, characterization and interaction of ZnO graphene nanocomposite with bovine serum albumin protein. *Journal of Molecular Liquids*, *237*, 113–119. doi:10.1016/j.molliq.2017.04.074

Natesan, S., Sugumaran, A., Ponnusamy, C., Thiagarajan, V., Palanichamy, R., & Kandasamy, R. (2017). Chitosan stabilized camptothecin nanoemulsions: Development, evaluation and biodistribution in preclinical breast cancer animal mode. *International Journal of Biological Macromolecules*, S0141-8130(16)32673-3.

Nayerossadat, N., Maedeh, T., & Ali, P. A. (2012). Viral and nonviral delivery systems for gene delivery. *Advanced Biomedical Research*, *1*(1), 27. doi:10.4103/2277-9175.98152 PMID:23210086

Nazaruk, E., Majkowska-Pilip, A., & Bilewicz, R. (2017). Lipidic Cubic-Phase Nanoparticles—Cubosomes for Efficient Drug Delivery to Cancer Cells. *ChemPlusChem*, *82*(4), 570–575. doi:10.1002/cplu.201600534

Nechipadappu, S. K., Tekuri, V., & Trivedi, D. R. (2017). Pharmaceutical Co-Crystal of Flufenamic Acid: Synthesis and Characterization of Two Novel Drug-Drug Co-Crystal. *Journal of Pharmaceutical Sciences*, *106*(5), 1384–1390. doi:10.1016/j.xphs.2017.01.033 PMID:28185907

Nedyalkova, M., Donkova, B., Romanova, J., Tzvetkov, G., Madurga, S., & Simeonov, V. (2017). Iron oxide nanoparticles - In vivo/in vitro biomedical applications and in silico studies. *Advances in Colloid and Interface Science*, *249*, 192–212. doi:10.1016/j.cis.2017.05.003 PMID:28499604

Nguyen, C. T., Webb, R. I., Lambert, L. K., Strounina, E., Lee, E. C., Parat, M.-O., ... Ross, B. P. (2017). Bifunctional Succinylated ε-Polylysine-Coated Mesoporous Silica Nanoparticles for pH-Responsive and Intracellular Drug Delivery Targeting the Colon. *ACS Applied Materials & Interfaces*, *9*(11), 9470–9483. doi:10.1021/acsami.7b00411 PMID:28252278

Nguyen, J., Steele, T. W. J., Merkel, O., Reul, R., & Kissel, T. (2008). Fast degrading polyesters as siRNA nano-carriers for pulmonary gene therapy. *Journal of Controlled Release*, *132*(3), 243–251. doi:10.1016/j.jconrel.2008.06.010 PMID:18619502

Nidhi, K., Indrajeet, S., Khushboo, M., Gauri, K., & Sen, D. J. (2011). Hydrotropy: A promising tool for solubility enhancement: A review. *Int J Drug Dev Res.*, *3*(2), 26–33.

Niemela, E., Desai, D., Nkizinkiko, Y., Eriksson, J. E., & Rosenholm, J. M. (2015). Sugar-decorated mesoporous silica nanoparticles as delivery vehicles for the poorly soluble drug celastrol enables targeted induction of apoptosis in cancer cells. *European Journal of Pharmaceutics and Biopharmaceutics*, *96*, 11–21. doi:10.1016/j.ejpb.2015.07.009 PMID:26184689

Nigam, P. W. S., Louis, M., Wangnoo, S., Chavanb, P., & Sarkar, D. (2014). Graphene quantum dots conjugated albumin nanoparticles for targeted drug delivery and imaging of pancreatic cancer. *Journal of Materials Chemistry. B, Materials for Biology and Medicine*, *2*(21), 3190–3195. doi:10.1039/C4TB00015C

Nikalje, A. P. (2015). Nanotechnology and its Applications in Medicine. *Medicinal Chemistry (Shariqah, United Arab Emirates)*, *5*(2), 81–89.

Nımesh, S. (2013). Cyclodextrin and cyclodextrin containing polymers. In Gene theraphy: Potentail Application Of Nanotechnology (pp. 287-304). UK Woodhead Publishing Limited. doi:10.1533/9781908818645.287

Nnamani, P. O., Attama, A. A., Ibezim, E. C., & Adikwu, M. U. (2010). SRMS142-based solid lipid microparticles: Application in oral delivery of glibenclamide to diabetic rats. *European Journal of Pharmaceutics and Biopharmaceutics*, *76*(1), 68–74. doi:10.1016/j.ejpb.2010.06.002 PMID:20554020

Nokhodchi, A., Jelvehgari, M., & Mozafari, M. (2007). Factors affecting the morphology of benzoyl peroxide microsponges. *Micron (Oxford, England)*, *38*(8), 834–840. doi:10.1016/j.micron.2007.06.012 PMID:17692528

Nourbakhsh, M., Jaafari, M. R., Lage, H., Abnous, K., Mosaffa, F., Badiee, A, & ... . (2015). Nanolipoparticles-mediated MDR1 siRNA delivery reduces doxorubicin resistance in breast cancer cells and silences MDR1 expression in xenograft model of human breast cancer. *Iran J Basic Med Sci*, *18*(4), 385–392. doi:10.1038/nbt.1602 PMID:26019802

Novicki, D. L. (2005). DNA vaccines. In H. V. Vohr (Ed.), *Encyclopedic reference of immunotoxicology* (pp. 212–215). Berlin: Springer. doi:10.1007/3-540-27806-0_396

O' Driscoll, C. M., & Griffin, B. T. (2008). Biopharmaceutical challenges associated with drugs with low aqueous solubility—The potential impact of lipid-based formulations. *Advanced Drug Delivery Reviews*, *60*(6), 617–624. doi:10.1016/j.addr.2007.10.012 PMID:18155800

O'Driscol, C. M. (1992). Anatomy and physiology of the lymphatics. In W. N. Charman & V. J. Stella (Eds.), *Lymphatic Transport of Drugs*. Boca Raton, FL: CRC Press Inc.

O'Hagan, D. T. (2007). MF59 is a safe and potent vaccine adjuvant that enhances protection against influenza virus infection. *Expert Review of Vaccines*, *6*(5), 699–710. doi:10.1586/14760584.6.5.699 PMID:17931151

Ochiya, T., & … . (1999). New delivery system for plasmid DNA in vivo using atelocollagen as a carrier material: The Minipellet. *Nature Medicine*, *5*(6), 707–710. doi:10.1038/9560 PMID:10371512

Ochiya, T., Nagahara, S., Sano, A., Itoh, H., & Terada, M. (2001). Biomaterials for gene delivery atelocollagen-mediated controlled release of molecular medicines. *Current Gene Therapy*, *1*(1), 31–52. doi:10.2174/1566523013348887 PMID:12109137

Ogaji, I. J., Nep, E. I., & Audu-Peter, J. D. (2012). *Advances in natural polymers as pharmaceutical excipients*. Academic Press.

Ogawa, K., Hirano, S., Miyanishi, T., Yui, T., & Watanabe, T. (1984). A new polymorph of chitosan. *Macromolecules*, *17*(4), 973–975. doi:10.1021/ma00134a076

Ogle, O. E., & Byles, N. (2014). Nanotechnology in Dentistry Today. *The West Indian Medical Journal*, *63*(4), 344–348. PMID:25429479

Ogris, M., Brunner, S., Schüller, S., Kircheis, R., & Wagner, E. (1999). PEGylated DNA/transferrin-PEI complexes: Reduced interaction with blood components, extended circulation in blood and potential for systemic gene delivery. *Gene Therapy*, *6*(4), 595–605. doi:10.1038j.gt.3300900 PMID:10476219

Oguzhan, P., & Yangilar, F. (2013). Pullulan: Production and usage in food industry. *African Journal of Food Science and Technology*, *4*(3), 57–63.

Oh, K. T., Lee, E. S., Kim, D., & Bae, Y. H. (2008). L-histidine-based pH-sensitive anticancer drug carrier micelle: Reconstitution and brief evaluation of its systemic toxicity. *International Journal of Pharmaceutics*, *358*(1), 177–183. doi:10.1016/j.ijpharm.2008.03.003 PMID:18407443

Oh, N., & Park, J.-H. (2014). Endocytosis and exocytosis of nanoparticles in mammalian cells. *International Journal of Nanomedicine*, *9*(Suppl 1), 51–63. PMID:24872703

Ohtsuki, C., Kokubo, T., & Yamamuro, T. (1992). Mechanism of apatite formation on CaOSiO2P2O5 glasses in a simulated body fluid. *Journal of Non-Crystalline Solids*, *143*, 84–92. doi:10.1016/S0022-3093(05)80556-3

Ojeda, E., Puras, G., Agirre, M., Zárate, J., Grijalvo, S., Pons, R., ... Pedraz, J. L. (2015). Niosomes based on synthetic cationic lipids for gene delivery: The influence of polar head-groups on the transfection efficiency in HEK-293, ARPE-19 and MSC-D1 cells. *Organic & Biomolecular Chemistry*, *13*(4), 1068–1081. doi:10.1039/C4OB02087A PMID:25412820

Okore, V. C., Attama, A. A., Ofokansi, K. C., Esimone, C. O., & Onuigbo, E. B. (2011). Formulation and evaluation of niosomes. *Indian Journal of Pharmaceutical Sciences*, *73*(3), 323–328. PMID:22457561

Oliveira, M. S., Mussi, S. V., Gomes, D. A., Yoshida, M. I., Frezard, F., Carregal, V. M., & Ferreira, L. A. (2016). α-Tocopherol succinate improves encapsulation and anticancer activity of doxorubicin loaded in solid lipid nanoparticles. *Colloids and Surfaces. B, Biointerfaces*, *140*, 246–253. doi:10.1016/j.colsurfb.2015.12.019 PMID:26764108

Olubummo, A., Schulz, M., Lechner, B., Scholtysek, P., Bacia, K., & Blume, A. (2012). Controlling the Localization of in Mixed Lipid / Polymer Membranes. *ACS Nano*, (10), 8713–8727. doi:10.1021/nn3023602 PMID:22950802

Onishi, H., & Machida, Y. (1999). Biodegradation and distribution of water-soluble chitosan in mice. *Biomaterials*, *20*(2), 175–182. doi:10.1016/S0142-9612(98)00159-8 PMID:10022787

Orlu, M., Cevher, E., & Araman, A. (2006). Design and evaluation of colon specific drug delivery system containing flurbiprofen microsponges. *International Journal of Pharmaceutics*, *318*(1-2), 103–117. doi:10.1016/j.ijpharm.2006.03.025 PMID:16687222

Ortega, M. M. D., Lorenzo, A. C., Concheiro, A., & Loftsson, T. (2012, May). Cyclodextrin-based nanogels for pharmaceutical and biomedical applications. *International Journal of Pharmaceutics*, *428*(1-2), 152–163. doi:10.1016/j.ijpharm.2012.02.038 PMID:22388054

Paillard, A., Hindré, F., Vignes-Colombeix, C., Benoit, J. P., & Garcion, E. (2010). The importance of endo-lysosomal escape with lipid nanocapsules for drug subcellular bioavailability. *Biomaterials*, *31*(29), 7542–7554. doi:10.1016/j.biomaterials.2010.06.024 PMID:20630585

Pajula, K., Wittoek, L., Lehto, V.-P., Ketolainen, J., & Korhonen, O. (2014). Phase Separation in Coamorphous Systems: In Silico Prediction and the Experimental Challenge of Detection. *Molecular Pharmaceutics*, *11*(7), 2271–2279. doi:10.1021/mp400712m PMID:24824610

Palakurthi, S., Yellepeddi, V. K., & Kumar, A. (2011). Nanocarriers for Cytosolic Drug and Gene Delivery in Cancer Therapy. In M. Anna & S. Olsztynska (Eds.), *Biomedical engineering, trends, research and technologies* (pp. 245–272). Croatia: InTech. doi:10.5772/12918

Paliwal, R., Rai, S., & Vyas, S. P. (2011). Lipid drug conjugate (LDC) nanoparticles as autolymphotrophs for oral delivery of methotrexate. *Journal of Biomedical Nanotechnology*, *7*(1), 130–131. doi:10.1166/jbn.2011.1235 PMID:21485837

Pal, M., Bera, S., Sarkar, S., & Jana, S. (2014). Influence of Al doping on microstructural, optical and photocatalytic properties of sol–gel based nanostructured zinc oxide films on glass. *RSC Advances*, *4*(23), 11552–11563. doi:10.1039/C3RA44612C

Pal, N., & Bhaumik, A. (2013). Soft templating strategies for the synthesis of mesoporous materials: Inorganic, organic-inorganic hybrid and purely organic solids. *Advances in Colloid and Interface Science*, *189-190*, 21–41. doi:10.1016/j.cis.2012.12.002 PMID:23337774

Pan, B., Cui, D., Xu, P., Ozkan, C., Feng, G., Ozkan, M., & He, R. (2009). Synthesis and characterization of polyamidoamine dendrimer-coated multi-walled carbon nanotubes and their application in gene delivery systems. *Nanotechnology*, *20*(12), 125101. doi:10.1088/0957-4484/20/12/125101 PMID:19420458

Pancholi, K., Ahras, N., Stride, E., Edirisinghe, M. J., & Samarasinghe, S. (2009). Novel electrohydrodynamic preparation of porous chitosan particles for drug delivery. *Journal of Materials Science. Materials in Medicine*, *20*(4), 917–923. doi:10.100710856-008-3638-4 PMID:19034624

Pandi, P., Jain, A., Raju, S., & Khan, W. (2017). Therapeutic approaches for the delivery of TNF-α siRNA. *Therapeutic Delivery*, *8*(5), 343–355. doi:10.4155/tde-2017-0011 PMID:28361614

Pandita, A., & Sharma, P. (2013). Pharmacosomes: An emerging novel vesicular drug delivery system for poorly soluble synthetic and herbal drugs. *ISRN Pharmaceutics*, *2013*(3), 1–10. doi:10.1155/2013/348186 PMID:24106615

Pandita, D., & Lather, V. (2015). Silica-Based Nanoparticles for Theranostic Applications. In B. Singh, M. S. Sachdeva, & A. Liopo (Eds.), *NanoBioMedicine* (Vol. 3, pp. 383–422). Houston, TX: Studium Press, LLC.

Pandita, D., Poonia, N., & Lather, V. (2015). Mesoporous Silica Nanoparticles in Drug Delivery and Targeting. In B. Singh, J. R. Kanwar, & O. P. Katare (Eds.), *NanoBioMedicine* (Vol. 1, pp. 267–336). Houston, TX: Studium Press, LLC.

Pantel, K., & Brakenhoff, R. H. (2004). Dissecting the metastatic cascade. *Nature Reviews. Cancer*, *4*(6), 448–456. doi:10.1038/nrc1370 PMID:15170447

Panyam, J., Dali, M. M., Sahoo, S. K., Ma, W., Chakravarthi, S. S., Amidon, G. L., ... Labhasetvar, V. (2003). Polymer degradation and *in vitro* release of a model protein from poly(D,L-lactideco- glycolide) nano- and microparticles. *Journal of Controlled Release*, *92*(1-2), 173–187. doi:10.1016/S0168-3659(03)00328-6 PMID:14499195

Panyam, J., & Labhasetwar, V. (2003). Biodegradable nanoparticles for drug and gene delivery to cells and tissue. *Advanced Drug Delivery Reviews*, *55*(3), 329–347. doi:10.1016/S0169-409X(02)00228-4 PMID:12628320

Papahadjopoulos, D., Vail, W. J., Jacobson, K., & Poste, G. (1975). Cochleate lipid cylinders: Formation by fusion of unilamellar lipid vesicles. *Biochimica et Biophysica Acta*, *394*(3), 483–491. doi:10.1016/0005-2736(75)90299-0 PMID:805602

Papanicolaou, I., Briggs, S., & Alpar, H. O. (2004). Increased Resistance of DNA Lipoplexes to Protein Binding In Vitro by Surface-modification with a Multivalent Hydrophilic Polymer. *Journal of Drug Targeting*, *12*(8), 541–547. doi:10.1080/10611860400011950 PMID:15621679

Pappinen, S., & Urtti, A. (2016). Microemulsions. In *Percutaneous Penetration Enhancers Chemical Methods in Penetration Enhancement* (pp. 253–262). Berlin: Springer Berlin Heidelberg; doi:10.1007/978-3-662-47862-2_16

Pardakhty, A., & Moazeni, E. (2013). Nano-niosomes in drug, vaccine and gene delivery: A rapid overview. *Nanomedicine Journal*, *1*(1), 1–12.

Parhi, P., Mohanty, C., & Sahoo, S. K. (2012). Nanotechnology-based combinational drug delivery: An emerging approach for cancer therapy. *Drug Discovery Today*, *17*(17-18), 1044–1052. doi:10.1016/j.drudis.2012.05.010 PMID:22652342

Park, B. K., & Kim, M. M. (2010). Applications of chitin and its derivatives in biological medicine. *International Journal of Molecular Sciences*, *11*(12), 5152–5164. doi:10.3390/ijms11125152 PMID:21614199

Parker, A. L., Newman, C., Briggs, S., Seymour, L., & Sheridan, P. J. (2003). Nonviral gene delivery: Techniques and implications for molecular medicine. *Expert Reviews in Molecular Medicine*, *5*(22). doi:10.1017/S1462399403006562 PMID:14585173

Park, I. K., Ng, C. P., Wang, J., Chu, B., Yuan, C., Zhang, S., & Pun, S. H. (2008). Determination of nanoparticle vehicle unpackaging by MR imaging of a T 2 magnetic relaxation switch. *Biomaterials*, *29*(6), 724–732. doi:10.1016/j.biomaterials.2007.10.018 PMID:18006052

Park, J. H., Gu, L., Von Maltzahn, G., Ruoslahti, E., Bhatia, S. N., & Sailor, M. J. (2009). Biodegradable luminescent porous silicon nanoparticles for in vivo applications. *Nature Materials*, *8*(4), 331–336. doi:10.1038/nmat2398 PMID:19234444

Park, J., & Lakes, R. S. (2007). *Biomaterials: An introduction*. Springer Science & Business Media.

Park, K., Lee, S., Kang, E., Kim, K., Choi, K., & Kwon, I. C. (2009). New generation of multifunctional nanoparticles for cancer imaging and therapy. *Advanced Functional Materials*, *19*(10), 1553–1566. doi:10.1002/adfm.200801655

Parvanian, S., Mostafavi, S. M., & Aghashiri, M. (2017). Multifunctional nanoparticle developments in cancer diagnosis and treatment. *Sensing and Bio-Sensing Research*, *13*, 81–87. doi:10.1016/j.sbsr.2016.08.002

Parveen, S., & Sahoo, S. K. (2008). Polymeric nanoparticles for cancer therapy. *Journal of Drug Targeting*, *16*(2), 108–123. doi:10.1080/10611860701794353 PMID:18274932

Patel, J. N. (2009). Chitosan based Nanoparticles inDrug Delivery. *International Journal of Pharmaceutical Sciences and Nanotechnology, 2*(2).

Patel, M., Patel, S., & Patel, N. (2011). A review: novel oral lipid based formulation for poorly soluble drugs. *International Journal of Pharmaceutical Sciences and Technology, 3*(4), 1181-1192.

Patel, G. B., & Sprott, G. D. (1999). Archaeobacterial ether lipid liposomes (archaeosomes) as novel vaccine and drug delivery systems. *Critical Reviews in Biotechnology, 19*(4), 317–357. doi:10.1080/0738-859991229170 PMID:10723627

Patel, H. K., Gajbhiye, V., Kesharwani, P., & Jain, N. K. (2016). Ligand anchored poly (propyleneimine) dendrimers for brain targeting: Comparative in vitro and in vivo assessment. *Journal of Colloid and Interface Science, 482*, 142–150. doi:10.1016/j.jcis.2016.07.047 PMID:27501037

Patel, K., Angelos, S., Dichtel, W. R., Coskun, A., Yang, Y. W., Zink, J. I., & Stoddart, J. F. (2008). Enzyme-responsive snap-top covered silica nanocontainers. *Journal of the American Chemical Society, 130*(8), 2382–2383. doi:10.1021/ja0772086 PMID:18232687

Pathak, C., Savjani, K., Gajjar, A. K., & Savjani, J. K. (2013). cocrystal formation of paracetamol with indomethacin and mefenamic acid: An efficient approach to enhance solubility. *International Journal of Pharmacy and Pharmaceutical Sciences, 5*(4), 414–419.

Patidar, A., Thakur, D. S., Kumar, P., & Verma, J. (2010). A review on novel lipid based nanocarriers. *International Journal of Pharmacy and Pharmaceutical Sciences, 2*(4), 30–35.

Patil, M., Mehta, D., & Guvva, S. (2008). Future impact of nanotechnology on medicine and dentistry. *Journal of Indian Society of Periodontology, 12*(2), 34–40. doi:10.4103/0972-124X.44088 PMID:20142942

Patil, Y. B., Swaminathan, S. K., Sadhukha, T., Ma, L., & Panyam, J. (2010). The use of nanoparticle-mediated targeted gene silencing and drug delivery to overcome tumor drug resistance. *Biomaterials, 31*(2), 358–365. doi:10.1016/j.biomaterials.2009.09.048 PMID:19800114

Patil, Y., & Panyam, J. (2009). Polymeric nanoparticles for siRNA delivery and gene silencing. *International Journal of Pharmaceutics, 367*(1), 195–203. doi:10.1016/j.ijpharm.2008.09.039 PMID:18940242

Patnaik, S., Aggarwal, A., Nimesh, S., Goel, A., Ganguli, M., Saini, N., ... Gupta, K. C. (2006). PEI-alginate nanocomposites as efficient in vitro gene transfection agents. *Journal of Controlled Release, 114*(3), 398–409. doi:10.1016/j.jconrel.2006.06.025 PMID:16891026

Patnaik, S., Arif, M., Pathak, A., Singh, N., & Gupta, K. C. (2010). PEI-alginate nanocomposites: Efficient non-viral vectors for nucleic acids. *International Journal of Pharmaceutics, 385*(1), 194–202. doi:10.1016/j.ijpharm.2009.10.041 PMID:19874879

Patnaik, S., & Gupta, K. C. (2013). Novel polyethylenimine-derived nanoparticles for *in vivo* gene delivery. *Expert Opinion on Drug Delivery, 10*(2), 215–228. doi:10.1517/17425247.2013.744964 PMID:23252504

Paudel, A., Worku, Z. A., Meeus, J., Guns, S., & Van den Mooter, G. (2013). Manufacturing of solid dispersions of poorly water soluble drugs by spray drying: Formulation and process considerations. *International Journal of Pharmaceutics, 453*(1), 253–284. doi:10.1016/j.ijpharm.2012.07.015 PMID:22820134

Paula, A. J., Martinez, D. S. T., Araujo Júnior, R. T., Souza Filho, A. G., & Alves, O. L. (2012). Suppression of the hemolytic effect of mesoporous silica nanoparticles after protein corona interaction: Independence of the surface microchemical environment. *Journal of the Brazilian Chemical Society, 23*(10), 1807–1814. doi:10.1590/S0103-50532012005000048

Paveli, Z., & Skalko-Basnet, N. (2005). Development and in vitro evaluation of a liposomal vaginal delivery system for acyclovir. *Journal of Controlled Release*, *106*(1-2), 34–43. doi:10.1016/j.jconrel.2005.03.032 PMID:15979189

Pawar, V. K., Meher, J. G., Singh, Y., Chaurasia, M., Surendar Reddy, B., & Chourasia, M. K. (2014). Targeting of gastrointestinal tract for amended delivery of protein/peptide therapeutics: Strategies and industrial perspectives. *Journal of Controlled Release*, *196*, 168–183. doi:10.1016/j.jconrel.2014.09.031 PMID:25305562

Pawar, V. K., Panchal, S. B., Singh, Y., Meher, J. G., Sharma, K., Singh, P., ... Chourasia, M. K. (2014). Immunotherapeutic vitamin E nanoemulsion synergies the antiproliferative activity of paclitaxel in breast cancer cells via modulating Th1 and Th2 immune response. *Journal of Controlled Release*, *196*, 295–306. doi:10.1016/j.jconrel.2014.10.010 PMID:25459427

Pelkmans, L., Kartenbeck, J., & Helenius, A. (2001). Caveolar endocytosis of simian virus 40 reveals a new two-step vesicular-transport pathway to the ER. *Nature Cell Biology*, *3*(5), 473–483. doi:10.1038/35074539 PMID:11331875

Peng, S., He, Y., Er, M., Sheng, Y., Gu, Y. & Chen, H. (2017). Biocompatible CuS-based nanoplatforms for efficient photothermal therapy and chemotherapy in vivo. *Biomater Sci*, *5*(3), 475-484.

Peng, H., Dong, R., Wang, S., Zhang, Z., Luo, M., Bai, C., ... Xiong, H. (2013). A pH-responsive nano-carrier with mesoporous silica nanoparticles cores and poly(acrylic acid) shell-layers: Fabrication, characterization and properties for controlled release of salidroside. *International Journal of Pharmaceutics*, *446*(1-2), 153–159. doi:10.1016/j.ijpharm.2013.01.071 PMID:23395877

Peng, L., Peng, X., Liu, B., Wu, C., Xie, Y., & Yu, G. (2013). Ultrathin Two-Dimensional MnO_2/Graphene Hybrid Nanostructures for High-Performance. *Flexible Planar Supercapacitors. Nano Lett.*, *13*, 2151–2157. PMID:23590256

Peng, S., He, Y., Er, M., Sheng, Y., & Chen, H. (2017). Biocompatible Cu S-based nanoplatforms for efficient photothermal therapy and chemotherapy *in vivo*. *Biomaterials Science*, *5*(3), 475–484. doi:10.1039/C6BM00626D PMID:28078340

Peng, X. H., Qian, X., Mao, H., Wang, A. Y., Chen, Z. G., & Nie, S. (2008). Targeted magnetic iron oxide nanoparticles for tumor imaging and therapy. *International Journal of Nanomedicine*, *3*(3), 311–321. PMID:18990940

Pereira, S., Egbu, R., Jannati, G., & Al-Jamal, W. T. (2016). Docetaxel-loaded liposomes: The effect of lipid composition and purification on drug encapsulation and in vitro toxicity. *International Journal of Pharmaceutics*, *514*(1), 150–159. doi:10.1016/j.ijpharm.2016.06.057 PMID:27863659

Perera, G., & Bernkop-Schnürch, A. (2012). Pharmaceutical non-viral formulations for gene vaccines. In J. Thalhamer, R. Weiss, & S. Scheiblhofer (Eds.), *Gene Vaccine* (pp. 109–127). New York: Springer. doi:10.1007/978-3-7091-0439-2_5

Peres, L. B., Peres, L. B., de Araújo, P. H. H., & Sayer, C. (2016). Solid lipid nanoparticles for encapsulation of hydrophilic drugs by an organic solvent free double emulsion technique. *Colloids and Surfaces. B, Biointerfaces*, *140*, 317–323. doi:10.1016/j.colsurfb.2015.12.033 PMID:26764112

Perez-Herrero, E., & Fernandez-Medarde, A. (2015). Advanced targeted therapies in cancer: Drug nanocarriers, the future of chemotherapy. *European Journal of Pharmaceutics and Biopharmaceutics*, *93*, 52–79. doi:10.1016/j.ejpb.2015.03.018 PMID:25813885

Pérez, O., Bracho, G., Lastre, M., Zayas, C., González, D., Gil, D., & Solís, R. L. (2006). Proteliposome-derived Cochleate as an immunomodulator for nasal vaccine. *Vaccine*, *24*(2), S52–S53. doi:10.1016/j.vaccine.2005.01.127 PMID:16823925

Perigo, E. A., Hemery, G., Sandre, O., Ortega, D., Garaio, E., Plazaola, F., & Teran, F. J. (2015). Fundamentals and advances in magnetic hyperthermia. *Applied Physics Reviews*, *2*(4), 041302. doi:10.1063/1.4935688

Perinelli, D. R., Cespi, M., Pucciarelli, S., Vincenzetti, S., Casettari, L., & Lam, J. K. W. ... Palmieri, G. F. (2017). Microemulsions for protein delivery: Loading optimization and stability. *Current Pharmaceutical Biotechnology*. doi:10.2174/1389201018666170508112947

Perreault, F., de Faria, A. F., Nejati, S., & Elimelech, M. (2015). Antimicrobial Properties of Graphene Oxide Nanosheets: Why Size Matters. *ACS Nano*, *9*(7), 7226–7236. doi:10.1021/acsnano.5b02067 PMID:26091689

Petros, R. A., & DeSimone, J. M. (2010). Strategies in the design of nanoparticles for therapeutic applications. *Nature Reviews. Drug Discovery*, *9*(8), 615–627. doi:10.1038/nrd2591 PMID:20616808

Pham, M. N. Van, Vo, T., Tran, V. T., Tran, P. H., & Tran, T. T. (2017). Microemulsion-based mucoadhesive buccal wafers: wafer formation, in vitro release, and ex vivo evaluation. *AAPS PharmSciTech*. doi:10.120812249-017-0754-9

Philosof-Mazor, L., Dakwar, G. R., Popov, M., Kolusheva, S., Shames, A., Linder, C., ... Jelinek, R. (2013). Bolaamphiphilic vesicles encapsulating iron oxide nanoparticles: New vehicles for magnetically targeted drug delivery. *International Journal of Pharmaceutics*, *450*(1), 241–249. doi:10.1016/j.ijpharm.2013.04.017 PMID:23623794

Pidaparthi, K., & Suares, D. (2016). Comparison of Nanoemulsion and Aqueous Micelle Systems of Paliperidone for Intranasal Delivery. *AAPS PharmSciTech*, 1–10. PMID:27714701

Pike, L. J. (2006). Rafts defined: A report on the Keystone Symposium on Lipid Rafts and Cell Function. *Journal of Lipid Research*, *47*(7), 1597–1598. doi:10.1194/jlr.E600002-JLR200 PMID:16645198

Pinhassi, R. I., Assaraf, Y. G., Farber, S., Stark, M., Ickowicz, D., Drori, S., ... Livney, Y. D. (2010). Arabinogalactan-folic acid-drug conjugate for targeted delivery and target-activated release of anticancer drugs to folate receptor-overexpressing cells. *Biomacromolecules*, *11*(1), 294–303. doi:10.1021/bm900853z PMID:20014825

Pinto Vitorino, G., Sperandeo, N. R., Caira, M. R., & Mazzieri, M. R. (2013). A supramolecular assembly formed by heteroassociation of ciprofloxacin and norfloxacin in the solid state: Co-crystal synthesis and characterization. *Crystal Growth & Design*, *13*(3), 1050–1058. doi:10.1021/cg301299e

Plank, C., & Rosenecker, J. (2009). Magnetofection: the use of magnetic nanoparticles for nucleic acid delivery. *Cold Spring Harbor Protocols, 2009*(6), pdb-prot5230.

Plank, C., Scherer, F., Schillinger, U., & Anton, M. (2000). Magnetofection: enhancement and localization of gene delivery with magnetic particles under the influence of a magnetic field. *J Gene Med, 2*(5), S24.

Plank, C., Vlaskou, D., Sanchez-Antequera, Y., & Mykhaylyk, O. (2015). Magnetofection: Using Magnetic Particles and Magnetic Force to Enhance and Target Nucleic Acid Delivery. In Gene and Cell Therapy: Therapeutic Mechanisms and Strategies, Fourth Edition (pp. 347-420). CRC Press.

Plank, C., Zelphati, O., & Mykhaylyk, O. (2011). Magnetically enhanced nucleic acid delivery. Ten years of magnetofection—Progress and prospects. *Advanced Drug Delivery Reviews*, *63*(14), 1300–1331. doi:10.1016/j.addr.2011.08.002 PMID:21893135

Plapied, L., Duhem, N., des Rieux, A., & Préat, V. (2011). Fate of polymeric nanocarriers for oral drug delivery. *Curr Opin Colloid Interface Sci., 16*(3), 228–37. Available from: 10.1016/j.cocis.2010.12.005

Pohl, M., & Braz, J. (2001). Gene therapy of pain: Emerging strategies and future directions. *European Journal of Pharmacology*, *429*(1–3), 39–48. doi:10.1016/S0014-2999(01)01304-8 PMID:11698025

Polyak, B., & Friedman, G. (2009). Magnetic targeting for site-specific drug delivery: Applications and clinical potential. *Expert Opinion on Drug Delivery*, *6*(1), 53–70. doi:10.1517/17425240802662795 PMID:19236208

Porteous, D. J., Dorin, J. R., McLachlan, G., Davidson-Smith, H., Davidson, H., Stevenson, B. J., ... Innes, J. A. (1997). Evidence for safety and efficacy of DOTAP cationic liposome mediated CFTR gene transfer to the nasal epithelium of patients with cystic fibrosis. *Gene Therapy*, *4*(3), 210–218. doi:10.1038j.gt.3300390 PMID:9135734

Porter, C. J. H., Pouton, C. W., Cuine, J. F., & Charman, W. N. (2008). Enhancing intestinal drug solubilisation using lipid-based delivery systems. *Advanced Drug Delivery Reviews*, *60*(6), 673–691. doi:10.1016/j.addr.2007.10.014 PMID:18155801

Porter, C. J., & Charman, W. N. (2001). In vitro assessment of oral lipid based formulations. *Advanced Drug Delivery Reviews*, *50*(Suppl. 1), 127–147. doi:10.1016/S0169-409X(01)00182-X PMID:11576699

Portnov, T., Shulimzon, T., & Zilberman, M. (2016). Injectable hydrogel-based scaffolds for tissue engineering applications. *Reviews in Chemical Engineering*, *33*(1), 91–107. doi:10.1515/revce-2015-0074

Pouton, C. W. (2000). Lipid formulations for oral administration of drugs: Non emulsifying, self-emulsifying and 'self-microemulsifying' drug delivery systems. *European Journal of Pharmaceutical Sciences*, *11*(Suppl. 2), 93–98. doi:10.1016/S0928-0987(00)00167-6 PMID:11033431

Pouton, C. W. (2006). Formulation of poorly water-soluble drugs for oral administration: Physicochemical and physiological issues and the lipid formulation classification system. *European Journal of Pharmaceutical Sciences*, *29*(3-4), 278–287. doi:10.1016/j.ejps.2006.04.016 PMID:16815001

Prabaharan, M. (2011). Prospective of guar gum and its derivatives as controlled drug delivery systems. *International Journal of Biological Macromolecules*, *49*(2), 117–124. doi:10.1016/j.ijbiomac.2011.04.022 PMID:21596058

Prabhu, P., & Patravale, V. (2014). Lipid based drug delivery systems. In N. Udupa & S. Mutalik (Eds.), *Recent Trends in Novel Drug Delivery* (pp. 80–167). Prism Books Pvt. Ltd.

Prabhu, P., Suryavanshi, S., Pathak, S., Patra, A., Sharma, S., & Patravale, V. (2016). Nanostructured lipid carriers of artemether-lumefantrine combination for intravenous therapy of cerebral malaria. *International Journal of Pharmaceutics*, *513*(1-2), 504–517. doi:10.1016/j.ijpharm.2016.09.008 PMID:27596113

Prabhu, P., Suryavanshi, S., Pathak, S., Sharma, S., & Patravale, V. (2016). Artemether-lumefantrine nanostructured lipid carriers for oral malaria therapy: Enhanced efficacy at reduced dose and dosing frequency. *International Journal of Pharmaceutics*, *511*(1), 473–487. doi:10.1016/j.ijpharm.2016.07.021 PMID:27421912

Prabhu, S., Ortega, M., & Ma, C. (2005). Novel lipid-based formulations enhancing the *in vitro* dissolution and permeability characteristics of a poorly water-soluble model drug, piroxicam. *International Journal of Pharmaceutics*, *301*(1-2), 209–216. doi:10.1016/j.ijpharm.2005.05.032 PMID:16046087

Prabhu, S., & Poulose, E. K. (2012). Silver nanoparticles: Mechanism of antimicrobial action,synthesis, medical applications, and toxicity effects. *International Nano Letters*, *2*(1), 32–42. doi:10.1186/2228-5326-2-32

Pradhan, G. C., Dash, S., & Swain, S. K. (2015). Barrier properties of nano silicon carbide designed chitosan nanocomposites. *Carbohydrate Polymers*, *134*, 60–65. doi:10.1016/j.carbpol.2015.06.081 PMID:26428100

Pradhan, P., Giri, J., Rieken, F., Koch, C., Mykhaylyk, O., Döblinger, M., ... Plank, C. (2010). Targeted temperature sensitive magnetic liposomes for thermo-chemotherapy. *Journal of Controlled Release*, *142*(1), 108–121. doi:10.1016/j.jconrel.2009.10.002 PMID:19819275

Prajapati, N. H., Patel, D. P., Patel, N. G., Dalrymple, D. M., & Serajuddin, A. T. (2011). Effect of difference in fatty acid chain lengths of medium chain lipids on lipid/surfactant/water phase diagrams and drug Solubility. *Journal of Excipients and Food Chemicals*, *2*, 73.

Prasad, P., Shuhendler, A., Cai, P., Rauth, A. M., & Wu, X. Y. (2013). Doxorubicin and mitomycin C co-loaded polymer-lipid hybrid nanoparticles inhibit growth of sensitive and multidrug resistant human mammary tumor xenografts. *Cancer Lett, 334*(2), 263–273. doi:10.1016/j.canlet.2012.08.008 PMID:22902994

Prausnitz, M. R., Mitragotri, S., & Langer, R. (2004). Transdermal and Topical Drug Delivery, Current status and future potential of transdermal drug delivery. *Nature Reviews. Drug Discovery, 3*(2), 115–124. doi:10.1038/nrd1304 PMID:15040576

Probst, C. E., Zrazhevskiy, P., Bagalkot, V., & Gao, X. (2013). Quantum dots as a platform for nanoparticle drug delivery vehicle design. *Advanced Drug Delivery Reviews, 65*(5), 703–718. doi:10.1016/j.addr.2012.09.036 PMID:23000745

Pruthi, J., Mehra, N. K., & Jain, N. K. (2012). Macrophages targeting of amphotericin B through mannosylated multiwalled carbon nanotubes. *Journal of Drug Targeting, 20*(7), 593–604. doi:10.3109/1061186X.2012.697168 PMID:22690657

Pujals, S., & Giralt, E. (2008). Proline-rich, amphipathic cell-penetrating peptides. *Advanced Drug Delivery Reviews, 60*(4-5), 473–484. doi:10.1016/j.addr.2007.09.012 PMID:18187229

Puras, G., Mashal, M., Zárate, J., Agirre, M., Ojeda, E., Grijalvo, S., ... Pedraz, J. L. (2014). A novel cationic niosome formulation for gene delivery to the retina. *Journal of Controlled Release, 174*, 27–36. doi:10.1016/j.jconrel.2013.11.004 PMID:24231407

Puri, A., Loomis, K., Smith, B., Lee, J. H., Yavlovich, A., Heldman, E., & Blumenthal, R. (2009). Lipid-based nanoparticles as pharmaceutical drug carriers: from concepts to clinic. *Critical Reviews™ in Therapeutic Drug Carrier Systems, 26*(6),523-580.

Putra, O. D., Furuishi, T., Yonemochi, E., Terada, K., & Uekusa, H. (2016). Drug–Drug Multicomponent Crystals as an Effective Technique to Overcome Weaknesses in Parent Drugs. *Crystal Growth & Design, 16*(7), 3577–3581. doi:10.1021/acs.cgd.6b00639

Qi, L., & Gao, X. (2008). Emerging application of quantum dots for drug delivery and therapy. *Expert Opinion on Drug Delivery, 5*(3), 263–267. doi:10.1517/17425247.5.3.263 PMID:18318649

Qi, S., McAuley, W. J., Yang, Z., & Tipduangta, P. (2014). Physical stabilization of low-molecular-weight amorphous drugs in the solid state: A material science approach. *Therapeutic Delivery, 5*(7), 817–841. doi:10.4155/tde.14.39 PMID:25287388

Qiu, Y., Wu, C., Jiang, J., Hao, Y., Zhao, Y., Xu, J., ... Ji, P. (2017). Lipid-coated hollow mesoporous silica nanospheres for co-delivery of doxorubicin and paclitaxel: Preparation, sustained release, cellular uptake and pharmacokinetics. *Materials Science and Engineering C, 71*, 835–843. doi:10.1016/j.msec.2016.10.081 PMID:27987779

Qu, D., Ma, Y., Sun, W., Chen, Y., Zhou, J., Liu, C., & Huang, M. (2015). Microemulsion-based synergistic dual-drug codelivery system for enhanced apoptosis of tumor cells. *International Journal of Nanomedicine, 10*, 1173–1187. PMID:25709440

Qu, W., Meng, B., Yu, Y., & Wang, S. (2017). EpCAM antibody-conjugated mesoporous silica nanoparticles to enhance the anticancer efficacy of carboplatin in retinoblastoma. *Materials Science and Engineering C, 76*, 646–651. doi:10.1016/j.msec.2017.03.036 PMID:28482574

Qu, Y., Feng, L., Tong, C., Liu, B., & Lü, C. (2013). Poly(p-phenylenevinylene) functionalized fluorescent mesoporous silica nanoparticles for drug release and cell imaging. *Microporous and Mesoporous Materials, 182*, 155–164. doi:10.1016/j.micromeso.2013.08.045

Radtke, M., & Müller, R. (2001). Nanostructured lipid drug carriers. *New Drugs,* 1–4. Retrieved from http://www.pharmasol-berlin.de/files/nlc.pdf

Raghuvanshi, S., & Pathak, K. (2016). Bioadhesive floating microsponges of cinnarizine as novel gastroretentive delivery: Capmul GMO bioadhesive coating and acconon MC 8-2 EP/NF as bioadhesive raw material. *International Journal of Pharmaceutical Investigation*, *6*(4), 181–193. doi:10.4103/2230-973X.195923 PMID:28123987

Ragusa, A., García, I., & Penadés, S. (2007). Nanoparticles as Nonviral Gene Delivery Vectors. *Transactions on Nanobioscience*, *6*(4), 319–330. doi:10.1109/TNB.2007.908996 PMID:18217625

Rahimnejad,, M., & Najafpour. (2006). Production of biological nanoparticles from bovine serum albumin for drug delivery. *African Journal of Biotechnology*, *5*(20), 1918–1923.

Rahman, Z., Siddiqui, A., Gupta, A., & Khan, M. (2014). Regulatory considerations in development of amorphous solid dispersions. In *Amorphous Solid Dispersions* (pp. 545–563). Springer. doi:10.1007/978-1-4939-1598-9_17

Rai, G., Yadav, A. K., Jain, N. K., & Agrawal, G. P. (2015). Enteric-coated epichlorohydrin crosslinked dextran microspheres for site-specific delivery to colon. *Drug Development and Industrial Pharmacy*, *41*(12), 2018–2028. doi:10.3109/03639045.2015.1044901 PMID:26006331

Rajanna, K. (2013). Packaging of Polyvinylidene fluoride nasal sensor for biomedical applications. *8th International Conference on Microsystems, Packaging, Assembly and Circuits Technology*, 356 – 358.

Rajera, R., Nagpal, K., Singh, S. K., & Mishra, D. N. (2011). Niosomes: A controlled and novel drug delivery system. *Biological & Pharmaceutical Bulletin*, *34*(7), 945–953. doi:10.1248/bpb.34.945 PMID:21719996

Ramachandran, R., Krishnaraj, C., Sivakumar, A. S., Prasannakumar, P., Kumar, V. A., Shim, K. S., ... Yun, S.-I. (2017). Anticancer activity of biologically synthesized silver and gold nanoparticles on mouse myoblast cancer cells and their toxicity against embryonic zebrafish. *Materials Science and Engineering C*, *73*, 674–683. doi:10.1016/j.msec.2016.12.110 PMID:28183660

Ramamoorth, M., & Narvekar, A. (2015). Non viral vectors in gene therapy- An overview. *Journal of Clinical and Diagnostic Research: JCDR*, *9*(1), 1–6. PMID:25738007

Ramamoorth, M., & Narvekar, A. (2015). Non viral vectors in gene therapy-an overview. *Journal of Clinical and Diagnostic Research: JCDR*, *9*(1), GE01. PMID:25738007

Ramishetti, S., Kedmi, R., Goldsmith, M., Leonard, F., Sprague, A. G., Godin, B., ... Peer, D. (2015). Systemic gene silencing in primary T lymphocytes using targeted lipid nanoparticles. *ACS Nano*, *9*(7), 6706–6716. doi:10.1021/acsnano.5b02796 PMID:26042619

Ranucci, E., Ferruti, P., Manfredi, A., & Cavalli, R. (2012). Cross-linked resins by stepwise polyaddition of β-cyclodextrin with bisacrylamides and assessment of their potential as ph-sensitive NPs for site-specific protein delivery. *Proceedings CRS 2012*, 99.

Rao, M., Bajaj, A., Khole, I., Mumjapara, G., & Trotta, F. (2013). In vitro and in vivo evaluation of β-cyclodextrin based nanosponges of telmisartan. *Journal of Inclusion Phenomena and Macrocyclic Chemistry*, *77*(1-4), 135–145. doi:10.100710847-012-0224-7

Rao, S., & Houska, C. R. (1986). X-ray particle-size broadening. *Acta Crystallographica. Section A, Foundations of Crystallography*, *42*(1), 6–13. doi:10.1107/S0108767386099981

Rao, S., & Prestidge, C. A. (2016). Polymer-lipid hybrid systems: Merging the benefits of polymeric and lipid-based nanocarriers to improve oral drug delivery. *Expert Opinion on Drug Delivery*, *13*(5), 691–707. doi:10.1517/17425247.2016.1151872 PMID:26866382

Ravi Sankar, V., & Dastagiri Reddy, Y. (2010). Nanocochleate - A new approach in lipid drug delivery. *International Journal of Pharmacy and Pharmaceutical Sciences*, *2*(4), 3.

Ravi, K., Shivjee, K., Shyam, S., & Amit, K. J. (2011). Vesicular system-carrier for drug delivery. Der. *Der Pharmacia Sinica*, *2*(4), 192–202.

Ravikumar, N., Gaddamanugu, G., & Solomon, K. A. (2013). Structural, spectroscopic (FT-IR, FT-Raman) and theoretical studies of the 1: 1 cocrystal of isoniazid with p-coumaric acid. *Journal of Molecular Structure*, *1033*, 272–279. doi:10.1016/j.molstruc.2012.10.029

Rawat, A., Majumder, Q. H., & Ahsan, F. (2008). Inhalable large porous microspheres of low molecular weight heparin: In vitro and in vivo evaluation. *Journal of Controlled Release*, *128*(3), 224–232. doi:10.1016/j.jconrel.2008.03.013 PMID:18471921

Rawat, M., Singh, D., Saraf, S., & Saraf, S. (2006). Nanocarriers: Promising vehicle for bioactive drugs. *Biological & Pharmaceutical Bulletin*, *29*(9), 1790–1798. doi:10.1248/bpb.29.1790 PMID:16946487

Reddy, L. H., Arias, J. L., Nicolas, J., & Couvreur, P. (2012). Magnetic nanoparticles: Design and characterization, toxicity and biocompatibility, pharmaceutical and biomedical applications. *Chemical Reviews*, *112*(11), 5818–5878. doi:10.1021/cr300068p PMID:23043508

Rehman, Z. U., Hoekstra, D., & Zuhorn, I. S. (2013). Mechanism of polyplex-and lipoplex-mediated delivery of nucleic acids: Real-time visualization of transient membrane destabilization without endosomal lysis. *ACS Nano*, *7*(5), 3767–3777. doi:10.1021/nn3049494 PMID:23597090

Reichmuth, A. M., Oberli, M. A., Jaklenec, A., Langer, R., & Blankschtein, D. (2016). mRNA vaccine delivery using lipid nanoparticles. *Therapeutic Delivery*, *7*(5), 319–334. doi:10.4155/tde-2016-0006 PMID:27075952

Rejman, J., Bragonzi, A., & Conese, M. (2005). Role of clathrin-and caveolae-mediated endocytosis in gene transfer mediated by lipo-and polyplexes. *Molecular Therapy*, *12*(3), 468–474. doi:10.1016/j.ymthe.2005.03.038 PMID:15963763

Remy, J.-S., Sirlin, C., Vierling, P., & Behr, J.-P. (1994). Gene transfer with a series of lipophilic DNA-binding molecules. *Bioconjugate Chemistry*, *5*(6), 647–654. doi:10.1021/bc00030a021 PMID:7873668

Ren, L. L., Chen, S. Z., Li, H. D., Zhang, Z. Y., Ye, C. H., Liu, M. L., & Zhou, X. (2015). MRI-visible liposome nanovehicles for potential tumor-targeted delivery of multimodal therapies. *Nanoscale*, *7*(30), 12843–12850. doi:10.1039/C5NR02144H PMID:26022345

Ren, M., Han, Z., Li, J., Feng, G., & Ouyang, S. (2015). Ascorbic acid delivered by mesoporous silica nanoparticles induces the differentiation of human embryonic stem cells into cardiomyocytes. *Materials Science and Engineering C*, *56*, 348–355. doi:10.1016/j.msec.2015.06.048 PMID:26249600

Ren, N., Wang, B., Yang, Y. H., Zhang, Y. H., Yang, W. L., Yue, Y. H., ... Tang, Y. (2005). General Method for the Fabrication of Hollow Microcapsules with Adjustable Shell Compositions. *Chemistry of Materials*, *17*(10), 2582–2587. doi:10.1021/cm0502828

Renuka, Singh, S. K., Gulati, M., & Narang, R. (2015). Stable amorphous binary systems of glipizide and atorvastatin powders with enhanced dissolution profiles: Formulation and characterization. *Pharmaceutical Development and Technology*, 1–13. PMID:26708555

Ren, Y., Mu, Y., Song, Y., Xie, J., Yu, H., Gao, S., ... Lu, W. (2016). A new peptide ligand for colon cancer targeted delivery of micelles. *Drug Delivery*, *23*(5), 1763–1772. doi:10.3109/10717544.2015.1077293 PMID:26289214

Rescignano, N., Amelia, M., Credi, A., Kenny, J. M., & Armentano, I. (2012). Morphological and thermal behavior of porous biopolymeric nanoparticle. *European Polymer Journal*, *48*(7), 1152–1159. doi:10.1016/j.eurpolymj.2012.05.005

Rescignano, N., Hernández, R., Armentano, I., Puglia, D., Mijangos, C., & Kenny, J. M. (2014). Inclusion of PLLA nanoparticles in thermosensitive semi-interpenetrating polymer. *Networks. Polymer Degradation & Stability*, *108*, 280–287. doi:10.1016/j.polymdegradstab.2014.03.007

Rezwan, K., Chen, Q. Z., Blaker, J. J., & Boccaccini, A. R. (2006). Biodegradable and bioactive porous polymer/inorganic composite scaffolds for bone tissue engineering. *Biomaterials*, *27*(18), 3413–3431. doi:10.1016/j.biomaterials.2006.01.039 PMID:16504284

Ribeiro, L. N., Alcântara, A. C., Darder, M., Aranda, P., Araújo-Moreira, F. M., & Ruiz-Hitzky, E. (2014). Pectin-coated chitosan–LDH bionanocomposite beads as potential systems for colon-targeted drug delivery. *International Journal of Pharmaceutics*, *463*(1), 1–9. doi:10.1016/j.ijpharm.2013.12.035 PMID:24374607

Richard, T. C., Dos Santos, R., Rolland, V. H., & Benoit, J. P. (2003). A supercritical fluid-based coating technology 1: Process considerations. *Journal of Microencapsulation*, *20*(1), 87–96. doi:10.3109/02652040309178051 PMID:12519704

Riehemann, K., Schneider, S. W., Luger, T. A., Godin, B., Ferrari, M., & Fuchs, H. (2009). Nanomedicine--challenge and perspectives. *Angewandte Chemie International Edition in English*, *48*(5), 872–897. doi:10.1002/anie.200802585 PMID:19142939

Rivera, E. (2003). Current status of liposomal anthracycline therapy in metastatic breast cancer. *Clinical Breast Cancer*, *4*(Suppl 2), S76–S83. doi:10.3816/CBC.2003.s.019 PMID:14667278

Rivolta, I., Panariti, A., Lettiero, B., Sesana, S., Gasco, P., Gasco, M. R., ... Miserocchi, G. (2011). Cellular uptake of coumarin-6 as a model drug loaded in solid lipid nanoparticles. *Journal of Physiology and Pharmacology*, *62*(1), 45–53. PMID:21451209

Rizkalla, C. M. Z., Aziz, R. L., & Soliman, I. I. (2011). In vitro and in vivo evaluation of hydroxyzine hydrochloride microsponges for topical delivery. *AAPS Pharma Scitech*, *12*(3), 989–1001. doi:10.120812249-011-9663-5 PMID:21800216

Roberts, C. M., Shahin, S. A., Wen, W., Finlay, J. B., Dong, J., Wang, R., ... Glackin, C. A. (2017). Nanoparticle delivery of siRNA against TWIST to reduce drug resistance and tumor growth in ovarian cancer models. *Nanomedicine; Nanotechnology, Biology, and Medicine*, *13*(3), 965–976. doi:10.1016/j.nano.2016.11.010 PMID:27890656

Rogers, J.A., & Anderson, K.E. (1998). The Potential of Liposomes in Oral Drug Delivery. *Critical Reviews™ in Therapeutic Drug Carrier Systems*.

Roggers, R. A., Joglekar, M., Valenstein, J. S., & Trewyn, B. G. (2014). Mimicking Red Blood Cell Lipid Membrane To Enhance the Hemocompatibility of Large-Pore Mesoporous Silica. *ACS Applied Materials & Interfaces*, *6*(3), 1675–1681. doi:10.1021/am4045713 PMID:24417657

Rohrer, M., Bauer, H., Mintorovitch, J., Requardt, M., & Weinmann, H. J. (2005). Comparison of magnetic properties of MRI contrast media solutions at different magnetic field strengths. *Investigative Radiology*, *40*(11), 715–724. doi:10.1097/01.rli.0000184756.66360.d3 PMID:16230904

Rosenthal, E., Poizot-Martin, I., Saint-Marc, T., Spano, J. P., Cacoub, P., & Group, D. N. X. S. (2002). Phase IV study of liposomal daunorubicin (DaunoXome) in AIDS-related Kaposi sarcoma. *American Journal of Clinical Oncology*, *25*(1), 57–59. doi:10.1097/00000421-200202000-00012 PMID:11823698

Rowe, R. C., Sheskey, P. J., & Owen, S. C. (2006). Handbook of pharmaceutical excipients (5th ed.). Washington, DC: American Pharmaceutical Association.

Royal Society of Chemistry. (2015). Nanoceramics in Clinical Use: From Materials to Applications (2nd ed.). Cambridge, UK: Author.

Royce, A., Suryawanshi, J., Shah, J., & Vishnupad, K. (1996). Alternative granulation technique: Melt granulation. *Drug Development and Industrial Pharmacy*, *22*(9-10), 917–924. doi:10.3109/03639049609065921

Roy, I., Kumar, P., Kumar, R., Ohulchanskyy, T. Y., Yong, K. T., & Prasad, P. N. (2014). Ormosil nanoparticles as a sustained-release drug delivery vehicle. *RSC Advances*, *4*(96), 53498–53504. doi:10.1039/C4RA10293B

Ruiz-Hernández, E., López-Noriega, A., Arcos, D., Izquierdo-Barba, I., Terasaki, O., & Vallet-Regí, M. (2007). Aerosol-assisted synthesis of magnetic mesoporous silica spheres for drug targeting. *Chemistry of Materials*, *19*(14), 3455–3463. doi:10.1021/cm0705789

Russo, M. G., Sancho, M. I., Silva, L. M., Baldoni, H. A., Venancio, T., Ellena, J., & Narda, G. E. (2016). Looking for the interactions between omeprazole and amoxicillin in a disordered phase. An experimental and theoretical study. *Spectrochimica Acta. Part A: Molecular and Biomolecular Spectroscopy*, *156*, 70–77. doi:10.1016/j.saa.2015.11.021 PMID:26654963

Ryou, S. M., Park, M., Kim, J. M., Jeon, C. O., Yun, C. H., Han, S. H., ... Lee, K. (2011). Inhibition of xenograft tumor growthin mice by gold nanoparticle-assisted delivery of short hairpin RNAs against Mcl-1L. *Journal of Biotechnology*, *156*(2), 89–94. doi:10.1016/j.jbiotec.2011.07.037 PMID:21906638

Rytkonen, J., Miettinen, R., Kaasalainen, M., Lehto, V., Salonen, J., & Narvanen, A. (2012). Functionalization of mesoporous silicon nanoparticles for targeting and bioimaging purposes. *Journal of Nanomaterials*, *2012*, 1–9. doi:10.1155/2012/896562

Saad, M., Garbuzenko, O. B., & Minko, T. (2008). Co-delivery of siRNA and an anticancer drug for treatment of multidrug-resistant cancer. *Nanomedicine (London)*, *3*(6), 761–776. doi:10.2217/17435889.3.6.761 PMID:19025451

Sachan, R., Khatri, K., & Kasture, S. (2010). Self-emulsifying drug delivery system a novel approach for enhancement of bioavailability. *International Journal of Pharm Tech Research*, *2*, 1738–1745.

Sadeghi, M., & Lynch, C. D. (2009). The Effect of Flowable Materials on the Microleakage of Class II Composite Restorations That Extend Apical to the Cemento-enamel Junction. *Operative Dentistry*, *34*(3), 306–311. doi:10.2341/08-91 PMID:19544820

Sadeghi, M., Lynch, C. D., & Shahamat, N. (2010). Eighteen-month clinical evaluation of microhybrid, packable and nanofilled resin composites in Class I restorations. *Journal of Oral Rehabilitation*, *37*(7), 532–537. doi:10.1111/j.1365-2842.2010.02073.x PMID:20202097

Sadhukha, T., Wiedmann, T. S., & Panyam, J. (2013). Inhalable magnetic nanoparticles for targeted hyperthermia in lung cancer therapy. *Biomaterials*, *34*(21), 5163–5171. doi:10.1016/j.biomaterials.2013.03.061 PMID:23591395

Saffari, M., Moghimi, H. R., & Dass, C. R. (2016). Barriers to liposomal gene delivery: From application site to the target. *Iranian Journal of Pharmaceutical Research*, *15*(Suppl), 3–17. PMID:28228799

Sahay, G., Alakhova, D. Y., & Kabanov, A. V. (2010). Endocytosis of Nanomedicines. *Journal of Controlled Release*, *145*(3), 182–195. doi:10.1016/j.jconrel.2010.01.036 PMID:20226220

Sahay, G., Kim, J. O., Kabanov, A. V., & Bronich, T. K. (2010). The exploitation of differential endocytic pathways in normal and tumor cells in the selective targeting of nanoparticulate chemotherapeutic agents. *Biomaterials*, *31*(5), 923–933. doi:10.1016/j.biomaterials.2009.09.101 PMID:19853293

Sahdev, P., Ochyl, L. J., & Moon, J. J. (2014). Biomaterials for nanoparticle vaccine delivery systems. *Pharmaceutical Research*, *31*(10), 2563–2582. doi:10.100711095-014-1419-y PMID:24848341

Sahoo, B., Devi, K. S. P., Dutta, S., Maiti, T. K., Pramanik, P., & Dhara, D. (2014). Biocompatible mesoporous silica-coated superparamagnetic manganese ferrite nanoparticles for targeted drug delivery and MR imaging applications. *Journal of Colloid and Interface Science*, *431*, 31–41. doi:10.1016/j.jcis.2014.06.003 PMID:24980623

Sahoo, S. K., & Labhasetwar, V. (2003). Nanotech approaches to drug delivery and imaging. *Drug Discovery Today*, *8*(24), 1112–1120. doi:10.1016/S1359-6446(03)02903-9 PMID:14678737

Sahoo, Y., Goodarzi, A., Swihart, M. T., Ohulchanskyy, T. Y., Kaur, N., Furlani, E. P., & Prasad, P. N. (2005). Aqueous ferrofluid of magnetite nanoparticles: Fluorescence labeling and magnetophoretic control. *The Journal of Physical Chemistry B*, *109*(9), 3879–3885. doi:10.1021/jp045402y PMID:16851439

Saito, G., Swanson, J. A., & Lee, K. D. (2003). Drug delivery strategy utilizing conjugation via reversible disulfide linkages: Role and site of cellular reducing activities. *Advanced Drug Delivery Reviews*, *55*(2), 199–215. doi:10.1016/S0169-409X(02)00179-5 PMID:12564977

Sala, M., Miladi, K., Agusti, G., Elaissari, A., & Fessi, H. (2017). Preparation of liposomes: A comparative study between the double solvent displacement and the conventional ethanol injection—From laboratory scale to large scale. *Colloids and Surfaces. A, Physicochemical and Engineering Aspects*, *524*, 71–78. doi:10.1016/j.colsurfa.2017.02.084

Salimzadeh, L., Jaberipour, M., Hosseini, A., & Avicenna, A. G. (2013). Non-viral transfection methods optimized for gene delivery to a lung cancer cell line. *Avicenna Journal of Medical Biotechnology*, *5*(2), 68–77. PMID:23799175

Salvador-Morales, C., Zhang, L., Langer, R., & Farokhzad, O.C. (2009). Immunocompatibility properties of lipid-polymer hybrid nanoparticles with heterogeneous surface functional groups. *Biomaterials, 30*(12), 2231–40. 10.1016/j.biomaterials.2009.01.005

Samba, I., Hernandez, R., Rescignano, N., Mijangos, C., & Kenny, J. M. (2015). Nanocomposite hydrogels based on embedded PLGA nanoparticles in gelatin. *Nanocomposites.*, *1*(1), 46–50. doi:10.1179/2055033214Y.0000000006

Sanchez, C., Belleville, P., Popall, M., & Nicole, L. (2011). Applications of advanced hybrid organic-inorganic nanomaterials: From laboratory to market. *Chemical Society Reviews*, *40*(2), 696–753. doi:10.1039/c0cs00136h PMID:21229132

Sanna, V., Pala, N., & Sechi, M. (2014). Targeted therapy using nanotechnology: Focus on cancer. *International Journal of Nanomedicine*, *9*, 467–483. PMID:24531078

Sano, A. (2003). Atelocollagen for protein and gene delivery. *Advanced Drug Delivery Reviews*, *55*(12), 1651–1677. doi:10.1016/j.addr.2003.08.005 PMID:14623406

Sanphui, P., Goud, N. R., Khandavilli, U. R., & Nangia, A. (2011). Fast dissolving curcumin cocrystals. *Crystal Growth & Design*, *11*(9), 4135–4145. doi:10.1021/cg200704s

Santos Akkari, A. C., Ramos Campos, E. V., Keppler, A. F., Fraceto, L. F., de Paula, E., Tofoli, G. R., & de Araujo, D. R. (2016). Budesonide-hydroxypropyl-beta-cyclodextrin inclusion complex in binary poloxamer 407/403 system for ulcerative colitis treatment: A physico-chemical study from micelles to hydrogels. *Colloids and Surfaces. B, Biointerfaces*, *138*, 138–147. doi:10.1016/j.colsurfb.2015.11.048 PMID:26674842

Sapino, S., Carlotti, M. E., Cavalli, R., Ugazio, E., Berlier, G., Gastaldi, L., & Morel, S. (2013). Photochemical and antioxidant properties of gamma-oryzanol in beta-cyclodextrin-based nanosponges. *Journal of Inclusion Phenomena and Macrocyclic Chemistry*, *75*(1-2), 69–76. doi:10.100710847-012-0147-3

Sapino, S., Ugazio, E., Gastaldi, L., Miletto, I., Berlier, G., Zonari, D., & Oliaro-Bosso, S. (2015). Mesoporous silica as topical nanocarriers for quercetin: Characterization and in vitro studies. *European Journal of Pharmaceutics and Biopharmaceutics*, *89*, 116–125. doi:10.1016/j.ejpb.2014.11.022 PMID:25478737

Saraf, S., Jain, A., Hurkat, P., & Jain, S. K. (2016). Topotecan Liposomes: A Visit from a Molecular to a Therapeutic Platform. *Critical Reviews in Therapeutic Drug Carrier Systems*, *33*(5), 401–432. doi:10.1615/CritRevTherDrugCarrierSyst.2016015926 PMID:27910741

Saraswathy, A., Nazeer, S. S., Nimi, N., Arumugam, S., Shenoy, S. J., & Jayasree, R. S. (2014). Synthesis and characterization of dextran stabilized superparamagnetic iron oxide nanoparticles for in vivo MR imaging of liver fibrosis. *Carbohydrate Polymers*, *101*, 760–768. doi:10.1016/j.carbpol.2013.10.015 PMID:24299836

Sardone, N., Bettinetti, G., & Sorrenti, M. (1997). Trimethoprim–Sulfadimidine 1: 2 Molecular Complex Monohydrate. *Acta Crystallographica. Section C, Structural Chemistry*, *53*(9), 1295–1299. doi:10.1107/S0108270197000425

Sareen, R., Nath, K., Jain, N., & Dhar, K. L. (2014). Curcumin loaded microsponges for colon targeting in inflammatory bowel disease: Fabrication, optimization, and *in vitro* and pharmacodynamic evaluation. *BioMed Research International*, *2014*, 1–8. doi:10.1155/2014/340701 PMID:25093165

Sarmento, B., Ribeiro, A., Veiga, F., Sampaio, P., Neufeld, R., & Ferreira, D. (2007). Alginate/chitosan nanoparticles are effective for oral insulin delivery. *Pharmaceutical Research*, *24*(12), 2198–2206. doi:10.100711095-007-9367-4 PMID:17577641

Sarpal, K., Pawar, Y.B., & Bansal, A.K. (2010). Self-emulsifying drug delivery systems: A strategy to improve oral bioavailablity. *Current Research and Information on Pharmaceutical Sciences, 11*(3), 42-49.

Sarrett, D. C. (2005). Clinical challenges and the relevance of materials testing for posterior composite restorations. *Dental Materials*, *21*(1), 9–20. doi:10.1016/j.dental.2004.10.001 PMID:15680997

Saupe, A., & Rades, R. (2006). Solid lipid nanoparticles. In M. R. Mozafari (Ed.), *Nanocarrier technologies frontiers of nanotherapy* (pp. 41–43). Springer, Netherlands. doi:10.1007/978-1-4020-5041-1_3

Sawant, R. R., & Torchilin, V. P. (2010). Liposomes as "smart" pharmaceutical nanocarriers. *Soft Matter*, *6*(17), 4026. doi:10.1039/b923535n

Sawant, R. R., & Torchilin, V. P. (2010). Multifunctionality of lipid-core micelles for drug delivery and tumour targeting. *Molecular Membrane Biology*, *27*(7), 232–246. doi:10.3109/09687688.2010.516276 PMID:20929339

Sayar, F., Güven, G., & Pişkin, E. (2006). Magnetically loaded poly (methyl methacrylate-co-acrylic acid) nano-particles. *Colloid & Polymer Science*, *284*(9), 965–978. doi:10.100700396-005-1383-5

Schick, M. J. (1987). *Surfactant science series* (Vol. 23). NewYork: Marcel Dekker.

Schmidt, H. (2000). The Sol - Gel Process as a basic technology for nano particle - dispersed inorganic - organic composites. *Journal of Sol - Gel Science and Technology*, *19*, 39–51.

Schmidt, N., Mishra, A., Lai, G. H., & Wong, G. C. L. (2010). Arginine-rich cell-penetrating peptides. *Federation of European Biochemical Societies*, *584*(9), 1806–1813. doi:10.1016/j.febslet.2009.11.046 PMID:19925791

Schultheiss, N., Roe, M., & Boerrigter, S. X. (2011). Cocrystals of nutraceutical p-coumaric acid with caffeine and theophylline: Polymorphism and solid-state stability explored in detail using their crystal graphs. *CrystEngComm*, *13*(2), 611–619. doi:10.1039/C0CE00214C

Seeballuck, F., Ashford, M. B., & O'Driscoll, C. M. (2003). The effects of Pluronic block copolymers and Cremophor EL on intestinal lipoprotein processing and the potential link with P-glycoprotein in Caco-2 cells. *Pharmaceutical Research, 20*(7), 1085–1092. doi:10.1023/A:1024422625596 PMID:12880295

Seeli, D. S., & Prabaharan, M. (2016). Guar gum succinate as a carrier for colon-specific drug delivery. *International Journal of Biological Macromolecules, 84*, 10–15. doi:10.1016/j.ijbiomac.2015.12.002 PMID:26675135

Sekiguchi, K., & Obi, N. (1961). Studies on Absorption of Eutectic Mixture. I. A Comparison of the Behavior of Eutectic Mixture of Sulfathiazole and that of Ordinary Sulfathiazole in Man. *Chemical & Pharmaceutical Bulletin, 9*(11), 866–872. doi:10.1248/cpb.9.866

Sekiguchi, K., Obi, N., & Ueda, Y. (1964). Studies on Absorption of Eutectic Mixture. II. Absorption of fused Conglomerates of Chloramphenicol and Urea in Rabbits. *Chemical & Pharmaceutical Bulletin, 12*(2), 134–144. doi:10.1248/cpb.12.134 PMID:14126741

Selvamuthukumar, S., Anandam, S., Krishnamoorthy, K., & Rajappan, M. (2012). Nanosponges: A novel class of drug delivery system—review. *Journal of Pharmacy & Pharmaceutical Sciences, 15*(1), 103–111. doi:10.18433/J3K308 PMID:22365092

Selvestrel, F., Moret, F., Segat, D., Woodhams, J. H., Fracasso, G., Echevarria, I. M., ... Mancin, F. (2013). Targeted delivery of photosensitizers: Efficacy and selectivity issues revealed by multifunctional ORMOSIL nanovectors in cellular systems. *Nanoscale, 5*(13), 6106–6116. doi:10.1039/c3nr00402c PMID:23728482

Semalty, A., Semalty, M., Rawat, B. S., Singh, D., & Rawat, M. (2009). Pharmacosomes: The lipid-based new drug delivery system. *Expert Opinion on Drug Delivery, 6*(6), 599–612. doi:10.1517/17425240902967607 PMID:19519287

Şenel, B., Büyükköroğlu, G., & Yazan, Y. (2015). Solid lipid and chitosan particulate systems for delivery of siRNA. *Die Pharmazie, 70*, 698–705. PMID:26790185

Sengupta, S., Eavarone, D., Capila, I., Zhao, G., Watson, N., Kiziltepe, T., & Sasisekharan, R. (2005). Temporal targeting of tumour cells and neovasculature with a nanoscale delivery system. *Nature, 436*(7050), 568–572. doi:10.1038/nature03794 PMID:16049491

Sensenig, R., Sapir, Y., MacDonald, C., Cohen, S., & Polyak, B. (2012). Magnetic nanoparticle-based approaches to locally target therapy and enhance tissue regeneration in vivo. *Nanomedicine (London), 7*(9), 1425–1442. doi:10.2217/nnm.12.109 PMID:22994959

Seo, A., & Schæfer, T. (2001). Melt agglomeration with polyethylene glycol beads at a low impeller speed in a high shear mixer. *European Journal of Pharmaceutics and Biopharmaceutics, 52*(3), 315–325. doi:10.1016/S0939-6411(01)00183-7 PMID:11677074

Sercombe, L., Veerati, T., Moheimani, F., Wu, S. Y., Sood, A. K., & Hua, S. (2015). Advances and challenges of liposome assisted drug delivery. *Frontiers in Pharmacology, 6*, 286. doi:10.3389/fphar.2015.00286 PMID:26648870

Sergio, C., Elena, B. P., Fernando, N. V., Judith, L., Marta, N., Luis, M. L. M., & María, C. M. B. (2016). Multibranched Gold–Mesoporous Silica Nanoparticles Coated with a Molecularly Imprinted Polymer for Label-Free Antibiotic Surface-Enhanced Raman Scattering Analysis. *Chemistry of Materials, 28*(21), 7947–7954. doi:10.1021/acs.chemmater.6b03613

Sessa, G., & Weissmann, G. (1968). Phospholipid spherules (liposomes) as a model for biological membranes. *Journal of Lipid Research, 9*(3), 310–318. Retrieved from http://www.ncbi.nlm.nih.gov/pubmed/5646182 PMID:5646182

Sethia, S., & Squillante, E. (2002). Physicochemical characterization of solid dispersions of carbamazepine formulated by supercritical carbon dioxide and conventional solvent evaporation method. *Journal of Pharmaceutical Sciences*, *91*(9), 1948–1957. doi:10.1002/jps.10186 PMID:12210042

Sethia, S., & Squillante, E. (2004). *In vitro-in vivo* evaluation of supercritical processed solid dispersions: Permeability and viability assessment in Caco-2 cells. *Journal of Pharmaceutical Sciences*, *93*(12), 2985–2993. doi:10.1002/jps.20199 PMID:15468328

Shahbazi, M. A., Herranz, B., & Santos, H. A. (2012). Nanostructured porous Si-based nanoparticles for targeted drug delivery. *Biomatter*, *2*(4), 296–312. doi:10.4161/biom.22347 PMID:23507894

Shah, D. S., Sakthivel, T., Toth, I., Florence, A. T., & Wilderspin, A. F. (2000). DNA transfection and transfected cell viability using amphipathic asymmetric dendrimers. *International Journal of Pharmaceutics*, *208*(1), 41–48. doi:10.1016/S0378-5173(00)00534-2 PMID:11064210

Shah, V. P., Elkins, J., Lam, S.-Y., & Skelly, J. P. (1989). Determination of *in-vitro* release from hydrocortisone creams. *International Journal of Pharmaceutics*, *53*(1), 53–59. doi:10.1016/0378-5173(89)90361-X

Shang, L., Nienhaus, K., & Nienhaus, G. U. (2014). Engineered nanoparticles interacting with cells: Size matters. *Journal of Nanobiotechnology*, *12*(1), 5. doi:10.1186/1477-3155-12-5 PMID:24491160

Shanmugam, V., Selvakumar, S., & Yeh, C. S. (2014). Near-infrared light-responsive nanomaterials in cancer therapeutics. *Chemical Society Reviews*, *43*(17), 6254–6287. doi:10.1039/C4CS00011K PMID:24811160

Shariatinia, Z., & Zahraee, Z. (2017). Controlled release of metformin from chitosan–based nanocomposite films containing mesoporous MCM-41 nanoparticles as novel drug delivery systems. *Journal of Colloid and Interface Science*, *501*, 60–76. doi:10.1016/j.jcis.2017.04.036 PMID:28433886

Sharma, M., Sharma, S., Sharma, V., Sharma, K., Yadav, S. K., Dwivedi, P., ... Rawat, A. K. S. (2017). Oleanolic-bioenhancer coloaded chitosan modified nanocarriers attenuate breast cancer cells by multimode mechanism and preserve female fertility. *International Journal of Biological Macromolecules*, *104*, 1345–1358. doi:10.1016/j.ijbiomac.2017.06.005 PMID:28591594

Sharma, P., Dube, B., & Sawant, K. (2012). Synthesis of cytarabine lipid drug conjugate for treatment of meningeal leukemia: Development, characterization and in vitro cell line studies. *Journal of Biomedical Nanotechnology*, *8*(6), 928–937. doi:10.1166/jbn.2012.1464 PMID:23030001

Sharma, R., & Pathak, K. (2011). Polymeric nanosponges as an alternative carrier for improved retention of econazole nitrate on to the skin through topical hydrogel formulation. *Pharmaceutical Development and Technology*, *16*(4), 367–376. doi:10.3109/10837451003739289 PMID:20367024

Shayanfar, A., & Jouyban, A. (2013). Drug–Drug Coamorphous Systems: Characterization and Physicochemical Properties of Coamorphous Atorvastatin with Carvedilol and Glibenclamide. *Journal of Pharmaceutical Innovation*, *8*(4), 218–228. doi:10.100712247-013-9162-1

Shegokar, R., & Müller, R. H. (2010). Nanocrystals: Industrially feasible multifunctional formulation technology for poorly soluble actives. *International Journal of Pharmaceutics*, *399*(1), 129–139. doi:10.1016/j.ijpharm.2010.07.044 PMID:20674732

Sheikhpour, M., Golbabaie, A., & Kasaeian, A. (2017). Carbon nanotubes: A review of novel strategies for cancer diagnosis and treatment. *Materials Science and Engineering C*, *76*, 1289–1304. doi:10.1016/j.msec.2017.02.132 PMID:28482496

Shen, C., Li, J., Zhang, Y., Li, Y., Shen, G., Zhu, J., & Tao, J. (2017). Polyethylenimine-based micro/nanoparticles as vaccine adjuvants. *International Journal of Nanomedicine*, *12*, 5443–5460. doi:10.2147/IJN.S137980 PMID:28814862

Shen, K., Li, D., Guan, J., Ding, J., Wang, Z., Gu, J., ... Chen, X. (2017). Targeted sustained delivery of antineoplastic agent with multicomponent polylactide stereocomplex micelle. *Nanomedicine (London)*, *13*(3), 1279–1288. doi:10.1016/j.nano.2016.12.022 PMID:28064009

Shen, R., Kim, J. J., Yao, M., & Elbayoumi, T. A. (2016). Development and evaluation of vitamin E d-α-tocopheryl polyethylene glycol 1000 succinate-mixed polymeric phospholipid micelles of berberine as an anticancer nanopharmaceutical. *International Journal of Nanomedicine*, *11*, 1687–1700. PMID:27217747

Shen, S., & .... (2007). *Nanocomposites for drug delivery*. Nanotechnologies for the Life Sciences.

Sher, Y.-P., Chang, C.-M., Juo, C.-G., Chen, C.-T., Hsu, J. L., Lin, C.-Y., ... Hung, M.-C. (2013). Targeted endostatin-cytosine deaminase fusion gene therapy plus 5-fluorocytosine suppresses ovarian tumor growth. *Oncogene*, *32*(9), 1082–1090. doi:10.1038/onc.2012.134 PMID:22562248

Shetake, N. G., Balla, M. M., Kumar, A., & Pandey, B. N. (2016). Magnetic hyperthermia therapy: An emerging modality of cancer treatment in combination with radiotherapy. *Journal of Radiation and Cancer Research*, *7*(1), 13. doi:10.4103/0973-0168.184606

Shetake, N. G., Kumar, A., Gaikwad, S., Ray, P., Desai, S., Ningthoujam, R. S., ... Pandey, B. N. (2015). Magnetic nanoparticle-mediated hyperthermia therapy induces tumour growth inhibition by apoptosis and Hsp90/AKT modulation. *International Journal of Hyperthermia*, *31*(8), 909–919. doi:10.3109/02656736.2015.1075072 PMID:26416812

Shete, H., Chatterjee, S., De, A., & Patravale, V. (2013). Long chain lipid based tamoxifen NLC. Part II: Pharmacokinetic, biodistribution and in vitro anticancer efficacy studies. *International Journal of Pharmaceutics*, *454*(1), 584–592. doi:10.1016/j.ijpharm.2013.03.036 PMID:23535344

She, X., Chen, L., Velleman, L., Li, C., Zhu, H., He, C., ... Kong, L. (2015). Fabrication of high specificity hollow mesoporous silica nanoparticles assisted by Eudragit for targeted drug delivery. *Journal of Colloid and Interface Science*, *445*, 151–160. doi:10.1016/j.jcis.2014.12.053 PMID:25617610

Shih, Y. H., Luo, T. Y., Chiang, P. F., Yao, C. J., Lin, W. J., Peng, C. L., & Shieh, M. J. (2017). EGFR-targeted micelles containing near-infrared dye for enhanced photothermal therapy in colorectal cancer. *Journal of Controlled Release*, *258*, 196–207. doi:10.1016/j.jconrel.2017.04.031 PMID:28445743

Shi, J., Votruba, A. R., Farokhzad, O. C., & Langer, R. (2010). Nanotechnology in drug delivery and tissue engineering: From discovery to applications. *Nano Letters*, *10*(9), 3223–3230. doi:10.1021/nl102184c PMID:20726522

Shi, J., Xiao, Z., Votruba, A. R., Vilos, C., & Farokhzad, O. C. (2011). Differentially Charged Hollow Core / Shell Lipid – Polymer – Lipid Hybrid Nanoparticles for Small Interfering RNA Delivery. *Angewandte Chemie International Edition*, *50*(31), 7027–7031. doi:10.1002/anie.201101554 PMID:21698724

Shimizu, K., Ito, A., Lee, J. K., Yoshida, T., Miwa, K., Ishiguro, H., ... Honda, H. (2007). Construction of multi-layered cardiomyocyte sheets using magnetite nanoparticles and magnetic force. *Biotechnology and Bioengineering*, *96*(4), 803–809. doi:10.1002/bit.21094 PMID:16865728

Shin, H.-C., Alani, A. W., Rao, D. A., Rockich, N. C., & Kwon, G. S. (2009). Multi-drug loaded polymeric micelles for simultaneous delivery of poorly soluble anticancer drugs. *Journal of Controlled Release*, *140*(3), 294–300. doi:10.1016/j.jconrel.2009.04.024 PMID:19409432

Shi, S., Chen, F., & Cai, W. (2013). Biomedical applications of functionalized hollow mesoporous silica nanoparticles: Focusing on molecular imaging. *Nanomedicine (London)*, *8*(12), 2027–2039. doi:10.2217/nnm.13.177 PMID:24279491

Shi, T. (2015). Why Sn doping significantly enhances the dielectric properties of Ba (Ti 1 - x Sn x) O3. Nature Communications, 5(8606). doi:10.1038rep08606 PMID:25721479

Shi, X., Wang, S. H., Shen, M., Antwerp, M. E., Chen, X., Li, C., ... Baker, J. R. Jr. (2009). Multifunctional dendrimer-modified multiwalled carbon nanotubes: Synthesis, characterization, and in vitro cancer cell targeting and imaging. *Biomacromolecules*, *10*(7), 1744–1750. doi:10.1021/bm9001624 PMID:19459647

Shrestha, H., Bala, R., & Arora, S. (2014). Lipid-Based Drug Delivery Systems. *Journal of Pharmaceutics*, 1-10.

Shukla, R. K., & Tiwari, A. (2012). Carbohydrate polymers: Applications and recent advances in delivering drugs to the colon. *Carbohydrate Polymers*, *88*(2), 399–416. doi:10.1016/j.carbpol.2011.12.021

Siddiqui, R. A., Harvey, K. A., Xu, Z., Natarajan, S. K., & Davisson, V. J. (2014). Characterization of lovastatin-docosahexaenoate anticancer properties against breast cancer cells. *Bioorganic & Medicinal Chemistry*, *22*(6), 1899–1908. doi:10.1016/j.bmc.2014.01.051 PMID:24556504

Siler-Marinkovic, S. (2016). Liposomes as drug delivery systems in dermal and transdermal drug delivery. In *Percutaneous Penetration Enhancers Chemical Methods in Penetration Enhancement* (pp. 15–38). Berlin: Springer Berlin Heidelberg; doi:10.1007/978-3-662-47862-2_2

Silva, S. M., Tavallaie, R., Sandiford, L., Tilley, R. D., & Gooding, J. J. (2016). Gold coated magnetic nanoparticles: From preparation to surface modification for analytical and biomedical applications. *Chemical Communications*, *52*(48), 7528–7540. doi:10.1039/C6CC03225G PMID:27182032

Simons, K., & Gerl, M. J. (2010). Revitalizing membrane rafts: New tools and insights. *Nature Reviews. Molecular Cell Biology*, *11*(10), 688–699. doi:10.1038/nrm2977 PMID:20861879

Singh, A., & Sahoo, S. K. (2014). Magnetic nanoparticles: A novel platform for cancer theranostics. *Drug Discovery Today*, *19*(4), 474–481. doi:10.1016/j.drudis.2013.10.005 PMID:24140592

Singh, B., Chauhan, N., & Kumar, S. (2008). Radiation crosslinked psyllium and polyacrylic acid based hydrogels for use in colon specific drug delivery. *Carbohydrate Polymers*, *73*(3), 446–455. doi:10.1016/j.carbpol.2007.12.009

Singh, D., Minz, A. P., & Sahoo, S. K. (2017). Nanomedicine-mediated drug targeting of cancer stem cells. *Drug Discovery Today*, *22*(6), 952–959. doi:10.1016/j.drudis.2017.04.005 PMID:28435061

Singh, H. D., Wang, G., Uludağ, H., & Unsworth, L. D. (2010). Poly-L-lysine-coated albumin nanoparticles: Stability, mechanism for increasing in vitro enzymatic resilience, and siRNA release characteristics. *Acta Biomaterialia*, *6*(11), 4277–4284. doi:10.1016/j.actbio.2010.06.017 PMID:20601248

Singh, R. (2016). Confirmation of gum polysaccharide structure from Moringa oleifera Lam. plant by periodate oxidation studies. *IJCS*, *4*(2), 40–41.

Singh, R. K., & Kim, H. W. (2013). Inorganic nanobiomaterial drug carriers for medicine. *Tissue Engineering and Regenerative Medicine*, *10*(6), 296–309. doi:10.100713770-013-1092-y

Singh, R. K., Patel, K. D., Leong, K. W., & Kim, H. W. (2017). Progress in Nanotheranostics Based on Mesoporous Silica Nanomaterial Platforms. *ACS Applied Materials & Interfaces*, *9*(12), 10309–10337. doi:10.1021/acsami.6b16505 PMID:28274115

Singh, R. P., Sharma, G., Kumari, L., Koch, B., Singh, S., Bharti, S., ... Muthu, M. S. (2016). RGD-TPGS decorated theranostic liposomes for brain targeted delivery. *Colloids and Surfaces. B, Biointerfaces*, *147*, 129–141. doi:10.1016/j.colsurfb.2016.07.058 PMID:27497076

Singh, R. P., Sharma, G., Singh, S., Bharti, S., Pandey, B. L., Koch, B., & Muthu, M. S. (2017). Chitosan-folate decorated carbon nanotubes for site specific lung cancer delivery. *Materials Science and Engineering C*, *77*, 446–458. doi:10.1016/j.msec.2017.03.225 PMID:28532051

Singh, R. P., Sharma, G., Singh, S., Kumar, M., Pandey, B. L., Koch, B., & Muthu, M. S. (2016). Vitamin E TPGS conjugated carbon nanotubes improved efficacy of docetaxel with safety for lung cancer treatment. *Colloids and Surfaces. B, Biointerfaces*, *141*, 429–442. doi:10.1016/j.colsurfb.2016.02.011 PMID:26895505

Singh, R. P., Sharma, G., Singh, S., Patne, S. C., Pandey, B. L., Koch, B., & Muthu, M. S. (2016). Effects of transferrin conjugated multi-walled carbon nanotubes in lung cancer delivery. *Materials Science and Engineering C*, *67*, 313–325. doi:10.1016/j.msec.2016.05.013 PMID:27287127

Singh, R., Mehra, N. K., Jain, V., & Jain, N. K. (2013). Gemcitabine-loaded smart carbon nanotubes for effective targeting to cancer cells. *Journal of Drug Targeting*, *21*(6), 581–592. doi:10.3109/1061186X.2013.778264 PMID:23484494

Singh, S., & Pathak, K. (2016). Assessing the bioadhesivity of Acconon MC 8-2 EP/NF for gastroretention of floating microsponges of loratadine and achieving controlled drug delivery. *Pharmaceutical and Biomedical Research*, *2*(2), 58–74. doi:10.18869/acadpub.pbr.2.2.58

Singh, Y., Meher, J. G., Raval, K., Khan, F. A., Chaurasia, M., Jain, N. K., & Chourasia, M. K. (2017). Nanoemulsion: Concepts, development and applications in drug delivery. *Journal of Controlled Release*, *252*, 28–49. doi:10.1016/j.jconrel.2017.03.008 PMID:28279798

Sinha, A. S., Khandavilli, U. R., O'Connor, E. L., Deadman, B. J., Maguire, A. R., & Lawrence, S. E. (2015). Novel co-crystals of the nutraceutical sinapic acid. *CrystEngComm*, *17*(26), 4832–4841. doi:10.1039/C5CE00777A

Sinha, R., Kim, G. J., Nie, S., & Shin, D. M. (2006). Nanotechnology in cancer therapeutics: Bioconjugated nanoparticles for drug delivery. *Molecular Cancer Therapeutics*, *5*(8), 1909–1917. doi:10.1158/1535-7163.MCT-06-0141 PMID:16928810

Sinha, V. R., & Kumar, A. (2002). Multiple emulsions: An overview of formulation, characterization-stability and applications. *Indian Journal of Pharmaceutical Sciences*, *64*(3), 191–199.

Sirousazar, M. (2013). Mechanism of gentamicin sulphate release in nanocomposite hydrogel drug delivery systems. *Journal of Drug Delivery Science and Technology*, *23*(6), 619–621. doi:10.1016/S1773-2247(13)50094-3

Sivapragasam, N., Thavarajah, P., Ohm, J. B., Ohm, J. B., Margaret, K., & Thavarajah, D. (2014). Novel starch based nano scale enteric coatings from soybean meal for colon-specific delivery. *Carbohydrate Polymers*, *111*, 273–279. doi:10.1016/j.carbpol.2014.04.091 PMID:25037352

Skidan, I., Miao, B., Thekkedath, R. V., Dholakia, P., Degterev, A., & Torchilin, V. (2009). In vitro cytotoxicity of novel pro-apoptotic agent DM-PIT-1 in PEG-PE-based micelles alone and in combination with TRAIL. *Drug Delivery*, *16*(1), 45–51. doi:10.1080/10717540802517951 PMID:19555308

Skrtic, D., Antonucci, J. M., Eanes, E. D., Eichmiller, F. C., & Schumacher, G. E. (2000). Physicochemical evaluation of bioactive polymeric composites based on hybrid amorphous calcium phosphates. *Journal of Biomedical Materials Research*, *53*(4), 381–391. doi: PMID:10898879

Sleeman, J. P. (2000). The lymph node as a bridgehead in the metastatic dissemination of tumors. *Recent Results in Cancer Research. Fortschritte der Krebsforschung. Progres Dans les Recherches Sur le Cancer*, *157*, 55–81. doi:10.1007/978-3-642-57151-0_6 PMID:10857162

Sleeman, J. P. (2006). The relationship between tumors and the lymphatics: What more is there to know. *Lymphology*, *39*, 62–68. PMID:16910096

Slowing, I. I., Trewyn, B. G., Giri, S., & Lin, V. S. Y. (2007). Mesoporous silica nanoparticles for drug delivery and biosensing applications. *Advanced Functional Materials*, *17*(8), 1225–1236. doi:10.1002/adfm.200601191

Slowing, I. I., Vivero-Escoto, J. L., Wu, C. W., & Lin, V. S. Y. (2008). Mesoporous silica nanoparticles as controlled release drug delivery and gene transfection carriers. *Advanced Drug Delivery Reviews*, *60*(11), 1278–1288. doi:10.1016/j.addr.2008.03.012 PMID:18514969

Smith, A., Perelman, M., & Hinchcliffe, M. (2014). Chitosan: A promising safe and immune-enhancing adjuvant for intranasal vaccines. *Human Vaccines & Immunotherapeutics*, *10*(3), 797–807. doi:10.4161/hv.27449 PMID:24346613

Smith, S., Morhenn, V., & Webster, G. (2006). The characteristics and utility of solid phase porous microspheres: A review. *Journal of Drugs in Dermatology*, *5*(10), 969–974. PMID:17373146

Smyth Templeton, N. (2002). Liposomal delivery of nucleic acids in vivo. *DNA and Cell Biology*, *21*(12), 857–867. doi:10.1089/104454902762053828 PMID:12573046

Sokal, A., Pindelska, E., Szeleszczuk, L., & Kolodziejski, W. (2017). Pharmaceutical properties of two ethenzamide-gentisic acid cocrystal polymorphs: Drug release profiles, spectroscopic studies and theoretical calculations. *International Journal of Pharmaceutics*, *522*(1), 80–89. doi:10.1016/j.ijpharm.2017.03.004 PMID:28274662

Sokolova, V., & Epple, M. (2007). Inorganic nanoparticles as carriers of nucleic acids into cells. *Angewandte Chemie International Edition in English*, *46*, 2–16.

Solanki, A., & Thakore, S. (2015). Cellulose crosslinked pH-responsive polyurethanes for drug delivery: A-hydroxy acids as drug release modifiers. *International Journal of Biological Macromolecules*, *80*, 683–691. doi:10.1016/j.ijbiomac.2015.07.003 PMID:26188306

Solanki, B., Patel, R., Barot, B., Parijiya, P., & Shelat, P. (2012). Multiple unit dosage form: A review. *Ph Tech Med*, *1*, 11–21.

Solanki, S. S., Sarkar, B., & Dhanwani, R. K. (2012). Microemulsion drug delivery system: For bioavailability enhancement of ampelopsin. *ISRN Pharmaceutics*. PMID:22830055

Son, D. I., Kwon, B. W., Park, D. H., Seo, W. S., Yi, Y., Angadi, B., ... Choi, W. K. (2012). Emissive ZnO-graphene quantum dots for white-light-emitting diodes. *Nature Nanotechnology*, *7*(7), 465–471. doi:10.1038/nnano.2012.71 PMID:22635098

Song, Y. K., Liu, F., Chu, S., & Liu, D. (1997). Characterization of cationic liposome-mediated gene transfer in vivo by intravenous administration. *Human Gene Therapy*, *8*(13), 1585–1594. doi:10.1089/hum.1997.8.13-1585 PMID:9322091

Soni, K., Mujtaba, A., & Kohli, K. (2017). Lipid drug conjugate nanoparticle as a potential nanocarrier for the oral delivery of pemetrexeddiacid: Formulation design, characterization, ex vivo, and in vivo assessment. *International Journal of Biological Macromolecules*, *103*, 139–151. doi:10.1016/j.ijbiomac.2017.05.015 PMID:28499946

Soni, N., Soni, N., Pandey, H., Maheshwari, R., Kesharwani, P., & Tekade, R. K. (2016). Augmented delivery of gemcitabine in lung cancer cells exploring mannose anchored solid lipid nanoparticles. *Journal of Colloid and Interface Science*, *481*, 107–116. doi:10.1016/j.jcis.2016.07.020 PMID:27459173

Soppimath, K. S., Aminabhavi, T. M., Kulkarni, A. R., & Rudzinski, W. E. (2001). Biodegradable polymeric nanoparticles as drug delivery devices. *Journal of Controlled Release*, *70*(1), 1–20. doi:10.1016/S0168-3659(00)00339-4 PMID:11166403

Sorscher, E. J., Logan, J. J., Frizzell, R. A., Lyrene, R. K., Bebok, Z., Dong, J. Y., ... Wiatrak, B. J. (1994). Gene Therapy for Cystic Fibrosis Using Cationic Liposome Mediated Gene Transfer: A Phase I Trial of Safety and Efficacy in the Nasal Airway. University of Alabama at Birmingham, Birmingham, Alabama. *Human Gene Therapy*, *5*(10), 1259–1277. doi:10.1089/hum.1994.5.10-1259 PMID:7531503

Soumya, S., Doney, A. B., & Sabitha, M. (2012). Current trends in lipid based delivery systems and its applications in drug delivery. *Asian J. Pharm. Clin. Res.*, *5*(3), 4–9.

Soundrapandian, C., Bharati, S., Basu, D., & Datta, S. (2011). Studies on novel bioactive glasses and bioactive glass–nano-HAp composites suitable for coating on metallic implants. *Ceramics International*, *37*(3), 759–769. doi:10.1016/j.ceramint.2010.10.025

Souto, E. B., & Doktorovová, S. (2009). Chapter Six-Solid Lipid Nanoparticle Formulations: Pharmacokinetic and Biopharmaceutical Aspects in Drug Delivery. *Methods in Enzymology*, *464*, 105–129. doi:10.1016/S0076-6879(09)64006-4 PMID:19903552

Spagnou, S., Miller, A. D., & Keller, M. (2004). Lipidic carriers of siRNA: Differences in the formulation, cellular uptake, and delivery with plasmid DNA. *Biochemistry*, *43*(42), 13348–13356. doi:10.1021/bi048950a PMID:15491141

Spirin, M. G., Brichkin, S. B., & Razumov, V. F. (2005). Synthesis and stabilization of gold nanoparticles in reverse micelles of aerosol OT and Triton X-100. *Colloid Journal*, *67*(4), 485–490. doi:10.100710595-005-0122-4

Sreekanth, V., Bansal, S., Motiani, R. K., Kundu, S., Muppu, S. K., Majumdar, T. D., ... Bajaj, A. (2013). Design, synthesis, and mechanistic investigations of bile acid-tamoxifen conjugates for breast cancer therapy. *Bioconjugate Chemistry*, *24*(9), 1468–1484. doi:10.1021/bc300664k PMID:23909664

Sridhar, R., Sundarrajan, S., Venugopal, J. R., Ravichandran, R., & Ramakrishna, S. (2013). Electrospun inorganic and polymer composite nanofibers for biomedical applications. *Journal of Biomaterials Science. Polymer Edition*, *24*(4), 365–385. doi:10.1080/09205063.2012.690711 PMID:23565681

Srivalli, K. M. R., & Mishra, B. (2015). Preparation and pharmacodynamic assessment of ezetimibe nanocrystals: Effect of P-gp inhibitory stabilizer on particle size and oral absorption. *Colloids and Surfaces. B, Biointerfaces*, *135*, 756–764. doi:10.1016/j.colsurfb.2015.08.042 PMID:26342321

Srivalli, K. M. R., & Mishra, B. (2016). Drug nanocrystals: A way toward scale-up. *Saudi Pharmaceutical Journal*, *24*(4), 386–404. doi:10.1016/j.jsps.2014.04.007 PMID:27330370

Srivastava, R., Kumar, D., & Pathak, K. (2010). Colonic luminal surface retention of meloxicam microsponges delivered by erosion based colon targeted matrix tablet. *International Journal of Pharmaceutics*, *427*(2), 153–162. doi:10.1016/j.ijpharm.2012.01.036 PMID:22306039

Srivastava, R., & Pathak, K. (2012). Microsponges: A futuristic approach for drug delivery. *Expert Opinion on Drug Delivery*, *9*(7), 863–878. doi:10.1517/17425247.2012.693072 PMID:22663167

Steichen, S. D., Caldorera-Moore, M., & Peppas, N. A. (2013). A review of current nanoparticle and targeting moieties for the delivery of cancer therapeutics. *European Journal of Pharmaceutical Sciences*, *48*(3), 416–427. doi:10.1016/j.ejps.2012.12.006 PMID:23262059

Steinmetz, N. F. (2013). Viral nanoparticles in drug delivery and imaging. *Molecular Pharmaceutics*, *10*(1), 1–2. doi:10.1021/mp300658j PMID:23294244

Stenzel, K. H., Miyata, T., & Rubin, A. L. (1974). Collagen as a biomaterial. *Annual Review of Biophysics and Bioengineering*, *3*(1), 231–253. doi:10.1146/annurev.bb.03.060174.001311 PMID:4607533

Stepanovs, D., & Mishnev, A. (2012). Multicomponent pharmaceutical cocrystals: Furosemide and pentoxifylline. *Acta Crystallographica. Section C, Structural Chemistry*, *68*(12), o488–o491. doi:10.1107/S0108270112045866 PMID:23221253

Stephen, Z. R., Kievit, F. M., & Zhang, M. (2011). Magnetite nanoparticles for medical MR imaging. *Materials Today*, *14*(7), 330–338. doi:10.1016/S1369-7021(11)70163-8 PMID:22389583

Stöber, W., Fink, A., & Bohn, E. (1968). Controlled growth of monodisperse silica spheres in the micron size range. *Journal of Colloid and Interface Science*, *26*(1), 62–69. doi:10.1016/0021-9797(68)90272-5

Stollman, N., & Raskin, J. B. (2004). Diverticular disease of the colon. *Lancet*, *363*(9409), 631–639. doi:10.1016/S0140-6736(04)15597-9 PMID:14987890

Stopeck, A. T. (2001). Phase II study of direct intralesional gene transfer of Allovectin-7, an HLA-B7/β2-microglobulin DNA-liposome complex, in patients with metastatic melanoma. *Clinical Cancer Research*, *7*(8), 2285–2291. PMID:11489803

Storni, T., Kündig, T. M., Senti, G., & Johansen, P. (2005). Immunity in response to particulate antigen-delivery systems. *Advanced Drug Delivery Reviews*, *57*(3), 333–355. doi:10.1016/j.addr.2004.09.008 PMID:15560945

Streicher, R. M., Schmidt, M., & Fiorito, S. (2007). Nanosurfaces and nanostructures for artificial orthopedic implants. *Nanomedicine (London)*, *2*(6), 861–874. doi:10.2217/17435889.2.6.861 PMID:18095851

Strickley, R. G. (2004). Solubilizing excipients in oral and injectable formulations. *Pharmaceutical Research*, *21*(2), 201–230. doi:10.1023/B:PHAM.0000016235.32639.23 PMID:15032302

Strickley, R. G. (2007). Currently marketed oral lipid-based dosage forms: drugs products and excipients. In D. J. Hauss (Ed.), *Oral lipid-based formulations: enhancing the bioavailability of poorly water soluble drugs* (pp. 1–31). New York: Informa Healthcare.

Suares, D., & Prabhakar, B. (2016). Oral delivery of rosuvastatin lipid nanocarriers: Investigation of *in vitro* and *in vivo* profile. *International Journal of Pharmaceutical Sciences and Research*, *7*(12), 4856.

Su, B., Cengizeroglu, A., Farkasova, K., Viola, J. R., Anton, M., Ellwart, J. W., ... Ogris, M. (2013). Systemic TNFα gene therapy synergizes with liposomal doxorubicine in the treatment of metastatic cancer. *Molecular Therapy*, *21*(2), 300–308. doi:10.1038/mt.2012.229 PMID:23299796

Subedi, R. K., Oh, S. Y., Chun, M. K., & Choi, H. K. (2010). Recent advances in transdermal drug delivery. *Archives of Pharmacal Research*, *33*(3), 339–351. doi:10.100712272-010-0301-7 PMID:20361297

Subudhi, M., Jain, A., Jain, A., Hurkat, P., Shilpi, S., Gulbake, A., & Jain, S. (2015). Eudragit S100 Coated Citrus Pectin Nanoparticles for Colon Targeting of 5-Fluorouracil. *Materials (Basel)*, *8*(3), 832–849. doi:10.3390/ma8030832 PMID:28787974

Sumio, I. (1991). Helical microtubules of graphitic carbon. *Nature*, 354.

Summary Basis of Approval Retin-A Micro 0.1%. (n.d.). Available at: www.accessdata.FDA.com

Sun, D. (2010). Nanotheranostics: Integration of Imaging and Targeted Drug Delivery. *Molecular Pharmaceutics*, *7*(6), 1879–1879. doi:10.1021/mp1003652 PMID:21128687

Sun, J. T., Piao, J. G., Wang, L. H., Javed, M., Hong, C. Y., & Pan, C. Y. (2013). One-pot synthesis of redox-responsive polymers-coated mesoporous silica nanoparticles and their controlled drug release. *Macromolecular Rapid Communications*, *34*(17), 1387–1394. doi:10.1002/marc.201300477 PMID:23881541

Sun, J., Bi, C., Chan, H. M., Sun, S., Zhang, Q., & Zheng, Y. (2013). Curcumin-loaded solid lipid nanoparticles have prolonged in vitro antitumour activity, cellular uptake and improved in vivo bioavailability. *Colloids and Surfaces. B, Biointerfaces*, *111*, 367–375. doi:10.1016/j.colsurfb.2013.06.032 PMID:23856543

Sun, L., Wang, D., Chen, Y., Wang, L., Huang, P., Li, Y., ... Shi, J. (2017). Core-shell hierarchical mesostructured silica nanoparticles for gene/chemo-synergetic stepwise therapy of multidrug-resistant cancer. *Biomaterials*, *133*, 219–228. doi:10.1016/j.biomaterials.2017.04.028 PMID:28441616

Sun, L., Zhang, X., Zheng, C., Wu, Z., & Li, C. (2013). A pH gated, glucose-sensitive nanoparticle based on worm-like mesoporous silica for controlled insulin release. *The Journal of Physical Chemistry B*, *117*(14), 3852–3860. doi:10.1021/jp400442x PMID:23517533

Sun, L., Zhou, S., Wang, W., Li, X., Wang, J., & Weng, J. (2009). Preparation and characterization of porous biodegradable microspheres used for controlled protein delivery. *Colloids and Surfaces. A, Physicochemical and Engineering Aspects*, *345*(1-3), 173–181. doi:10.1016/j.colsurfa.2009.04.053

Sun, N. F., Liu, Z. A., & Hu, S. Y. (2013). The application of nanoparticles for gene vector in tumor gene therapy. *Journal of Tumor*, *1*(5), 24–27.

Sun, Q., You, Q., Pang, X., Tan, X., Wang, J., Liu, L., ... Li, N. (2017). A photoresponsive and rod-shape nanocarrier: Single wavelength of light triggered photothermal and photodynamic therapy based on AuNRs-capped & Ce6-doped mesoporous silica nanorods. *Biomaterials*, *122*, 188–200. doi:10.1016/j.biomaterials.2017.01.021 PMID:28131043

Sun, S., & Zeng, H. (2002). Size-controlled synthesis of magnetite nanoparticles. *Journal of the American Chemical Society*, *124*(28), 8204–8205. doi:10.1021/ja026501x PMID:12105897

Sun, T.-M., Du, J.-Z., Yao, Y.-D., Mao, C.-Q., Dou, S., Huang, S.-Y., ... Wang, J. (2011). Simultaneous delivery of siRNA and paclitaxel via a "two-in-one" micelleplex promotes synergistic tumor suppression. *ACS Nano*, *5*(2), 1483–1494. doi:10.1021/nn103349h PMID:21204585

Sun, W., Hu, Q., Ji, W., Wright, G., & Gu, Z. (2017). Leveraging Physiology for Precision Drug Delivery. *Physiological Reviews*, *97*(1), 189–225. doi:10.1152/physrev.00015.2016

Suresh, K., Mannava, M. C., & Nangia, A. (2014). A novel curcumin–artemisinin coamorphous solid: Physical properties and pharmacokinetic profile. *RSC Advances*, *4*(102), 58357–58361. doi:10.1039/C4RA11935E

Surov, A. O., Voronin, A. P., Manin, A. N., Manin, N. G., Kuzmina, L. G., Churakov, A. V., & Perlovich, G. L. (2014). Pharmaceutical cocrystals of diflunisal and diclofenac with theophylline. *Molecular Pharmaceutics*, *11*(10), 3707–3715. doi:10.1021/mp5004652 PMID:25184906

Su, X., Gao, C., Shi, F., Feng, X., Liu, L., Qu, D., & Wang, C. (2017). A microemulsion co-loaded with Schizandrin A–docetaxel enhances esophageal carcinoma treatment through overcoming multidrug resistance. *Drug Delivery*, *24*(1), 10–19. doi:10.1080/10717544.2016.1225854 PMID:28155336

Swaminathan, S., Pastero, L., Serpe, L., Trotta, F., Vavia, P., Aquilano, D., ... Cavalli, R. (2010). Cyclodextrin-based nanosponges encapsulating camptothecin: Physicochemical characterization, stability and cytotoxicity. *European Journal of Pharmaceutics and Biopharmaceutics*, *74*(2), 193–201. doi:10.1016/j.ejpb.2009.11.003 PMID:19900544

Swaminathan, S., Vavia, P. R., Trotta, F., & Roberta, C. (2013, June 01). Nanosponges encapsulating dexamethasone for ocular delivery: Formulation design, physicochemical characterization, safety and corneal permeability assessment. *Journal of Biomedical Nanotechnology*, *9*(6), 998–1007. doi:10.1166/jbn.2013.1594 PMID:23858964

Swaminathan, S., Vavia, P. R., Trotta, F., & Torne, S. (2007). Formulation of betacyclodextrin based nanosponges of itraconazole. *Journal of Inclusion Phenomena and Macrocyclic Chemistry*, *57*(1-4), 89–94. doi:10.100710847-006-9216-9

Swami, R., Singh, I., Khan, W., & Ramakrishna, S. (2013). Diseases originate and terminate by genes: Unraveling nonviral gene delivery. *Drug Delivery and Translational Research*, *3*(6), 593–610. doi:10.100713346-013-0159-6 PMID:25786377

Szejtli, J., & Osa, T. (1996). *Comprehensive Supramolecular Chemistry: Cyclodextrins* (Vol. 3). Oxford: Elsevier.

Szymański, P., Markowicz, M., & Mikiciuk-Olasik, E. (2011). Nanotechnology in pharmaceutical and biomedical applications: Dendrimers. *Nano*, *6*(06), 509–539. doi:10.1142/S1793292011002871

Tagami, T., Ando, Y., & Ozeki, T. (2017). Fabrication of liposomal doxorubicin exhibiting ultrasensitivity against phospholipase A 2 for efficient pulmonary drug delivery to lung cancers. *International Journal of Pharmaceutics*, *517*(1), 35–41. doi:10.1016/j.ijpharm.2016.11.039 PMID:27865984

Taghdisi, S. M., Danesh, N. M., Ramezani, M., Lavaee, P., Jalalian, S. H., Robati, R. Y., & Abnous, K. (2016). Double targeting and aptamer-assisted controlled release delivery of epirubicin to cancer cells by aptamers-based dendrimer in vitro and in vivo. *European Journal of Pharmaceutics and Biopharmaceutics*, *102*, 152–158. doi:10.1016/j.ejpb.2016.03.013 PMID:26987703

Taheri, A., Dinarvand, R., Atyabi, F., Ghahremani, M. H., & Ostad, S. N. (2012). Trastuzumab decorated methotrexate–human serum albumin conjugated nanoparticles for targeted delivery to HER2 positive tumor cells. *European Journal of Pharmaceutical Sciences*, *47*(2), 331–340. doi:10.1016/j.ejps.2012.06.016 PMID:22771547

Taneja, K., Pareeka, A., Vermaa, P., Jaina, V., Yashumati Ratana, Y., & Ashawatb, M. S. (2012). Nanocomposite: An emerging tool for bone tissue transplantation and drug delivery. *Indian Journal of Transplantation.*, *6*(3), 88–96. doi:10.1016/j.ijt.2012.07.002

Tang, Y., Hu, H., Zhang, M.G., Song, J., Nie, L., Wang, S., … Chen X. (2015). An aptamer-targeting photoresponsive drug delivery system using "off-on" graphene oxide wrapped mesoporous silica nanoparticles. *Nanoscale*, *7*(14), 6304-10.

Tang, Y., Hu, H., Zhang, M.H., Song, J., Nie, L., Wang, S., … Xiaoyuan, C. (2015). An aptamer-targeting photoresponsive drug delivery system using "off–on" graphene oxide wrapped mesoporous silica nanoparticles. *Nanoscale, 7*(14), 6304–6310.

Tang, C., Qiu, F., & Zhao, X. (2013). Molecular design and applications of self-assembling surfactant-like peptides. *Journal of Nanomaterials*, *2013*, 15. doi:10.1155/2013/469261

Tang, F., Li, L., & Chen, D. (2012). Mesoporous Silica Nanoparticles: Synthesis, Biocompatibility and Drug Delivery. *Advanced Materials*, *24*(12), 1504–1534. doi:10.1002/adma.201104763 PMID:22378538

Tang, H., Guo, J., Sun, Y., Chang, B., Ren, Q., & Yang, W. (2011). Facile synthesis of pH sensitive polymer-coated mesoporous silica nanoparticles and their application in drug delivery. *International Journal of Pharmaceutics*, *421*(2), 388–396. doi:10.1016/j.ijpharm.2011.10.013 PMID:22001840

Tang, H., Xiang, D., Wang, F., Mao, J., Tan, X., & Wang, Y. (2017). 5-ASA-loaded SiO2 nanoparticles-a novel drug delivery system targeting therapy on ulcerative colitis in mice. *Molecular Medicine Reports*, *15*(3), 1117–1122. doi:10.3892/mmr.2017.6153 PMID:28138699

Tang, M. X., Redemann, C. T., & Szoka, F. C. (1996). In vitro gene delivery by degraded polyamidoamine dendrimers. *Bioconjugate Chemistry*, *7*(6), 703–714. doi:10.1021/bc9600630 PMID:8950489

Tang, T. T., Hu, X. B., Liao, D. H., Liu, X. Y., & Xiang, D. X. (2013). Mechanisms of microemulsion enhancing the oral bioavailability of puerarin: Comparison between oil-in-water and water-in-oil microemulsions using the single-pass intestinal perfusion method and a chylomicron flow blocking approach. *International Journal of Nanomedicine*, *8*, 4415–4426. doi:10.2147/IJN.S51469 PMID:24277986

Tang, Y., Hu, H., Zhang, M. G., Song, J., Nie, L., Wang, S., ... Chen, X. (2015, April 14). An aptamer-targeting photo-responsive drug delivery system using "off-on" graphene oxide wrapped mesoporous silica nanoparticles. *Nanoscale*, *7*(14), 6304–6310. doi:10.1039/C4NR07493A PMID:25782595

Tang, Y., Li, Z., He, N., Zhang, L., Ma, C., Li, X., ... He, L. (2013). Preparation of functional magnetic nanoparticles mediated with PEG-4000 and application in Pseudomonas Aeruginosa rapid detection. *Journal of Biomedical Nanotechnology*, *9*(2), 312–317. doi:10.1166/jbn.2013.1493 PMID:23627062

Tan, L., Wu, T., Tang, Z. W., Xiao, J. Y., Zhuo, R. X., Shi, B., & Liu, C. J. (2016). Water-soluble photoluminescent fullerene capped mesoporous silica for pH-responsive drug delivery and bioimaging. *Nanotechnology*, *27*(31), 315104. doi:10.1088/0957-4484/27/31/315104 PMID:27346782

Tannock, I. F., & Rotin, D. (1989). Acid pH in tumors and its potential for therpeutic exploitation. [Internet]. *Cancer Research*, *49*(16), 4373–4384. Available from http://www.scopus.com/inward/record.url?eid=2-s2.0-0024379967&partnerID=40&md5=9790fdf29f52b21920045c832198f74c PMID:2545340

Tao, C., Zhu, Y., Li, X., & Hanagata, N. (2015). Binding of CpG oligodeoxynucleotides to mesoporous silica nanoparticles for enhancing delivery efficiency. *Microporous and Mesoporous Materials*, *204*, 91–98. doi:10.1016/j.micromeso.2014.11.007

Tarn, D., Ashley, C. E., Xue, M., Carnes, E. C., Zink, J. I., & Brinker, C. J. (2013). Mesoporous Silica Nanoparticle Nanocarriers: Biofunctionality and Biocompatibility. *Accounts of Chemical Research*, *46*(3), 792–801. doi:10.1021/ar3000986 PMID:23387478

Tartaj, P., Veintemillas-Verdaguer, S., & Serna, C. J. (2003). The preparation of magnetic nanoparticles for applications in biomedicine. *Journal of Physics. D, Applied Physics*, *36*(13), R182–R197. doi:10.1088/0022-3727/36/13/202

Taton, T. A. (2001). Nanotechnology: Boning up on biology. *Nature*, *412*(6846), 491–492. doi:10.1038/35087687 PMID:11484032

Taylor, K. M. L., Kim, J. S., Rieter, W. J., An, H., Lin, W., & Lin, W. (2008). Mesoporous Silica Nanospheres as Highly Efficient MRI Contrast Agents. *Journal of the American Chemical Society*, *130*(7), 2154–2155. doi:10.1021/ja710193c PMID:18217764

Teja, A., Musmade, P. B., Khade, A. B., & Dengale, S. J. (2015). Simultaneous improvement of solubility and permeability by fabricating binary glassy materials of Talinolol with Naringin: Solid state characterization, in-vivo in-situ evaluation. *European Journal of Pharmaceutical Sciences*, *78*, 234–244. doi:10.1016/j.ejps.2015.08.002 PMID:26253355

Teng, X., Black, D., Watkins, N. J., Gao, Y., & Yang, H. (2003). Platinum-maghemite core– shell nanoparticles using a sequential synthesis. *Nano Letters*, *3*(2), 261–264. doi:10.1021/nl025918y

Teow, H. M., Zhou, Z., Najlah, M., Yusof, S. R., Abbott, N. J., & D'Emanuele, A. (2013). Delivery of paclitaxel across cellular barriers using a dendrimer-based nanocarrier. *International Journal of Pharmaceutics*, *441*(1), 701–711. doi:10.1016/j.ijpharm.2012.10.024 PMID:23089576

Termeer, C., Averbeck, M., Hara, H., Eibel, H., Herrlich, P., Sleeman, J., & Simon, J. C. (2003). Targeting dendritic cells with CD44 monoclonal antibodies selectively inhibits the proliferation of naive $CD4^+$ T-helper cells by induction of FAS-independent T-cell apoptosis. *Immunology*, *109*(1), 32–40. doi:10.1046/j.1365-2567.2003.01617.x PMID:12709015

Terry, D. A. (2004). Applications of nanotechnology. *Pract Proced Aesthet Dent*, *16*(3), 220–222. PMID:15199697

Thapa, B., & Narain, R. (2016). Mechanism, current challanges and new approaches for non viral gene delivery. In R. Narain (Ed.), *Polymer and Nanomaterials for gene therapy* (pp. 1–28). Elsevier. doi:10.1016/B978-0-08-100520-0.00001-1

Theiss, F. L., Ayoko, G. A., & Frost, R. L. (2016). Synthesis of layered double hydroxides containing Mg^{2+}, Zn^{2+}, Ca^{2+} and Al^{3+} layer cations by co-precipitation methods—A review. *Applied Surface Science*, *383*, 200–213. doi:10.1016/j.apsusc.2016.04.150

Thenmozhi, S., Dharmaraj, N., Kadirvelu, K., & Kim, H. Y. (2017). Electrospun nanofibers: New generation materials for advanced applications. *Materials Science and Engineering B*, *217*, 36–48. doi:10.1016/j.mseb.2017.01.001

Thevenot, J., Troutier, A. L., David, L., Delair, T., & Ladavière, C. (2007). Steric stabilization of lipid/polymer particle assemblies by poly(ethylene glycol)-lipids. *Biomacromolecules*, *8*(11), 3651–3660. doi:10.1021/bm700753q PMID:17958441

Thipparaboina, R., Chavan, R. B., Kumar, D., Modugula, S., & Shastri, N. R. (2015). Micellar carriers for the delivery of multiple therapeutic agents. *Colloids and Surfaces. B, Biointerfaces*, *135*, 291–308. doi:10.1016/j.colsurfb.2015.07.046 PMID:26263217

Thipparaboina, R., Kumar, D., Chavan, R. B., & Shastri, N. R. (2016). Multidrug co-crystals: Towards the development of effective therapeutic hybrids. *Drug Discovery Today*, *21*(3), 481–490. doi:10.1016/j.drudis.2016.02.001 PMID:26869329

Thipparaboina, R., Thumuri, D., Chavan, R., Naidu, V., & Shastri, N. R. (2017). Fast dissolving drug-drug eutectics with improved compressibility and synergistic effects. *European Journal of Pharmaceutical Sciences*, *104*, 82–89. doi:10.1016/j.ejps.2017.03.042 PMID:28366649

Thomas, M. J., Slipper, I., Walunj, A., Jain, A., Favretto, M. E., Kallinteri, P., & Douroumis, D. (2010). Inclusion of poorly soluble drugs in highly ordered mesoporous silica nanoparticles. *International Journal of Pharmaceutics*, *387*(1-2), 272–277. doi:10.1016/j.ijpharm.2009.12.023 PMID:20025947

Tian, Z. F., Yi, X. & Zhu, Y. (2017). Aldehyde-functionalized dendritic mesoporous silica nanoparticles as potential nanocarriers for pH-responsive protein drug delivery. *Materials Science & Engineering CInt J Nanomedicine*, *12*, 2733-2748.

Tian, B., Ding, Y., Han, J., Zhang, J., Han, Y., & Han, J. (2015). N-Acetyl-D-glucosamine decorated polymeric nanoparticles for targeted delivery of doxorubicin: Synthesis, characterization and in vitro evaluation. *Colloids and Surfaces. B, Biointerfaces*, *130*, 246–254. doi:10.1016/j.colsurfb.2015.04.019 PMID:25921641

Tian, B., Liu, S., Wu, S., Lu, W., Wang, D., Jin, L., ... Quan, Z. (2017). pH-responsive poly (acrylic acid)-gated mesoporous silica and its application in oral colon targeted drug delivery for doxorubicin. *Colloids and Surfaces. B, Biointerfaces*, *154*, 287–296. doi:10.1016/j.colsurfb.2017.03.024 PMID:28351801

Tian, J., Yan, C., Liu, K., Tao, J., Guo, Z., Liu, J., ... Gu, N. (2017). Paclitaxel-Loaded Magnetic Nanoparticles: Synthesis, Characterization, and Application in Targeting. *Journal of Pharmaceutical Sciences*, *106*(8), 2115–2122. doi:10.1016/j.xphs.2017.04.023 PMID:28456728

Tiera, M. J., Winnik, F. O., & Fernandes, J. C. (2006). Synthetic and natural polycations for gene therapy: State of the art and new perspectives. *Current Gene Therapy*, *6*(1), 59–71. doi:10.2174/156652306775515510 PMID:16475946

Tiwari, A., Jain, A., Verma, A., & Jain, S. K. (2017). Exploitable Signaling Pathways for the treatment of Inflammatory Bowel Disease. *Current Signal Transduction Therapy*, 12.

Tkachenko, A. G., Xie, H., Coleman, D., Glomm, W., Ryan, J., Anderson, M. F., ... Feldheim, D. L. (2003). Multifunctional Gold Nanoparticle−Peptide Complexes for Nuclear Targeting. *Journal of the American Chemical Society*, *125*(16), 4700–4701. doi:10.1021/ja0296935 PMID:12696875

Tong, H., Shi, Q., Fernandes, J., Liu, L., Dai, K., & Zhang, X. (2009). Progress and prospects of chitosan and its derivatives as non-viral gene vectors in gene therapy. *Current Gene Therapy*, *9*(6), 495–502. doi:10.2174/156652309790031111 PMID:19807649

Torchilin, V. P. (2005). Lipid-core micelles for targeted drug delivery. *Current Drug Delivery*, *2*(4), 319–327. doi:10.2174/156720105774370221 PMID:16305435

Torchilin, V. P. (2007). Targeted pharmaceutical nanocarriers for cancer therapy and imaging. *The AAPS Journal*, *9*(2), E128–E147. doi:10.1208/aapsj0902015 PMID:17614355

Torchilin, V. P. (2014). Multifunctional, stimuli-sensitive nanoparticulate systems for drug delivery. *Nature Reviews. Drug Discovery*, *13*(11), 813–827. doi:10.1038/nrd4333 PMID:25287120

Torne, S. J., Ansari, K. A., Vavia, P. R., Trotta, F., & Cavalli, R. (2010). Enhanced oral paclitaxel bioavailability after administration of paclitaxel-loaded nanosponges. *Drug Delivery*, *17*(6), 419–425. doi:10.3109/10717541003777233 PMID:20429848

Torne, S., Darandale, S., Vavia, P., Trotta, F., & Cavalli, R. (2013). Cyclodextrin-based nanosponges: Effective nanocarrier for tamoxifen delivery. *Pharmaceutical Development and Technology*, *18*(3), 619–625. doi:10.3109/10837450.2011.649855 PMID:22235935

Toth, I. (1999). Novel cationic lipidic peptide dendrimer vectors in vitro gene delivery. *STP Pharma Sciences, 9*(1), 93-99.

Towner, R. A., Smith, N., Asano, Y., He, T., Doblas, S., Saunders, D., ... Seeney, C. E. (2009). Molecular magnetic resonance imaging approaches used to aid in the understanding of angiogenesis in vivo: Implications for tissue engineering. *Tissue Engineering. Part A*, *16*(2), 357–364. doi:10.1089/ten.tea.2009.0233 PMID:19663584

Toy, R., Peiris, P. M., Ghaghada, K. B., & Karathanasis, E. (2014). Shaping cancer nanomedicine: The effect of particle shape on the in vivo journey of nanoparticles. *Nanomedicine (London)*, *9*(1), 121–134. doi:10.2217/nnm.13.191 PMID:24354814

Toy, R., & Roy, K. (2016). Engineering nanoparticles to overcome barriers to immunotherapy. *Bioengineering & Translational Medicine*, *1*(1), 47–62. doi:10.1002/btm2.10005 PMID:29313006

Tran, N., & Webster, T. J. (2010). Magnetic nanoparticles: Biomedical applications and challenges. *Journal of Materials Chemistry*, *20*(40), 8760–8767. doi:10.1039/c0jm00994f

Treenate, P., & Monvisade, P. (2017). In vitro drug release profiles of pH-sensitive hydroxyethylacryl chitosan/sodium alginate hydrogels using paracetamol as a soluble model drug. *International Journal of Biological Macromolecules*, *99*, 71–78. doi:10.1016/j.ijbiomac.2017.02.061 PMID:28219689

Trewyn, B. G., Giri, S., Slowing, I. I., & Lin, V. S. (2007). Mesoporous silica nanoparticle based controlled release, drug delivery, and biosensor systems. *Chemical communications (Cambridge, England)*, *31*(31), 3236–3245. doi:10.1039/b701744h PMID:17668088

Trewyn, B. G., Slowing, I. I., Giri, S., Chen, H.-T., & Lin, V. S. Y. (2007). Synthesis and functionalization of a mesoporous silica nanoparticle based on the sol-gel process and applications in controlled release. *Accounts of Chemical Research*, *40*(9), 846–853. doi:10.1021/ar600032u PMID:17645305

Trewyn, B. G., Whitman, C. M., & Lin, V. S. Y. (2004). Morphological Control of Room-Temperature Ionic Liquid Templated Mesoporous Silica Nanoparticles for Controlled Release of Antibacterial Agents. *Nano Letters*, *4*(11), 2139–2143. doi:10.1021/nl048774r

Trotta, F., & Tumiatti, W. (2003). Cross-linked polymers based on cyclodextrins for removing polluting agents. *WO 03/085002 A1*.

Trotta, F., Cavalli, R., Tumiatti, W., Zerbinati, O., Roggero, C., & Vallero, R. (2006). Ultrasound assisted synthesis of cyclodextrin based nanosponges. *WO 0002814 A1*.

Trotta, F., & Cavalli, R. (2009). Characterization and application of new hyper-cross-linked cyclodextrins. *Composite Interfaces*, *16*(1), 39–48. doi:10.1163/156855408X379388

Trotta, F., Zanetti, M., & Cavalli, R. (2012). Cyclodextrin-based nanosponges as drug carriers. *Beilstein Journal of Organic Chemistry*, *8*, 2091–2099. doi:10.3762/bjoc.8.235 PMID:23243470

Truzzi, E., Bongio, C., Sacchetti, F., Maretti, E., Montanari, M., Iannuccelli, V., ... Leo, E. (2017). Self-Assembled Lipid Nanoparticles for Oral Delivery of Heparin-Coated Iron Oxide Nanoparticles for Theranostic Purposes. *Molecules (Basel, Switzerland)*, *22*(6), 963. doi:10.3390/molecules22060963 PMID:28598368

Tsai, C. H., Vivero-Escoto, J. L., Slowing, I. I., Fang, I. J., Trewyn, B. G., & Lin, V. S. Y. (2011). Surfactant-assisted controlled release of hydrophobic drugs using anionic surfactant templated mesoporous silica nanoparticles. *Biomaterials*, *32*(26), 6234–6244. doi:10.1016/j.biomaterials.2011.04.077 PMID:21684000

Tyagi, L. K., Kumar, S., Maurya, S. S., & Kori, M. L. (2013). Ethosomes : Novel vesicular carrier for enhanced transdermal drug delivery system. *Bulletin of Pharmaceutical Research*, *3*(1), 6–13.

Ueda, H., Kadota, K., Imono, M., Ito, T., Kunita, A., & Tozuka, Y. (2017). Co-amorphous formation induced by combination of tranilast and diphenhydramine hydrochloride. *Journal of Pharmaceutical Sciences*, *106*(1), 123–128. doi:10.1016/j.xphs.2016.07.009 PMID:27539557

Ueda, H., Muranushi, N., Sakuma, S., Ida, Y., Endoh, T., Kadota, K., & Tozuka, Y. (2016). A strategy for co-former selection to design stable co-amorphous formations based on physicochemical properties of non-steroidal inflammatory drugs. *Pharmaceutical Research*, *33*(4), 1018–1029. doi:10.100711095-015-1848-2 PMID:26700604

Ugazio, E., Gastaldi, L., Brunella, V., Scalarone, D., Jadhav, S. A., Oliaro-Bosso, S., ... Sapino, S. (2016). Thermoresponsive mesoporous silica nanoparticles as a carrier for skin delivery of quercetin. *International Journal of Pharmaceutics*, *511*(1), 446–454. doi:10.1016/j.ijpharm.2016.07.024 PMID:27421910

Ukita, K., Kuroda, M., Honda, H., & Koishi, M. (1989). Characterization of powder coated microsponge prepared by dry impact blending method. *Chemical & Pharmaceutical Bulletin*, *37*(12), 3367–3371. doi:10.1248/cpb.37.3367

Ulery, B. D., Nair, L. S., & Laurencin, C. T. (2011). Biomedical applications of biodegradable polymers. *Journal of Polymer Science. Part B, Polymer Physics*, *49*(12), 832–864. doi:10.1002/polb.22259 PMID:21769165

Ulman, A. (1996). Formation and structure of self-assembled monolayers. *Chemical Reviews*, *96*(4), 1533–1554. doi:10.1021/cr9502357 PMID:11848802

Umeyor, C. E., Kenechukwu, F. C., Uronnachi, E. M., Osonnwa, U. E., & Nwakile, C. D. (2012). Solid lipid microparticles (SLMs): An effective lipid based technology for controlled drug delivery. *Am J PharmTech Res.*, *2*, 1–18.

Vahed, S. Z., Salehi, R., Davaran, S., & Sharifi, S. (2016). Liposome-based drug co-delivery systems in cancer cells. *Materials Science and Engineering C*, *71*, 1327–1341. doi:10.1016/j.msec.2016.11.073 PMID:27987688

Valencia, P. M., Basto, P. A., Zhang, L., Rhee, M., Langer, R., Farokhzad, O. C., & Karnik, R. (2010). Single-step assembly of homogenous lipid-polymeric and lipid-quantum dot nanoparticles enabled by microfluidic rapid mixing. *ACS Nano*, *4*(3), 1671–1679. doi:10.1021/nn901433u PMID:20166699

Vallet-Reg. (2012). *Mesoporous Silica Nanoparticles: Their Projection in Nanomedicine. Materials Science.*

Vallet-Regí, M., Manzano, M., & Colilla, M. (2012). Biomedical Applications of Mesoporous Ceramics: Drug Delivery, Smart Materials and Bone Tissue Engineering. CRC Press.

Vallet-Regi, M. (2014). *Bio-ceramics with clinical applications.* John Wiley & Sons Ltd. doi:10.1002/9781118406748

Vallet-Regí, M., Balas, F., & Arcos, D. (2007). Mesoporous materials for drug delivery. *Angewandte Chemie International Edition*, *46*(40), 7548–7558. doi:10.1002/anie.200604488 PMID:17854012

Vallet-Regi, M., Rámila, A., del Real, R. P., & Pérez-Pariente, J. (2001). A New Property of MCM-41: Drug Delivery System. *Chemistry of Materials*, *13*(2), 308–311. doi:10.1021/cm0011559

Vallet-Regí, M., & Ruiz-Hernandez, E. (2011). Bioceramics: From bone regeneration to cancer nanomedicine. *Advanced Materials*, *23*(44), 5177–5218. doi:10.1002/adma.201101586 PMID:22009627

van Elk, M., Murphy, B. P., Eufrásio-da-Silva, T., O'Reilly, D. P., Vermonden, T., Hennink, W. E., ... Ruiz-Hernández, E. (2016). Nanomedicines for advanced cancer treatments: Transitioning towards responsive systems. *International Journal of Pharmaceutics*, *515*(1), 132–164. doi:10.1016/j.ijpharm.2016.10.013 PMID:27725268

van Oirschot, B. A. (2014). A.H., Närhi TO, Anil S, Al Farraj Aldosari A, van den Beucken JJ, Jansen JA, *In vivo evaluation of bioactive glassbased coatings on dental implants in a dog implantation model. Clinical Oral Implants Research.* doi:10.1111/clr.12060

Vandervoort, J., & Ludwig, A. (2004). Preparation and evaluation of drug-loaded gelatin nanoparticles for topical ophthalmic use. *European Journal of Pharmaceutics and Biopharmaceutics*, *57*(2), 251–261. doi:10.1016/S0939-6411(03)00187-5 PMID:15018982

Vasconcelos, T., Marques, S., das Neves, J., & Sarmento, B. (2016). Amorphous solid dispersions: Rational selection of a manufacturing process. *Advanced Drug Delivery Reviews*, *100*, 85–101. doi:10.1016/j.addr.2016.01.012 PMID:26826438

Vavia, P. R., Swaminathan, S., Trotta, F., & Cavalli, R. (2006). Applications of nanosponges in drug delivery. *Proceedings XIII International Cyclodextrin Symposium*, p. 207.

Veiseh, O., Gunn, J. W., & Zhang, M. (2010). Design and fabrication of magnetic nanoparticles for targeted drug delivery and imaging. *Advanced Drug Delivery Reviews*, *62*(3), 284–304. doi:10.1016/j.addr.2009.11.002 PMID:19909778

Venkata Ramana Rao, S., & Shao, J. (2008). Self-nanoemulsifying drug delivery systems (SNEDDS) for oral delivery of protein drugs. *International Journal of Pharmaceutics*, *362*(1–2), 2–9. doi:10.1016/j.ijpharm.2008.05.018 PMID:18650038

Venkatesan, N., Yoshimitsu, J., Ito, Y., Shibata, N., & Takada, K. (2005). Liquid filled nanoparticles as a drug delivery tool for protein therapeutics. *Biomaterials*, *26*(34), 7154–7163. doi:10.1016/j.biomaterials.2005.05.012 PMID:15967493

Venkatesan, N., Yoshimitsu, J., Ohashi, Y., Ito, Y., Sugioka, N., Shibata, N., & Takada, K. (2006). Pharmacokinetic and pharmacodynamic studies following oral administration of erythropoietin mucoadhesive tablets to beagle dogs. *International Journal of Pharmaceutics*, *310*(1-2), 46–52. doi:10.1016/j.ijpharm.2005.11.014 PMID:16439074

Venugopal, B., Awada, A., Evans, T. R., Dueland, S., Hendlisz, A., Rasch, W., ... Aamdal, S. (2015). A first-in-human phase I and pharmacokinetic study of CP-4126 (CO-101), a nucleoside analogue, in patients with advanced solid tumours. *Cancer Chemotherapy and Pharmacology*, *76*(4), 785–792. doi:10.100700280-015-2846-0 PMID:26289594

Verissimo, L. M., Lima, L. F. A., Egito, L. C. M., de Oliveira, A. G., & do Egito, E. S. T. (2010). Pharmaceutical emulsions: A new approach for gene therapy. *Journal of Drug Targeting*, *18*(5), 333–342. doi:10.3109/10611860903434019 PMID:19958051

Verma, A., & Stellacci, F. (2010). Effect of surface properties on nanoparticle–cell interactions. *Small*, *6*(1), 12–21. doi:10.1002mll.200901158 PMID:19844908

Verma, D. D., Verma, S., Blume, G., & Fahr, A. (2003a). Particle size of liposomes influences dermal delivery of substances into skin. *International Journal of Pharmaceutics*, *258*(1-2), 141–151. doi:10.1016/S0378-5173(03)00183-2 PMID:12753761

Verma, I. M., & Somia, N. (1997). Gene therapy-promises, problems and prospects. *Nature*, *389*(6648), 239–242. doi:10.1038/38410 PMID:9305836

Verron, E., Gauthier, O., Janvier, P., Pilet, P., Lesoeur, J., Bujoli, B., ... Bouler, J.-M. (2010). In vivo bone augmentation in an osteoporotic environment using bisphosphonate-loaded calcium deficient apatite. *Biomaterials*, *31*(30), 7776–7784. doi:10.1016/j.biomaterials.2010.06.047 PMID:20643480

Verwey, E. J. W., Overbeek, J. T. G., & Overbeek, J. T. G. (1999). *Theory of the stability of lyophobic colloids*. Courier Corporation.

Vestal, C. R., & Zhang, Z. J. (2003). Synthesis and magnetic characterization of Mn and Co spinel ferrite-silica nanoparticles with tunable magnetic core. *Nano Letters*, *3*(12), 1739–1743. doi:10.1021/nl034816k

Vikas, S., Seema, S., Gurpreet, S., Rana, A. C., & Baibhav, J. (2011). Penetration enhancers: A novel strategy for enhancing transdermal drug delivery. *Int. Res. J. Pharm.*, *2*, 32–36.

Villa, C. H., Dao, T., Ahearn, I., Fehrenbacher, N., Casey, E., Rey, D. A., ... Philips, M. R. (2011). Single-walled carbon nanotubes deliver peptide antigen into dendritic cells and enhance IgG responses to tumor-associated antigens. *ACS Nano*, *5*(7), 5300–5311. doi:10.1021/nn200182x PMID:21682329

Vishweshwar, P., McMahon, J. A., Peterson, M. L., Hickey, M. B., Shattock, T. R., & Zaworotko, M. J. (2005). Crystal engineering of pharmaceutical co-crystals from polymorphic active pharmaceutical ingredients. *Chemical Communications*, (36): 4601–4603. doi:10.1039/b501304f PMID:16158128

Vivero-Escoto, J. L., Slowing, I. I., Wu, C. W., & Lin, V. S. (2009). Photoinduced intracellular controlled release drug delivery in human cells by gold-capped mesoporous silica nanosphere. *Journal of the American Chemical Society*, *131*(10), 3462–3463. doi:10.1021/ja900025f PMID:19275256

Vo, C. L. N., Park, C., & Lee, B. J. (2013). Current trends and future perspectives of solid dispersions containing poorly water-soluble drugs. *European Journal of Pharmaceutics and Biopharmaceutics*, *85*(3), 799–813. doi:10.1016/j.ejpb.2013.09.007 PMID:24056053

Vogt, F. G., Clawson, J. S., Strohmeier, M., Edwards, A. J., Pham, T. N., & Watson, S. A. (2008). Solid-state NMR analysis of organic cocrystals and complexes. *Crystal Growth & Design*, *9*(2), 921–937. doi:10.1021/cg8007014

Vold, I. M. N., Kristiansen, K. A., & Christensen, B. E. (2006). A study of the chain stiffness and extension of alginates, in vitro epimerized alginates, and periodate-oxidized alginates using size-exclusion chromatography combined with light scattering and viscosity detectors. *Biomacromolecules*, *7*(7), 2136–2146. doi:10.1021/bm060099n PMID:16827580

Von Hoff, D. D., Mita, M. M., Ramanathan, R. K., Weiss, G. J., Mita, A. C., LoRusso, P. M., ... Sachdev, J. C. (2016). Phase I Study of PSMA-Targeted Docetaxel-Containing Nanoparticle BIND-014 in Patients with Advanced Solid Tumors. *Clinical Cancer Research*, *22*(13), 3157–3163. doi:10.1158/1078-0432.CCR-15-2548 PMID:26847057

Vonarbourg, A., Passirani, C., Saulnier, P., Simard, P., Leroux, J. C., & Benoit, J. P. (2006). Evaluation of pegylated lipid nanocapsules versus complement system activation and macrophage uptake. *Journal of Biomedical Materials Research. Part A*, *78*(3), 620–628. doi:10.1002/jbm.a.30711 PMID:16779767

Vong, L. B., Kimura, S., & Nagasaki, Y. (2017). Newly Designed Silica-Containing Redox Nanoparticles for Oral Delivery of Novel TOP2 Catalytic Inhibitor for Treating Colon Cancer. *Adv Healthc Mater.*

Voyles, P. M., Zotov, N., Nakhmanson, S. M., Drabold, D. A., Gibson, J. M., Treacy, M. M. J., & Keblinski, P. (2001). Structure and physical properties of paracrystalline atomistic models of amorphous silicon. *Journal of Applied Physics*, *90*(9), 4437–4451. doi:10.1063/1.1407319

Vyas, S. P., & Khar, R. K. (2002). Controlled drug delivery concepts and advances. *Vallabh prakashan, 1*, 411-447.

Wadhwa, M. S., Collard, W. T., Adami, R. C., McKenzie, D. L., & Rice, K. G. (1997). Peptide-mediated gene delivery: Influence of peptide structure on gene expression. *Bioconjugate Chemistry*, *8*(1), 81–88. doi:10.1021/bc960079q PMID:9026040

Wagnera, D., Langguth, H. S., Hanafy, A., Koggela, A., & Langguth, P. (2001). Intestinal drug efflux: Formulation and food effects. *Advanced Drug Delivery Reviews*, *50*(Suppl. 1), 113–131. PMID:11576693

Wairkar, S., & Gaud, R. (2015). Co-Amorphous Combination of Nateglinide-Metformin Hydrochloride for Dissolution Enhancement. *AAPS PharmSciTech*, 1–9. PMID:26314243

Wang, H. (2015). Enhanced Dielectric Performance of BaTiO3 / PVDF Composites Prepared by Modified Process for Energy Storage Applications. *IEEE Transactions on Ultrasonics, Ferroelectrics, and Frequency Control, 62*(1).

Wang, J. (2011). Porous microbeads as three-dimensional scaffold for tissue engineering. *NNIN Reu Research Accomplished*, 32-33.

Wang, J., Byrne, J. D., Napier, M. E., & DeSimone, J. M. (2011). More Effective Nanomedicines through Particle Design. *Small (Weinheim an Der Bergstrasse, Germany)*, *7*(14), 1919–1931.

Wang, A. Z., Yuet, K., Zhang, L., Gu, F. X., Huynh-Le, M., Radovic-Moreno, A. F., ... Farokhzad, O. C. (2010). ChemoRad nanoparticles: A novel multifunctional nanoparticle platform for targeted delivery of concurrent chemoradiation. *Nanomedicine (London)*, *5*(3), 361–368. doi:10.2217/nnm.10.6 PMID:20394530

Wang, A., Guo, M., Wang, N., Zhao, J., Qi, W., Muhammad, F., ... Zhu, G. (2014). Redox-mediated dissolution of paramagnetic nanolids to achieve a smart theranostic system. *Nanoscale*, *6*(10), 5270–5278. doi:10.1039/C3NR05687B PMID:24695417

Wang, D., Fei, B., Halig, L. V., Qin, X., Hu, Z., Xu, H., ... Chen, Z. (2014). Targeted iron-oxide nanoparticle for photodynamic therapy and imaging of head and neck cancer. *ACS Nano*, *8*(7), 6620–6632. doi:10.1021/nn501652j PMID:24923902

Wang, F., Chen, L., Zhang, R., Chen, Z., & Zhu, L. (2014). RGD peptide conjugated liposomal drug delivery system for enhance therapeutic efficacy in treating bone metastasis from prostate cancer. *Journal of Controlled Release*, *196*, 222–233. doi:10.1016/j.jconrel.2014.10.012 PMID:25456829

Wang, F., Li, L., Liu, B., Chen, Z., & Li, C. (2017). Hyaluronic acid decorated pluronic P85 solid lipid nanoparticles as a potential carrier to overcome multidrug resistance in cervical and breast cancer. *Biomedicine and Pharmacotherapy*, *86*, 595–604. doi:10.1016/j.biopha.2016.12.041 PMID:28027535

Wang, F., Zhang, B., Zhou, L., Shi, Y., Li, Z., Xia, Y., & Tian, J. (2016). Imaging Dendrimer-Grafted Graphene Oxide Mediated Anti-miR-21 Delivery With an Activatable Luciferase Reporter. *ACS Applied Materials & Interfaces*, *8*(14), 9014–9021. doi:10.1021/acsami.6b02662 PMID:27010367

Wang, H., Agarwal, P., Zhao, S., Yu, J., Lu, X., & He, X. (2016). Combined cancer therapy with hyaluronan-decorated fullerene-silica multifunctional nanoparticles to target cancer stem-like cells. *Biomaterials*, *97*, 62–73. doi:10.1016/j.biomaterials.2016.04.030 PMID:27162075

Wang, H., Li, Y., Zuo, Y., Li, J., Ma, S., & Cheng, L. (2007). Biocompatibility and osteogenesis of biomimetic nano-hydroxyapatite/polyamide composite scaffolds for bone tissue engineering. *Biomaterials*, *28*(22), 3338–3348. doi:10.1016/j.biomaterials.2007.04.014 PMID:17481726

Wang, J.-R., Yu, Q., Dai, W., & Mei, X. (2016). Drug–drug co-crystallization presents a new opportunity for the development of stable vitamins. *Chemical Communications (Cambridge)*, *52*(17), 3572–3575. doi:10.1039/C5CC10297A PMID:26845759

Wang, K., Yao, H., Meng, Y., Wang, Y., Yan, X., & Huang, R. (2015). Specific aptamer-conjugated mesoporous silica-carbon nanoparticles for HER2-targeted chemo-photothermal combined therapy. *Acta Biomaterialia*, *16*, 196–205. doi:10.1016/j.actbio.2015.01.002 PMID:25596325

Wang, L. L., Huang, S., Guo, H. H., Han, Y. X., Zheng, W. S., & Jiang, J. D. (2016). In situ delivery of thermosensitive gel-mediated 5-fluorouracil microemulsion for the treatment of colorectal cancer. *Drug Design, Development and Therapy*, *10*, 2855–2867. doi:10.2147/DDDT.S111351 PMID:27660416

Wang, L. V., & Hu, S. (2012). Photoacoustic Tomography: In Vivo Imaging from Organelles to Organs. *Science*, *335*(6075), 1458–1462. doi:10.1126cience.1216210 PMID:22442475

Wang, M. (2003). Developing bioactive composite materials for tissue replacement. *Biomaterials*, *24*(13), 2133–2151. doi:10.1016/S0142-9612(03)00037-1 PMID:12699650

Wang, Q., Yan, J., Yang, J., & Li, B. (2016). Nanomaterials promise better bone repair. *Materials Today*, *19*(8), 451–463. doi:10.1016/j.mattod.2015.12.003

Wang, Q., Ye, J., Zhoua, X., & Zhang, N. (2008). Injectable loaded solid lipid nanoparticles as passive targeting therapeutic agents for rheumatoid arthritis. *International Journal of Pharmaceutics*, *352*(1-2), 273–279. doi:10.1016/j.ijpharm.2007.10.014 PMID:18054182

Wang, W., Liao, S., Liu, M., Zhao, Q., & Zhu, Y. (2014). Polymer Composites Reinforced by Nanotubes as Scaffolds for Tissue Engineering. *International Journal of Polymer Science*, *2014*, 14. doi:10.1155/2014/805634

Wang, X., Li, C., Fan, N., Li, J., He, Z., & Sun, J. (2017). Multimodal nanoporous silica nanoparticles functionalized with aminopropyl groups for improving loading and controlled release of doxorubicin hydrochloride. *Materials Science and Engineering C*, *78*, 370–375. doi:10.1016/j.msec.2017.04.060 PMID:28575997

Wang, X., Liu, Y., Wang, S., Shi, D., Zhou, X., Wang, C., ... Lu, G. (2015). CD44-engineered mesoporous silica nanoparticles for overcoming multidrug resistance in breast cancer. *Applied Surface Science*, *332*, 308–317. doi:10.1016/j.apsusc.2015.01.204

Wang, X., Niu, D., Hu, C., & Li, P. (2015). Polyethyleneimine-based nanocarriers for gene delivery. *Current Pharmaceutical Design*, *21*(42), 6140–6156. doi:10.2174/1381612821666151027152907 PMID:26503146

Wang, X., Wang, L., He, X., Zhang, Y., & Chen, L. (2009). A molecularly imprinted polymer-coated nanocomposite of magnetic nanoparticles for estrone recognition. *Talanta*, *78*(2), 327–332. doi:10.1016/j.talanta.2008.11.024 PMID:19203590

Wang, Y., Cui, Y., Huang, J., Di, D., Dong, Y., Zhang, X., ... Wang, S. (2015a). Redox and pH dual-responsive mesoporous silica nanoparticles for site-specific drug delivery. *Applied Surface Science*, *356*, 1282–1288. doi:10.1016/j.apsusc.2015.07.151

Wang, Y., Gao, S., Ye, W.-H., Yoon, H. S., & Yang, Y.-Y. (2006). Co-delivery of drugs and DNA from cationic core–shell nanoparticles self-assembled from a biodegradable copolymer. *Nature Materials*, *5*(10), 791–796. doi:10.1038/nmat1737 PMID:16998471

Wang, Y., Han, N., Zhao, Q., Bai, L., Li, J., Jiang, T., & Wang, S. (2015b). Redox-responsive mesoporous silica as carriers for controlled drug delivery: A comparative study based on silica and PEG gatekeepers. *European Journal of Pharmaceutical Sciences*, *72*, 12–20. doi:10.1016/j.ejps.2015.02.008 PMID:25701727

Wang, Y.-L., Lee, B.-S., Chang, K.-C., Chiu, H.-C., Lin, F.-H., & Lin, C.-P. (2007). Characterization, fluoride release and recharge properties of polymer–kaolinite nanocomposite resins. *Composites Science and Technology*, *67*(15), 3409–3416. doi:10.1016/j.compscitech.2007.03.018

Wang, Y., Rajala, A., & Rajala, R. V. S. (2015). Lipid nanoparticles for ocular gene delivery. *Journal of Functional Biomaterials*, *6*(2), 379–394. doi:10.3390/jfb6020379 PMID:26062170

Wang, Y., Shen, W., Shi, X., Fu, F., Fan, Y., Shen, W., ... Qi, R. (2017). Alpha-Tocopheryl Succinate-Conjugated G5 PAMAM Dendrimer Enables Effective Inhibition of Ulcerative Colitis. *Advanced Healthcare Materials*, *6*(14), 1700276. doi:10.1002/adhm.201700276 PMID:28474434

Wang, Y., Shi, W., Wang, S., Li, C., Qian, M., Chen, J., & Huang, R. (2016). Facile incorporation of dispersed fluorescent carbon nanodots into mesoporous silica nanosphere for pH-triggered drug delivery and imaging. *Carbon*, *108*, 146–153. doi:10.1016/j.carbon.2016.07.009

Wang, Y., Strohm, E. M., Sun, Y., Wang, Z., Zheng, Y., Wang, Z., & Kolios, M. C. (2016). Biodegradable polymeric nanoparticles containing gold nanoparticles and Paclitaxel for cancer imaging and drug delivery using photoacoustic methods. *Biomedical Optics Express*, *7*(10), 4125–4138. doi:10.1364/BOE.7.004125 PMID:27867720

Wang, Y., Yang, T., Ke, H., Zhu, A., Wang, Y., Wang, J., ... Chen, H. (2015). Smart Albumin-Biomineralized Nanocomposites for Multimodal Imaging and Photothermal Tumor Ablation. *Advanced Materials*, *27*(26), 3874–3882. doi:10.1002/adma.201500229 PMID:25997571

Wang, Z., Xu, Y., Meng, X., Watari, F., Liu, H., & Chen, X. (2015). Suppression of c-Myc is involved in multi-walled carbon nanotubes' down-regulation of ATP-binding cassette transporters in human colon adenocarcinoma cells. *Toxicology and Applied Pharmacology*, *282*(1), 42–51. doi:10.1016/j.taap.2014.11.002 PMID:25461681

Wan, Y., Dai, W., Nevagi, R. J., Toth, I., & Moyle, P. M. (2017). Multifunctional peptide-lipid nanocomplexes for efficient targeted delivery of DNA and siRNA into breast cancer cells. *Acta Biomaterialia*, *59*, 257–268. doi:10.1016/j.actbio.2017.06.032 PMID:28655658

Ward, M. A., & Georgiou, T. K. (2011). Thermoresponsive Polymers for Biomedical Applications. *Polymers*, *3*(4), 1215–1242. doi:10.3390/polym3031215

Watson, B., Meldrum, S., Riddle, H., Brown, R., & Sladen, G. (1972). pH profile of gut as measured by radiotelemetry capsule. *British Medical Journal*, *2*(5805), 104–106. doi:10.1136/bmj.2.5805.104 PMID:5018285

Waugh, A., & Grant, A. (2010). *Ross & Wilson anatomy and physiology in health and illness*. Elsevier Health Sciences.

Webster, T. J., Ergun, C., Doremus, R. H., Siegel, R. W., & Bizios, R. (2000). Specific proteins mediate enhanced osteoblast adhesion on nanophase ceramics. *Journal of Biomedical Materials Research. Part A*, *51*(3), 475–483. doi: PMID:10880091

Wegmann, F., Gartlan, K. H., Harandi, A. M., Brinckmann, S. A., Coccia, M., Hillson, W. R., ... Settantau, Q. J. (2012). Polyethyleneimine is a potentmucosal adjuvant for viral glycoprotein antigens. *Nature Biotechnology*, *30*(9), 883–888. doi:10.1038/nbt.2344 PMID:22922673

Wei, G., & Ma, P. X. (2004). Structure and properties of nano-hydroxyapatite/polymer composite scaffolds for bone tissue engineering. *Biomaterials*, *25*(19), 4749–4757. doi:10.1016/j.biomaterials.2003.12.005 PMID:15120521

Wei, L., Cai, C., Lin, J., & Chen, T. (2009). Dual-drug delivery system based on hydrogel/micelle composites. *Biomaterials*, *30*(13), 2606–2613. doi:10.1016/j.biomaterials.2009.01.006 PMID:19162320

Wei, L., Shi, D., Zhou, Z., Ye, P., Wang, J., Zhao, J., ... Zhang, Y. (2012). Functionalized self-assembled monolayers on mesoporous silica nanoparticles with high surface coverage. *Nanoscale Research Letters*, *7*(1), 334. doi:10.1186/1556-276X-7-334 PMID:22720819

Wei, L., Sun, P., Nie, S., & Pan, W. (2005). Preparation and evaluation of SEDDS and SMEDDS containing carvedilol. *Drug Development and Industrial Pharmacy*, *31*(8), 785–794. doi:10.1080/03639040500216428 PMID:16221613

Weissleder, R., Kelly, K., Sun, E. Y., Shtatland, T., & Josephson, L. (2005). Cell-specific targeting of nanoparticles by multivalent attachment of small molecules. *Nature Biotechnology*, *23*(11), 1418–1423. doi:10.1038/nbt1159 PMID:16244656

Wei, Y., Gao, L., Wang, L., Shi, L., Wei, E., Zhou, B., ... Ge, B. (2017). Polydopamine and peptide decorated doxorubicin-loaded mesoporous silica nanoparticles as a targeted drug delivery system for bladder cancer therapy. *Drug Delivery*, *24*(1), 681–691. doi:10.1080/10717544.2017.1309475 PMID:28414557

Wen, R., Umeano, A. C., Francis, L., Sharma, N., Tundup, S., & Dhar, S. (2016). Mitochondrion: A promising target for nanoparticle-based vaccine delivery systems. *Vaccines*, *4*(18), 1–25. PMID:27258316

Wenson, E. S., & Curtalo, W. J. (1992). Article. *Advanced Drug Delivery Reviews*, *8*, 39. doi:10.1016/0169-409X(92)90015-I

Wester, R., Patel, R., Natch, S., Leyden, J., Melendres, J., & Maibach, H. (1991). Controlled release of benzoyl peroxide from a porous microsphere polymeric system can reduce topical irritancy. *Journal of the American Academy of Dermatology*, *24*(5), 720–726. doi:10.1016/0190-9622(91)70109-F PMID:1869643

Wicki, A., Witzigmann, D., Balasubramanian, V., & Huwyler, J. (2015). Nanomedicine in cancer therapy: Challenges, opportunities, and clinical applications. *Journal of Controlled Release*, *200*, 138–157. doi:10.1016/j.jconrel.2014.12.030 PMID:25545217

Wiechers, J. W. (1989). The barrier functions of the skin in relation to percutaneous absorption of drugs. *Pharmaceutisch Weekblad. Scientific Edition*, *11*(6), 185–198. doi:10.1007/BF01959410 PMID:2694089

Winstanley, P. A., & Orme, M. L. E. (1989). The effects of food on drug bioavailability. *British Journal of Clinical Pharmacology*, *28*(6), 621–628. doi:10.1111/j.1365-2125.1989.tb03554.x PMID:2692684

Wiwattanapatapee, R., Lomlim, L., & Saramunee, K. (2003). Dendrimers conjugates for colonic delivery of 5-aminosalicylic acid. *Journal of Controlled Release*, *88*(1), 1–9. doi:10.1016/S0168-3659(02)00461-3 PMID:12586498

Wolfert, M., & Seymour, L. (1998). Chloroquine and amphipathic peptide helices show synergistic transfection in vitro. *Gene Therapy*, *5*(3), 409–414. doi:10.1038j.gt.3300606 PMID:9614562

Wong, H. L., Bendayan, R., Rauth, A. M., Li, Y., & Wu, X. Y. (2007). Chemotherapy with anticancer drugs encapsulated in solid lipid nanoparticles. *Advanced Drug Delivery Reviews*, *59*(6), 491–504. doi:10.1016/j.addr.2007.04.008 PMID:17532091

Wong, H. L., Bendayan, R., Rauth, A. M., & Wu, X. Y. (2004). Development of solid lipid nanoparticles containing ionically complexed chemotherapeutic drugs and chemosensitizers. *Journal of Pharmaceutical Sciences*, *93*(8), 1993–2008. doi:10.1002/jps.20100 PMID:15236449

Wu, B., Wan, B., Lu, S. T., Deng, K., Li, X. Q., Wu, B. L., ... Xu, H.-B. (2017). Near-infrared light-triggered theranostics for tumor-specific enhanced multimodal imaging and photothermal therapy. *International Journal of Nanomedicine*, *12*, 4467–4478. doi:10.2147/IJN.S137835 PMID:28670120

Wu, C. Y., & Benet, L. Z. (2005). Predicting drug disposition via application of BCS: Transport/absorption/ elimination interplay and development of a biopharmaceutics drug disposition classification system. *Pharmaceutical Research*, *22*(1), 11–23. doi:10.100711095-004-9004-4 PMID:15771225

Wu, L. G. U., & Boker, A. (2016). Synthesis of Hybrid Silica Nanoparticles Densely Grafted with Thermo and pH Dual-Responsive Brushes via Surface-Initiated ATRP. *Macromolecules*, *49*(24), 9586–9596. doi:10.1021/acs.macromol.6b01792

Wunder, A., Müller-Ladner, U., Stelzer, E. H., Funk, J., Neumann, E., Stehle, G., ... Fiehn, C. (2003). Albumin-based drug delivery as novel therapeutic approach for rheumatoid arthritis. *Journal of Immunology (Baltimore, Md.: 1950)*, *170*(9), 4793–4801. doi:10.4049/jimmunol.170.9.4793 PMID:12707361

Wu, Q., Xu, Y., Yao, Z., Liu, A., & Shi, G. (2010). Supercapacitors Based on Flexible Graphene/Polyaniline Nanofiber Composite Films. *ACS Nano*, *4*(4), 1963–1970. doi:10.1021/nn1000035 PMID:20355733

Wu, S. H., Mou, C. Y., & Lin, H. P. (2013). Synthesis of mesoporous silica nanoparticles. *Chemical Society Reviews*, *42*(9), 3862–3875. doi:10.1039/c3cs35405a PMID:23403864

Wu, W., He, Q., & Jiang, C. (2008). Magnetic iron oxide nanoparticles: Synthesis and surface functionalization strategies. *Nanoscale Research Letters*, *3*(11), 397–415. doi:10.100711671-008-9174-9 PMID:21749733

Wu, X. Y. (2016). Strategies for optimizing polymer-lipid hybrid nanoparticle-mediated drug delivery. [Internet]. *Expert Opinion on Drug Delivery*, *13*(5), 609–612. doi:10.1517/17425247.2016.1165662 PMID:26978527

Wu, X., Han, Z., Schur, R. M., & Lu, Z. R. (2016). Targeted Mesoporous Silica Nanoparticles Delivering Arsenic Trioxide with Environment Sensitive Drug Release for Effective Treatment of Triple Negative Breast Cancer. *ACS Biomaterials Science & Engineering*, *2*(4), 501–507. doi:10.1021/acsbiomaterials.5b00398

Wu, Y. Z., Sun, J., Zhang, Y., Pu, M., Zhang, G., He, N., & Zeng, X. (2017). Effective Integration of Targeted Tumor Imaging and Therapy Using Functionalized InP QDs with VEGFR2 Monoclonal Antibody and miR-92a Inhibitor. *ACS Applied Materials & Interfaces*, *9*(15), 13068–13078. doi:10.1021/acsami.7b02641 PMID:28358188

Wu, Z. S., Ren, W., Wen, L., Gao, L., Zhao, J., Chen, Z., ... Cheng, H. M. (2010). Graphene Anchored with Co_3O_4 Nanoparticles as Anode of Lithium Ion Batteries with Enhanced Reversible Capacity and Cyclic Performance. *ACS Nano*, *4*(6), 3187–3194. doi:10.1021/nn100740x PMID:20455594

Wu, Z., Tang, T., Guo, H., Tang, S., Niu, Y., Zhang, J., ... Wei, J. (2014). In vitro degradability, bioactivity and cell responses to mesoporous magnesium silicate for the induction of bone regeneration. *Colloids and Surfaces. B, Biointerfaces*, *120*, 38–46. doi:10.1016/j.colsurfb.2014.04.010 PMID:24905677

Xiao, Y., Jaskula-Sztul, R., Javadi, A., Xu, W., Eide, J., Dammalapati, A., ... Gong, S. (2012). Co-delivery of doxorubicin and siRNA using octreotide-conjugated gold nanorods for targeted neuroendocrine cancer therapy. *Nanoscale*, *4*(22), 7185–7193. doi:10.1039/c2nr31853a PMID:23070403

Xia, W., & Chang, J. (2006). Well-ordered mesoporous bioactive glasses (MBG): A promising bioactive drug delivery system. *Journal of Controlled Release*, *110*(3), 522–530. doi:10.1016/j.jconrel.2005.11.002 PMID:16375986

Xia, W., Chang, J., Lin, J., & Zhu, J. (2008). The pH-controlled dual-drug release from mesoporous bioactive glass/polypeptide graft copolymer nanomicelle composites. *European Journal of Pharmaceutics and Biopharmaceutics*, *69*(2), 546–552. doi:10.1016/j.ejpb.2007.11.018 PMID:18248801

Xia, Y., Yang, P., Sun, Y., Wu, Y., Mayers, B., Gates, B., ... Yan, H. (2003). One-dimensional nanostructures: Synthesis, characterization, and applications. *Advanced Materials*, *15*(5), 353–389. doi:10.1002/adma.200390087

Xie, J., Lee, S., & Chen, X. (2010). Nanoparticle-based theranostic agents. *Advanced Drug Delivery Reviews*, *62*(11), 1064–1079. doi:10.1016/j.addr.2010.07.009 PMID:20691229

Xie, J., Liu, G., Eden, H. S., Ai, H., & Chen, X. (2011). Surface-engineered magnetic nanoparticle platforms for cancer imaging and therapy. *Accounts of Chemical Research*, *44*(10), 883–892. doi:10.1021/ar200044b PMID:21548618

Xie, J., Zheng, Y., & Ying, J. Y. (2009). Protein-directed synthesis of highly fluorescent gold nanoclusters. *Journal of the American Chemical Society*, *131*(3), 888–889. doi:10.1021/ja806804u PMID:19123810

Xie, M., Shi, H., Ma, K., Shen, H., Li, B., Shen, S., ... Jin, Y. (2013). Hybrid nanoparticles for drug delivery and bioimaging: Mesoporous silica nanoparticles functionalized with carboxyl groups and a near-infrared fluorescent dye. *Journal of Colloid and Interface Science*, *395*, 306–314. doi:10.1016/j.jcis.2013.01.001 PMID:23394807

Xie, M., Xu, Y., Shen, H., Shen, S., Ge, Y., & Xie, J. (2014). Negative-charge-functionalized mesoporous silica nanoparticles as drug vehicles targeting hepatocellular carcinoma. *International Journal of Pharmaceutics*, *474*, 223–231. PMID:25149125

Xie, X.-H., Wang, X.-L., He, Y.-X., Liu, Z., Sheng, H., Zhang, G., & Qin, L. (2012). Promotion of bone repair by implantation of cryopreserved bone marrow–derived mononuclear cells in a rabbit model of steroid-associated osteonecrosis. *Arthritis and Rheumatism*, *64*(5), 1562–1571. doi:10.1002/art.34525 PMID:22544527

Xie, X., Li, F., Zhang, H., Lu, Y., Lian, S., Lin, H., ... Jia, L. (2016). EpCAM aptamer-functionalized mesoporous silica nanoparticles for efficient colon cancer cell-targeted drug delivery. *European Journal of Pharmaceutical Sciences*, *83*, 28–35. doi:10.1016/j.ejps.2015.12.014 PMID:26690044

Xiong, X.-B., & Lavasanifar, A. (2011). Traceable multifunctional micellar nanocarriers for cancer-targeted co-delivery of MDR-1 siRNA and doxorubicin. *ACS Nano*, *5*(6), 5202–5213. doi:10.1021/nn2013707 PMID:21627074

Xu, C., & Teja, A. S. (2008). Continuous hydrothermal synthesis of iron oxide and PVA-protected iron oxide nanoparticles. *The Journal of Supercritical Fluids*, *44*(1), 85–91. doi:10.1016/j.supflu.2007.09.033

Xu, F., Ding, L., Tao, W., Yang, X. Z., Qian, H. S., & Yao, R. S. (2016). Mesoporous-silica-coated upconversion nanoparticles loaded with vitamin B12 for near-infrared-light mediated photodynamic therapy. *Materials Letters*, *167*, 205–208. doi:10.1016/j.matlet.2015.12.105

Xu, G., Shi, C., Guo, D., Wang, L., Ling, Y., Han, X., & Luo, J. (2015). Functional-segregated coumarin-containing telodendrimer nanocarriers for efficient delivery of SN-38 for colon cancer treatment. *Acta Biomaterialia*, *21*, 85–98. doi:10.1016/j.actbio.2015.04.021 PMID:25910639

Xu, G., Zeng, S., Zhang, B., Swihart, M. T., Yong, K. T., & Prasad, P. N. (2016). New Generation Cadmium-Free Quantum Dots for Biophotonics and Nanomedicine. *Chemical Reviews*, *116*(19), 12234–12327. doi:10.1021/acs.chemrev.6b00290 PMID:27657177

Xu, H. H., Moreau, J. L., Sun, L., & Chow, L. C. (2008). Strength and fluoride release characteristics of a calcium fluoride based dental nanocomposite. *Biomaterials*, *29*(32), 4261–4267. doi:10.1016/j.biomaterials.2008.07.037 PMID:18708252

Xu, H. H., Weir, M. D., & Sun, L. (2007). Nanocomposites with Ca and PO 4 release: Effects of reinforcement, dicalcium phosphate particle size and silanization. *Dental Materials*, *23*(12), 1482–1491. doi:10.1016/j.dental.2007.01.002 PMID:17339048

Xu, H. H., Weir, M. D., & Sun, L. (2009). Calcium and phosphate ion releasing composite: Effect of pH on release and mechanical properties. *Dental Materials*, *25*(4), 535–542. doi:10.1016/j.dental.2008.10.009 PMID:19101026

Xu, H. H., Weir, M. D., Sun, L., Moreau, J. L., Takagi, S., Chow, L. C., & Antonucci, J. M. (2010). Strong nanocomposites with Ca, PO(4), and F release for caries inhibition. *Journal of Dental Research*, *89*(1), 19–28. doi:10.1177/0022034509351969 PMID:19948941

Xu, H., Sun, L., Weir, M. D., Antonucci, J. M., Takagi, S., Chow, L. C., & Peltz, M. (2006). Nano DCPA-whisker composites with high strength and Ca and PO4 release. *Journal of Dental Research*, *85*(8), 722–727. doi:10.1177/154405910608500807 PMID:16861289

Xu, H., Weir, M. D., Sun, L., Takagi, S., & Chow, L. C. (2007). Effects of calcium phosphate nanoparticles on Ca-PO4 composite. *Journal of Dental Research*, *86*(4), 378–383. doi:10.1177/154405910708600415 PMID:17384036

Xu, Q., Huang, W., Jiang, L., Lei, Z., Li, X., & Deng, H. (2013). KGM and PMAA based pH-sensitive interpenetrating polymer network hydrogel for controlled drug release. *Carbohydrate Polymers*, *97*(2), 565–570. doi:10.1016/j.carbpol.2013.05.007 PMID:23911486

Xu, W., Gao, Q., Xu, Y., Wu, D., Sun, Y., Shen, W., & Deng, F. (2009). Controllable release of ibuprofen from size-adjustable and surface hydrophobic mesoporous silica spheres. *Powder Technology*, *191*(1-2), 13–20. doi:10.1016/j.powtec.2008.09.001

Xu, W., Riikonen, J., & Lehto, V. P. (2013). Mesoporous systems for poorly soluble drugs. *International Journal of Pharmaceutics*, *453*(1), 181–197. doi:10.1016/j.ijpharm.2012.09.008 PMID:22990124

Xu, X., Lü, S., Gao, C., Wang, X., Bai, X., Gao, N., & Liu, M. (2015). Facile preparation of pH-sensitive and self-fluorescent mesoporous silica nanoparticles modified with PAMAM dendrimers for label-free imaging and drug delivery. *Chemical Engineering Journal*, *266*, 171–178. doi:10.1016/j.cej.2014.12.075

Yalkowsky, S.H. (2000). *Solubility and solubilization in aqueous media*. Washington, DC: American Chemical Society.

Yamada, H., Urata, C., Aoyama, Y., Osada, S., Yamauchi, Y., & Kuroda, K. (2012). Preparation of Colloidal Mesoporous Silica Nanoparticles with Different Diameters and Their Unique Degradation Behavior in Static Aqueous Systems. *Chemistry of Materials*, *24*(8), 1462–1471. doi:10.1021/cm3001688

Yamamoto, M., Ikada, Y., & Tabata, Y. (2001). Controlled release of growth factors based on biodegradation of gelatin hydrogel. Biomater. *Sci. Polym. Ed.*, *12*(1), 77–88. PMID:11334191

Yamamoto, M., Takahashi, Y., & Tabata, Y. (2003). Controlled release by biodegradable hydrogels enhances the ectopic bone formation of bone morphogenetic protein. *Biomaterials*, *24*(24), 4375–4383. doi:10.1016/S0142-9612(03)00337-5 PMID:12922150

Yamamura, S., Gotoh, H., Sakamoto, Y., & Momose, Y. (2000). Physicochemical properties of amorphous precipitates of cimetidine–indomethacin binary system. *European Journal of Pharmaceutics and Biopharmaceutics*, *49*(3), 259–265. doi:10.1016/S0939-6411(00)00060-6 PMID:10799818

Yamamura, S., Gotoh, H., Sakamoto, Y., & Momose, Y. (2002). Physicochemical properties of amorphous salt of cimetidine and diflunisal system. *International Journal of Pharmaceutics*, *241*(2), 213–221. doi:10.1016/S0378-5173(02)00195-3 PMID:12100849

Yameen, B., Choi, W. I., Vilos, C., Swami, A., Shi, J., & Farokhzad, O. C. (2014). Insight into nanoparticle cellular uptake and intracellular targeting. *Journal of Controlled Release*, *190*, 485–499. doi:10.1016/j.jconrel.2014.06.038 PMID:24984011

Yanagisawa, T., Shimizu, T., Kuroda, K., & Kato, C. (1990). The Preparation of Alkyltrimethylammonium-Kanemite Complexes and Their Conversion to Microporous Materials. *Bulletin of the Chemical Society of Japan*, *63*(4), 988–992. doi:10.1246/bcsj.63.988

Yang, Y., Leonand, M., & Gan, H. (n.d.). Viral and Non-Viral Cancer Gene Therapy. In D. Shi (Ed.), The World Scientific Encyclopedia of Nanomedicine and Bioengineering I: Nanotechnology for Translational Medicine: Tissue Engineering, Biological Sensing, Medical Imaging, and Therapeutics, Volume 3 Nanotechnology in Gene Delivery (pp. 1-33). Singapoure: World Scientific.

Yang, H., Zhao, F., Li, Y., Xu, M., Li, L., Wu, C., ... Liu, Y. (2013). VCAM-1-targeted core/shell nanoparticles for selective adhesion and delivery to endothelial cells with lipopolysaccharide-induced inflammation under shear flow and cellular magnetic resonance imaging in vitro. *International Journal of Nanomedicine*, *8*, 1897–1906. PMID:23696701

Yang, L., Liu, M., Huang, K., Ai, X., Li, C., Ma, J., ... Liu, X. (2017). Folate-targeted single-wall metal-organic nanotubes used as multifunctional drug carriers. *Applied Surface Science*, *392*, 189–195. doi:10.1016/j.apsusc.2016.09.030

Yang, P., Gai, S., & Lin, J. (2012). Functionalized mesoporous silica materials for controlled drug delivery. *Chemical Society Reviews*, *41*(9), 3679–3698. doi:10.1039/c2cs15308d PMID:22441299

Yang, P., Quan, Z., Hou, Z., Li, C., Kang, X., Cheng, Z., & Lin, J. (2009). A magnetic, luminescent and mesoporous core–shell structured composite material as drug carrier. *Biomaterials*, *30*(27), 4786–4795. doi:10.1016/j.biomaterials.2009.05.038 PMID:19520428

Yang, P., Quan, Z., Lu, L., Huang, S., & Lin, J. (2008). Luminescence functionalization of mesoporous silica with different morphologies and applications as drug delivery systems. *Biomaterials*, *29*(6), 692–702. doi:10.1016/j.biomaterials.2007.10.019 PMID:17996294

Yang, P., Yang, P., Teng, X., Lin, J., & Huang, L. (2011). A novel luminescent mesoporous silica/apatite composite for controlled drug release. *Journal of Materials Chemistry*, *21*(14), 5505–5510. doi:10.1039/c0jm03878d

Yang, X., & ... . (2012). Anterior reconstruction with nano-hydroxyapatite/polyamide-66 cage after thoracic and lumbar corpectomy. *Orthopedics*, *35*(1), 01477447–20111122. PMID:22229617

Yang, Y., Wang, J. C., Zhang, X., Lu, W. L., & Zhang, Q. (2009). A novel mixed micelle gel with thermo-sensitive property for the local delivery of docetaxel. *Journal of Controlled Release*, *135*(2), 175–182. doi:10.1016/j.jconrel.2009.01.007 PMID:19331864

Yan, J., Su, T., Cheng, F., Cao, J., Zhang, H., & He, B. (2017). Multifunctional nanoparticles self-assembled from polyethylenimine-based graft polymers as efficient anticancer drug delivery. *Colloids and Surfaces. B, Biointerfaces*, *155*, 118–127. doi:10.1016/j.colsurfb.2017.02.030 PMID:28415029

Yan, Y., Fu, J., Wang, T., & Lu, X. (2017). Controlled release of silyl ether camptothecin from thiol-ene click chemistry-functionalized mesoporous silica nanoparticles. *Acta Biomaterialia*, *51*, 471–478. doi:10.1016/j.actbio.2017.01.062 PMID:28131940

Yan, Y., Zhang, H., Sun, J., Wang, P., Dong, K., Dong, Y., & Xing, J. (2016). Enhanced transdermal delivery of sinomenine hydrochloride by ethosomes for anti-inflammatory treatment. *Journal of Drug Delivery Science and Technology*, *36*, 201–207. doi:10.1016/j.jddst.2016.10.013

Yao, Feng, & Chen. (2016). External-stimuli responsive systems for cancer theranostic. *Asian Journal of Pharmaceutical Sciences, 11*(5), 585-595.

Yao, H. J., Sun, L., Liu, Y., Jiang, S., Pu, Y., Li, J., & Zhang, Y. (2016). Monodistearoylphosphatidylethanolamine-hyaluronic acid functionalization of single-walled carbon nanotubes for targeting intracellular drug delivery to overcome multidrug resistance of cancer cells. *Carbon*, *96*, 362–376. doi:10.1016/j.carbon.2015.09.037

Yao, X., Chen, X., He, C., Chen, L., & Chen, X. (2015). Dual pH-responsive mesoporous silica nanoparticles for efficient combination of chemotherapy and photodynamic therapy. *Journal of Materials Chemistry. B, Materials for Biology and Medicine*, *3*(23), 4707–4714. doi:10.1039/C5TB00256G

Yasir, M., Gaur, P. K., Puri, D., Shekar, P., & Kumar, S. S. (2017). Solid lipid nanoparticles approach for lymphatic targeting through intraduodenal delivery of quetiapine fumarate. *Current Drug Delivery*, *14*(999), 1. doi:10.2174/1567201814666170525121049 PMID:28545354

Yassin, A. E., Alsarra, I. A., Alanazi, F. K., Al-Mohizea, A. M., Al-Robayan, A. A., & Al-Obeed, O. A. (2010). New targeted-colon delivery system: In vitro and in vivo evaluation using X-ray imaging. *Journal of Drug Targeting*, *18*(1), 59–66. doi:10.3109/10611860903165022 PMID:19653868

Yeh, C.-C., Su, Y.-H., Lin, Y.-J., Chen, P.-J., Shi, C.-S., Chen, C.-N., & Chang, H.-I. (2015). Evaluation of the protective effects of curcuminoid (curcumin and bisdemethoxycurcumin)-loaded liposomes against bone turnover in a cell-based model of osteoarthritis. *Drug Design, Development and Therapy*, *9*, 2285–2300. PMID:25945040

Yeung, T., Gilbert, G. E., Shi, J., Silvius, J., Kapus, A., & Grinstein, S. (2008). Membrane phosphatidylserine regulates surface charge and protein localization. *Science*, *319*(5860), 210–213. doi:10.1126cience.1152066 PMID:18187657

Yin, H., & Bae, Y. H. (2009). Physicochemical aspects of doxorubicin-loaded pH-sensitive polymeric micelle formulations from a mixture of poly (L-histidine)-b-poly (L-lactide)-b-poly (ethylene glycol). *European Journal of Pharmaceutics and Biopharmaceutics*, *71*(2), 223–230. doi:10.1016/j.ejpb.2008.08.013 PMID:18782616

Yin, H., Kanasty, R. L., Eltoukhy, A. A., Vegas, A. J., Dorkin, J. R., & Anderson, D. G. (2014). Non-viral vectors for gene-based therapy. *Nature Reviews. Genetics*, *15*(8), 541–555. doi:10.1038/nrg3763 PMID:25022906

Yin, Q., Shen, J., Chen, L., Zhang, Z., Gu, W., & Li, Y. (2012). Overcoming multidrug resistance by co-delivery of Mdr-1 and survivin-targeting RNA with reduction-responsible cationic poly (β-amino esters). *Biomaterials*, *33*(27), 6495–6506. doi:10.1016/j.biomaterials.2012.05.039 PMID:22704597

Yin, T., Cai, H., Liu, J., Cui, B., Wang, L., Yin, L., ... Huo, M. (2016). Biological evaluation of PEG modified nanosuspensions based on human serum albumin for tumor targeted delivery of paclitaxel. *European Journal of Pharmaceutical Sciences*, *83*, 79–87. doi:10.1016/j.ejps.2015.12.019 PMID:26699227

Yi, X., Shi, X., & Gao, H. (2011). Cellular uptake of elastic nanoparticles. *Physical Review Letters*, *107*(9), 098101. doi:10.1103/PhysRevLett.107.098101 PMID:21929271

Yoncheva, K., Popova, M., Szegedi, A., Mihaly, J., Tzankov, B., Lambov, N., ... Valoti, M. (2014). Functionalized mesoporous silica nanoparticles for oral delivery of budesonide. *Journal of Solid State Chemistry*, *211*, 154–161. doi:10.1016/j.jssc.2013.12.020

Yoon, G., Park, J. W., & Yoon, I. S. (2013). Solid lipid nanoparticles (SLNs) and nanostructured lipid carriers (NLCs): Recent advances in drug delivery. *Journal of Pharmaceutical Investigation*, *43*(5), 353–362. doi:10.100740005-013-0087-y

Young, S., Wong, M., Tabata, Y., & Mikos, A. G. (2005). Gelatin as a delivery vehicle for the controlled release of bioactive molecules. *J. Controll. Rel.*, *109*(1-3), 256–274. doi:10.1016/j.jconrel.2005.09.023 PMID:16266768

Yuan, H., Miao, J., Du, Y. Z., You, J., Hu, F. Q., & Zeng, S. (2008). Cellular uptake of solid lipid nanoparticles and cytotoxicity of encapsulated paclitaxel in A549 cancer cells. *International Journal of Pharmaceutics*, *348*(1), 137–145. doi:10.1016/j.ijpharm.2007.07.012 PMID:17714896

Yuan, Q., Han, J., Cong, W., Ge, Y., Ma, D., Dai, Z., ... Bi, L. (2014). Docetaxel-loaded solid lipid nanoparticles suppress breast cancer cells growth with reduced myelosuppression toxicity. *International Journal of Nanomedicine*, *9*, 4829–4846. PMID:25378924

Yu, E., Lo, A., Jiang, L., Petkus, B., Ileri Ercan, N., & Stroeve, P. (2017). Improved controlled release of protein from expanded-pore mesoporous silica nanoparticles modified with co-functionalized poly(n-isopropylacrylamide) and poly(ethylene glycol) (PNIPAM-PEG). *Colloids and Surfaces. B, Biointerfaces*, *149*, 297–300. doi:10.1016/j.colsurfb.2016.10.033 PMID:27776334

Yu, F., Huang, J., Yu, Y., Lu, Y., Chen, Y., Zhang, H., ... Zhong, Y. (2016). Glutathione-responsive multilayer coated gold nanoparticles for targeted gene delivery. *Journal of Biomedical Nanotechnology*, *12*(3), 503–515. doi:10.1166/jbn.2016.2177 PMID:27280248

Yu, J., Zhang, Y., Bomba, H., & Gu, Z. (2016). Stimuli-responsive delivery of therapeutics for diabetes treatment. *Bioengineering & Translational Medicine*, *1*(3), 323–337. doi:10.1002/btm2.10036 PMID:29147685

Yu, M., Niu, Y., Zhang, J., Zhang, H., Yang, Y., Taran, E., ... Yu, C. (2016). Size-dependent gene delivery of amine-modified silica nanoparticles. *Nano Research*, *9*(2), 291–305. doi:10.100712274-015-0909-5

Yun, L., Xingwei, D., Jinghua, L., Zhong, L., Yan, H., Junjie, L., ... Kaiyong, C. (2015). Enzyme responsive drug delivery system based on mesoporous silica nanoparticles for tumor therapy in vivo. *Nanotechnology*, *26*(14), 145102. doi:10.1088/0957-4484/26/14/145102 PMID:25789511

Yu, X., Du, L., Li, Y., Fu, G., & Jin, Y. (2015). Improved anti-melanoma effect of a transdermal mitoxantrone ethosome gel. *Biomedicine and Pharmacotherapy*, *73*, 6–11. doi:10.1016/j.biopha.2015.05.002 PMID:26211575

Yu, Y. H., Kim, E., Park, D. E., Shim, G., Lee, S., Kim, Y. B., ... Oh, Y.-K. (2012). Cationic solid lipid nanoparticles for co-delivery of paclitaxel and siRNA. *European Journal of Pharmaceutics and Biopharmaceutics*, *80*(2), 268–273. doi:10.1016/j.ejpb.2011.11.002 PMID:22108492

Zackova Suchanova, J., Neburkova, J., Spanielova, H., Forstova, J., & Cigler, P. (2017). Retargeting Polyomavirus-Like Particles to Cancer Cells by Chemical Modification of Capsid Surface. *Bioconjugate Chemistry*, *28*(2), 307–313. doi:10.1021/acs.bioconjchem.6b00622 PMID:28035816

Zaitu, S., Miwa, Y., & Taga, T. (1995). A 2: 1 molecular complex of theophylline and 5-fluorouracil as the monohydrate. *Acta Crystallographica. Section C, Structural Chemistry*, *51*(9), 1857–1859. doi:10.1107/S0108270195003295

Zakerzadeh, E., Alizadeh, E., Kafil, H. S., Hassanzadeh, A. M., Salehi, R., & Mahkam, M. (2016). Novel antibacterial polymeric nanocomposite for smart co-delivery of anticancer drugs. Artifical Cells [volume?]. *NanoBiotechnology*, *3*, 1–12. doi:10.1080/21691401.2016.1260576

Zanotto-Filho, A., Coradini, K., Braganhol, E., Schröder, R., De Oliveira, C. M., Simões-Pires, A., ... Beck, R. C. R. (2013). Curcumin-loaded lipid-core nanocapsules as a strategy to improve pharmacological efficacy of curcumin in glioma treatment. *European Journal of Pharmaceutics and Biopharmaceutics*, *83*(2), 156–167. doi:10.1016/j.ejpb.2012.10.019 PMID:23219677

Zare, Y., Rhee, K. Y., & Hui, D. (2017). Influences of nanoparticles aggregation/agglomeration on the interfacial/interphase and tensile properties of nanocomposites. *Composites. Part B, Engineering*, *122*, 41–46. doi:10.1016/j.compositesb.2017.04.008

Zarif, L., Graybill, J. R., Perlin, D., & Manninoa, R. J. (2000). *Cochleates: New lipid-based drug delivery system.* Academic Press.

Žegarac, M., Lekšić, E., Šket, P., Plavec, J., Bogdanović, M. D., Bučar, D.-K., ... Meštrović, E. (2014). A sildenafil cocrystal based on acetylsalicylic acid exhibits an enhanced intrinsic dissolution rate. *CrystEngComm*, *16*(1), 32–35. doi:10.1039/C3CE42013B

Zeiderman, M. R., Morgan, D. E., Christein, J. D., Grizzle, W. E., McMasters, K. M., & McNally, L. R. (2016). Acidic pH-targeted chitosan capped mesoporous silica coated gold nanorods facilitate detection of pancreatic tumors via multispectral optoacoustic tomography. *ACS Biomater Sci Eng*, *2*(7), 1108–1120. doi:10.1021/acsbiomaterials.6b00111 PMID:28626793

Zha, M. X., & Zhu, B. J. (2016). The research and applications of quantum dots as nano-carriers for targeted drug delivery and cancer therapy. *Nanoscale Research Letters*, *11*(207), 1–9. PMID:26729219

Zhang, J. (2015). Unfolding grain size effects in barium titanate ferroelectric ceramics. *Nature Communications, 5*(9953).

Zhang, L., & Zhang, L. (2010). Lipid–Polymer Hybrid Nanoparticles: Synthesis, Characterization and Applications. *Nano Life, 1*(1-2), 163–73. Available from: http://www.worldscientific.com/doi/abs/10.1142/S179398441000016X

Zhang, L., Chan, J.M., Gu, F.X., Rhee, J., Wang, A.Z., & Radovic-moreno, A.F. (2008). Self-Assembled Lipid Polymer Hybrid Nanoparticles: A Robust Drug Delivery Platform. *ACS Nano, 2*(8), 1696–702.

Zhang, T. (2014). Low - Loss Composite NiCuZnCo – BaTiO3 with Matched Permeability and Permittivity in High Frequency Range. *IEEE Transactions on Magnetic, 50*(11).

Zhang, T. (2014). Low - Loss Composite NiCuZnCo – BaTiO3 With Matched Permeability and Permittivity in High Frequency Range. *IEEE Transactions on Magnetics, 50*(11).

Zhang, B., Chen, Q., Tang, H., Xie, Q., Ma, M., Tan, L., ... Yao, S. (2010). Characterization of and biomolecule immobilization on the biocompatible multi-walled carbon nanotubes generated by functionalization with polyamidoamine dendrimers. *Colloids and Surfaces. B, Biointerfaces*, *80*(1), 18–25. doi:10.1016/j.colsurfb.2010.05.023 PMID:20542415

Zhang, B., Luo, Z., Liu, J., Ding, X., Li, J., & Cai, K. (2014). Cytochrome c end-capped mesoporous silica nanoparticles as redox-responsive drug delivery vehicles for liver tumor-targeted triplex therapy in vitro and in vivo. *Journal of Controlled Release*, *192*, 192–201. doi:10.1016/j.jconrel.2014.06.037 PMID:25034575

Zhang, J., Sun, Y., Tian, B., Li, K., Wang, L., Liang, Y., & Han, J. (2016). Multifunctional mesoporous silica nanoparticles modified with tumor-shedable hyaluronic acid as carriers for doxorubicin. *Colloids and Surfaces. B, Biointerfaces*, *144*, 293–302. doi:10.1016/j.colsurfb.2016.04.015 PMID:27107383

Zhang, J., Yuan, Z. F., Wang, Y., Chen, W. H., Luo, G. F., Cheng, S. X., ... Zhang, X. Z. (2013). Multifunctional Envelope-Type Mesoporous Silica Nanoparticles for Tumor-Triggered Targeting Drug Delivery. *Journal of the American Chemical Society*, *135*(13), 5068–5073. doi:10.1021/ja312004m PMID:23464924

Zhang, M., Liu, J., Kuang, Y., Li, Q., Zheng, D. W., Song, Q., ... Jiang, B. (2017). Ingenious pH-sensitive dextran/mesoporous silica nanoparticles based drug delivery systems for controlled intracellular drug release. *International Journal of Biological Macromolecules*, *98*, 691–700. doi:10.1016/j.ijbiomac.2017.01.136 PMID:28174081

Zhang, M., Xu, C., Wen, L., Han, M. K., Xiao, B., Zhou, J., ... Merlin, D. (2016). A Hyaluronidase-Responsive Nanoparticle-Based Drug Delivery System for Targeting Colon Cancer Cells. *Cancer Research*, *76*(24), 7208–7218. doi:10.1158/0008-5472.CAN-16-1681 PMID:27742685

Zhang, Q., Li, J., Zhang, W., An, Q., Wen, J., Wang, A., ... Chen, S. (2015). Acute and sub-chronic toxicity studies of honokiol microemulsion. *Regulatory Toxicology and Pharmacology*, *71*(3), 428–436. doi:10.1016/j.yrtph.2014.11.007 PMID:25481277

Zhang, Q., Liu, F., Nguyen, K. T., Ma, X., Wang, X., Xing, B., & Zhao, Y. (2012). Multifunctional Mesoporous Silica Nanoparticles for Cancer-Targeted and Controlled Drug Delivery. *Advanced Functional Materials*, *22*(24), 5144–5156. doi:10.1002/adfm.201201316

Zhang, Q., Ye, X., Wang, L., Peng, B., Zhang, Y., Bao, J., ... Chen, S. (2016). Embryo-fetal development toxicity of honokiol microemulsion intravenously administered to pregnant rats. *Regulatory Toxicology and Pharmacology*, *74*, 117–122. doi:10.1016/j.yrtph.2015.11.012 PMID:26619782

Zhang, Q., Zhao, H., Li, D., Liu, L., & Du, S. (2017). A surface-grafted ligand functionalization strategy for coordinate binding of doxorubicin at surface of PEGylated mesoporous silica nanoparticles: Toward pH-responsive drug delivery. *Colloids and Surfaces. B, Biointerfaces*, *149*, 138–145. doi:10.1016/j.colsurfb.2016.10.018 PMID:27750088

Zhang, R. X., Ahmed, T., Li, L. Y., Li, J., Abbasi, A. Z., & Wu, X. Y. (2017). Design of nanocarriers for nanoscale drug delivery to enhance cancer treatment using hybrid polymer and lipid building blocks. *Nanoscale*, *9*(4), 1334–1355. doi:10.1039/C6NR08486A PMID:27973629

Zhang, R. X., Cai, P., Zhang, T., Chen, K., Li, J., & Cheng, J. (2016). Polymer-lipid hybrid nanoparticles synchronize pharmacokinetics of co-encapsulated doxorubicin-mitomycin C and enable their spatiotemporal co-delivery and local bioavailability in breast tumor. *Nanomedicine Nanotechnology, Biol Med*, *12*(5), 1279–1290. doi:10.1016/j.nano.2015.12.383

Zhang, R. X., Wong, H. L., Xue, H. Y., Eoh, J. Y., & Wu, X. Y. (2016). Nanomedicine of synergistic drug combinations for cancer therapy??? Strategies and perspectives. *J Control Release*, *240*, 489–503. doi:10.1016/j.jconrel.2016.06.012 PMID:27287891

Zhang, S., Xu, Y., Wang, B., Qiao, W., Liu, D., & Li, Z. (2004). Cationic compounds used in lipoplexes and polyplexes for gene delivery. *Journal of Controlled Release*, *100*(2), 165–180. doi:10.1016/j.jconrel.2004.08.019 PMID:15544865

Zhang, X., Hui, Z., Wan, D., Huang, H., Huang, J., Yuan, H., & Yu, J. (2010). Alginate microsphere filled with carbon nanotube as drug carrier. *International Journal of Biological Macromolecules*, *47*(3), 389–395. doi:10.1016/j.ijbiomac.2010.06.003 PMID:20600269

Zhang, X., Li, F., Guo, S., Chen, X., Wang, X., Li, J., & Gan, Y. (2014). Biofunctionalized polymer-lipid supported mesoporous silica nanoparticles for release of chemotherapeutics in multidrug resistant cancer cells. *Biomaterials*, *35*(11), 3650–3665. doi:10.1016/j.biomaterials.2014.01.013 PMID:24462359

Zhang, X.-X., McIntosh, T. J., & Grinstaff, M. W. (2012). Functional lipids and lipoplexes for improved gene delivery. *Biochimie*, *94*(1), 42–58. doi:10.1016/j.biochi.2011.05.005 PMID:21621581

Zhang, X., Yang, P., Dai, Y., Ma, P. A., Li, X., Cheng, Z., ... Lin, J. (2013). Multifunctional up-converting nanocomposites with smart polymer brushes gated mesopores for cell imaging and thermo/pH dual-responsive drug controlled release. *Advanced Functional Materials*, *23*(33), 4067–4078. doi:10.1002/adfm.201300136

Zhang, Y. T., Huang, Z. B., Zhang, S. J., Zhao, J. H., Wang, Z., Liu, Y., & Feng, N. P. (2012). In vitro cellular uptake of evodiamine and rutaecarpine using a microemulsion. *International Journal of Nanomedicine*, *7*, 2465–2472. PMID:22679361

Zhang, Y., Ang, C. Y., Li, M., Tan, S. Y., Qu, Q., Luo, Z., & Zhao, Y. (2015a). Polymer-Coated Hollow Mesoporous Silica Nanoparticles for Triple-Responsive Drug Delivery. *ACS Applied Materials & Interfaces*, *7*(32), 18179–18187. doi:10.1021/acsami.5b05893 PMID:26221866

Zhang, Y., Guo, J., Zhang, X. L., Li, D. P., Zhang, T. T., Gao, F. F., ... Sheng, X. G. (2015b). Antibody fragment-armed mesoporous silica nanoparticles for the targeted delivery of bevacizumab in ovarian cancer cells. *International Journal of Pharmaceutics*, *496*(2), 1026–1033. doi:10.1016/j.ijpharm.2015.10.080 PMID:26541303

Zhang, Y., He, L., Yue, S., Huang, Q., Zhang, Y., & Yang, J. (2017). Characterization and evaluation of a self-microemulsifying drug delivery system containing tectorigenin, an isoflavone with low aqueous solubility and poor permeability. *Drug Delivery*, *24*(1), 632–640. doi:10.1080/10717544.2017.1284946 PMID:28283000

Zhang, Y., Satterlee, A., & Huang, L. (2012). *In vivo* gene delivery by nonviral vectors: Overcoming hurdles? *Molecular Therapy*, *20*(7), 1298–1304. doi:10.1038/mt.2012.79 PMID:22525514

Zhang, Y., Zhi, Z., Jiang, T., Zhang, J., Wang, Z., & Wang, S. (2010). Spherical mesoporous silica nanoparticles for loading and release of the poorly water-soluble drug telmisartan. *Journal of Controlled Release*, *145*(3), 257–263. doi:10.1016/j.jconrel.2010.04.029 PMID:20450945

Zhang, Z., Balogh, D., Wang, F., Sung, S. Y., Nechushtai, R., & Willner, I. (2013). Biocatalytic Release of an Anticancer Drug from Nucleic-Acids-Capped Mesoporous SiO2 Using DNA or Molecular Biomarkers as Triggering Stimuli. *ACS Nano*, *7*(10), 8455–8468. doi:10.1021/nn403772j PMID:23985013

Zhan, J., Ma, Z., Wang, D., Li, X., Li, X., Le, L., ... Yang, F. (2017). Li, x., Le, li., Hu, P., She, L., & Yan, F.(2017) Magnetic and pH dual-responsive mesoporous silica nanocomposites for effective and low-toxic photodynamic therapy. *International Journal of Nanomedicine*, *12*, 2733–2748. doi:10.2147/IJN.S127528 PMID:28442903

Zhan, Z., Zheng, L., Pan, Y., Sun, G., & Li, L. (2012). Self-powered, visible-light photodetector based on thermally reduced graphene oxide–ZnO (rGO–ZnO) hybrid nanostructure. *Journal of Materials Chemistry*, *22*(6), 2589–2595. doi:10.1039/C1JM13920G

Zhao, Y.Z., Dai, D.D., Lu, C.T., Chen, L.J., Lin, M., … Shen, X.T. (2013). Epirubicin loaded with propyleneglycol liposomes significantly overcomes multidrug resistance in breast cancer. *Cancer Lett*, *330*, 74–83.

Zhao, Z., Meng, H., Wang, N., Donovan, M. J., Fu, T., You, M., . . . Tan, W. A. (2013). Controlled-release nanocarrier with extracellular pH value driven tumor targeting and translocation for drug delivery. Angew. Chem. Int., 52, 7487-7491.

Zhao, D., Feng, J., Huo, Q., Melosh, N., Fredrickson, G. H., Chmelka, B. F., & Stucky, G. D. (1998). Triblock Copolymer Syntheses of Mesoporous Silica with Periodic 50 to 300 Angstrom Pores. *Science*, *279*(5350), 548–552. doi:10.1126cience.279.5350.548 PMID:9438845

Zhao, H., Chao, Y., Liu, J., Huang, J., Pan, J., Guo, W., ... Liu, Z. (2016). Polydopamine Coated Single-Walled Carbon Nanotubes as a Versatile Platform with Radionuclide Labeling for Multimodal Tumor Imaging and Therapy. *Theranostics*, *6*(11), 1833–1843. doi:10.7150/thno.16047 PMID:27570554

Zhao, J., He, Z., Li, B., Cheng, T., & Liu, G. (2017). AND logic-like pH- and light-dual controlled drug delivery by surface modified mesoporous silica nanoparticles. *Materials Science and Engineering C*, *73*, 1–7. doi:10.1016/j.msec.2016.12.056 PMID:28183586

Zhao, L., Seth, A., Wibowo, N., Zhao, C. X., Mitter, N., Yu, C., & Middelberg, A. P. J. (2014). Nanoparticle vaccines. *Vaccine*, *32*(3), 327–337. doi:10.1016/j.vaccine.2013.11.069 PMID:24295808

Zhao, L., Wei, Y., Huang, Y., He, B., Zhou, Y., & Fu, J. (2013). Nanoemulsion improves the oral bioavailability of baicalin in rats: In vitro and in vivo evaluation. *International Journal of Nanomedicine*, *8*, 3769–3779. doi:10.2147/IJN.S51578 PMID:24124365

Zhao, L., Zhu, J., Cheng, Y., Xiong, Z., Tang, Y., Guo, L., ... Zhao, J. (2015). Chlorotoxin-Conjugated Multifunctional Dendrimers Labeled with Radionuclide 131I for Single Photon Emission Computed Tomography Imaging and Radiotherapy of Gliomas. *ACS Applied Materials & Interfaces*, *7*(35), 19798–19808. doi:10.1021/acsami.5b05836 PMID:26291070

Zhao, Q., Liu, J., Zhu, W., Sun, C., Di, D., Zhang, Y., ... Wang, S. (2015). Dual-stimuli responsive hyaluronic acid-conjugated mesoporous silica for targeted delivery to CD44-overexpressing cancer cells. *Acta Biomaterialia*, *23*, 147–156. doi:10.1016/j.actbio.2015.05.010 PMID:25985912

Zhao, Q., Wang, L., Cheng, R., Mao, L., Arnold, R. D., Howerth, E. W., ... Platt, S. (2012). Magnetic nanoparticle-based hyperthermia for head & neck cancer in mouse models. *Theranostics*, *2*(1), 113–121. doi:10.7150/thno.3854 PMID:22287991

Zhao, Q., Wang, S., Yang, Y., Li, X., Di, D., Zhang, C., ... Wang, S. (2017). Hyaluronic acid and carbon dots-gated hollow mesoporous silica for redox and enzyme-triggered targeted drug delivery and bioimaging. *Materials Science and Engineering C*, *78*, 475–484. doi:10.1016/j.msec.2017.04.059 PMID:28576012

Zhao, W., Zhang, H., He, Q., Li, Y., Gu, J., Li, L., ... Shi, J. (2011). A glucose-responsive controlled release of insulin system based on enzyme multilayers-coated mesoporous silica particles. *Chemical Communications*, *47*(33), 9459–9461. doi:10.1039/c1cc12740c PMID:21779606

Zhao, X., Li, H., & Lee, R. J. (2008). Targeted drug delivery via folate receptors. *Expert Opinion on Drug Delivery*, *5*(3), 309–319. doi:10.1517/17425247.5.3.309 PMID:18318652

Zhao, Y., Chang, Y. X., Hu, X., Liu, C. Y., Quan, L. H., & Liao, Y. H. (2016). Solid Lipid Nanoparticles for Sustained Pulmonary Delivery of Yuxingcao Essential Oil: Preparation, Characterization and in Vivo Evaluation. *International Journal of Pharmaceutics*, *516*(1-2), 364–371. doi:10.1016/j.ijpharm.2016.11.046 PMID:27884712

Zhao, Y., & Huang, L. (2014). Lipid nanoparticles for gene delivery. *Advances in Genetics*, *88*, 13–36. doi:10.1016/B978-0-12-800148-6.00002-X PMID:25409602

Zhao, Y., Sun, X., Zhang, G., Trewyn, B. G., Slowing, I. I., & Lin, V. S. Y. (2011). Interaction of Mesoporous Silica Nanoparticles with Human Red Blood Cell Membranes: Size and Surface Effects. *ACS Nano*, *5*(2), 1366–1375. doi:10.1021/nn103077k PMID:21294526

Zhao, Y., Trewyn, B. G., Slowing, I. I., & Lin, V. S. Y. (2009). Mesoporous Silica Nanoparticle-Based Double Drug Delivery System for Glucose-Responsive Controlled Release of Insulin and Cyclic AMP. *Journal of the American Chemical Society*, *131*(24), 8398–8400. doi:10.1021/ja901831u PMID:19476380

Zhao, Z. X., Huang, Y. Z., Shi, S. G., Tang, S. H., Li, D. H., & Chen, X. L. (2014). Cancer therapy improvement with mesoporous silica nanoparticles combining photodynamic and photothermal therapy. *Nanotechnology*, *25*(28), 285701. doi:10.1088/0957-4484/25/28/285701 PMID:24971525

Zheng, J., Tian, X., Sun, Y., Lu, D., & Yang, W. (2013). pH-sensitive poly(glutamic acid) grafted mesoporous silica nanoparticles for drug delivery. *International Journal of Pharmaceutics*, *450*(1-2), 296–303. doi:10.1016/j.ijpharm.2013.04.014 PMID:23598077

Zheng, Q., Lin, T., Wu, H., Guo, L., Ye, P., Hao, Y., ... Chen, G. (2014). Mussel-inspired polydopamine coated mesoporous silica nanoparticles as pH-sensitive nanocarriers for controlled release. *International Journal of Pharmaceutics*, *463*(1), 22–26. doi:10.1016/j.ijpharm.2013.12.045 PMID:24393764

Zheng, X. F., Lian, Q., Yang, H., & Wang, X. (2016). Surface Molecularly Imprinted Polymer of Chitosan Grafted Poly(methyl methacrylate) for 5-Fluorouracil and Controlled Release. *Scientific Reports*, *6*(1), 21409. doi:10.1038rep21409 PMID:26892676

Zheng, Y., Yu, B., Weecharangsan, W., Piao, L., Darby, M., Mao, Y., & … . (2010). Transferrin-conjugated lipid-coated PLGA nanoparticles for targeted delivery of aromatase inhibitor 7α-APTADD to breast cancer cells. *Int J Pharm*, *390*(2), 234–241. doi:10.1016/j.ijpharm.2010.02.008 PMID:20156537

Zhong, Q., Chinta, D., Pamujula, S., Wang, H., Yao, X., Mandal, T. K., & Luftig, R. B. (2010). Optimization of DNA delivery by three classes of hybrid nanoparticle/DNA complexes. *Journal of Nanobiotechnology*, *8*(1), 6. doi:10.1186/1477-3155-8-6 PMID:20181278

Zhou, G., Wang, D. W., Li, F., Zhang, L., Li, N., Wu, Z. S., ... Cheng, H. M. (2010). Graphene-Wrapped Fe_3O_4 Anode Material with Improved Reversible Capacity and Cyclic Stability for Lithium Ion Batteries Chem. *Mater.*, *22*, 5306–5313.

Zhou, H., Lee, J., Park, T. J., Lee, S. J., Park, J. Y., & Lee, J. (2012). Ultrasensitive DNA monitoring by Au–Fe 3 O 4 nanocomplex. *Sensors and Actuators. B, Chemical*, *163*(1), 224–232. doi:10.1016/j.snb.2012.01.040

Zhou, M., Peng, Z., Liao, S., Li, P., & Li, S. (2014). Design of microencapsulated carbon nanotube-based microspheres and its application in colon targeted drug delivery. *Drug Delivery*, *21*(2), 101–109. doi:10.3109/10717544.2013.834413 PMID:24044613

Zhou, X., Chen, L., Nie, W., Wang, W., Qin, M., Mo, X., ... He, C. (2016). Dual-Responsive Mesoporous Silica Nanoparticles Mediated Codelivery of Doxorubicin and Bcl-2 SiRNA for Targeted Treatment of Breast Cancer. *The Journal of Physical Chemistry C*, *120*(39), 22375–22387. doi:10.1021/acs.jpcc.6b06759

Zhu, C. L., Wang, X. W., Lin, Z. Z., Xie, Z. H., & Wang, X. R. (2014). Cell microenvironment stimuli-responsive controlled-release delivery systems based on mesoporous silica nanoparticles. *Journal of Food and Drug Analysis*, *22*(1), 18–28. doi:10.1016/j.jfda.2014.01.002 PMID:24673901

Zhu, D., Liu, F., Ma, L., Liu, D., & Wang, Z. (2013). Nanoparticle-based systems for t1-weighted magnetic resonance imaging contrast agents. *International Journal of Molecular Sciences*, *14*(5), 10591–10607. doi:10.3390/ijms140510591 PMID:23698781

Zhu, M., Nie, G., Meng, H., Xia, T., Nel, A., & Zhao, Y. (2012). Physicochemical properties determine nanomaterial cellular uptake, transport, and fate. *Accounts of Chemical Research*, *46*(3), 622–631. doi:10.1021/ar300031y PMID:22891796

Zou, H., Wu, S., & Shen, J. (2008). Polymer/silica nanocomposites: Preparation, characterization, properties, and applications. *Chemical Reviews*, *108*(9), 3893–3957. doi:10.1021/cr068035q PMID:18720998

Zou, L., Wang, H., He, B., Zeng, L., Tan, T., Cao, H., ... Li, Y. (2016). Current approaches of photothermal therapy in treating cancer metastasis with nanotherapeutics. *Theranostics*, *6*(6), 762–772. doi:10.7150/thno.14988 PMID:27162548

Zuhorn, I. S., Kalicharan, R., & Hoekstra, D. (2002). Lipoplex-mediated transfection of mammalian cells occurs through the cholesterol-dependent clathrin-mediated pathway of endocytosis. *The Journal of Biological Chemistry*, *277*(20), 18021–18028. doi:10.1074/jbc.M111257200 PMID:11875062

About the Contributors

Md Abul Barkat has received his PhD in Pharmaceutical Sciences (Pharmaceutics) from Integral University Lucknow, India, in the year 2017. He has completed his Masters in Pharmaceutical Sciences from Hamdard University, New Delhi, India. He has more than 6 years of research experience in the field of Pharmaceutics. His major areas of research interest include herbal and silver based development and characterization of diverse nanostructured systems, controlled release drug delivery systems, bioenhanced drug delivery systems, nanomaterials and nanocomposites. Till date he has authored more than 14 publications in various peer-reviewed journals, 3 book chapters, 2 books and 1 Indian patent application to his credit. Dr Barkat has also participated and presented his research work at conferences in India, Canada, and Spain.

Sarwar Beg has over 7 years of research experience in the field of pharmaceutics, especially systematic development and characterization of diverse nanostructured drug delivery systems, controlled release drug delivery systems, bioenhanced drug delivery systems, nanomaterials and nanocomposites employing Quality by Design and Design of Experiments approaches. Currently, he working as the Research Scientist at Jubilant Generics Limited, Noida, U.P., India. Till date he has authored over 110 publications in various high impact peer-reviewed journals, 25 book chapters, 7 books and 3 Indian patent applications to his credit. He is also serving as an Editorial Board Member of the journal "Current Nanomedicine" and "Nanotech Research Letters", besides "JSM-Bioavailability and Bioequivalence" Journal. Overall, he has earned highly impressive published and cited record (Google Scholar H-Index: 18). Dr Beg has also participated and presented his research work at over ten conferences in India, USA, Canada, and bagged several best paper awards and young scientist awards to his credit.

* * *

Mohd Aleem had completed his masters in chemistry from JamiaMilliaIslamia, Delhi, India. Currently working as a research intern at Institute of Nuclear Medicine and Allied Sciences. Mr. Aleem has research interest on the targeted drug delivery systems.

Gülay Büyükköroğlu has completed her Ph.D at 2005 from Anadolu University and postdoctoral studies from University of London The School of Pharmacy on transcutaneous DNA vaccination at 2009. She is head of Pharmaceutical Biotechnology at Anadolu University Faculty of Pharmacy. She is working on gene delivery systems such as cancer treatment with siRNA loaded albumin based and lipidic carrier systems and DNA vaccination for pulmonary, and specific antibodies conjugated drug delivery systems for targeting therapy.

Rahul Chavan was born in Ahmedpur, India. He obtained his Bachelor of Pharmacy degree from Sant Gadge Baba University, Amravati (India). After, he joined National Institute of Pharmaceutical Education and Research (NIPER), S.A.S. Nagar where he completed his master's in pharmaceutics subject under the guidance of Dr. Arvind K Bansal. Currently he is a PhD student at NIPER- Hyderabad, supervised by Dr. Nalini Shastri. His current research aims toward development of supersaturated drug delivery system, with particular emphasis on screening of polymers for precipitation inhibition, nucleation and crystal growth. His broad research interests include crystal engineering, preformulation, formulations, developing oral dosage forms and drug delivery.

Dimple Sethi Chopra is presently working as Senior Assistant Professor (Pharmaceutics) in Department of Pharmaceutical Sciences and Drug Research, Punjabi University, Patiala. Her present areas of interest are molecular nanotechnology, targeted drug delivery, nanobiotechnology and nanomedicine. She has expertise in teaching wide variety of subjects like mathematics, statistics, computer applications, cosmeticology, physical pharmacy, dispensing pharmacy, unit operations, advanced pharmacokinetics and biopharmaceutics at undergraduate and postgraduate level. She has supervised 17 M.Pharm students for their thesis work and presently 2 Ph.D students are enrolled under her. Her research interest includes exploring different types of nanoparticles for treatment of dementia related to various neurodegenerative disorders like Alzheimer's disease. She is also actively engaged in developing nanocarrier systems for treatment of rheumatoid arthritis and osteoarthritis. She has also worked on other particulate systems like microspheres and niosomes for development of controlled drug delivery systems for oral as well as topical use. She has published several research papers in national and international journals of repute. She has presented her work at several national and international conferences. She won the best presentation award at National Seminar on current trends and Future challenges in Pharmaceutics held at UIPS, PU, Chandigarh. She is an invited manuscript reviewer of many international journals like Drug Discovery today, Journal of Nanoparticle Research, drug delivery, seizure, Open Access Rheumatology: Research and Reviews, International Journal of Nanomedicine, Drug Design, Development and Therapy. She is a member of American Nano Society. She has recently been granted two Indian Patents on Brain Permeable Nanoparticles. She has successfully published four chapters with publishing houses like INTECH OPEN, Studium Press LLC, USA, McGraw Hill Education (India) Private Limited, New Delhi. All the book chapters are on nanoparticles. The chapter with INTECH OPEN has reached 3000 downloads.

Preshita Desai has completed her Ph.D. (Tech.) Degree in Pharmaceutical Sciences (Pharmaceutics) as an INSPIRE Fellow and UKIERI Visiting Fellow (UK-India Education and Research Initiative) from Institute of Chemical Technology, India. She is a passionate researcher and formulation scientist with over a decade of experience in Pharmaceutical and biopharmaceutical sector with specialized in 'nanotechnology based targeted delivery systems'. Her research background includes Quality by Design (QbD) assisted strategic designing, development, optimization, scale up and characterization of novel pharmaceutical formulations for targeted nano drug delivery and enhanced bioavailability of therapeutic actives. Briefly, she has worked on design (Computer aided design), synthesis of novel bioconjugates (patent filed) and formulation thereof to achieve active targeted nanodelivery system for enhanced delivery of drugs across the blood brain barrier via various routes of delivery. Her area of research and expertise also include exploring hot melt extrusion, high pressure homogenizer and Microfluidiser technology to achieve bioenhancement of poorly bioavailable BCS class II and IV drugs by developing nanoformulations and hydrophilic matrices upon oral administration. She is an expert in in vitro cell culture models, imaging studies and in vivo preclinical studies in rodent models. Till date, she has filed 2 patent applications and have published 6 peer reviewed articles in international journals. She has been rewarded with over 15 National and International Awards for paper presentations. She holds a teaching experience of over 3 years to undergraduate students. Also, she has authored 5 chapters in the book entitled, 'Pharmaceutical Product Development: Insights into Pharmaceutical Processes, Management and Regulatory Affairs' by CRC press (2016). With this diverse academic and research experience of over a decade, she is interested in continuing her translational research especially in the pertinent areas of neural ailments and cancer therapeutics.

Vivek Dhawan has completed his Masters Degree in Pharmaceutics from Bombay College of Pharmacy, Mumbai and is currently working as Assistant Professor at Shobhaben Pratapbhai Patel School of Pharmacy and Technology Management, SVKM's NMIMS deemed-to-be University. His research interests include lipid based nano drug delivery systems for targeted therapy and augmentation of bioavailability. He has authored 10 publications in the field of lipid based drug delivery and co-authored one book chapter on in vitro release methodology of novel drug delivery systems.

A. R. Fernandes is a PhD student and researcher in the pharmaceutical technology department of Faculty of Pharmacy of University of Coimbra.

Clara Fernandes is currently working as Assistant Professor in Department of Pharmacognosy at Shobhaben Pratapbhai Patel School of Pharmacy and Technology Management, SVKM's NMIMS deemed-to-be University. She obtained her Ph. D (Tech.) degree in Pharmaceutics from Institute of Chemical Technology in 2013. She has authored 3 research papers, 1 book chapter, and 3 review articles till date. She has filed 3 Indian patents in the area of innovative drug delivery. Her research interests include designing innovative strategies to tackle infections, biofilms, cancer, and autoimmune disorders. Further, her research includes exploring indigenous polysaccharides for wound healing, drug delivery and water purification.

J. Dias Ferreira received his MSc in Pharmaceutical Sciences from Faculty of Pharmacy, University of Coimbra, in 2017. He has work experience in the fields of Pharmaceutical Chemistry - steroid synthesis for breast and prostatic cancer purposes - and Pharmaceuticals, on nanoformulations with multiple purposes. During the last two years of his degree he also worked with new photosensitizer molecules in Photodynamic Therapy applied to melanoma treatment, which culminated on his master thesis. Currently, he holds a research fellowship at the Pharmaceutical Technology Department of the same faculty under the supervision of Professor Eliana B. Souto.

Laxmikant Gautam is pursuing his Ph.D. under the supervision of Prof. S. P. Vyas at Drug Delivery Research Laboratory, Department of Pharmaceutical Sciences, Dr. H.S. Gour University, Sagar (MP) INDIA. He is currently working on the targeted drug delivery and cancer immunotherapy.

Anamika Jain is pursuing her Ph.D. under the supervision of Prof. S. P. Vyas at Drug Delivery Research Laboratory, Department of Pharmaceutical Sciences, Dr. H.S. Gour University, Sagar (MP) INDIA. She is currently working on the targeted drug delivery system(s).

Ankit Jain, with a breakthrough out of his diligence, cracked GATE-2008 (99.34 percentile). He completed his B. Pharm. (70%, First division), M. Pharm. (Pharmaceutics, 8.26 CGPA with A+ Grade) and PhD from Depart. Pharm. Sci., Dr. H. S. Gour Central University, Sagar (M.P.), India. He is a recipient of valuable scholarships (JRF-UGC, UGC-RFSMS and CSIR-SRF) and rewards (SASS and YJA). He has number of best paper awards (more than 10) in national and international level seminars to his credit. He has published more than 45 international high repute publications (total impact factor above 90) including book chapters. He has been invited to present his research work at ESGO-2013 (Liverpool, UK) and Cancer Science and Therapy-2014 (Chicago, USA) with travel grant supports from DST (New Delhi) and ICMR (New Delhi), respectively. Recently, he has received "Young Scientist Award" in 32nd M.P. Young Scientists Congress – 2017 (10-11 March), Bhopal (M.P.). Currently, he is working as an Assistant Professor in Pharmaceutics at Institute of Pharmaceutical Research, GLA University, Mathura (U.P.), India. His area of research is exploration of smart tactics for targeting cancer using "In/On" fabricated nanocarriers.

Sanjay K. Jain has obtained B. Pharm. (1981) and M. Pharm. (1983) in Pharmaceutics both from Dr. Harisingh Gour University Sagar (MP) and completed his Doctoral Degree from the same University in 1992. Currently, he is a professor in Pharmaceutics in the Department of Pharmaceutical Sciences, Dr. Harisingh Gour Central University, Sagar (M.P.). He has over 30 years of teaching and research experience. He also possesses 2 years of industrial experience. Dr. Jain has more than 167 research papers published in National and International journals of high impact to his credit. He has written a book published by Elsevier Publisher and 14 Book Chapters in different reference books. Dr. Jain has presented number of research papers in various conferences. He has 1 US, 1 European patent and 1 Indian Patent to his credit. He has been awarded 3 times the IDMA award for best research paper in 1992, 2003 and 2006. He is the recipient of M L Khurana award 2003 and Best Research Poster Award in Pharmaceutical Technology 2005 in 57th IPC. He has been conferred the prestigious 2004 CRS-Capsugel/Pfizer innovation aspects of oral drug delivery and absorption graduate/post-doc award a 31st Annual Meeting and Exposition of Controlled Release Society, USA which represents his potential of academic excellence and scientific venture. Dr Jain has also been conferred the Dr. R. K. Upadhyay National Teachers Excellence Award in the field of Pharmaceutical Sciences Education 2012 by IES Group of Institutions, Bhopal, which was graced by Hon. Shri Ram Naresh YadavJi, H.E. Governor of M.P. Department of Science and Technology, Government of India has found and recorded as Rank 3 (Citation Repository on National Level) under subject scheme of Pharmacology and Pharmaceutics with SCOPUS citation domain during academic year 2015-16. Dr. Jain has completed 6 major research projects funded by UGC and AICTE. His areas of interest include Colon specific and Brain targeted drug delivery. He has 22 PhD awarded under his supervision and his research team consists of 6 PhD scholars working under his able guidance. He is Editor in Chief of the Department of Annual magazine "Pharmakon" and member of editorial board of Critical Reviews™ in Therapeutic Drug Carrier Systems, Begell House, UK. He is also referee of various National and International Journals of repute. Dr. Jain has delivered invited lectures in various conferences on different topics. He is also chairman of University technical committee and member of board of studies of various Universities. He is a life member of many learned societies and organized many training programme and conferences. Recently, he has been appointed as the "Bentham Ambassador" in India.

Sabna Kotta is an Assistant Professor of Pharmaceutics in Buraidah college of Pharmacy and Dentistry, KSA. She received her doctorate in Pharmaceutics from Hamdard University, New Delhi, India and M Pharm in pharmaceutics from Kerala University, India. The topic of her PhD thesis was "Development of an Oral Nanoemulsion of Efavirenz- an Anti-HIV Agent for its Bioavailability Enhancement". She has more than 13 international publications out of her research work and her areas of research interest are nanotechnology based drug delivery and tumor targeted gene delivery.

Viney Lather is working as a Professor & Principal, JCDM College of Pharmacy, Sirsa since August, 2010. Earlier he worked as a Postdoc Fellow at Centro de Quimica da Madeira, University of Madeira, Portugal on a project funded by Faculty of Science and Technology, Portugal for a span of 03 years. His research work focused on the design of scaffolds with specificity amongst their therapeutic targets utilizing computational tools i.e. Rigid and flexible docking, shape comparisons, substrate envelope, molecular mechanics and dynamics, virtual screening, and chemoinformatics (QSAR & QSPR) etc. He achieved his PhD in Computational Chemistry from Maharshi Dayanand University, Rohtak. Dr. Lather was awarded with DST Young Scientist Award under FAST TRACK scheme in 2006. Post PhD he joined as Research Scientist in Jubilant Biosys Ltd., Bangalore for 2 years and worked on Drug Discovery Projects in areas of Kinases like CDKs & CHK-1, Alzheimer's disease targeting BACE enzyme, G-protein coupled receptors. He has received the best scientist award during his work in Jubilant Biosys. He has 04 book chapters, 07 National and 53 International publications to his credit in Journals with an average I. F. of more than 2.5. The h-index for his publications is presently more than 15 and total citations include more than 750. He has presented oral as well as poster presentations in more than 20 National and International Conferences. He received travel grants award from AICTE and DST for his oral presentation in Pharmaceutical World Congress, 2004, Kyoto, Japan and from DST for presenting his work in Pharmatech 2014, Bangkok. His present areas of research include structure based drug design of Matrix Metallo Proteinase Inhibitors as anticancer agents, computational and synthetic approaches for antibacterial drug resistance, Glucokianse activators as anti-diabetic agents, PPAR agonists for metabolic disorders, novel drug delivery particularly using dendrimers and SLNs. He is the reviewer of several peer reviewed journals like Chemical Biology Drug Design, QSAR and Combinatorial Science presently Molecular Informatics, Bioorganic and Medicinal Chemistry, Medicinal Chemistry Research and European Journal of Pharmaceutical Sciences. He has received grants worth Rupees Forty Six Lacs under Research Promotion Schemes, Faculty Development Program and Seminar Schemes of AICTE. He has supervised 26 M.Pharm theses and currently supervising 06 PhD and 06 M. Pharm students. He is a Life member of IPGA, APTI, and IPA.

Anurag Loodagekar was born in Nilanga, India. He obtained his Bachelor of Pharmacy degree from Swami Ramanand Teerth Marathwada University, Nanded (India). After, he joined National Institute of Pharmaceutical Education and Research (NIPER), Hyderabad where he completed his master's in pharmaceutics subject under the guidance of Dr. Naveen Chella. Currently he is a PhD student at NIPER- Hyderabad, supervised by Dr. Nalini Shastri. His current research aims toward development of high energy and rapidly dissolving solid forms to improve pharmaceutical attributes of small molecules, with particular emphasis on screening of small molecules and nutraceuticals for precipitation inhibition, nucleation and crystal growth. His broad research interests include, preformulation, formulations, developing oral dosage forms and drug delivery.

Sanyat Mapara is an undergraduate student pursuing Bachelor of Technology in Pharmaceutical Sciences and Technology at Institute of Chemical Technology. He has over 3 years of research experience and has published one peer reviewed paper. He has received the prestigious ETH Zurich Excellence Scholarship and Opportunity Award. He has been bestowed as the "Best Student of the Year" for consecutive two years by Institute of Chemical Technology. He has been awarded the "Narotam Sekhsaria Excellence Award" which is granted to the excellent student among thirteen engineering colleges in Mumbai. He was also awarded the Bal G. Joshi Endowment Award for Innovation, Creativity and Thinking in 2016. His research interests include advanced drug delivery systems, targeted drug delivery and crystal engineering.

Carlos Martins-Gomes graduated in Biochemistry in 2015 and received his MSc degree in Biochemistry in 2017 from University of Trás-os-Montes and Alto Douro (UTAD), Portugal. He has experience in extraction and analysis of plant extracts composition by liquid and gas chromatography, phytochemicals isolation and study of their bioactivities using cell cultures. Has expertise in cell culture, studies on biochemistry, molecular biology and toxicology (using technics as western-blot, flow-cytometry, immunocytochemistry, and others). Currently, C. Martins-Gomes is a researcher at the Department of Biology and Environment, UTAD, Portugal, as part of the team of an undergoing project. C. Martins-Gomes has already participated in national and international meetings in which presented/authored several communications (proceedings, oral and poster) and is author/co-author of some book chapters that are in press.

Aliva Prity Minz received a B.S. in Biotechnology from Orissa University of agriculture and Technology in year 2013 and M.Sc. from National Institute of Technology, Rourkela, from the department of life sciences, in year 2015. Currently she is pursuing her Ph.D in the laboratory of tumour microenvironment and animal model, Institute of life Sciences, Odisha.

Brahmeshwar Mishra received his B.Pharm, M.Pharm and Ph.D Degrees from Banaras Hindu University (BHU). He also obtained Diploma in German and Diploma in Yoga from BHU. He has 33 years of teaching and research experience. Currently he is working as Professor of Pharmaceutics at the Department of Pharmaceutical Engineering & Technology, IIT (BHU) and is a senior most faculty in the department. He was Head of the Department also there for 4 years in recent past. His research area is development of novel drug delivery systems, including nanoformulations. He has produced 17 Ph.D and 62 M.Pharm students, published more than 200 research/ review articles and 9 book chapters, honoured with several awards and affiliated as editorial board member and reviewer for many reputed journals. He has delivered lectures in India and abroad at various platforms.

Nishi Mody is pursuing her Ph.D. as DST Inspire fellow (SRF) under the supervision of Prof. S. P. Vyas at Drug Delivery Research Laboratory, Department of Pharmaceutical Sciences, Dr. H.S. Gour University, Sagar (MP) INDIA. She is currently working on the bioligand for targeting of bioactive and drug moiety and includes biopolymers.

Deepti Pandita is working as Prof. & Head, Dept. of Pharmaceutics, JCDM College of Pharmacy, JCD Vidyapeeth, Sirsa. Earlier she was associated with Centro de Quimica da Madeira, University of Madeira, Portugal as a research scientist. She obtained her B. Pharm., M. Pharm. and Ph.D. in top honors from Mysore University, Manipal University and Jamia Hamdard respectively. Dr. Pandita's present areas of research include development of functionalized nanoparticulate systems for anti-cancer agents and oral bioavailability enhancement of poorly water soluble drugs. She holds to her credit research grants worth 45 lacs from various government funding agencies of India i.e. AICTE; Science and Engineering Research Board, DST, Government of India under Research Promotion, Young Scientist schemes, etc. She has earned to her credit 50 publications in peer-reviewed journals like Journal of Controlled Release, Drug Delivery, Drug Discovery Today, Molecular Pharmaceutics, Biomacromolecules, Current Gene Therapy, Nanotoxicology, Nanomedicine etc.; two Indian Patents and 50 abstracts in national and international conferences. She has also received International Travel Grants from DST and ICMR for presenting research papers in PharmaTech 2012 Malaysia and PharmaTech 2014 Bangkok. She has organized AICTE sponsored Faculty Development Programme and short-term training courses. Her work has fetched several awards and accolades like, Best Pharmaceutical Scientist Award-2014 by Association of Pharmaceutical Teachers of India, Haryana State Branch; Best Paper Awards at 5th European Symposium on Biopolymers, Portugal, 2009 and at 58th Indian Pharmaceutical Congress, 2006. She has guided/guiding 02 Ph.D.'s and 44 M. Pharm. Scholars. She is a Life member of Indian Pharmaceutical Association, Indian Pharmacy Graduates Association, Association of Pharmaceutical Teachers' of India, and Indian Pharmacological Society.

Kamla Pathak, graduate and post graduate from University Institute of Pharmaceutical sciences Panjab University Chandigarh earned her Doctorate in Pharmaceutics in the year 1991 from the same institute. With a teaching and research experience of more than 27 years, is currently working as Professor, Pharmacy College Saifai, Uttar Pradesh University of Medical Sciences, Saifai, Etawah, India; is a member of various professional bodies. Actively engaged in research on oral controlled /modulated/ targeted and topical drug delivery systems has over 235 publications in journals of international and national repute, 3 patents, authored book chapters and more than 180 abstracts of the papers presented in scientific forums to her credit. Credited as reviewer of national and international journals of repute in the field of Pharmaceutics, has a h-index of 25. She has handled various research projects and has guided Ph. Ds, 120+ postgraduate theses. Awards bestowed upon include Dr. R.L. Nicore award 2012, for Best Research paper in Pharmaceutics; Motan Devi Dandiya prize for best research publications in Pharmacy (2012 and 2013); Eminent Teacher Award, 2012 for various poster presentations at National Pharmacy conferences held in India. She has delivered lectures on various platforms and is associated to pharmaceutical industry in the capacity of scientific consultant. Credited as reviewer of scientific projects, Knowledge Foundation, Sweden; Israel Science foundation, is an invited member of American Nano Society.

Vandana Patravale is currently a Professor of Pharmaceutics at Department of Pharmaceutical Sciences and Technology of the Institute of Chemical Technology, India. She has over 100 refereed publications, 250 research presentations, 9 book chapters, 4 granted patents, 24 patents in pipeline and 2 trademark registries to her credit. She has guided over 75 postgraduate students. Her areas of expertise include medical device development viz. coronary stents, intrauterine devices etc., nanodiagnostics and novel nanocarriers for pertinent areas of national relevance with major emphasis on malaria, cancer and neurodegenerative disorders. She has published two books entitled, 'Nanotechnology in drug delivery- a perspective on transition from laboratory to market' by Woodhead Publishing house (now Elsevier) and 'Pharmaceutical product development: insights into pharmaceutical processes, management and regulatory affairs' by CRC Press, Taylor and Francis group. Dr. Patravale has been active in teaching, research and service throughout her career. In recognition to that she was awarded OPPI women scientist award 2015, Best pharmaceutical scientist award 2014, VASVIK award 2013, Veneto nanotech award 2013, APTI best teacher award 2012, state level recognition-Fellowship of Maharashtra Academy of Sciences for outstanding contributions in drug delivery research 2011 and K.H. Garda Distinguished researcher award 2009. She is also a recipient of prestigious Bill and Melinda Gates Foundation grant to develop the first ever eco-friendly nanovaccine for nasal immunization.

Neelam Poonia is working as Assistant Professor in Department of Pharmaceutics, JCDM College of Pharmacy, Sirsa (Haryana), India. She has co-supervised 6 post graduate research projects. She has 10 publications in National and International journals of repute and 3 book chapters to her credit. She has also presented her research at various National and International Conferences. Ms Poonia is presently pursuing her doctoral studies in Pharmaceutical Sciences on the development of targeted nanosystems for delivery of anticancer agents, from I.K. Gujral Punjab Technical University, Jalandhar. Her interest areas of research include development of nanotechnology based drug delivery systems viz. solid lipid nanoparticles, nanostructured lipid carriers, mesoporous silica nanoparticles etc. for combating solubility, stability, toxicity, MDR related issues associated with drugs.

Sanjeeb Sahoo is a scientist at the Institute of Life Sciences, Bhubaneswar, India since 2005. He received his M.Sc. degree in 1994 and Ph. D in 1999 from the University of Delhi, Delhi. He served as a JSPS Postdoctoral fellow at the Department of Microbiology, School of Medicine, Kumamoto University, Kumamoto, Japan from 1999-2001. This was followed by a four-year postdoctoral fellowship at the Nebraska Medical Centre, Omaha, USA from 2001-2005 including a 2 years' fellowship from American Heart Association. Scientific Contributions include over more than 90 peer reviewed research papers including review articles and book chapters in leading scientific journals of the utmost quality in this field, such as Biomaterials, Future Nanomedicine, Molecular Pharmaceutics, Cancer Research, International Journal of Cancer, Journal of Controlled Release and many more. Dr Sahoo has been granted 4 US patents; one EU patent on Nanotechnology based targeted drug and gene delivery. He is one of the experts in the field of Nanotechnology based drug delivery system mainly in the field of Cancer. Scientific and Professional Activities includes, Editorial board member of Current Nanomedicine, Clinical & Experimental Pharmacology, Serving Section Editor (cancer section) of Current Pharmaceutical Biotechnology and members of different scientific organizations.

Behiye Şenel is research assistant at Anadolu University, Faculty of Pharmacy, Department of Pharmaceutical Biotechnology. She has completed M.Sc. on medical genetics and PhD on developing of siRNA delivery systems at Anadolu University. She works in the fields of gene delivery systems, developing polymeric and lipidic nanoparticulate systems, gene therapy, targeting systems to the lung and vagina. Has done a lot of research on human genetics. Up to this day, 14 research articles have been published in scientific journals and she has many posters and oral presentations at various international and national conferences. And also there are three best presentation awards. Behiye Şenel is an Editorial Board Member of International Journal of Drug Discovery, International Journal of Respiratory Disease, Care & Medicine (IJRDM) and Journal of Pharmaceutical Sciences and Experimental Pharmacology which are an international journal.

P. Severino has a Degree in Pharmacy from the Methodist University of Piracicaba - Unimep (2005). Master and PhD from the School of Chemical Engineering, State University of Campinas - Unicamp (2005 and 2012). In the master made the sandwich program at the Faculty of Pharmacy of the Federal University of Rio Grande do Sul - UFRGS (2007-2008), and held a doctorate sandwich program at the Faculty of Pharmacy, University Fernando Pessoa - UFP in Porto, Portugal (2010-2011). She is currently professor Program in Industrial Biotechnology and pharmacy Institute at University Tiradentes and researcher at the Institute of Technology and Research. She has extensive experience area of drugs and cosmetics, mainly in: pharmacological, pharmacokinetic, pharmaceutical technology, industrial pharmaceutical technology, nano and polymeric and lipid microparticles.

Navneet Sharma is a senior research fellow at the Institute of Nuclear Medicine & Allied Sciences (INMAS-DRDO), New Delhi, India and pursuing his PhD on the development and evaluation of topical nanoformulation for CBRN decontamination under the advisement of Dr. Rakesh Kumar Sharma. Mr. Sharma graduated in Pharmaceutical Science from the UP Technical University Lucknow, India in 2011. He had completed his masters in Pharmaceutics from the JSS University, Mysore, Karnataka, India. He has acclaimed AICTE GPAT and DRDO Research fellowship for his masters and PhD respectively. He is the recipient of the International travel grant from DST-2014 and ICMR-2017. He had filed 3 patents and more than 20 publications in his credit. His research interests include the applications of the nanomaterials and their use in drug delivery systems.

Rajeev Sharma is pursuing his Ph.D. as a research fellow (CSIR- Research Associate) under the supervision of Prof. S. P. Vyas at Drug Delivery Research Laboratory, Department of Pharmaceutical Sciences, Dr. H.S. Gour University, Sagar (MP) INDIA. He is currently working on the targeted drug delivery and cancer immunotherapy.

Rakesh Kumar Sharma, Scientist ‘G’, is the Director of the Defence Food Research Laboratory (DFRL), Mysore. Dr. Sharma did his M. Pharmacy from Panjab University and acquired PhD from University of Delhi. He has acclaimed various honors/awards including Young Scientist Award (1993), Laboratory Scientist of the Year Award (2001), INMAS Team Leadership Awards for the years 2003, 2004, 2011& 2015. Chandra KantaDandiya Prize in Pharmacology (2004), Jaipur Prize (2005) of the Indian Pharmacological Society, ICMR International Fellowship award for Senior Biomedical Scientist (2008), AAPS PharmSciTech Outstanding Manuscript Award (2008), Acharya PC Ray Memorial Gold Medal Award (2013) and Dr. HAB Parpia Memorial Lecture Award (2016). Dr. Sharma applied 20 patents and has more than 300 publications to his credit besides contributing 50 chapters in books. Seven technologies developed by him have been successfully transferred to Industry and are at the production or final stages of trial.

Nalini Shastri has rendered more than two and half decades of service towards pharmaceutical education and research. She is presently working as an Associate Professor at NIPER, Hyderabad since Oct 2009. She has completed her PhD from Bombay College of Pharmacy, Mumbai, with Pharmaceutics specialization. She is a certified six sigma green belt with a post graduate diploma in statistical quality control. She also holds a post graduate diploma in Computer programming, system analysis and design. She has worked in various pharmaceutical companies like E.Merck Ltd, Meyer Organics Ltd, Pfimex Pharmaceuticals Ltd, Armour Pharmaceuticals Ltd and Natco Pharma at Managerial level. She established a Solid State Pharmaceutical Group (SSPRG) which focuses on solid state formulations, crystal engineering, cocrystals and polymorphs. The group also undertakes various projects on use of various software tools for formulation development and crystal/polymorph designing. The group contribution has resulted in many national and international awards. She has guided 4 PhD students, 30 Master students, published more than 50 papers in international peer reviewed journals, 7 invited international book chapters and authored a text book on Instrumental Analysis for Dr. Ambedkar OU, AP. Her two clinical trials have been successfully completed and registered at CTRI. She also has 2 patents to her credit. Her area of expertise include solid state pharmaceutics, crystal engineering, mesoporous drug delivery systems, IVIVC, QbD, chemometry, six sigma implementation and utilization of software tools for formulation development and optimization.

Saritha R. Shetty is currently working as Assistant Professor in Department of Pharmaceutics at Shobhaben Pratapbhai Patel School of Pharmacy and Technology Management, SVKM's NMIMS deemed-to-be University, India. She completed her Ph.D. from SVKM's NMIMS University, India. Before pursuing her Ph.D. she worked as a scientist in Syngene International Pvt.Ltd. (A Biocon Company) in Research and Development department. Her areas of research interests include exploring novel excipients in drug delivery systems, development of topical, transdermal and muco-adhesive drug delivery system and cosmeticology.

Amelia M. Silva (AM Silva) is affiliated to the Department of Biology and Environment, University of Trás-os-Montes and Alto Douro, Portugal and to the Centre for the Research and Technology of Agro Environmental and Biological Sciences (CITAB-UTAD). AM Silva graduated in Biochemistry (1992), has MSc degree in Cell Biology (1995) and PhD in Biochemistry/Cellular Biophysics (2003), Faculty of Science and Technology, Coimbra University, Portugal. AM Silva leads scientific research in the area of: characterization of plant derived bioactive compounds and its effects on cell metabolism and toxicology; encapsulation of compounds with resource to nanotechnology (effects on cell physiology/toxicology). She has expertise in several methodologies to study cell physiology, biochemistry, toxicology and pharmacology. A. Silva has 70 JCR publications, Scopus H-factor=18 (S. Author ID: 35578752300), authored/co-authored 15 book chapters, 8 non-JCR articles, and about 150 communications (national/international meetings). A. Silva has long experience supervising student (PhD, Master and undergraduate), in national/international teaching (undergraduate, Master and PhD courses) and as referee.

Deepika Singh has completed her Masters in Biotechnology from Barkatullah University, Bhopal in 2014. She qualified CSIR NET LS in 2015. Presently she is pursuing her Doctorate Degree from Institute of Life Sciences, Bhubaneswar, India under the supervision of Dr. Sanjeeb Kumar Sahoo. Her area of interest is nanomedicinal approach for targeting Breast Cancer Stem Cells.

Priya Singh is a Ph.D scholar at Institute of Life Sciences, Bhubaneswar, India. She has completed her Master of Pharmacy in Pharmaceutical Chemistry from Dr. Hari Singh Gour Vishwavidyalaya, Sagar. She received Nagarjun Gold medal during her post graduation. Her Bachelor of Pharmacy is from Banasthali Vidyapith University, Rajasthan during which she secured 81%. She has completed a project on "A brief learning of the drug discovery process with emphasis on the techniques of synthesis" under Vice President Dr. Laxmikant Gharat, Glenmark Pharmaceuticals, Mumbai. She has qualified two national exams, TIFR -2017(Tata Institute of Fundamental Research) and GPAT-2014 (Graduate Pharmacy Aptitude Test).

Shubham Singh had completed his masters in chemistry from the department of chemistry, University of Delhi and currently working as a research intern at Institute of Nuclear Medicine and Allied Sciences. His research interest includes the preparation and evaluation of the Novel Drug Delivery Systems.

Eliana Souto (Souto, E.B.) is affiliated with the Department of Pharmaceutical Technology of the Faculty of Pharmacy, University of Coimbra, Portugal. Eliana is graduated in Pharmaceutical Sciences from the same University. She holds a Master in Science degree in Pharmaceutical Technology and Pharmacotechnique from the Faculty of Pharmacy, University of Porto, and the PhD in Pharmaceutical Technology, Biopharmaceutics and Biotechnology from the Institut fuer Pharmazie der Freie Universitaet Berlin, Germany. Since August 2012, Eliana Souto holds the dr. Habil. from the University Fernando Pessoa. Her research lines focus on the design, development, and characterization of new drug delivery systems. Other research interests include the controlled delivery of drugs across biological barriers, e.g. skin, gastrointestinal tract and blood-brain-barrier. Eliana Souto is Associate Editor, member of the Editorial Board, and reviewer of several international scientific journals.

Divya Suares is currently working as Assistant Professor in Department of Pharmaceutics at Shobhaben Pratapbhai Patel School of Pharmacy and Technology Management, SVKM's NMIMS deemed-to-be University. She got her Ph. D. degree in Pharmaceutical Sciences from NMIMS deemed-to-be-University in 2017. She has authored 7 research papers and 2 review articles till date. Her research interests include development of lipid based delivery system, nanotechnology, cosmeticology and wound healing.

Sathish Thokala is currently working as a Teaching Assistant (TA) and pursuing research for Ph.D Degree at Department of Pharmaceutical Engineering & Technology in Indian Institute of Technology (Banaras Hindu University), Varanasi, India. He has received his B. Pharm from Osmania University, Hyderabad and M. Pharm in Pharmaceutics from Kakatiya University, Warangal. He also obtained Post Graduated Diploma in Intellectual Property Rights (PGDIPR) from Osmania University, Hyderabad. Prior to his TA assignment, he worked as an officer in Formulation and Development Division of a Pharmaceutical Company, (Plethico Pharmaceutical Ltd) at Indore, India. And his current research area is development of novel drug delivery systems.

Ankita Tiwari, with an assiduous performance in her academic career, she secured 83.2% in Secondary School examination and 84.2% in Senior School examination. She completed her B. Pharm. (81.2%, College topper) from Sagar Institute of Pharmaceutical Sciences, Sagar (M.P.) and cracked GPAT-2011 (AIR 357). She pursued her M. Pharm. (Pharmaceutics, 7.92 CGPA) from Rajiv Gandhi Proudyogiki Vishwavidyalaya, Sagar (M.P.), India. She is a recipient of valuable scholarships (JRF-AICTE, Non-NET UGC). She has been awarded with Late Phoolwasa Devi Dubey Memorial Award 2012 in 1st Annual National Convention of Association of Pharmacy Professionals held at Bhopal on 7 April 2012. She has few best poster awards in national level seminars to her credit. She has published more than 3 international high repute publications including book chapters. Currently, she is working as a PhD Scholar in Department of Pharmaceutical Sciences, Dr. H. S. Gour Central University, Sagar (M.P.) India. Her area of research is nanocarriers based colorectal cancer targeting.

Archana Upadhya is currently working as an Assistant Professor at Shobhaben Pratapbhai Patel School of Pharmacy & Technology Management, Mumbai. She was a master's student in the stream of bioprocess technology from Institute of Chemical Technology. She graduated in pharmacy from Bombay College of Pharmacy. She has completed her PhD in Pharmaceutical Sciences, from Shobhaben Pratapbhai Patel School of Pharmacy & Technology Management, SVKM'S NMIMS on the topic "Solid Tumour Therapy with peptide-DNA complexes". She has six publications to her credit. Her research interests are downstream processing, molecular biology, cell biology and oncology.

Amit Verma, with a breakthrough out of his diligence, cracked GATE-2008 (98.39 percentile). He completed his B. Pharm. (65.153%, First division), M. Pharm. (Pharmaceutics, 7.76 CGPA with A Grade) and engaging in PhD at Depart. Pharm. Sci., Dr. H. S. Gour Central University, Sagar (M.P.), India. He is a recipient of valuable scholarships (JRF-AICTED, UGC-Non-NET. He has published more than 5 international high repute publications including book chapters. Currently, he is working as a Ph. D Scholar in Department of Pharmaceutical Sciences, Dr. H. S. Gour Central University, Sagar (M.P.) India. His area of research is exploration of topical delivery at the ocular site for the treatment of fungal infection.

Nikhar Vishwakarma is pursuing his Ph.D. under the supervision of Prof. S. P. Vyas at Drug Delivery Research Laboratory, Department of Pharmaceutical Sciences, Dr. H.S. Gour University, Sagar (MP), India. He is currently working on the bioligand for targeting of bioactive and drug moiety and includes biopolymers.

Suresh P. Vyas is a senior most professor (Department of Pharmaceutical Sciences) in Dr. Hari Singh Gour Vishwavidyalaya, Sagar, India. He has about 35 years of teaching and research experience at postgraduate level. He is pioneer scientist in the field of nano-biotechnology and immunology. He has supervised 52 PhD's and more than 139 M. Pharm students. He has over 317 research publications to his credit published in journals of high scientific impact. His research work is cross cited and referenced internationally. He authored 18 reference books including Pharmaceutical Biotechnology, Liposomal Therapeutics, Novel Controlled Drug Delivery Systems, Targeted Drug Delivery Systems, Theory and Practices in Novel Drug Delivery Systems and contributed many chapters in various renowned books. He is a commonwealth postdoctoral fellowship awardee and has worked under fellowship at School of Pharmacy University of London (U.K.). Prof. Vyas is a recipient of Best Scientist award by Association of Pharmacy Professionals (APP) 2014, National Teacher Excellence Award by IES group of Institution, 2014, Pandit Lajja Shankar Jha award, Best Pharmacy Teacher of the year 2001 by Association of Pharmaceutical Teachers of India, Received First position in India for their research impact, citation and H- index by Department of Science and Technology, 2016; Nominated as a subject expert in the area of Noval drug delivery for new drug approval by Ministry of health & Family welfare, India 2016; Nominated for Prof. Rudolph A. Marcus Award 2016 (Prof. Rudolph A. Marcus received the 1992 Nobel Prize in Chemistry) given by Publishing Division of Cognizure and LOGNOR and many more. He has been on various administrative positions of the university including Dean Faculty of technology; Head, Department of Pharmaceutical Sciences and Department of Biotechnology, Chairman, board of studies and Vice Chancellor of University (15 Sep 2014 to 15th March 2015) etc. He serves on the editorial board of International Journal of Pharmaceutics (Elsevier), Recent Patents on Drug Delivery and Formulation (Bentham Science Publishers), Therapeutic Delivery (Future Science Groups), Journal of Drug Delivery (Hindawi) and Journal of Nanoscience Letters (Simplex publishers). Prof. Vyas is widely visited scientist and delivered invited/popular/keynote addresses in national and international conferences in India and abroad.

Balvant Yadav was born in Azamgarh (Uttar Pradesh), India. He obtained his Bachelor of Pharmacy degree from Bombay College of Pharmacy (India). He had completed his M.S. (Pharm.) in Pharmaceutics under the guidance of Dr. Sanyog Jain from National Institute of Pharmaceutical Education and Research (NIPER), S.A.S. Nagar Mohali (India). At present, he is Ph.D. Scholar at NIPER Hyderabad under the guidance of Dr. Nalini Shastri. His current research area includes development of novel cocrystals for improvement of drug properties. His broad research includes crystal engineering, multicomponent system, pre-formulation, formulations, developing oral dosage forms, and drug delivery.

Index

A

B

C

D

E

F

G

H

I

L

M

N

Purchase Print, E-Book, or Print + E-Book

IGI Global books can now be purchased from three unique pricing formats: Print Only, E-Book Only, or Print + E-Book. Shipping fees apply.

www.igi-global.com

Recommended Reference Books

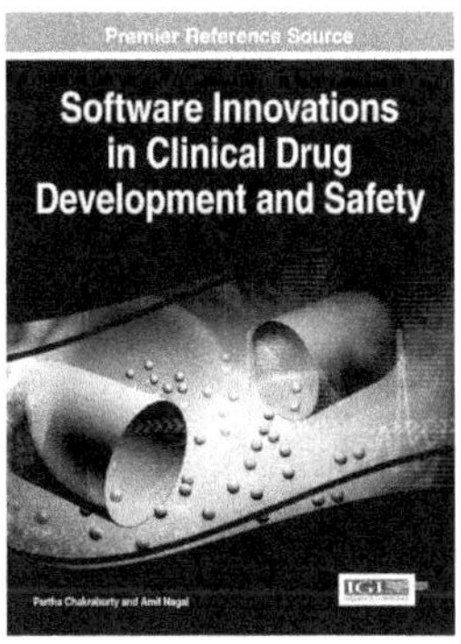

ISBN: 978-1-4666-8726-4
© 2016; 305 pp.
List Price: $225

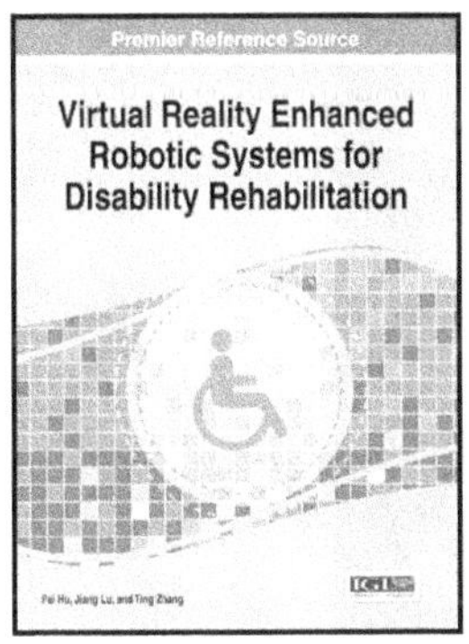

ISBN: 978-1-4666-9740-9
© 2016; 383 pp.
List Price: $210

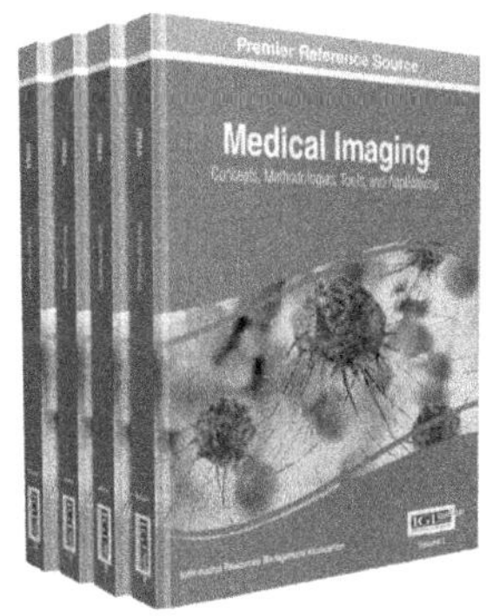

ISBN: 978-1-5225-0571-6
© 2017; 2,081 pp.
List Price: $2,150

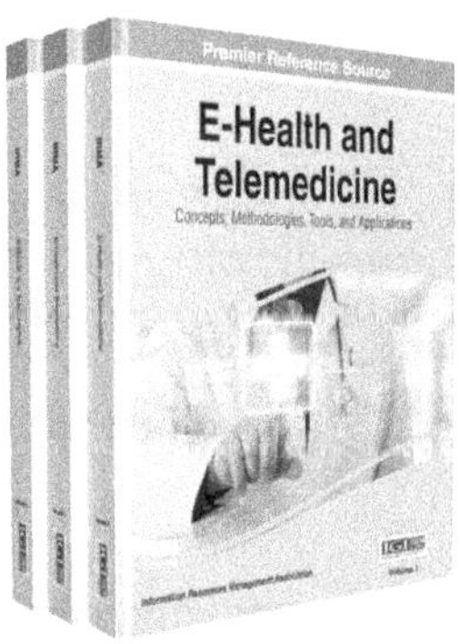

ISBN: 978-1-4666-8756-1
© 2016; 1,759 pp.
List Price: $2,435

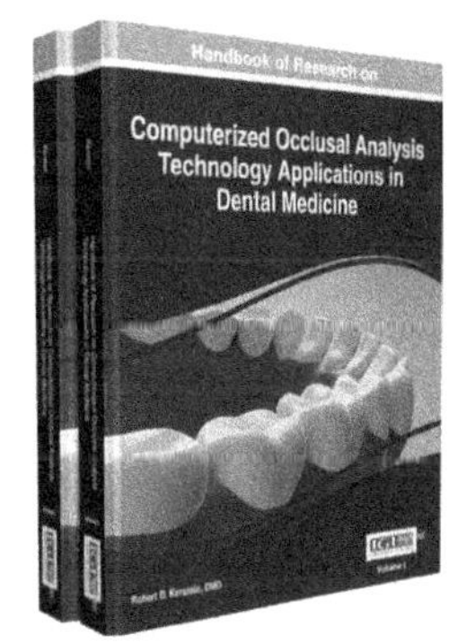

ISBN: 978-1-4666-6587-3
© 2015; 973 pp.
List Price: $475

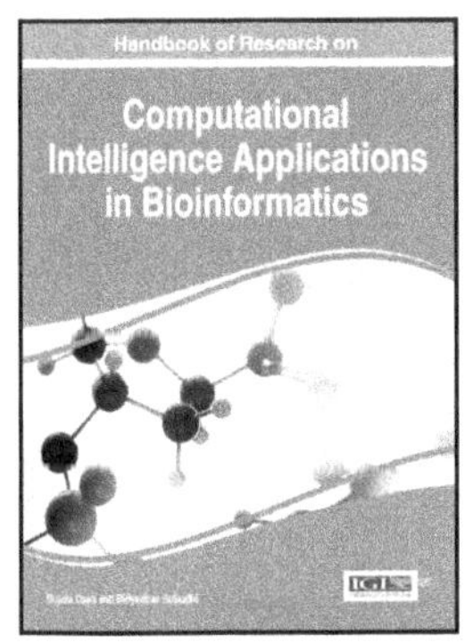

ISBN: 978-1-5225-0427-6
© 2016; 514 pp.
List Price: $230

Looking for free content, product updates, news, and special offers?
Join IGI Global's mailing list today and start enjoying exclusive perks sent only to IGI Global members.
Add your name to the list at **www.igi-global.com/newsletters.**

Publishing Information Science and Technology Research Since 1988

IGI Global
DISSEMINATOR OF KNOWLEDGE

www.igi-global.com | Sign up at www.igi-global.com/newsletters | facebook.com/igiglobal | twitter.com/igiglobal

Stay Current on the Latest Emerging Research Developments

Become an IGI Global Reviewer for Authored Book Projects

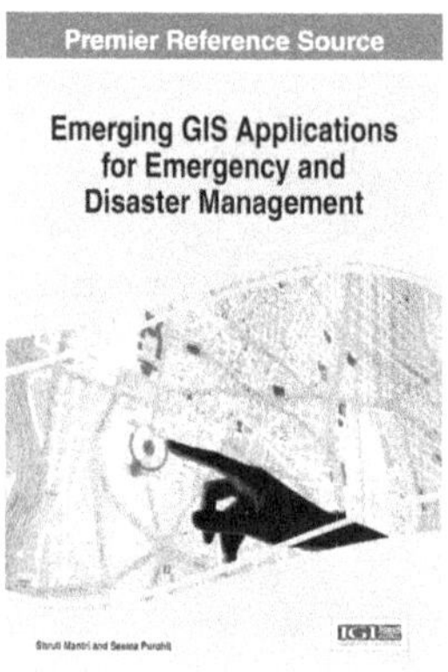

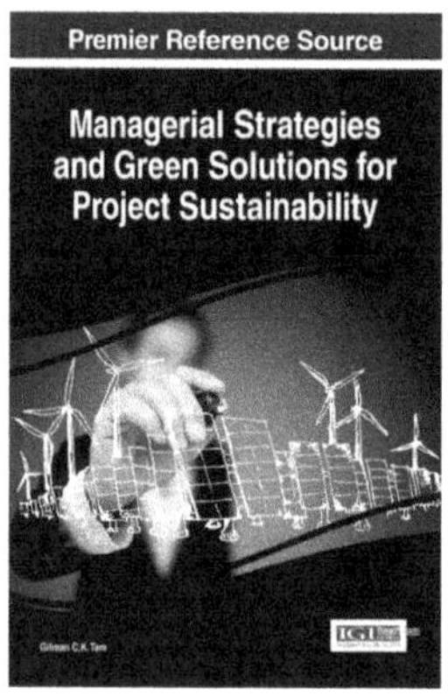

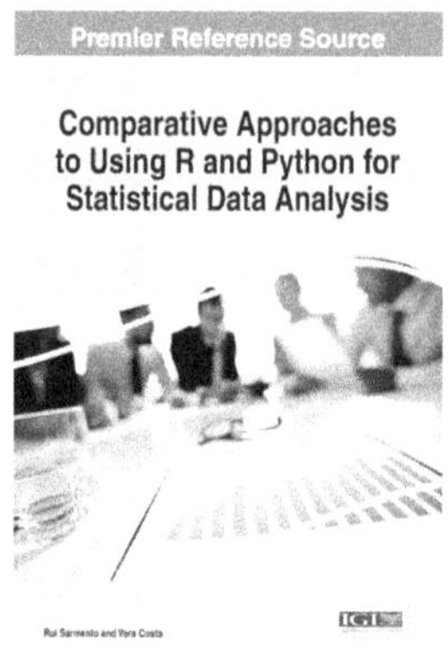

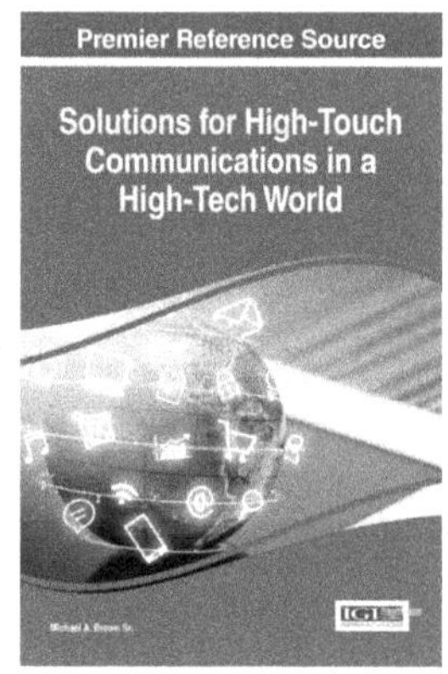

The overall success of an authored book project is dependent on quality and timely reviews.

In this competitive age of scholarly publishing, constructive and timely feedback significantly decreases the turnaround time of manuscripts from submission to acceptance, allowing the publication and discovery of progressive research at a much more expeditious rate. Several IGI Global authored book projects are currently seeking highly qualified experts in the field to fill vacancies on their respective editorial review boards:

Applications may be sent to:
development@igi-global.com

Applicants must have a doctorate (or an equivalent degree) as well as publishing and reviewing experience. Reviewers are asked to write reviews in a timely, collegial, and constructive manner. All reviewers will begin their role on an ad-hoc basis for a period of one year, and upon successful completion of this term can be considered for full editorial review board status, with the potential for a subsequent promotion to Associate Editor.

If you have a colleague that may be interested in this opportunity,
we encourage you to share this information with them.

www.igi-global.com

InfoSci®-Books

A Database for Information Science and Technology Research

Maximize Your Library's Book Collection!

Invest in IGI Global's InfoSci®-Books database and gain access to hundreds of reference books at a fraction of their individual list price.

The InfoSci®-Books database offers unlimited simultaneous users the ability to precisely return search results through more than 80,000 full-text chapters from nearly 3,900 reference books in the following academic research areas:

Business & Management Information Science & Technology • Computer Science & Information Technology
Educational Science & Technology • Engineering Science & Technology • Environmental Science & Technology
Government Science & Technology • Library Information Science & Technology • Media & Communication Science & Technology
Medical, Healthcare & Life Science & Technology • Security & Forensic Science & Technology • Social Sciences & Online Behavior

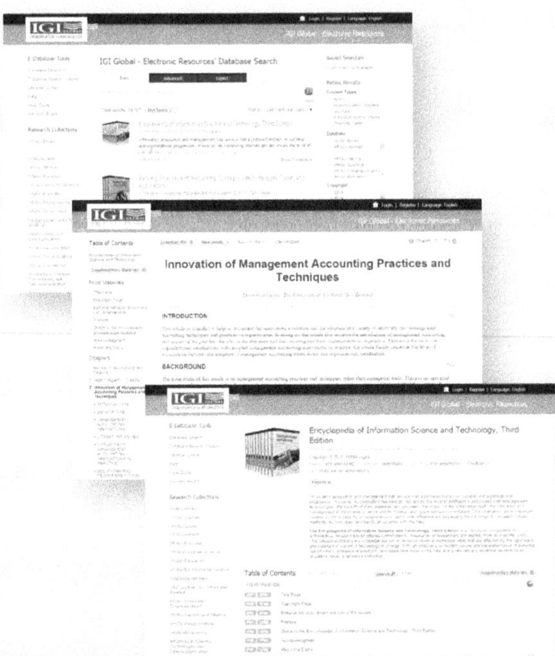

Peer-Reviewed Content:
- Cutting-edge research
- No embargoes
- Scholarly and professional
- Interdisciplinary

Award-Winning Platform:
- Unlimited simultaneous users
- Full-text in XML and PDF
- Advanced search engine
- No DRM

Librarian-Friendly:
- Free MARC records
- Discovery services
- COUNTER4/SUSHI compliant
- Training available

To find out more or request a free trial, visit:
www.igi-global.com/eresources

IGI Global
DISSEMINATOR OF KNOWLEDGE
www.igi-global.com

IGI Global
DISSEMINATOR OF KNOWLEDGE
www.igi-global.com

IGI Global Proudly Partners with

eContent Pro International

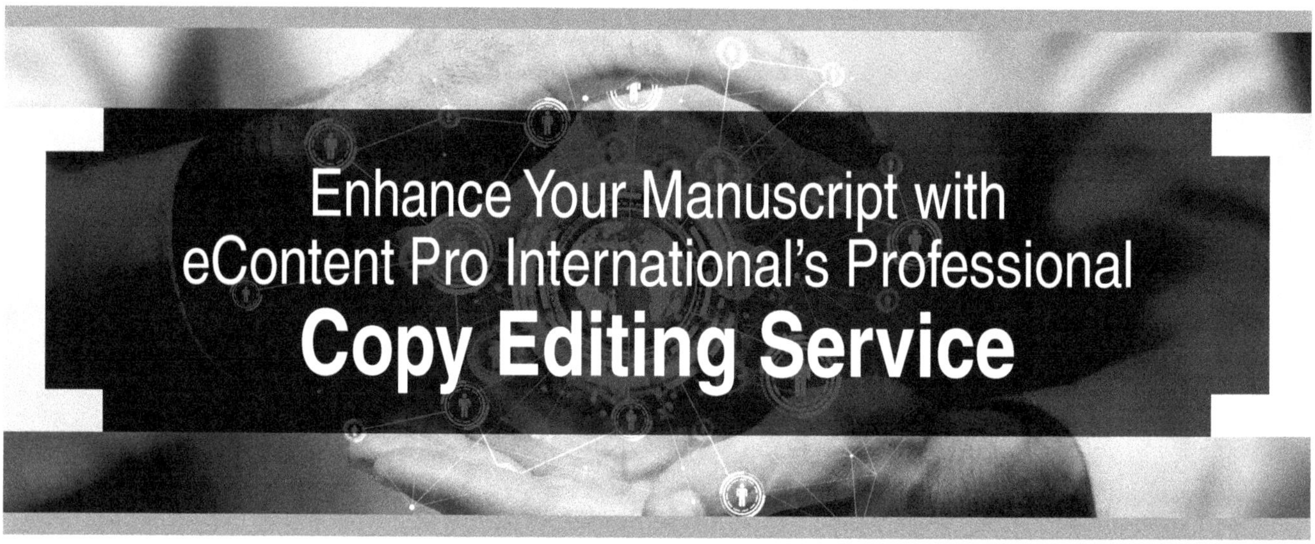

Expert Copy Editing

eContent Pro International copy editors, with over 70 years of combined experience, will provide complete and comprehensive care for your document by resolving all issues with spelling, punctuation, grammar, terminology, jargon, semantics, syntax, consistency, flow, and more. In addition, they will format your document to the style you specify (APA, Chicago, etc.). All edits will be performed using Microsoft Word's Track Changes feature, which allows for fast and simple review and management of edits.

Additional Services

eContent Pro International also offers fast and affordable proofreading to enhance the readability of your document, professional translation in over 100 languages, and market localization services to help businesses and organizations localize their content and grow into new markets around the globe.

IGI Global Authors Save 25% on eContent Pro International's Services!

Scan the QR Code to Receive Your 25% Discount

The 25% discount is applied directly to your eContent Pro International shopping cart when placing an order through IGI Global's referral link. Use the QR code to access this referral link. eContent Pro International has the right to end or modify any promotion at any time.

Email: customerservice@econtentpro.com

econtentpro.com

Information Resources Management Association

IRMA INTERNATIONAL EST. 1987

Advancing the Concepts & Practices of Information Resources Management in Modern Organizations

Become an IRMA Member

Members of the **Information Resources Management Association (IRMA)** understand the importance of community within their field of study. The Information Resources Management Association is an ideal venue through which professionals, students, and academicians can convene and share the latest industry innovations and scholarly research that is changing the field of information science and technology. Become a member today and enjoy the benefits of membership as well as the opportunity to collaborate and network with fellow experts in the field.

IRMA Membership Benefits:

- **One FREE Journal Subscription**
- **30% Off Additional Journal Subscriptions**
- **20% Off Book Purchases**
- Updates on the latest events and research on Information Resources Management through the IRMA-L listserv.
- Updates on new open access and downloadable content added to Research IRM.
- A copy of the Information Technology Management Newsletter twice a year.
- A certificate of membership.

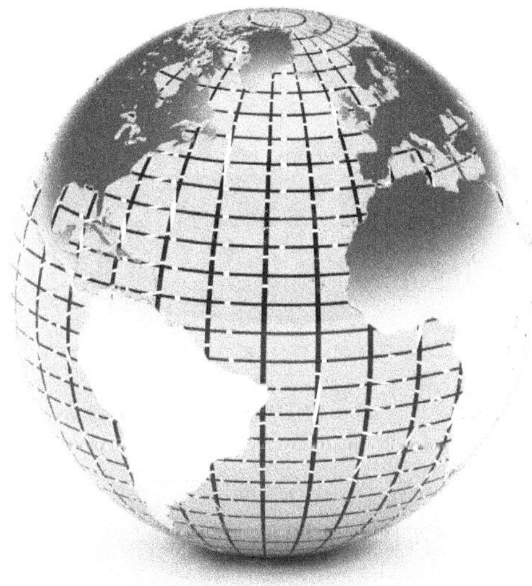

IRMA Membership $195

Scan code or visit **irma-international.org** and begin by selecting your free journal subscription.

Membership is good for one full year.

www.irma-international.org

IGI Global
DISSEMINATOR OF KNOWLEDGE
www.igi-global.com

Available to Order Now

Order through www.igi-global.com with **Free Standard Shipping**.

The Premier Reference for Information Science & Information Technology

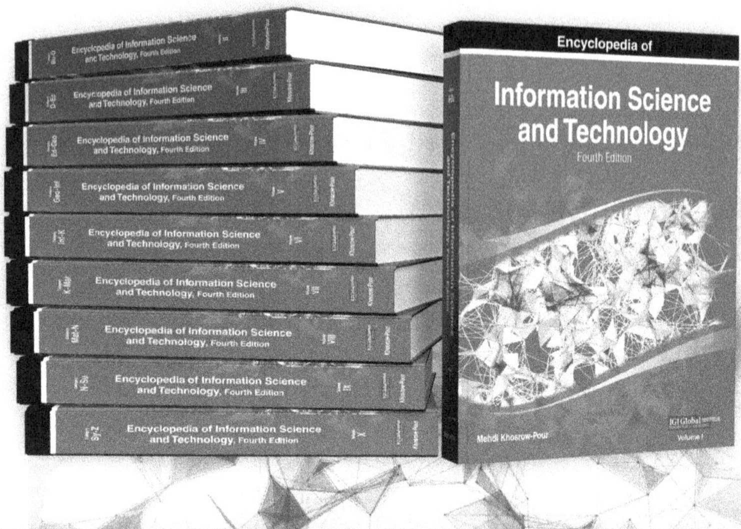

100% Original Content
Contains 705 new, peer-reviewed articles with color figures covering over 80 categories in 11 subject areas

Diverse Contributions
More than 1,100 experts from 74 unique countries contributed their specialized knowledge

Easy Navigation
Includes two tables of content and a comprehensive index in each volume for the user's convenience

Highly-Cited
Embraces a complete list of references and additional reading sections to allow for further research

Included in:
InfoSci®-Books

Encyclopedia of Information Science and Technology Fourth Edition

A Comprehensive 10-Volume Set

Mehdi Khosrow-Pour, D.B.A. (Information Resources Management Association, USA)
ISBN: 978-1-5225-2255-3; © 2018; Pg: 8,104; Release Date: July 2017

The **Encyclopedia of Information Science and Technology, Fourth Edition** is a 10-volume set which includes 705 original and previously unpublished research articles covering a full range of perspectives, applications, and techniques contributed by thousands of experts and researchers from around the globe. This authoritative encyclopedia is an all-encompassing, well-established reference source that is ideally designed to disseminate the most forward-thinking and diverse research findings. With critical perspectives on the impact of information science management and new technologies in modern settings, including but not limited to computer science, education, healthcare, government, engineering, business, and natural and physical sciences, it is a pivotal and relevant source of knowledge that will benefit every professional within the field of information science and technology and is an invaluable addition to every academic and corporate library.

Scan for Online Bookstore

Pricing Information

Hardcover: **$5,695** E-Book: **$5,695** Hardcover + E-Book: **$6,895**

Recommend this Title to Your Institution's Library: www.igi-global.com/books

www.igi-global.com/infosci-ondemand

InfoSci®-OnDemand

Continuously updated with new material on a weekly basis, InfoSci®-OnDemand offers the ability to search through thousands of quality full-text research papers. Users can narrow each search by identifying key topic areas of interest, then display a complete listing of relevant papers, and purchase materials specific to their research needs.

Comprehensive Service

- Over 81,600+ journal articles, book chapters, and case studies.
- All content is downloadable in PDF format and can be stored locally for future use.

No Subscription Fees

- One time fee of $37.50 per PDF download.

Instant Access

- Receive a download link immediately after order completion!

"It really provides an excellent entry into the research literature of the field. It presents a manageable number of highly relevant sources on topics of interest to a wide range of researchers. The sources are scholarly, but also accessible to 'practitioners'."

- Lisa Stimatz, MLS, University of North Carolina at Chapel Hill, USA

"It is an excellent and well designed database which will facilitate research, publication and teaching. It is a very very useful tool to have."

- George Ditsa, PhD, University of Wollongong, Australia

"I have accessed the database and find it to be a valuable tool to the IT/IS community. I found valuable articles meeting my search criteria 95% of the time."

- Lynda Louis, Xavier University of Louisiana, USA

Database Platform Features:

- Comprehensive Pay-Per-View Service
- Written by Prominent International Experts/Scholars
- Precise Search and Retrieval
- Updated With New Material on a Weekly Basis
- Immediate Access to Full-Text PDFs
- No Subscription Needed
- Purchased Research Can Be Stored Locally for Future Use

Recommended for use by researchers who wish to immediately download PDFs of individual chapters or articles.

www.igi-global.com/e-resources/infosci-ondemand

IGI Global
DISSEMINATOR OF KNOWLEDGE
www.igi-global.com

www.ingramcontent.com/pod-product-compliance
Lightning Source LLC
LaVergne TN
LVHW080403011026
849161LV00009B/2341